IMMUNOLOGY AND INFLAMMATION
Basic Mechanisms and Clinical Consequences

NOTICE

Medicine is an ever-changing science. As new research and clinical experience broaden our knowledge, changes in treatment and drug therapy are required. The editors and the publisher of this work have checked with sources believed to be reliable in their efforts to provide information that is complete and generally in accord with the standards accepted at the time of publication. However, in view of the possibility of human error or changes in medical sciences, neither the editors nor the publisher nor any other party who has been involved in the preparation or publication of this work warrants that the information contained herein is in every respect accurate or complete, and they are not responsible for any errors or omissions or for the results obtained from use of such information. Readers are encouraged to confirm the information contained herein with other sources. For example and in particular, readers are advised to check the product information sheet included in the package of each drug they plan to administer to be certain that the information contained in this book is accurate and that changes have not been made in the recommended dose or in the contraindications for administration. This recommendation is of particular importance in connection with new or infrequently used drugs.

IMMUNOLOGY AND INFLAMMATION
Basic Mechanisms and Clinical Consequences

EDITORS

LEONARD H. SIGAL, M.D.
Chief, Division of Rheumatology and
*   Connective Tissue Research*
Associate Professor, Departments of Medicine and Molecular Genetics and
*   Microbiology*
UMDNJ-Robert Wood Johnson Medical School

YACOV RON, Ph.D.
Assistant Professor, Department of Molecular Genetics and Microbiology
UMDNJ-Robert Wood Johnson Medical School

McGRAW-HILL, INC.
Health Professions Division
New York   St. Louis   San Francisco   Auckland   Bogotá
Caracas   Lisbon   London   Madrid   Mexico City   Milan   Montreal
New Delhi   Paris   San Juan   Singapore   Sydney   Tokyo   Toronto

IMMUNOLOGY AND INFLAMMATION
Basic Mechanisms and Clinical Consequences

1 2 3 4 5 6 7 8 9 0 DOC DOC 9 8 7 5 4 3

ISBN 0-07-057386-7

This book was set in Trump Medieval by
   J.M. Post Graphics, A Division of Cardinal
   Communications Group.
The editors were Edward M. Bolger and
   Peter McCurdy;
the production supervisor was Richard Ruzycka;
the cover designer was Joan O'Connor.
R. R. Donnelley and Sons Company was printer
   and binder.
This book is printed on acid-free paper.

**Library of Congress Cataloging-in-Publication
   Data**

Immunology and inflammation : basic
   mechanisms and clinical
   consequences / [edited by] Leonard H. Sigal,
   Yacov Ron.
         p.   cm.
      Includes bibliographical references and
   index.
      ISBN 0-07-057386-7
      1. Immunology.   2. Clinical
   immunology.   3. Inflammation.
   I.   Sigal, Leonard H.   II. Ron, Yacov.
      [DNLM: 1. Immunity, Cellular. 2.
   Inflammation—immunology.
   3.   Immunologic Diseases. QW 700 I3345
   1993]
   QR181.I427   1993
   616.07'9—dc20
   DNLM/DLC
   for Library of Congress   93-18419
                                                    CIP

CONTENTS

PART II: BASIC MECHANISMS OF INFLAMMATION

PART III: CLINICAL CONSEQUENCES

APPENDICES

CONTRIBUTORS

Robert Ader, Ph.D. [23]
Department of Psychiatry
Center for Psychoneuroimmunology Research
University of Rochester Medical Center
Rochester, NY

Hugh R. Brady, M.D. [15]
Department of Medicine
Brigham and Women's Hospital
Harvard Medical School
Boston, MA

Mitchell S. Cappell, M.D., Ph.D. [22b]
Division of Gastroenterology
Department of Medicine
UMDNJ–Robert Wood Johnson Medical School
New Brunswick, NJ

Marc Sin-chye Cheah, M.D. [17]
Division of Hematology/Oncology
Department of Pediatrics
University of Texas Health Sciences Center at San Antonio
San Antonio, TX

David A. Clark, M.D., Ph.D. [27]
McMaster University
Hamilton, Ontario, Canada

Philip J. Clements, M.D. [33a]
Department of Medicine
UCLA School of Medicine
Los Angeles, CA

Nicholas Cohen, Ph.D. [23]
Department of Microbiology and Immunology
Center for Psychoneuroimmunology Research
University of Rochester Medical Center
Rochester, NY

Robert W. Colman, M.D. [14]
Director, Thrombosis Research Center
Temple University Health Science Center
Philadelphia, PA

Kiron M. Das, M.D., Ph.D. [22b, 35c]
Chief, Division of Gastroenterology
Department of Medicine
UMDNJ–Robert Wood Johnson Medical School
New Brunswick, NJ

Salim Daya, M.B., M.Sc. [27]
McMaster University
Hamilton, Ontario, Canada

David B. Duggan, M.D. [10]
Division of Hematology and Oncology
Department of Medicine
SUNY Syracuse Health Science Center
Syracuse, NY

John M. Dwyer, M.D., Ph.D. [1, 34]
Professor and Head, Department of Medicine
School of Medicine
The Prince of Wales Hospital
The University of New South Wales
Randwick, New South Wales, Australia

Lawrence F. Eichenfield, M.D. [13]
Chief, Division of Dermatology
Department of Pediatrics
University of California San Diego School of Medicine
Children's Hospital and Health Center
San Diego, CA

Joseph C. Fantone, M.D. [20]
Department of Pathology
University of Michigan Medical School
Ann Arbor, MI

David L. Felten, M.D., Ph.D. [23]
Department of Neurobiology and Anatomy
Center for Psychoneuroimmunology Research
University of Rochester Medical Center
Rochester, NY

Patrick Flood, Ph.D. [9, 25]
Department of Periodontics
UNC-Chapel Hill
Chapel Hill, NC

Arthur J. Geller, M.D. [35c]
Division of Gastroenterology and Nutrition
Department of Medicine
University of Florida Health Science Center
Jacksonville, FL

I. Michael Goonewardene, Ph.D. [24a]
Department of Microbiology and Immunology
The Medical College of Pennsylvania
Philadelphia, PA

Douglas R. Green, Ph.D. [4]
La Jolla Institute of Allergy and Immunology
La Jolla, CA

Barry L. Gruber, M.D. [19a]
Division of Allergy, Rheumatology, and Clinical Immunology
Department of Medicine
SUNY at Stony Brook
Northport Veterans Administration
Stony Brook, NY

Ian B. Hoffman, M.D. [14]
Department of Medicine
University of Maryland
Baltimore, MD

Norman Ilowite, M.D. [28]
Chief, Pediatric Rheumatology
Schneider Children's Hospital of LIJ-Hillside Medical Center
Associate Professor of Pediatrics
Albert Einstein College of Medicine
New Hyde Park, NY

Stephen P. James, M.D. [11]
Chief, Division of Gastroenterology
Department of Medicine
University of Maryland
Baltimore, MD

Richard B. Johnston, Jr., M.D. [13]
Medical Director, March of Dimes Birth Defects Foundation
White Plains, NY
Department of Pediatrics
Yale University School of Medicine
New Haven, CT

Hidenori Kawanishi, M.D., Ph.D. [22b]
Division of Gastroenterology
Department of Medicine
UMDNJ–Robert Wood Johnson Medical School
New Brunswick, NJ

CONTRIBUTORS

Neil E. Kay, M.D. [30]
Department of Medicine
University of Kentucky
Lexington, KY

Charles H. Kirkpatrick, M.D. [33b]
Staff Physician
National Jewish Hospital
Professor, Department of Medicine
University of Colorado Health Sciences Center
Denver, CO

Catherine Monteleone, M.D. [29]
Division of Allergy, Immunology, and Infectious Diseases
Department of Medicine
UMDNJ–Robert Wood Johnson Medical School
New Brunswick, NJ

Donna Marie Murasko, Ph.D. [24a]
Department of Microbiology and Immunology
The Medical College of Pennsylvania
Philadelphia, PA

Andrew R. Pachner, M.D. [35d]
Department of Neurology
Georgetown University Hospital
Washington, DC

Suehiro Pan, Ph.D. [5]
Department of Pathology
UMDNJ-Robert Wood Johnson Medical School
Piscataway, NJ

Richard T. Parmley, M.D. [17]
Chief, Division of Hematology/Oncology
Department of Pediatrics
University of Texas Health Sciences Center at San Antonio
San Antonio, TX

Nicholas M. Ponzio, Ph.D. [2]
Department of Laboratory Medicine and Pathology
UMDNJ–Robert Wood Johnson Medical School
New Brunswick, NJ

Otto J. Plescia, Ph.D. [3]
Waksman Institute of Microbiology
Piscataway, NJ

Karel Raška, Jr., M.D., Ph.D. [2]
Institute for Molecular Diagnostics and Pathology
St. Peter's Medical Center
New Brunswick, NJ

Helen V. Ratajczak, Ph.D. [32]
Life Sciences Department
I.I.T. Research Institute
Chicago, IL

Yacov Ron, Ph.D. [6, 7]
Assistant Professor, Department of Molecular Genetics and Microbiology
UMDNJ–Robert Wood Johnson Medical School
New Brunswick, NJ

Robert A. Schwartz, M.D. [26]
Department of Surgery
SUNY-HSC-Syracuse
Syracuse, NY

Charles N. Serhan, Ph.D. [15]
Department of Medicine
Brigham and Women's Hospital
Harvard Medical School
Boston, MA

Leonard H. Sigal, M.D. [3, 16, 19b, 21, 22a, 24b, 31, App. A, App. B]
Chief, Division of Rheumatology and Connective Tissue Research
Associate Professor, Departments of Medicine and Molecular Genetics and
  Microbiology
UMDNJ–Robert Wood Johnson Medical School
New Brunswick, NJ

Barbara K. Snyder, M.D. [24b]
Division of Adolescent Medicine
Department of Pediatrics
UMDNJ–Robert Wood Johnson Medical School
New Brunswick, NJ

Kirk Sperber, M.D. [18]
Division of Clinical Immunology
Department of Medicine
Mt. Sinai Hospital
New York, NY

Randall M. Stevens, M.D. [App. C]
Division of Rheumatology and Connective Tissue Research
Department of Medicine
UMDNJ–Robert Wood Johnson Medical School
New Brunswick, NJ

Philip R. Streeter, Ph.D. [12]
Monsanto Company
St. Louis, MO

Natalie Sutkowski, B.S. [6]
Department of Molecular Genetics and Microbiology
UMDNJ–Robert Wood Johnson Medical School
New Brunswick, NJ

Rosa M. Ten, M.D. [35a]
Division of Nephrology and Internal Medicine
Mayo Clinic
Rochester, MN

Diane G. Tice, Ph.D. [26]
Department of Surgery
SUNY–HSC–Syracuse
Syracuse, NY

Vicente E. Torres, M.D. [35a]
Division of Nephrology and Internal Medicine
Mayo Clinic
Rochester, MN

C. Reynold Verret, Ph.D. [8]
Department of Chemistry
Clark-Atlanta University
Atlanta, GA

Yanina T. Wachtfogel [14]
Thrombosis Research Center
Department of Medicine
Temple University Health Science Center
Philadelpia, PA

Blair A.M. Walker, M.D. [20]
Department of Pathology
University of Michigan Medical School
Ann Arbor, MI

Ruth S. Weinstock, M.D., Ph.D. [35b]
VAMC Syracuse
SUNY–Health Science Center at Syracuse
Department of Medicine
Syracuse, NY

PREFACE

How can one successfully teach immunology in an era when the field is rapidly expanding into all aspects of medical practice? What is needed is a text which represents all of the necessary basic concepts and mechanisms of immunology presented in the proper contexts. First, it must be clear how these facts are of relevance to the practice of medicine; medical students want to see the clinical relevance of the facts they learn, the promise at the end of the seemingly endless course work, reading, and studying. Second, immunology is ineluctably wed to the process of inflammation, so that any course teaching immunology must also show how specific immunity and non-specific inflammation cooperate in healing and in defense from pathogens and neoplasia. Finally, the immune system is but one part of the human body. Immunologic processes interact with many other parts of the body, including the nervous, endocrine, gastrointestinal, and pulmonary systems, as well as with the psyche; any forward looking approach to immunology must address these interactions. This, then, describes the task we set for ourselves: to produce a text which meets the needs of medical students and will serve them well when they are in the practice of the clinical or basic science field of their choice.

The text is divided into three parts; the first describes immunology, the second presents the various components of the inflammatory process, and the third shows how these interact to provide defenses and occasionally to produce disease.

Interspersed within many of the chapters are self-contained sections of text labeled "Clinical Asides." These are, in essence, tangents to the flow of the text; Asides provide another insight into the subject or offer a related idea. Many of them are descriptions of the clinical consequences of the processes being described in the text. We ask that you not read the Asides during your first reading of the text—they are to some degree tangential and may interfere with the momentum of the chapter. Go back to look them over in subsequent readings of the chapter, at a time when you can reflect on them having already assimilated the material in the chapter. The Asides may then be viewed as a new idea or facet of interest.

At the end of each chapter are selected references and questions. The references are designed to give you a more in-depth review of the material presented in the text, after your curiosity has been tickled. The questions, usually multiple choice or other board-type questions, are designed as a study guide. The authors have written questions which will allow you to focus on the most important points made in the chapter; use them as a study guide rather than as isolated quiz questions. In some cases, the material of the chapter does not lend itself to this kind of question, and essay-type questions are provided instead, again as a guide to the important issues covered in the chapter.

This is a text for medical students, soon to become physicians. The chapters on the feto-maternal interaction, the immune system of the newborn, psychoneuroimmunology, aging and nutrition and the immune system, immunotoxicology, and immunopharmacology, to name a few, may not fall within the confines of your current course in immunology. We offer these chapters because they represent the use to which you will put the basic principles in any immunology course. We hope that they will be of use to you when you enter the final two years of medical school and beyond, when you take on the role of a clinician. We hope that when you see patients you will think of the immune and inflammatory mechanisms which may underlie the patients' pathology. With the mechanism in mind, your understanding of the patient will be enhanced, and therapeutic decisions will make more sense. Some of these same chapters may seem on the verge of science fiction today but will surely be part of the routine practice of medicine in the near future. At the turn of the 19th century, who would have believed that there is more than one kind of white blood cell and that inert compounds are produced to recognize any constituent of an invading micro-organism? We are nearing the turn of another century; it is probably worthwhile to think of the future, and what better way than in the study of the evolving field of immunology?

INTRODUCTORY NOTES ON THE TEXT:
A statement of approach

Recent medical history has seen a revolution in our understanding of the mechanisms of disease and defense mechanisms. Now that we know some of the details it is increasingly important to approach clinical medicine with an appreciation of how immunologic mechanisms might be at the root of the disease or the response to the disease. With this insight, it becomes clear that an understanding of immunology is crucial to the practice of medicine, in diagnosis, understanding pathophysiology, and in determining an appropriate therapeutic regimen. Thus, teaching immunology represents a linchpin in medical education. We have carefully looked at the fields of basic and clinical immunology and inflammation and designed this book to help you learn the basic mechanisms and the clinical significance of this machinery.

The design of this text is a bit different from the others available. We think that immunology, with the potential for antigen-specific reactivity by cells and antibody, and inflammation, a series of non-specific mechanisms involved in resistance to and destruction of pathogens (and of host) and the repair of host tissues, cannot be taught as if unrelated. One must understand both and how the two are inextricably interwoven before one can appreciate their roles in human health and disease. Thus, we have assembled the book into three sections.

The first part deals with what is classically called immunology, the second with the variety of processes which constitute inflammation, and the third with how all of these mechanisms are related to human disease. The intent of the first two-thirds of this text is to prepare you for the final part and, by extension, for the practice of an immunologically enlightened style of medicine. We hope that this book will find a place in your locker while you are on your clinical rotations as student and house staff trainee and in your office when you finish your formal training.

Chapters on the interaction of immune function with stress, aging and/or diet, and reproduction are descriptions of new areas in immunology research. The final answers are not now available, but these chapters will hopefully give you a slightly different perspective on these and other clinical concerns, and demonstrate the range of processes in which immune mechanisms play a role.

Our aims are

  to prepare you to understand the basic principles of immunology
  to demonstrate how immunologic mechanisms are active in preventing and producing human diseases and how these diseases may be modified
  to encourage independent thinking and problem solving skills, especially as they pertain to clinical medicine
  to expose you to the new technology in use in all major research laboratories and help you understand how it can be applied.

The text includes two features with which you may have little previous experience. You will find occasional questions within the text. When you come across such a question, please pause and consider it; the question is designed to make you think, either about mechanisms, analogies with other immunologic or non-immunologic physiology, or the clinical relevance of the principles being described in the text. By addressing the question, you will make use of the information you are reading and hopefully find ways of retaining the information rather than simply memorizing a fact or two.

The second feature, mentioned previously, is the occasional boxed-in text, labeled "Aside" or "Clinical Aside." On your first reading of the text, please do not stop your reading in order to read the Asides. When you come back to the text for the second go-round, then please refer to the Asides. The Asides are usually somewhat tangential to the text. They are designed to give you a more in-depth explanation of a phenomenon or provide a clinical example of how the immunologic principles you are reading about are of clinical relevance. Thus, to stop during your first reading would interfere with the momentum of the text. Such ancillary information can best be appreciated and assimilated with a little more perspective, hopefully achieved after your first time through the section.

We hope that we have been able to communicate our fascination and excitement with immunology to you. We also hope that you will find this book useful when you start on your clinical rotations, so that you will be able to bring your basic science education directly into your practice of medicine. Good luck—your adventure has just begun!

INTRODUCTION

The purpose of the immune response is, basically, to keep us safe from microscopic invaders, whether they originate internally (e.g., malignant cells) or externally (e.g., bacterial, fungal, parasitic, or viral infections). The term originates with the root *munis*, referring to the city; thus immunity is a means by which to avoid the responsibilities incumbent upon a citizen (e.g., granting immunity to one of the watergate criminals in return for testimony), or it may be a means by which to avoid microscopic problems, as noted above.

The original problem confronting microscopic multicellular organisms was to differentiate "self" from "non-self"; non-self includes potential pathogens, effete or dead components of "self," and food. The primordial "immune" system sought to provide nutrition as well as defend the host; the separation of these two functions is recent enough that one can see significant homologies between various digestive enzymes and molecules active in the immune system (trypsin and thrombin are two such related molecules).

In order to efficiently study and understand the immune system a few guidelines or philosophic points are valuable. The first of these is the seemingly unnecessary assertion that the immune system is truly part of the body. As will be seen below, the immune system interacts continuously with the other organ systems of the body, in direct opposition to the old feeling that the immune system was somehow different, separate from the rest of the body, and non-interactive; nothing could be further from the truth. What affects the other "organs" usually affects the immune system (if thinking of the immune system as an organ spread widely around the body is confusing to you, think of the very covering of the body, the skin, as another non-centralized, very metabolically and immunologically active "organ"). Aspects of diet and the intake of toxins are environmental factors which affect the immune system. The status of the endocrine milieu has an effect on (and in turn, is affected by) the immune system. The various hormonal circadian rhythms actively interact with immunologic readiness, as does the neuropsychiatric status of the individual.

The immune system serves as a sensory organ, detecting danger and responding to this in just the way the neurologic system allows us to avoid walking into walls and open manhole covers. In ways that are not yet clear, this set of sensory inputs may affect us in a profound fashion (mice are capable of perceiving the genetic type of potential mates by sense of smell, the genetic type being determined by the immunologically important molecules found on all nucleated cells in their bodies).

Our understanding of the immune system is in its infancy and changing even as you read these words. Learning this set of topics demands acquiring what amounts to a new language, so your lack of fluency is not surprising. One of the major goals of this text will be to present the most up to date "truth"; there will be times when this text and older textbooks and journal articles may be directly contradictory. These contradictions may be so profound as to suggest that the fields are totally different, but they are not. These changes are to be expected in such a rapidly changing discipline. Techniques frequently have been borrowed from other disciplines, often revealing new insights of profound importance. Occasionally, revolutions in immunologic understanding have resulted. These techniques will be reviewed so that their true power will be clear, and their use as diagnostic tests will be discussed.

The systems which are included in immune responses appear complex and confusing at first. On closer observation, one can perceive a multilayered and intricately interactive pattern; the image of an archaeologic "dig" may be helpful in thinking about the study of immunology. The immune system is ancient, the first components appearing in multicellular organisms hundreds of millions of years ago. Many of the mechanisms in place at that time remain, some quite recognizable, others having taken on new guises. For this reason there are many sets of homologous molecules, a legacy of this long phylogenetic trial. Different functions are served by (a) the cell surface molecules which define "self," in an immunologic sense, (b) those molecules, known as antibodies, which recognize pathogens in the blood and tissue, and (c) those which define the function of certain cells, and yet all these molecules are clearly derived from a common ancestor. All of these molecules are quite polymorphic and their common ancestry is demonstrated clearly when one examines the means by which this heterogeneity is generated. In like fashion, with the evolution of these molecules to suit a variety of specific purposes, one finds homologous proteins serving very different purposes (recall, above, the fact that some digestive enzymes and pro-inflammatory molecules are quite similar).

Another manifestation of the phylogeny of the immune system is the presence of a variety of *non-specific* mechanisms which seem to function in parallel with the very *specific* mechanisms seen in the "modern" immune response. The responses seen in less advanced vertebrates and invertebrates are often non-specific, responding to a threat, every threat, in the same way. Some of these responses have been well studied and are termed "quasi-immune," since they are not truly *immune* (that is, do not demonstrate the ability to become more efficient with subsequent interactions with the same invader, and thus have "memory"), but do appear to serve an immune function. A good example of this is the "acute phase response" seen during the process of inflammation; a variety of serum proteins, including C-reactive protein, are produced by the liver in response to molecules which are made by inflammatory cells. The exact function of C-reactive protein is not clear; it may be a molecule which cleans up the debris left after an inflammatory process has occurred, or it may provide non-specific local defense from infections while the specific immune response begins to develop. Many of these quasi-immune mechanisms remain in the human repertoire, usually obscured by the vastly more effective and specific true immune response.

In general, nature is not wasteful, a concept known as the parsimony of nature (or "if it's not broke, don't fix it; if it works, keep it"). Once a molecule has been proven effective, it is retained, often improved and then applied for other purposes. Therefore, it is common to find a single molecule or class of molecules acting on a number of different cell types or active in a variety of pathways. In addition, it is common to find that multiple molecules may do what appears to be the same thing to a single cell type or organ.

There is virtually always a set of competing influences on any immune mechanism, positive and negative, helper/inducer and suppressor, yin and yang. In certain cases, there are multiple influences at work at the same time. And these influences are under controls of their own. And so on.

These very immune control systems, so vital for organized responses, may also cause or mediate tissue damage in various diseases. In certain circumstances the immune system turns on the host, causing auto-immunity. Current theories suggest that auto-immune reactivity, once thought to always be an aberrancy, may be a crucial part of normal housekeeping; only when immune self-recognition escapes from normal control does it cause disease. Poorly choreographed responses may be at the root of certain disease processes. Leprosy is due to an infection with *Mycobacterium leprae*; with a proper immune response to the organism, the host may experience no clinical problems at all (the only immune marker of preceding infection being the fact that there are immune blood cells in the person's body which can specifically recognize the organism). If the response is too great, the host suffers, with damage caused by the excess immune response. If the response is too feeble, uncontrolled growth of the organism will result and damage to the host occurs.

In the preceding and in subsequent discussions of immune response. The word *specific* is used. Strictly speaking the immune responses to an individual organism or tumor or to "self" are not directed solely to that target. There is almost always a certain amount of cross-reactivity involved; that is, the cell or antibody which recognizes one target may also recognize a second, similar, although occasionally unrelated, structure. These concepts of cross-reactivity and the true nature of "specific" should be kept in mind when trying to understand the immune system's role in defense from invasion and its ability to cause damage itself.

If medicine is the youngest science, then immunology is certainly the most junior discipline. In the last twenty years there has been an explosion of information and insight into the very finely tuned mechanisms which provide effective defense from infection and malignancy in the vast majority of individuals. The details of the immune response and the control mechanisms active in them will become clear during your careers. It is only through understanding these mechanisms that we can understand how the immune response has an effect on health and the practice of medicine.

The study of immunology should not be viewed as an end in itself but rather as a means to understanding the pathogenesis of diseases of virtually every organ system. Whether you decide to practice pediatrics or medicine, pathology or obstetrics and gynecology, surgery or neurology, immune mechanisms are active in the prevention and production of disease you will be studying and treating. The experimental tools you will learn about are being used in immunology and in other fields of medical research in order to understand the molecular pathogenesis of disease. The medical literature increasingly reports highly complex studies which you will have to evaluate, asking if the question is being answered and if the answer is relevant to your interests or those of your patients. Thus, an understanding of the body of information and the sharpening of your critical approach to this information will prove to be very useful in your future.

The remarkable fact is that the immune response works as well as it does, is as well behaved, well controlled, and efficient as it truly is. The application of our understanding of the immune systems to clinical situations is in its infancy. The truth as we know it changes every day. All of this may be viewed with alarm or it may be viewed as an adventure. It is, of course, the kind of challenge which drew you to medicine in the first place. The practice of good medicine is, in fact, a series of intellectual challenges, and it demands that we confront these tasks. Therefore, if challenge is your desire and delight, read on: the challenge of immunology awaits.

IMMUNOLOGY AND INFLAMMATION
Basic Mechanisms and Clinical Consequences

1

Immunology: A Historical Perspective

INTRODUCTION

On opening a new scientific text and finding that an early chapter discusses the historical perspectives of the discipline to be detailed, the reader may well be tempted to bypass the past and head toward the excitement of MHC restriction and the α and β chains of T-cell receptors. Resist! Wait, while a historical framework is reviewed on which a better understanding of immunology can be built.

Why is a historical perspective on science important? It would be enough to point out that it is as fascinating to look at the evolution of ideas as it is to look at the evolution of species, for here is the drama of missed opportunities, great mistakes, and brilliant intuition. But there are other compelling reasons for historical perspectives. History reminds us to encourage intellectual leaps and not to be satisfied with always moving from A to B to C. Time and time again, we can find an imaginative hypothesis being summarily dismissed by mainstream scientists, becoming firmly established as fact only many years later, after science has moved far away from the correct concept. History keeps us humble. When we examine how little was known about immunology a hundred years ago, we tend to forget that we must hope that our apparently sophisticated knowledge of the immune system will seem trivial to reviewers looking at our current perspectives this time next century.

The history of science reveals just how constructive and enjoyable passionate scientific debates can be, although pleasure is a motivation we seem to be losing in modern times. But a further and perhaps more important aspect of scientific history is being emphasized to the author as he writes this chapter in Berlin.

Berlin, more than any other city, can and does proclaim itself to have been the garden where the seeds of our knowledge about immunology were nurtured. It was in Berlin almost a hundred years ago that antibodies were discovered and serum institutes established. Brilliant teachers attracted brilliant students, and a discipline within medicine, destined to banish more suffering than any other, had life breathed into it after thousands of years of neglect.

Berlin is the city of Robert Koch, who identified the tubercle bacillus, and of his brilliant student, Paul Ehrlich, the first great immunologic thinker. It's the city where von Behring, Kitasato, Hoffman, Planck, and many others whom we will meet in the ensuing pages carried out some of their greatest experiments.

Looking at the history of immunology in Berlin reminds us that historical knowledge is indeed a vital factor in our attempts to understand the present behavior of human beings, both laudable and productive as well and shameful and wasteful, and our likely behavior in the future. Thus, it was in the spirit of "lest we forget" that the newly elected mayor of Berlin recently told those assembled for the opening ceremony of an immunology congress that Berliners were acutely aware that the famous Robert Koch Institute, whose founding scientists ignited the immunologic studies of this century, struggled through its period of shame when in 1933 many of its most famous scientists had to flee Germany because they were Jewish. In the years that followed many of the scientists in the institute disgraced themselves and, indeed, dishonored Koch and his pupils, as they participated in horrendous crimes against humanity in an evil and total distortion of all that is noble in medical research.

As scientific techniques develop ever greater capacities for the creation of happiness and misery in our world, we must diligently insist that science remain at the service of humanity. Remembering periods when the opposite was true is important in keeping science in its place. With those opening thoughts, let's examine the evolution of our understanding of the human defense system.

ANCIENT CONCEPTS

From the earliest clustering of human beings into primitive societal units, there must have been an appreciation of the obvious fact that survivors of certain diseases, characterizable by a set of specific features, were not visited by the same affliction a second time. Certainly, from the earliest periods of written history this fact was often noted. For example, we know from ancient Chinese writings that the observation of adaptive immunity led to an empirical approach to immunotherapy as long ago as 5000 B.C., even though there are no written speculations on the *mechanism* which might be involved. Very likely, the first significant (and dangerous) immunologic experiments involved attempts to protect individuals from the scourge that was smallpox. One did not suffer a second attack of the pox, and the healing scars of survivors were known to contain some material which could protect those not yet infected. The Chinese introduced a technique of inoculation of dust obtained from smallpox scars. The dust was blown through a silver tube into the left nostril of males and the right nostril of females; a protection could follow if the disease which ensued was itself not fatal. The procedure was associated with a death rate of about 4 percent, but the natural disease frequently burst upon communities killing more than 20 percent of its victims. We know that in many early societies, citizens would deliberately seek physical contact with an infected but recovering smallpox patient.

An appreciation of immunity was obvious in Thucydides' description of the plague which swept through Athens in 430 B.C. He noted that the sick and the dying found help and compassion most readily among those who had recovered from the disease: "These knew what it was from experience and had now no fear for themselves, for the same man

was never attacked twice—never at least fatally."

While smallpox forced early societies to think about immunity, the then-current concepts of disease and body function ensured that no understanding of the phenomenon was possible. For centuries, disease was seen as a punishment which destroyed health by interfering with the balance within the body of the vital fluids: blood, phlegm, and yellow and black bile.

DISEASE AS PESTILENCE

As early as 2000 B.C. the Babylonians were reporting the "visitation of pestilence." Disease was attributed in most early societies to the manipulation of health by demons, spirits, or gods, usually as punishment for sin. So ingrained was this concept in ancient Egypt that the Egyptians decided that there must be a god of disease. The Greeks accused an annoyed Apollo of firing plague arrows and were convinced that the misdeeds of Oedipus Rex resulted in the plague of Thebes.

In the Old Testament, God regularly "smited" the chosen people and their enemies with pestilence. Whether it was David annoying God by numbering the people or the Egyptians, Philistines, or Assyrians attacking his people, punishment by disease was at hand.

If disease was punishment, recovery must signal forgiveness. The bigger the sin the worse the disease, and recovery could only mean that a cleansing of the soul had occurred. After such an experience one would be unlikely to sin again and was thus "immune" to the recurrence of the process. So strong was this sentiment in the early Christian church that no other explanation for immunity would have been considered.

If religious conviction left the masses satisfied that they understood the extraordinary reality of immunity, the convictions of the Hippocratic school of medicine, passed on to physicians for century after century, very much restricted the framework within which early scientific minds could explore other possibilities. Body dynamics could only be viewed in terms of fluid changes. The sick vomited, had diarrhea, sweated, passed copious amounts of urine, bled profusely, etc. Thus, when the remarkable Islamic physician Rhazes approached the problem of immunity in the tenth century, he acknowledged that recovery from measles and smallpox (which he quite clearly differentiated) meant immunity to these diseases, but explained the phenomenon in terms of an "excessive moisture" theory. Smallpox was associated with fever, as a result of which blood would ferment and be expelled through pustules, the excessive fluid thought to be circulating in the body of the young. Smallpox was not a bad thing, as this fluid must be expelled if health was to be established for adult life. Once the excessive and therefore offensive fluid was removed, the problem was solved and one became immune to smallpox.

In the eleventh century another great early thinker, Avicenna, introduced the concept of germs, which he thought of as small seeds (*seminaria*) with special predilection for growing in this or that bodily region. Such seeds could be passed from one person to another, thus being agents of infection. In 1546 the Italian physician Fracastoro wrote *On Contagion*, a book in which he described how smallpox seeds best fermented in menstrual blood. He believed that all neonates were contaminated with menstrual blood which had to be expelled from their bodies if they were to become healthy. Smallpox seeds caused the menstrual blood to ferment, which then escaped through the pustules. Once free of this contaminating blood, one could not be troubled by smallpox seeds, which would subsequently be denied any appropriate substrate. Others picked up on this idea and proposed that certain germs were needed to rid the young of contaminating amniotic fluid and umbilical blood.

It is easy to understand the concentration in early writings on children with infectious diseases, for children were so often associated with skin manifestations not seen in the older, "purified," population.

Depletion theories of acquired immunity held their currency until the time of Louis Pasteur, but there evolved a number of variations on the theme. Inoculation procedures to protect one from smallpox gained favor in the Europe of the early eighteenth century; the popularity of inoculation was somewhat romantically attributed by Voltaire to the efforts of one Lady Mary Wortley Montagu, who had supposedly observed the procedure in Turkey. After the Prince of Wales allowed his children to be inoculated in 1722, the now-respectable technique was subjected to a more scientific scrutiny. Many considered that inoculation utilized all the available but irreplaceable substrate, thus cheating the natural disease of "those Humours in the Blood which the Invader makes a Seizure on."

During the seventeenth and eighteenth centuries it was hypothesized that every human being was born with all the seeds (or "ovula," as they were described by Thomas Fuller) necessary for every disease process. Once fertilized by a specific and contagious substrate, that particular germ would flourish and cause its disease, "and when these had been impregnated and delivered of their morbid fetus there is an end of them. Upon this account no man can possibly be infected with any of the respective distempers any more than once." With this historical perspective on acquired immunity, it is not surprising that after the discovery of real germs in the form of bacteria by Robert Koch, Hansen, and others, the great Louis Pasteur tried to explain his first great observation in substrate terms.

Pasteur was able to demonstrate that chickens could be protected from fowl cholera by exposure to an attenuated strain of organisms. Chance played into Pasteur's talented hands here. A cholera strain left in the laboratory during a vacation period lost its virulence; it could no longer cause disease, but could produce immunity when introduced into naive animals. "Chance favoring the prepared mind," as Pasteur himself noted, he was able to correctly interpret this result in terms of the protective capacity of attenuated organisms.

Because Pasteur had observed bacteria rapidly growing in culture for a period, then seemingly resting as the rate of growth slowed, he proposed that natural and attenuated organisms produced immunity by depletion of an essential trace element during the in vivo proliferation of the organism.

Soon, however, the contortions required to make acquired immunity fit substrate-depletion concepts ended with the scientifically shattering evidence produced by Theobald Smith that dead organisms were as good as live ones in producing immunity. Such theories were further brought into disrepute when von Behring and Kitasato demonstrated that even supernatants from diphtheria organisms could confer immunity.

With these observations, immunology came into its own as a science. Robert Koch and his team worked tirelessly to isolate and identify organisms, and Pasteur produced a series of attenuated vaccines. To honour Edward Jenner, Pasteur deliberately extended the term vaccination (Latin *vacca*, "cow") to include immunization with any attenuated strain.

The country general practitioner Edward Jenner (1749–1823) had published his report in 1798 that material obtained from cowpox pustules, when inoculated into the skin of individuals who had not had smallpox, produced protection against the dangerous disease with minimal side effects. Although Jenner was highly regarded in his own lifetime, and indeed within a few years of his 1796 observation Jenner's vaccination techniques were used throughout the world, he never speculated on the mechanisms by which those techniques produced protection. Perhaps he had been influenced by a remark reportedly made to him by one of his mentors, the famous teacher John Hunter: "Why think? Why not try the experiment?" Things were very different, however, 100 years later as more and more scientists observing the work of Pasteur and Koch wanted to know what

actually happens in the host exposed to an organism which renders the host invulnerable to further attacks by the same organism.

HUMORAL IMMUNITY

After the great fire of London in 1666, Samuel Pepys wrote in his invaluable diaries of an evening when two doctors, Lower and King, demonstrated blood transfusion from one animal to another using a needle specifically designed for the purpose by the great architect Sir Christopher Wren. After the successful demonstration, Lower turned to the friends gathered for the evening and in an excited fashion explained that with this experiment he foresaw an era in which there would be "the mending of bad blood by the borrowing of blood from a better body."

Undoubtedly those words were not ringing in the ears of Emil von Behring and Shibasuburo Kitasato in 1890 as they discovered that immunized animals produced something in their blood which neutralized the deadly diphtheria toxin. They observed the same phenomenon when experimenting with tetanus toxin. They immunized pigs and subsequently horses with diphtheria toxin isolated by Roux and Yersin in 1888. The toxin had been shown to produce all the worst features of the disease, an observation which explained why Pasteur had failed to produce a vaccine using whole organisms. One can now only imagine the excitement and trepidation with which they "borrowed blood from a better body," in this case their immunized horses, and administered the material to children with diphtheria. The results were dramatically positive, especially if the fluid was given during the early stage of the disease. Whatever it was they were administering, it was soon called "antitoxin" and then "antibody" to broaden the concept beyond bacterial toxins. With humoral substances to chase, it was time for chemists to take up the challenge presented by the observations of von Behring and Kitasato.

IMMUNOCHEMISTRY

It soon became obvious that antibodies were not substances made only in response to exposure to toxins or even bacteria. Antibodies to harmless substances could be made. The demonstration of such phenomena required a laboratory technique for visualizing the interaction of antigen and antibody. In 1896 Gruber and Durham discovered the agglutination reaction (initially using bacteria), and a year later Kraus discovered the precipitin reaction. Now quantitative work on antibodies could begin.

Paul Ehrlich was the genius who most advanced immunochemistry and immunology at this time. At the age of 20 Ehrlich had begun his studies with Robert Koch, and he was very much influenced by his friend August von Hoffmann, a famous chemist whose knowledge of dyes was unsurpassed. Ehrlich applied dye technology to the staining of organisms, and, among other things, established the acid-fast nature of mycobacteria. When he turned his attention to the problem of antibodies, he clearly stated that the principles of structural chemistry, including the lock-and-key metaphor used by chemists in describing enzyme combinations with substrate, must apply to antigen-antibody interactions. He talked about functional domains and binding sites, and established methods for quantifying the toxin-neutralizing capacity of antitoxin. But when in 1897 he was invited to London to give the Croonian Lecture before the Royal Society, he addressed the question of the origin of antibodies in cellular terms.

He disagreed with the prevailing theories that antibody specificity was determined by antigen which could somehow induce conformational changes in a passive chemical, that would subsequently retain such changes. Such thinking was the basis for "template," or "instructional," theories of antibody formation, which were to hold sway for many years to come. Ehrlich, however, argued that cells had side chains projecting from their surfaces. Although these side chains were primarily involved with absorbing nutrients required by the cell, individual chains were programmed prior to an encounter with an antigen to interact, key-in-lock fashion, with the specific foreign protein. Such antibodies could be released from the surface of cells bearing such structures once antigen-bound to some of these unique side chains.

This was an extraordinary conceptual leap for the time. Indeed, the essential element of Ehrlich's theory was correct, although he was wrong in two areas. First, he thought every cell in the body was capable of making antibodies. Such was his influence that few researchers bothered to hypothesize the existence of specific antibody-producing cells for another 50 years. Second, Ehrlich wrongly considered that antigen-antibody reactions were irreversible.

As the huge repertoire of antibodies became clearer, many began to doubt Ehrlich's concepts. Template theories reemerged and grew stronger. It would not be until 1941, when dissatisfaction with observations that antibody production could continue without the presence of antigen and that second immunizations resulted in the production of excessive and larger amounts of antibody with higher affinity for antigen, that Macfarlane Burnet would find it essential to modify template theories. Ehrlich would go on to cancer research and to the development of chemotherapy for a number of conditions, notably syphilis, but his theories on antibody formation established for posterity the genius of his intellect.

CELLULAR IMMUNITY

With the discovery of antibodies, most turn-of-the-century scientists thought that the complete solution to immunity was within their grasp. However, a vociferous minority insisted that specific cells in the body were equally important, if not more important, than antibodies. The chief proponent of cellular immunity was the brilliant Russian zoologist, Elie Metchnikoff (1845–1916), who was strongly influenced by the theories of Darwin circulating in the 1860s and 1870s. He was looking for a genetic and embryologic unity in phylogeny.

In a famous and spontaneous experiment, he recognized the importance of cellular defenses in the general scheme of inflammatory responses. He tells the story of his famous experiment thus. In 1883 Metchnikoff and his family were relaxing in the straits of Messina. One afternoon when the rest of the family had gone to the circus, he was looking through his microscope at transparent starfish, visualizing the incessant wandering of mobile cells around their bodies. Suddenly, the thought that such cells could play a role in defense flashed into his mind.

Previously, the observation of cells containing foreign matter had been interpreted as a phenomenon resulting from the invasion of the cell by an organism, and the foreign matter was regarded as deleterious. Now Metchnikoff came up with the idea that cells containing such matter might actually be "swallowing" an invader in an attempt to destroy it. In his garden in Messina was a little tangerine tree already decorated for Christmas. He took some thorns from the tree and introduced them under the skin of some "beautiful starfish as transparent as water." After a sleepless night, he was able to observe that, as he had predicted, the mobile cells of the starfish had swarmed to and subsequently engulfed his thorns.

Metchnikoff's observation became the basis for his theory of an active cellular defense mechanism. In 1884 Metchnikoff observed that the tiny transparent metazoan animal *Daphnia* was not killed by the spores of a certain fungus in cases in which *Daphnia*'s blood cells attacked, engulfed, and subsequently destroyed those spores. He demonstrated a similar phenomenon in rabbits, and introduced the term "phagocytosis" to describe it. He demonstrated that phagocytic ability was shared by two distinct cells in the body of higher species, the polymorphonuclear leukocyte and the monocyte, and established that these cells could move by diapedesis from blood vessels into tissues for the purpose of phagocytosis.

As Metchnikoff developed his theories, he so impressed Louis Pasteur that the latter convinced him to join his team in Paris. After so doing, Metchnikoff doggedly pursued the importance of phagocytosis for many years. However, the scientific sun was shining ever more brightly on the humoralists in Berlin, and few accepted primacy for any cellular theory. Who needed phagocytes after Nuttall, in 1888, showed that antibodies would kill bacteria and Bordet discovered complement. The young Belgian Jules Bordet was actually working in Metchnikoff's laboratory when, in 1895, he clearly demonstrated that for antibody to lyse bacteria (or blood cells, for that matter), a second and thermolabile factor or series of factors was needed. He grouped these substances under the name of *Alexine*, but Ehrlich thought that *complement* was a better term and indeed this soon became the accepted terminology. One can only imagine the heated debates which must have raged in Metchnikoff's laboratories as antibodies and complement were shown to form such a powerful team.

Metchnikoff fought back, however, and in a series of brilliant experiments showed that there was not often a good correlation between the bactericidal powers of blood and host resistance to infection. Organisms wrapped in filter paper and thus protected from phagocytosis remained virulent despite the presence of an antibody in certain circumstances. He was able to demonstrate that normally lethal injections of organisms into the peritoneal cavity of experimental animals could be rendered harmless by activating peritoneal macrophages prior to injection of the organisms.

Who was right, Metchnikoff or Ehrlich, wondered the scientific world? We know that both were right of course, and so did two Englishmen, Wright and Douglass, who tried to bring the two schools together with their demonstration of opsonization (from the Greek *opsonein*, "to render palatable"). They correctly showed that antibody-coated organisms were prepared for phagocytosis, but the methods they used were cumbersome, and few at the time could confirm their observations and therefore support them. In 1908 the argument was still raging, so the Nobel Prize for Medicine was awarded to both Metchnikoff and Ehrlich.

HYPERSENSITIVITY

As the twentieth century started, all manner of new observations were being made by more and more excited immunologists. In the early part of the century two crucial sets of experiments introduced the concept of hypersensitivity. Previously, it had been presumed by Ehrlich and others that immune responses were protective—occasionally useless when provoked by trivial antigens, but never harmful.

Robert Koch had experienced a difficult period in trying to prepare a vaccine against tuberculosis. Unlike Pasteur's success with rabies and anthrax, giving tuberculin to humans produced an altogether unwanted response, which became known as the Koch phenomenon. The more tuberculous material Koch injected into the skin, the more severe the provoked reaction. He incorrectly interpreted this as resulting from the presence of a toxin in his preparations.

Meanwhile out in the Mediterranean in the summer of 1902, two scientific friends of the Prince of Morocco, Richet and Portier, were working on ways of desensitizing animals to the sting of *Actiniaria*, a most unpleasant jellyfish. When they injected a glycerine extract of the toxic substance found in the tentacles of these creatures, their experimental dogs did not seem perturbed, and Richet and Portier concluded that after an appropriate time, the dogs would become immune to *Actiniaria's* sting. To their surprise, a second injection of the same material led to the sudden death of a number of the dogs. This phenomenon they called *anaphylaxis* (from the Greek word *ana*, meaning "excessive," and *phylassein*, meaning "to guard").

It remained for another towering figure of early twentieth century immunology to sort out the observations being made by Koch, Richet, and Portier. The famous Prussian pediatrician Clemens von Pirquet, working hard to explain the Koch phenomenon, noted that the skin reaction some 24 to 48 hours after the injection of tuberculin indicated the prior existence of a useful immune response. "Delayed hypersensitivity," he concluded, was useful, in contradistinction to the immediate hypersensitivity noted by Richet, Portier, and many others. These latter reactions were not only useless, they were dangerous. Von Pirquet was able to distinguish "useful" from "useless" on the basis of the timing of the reaction which followed introduction of the antigen. He noted that what was being observed in both cases was clearly an altered state of immunologic energy, and to cover both extremes, he coined the term "allergy," from the Greek *allergie*, a combination of *all-*, "altered," and *ergie*, from *ergon*, "work."

Von Pirquet tried to explain these phenomena in terms of antibodies. This of course was impossible, but it was now clear that some immunologic mechanisms could cause harm. Von Pirquet, one of the most complex, indeed, neurotic of immunologic pioneers, was to terminate his life whilst still in his intellectual prime in a suicide pact with his wife. He left a note saying that he could no longer tolerate the imperfection of the world in which he lived. Before he died, however, he had linked another form of hypersensitivity, the Arthus phenomenon, to serum sickness, a major problem for clinicians and patients in the heyday of serum therapy.

Arthus had demonstrated that simple proteins injected into the skin of immune animals could produce a reaction, the timing of which fell between the immediate-hypersensitivity-type reactions of anaphylaxis and the delayed reactions of the tuberculin test. Histologic examination of those lesions showed a profuse polymorphonuclear infiltrate which could result in necrosis of the skin. This phenomenology correlated well with the ever more frequently noted serum sickness.

In 1910 Schulz demonstrated that a strip of intestine from an immunized animal actually contracted when exposed to the sensitizing antigen. A better model was established by Dale in Switzerland, who demonstrated that histamine caused a similar response on uterine smooth muscle. Dale's observations enabled the establishment of the science of immunopharmacology.

That a specific chemical entity was responsible for anaphylactic phenomena was demonstrated in 1921 by the remarkable experiments of Prausnitz and Kustner. Serum from Kustner, who was allergic to certain fish, was injected into Prausnitz's skin. No reaction occurred after the initial injection. However, a classic wheal-and-flare response developed if fish extracts were subsequently introduced into his sensitized site. Prausnitz's local tissues had clearly been sensitized by an allergic factor in Kustner's serum.

If an "overenthusiastic" response to antigen could cause tissue damage, could some forms of pathology result from a reaction against self, that is, autoimmunity?

AUTOIMMUNITY

Paul Ehrlich had stated that our immune system should not react against components of self. He termed such a phenomenon, if it occurred, "horror autotoxicus." But Metchnikoff had noted that animals could make an immune response to an injection of their own sperm. Here, as with immediate hypersensitivity, was a situation wherein the immune system could embarrass an individual by participating in reactions which could be deleterious. Observations that injuries to an eye could be followed by a dangerous immunologic response against that damaged eye, and even the noninjured eye, were clear-cut demonstrations that autoimmune responses did in fact exist. It wasn't long before immunologic attacks on red cells, thyroid tissue, and even the brain were noted to occur, first in experimental and then in clinical situations.

THE ERA OF IMMUNOCHEMISTRY

During the first three decades of this century, vaccine production and serum therapy dominated clinical immunology. Immunochemical techniques concentrated on understanding and quantifying the antigen-antibody reaction. This was the period when template or instructional theories held sway. It was constantly argued that antigen must itself, in some way, transmit the information for specificity to a malleable substance. Ehrlich's prophecies slid into the background.

In 1930 Breinl and Haurowitz published their template theory, which was subsequently supported by the prestigious physicist Linus Pauling. Few had been deterred from this logical, if simplistic, approach by what Karl Landsteiner called "hapten phenomenology" in 1921. Landsteiner had demonstrated that a group of substances which by themselves could not provoke the formation of antibodies were definitely responsible for the production of antibodies to themselves when conjugated to a protein. Clearly, this was a difficult phenomenon for the instructionalist to explain.

The biologic inadequacies of the template theory led Macfarlane Burnet to look for a new explanation. He introduced an additional step. An antigen would instruct a series of adaptive enzymes, which would then produce a uniquely specific globulin. Replication of the cells producing these enzymes could allow antibody formation to persist beyond the presence of antigen itself, and explain the memory responses. This was the first clear proposal for clonal proliferation.

Shortly after Burnet's stimulating concepts were proposed, Niels Jerne in 1955 returned immunology to the ideas of Ehrlich. Jerne agreed with Ehrlich that the entire antibody repertoire was inherited and that small amounts of antibody would appear in the serum as "natural antibodies." When an antigen entered the body, these antibodies would transport it to the appropriate cell, which would then greatly increase its production of the specific antibody. This theory of natural selection incorporated Burnet's ideas on clonal expansion to explain the memory response of second exposures to an antigen, and offered an explanation for the emerging concepts of tolerance (see below). Reactions to self could not be amplified, as self-tissues would absorb out of the circulation "natural" self-antibodies, which would therefore not be available to present antigen to antibody-producing cells.

In a series of papers which most certainly would have delighted Ehrlich, Jerne's theory was modified by Burnet, Lederberg, and Talmadge. Antibodies would be present on the surface of specific cells (not all cells, as proposed by Ehrlich) and act as receptors for an antigen. In this way, an antigen would select a specific clone, which would then produce and secrete a specific antibody. With the development by Jerne of the Haemolytic Plaque Assay System, a tool was at last available for examining individual cells reacting to antigen. This, and the development of fluorescent antibody, soon allowed immunochemists to establish these pioneering theories as fact.

THE SECOND COMING OF CELLULAR IMMUNOLOGY

Von Pirquet had been well aware that all the immune phenomena he studied except delayed-type hypersensitivity could be transferred from one animal to another by serum; this exception troubled him greatly. The importance, therefore, of the demonstration by Landsteiner and Chase in 1942 that peripheral blood cells, but not serum, could transfer delayed-type hypersensitivity cannot be exaggerated. Cell-mediated immunity had arrived. Soon it was demonstrated that many of the experimental autoimmune diseases (for example, experimental allergic encephalomyelitis) could be transferred from one animal to another by cells but not by serum.

In our time of T-cell heterogeneity, which sees such cells dominating both in the in-

duction and regulation of an immune response, we can easily appreciate the enormous importance of the discovery that there was a powerful immune mechanism (occasionally capable of producing pathology) mediated by a cellular defense system independent of an antibody. But history tells us that the impact on the scientific world of the demonstration by Landsteiner and Chase of cell-mediated immunity was initially minimal. It would take another decade for cell-mediated immunity to be widely accepted as the vital force in immunology.

It is of interest that the requirements of military medicine in the early stages of World War II increased the momentum for immunologic research. Cohn's laboratory in the United States was working on fluid-replacement strategies for the wounded soldier when their research produced gammaglobulin preparations for therapeutic use. At the same time, a brilliant young scientist named Peter Medawar was at work on a quite different problem, that of tissue grafts for the severely wounded and/or burned. Medawar, a zoologist and pathologist, showed that skin-graft rejection followed all of the known immunologic laws for specificity and certainly involved a massive cellular infiltrate into the tissue as it was rejected.

In 1945 Ray Owen demonstrated a remarkable phenomenon observed in dizygotic twin cattle. The animals were true chimeras, immunologically tolerant of each other's tissues and serum.

This observation excited the theoretician Burnet, who in 1949 provided an intellectually appealing explanation of Owen's findings. During fetal life, he argued, the developing system catalogued all the antigenic determinants in its microenvironment. All noted were regarded as *self*, and tolerance to these "self-determinants" followed. Any new antigen introduced after cataloging was complete would be regarded as *nonself* and provoke an immune response. Later, Burnet refined these ideas; his clonal selection theory proposed that cells reacting to an antigen during the early formation of the immune system would be clonally aborted, thus ensuring nonreactivity to self. This theory in turn required refinement, but the debate Burnet's hypotheses generated moved cellular concepts to the forefront of immunologic research.

Medawar and his students Brent and Billingham, building on the theories of Burnet, were able to show that the introduction of an antigen to a fetal immune system did indeed produce a state of tolerance. Cellular concepts of immunology had arrived, but where were these invaluable cells generated?

In 1962 Jacques Miller was working in London studying leukemia which developed in AKR mice. It had been noted that leukemia usually started in the thymus gland of these mice, and Miller wondered if they would be protected from leukemia by thymectomy. In a brilliant series of experiments, he was able to demonstrate that thymectomy, done at a very early age in these mice, left them without the capacity to generate a cell-mediated immune system. The thymus was essential for the production of cells capable of organizing the complexity of a cellular immune defense. Simultaneously, Robert Good and his colleagues in Minnesota demonstrated the same phenomenon in rabbits. It was considerably later that the cells generated in the thymus gland were to be designated as T cells.

Shortly after the discovery of the role of the thymus, Noel Warner and his colleagues in Melbourne discovered, in a series of experiments with chickens, that the bursa of Fabricius is responsible for generating the cells capable of manufacturing antibodies in birds. Such cells were soon to be designated *B cells*. By coincidence, the major source of such antibody-producing cells in higher species is the bone marrow, so the B-cell label is equally applicable to human beings. With the somewhat serendipitous discovery in 1962 by Claman and his colleagues in Denver that B cells were in fact not efficient antibody producers unless helped by T cells, modern immunology was at last able to join the cellular and humoral aspects of immunology. The stage was set for three decades of extraordinarily productive research. It is the results of this exciting work which fill the pages of this book.

ADDITIONAL READINGS

Bordet J. *Studies on Immunity*, Gay F (trans.). New York: Wiley; 1990.

Burnet FM. *The Production of Antibodies*, 1st ed. Melbourne: Macmillan; 1941.

Burnet FM. *The Clonal Selection Theory of Acquired Immunity*. Cambridge: Cambridge University Press; 1959.

Burnet FM, Fenner F. *The Production of Antibodies*, 2nd ed. Melbourne: Macmillan; 1949.

Castiglioni A. *A History of Medicine*. New York: Knopf; 1947.

Ehrlich P. The Croonian lecture: On immunity. *Proc R Soc Lond* (Biol). 1900; 66:424.

Foster WD. *A History of Medical Bacteriology and Immunology*. London: Heinemann; 1970.

Kelly EC. *Encyclopedia of Medical Sources*. Baltimore: Williams & Wilkins; 1948.

Landsteiner K. *The Specificity of Serological Reactions*. Cambridge, Mass: Harvard University Press; 1945.

Metchnikoff E. *Lectures on the Comparative Pathology of Inflammation*. London: Kegan, Paul, Trench, Trubner; 1893.

Metchnikoff E. *Immunity in the Infectious Diseases*. New York: Macmillan; 1905.

Metchnikoff O. *Life of Elie Metchnikoff*. Boston: Houghton Mifflin; 1921.

Morton LT. *Medical Bibliography: An Annotated Checklist of Texts Illustrating the History of Medicine*, 3rd ed. Philadelphia: Lippincott; 1970.

Nuttall GHF. *Blood Immunity and Blood Relationships*. Cambridge: Cambridge University Press; 1904.

Schmidt JE. *Medical Discoveries: Who and When*. Springfield, Ill: Charles C Thomas; 1959.

von Pirquet C, Schick B. *Serum Sickness*. Baltimore: Williams & Wilkins; 1951.

Wilson D. *Science of Self: A Report of the New Immunology*. White Plains, NY: Longman; 1971.

PART

ONE

Basic Mechanisms of Immunology

One cannot fathom medicine as it will be practiced in the next century nor the current scientific and medical literature without understanding immunology. As was described in Chapter 1, "The History of Immunology", this is a young science, first appearing only after vaccination to prevent disease (1798), inoculation to elicit "antitoxins" (1890), and Ehrlich's rejection of the "template" theory (1897). The quality of plasticity intrinsic to such a model presaged all that was to come in the study of humoral and cellular immunity. It is plasticity, the ability to respond and tailor the host response to invading pathogens, that is the subject of Part I: Basic Mechanisms of Immunology.

In Part I antigen-specific mechanisms of the immune response will be described after you are introduced to the histologic frameworks that provide organization and structure for the immune system (Chapter 2, "Effector Cells and Tissues of the Immune System"). Three chapters will describe molecules capable of antigen-specific interactions, immunoglobulin (Chapter 3, "Antibodies: Structure and Function"), the molecules of the major histocompatibility complex (Chapter 4), and how a virtually limitless degree of antigen specificity can be programmed by a finite amount of genetic material (Chapter 5, "Generation of Diversity in the Acquired Immune Response"). Development and regulation are the themes of the final seven chapters of Part I. Chapters 6 and 7 describe the ontogeny and differentiation of the two immune cells capable of producing an antigen-specific response, the B cell (which gives rise to plasma cells, which produce antibody) and the T cell (different families of T cells having a variety of regulatory and effector functions, including cytotoxicity, described in Chapter 8, "Specific and Non-specific Cell Mediated Cytotoxicity"). Cell-cell and antibody-antibody regulatory interactions are described in Chapters 9 and 10 ("Regulation of the Immune System" and "Cytokines and the Immune System," respectively). Finally, we come to a description of organization and compartmentalization of antigen-specific responses in Chapters 11 and 12 ("The Mucosal Immune System" and "Mechanisms of Lymphocyte Recirculation and Homing"), where we discuss how the immune response can remain localized or become systemic, depending on the need.

Thus, in the space of 12 chapters, you will have started with the ancients, pondering bad blood and imbalances of bile and considering how much further to bleed patients in order to effect a cure, and proceeded all the way to the threshold of the twenty-first century, as we dissect the molecular biology of immune defenses and immune mechanisms of disease. A long road, to be sure, but a road which is about to lead to pathogenetic and therapeutic insights which would have brought a smile (and probably a knowing nod) to the faces of Pasteur, Metchnikoff, Ehrlich, Koch, and Jenner).

A final word: make free use of the Glossary (Appendix A) at the end of the book so that new terms are clear to you: learn the new language of immunology and the study of the subject will be vastly easier.

2

Cells and Tissues of the Immune System

INTRODUCTION

The major role of the immune system is to protect the individual from invasion by infectious organisms and other agents that can cause disease. The cells of the immune system include lymphocytes and different types of phagocytic cells organized in the lymphoid tissues (Fig. 2-1). These lymphoid tissues are in constant communication by virtue of lymphocyte traffic. Such traffic is possible through the blood and lymphatic networks of the body.

The phagocytic cells are the more primitive cellular elements of the immune system. In mammalian species one type of phagocytic cells, the mononuclear phagocytes, also act as antigen-presenting cells (APC). These cells ingest and partially degrade foreign substances and then express constituent parts (antigenic determinants) of phagocytized antigens on their membrane so that they can be recognized by lymphocytes. Lymphocytes then respond in a variety of ways to neutralize or destroy agents that express these determinants. There is a division of labor among different types of lymphocytes, and their responses vary with the type of antigen they encounter. There are two major types of lymphocytes.

The so-called *T lymphocytes* are responsible for cell-mediated immunity. Their specificity is controlled by antigen receptors on their surface, the T-cell receptors (TCRs). The TCR is composed of polypeptide chains, the N-terminal ends of which make up the antigen-combining site. The response of an individual T cell is initiated when it encounters an antigenic determinant (on the surface of an APC) for which its receptor is specific. T lymphocytes produce several types of molecules known as lymphokines. Lymphokines have various functions which serve to stimulate or amplify the responses of other lymphocytes by interaction with different specific receptors, and are produced primarily by a functional subset of helper T cells. A different type of T lymphocyte, called cytotoxic T cells or killer T cells, develops the capability to lyse specific cellular targets such as virally infected cells, tumor cells, or foreign cells transplanted into the body. Another type of T lymphocyte, called suppressor T cells, performs an immunoregulatory role for the immune system. When appropriately stimulated, suppressor T cells negatively influence the responses of other

Figure 2-1. *Origin and development of the cells involved in the immune response.*

The lymphoid progenitor cell is derived from the pluripotent stem cell, giving rise to three distinct types of cells. Lymphoid stem cells arrive in the thymus and develop into T cells (*T* stands for thymus). Once T cells have matured, they populate the T cell areas of lymph nodes and other lymphoid tissues, circulate in the lymph and blood, and provide *cellular immunity*, including immune control and effector function.

$$T_s = T \text{ suppressor cells}$$
$$T_C = T \text{ cytotoxic cells}$$
$$T_H = T \text{ helper cells}$$

Other stem cells arrive in the bone marrow and develop into B cells (*B* stands for the bursa of Fabricius, the organ in birds where B cell maturation was first described). B cells then populate the B cell areas of lymph nodes and other lymphoid organs. After they develop further, into plasma cells (which secrete immunoglobulin), they provide *humoral immunity*.

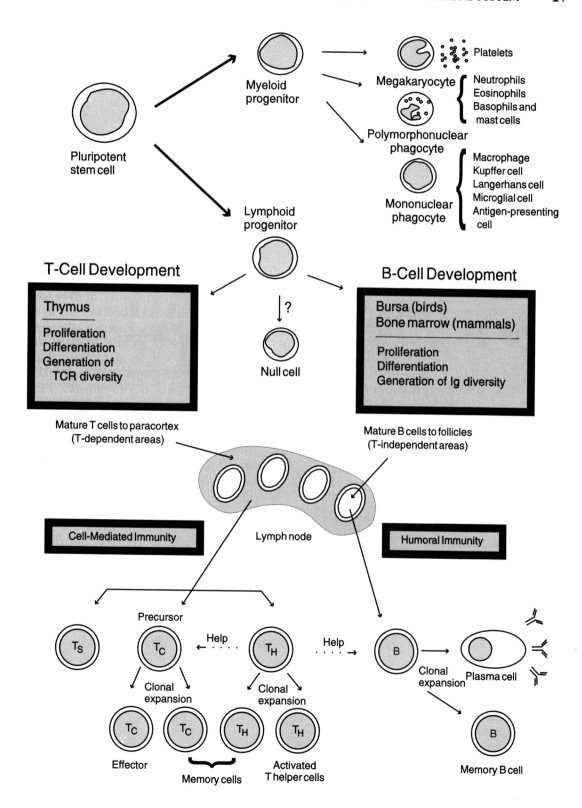

lymphocytes. Thus, suppressor T cells can, in effect, "turn off" the immune response. A newly defined population of lymphocytes known as contrasuppressor cells is believed to balance the action of suppressor cells.

Other lymphocytes, called *B cells*, are responsible for humoral immunity. Their surface receptors for antigen are the immunoglobulin (Ig) molecules. Ig molecules are composed of four polypeptides (two identical heavy chains of 50 kd each; and two identical light chains of 25 kd each) that are linked by disulfide bonds. Their N-terminal ends comprise what is called the variable region. The specificity of the Ig molecule for a particular antigenic determinant is determined by the amino acid sequence within the variable region. When a B cell encounters a specific antigenic determinant it can recognize through its Ig surface receptor, it is stimulated to divide, to produce more of the Ig molecules, and to secrete them. These secreted Ig molecules, now referred to as antibodies, have the same specificity as the original Ig membrane receptor on the B cell, and can bind to the same antigenic determinant. Interactions of antibodies with antigens can trigger secondary mechanisms involving other plasma proteins, such as the complement components.

The cells of the immune system are organized into the lymphoid organs. The primary (central) lymphoid organs provide the environment for lymphopoiesis and lymphocyte differentiation and maturation. In these organs the lymphocytes acquire their antigen-recognition capacity, but their proliferation there is not driven by antigenic stimulation. In mammals, the T lymphocytes are generated in the thymus and the B lymphocytes in the fetal liver and bone marrow. In birds, there is a specific organ for B-cell differentiation, the bursa of Fabricius.

The secondary (peripheral) lymphoid organs provide an environment useful for interaction of lymphocytes with antigens and other cell types required for an effective immune response. These organs consist of spleen, lymph nodes, and diffuse areas of lymphoid tissue associated with the mucosal surfaces in the body. The best-known examples of mucosa-associated lymphoid tissue are the aggregated lymphoid nodules in the ileum called Peyer's patches. Mature lymphocytes in peripheral lymphoid tissues proliferate in response to antigenic stimuli. There is a continuing communication between the lymphoid tissues by the pool of recirculating lymphocytes present in the blood and lymph.

LYMPHOCYTES AND THEIR DIFFERENTIATION IN PRIMARY LYMPHOID ORGANS

An adult human has about 10^{12} mature lymphocytes. Within this number are cells that express receptors which can recognize virtually every antigenic determinant that exists, not only in nature, but even those that are newly synthesized in the laboratory. The genetic mechanisms by which this diversity is produced have been the focus of one of the most fascinating scientific investigations of the past decade.

Resting lymphocytes, as they appear in a peripheral blood smear, show little heterogeneity in their morphology (Fig. 2-2a). They range in size from 6 to 10 μm; there is usually a high nucleus/cytoplasm ratio, and few cytoplasmic organelles are present. A minority of lymphocytes are slightly larger and possess azurophilic granules in their cytoplasm. These cells are referred to as *large granular lymphocytes* (Fig. 2-2b).

Once stimulated by the antigenic determinant for which it has a specific receptor, the morphology of the lymphocyte changes dramatically. The cell undergoes a process known as *blast transformation*. The cell increases in size due to activation of protein and DNA synthetic mechanisms. The antigen-stimulated lymphocyte proliferates and its progeny differentiate into mature effector cells, all of which have the same antigen specificity. This process of *clonal expansion* increases the number of lymphocytes

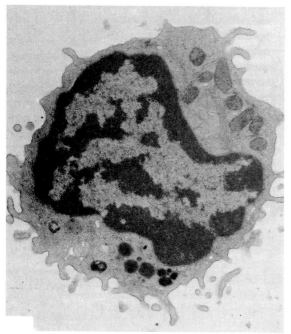

(a)

Figure 2-2 *Morphology of peripheral blood lymphocyte* (a) *and large granular lymphocyte* (b). Note that the large granular lymphocyte is larger, has a lower cytoplasm to nucleus ratio, and contains a large number of azurophilic granules in the cytoplasm, many close to the well-developed Golgi apparatus and others distributed throughout. (*From Williams WJ et al. (eds): Hematology, 4/e, McGraw-Hill, 1990, with permission.*)

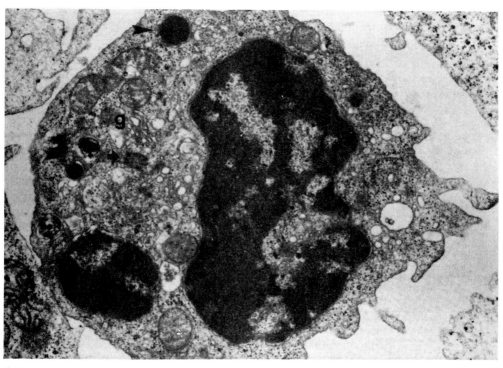

(b)

capable of producing antibody molecules (in the case of B cells) or lymphokines (in the case of helper T cells) (see Fig. 2-3). Since each cell within the clone of the antigen-stimulated population has identical antigenic specificity, the overall result of stimulation with antigen is an increase in the number of cells capable of reacting with this specific antigen.

Within the total lymphocyte population, only a limited number of cells will have receptors that bind determinants expressed by a particular antigen molecule. It is estimated that less than 0.1 percent of the total lymphocyte population will possess specific receptors for any given antigen. Therefore, the immune system relies on expansion of this small number of antigen-reactive lymphocyte clones in order to mount an effective immune response. There are, however, certain molecules, known as *lectins* or *mitogens*, which are polyclonal activators of lymphocyte populations. Polyclonal activators stimulate most, if not all, lymphocyte clones, regardless of their antigen specificity, by nonspecific interaction with cell surface membrane molecules. Some mitogens, such as concanavalin A (ConA) and phytohemagglutinin (PHA), preferentially activate T cells. Other mitogens, such as bacterial li-

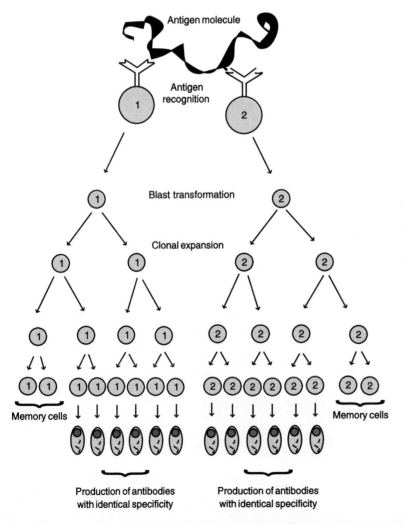

Figure 2-3   Clonal expansion of B (or T) lymphocytes after interaction of their surface, antigen-specific receptor, with that antigenic determinant. Recognition of a single antigenic determinant by a B cell with a receptor specific for this determinant causes that B cell to proliferate (*blast transformation*), which results in the production of a large number of daughter cells, a process known as *clonal expansion*. These B cells undergo differentiation into antibody-secreting plasma cells and B memory cells. Antigen-specific T cells undergo a similar process of clonal expansion.

popolysaccharide (LPS) or pokeweed mitogen (PWM), primarily stimulate B cells. These polyclonal activators are used diagnostically to evaluate the presence of functional lymphocyte subpopulations in suspected cases of immunodeficiency.

At distinct stages of their development, lymphocytes express different molecules within their cytoplasm or on their surface membrane, which allow immunologists to identify different subpopulations. These identifying "markers" are known as differentiation antigens, and antibodies can be produced against them. In 1982, an International Workshop on Human Leukocyte Differentiation Antigens was convened in Paris to compare the specificities of 139 different monoclonal antibodies to human differentiation antigens.

It was established that several purportedly unique antibodies in fact react with the same determinants. As a result of this meeting these lymphocyte markers are now grouped into *clusters of differentiation* (CD for short). Appendix D lists some of the CD determinants that are present on cells of the immune system. Using panels of monoclonal antibodies that are specific for these CD antigens, immunologists have been able to characterize the lineage and assign functional attributes to the various lymphocyte subsets.

T Lymphocytes

Within the fetal liver and bone marrow, the common lymphocyte progenitor cells give rise to stem cells which migrate to the thymus gland and differentiate into mature T cells. During this thymic phase of differentiation, the repertoire of T-cell antigen-receptor specificities is generated. Developing T cells rearrange the genes that code for the variable regions of the T-cell receptor (TCR) in order to establish the diversity of specificity that is present within the T-cell populations.

There are two major pathways in the development of the TCR repertoire. The majority of thymocytes differentiate into T cells that express dimeric antigen receptors (TCR-2) which are composed of polypeptide chains

that are designated as α (molecular mass = 45 kd) and β (molecular mass = 40 kd). A small fraction of thymocytes follows the other pathway of differentiation, which results in the expression of dimeric antigen receptors (TCR-1) composed of γ and δ chains (Fig. 2-4).

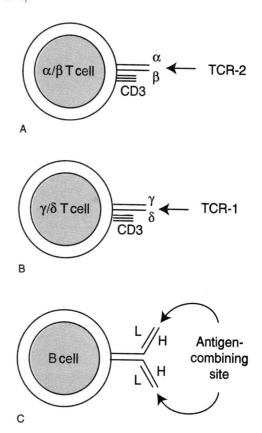

Figure 2-4 *Definition of antigen specificity of T and B lymphocytes by cell surface receptors.* Antigen specificity of T and B cells is defined by the presence on the cell surface of antigen-specific receptors. For T cells, one of two kinds of TCR (T-cell receptor) is expressed, either TCR-2 (*a*) or, less frequently, TCR-1 (*b*). These multimolecular complexes are made by the T cell and expressed on the surface, with transmembrane tails remaining within the cytoplasm. (*c*) In B cells, the antigen-specific receptor is an immunoglobulin molecule made by that B cell; the immunoglobulin molecule is extruded from the cell and expressed on its surface with a small cytoplasmic tail remaining within the cell.

The three subpopulations of mature T lymphocytes are defined on the basis of their function: *helper T cells, cytotoxic T cells,* and *suppressor T cells.* All three subpopulations express CD2 and CD3 surface markers. The expression of CD4 or CD8 surface markers defines nonoverlapping subsets of mature peripheral T cells. Generally speaking, helper T cells are CD4$^+$CD8$^-$, while cytotoxic T cells and suppressor T cells are CD4$^-$CD8$^+$. Currently, there is no surface marker which distinguishes cytotoxic T cells from suppressor T cells. However, this is not an absolute functional separation for T cells that express these markers. Some CD4$^+$CD8$^-$ T cells have been shown to mediate cytotoxic or suppressor activity. More precisely, CD4 and CD8 appear to be cell interaction molecules, which determine recognition by the T cell of major histocompatibility complex (MHC) determinants expressed by other cell types. Thus, the CD4 molecule interacts with a class II MHC determinant, and the CD8 molecule interacts with a class I MHC determinant.

The TCR in conjunction with CD3 and CD4 (known as the *TCR complex*) on helper T cells recognizes an antigenic determinant that is presented on APC in the context of the "self" class II MHC molecules which the APCs express. In order for the helper T cell to recognize the foreign antigen determinant, the class II MHC molecules on the APC must be the same as those encountered in the thymus during differentiation. In this way, the response of the helper T cell is said to be *restricted* by the MHC. Following antigen recognition, the helper T cell undergoes blast transformation and clonal expansion. As a result of this activation, responding helper T cells produce a variety of lymphokines that influence the response of other cellular elements of the immune system. Interleukin 2 (IL-2) acts as a major growth factor, which enhances the clonal expansion of activated T cells. The "help" that helper T cells provide to B cells is the production of IL-4 and IL-5 (and to a lesser extent IL-2), which act as B-cell growth and differentiation factors. These lymphokines promote both clonal expansion of antigen-activated B cells, and their differentiation into antibody-producing plasma cells. Interferon-gamma (IFN-γ) is also produced by antigen-stimulated helper T cells, and represents the major lymphokine which activates macrophages.

Resting cytotoxic T cells possess the potential to develop cytotoxic effector function following interaction with the antigen determinant for which they possess specific TCR. The TCR of cytotoxic T cells recognizes antigenic determinant in the context of class I MHC molecules, and in this way the cytotoxic T-cell response is also "restricted" by the MHC. One cytotoxic T cell can kill multiple targets cells that express the appropriate antigenic determinant. In performing its cytotoxic effector function, the cytotoxic T cell first binds to the determinant on the target cell and then causes membrane damage, which results in lysis of the target cell. The topic of cytotoxic cells is described in greater detail in Chap. 8.

Less is known about the requirements for antigen recognition and activation of suppressor T cells. Both antigen-specific and antigen-nonspecific activation of suppressor T cells have been described; however, the influence of the MHC in this activation process is not well defined. Under appropriate conditions, suppressor T cells have been shown to act on helper T cells as well as on B cells, and evidence indicates that the suppression is mediated by soluble factors that are secreted by activated suppressor T cells.

The central site in which differentiation of lymphocytes of T lineage takes place is the *thymus,* a bilobed lymphoepithelial organ located in front of the great vessels in the upper mediastinum (Fig. 2-5). It is derived primarily from the endoderm of the third pharyngeal pouches and lymphocytes which enter it from the blood. In humans it increases in size after birth, reaching a maximum weight of 30 to 40 g at puberty, and later involutes in adults.

The thymus consist of lymphocytes and epithelial cells organized into lobules separated by connective tissue septa. The thymic

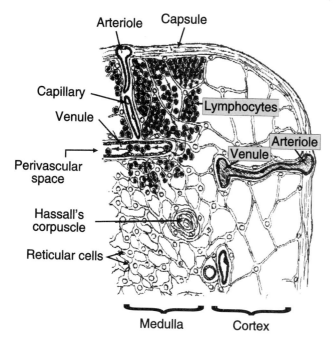

Figure 2-5   *Thymus: Structure and functional anatomy.* The lobules or follicles are organized into an outer cortex containing most of the immature thymocytes; the medulla is composed of more mature or differentiated cells. The many reticular and epithelial cells play a role in providing maturation signals for the thymocytes. The role of Hassall's corpuscles, structures unique to the thymic medulla, is not known, although there is evidence suggesting that they may be involved in intrathymic cell death. (*Adapted from Bellanti: Immunology in Medicine, 3/e. Philadelphia, Saunders, 1985, with permission.*)

epithelial cells play a role in differentiation of bone marrow stem cells into T lymphocytes and produce several humoral factors called thymic hormones.

More than 85 percent of the thymic lymphocytes (thymocytes) are located in the thymic cortex; only the more mature thymocyte forms are present in the medulla. The differentiation of thymocytes can be classified into three stages, with characteristic genotypic and phenotypic features. During this process the antigen-recognition repertoire of the TCR is generated.

A variety of cell surface markers and cellular enzymes have been defined in T cells and can be used to document stages in the maturation of T cells. In the early (stage I) thymocyte (Fig. 2-6), commitment to T-cell differentiation takes place and is associated with rearrangement of the gene for the β chain of the TCR-2. The stage I thymocytes express the CD2, CD5, and CD7 determinants, which are expressed during the later stages of the T-cell development as well. Tdt (terminal deoxyribonucleotidyl transferase) is an enzyme found only in stem cells and cortical, less mature thymocytes. Intermediate,

or common (stage II), thymocytes are characterized by rearrangement of the α chain of the TCR-2. During this stage of T-cell development, the cells express CD1 determinants together with the simultaneous presence of CD4 and CD8 molecules. The mature thymocytes also differentiate into nonoverlapping cell subsets expressing either CD4 or CD8 markers, but not both. Stage III thymocytes are phenotypically identical to the mature, recirculating T-lymphocyte population with its two major functional subsets, helper/inducer (CD2$^+$, CD3$^+$, and CD4$^+$) and suppressor/cytotoxic (CD2$^+$, CD3$^+$, and CD8$^+$), respectively. The T cells represent a major fraction of peripheral blood lymphocytes (> 70 percent) and migrate, or "home," to T cell-specific areas of peripheral lymphoid organs.

A small portion of thymocytes follows a TCR-1 (γ/δ) differentiation pathway. These cells ultimately express CD3 protein in the absence of CD4 or CD8 molecules. The TCR-1-bearing T cells appear to have distinct homing properties for mucosa-associated lymphoid tissue or epidermis.

Absence or hypoplasia of the thymus, seen

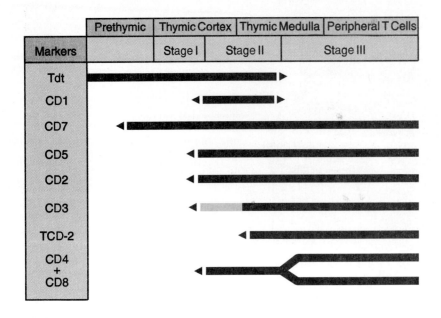

Markers	Prethymic	Thymic Cortex	Thymic Medulla	Peripheral T Cells
		Stage I	Stage II	Stage III
Tdt				
CD1				
CD7				
CD5				
CD2				
CD3				
TCD-2				
CD4 + CD8				

Figure 2-6 *Stages of T lymphocyte development.* Many markers are used to document the development of thymocytes into mature T lymphocytes. Some of these markers are expressed in the early stages but are lost as the cells mature, e.g., Tdt (terminal deoxyribonucleotidyl transferase) and CD1. At one stage of development T cells express both CD4 and CD8 on their surface; with further differentiation, only one of these markers is found on the cells. In early stages of development the γ, δ, and ε chains of the CD3 molecule are made but remain intracellular. Shortly thereafter, the cells begin to make T cell antigen receptor (TCR) β chain. Once the cells make the TCR α chain, the α/β TCR-CD3 complex is expressed on the surface of the cell. The purely intracellular status of CD3 during stage II of thymocyte development is denoted by the initial cross-hatching, whereas the solid denotes surface expression of the complex. (*From Roitt IM et al: Immunology, 2d ed. New York, Gower, 1989, with permission.*)

in various forms of III–IV pharyngeal pouch syndrome, is associated with profound defects of T-cell function and a paucity of lymphocytes in peripheral blood and T-cell regions of peripheral lymphoid tissues. This clinical syndrome, consisting of immune and nonimmune features, is called the DiGeorge Syndrome. (See Chap. 7 on T-cell development and Chap. 22a on immunodeficiencies.)

B Lymphocytes

In birds, B-lymphocyte differentiation is dependent on the primary lymphoid organ called the *bursa of Fabricius,* a lymphoepithelial appendage of the cloaca. In mammals, the development of the B lymphocytes takes place in fetal liver and later directly in bone marrow, which is the primary site of B lymphopoiesis. The bone marrow is located in the cavities of long bones and spongiosa of other bones including the flat bones of the skull and pelvis. It is a soft, highly cellular tissue containing the precursors of all blood cells. The development of B lymphocytes is associated with expression of immunoglobulin (Ig) genes. The Ig molecules are not only major products of B lymphocytes, but also serve in their membrane-associated form as antigen-specific receptors.

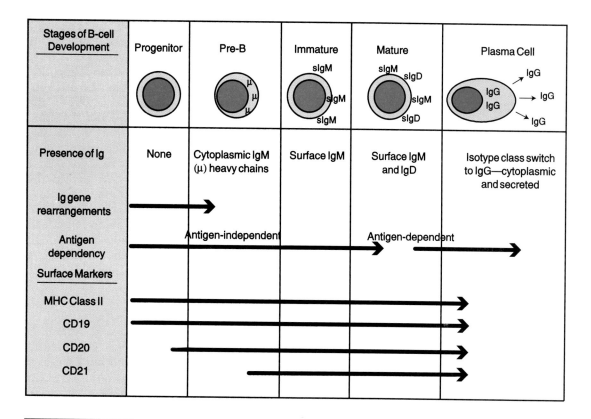

Stages of B-cell Development	Progenitor	Pre-B	Immature	Mature	Plasma Cell
Presence of Ig	None	Cytoplasmic IgM (μ) heavy chains	Surface IgM	Surface IgM and IgD	Isotype class switch to IgG—cytoplasmic and secreted
Ig gene rearrangements					
Antigen dependency		Antigen-independent		Antigen-dependent	
Surface Markers					
MHC Class II					
CD19					
CD20					
CD21					

Figure 2-7   *Stages of B lymphocyte development.* As progenitor cells mature into B cells and then into antibody-secreting plasma cells, one can document the presence, in the cytoplasm only, of μ chains, followed by the surface expression of IgM and then IgD molecules. All of this takes place in the absence of antigen and is part of the maturation of these cells. Upon exposure to antigens, such mature B cells will undergo blast tranformation and proliferation, as well as differentiation of the progeny into antibody-secreting plasma cells.

Differentiation of B cells (Fig. 2-7) occurs in two stages: before the B cell encounters antigen (*antigen-independent* stage), and after the B cell encounters antigen (*antigen-dependent* stage). During the early stages of differentiation, an individual precursor B cell rearranges the genes which code for the variable regions of the Ig heavy and light chains. This process of Ig gene rearrangement is the mechanism by which the diversity of the Ig antigen-receptor repertoire is generated in the total population of B cells. The Ig molecule is then assembled and inserted into the cell membrane, becoming the receptor for anti-

gen for that B cell. The specificity of all the surface Ig of a particular B cell is identical, and each B lymphocyte is committed to the antigen-binding specificity of its surface Ig molecule for its entire life. Following stimulation with the antigenic determinant for which the Ig receptor is specific, the antibody molecules produced by the clonal progeny of a particular B lymphocyte will be the same as those of its surface Ig receptor for antigen.

Pre-B cells, an early stage in differentiation of B lymphocytes, contain only μ heavy chains within their cytoplasm. As the pre-B cell produces light chains and assembles and inscrts IgM molecules into its cell membrane, it moves to the next stage of development and is referred to as an *immature* B cell. The immature B cell next begins to produce IgD molecules, which possess the same antigenic specificity as the IgM molecules already expressed by the B cell. These IgD molecules are also inserted into the B-cell membrane, and at this stage of development, with both IgD and IgM on its surface, the cell is referred to as a *mature* B lymphocyte.

Up to this point, the process of differentiation has moved in the complete absence of exogenous antigen. The mature B lymphocyte expresses surface Ig molecules which possess specificity for a particular antigenic determinant. When that B lymphocyte encounters that specific antigenic determinant, it enters the antigen-dependent phase of differentiation. The B-cell response to antigen involves (1) blast transformation and proliferation of the stimulated cell to increase the number of antigen-reactive B cells, and (2) the differentiation of this progeny to produce and secrete antibody molecules (Fig. 2-3). The majority of the progeny cells will differentiate to the terminal stage of differentiation for a B lymphocyte, that of a *plasma cell*. The plasma cell is an antibody-producing "factory," and has distinctive morphologic characteristics. These cells have an eccentric nucleus with a large amount of basophilic cytoplasm, except for the area of the Golgi apparatus. The cytoplasmic basophilia is due to the abundant rough endoplasmic reticulum in which the cisternae become dilated with antibody molecules.

During this response, the antigen-activated B cell first secretes antibody molecules of IgM isotype. However, the action of lymphokines that are produced by antigen-stimulated helper T cells causes what is known as "isotype switch" to occur. As a result of this phenomenon, further Ig gene rearrangements take place which result in a switch from IgM antibody production to another isotype (that is, IgG, IgA, IgE). It is important to note that despite the switch to another isotype, the antigen specificity of the secreted antibody molecules remains the same

during isotype switching. Thus, the gene rearrangements primarily involve the Ig heavy-chain genes. The phenomenon of Ig isotype switching is discussed in Chap. 5.

Not all of the cells within the antigen-stimulated clonal population follow the pathway to terminal plasma cell differentiation. Those clonal progeny that do not differentiate into plasma cells become memory cells, and are referred to as *follicular center cells* (because of their location within the follicles of the peripheral lymphoid tissues). They are morphologically distinct from non-stimulated B lymphocytes, being larger and possessing polyribosomes and some rough endoplasmic reticulum in their cytoplasm. These B memory cells are responsible for the characteristic *secondary* (or *anamnestic*) antibody response that occurs upon subsequent exposure of the host to the same antigen.

While endogenously produced surface Ig molecules are the characteristic B-cell markers, other cell membrane markers are also expressed by B lymphocytes. Some of them are of central importance in the interaction of the B cell with other elements of the immune system. Among them, class II MHC molecules are involved in the interaction of B cells with helper T cells in the antibody response to antigen. Most mature B lymphocytes also express receptors for some of the complement proteins, for example, C3b and C3d. A small population of human B cells is implicated in autoimmune phenomena. These cells express a T-cell determinant, CD5. B-cell ontogeny and differentiation are described in greater detail in Chap. 6.

Null Lymphocytes

Null cells are lymphoid cells that do not express the characteristic markers that define B lymphocytes (surface Ig) or T lymphocytes (TCR). The precursors for null cells are present in the fetal liver and bone marrow; however, it is unclear whether null cells are derived from the same precursors that give rise to T and B cells or represent an entirely separate lymphoid cell lineage. Thus, the term *third-population cells* has also been used to describe these cells. Unlike T lymphocytes, null cells do not require the microenvironment of the thymus in order to develop, as evidenced by the fact that they are present in nude mice that are congenitally athymic because of a genetic mutation (*nu/nu*).

The genetic mutation in these mice results in two characteristic traits—one internal and one external. The external trait is a complete lack of fur, hence the designation "nude." The internal trait is a lack of formation of the third and fourth pharyngeal pouches during embryogenesis, which results in failure of thymus gland development. Since this mouse is lacking an environment for T-cell differentiation and maturation, it has no mature T cells and is deficient in those immune responses for which T cells are required. This mouse model has been an important tool in understanding human T-cell immunodeficiency diseases, such as DiGeorge syndrome. Moreover, in the absence of T-cell immunity, nude mice have been used to propagate human tumor cells and to study the influence of the host response to tumors in vivo.

Morphologically, null cells are slightly larger than resting T or B lymphocytes, have a lower nucleus/cytoplasm ratio, and contain azurophilic granules in their cytoplasm (Fig. 2-2b). Based on their size, and the presence of these distinct cytoplasmic granules, the term *large granular lymphocyte* (LGL) has also been used to describe this cell population. Several CD determinants are present on LGL; however, these markers are not unique to this population, also being expressed on T cells or mononuclear phagocytes. These include CD2, CD7, CD11b, CD16 (receptor for Fc portion of IgG), and CD38. Determinants on null cells that are detected by several other monoclonal antibodies, such as Leu-7, Leu-19, and HNK-1, have also been described.

Functionally, null cells possess cytotoxic effector activity against a limited variety of cellular targets, including some tumor cells (primarily those of hematopoietic origin) and virally infected cells. However, unlike MHC-restricted cytotoxic T cells, which require a period of sensitization after exposure to antigen in order to develop their cytotoxic function, the killer activity of the null cell population can be detected in nonsensitized donors and is not MHC-restricted. Hence, these cells have also been termed *natural killer (NK)* cells. Null cells can also lyse target cells that are coated with IgG antibody, and this killer activity is known as *antibody-dependent cellular cytotoxicity* (ADCC). In this situation, the antibody molecule confers the apparent specificity of the killer cell by acting as a "bridge" between the target cell surface antigen (bound by the antigen-specific binding site) and the killer effector cell which has a receptor for the Fc portion of the IgG molecule (CD16). Cytotoxic cells are described in more detail in Chap. 8.

OTHER CELLS OF THE IMMUNE SYSTEM

Mononuclear Phagocyte System

Cells of the mononuclear phagocyte system are present throughout the body, and provide a number of functions of central importance to host defense mechanisms. Arising from the myeloid progenitor cells in the bone marrow, mononuclear phagocytes circulate in the blood as monocytes, and cells of mononuclear phagocyte lineage migrate to and take up residence in virtually every tissue of the body. Kupffer cells in the liver, Langerhans cells in the skin, microglial cells in the brain, and mesangial cells in the kidney all represent cells of the mononuclear phagocyte system.

Most of what is known about cells of the mononuclear phagocyte system has been obtained by studying the blood monocytes and the macrophages that migrate into sites of inflammation. Morphologically, monocytes and macrophages are 10 to 18 μm in diameter, with a high nucleus/cytoplasm ratio and a U-shaped nucleus. Monocytes have many intracytoplasmic lysosomes which contain peroxidase and acid hydrolases which are important for the cell's primary function of intracellular lysis and breakdown of phagocytized microorganisms and other antigens.

Phenotypically, monocytes and macrophages express receptors for the Fc portion of IgG and IgE, for some of the complement components, for example, C3b and C3d, and for carbohydrate moieties that are present on nonencapsulated microorganisms. These receptors serve to enhance the capability of macrophages to bind to and phagocytize microorganisms and particulate antigens. Some cells of the mononuclear phagocyte system also express class II MHC determinants. This combination of high efficiency in phagocytosis, intracellular digestion, and expression of class II MHC determinants makes these cells effective in their role as *antigen-presenting cells (APCs)*.

As part of the first line of defense against invasion by infectious organisms, mononuclear phagocytes are attracted from the circulation to sites of inflammation, arriving somewhat later than the polymorphonuclear leukocytes. Their primary function in this situation is to clean up the cellular debris that results from the initial encounter of the polymorphs with the agents that stimulate the inflammatory response.

A variety of other cell types located in the lymphoid tissues and in skin can also act as APCs. In the epidermis, Langerhans cells are APCs, and after contact with antigen these cells migrate via the afferent lymphatics to the draining lymph node. Here, they "interdigitate" among the T cells located in the diffuse cortex and act as APCs. In this capacity, they are referred to as antigen-presenting *interdigitating* cells. Similar to macrophage APCs, Langerhans cells and the interdigitating cells also express class II MHC molecules which are involved in the recognition of antigenic determinants by helper T cells.

Another type of APC is the dendritic cell which circulates in blood and lymphatic fluid. Dendritic cells share some properties with macrophage APCs (expression of class II MHC determinants), but not others (Fc receptor negative and nonphagocytic). Dendritic cells

are very efficient APCs for T cells, and may be related to the Langerhans APCs in the skin. B cells can also function as APCs; their antigen-specific surface IgM allows B cells to present specific antigens efficiently.

Cells of the mononuclear phagocyte system are also a source of a variety of soluble factors that are generically referred to as *monokines*. When appropriately stimulated, macrophages can produce IFN-α, IL-1, IL-6, and tumor necrosis factor alpha (TNF-α). They also produce some of the complement proteins, a variety of enzymes, plasma proteins, prostaglandins, and leukotrienes.

Functionally, macrophages are involved in both the initiation and the effector phases of the immune response. Some types of mononuclear phagocytes act as APCs. Following phagocytosis or endocytosis, the lysosomal enzymes break down an antigen into its component antigenic determinants. The APC then expresses these antigenic determinants on its cell membrane in association with class II MHC determinants (Fig. 2-8). As mentioned earlier, a helper T cell will recognize the antigenic determinant for which its TCR is specific only in the context of the class II MHC molecules of the APC.

Lymphokines, such as IFN-γ, that are produced by antigen-stimulated T cells can "activate" macrophages to become cytotoxic effector cells. The receptors for the Fc portion of IgG enable macrophages to act as effectors of ADCC. This cytotoxic function of macrophages is an important contribution to the other cellular immune defenses against tumor cells and virally infected cells. Mononuclear phagocytes are discussed at further length in Chap. 18.

Polymorphonuclear Leukocytes

The *polymorphonuclear leukocytes* are divided into three categories—neutrophils, eosinophils, and basophils—based on the histologic staining properties of the granules present in their cytoplasm. These cells, also known as *granulocytes*, share some common properties. They are derived from precursors

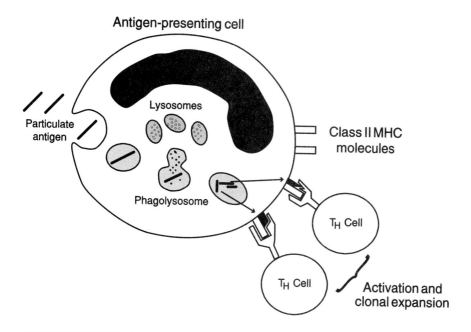

Figure 2-8   *Antigen processing by antigen-presenting cell (APC).* APCs ingest particulate matter, with subsequent formation of a phagosome and fusion of the phagosome with an enzyme-containing lysosome. Within the resulting acidic phagolysosome, the particle is degraded into smaller fragments that contain the individual antigenic determinant recognized by the immune response. The antigenic determinant is then associated with a class II MHC (major histocompatibility complex) marker for surface expression, so that, in this case, the appropriate T cell can be stimulated. MHC molecules are identifiers of "self," i.e., they vary between individuals and immunologically define an individual. Antigenic determinants are always "presented" by an APC to other cells in the context of "self," as defined by MHC.

that develop and mature in the bone marrow. Collectively, granulocytes are produced in high numbers, since they are relatively short-lived (2 to 3 days). Mature granulocytes represent the terminal stage of development for these cells and thus are unable to divide. Granulocytes represent 60 to 70 percent of the circulating white blood cells. However, they are also able to migrate from the blood into various tissues of the body, and are particularly attracted to sites of inflammation. In conjunction with antibodies and complement, granulocytes play an important role in defense against infection by microorganisms.

Neutrophils

Neutrophils account for 90 percent of the granulocytes found in peripheral blood. These cells are 10 to 20 μm in diameter, have a segmented (multilobulated) nucleus, and are phagocytic. Neutrophils contain two types of cytoplasmic granules (also known as *lysosomes*). The primary (or azurophilic) granules (0.4 μm in diameter) appear early in the cell's maturation and contain myeloperoxidase, arginine-rich basic proteins, sulfated mucopolysaccharides, acid phosphatase, and muramidase (lysozyme). The azurophilic granules are similar to the lysosomes present in cells of other tissues. The secondary (or specific) granules are smaller and less dense than the azurophilic granules. The specific granules contain alkaline phosphatase, aminopeptidase, and lactoferrin in addition to lysozyme. Both types of granules are present in neutrophils at the intermediate stage of development, but the specific granules predominate in mature neutrophils.

As part of the body's cellular defenses, neutrophils are the first cell type to appear at local sites of infection by microorganisms. Their function is to phagocytize these organisms into cytoplasmic phagosomes and, by virtue of their lysosomal enzymes, lyse and degrade the ingested organisms. Chaper 17 gives more details about these cells.

Eosinophils

Eosinophilic granulocytes (*eosinophils*) represent 2 to 5 percent of the peripheral blood leukocytes of healthy individuals. The nucleus of the eosinophil is usually bilobed, but can be multilobulated, and these cells contain large cytoplasmic granules that stain red with the histologic dye eosin. In electron micrographs, the eosinophilic granules have a unique appearance, with a crystalloid core surrounded by a matrix that is less electron dense. The granules are rich in acid phosphatase and peroxidase activity.

Like neutrophils, eosinophils are capable of phagocytosis and have been shown to ingest antigen-antibody complexes; however, this is not their primary function. Eosinophils can be triggered to degranulate and release a variety of enzymes that cause damage to parasitic organisms, helminths in particular. Eosinophils express Fc receptors, and thus can also participate in ADCC reactions against antibody-coated parasites, such as schistosomes. Parasitic infestations are often associated with an increased number of circulating eosinophils. Eosinophilia is also observed in people who suffer from allergic disease. How eosinophils help defeat parasites but also cause host tissue damage is discussed in Chap. 19b.

Basophils and Mast Cells

Basophilic granulocytes (*basophils*) make up less than 0.5 percent of circulating leukocytes. *Mast* cells are very similar in appearance to basophils, and are found primarily in the mucosal epithelium and in connective tissue. Although they have many characteristics in common, the exact relationship between basophils and mast cells is unclear. Basophils contain large granules that stain purple with histologic dyes and, ultrastructurally, are homogenous and electron-dense. These granules contain acid mucopolysaccharides, heparin and histamine, as well as other chemicals that are important mediators of allergic (type I hypersensitivity) reactions, such as slow-reacting substance of anaphylaxis (SRS-A) and eosinophil chemotactic factor of anaphylaxis (ECF-A).

Basophils and mast cells are nonphagocytic and, like eosinophils, can be triggered to degranulate, releasing the contents of the granules into the extracellular space. Basophils and mast cells express receptors for the Fc portion of the IgE molecules. Cross-linking of these Fc receptors by antigen-IgE antibody complexes can trigger degranulation. The release of the contents of the granules is responsible for increased vascular permeability (leading to edema and swelling) and smooth muscle contraction (leading to bronchoconstriction and respiratory distress) seen in allergic reactions. The role of these cell types in host defenses is described in more detail in Chap. 19a.

SECONDARY LYMPHOID ORGANS

Spleen

The *spleen* is an abdominal organ located under the diaphragm in the left subcostal space. It is the only lymphoid organ with a function to filter blood. It has a dense capsule from which extend collagenous trabeculae dividing the tissue into multiple communicating small spaces. Upon sectioning, two readily distinguishable types of soft parenchyma can be seen (Fig. 2-9). The red pulp is a pastelike red mass which consists of a network of branching venous tissues which drain into pulp veins. The sinuses are separated by splenic cellular cords containing various cell types including lymphocytes, monocytes, and reticular cells. (See Fig. 2-9.) It is in the splenic cords that destruction of senescent blood cells takes place.

The other type of parenchyma, the white pulp, is seen as small, rounded, grayish-white areas (0.2 to 0.7 mm in diameter) which contain typical lymphoid tissue. The white pulp has two distinct lymphoid components. The periarterial lymphocyte sheath (PALS) is a cylinder surrounding the central artery. Within the PALS are lymphatic nodules. Upon antigenic stimulation a central area containing large lymphocytes and macrophages, called germinal center, is easily identified in the nodules. The T lymphocytes are found around the central arteriole, while the B cells are in the nodules.

The PALS is surrounded by the second component of the white pulp, called the marginal zone, which serves as a barrier separating the PALS from the red pulp. It contains B cells, macrophages, and dendritic cells.

The filtering function of the spleen is enhanced by macrophage populations in the splenic cords. The intravascular antigens first localize in the macrophages of the marginal zone. These cells, together with dendritic cells, present the processed antigen to lymphocytes. The lymphocyte traffic in and out of PALS takes place through the capillaries of the central arteriole. The spleen has various immunologic functions. Its role in antibody production is particularly important in childhood, when other lymphoid elements are not fully developed. At any age, splenectomy has been shown to increase risk of overwhelming bacterial infections attributed to loss of filtering function of the spleen.

Splenomegaly—enlargement of the spleen—can be caused by lymphocytic neoplastic transformation (lymphoma) or chronic

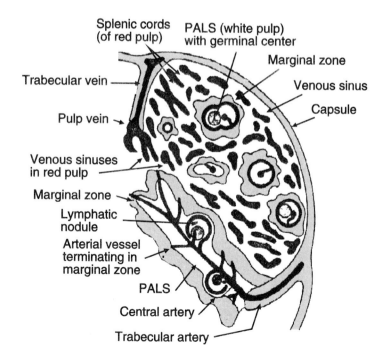

Figure 2-9 *Spleen: Structure and functional anatomy.* The spleen is made up of two distinguishable types of parenchyma. The first, called the *red pulp*, consists of a network of venous sinuses filled with red blood cells; this is where aging red cells are removed from the circulation. Separating these sinuses are cellular cords containing lymphocytes, monocytes, and reticular cells. The second type of parenchyma is called the *white pulp*, due to the large number of lymphocytes (white blood cells) present in this compartment. It surrounds the central arterioles. There are two distinct lymphoid components: the periarterial lymphocyte sheath (PALS) and the adjacent marginal zone. (*From Roitt et al, 1989, with permission.*)

inflammatory conditions. The spleen may be palpable below the left costal margin or enlargement may be obvious only by dullness to percussion in this area, known as *Traube's space.*

Lymph Nodes

Lymph nodes are encapsulated ovoid lymphoid bodies which function as filters of tissue fluid and lymph (Fig. 2-10). They are located between lymphatic vessels, and lymph passes through them as it moves to junctions of lymphatic vessels and veins. Lymph nodes are particularly concentrated at the neck, at the base of the upper and lower extremities,

in the retroperitoneum, and in the mediastinum. The lymph nodes are often kidney-shaped, with blood vessels entering and leaving at the indentation called the *hilus.*

The lymph node cells are arranged in a delicate meshwork of the reticulum surrounded by the capsule. In the periphery of a node there is a closely packed layer called the *cortex.* The cortical lymphocytes form spherical lymphatic nodules. Uniform and tightly packed nodules are called *primary follicles.* After encounter with antigen, *germinal centers* can be seen in the nodules, which are then identified as *secondary follicles.* The germinal center of each secondary follicle is surrounded by a zone of small lym-

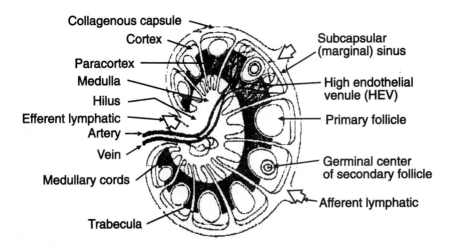

Figure 2-10 *Lymph nodes: Structure and functional anatomy.* Lymph nodes are 1 to 25 mm in size and are widely distributed around the body, along the path of the lymphatic vessels. Lymph, containing lymphocytes (and often antigens), enters the subcapsular sinus through the afferent lymphatics. Lymphocytes can also enter by way of the nutrient artery; egress of lymphocytes occurs through interaction with high endothelial venules (HEVs), venules whose lining cells have a different, more cuboidal structure and carry surface markers capable of interacting with certain lymphocytes. Lymphatic sinusoids then allow passage of the lymph into the cortex, with its follicles and paracortical areas, so that cells and molecules can interact with the immune cells of the lymph node. Lymph then passes into the medulla. Medullary sinuses then drain into the efferent lymphatics. Immune reactivity occurs within the lymphoid follicles; after an encounter with an antigen, a germinal center develops within what is now termed a *secondary follicle,* the site of current immune reactivity. (*From Roitt et al, 1989, with permission.*)

phocytes called the mantle. The cortex area in the lymph node is divided into the nodular cortex, containing the follicles and the diffuse cortex. The follicles contain the B lymphocytes, while the diffuse cortex is rich in T cells. The cortex also contains accessory cells which express class II MHC determinants on their surface and specialize in antigen-presenting function. Most plasma cells and phagocytic cells are located in the medulla. Upon antigenic stimulation, the regional lymph nodes show proliferation of T cells in the diffuse cortex and of B cells in the follicles. The secondary follicles with active germinal centers contain dendritic antigen-presenting cells, macrophages, and CD4$^+$ T lymphocytes.

The proliferative response in the lymph nodes is associated with lymph node enlargement—*lymphadenopathy*. It may result from infections or responses associated with either local or generalized antigenic stimulation. Such proliferations can also represent lymphocyte neoplastic transformation, such as in lymphomas or lymphatic leukemias. The filtering function of lymph nodes may also lead to enlargement due to involvement with tumor metastasis.

Mucosa-Associated Lymphoid Tissue

The epithelial linings of the alimentary, respiratory, and genitourinary tracts serve as a barrier to entry of pathogenic microorganisms and other antigens. In close proximity to these surfaces there often are aggregates of lymphoid cells. They may occur as diffuse collections of lymphocytes and macrophages or as more clearly organized lymphoid tissue with discernible follicles. Such unencapsulated areas of lymphoid tissue are collectively called *mucosa-associated lymphoid tissues (MALT)*. The significance of this type of lymphoid tissue was established by the discovery that IgA is the major antibody in external secretions. This immunoglobulin enters the secretory fluids by a specific transport mechanism through the epithelial cells

by means of interaction with a specific transport receptor of secretory component (described in Chap. 3).

In the intestine there are two types of MALT. In the small intestine the lamina propria contains specific lymphoid tissue called *Peyer's patches*, frequently associated with secondary follicles. The mucosa overlying the patches is devoid of villi and allows antigen transport into the lymphoid tissue and transport of specific antibody in the opposite direction, into the intestinal lumen. The lymphocytes in the follicles are primarily B cells, with T cells in the interfollicular areas. Antigen activation of lymphocytes in Peyer's patches depends on class-specific helper T cells, resulting in IgA-producing lymphoblasts. Proliferating cells enter lymphocyte traffic and reach distant mucosal surfaces in other mucosal systems, so that a local immune response can be of benefit elsewhere in the body.

In the lower portion of the gastrointestinal tract there are frequent isolated lymphoid nodules, predominantly in the colon. Lymphoid cells are also diffusely scattered in the lamina propria and also in the epithelium itself. The intraepithelial lymphocytes in the gut represent an unusual population, consisting predominantly (> 80 percent) of T lymphocytes of the CD8 phenotype.

Lymphoid tissue in humans is also well organized in the lingual, palatine, and pharyngeal tonsils. Tonsils usually show lymphoid tissue containing secondary follicles with prominent germinal centers. Lymphoid aggregates similar to those in the gastrointestinal tract are seen in the bronchi and also along the genitourinary tract. There is little direct information on normal lymphoid aggregates associated with other mucosal surfaces. Antigens enter the MALT across the epithelial lining and stimulate appropriate antigen-specific B lymphocytes. Locally produced IgA is an important component in the local defense at mucosal surfaces together with other humoral and cellular factors. The MALT is the subject of Chap. 11.

LYMPHOCYTE TRAFFIC

Prompt interactions of lymphocytes with antigens in the peripheral lymphoid organs depend on a recirculating pool of lymphocytes. More than 1 percent of the total lymphocyte pool recirculates each hour. Despite the large number of cells involved, this process of lymphocyte traffic is carefully regulated, and distinct patterns and control mechanisms are emerging. Different cell populations show distinct homing preferences for peripheral lymph nodes, the MALT, or the spleen. (See Fig. 2-11.)

The main exit of lymphocytes from the blood to the lymphoid tissue is through a specific section of the postcapillary venules called *high endothelial venules (HEV)*. The HEV in lymph nodes are located almost exclusively in the cortex, and lymphocytes enter the nodes through the cuboidal HEV cells. In nonencapsulated tissues such as Peyer's patches recirculating lymphocytes also enter through HEV and continue into the afferent lymphatics of the regional lymph nodes. Homing into the spleen involves the venous sinuses adjacent to the marginal zone. The

lymphocytes then pass through channels bridging the marginal zone into the sinuses of the red pulp.

The differential recirculating patterns of individual lymphocyte populations through peripheral lymph nodes and Peyer's patches have been attributed to putative homing receptors (HOR). These homing receptors have the ability to differentiate between the HEV of different lymphoid tissues. Lymphocyte surface recognition molecules for HEV in lymph nodes and/or Peyer's patches, with properties corresponding to HOR, have been identified in several mammalian species, including humans.

The specific traffic patterns depend not only on the lymphocyte subsets involved, but on their functional state as well. It has been established that expression of HOR is differentially modulated by different activation stimuli. The same stimulus thus may increase binding to HEV of peripheral lymph nodes, while binding in Peyer's patches is virtually abrogated. It also appears that blast cell populations have a decreased HEV-binding capacity.

The homing patterns are also dependent on the presence of accessory molecules on

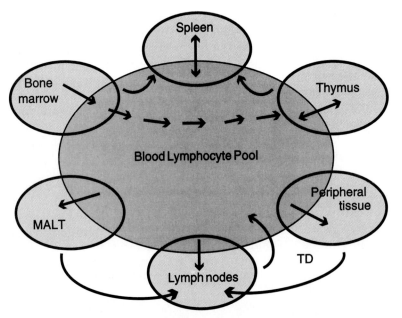

Figure 2-11 *Lymphocyte traffic.* There is free movement of lymphocytes between a variety of compartments, including the bone marrow, lymph nodes, spleen, thymus, peripheral tissues, and mucosa-associated lymphoid tissues (MALT). There are specialized surface molecules on lymphocytes and endothelial cells in certain lymphoid structures which provide some specificity in the travels of lymphocytes. *(From Roitt et al, 1989, with permission.)*

the cell surfaces. Some of these molecules can be induced by various cytokines released during inflammatory processes. These molecules also facilitate cell-to-cell interactions, such as in T-cell activation by APC, T-B cell cooperation, or binding of cytotoxic T lymphocytes to their targets. The best-studied factor in lymphocyte adhesion is the lymphocyte function antigen 1 (LFA-1). Experimental evidence suggests that this adhesion molecule plays a role in the context of weak but not strong interactions with HEV.

This highly regulated lymphocyte traffic allows recruitment of specific antigen-reactive cells at the sites of reaction with antigens. The recirculation of memory cells provides a more effective response upon future encounter with specific antigens. Such interactions result in a rapid depletion of specific antigen-reactive cells from the circulation. These cells are then trapped in the lymphoid tissues, draining the source of the specific antigen. Only after several days do the activated cells generated in response to the specific antigens reenter the recirculatory pool. The mechanisms of lymphocyte recirculation and homing are covered in Chap. 12.

SELF-TEST QUESTIONS*

For the following incomplete statements, choose the letter of the appropriate combination of correct completions.

    A. Only a, b, and c are correct.
    B. Only b and c are correct.
    C. Only b and d are correct.
    D. Only d is correct.
    E. All are correct.

1. The cell or cells of the immune system that function in antigen capture and/or presentation include:
    a. Helper T cells
    b. Dendritic cells
    c. Suppressor T cells
    d. Monocytes and macrophages

*Answers will be found in Appendix E.

2. Helper T lymphocytes:
    a. Recirculate in blood and lymph
    b. Express MHC class I surface determinants
    c. Produce IL-2 following appropriate stimulation
    d. Reside primarily in follicles and germinal centers of lymph nodes
3. Functional attributes of antigenically stimulated T lymphocytes may include:
    a. Development of cytotoxic potential
    b. Provision of "help" to antigen-stimulated B lymphocytes
    c. Secretion of IL-2
    d. Ability to "suppress" antibody production

For problems 4 through 6 select the lettered phrase which most correctly completes the preliminary statement or answers the question.

4. Mature T and B lymphocytes localize in different areas within lymphoid tissues of the body. T lymphocytes reside primarily in the:
    a. Germinal centers of lymph nodes and periarteriolar sheath of the spleen
    b. Follicles of lymph nodes and marginal zone of the spleen
    b. Follicles of lymph nodes and periarteriolar sheath of the spleen
    d. Diffuse cortex of lymph nodes and periarteriolar sheath of the spleen
    e. Diffuse cortex of lymph nodes and marginal zone of the spleen
5. The lymphocyte population that requires the microenvironment of the thymus in order to mature and differentiate into a functional cell type that expresses the CD4 membrane surface marker is the:
    a. B cell
    b. Suppressor T cell
    c. Cytotoxic T cell
    d. Helper T cell
    e. Null cell

6. The lymphocyte population that expresses surface immunoglobulin molecules as integral membrane components is the:
   a. Suppressor T cell
   b. B cell
   c. Helper T cell
   d. Null cell
   e. Cytotoxic T cell

7. What is the pathway traveled by a lymphocyte from the time of exposure to an antigen to its clonal expansion in a lymph node?

ADDITIONAL READINGS

T Lymphocytes
Moller G, ed. The T cell repertoire. *Immunol Rev.* 1988;101(special issue).

von Boehmer H. The developmental biology of T lymphocytes. *Ann Rev Immunol.* 1988;6:309–326.

B Lymphocytes
Hunkapiller T, Hood L. Diversity of the immunoglobulin gene superfamily. *Adv Immunol.* 1989; 44:1–64.

Kincade P. Experimental models for understanding B lymphocyte function. *Adv Immunol.* 1987; 41:181–268.

Moller G, ed. B cell lineages. *Immunol Rev.* 1986;93(special issue).

Antigen-Presenting Cells
Kosco MH, Tew JG. Microanatomy of lymphoid tissue during humoral immune responses: structure function relationship. *Ann Rev Immunol.* 1989;7:91–109.

Moller G, ed. Antigen processing. *Immunol Rev.* 1988;106(special issue).

Cellular Interactions
Vitetta ES, Fernandes-Botran R, Myers CD, Sanders VM. Cellular interactions in the humoral immune response. *Adv Immunol.* 1989;45:1–106.

Organization of Lymphoid Tissues and Lymphocyte Traffic
Moller G, ed. Lymphocyte homing. *Immunol Rev.* 1989;108(special issue).

Ponzio NM, Thorbecke GJ. Antigen-specific and nonspecific patterns of B lymphocyte localization, In: Husband AJ, ed. *Migration and Homing of Lymphoid Cells.* Boca Raton, FL: CRC Press; 1988:85–112.

Weiss L. *Cell and Tissue Biology: A Textbook of Histology.* Baltimore: Urban and Schwarzenberg; 1988.

Woodruff JJ, Clarke LM, Chin YH. Specific cell-adhesion mechanisms determining migration pathways of recirculating lymphocytes. *Ann Rev Immunol.* 1987;5:201–222.

CHAPTER

3

Antibodies: Structure and Function

INTRODUCTION

Long before the beginning of immunology as an experimental science, the implementation of immunization against smallpox established by Jenner in 1798, gave rise to the concept of innate and acquired resistance to diseases. Despite Jenner's successful use of infectious material from cows, essentially an attenuated form of virulent smallpox, to induce effective immunity in healthy individuals, it was not until the germ theory was firmly established nearly a century later with the isolation and characterization of infectious microorganisms that a concerted effort was made to develop prophylactic vaccines by notable bacteriologists, including Pasteur, von Behring, and Ehrlich.

As the efficacy of prophylactic vaccines became established, attention began to be directed to the determination of the essential ingredients of a vaccine and of the nature of host factors that might be produced in response to a vaccine and account for the observed resistance to infection. Factors associated with immunity were sought in the circulating blood, the plasma, and the cellular components. Two distinct schools of thought emerged. One argued on behalf of humoral immunity, believing that resistance to infectious diseases was due solely to soluble factors in serum. The other school, led primarily by Metchnikoff, argued just as strongly that immunity was cellular in nature, comprising specialized white cells capable of phagocytizing foreign material.

The analysis of serum was feasible, and certainly less involved than the isolation and functional characterization of the cellular components of blood. By 1900, functional analysis of serum from vaccinated individuals and experimental animals clearly established the validity of the theory of humoral immunity. Immune serum, in contrast to serum prior to vaccination, was capable of neutralizing bacterial toxins, agglutinating and killing bacteria, and precipitating soluble factors in bacterial cultures. Not all of these factors—the antitoxins and the agglutinating, bactericidal, and precipitating substances—were present in the preimmune serum, so they were obviously generated by the vaccinated host in response to certain ingredients of the vaccine. The latter substances are termed *antigens,* and the host factors in the immune serum are collectively described as *antibodies.* We now know that antibodies do not represent a unique response to bacterial antigens, but are generally produced by a competent host to "non-self" antigens derived from organisms of a different genotype. The structure and functions of antibodies are known. Antibodies are immunoglobulins, proteins which electrophoretically are classified as gammaglobulins; the different types of immunoglobulins are defined later in this chapter. They comprise a family of proteins, unique in their diversity to recognize and bind an extraordinarily large repertoire of antigens and to effect a finite set of different biologic functions.

Regardless of any biologic property associated with antibodies, they all shared the fundamental property of recognizing and binding antigens specifically. Accordingly, antibodies were at first defined functionally and operationally as proteins in immune serum induced by and reactive with antigens.

The early studies of antibodies were extended to include analysis of their physicochemical, chemical, and antigenic properties. Antibodies were characterized in terms of their solubility in water, salt solutions, and organic solvents, and also in terms of their size, shape, and charge. These results clearly indicated the heterogeneity of antibodies. Electrophoretically they migrated with the gammaglobulin fraction of serum proteins with disperse mobility and isoelectric points. Some antibodies were water-soluble, but others were not. Non-water-soluble antibodies were denoted as *euglobulins.* In terms of their size, based on sedimentation in an ultracentrifuge, antibodies could be divided into two major groups, 7 S and 19 S (S stands for *Svedberg units*, a measure of sedimentation in ultracentrifugation studies) antibodies. Antibodies in each group were heterogeneous with respect to their charge, although they were seemingly the same in size and shape. These differences resulted in the development of nonspecific physicochemical methods for the isolation and purification of antibodies.

Antibodies, being proteins, could be altered chemically through their constituent amino acid residues. Landsteiner took advantage of such chemical reactions to conjugate small molecules to antigenic proteins as carriers, and was thus able to study the specificity of antibodies. Coons conjugated fluorescent molecules to antibodies as probes, laying the groundwork for the development of powerful and versatile immunofluorescence assays.

Defined antigens could be used to precipitate specific antibodies from an immune serum, and these antibodies were used as antigens to generate anti-antibodies. Antibodies, despite their differences in specificity for antigens, were seemingly indistinguishable as antigens. In fact, anti-antibodies reacted equally well with nonimmune serum. In retrospect, this was evidence of the dual nature of antibodies. One portion of the antibody molecule, associated with the binding site for antigen, varied with its specificity. The second portion, associated with the biologic function of the molecule, was essentially constant and reflected species specificity as an antigen.

Analysis of antigen-specific antibodies revealed other essential features of antibodies. They were shown to be bivalent, having two epitope-binding sites per molecule, and highly diverse in their specificity for antigens. Trying to rationalize the basis of antibody diversity was a formidable problem and became a major focus. Antibodies were also shown to be heterogeneous in their biologic activity, such as activation of the complement system, promotion of phagocytosis, and crossing the placental barrier.

TERMINOLOGY

Concept of Antigens

Antigens, initially associated with infectious organisms, were defined operationally as foreign substances capable of generating antibodies when injected into a suitable vertebrate animal host. The use of defined molecules as antigens, and analysis of their reaction with antibodies, has resulted in a molecular definition of antigens. Antigens comprise chemical groupings, termed epitopes or antigenic determinants, that can elicit an immunoglobulin (or T-cell) immune response and can interact specifically with the antigen-binding site of the induced antibodies.

Antigens, Immunogens, and Haptens

Before we proceed, other terms commonly used in immunologic discussions need to be defined. Antigens, as described above, are *immunogens* (the suffix *-gen* is the same as in *genesis*); i.e., they can engender an immune response. Other substances, usually of low molecular weight, may be incapable of eliciting a response alone, but can do so when coupled to a larger molecule, termed a *carrier*. These small compounds are called *haptens*. So a hapten can become immunogenic only when attached to a carrier; once that is done, the result is an immunogen.

Epitopes, Paratopes, and Immune Complexes

The part of an antigen that is bound by the specific antibody produced in the immune response is known as the *antigenic determinant*; a synonymous term for the recognized part of the antigen is the *epitope*. The part of the antibody molecule that binds to the epitope is the *paratope.*

Picture an invading virus. It consists of a number of surface components, each capable of eliciting an immune response to one or more epitopes. If such an organism attempts to invade a person who has been previously exposed to such an organism (an *immune host*), many different kinds of antibodies will bind to the surface. Since antibodies have more than one antigen-binding site, they may be able to cross-link two or more virus particles. As this happens, there may be accretion of larger and larger collections of antibody and antigen(s), which are called *immune complexes.* Complex formation can occur around a microorganism, or an inert protein may be the nidus of such a process. Immune complexes small enough to remain soluble, and complexes bound by immune cells, will be removed from the circulation. However, if a complex should become large enough to become insoluble, it might deposit in tissues and cause damage. (See Clinical Aside 3-1.)

Clinical Aside 3-1
Immune Complex–Mediated Disease

Immune complexes consist of immunoglobulin, the antigen to which the antibody is bound, and other serum proteins. These can include fibronectin and other proinflammatory proteins, including members of the complement system.

Complement was originally described as an accessory factor responsible for the hemolytic and bacteriolytic activity of immune serum—it *complemented* other effector functions of the serum. We now know that the complement cascade is a complex system, comprising nine components and several regulatory proteins that are present in normal serum and are activated by antibody in the presence of the relevant antigen. As noted in the text, only IgG and IgM have the ability to activate or "fix" complement by the classical pathway. This is defined as initiation of the cascade by binding the first component (C1). C1 is itself a complex of three proteins: C1q, C1r, and C1s. Antibody, as an immune complex, binds C1q, which results in the activation of an esterase activity in C1s. This serine esterase then acts on the components C4 and C2 to produce fragments

C4b and C2a, respectively, with further proteolytic activity. C3, C5, C6, C7, C8, and C9 are then, in turn, modified, until the formation of the *membrane attack complex*, which is inserted into the target cell's membrane, producing holes and lysis of the cell. The alternate pathway for activation of complement bypasses C1 and C4 and directly modifies C3. Fragments of C5 and C3, known as C5a and C3a, are potent *chemoattractants* for polymorphonuclear cells. Once these cells are on the scene, they can be activated and may cause profound tissue damage through their own effector mechanisms.

The order of discovery of the complement components is reflected in the numeric label applied, resulting in the fact that activation of the first component is followed by number 4 and then number 2, before we get to number 3 and the logical sequence of 5 through 9, in order. The cascade and its control proteins are described in more detail in Chap. 13.

Immune complexes can activate the complement system and cause significant tissue damage. As noted in Chapter 1, "The History of Immunology," even before the discovery of any of these molecules, von Pirquet had suggested that antitoxin-toxin interaction might be the principle behind *serum sickness*, which included arthritis, glomerulonephritis, and vasculitis. Experimental serum-sickness can be induced by injecting an animal with a foreign protein; continuing exposure to the antigen(s) will ultimately lead to the formation of immune complexes.

Soluble immune complexes are cleared by host cells and pose no problem. In what appears to be a paradox, certain of the complement components (notably, C2 and C4) seem to be important in keeping immune complexes in solution. As noted previously, the size of the complex is also important. But size is not the only factor that determines if a complex will come out of solution and be deposited in tissue. Other factors are involved, as well. Immune complexes deposit more readily in areas of *turbulent blood flow or in vascular beds where filtration is taking place*, often an area of high pressure gradients. This can mean immune complex deposition at vessel bifurcations *(vasculitis)*, in the lining of joints *(synovitis or arthritis)*, in the renal glomerulus *(glomerulonephritis)*, and in the choroid plexus. These, in fact, are areas where immune complex–mediated damage may occur. The *charge* of the antigen and/or complex is important; cationic charged antigens may preferentially deposit on negatively charged surfaces, like the glomerular basement membrane.

However, if an immune complex deposits in tissues, complement and polymorphonuclear cells may cause serious damage. If immune complexes deposit on blood vessel walls, the result is inflammation of these vessels, called *vasculitis*. A syndrome with symptoms similar to those of serum sickness can occur in association with chronic infections, e.g., leprosy and some parasitic infections, as well as early in the course of infection

with hepatitis B virus. After a streptococcal infection, immune complexes made up of streptococcal antigens and antibodies to them may cause a glomerulonephritis.

Figure 3-A1 shows how serum levels of antigen, antibody, immune complexes, and complement vary during the initiation of the immunoglobulin response to hepatitis B virus with associated immune complex–mediated multisystem inflammatory disease.

Immune complex–mediated disease will be discussed in more detail in Chap. 31, autoimmune disorders.

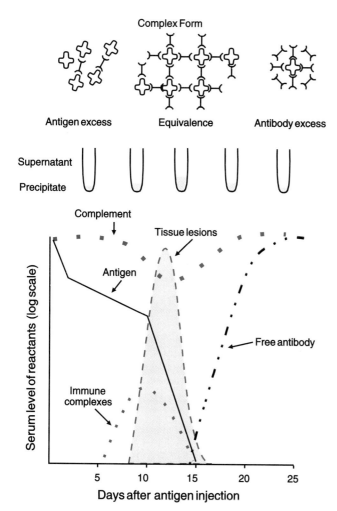

Figure 3-A1 Comparison of antigen elimination, precipitin reaction, and serum complement levels during experimental serum sickness. After a delay, antibody is secreted and binds to the antigen, thus removing it from circulation. The resulting immune (antibody-antigen) complexes can precipitate in blood vessels and fix complement, thereby causing damage to the endothelium, which can result in inflammation of the blood vessels (vasculitis). (*From Sell S: Immunology, Immunopathology, and Immunity, 4th ed. New York, Elsevier, with permission.*)

Description of Antigens

Various words are used to describe antigens; some of these are of major importance in understanding experiments where organs or tissue or cells are taken from a donor and placed in or on a recipient, a process known as *grafting;* transplantation immunology is discussed in more detail in Chapter 26. When an antigen is transplanted into an individual of a different species, the antigen is termed *xenogeneic* or *heterologous* (*hetero,* "other"). An example of this is the use of calf serum in the in vitro growth of human lymphocytes; this supplement is known as heterologous serum. When a graft is derived from another individual of the same species (a kidney transplanted from one human to another unrelated human), the transplant is known as *allogeneic* (*all,* "differing from the normal"), or *homologous.* When the donor and recipient in a graft are either identical twins or are genetically absolutely identical, e.g., the same genetically defined mouse strain, the graft is known as *autologous* (*auto-,* "self"), or *syngeneic.*

T-Dependent and T-Independent Antigens

The antibody response to certain antigens requires the help of T cells; these are called *T-dependent antigens.* Antigens that can elicit an antibody response in the absence of T-cell help are called *T-independent antigens.* The latter are typically polymeric and large in size, usually with repeating antigenic sequences. Occasionally, these are also capable of activating a large number of B cells nonspecifically; this is called *polyclonal B-cell activation.* This phenomenon can be caused by a number of infectious agents, including Epstein-Barr virus (the cause of infectious mononucleosis and nasopharyngeal carcinoma), *Plasmodium* (the cause of malaria), and *Borrelia burgdorferi* (the cause of Lyme disease). Perhaps the most widely used polyclonal B-cell activator in the laboratory setting is the lipopolysaccharide (LPS) found in the cell walls of gram-negative bacteria.

On closer analysis, T-independent antigens can be subdivided into two types. Type I is completely T-independent. These are usually polyclonal B-cell activators, like LPS, which are directly B-cell stimulatory. The antibody response to these antigens is almost entirely IgM.

Type II T-independent antigens need some, although very little, T-cell help. They are usually polysaccharides, like those found in bacterial cell walls. The repeating units on these large molecules can bind to a number of immunoglobulin molecules on the surface of a B cell, and thereby in a specific fashion stimulate B cells. Type II molecules are not polyclonal B-cell activators. The antibody produced is specific, and there may be some IgG present, possibly due to the small T-cell influence.

Adjuvants: Boosting the Immune Response to Inoculations

It is possible to boost the magnitude of an immune response by using an *adjuvant* to maintain the antigen in close proximity to immune cells and/or keep the antigen from dissipating from the inoculation site. Different types of adjuvants are available, such as alum (aluminum hydroxide gels, which keep the antigen from dissolving away) and microorganisms, e.g, whole *Bordetella pertussis.* Two commonly used preparations are Freund's incomplete (antigen in an emulsion of mineral oil and water) and Freund's complete (*complete* because it adds mycobacterial antigens to the emulsion).

Studies of protein haptens as antigens clearly show that haptens contain epitopes that bind to antibodies. But they cannot induce the formation of antibodies without the help of proteins as carriers, the reason being that induction of antibody formation generally requires the interaction of helper T lymphocytes with antibody-producing B lymphocytes. Interaction between these two types of cells is dependent upon each being able to recognize antigen through their antigen-specific membrane receptors. It is instructive and useful, therefore, to classify antigenic epitopes on the basis of their reactivity with T and B lymphocytes. Hapten epitopes can react with B lymphocytes, but not T lymphocytes, since they need to be conjugated to a carrier in order to induce antibody formation. Carrier-type epitopes, associated with the carrier of a protein-hapten conjugate, by definition are epitopes that bind to T-lymphocyte antigen receptors. Conceivably, carrier epitopes could also bind to B-lymphocyte antigen receptors, in which case their function would be that of a hapten.

Epitopes are relatively small in molecular dimension, and in the case of biomolecules such as proteins, polysaccharides, and polynucleotides, they comprise multiple monomeric units. The overall structural configuration of such epitopes depends on the sequence of individual monomers and their interactions, which result in secondary and tertiary structures reflecting differences in conformation. In basic terms an epitope is a constellation of atoms, in the form of amino acids, sugars, and nucleotides, with a fixed structural configuration.

In view of the above, it is useful to view and define an antigen as any substance, simple or complex, that is capable of inducing antibody formation or reacting with antibodies however they are induced. An antigen is termed an immunogen if it can induce antibody formation directly. It is termed a hapten if it requires help of a carrier to do so. Thus, a protein-hapten conjugate is an immunogen. Antigens which are structurally related although not identical but which react with the same antibodies are termed *cross-reacting antigens.*

MOLECULAR CHARACTERIZATION

Amino Acid Composition

After the specificity of antibodies for individual antigenic epitopes had been clearly established, a key question was whether or not this specificity was associated with differences in the composition and sequence of

amino acids in their antigen-binding site. Analysis of antibodies induced by structurally different haptens did in fact reveal significant differences in amino acid composition, suggesting variability in the antigen-binding site rather than differences in folding of antibody polypeptides. These antibodies were heterogeneous despite the fact that they were induced by a single haptenic epitope, thus precluding any analysis of amino acid sequence.

Enzymatic Digestion

Porter achieved a major breakthrough in elucidating the basic structural unit of antibodies. He subjected ovalbumin-specific rabbit antibodies to digestion by papain in the presence of cysteine as a reducing agent, and separated the resulting fragments chromatographically on carboxymethyl cellulose. Three fragments were obtained, each one-third the size of the original antibody molecule. Two of these no longer precipitated ovalbumin from solution, but they retained their ability to bind ovalbumin since they inhibited the precipitation of ovalbumin by the undigested control antibodies. Thus, they seemed to be monovalent fragments of the original bivalent antibody molecules. These fragments retained the antigen-binding sites intact, and were designated *Fab,* or *antigen-binding fragments.* The remaining fragment could be crystallized, suggesting that it had a greater degree of homogeneity than the Fab fragments and constancy in composition. It was designated *Fc.* It did not bind antigen, but it carried the complement-binding site and was considered to be the portion of the antibody molecule responsible for its biologic activity.

Nisonoff used pepsin, instead of papain-cysteine, to digest precipitating rabbit antibodies. He obtained one fragment, twice the size of Fab, that retained the precipitating activity of the original antibodies. On reduction with cysteine the new fragment bound antigen but no longer precipitated it from solution, and it was half of its original size, equivalent to Fab. Thus the pepsin-derived fragment was bivalent; it had both of the antibody-combining sites, each on a fragment joined by interchain disulfide bridges.

Enzymatic digestion of antibodies yielded a penetrating insight about the basic structural unit of antibodies. It consists of two equal portions, each having an epitope-binding site. Still to be determined were the number and kinds of polypeptide chains in each antibody molecule. Edelman obtained this information by subjecting antibody to selective reduction of any interchain disulfide bonds and subsequent separation of resultant polypeptides by chromatography. Polypeptides of two sizes were obtained, one 25 kd and the other 50 kd, and were designated light (L) and heavy (H) chains, respectively.

Together they added up to one-half the size of the original antibody molecule. Thus, it was concluded that antibody molecules consist of two L chains and two H chains. Further analysis showed that each L chain is linked to an H chain by a disulfide bond and that the two H chains are linked to each other by disulfide bonds. Thus, antibodies are symmetrical molecules consisting of pairs of L and H chains. Furthermore, it was shown that Fab fragments consist of the entire L chain, and about one-half of the H chain. On the basis of these studies, a schematic representation of the basic structural unit of antibodies can be formulated (Fig. 3-1). Proteins with this basic structure are termed *immu-*

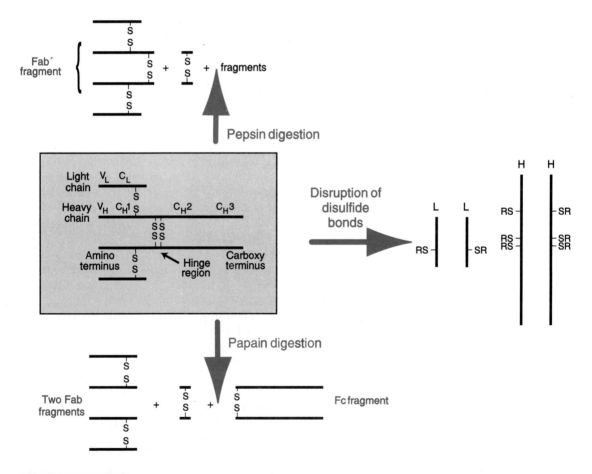

Figure 3-1   Schematic representation of the basic structural unit of antibodies. Enzymatic digestion yields fragments of value in research and in understanding the structure of immunoglobulins.

noglobulins since they are globulins with the immunologic activity of antibodies.

STRUCTURE

Characteristic Features

Bifunctional Molecule
Antibodies are unique among proteins in that they are designed to carry out two separate but coordinate functions. An essential feature of all antibodies is their ability to recognize and bind antigens through individual epitopes for the express purpose of eliminating them, which is the basis of host defense against infectious organisms and other potentially noxious antigens. The effector, or biologic, function of antibodies is mediated through binding sites located on the Fc fragment, whereas the antigen-binding sites are located on the Fab fragment.

Diversity
Another unique feature of antibodies is the vast number of antigenic epitopes against which they can be generated and with which they react. This feature posed two fundamental questions: namely, what is the molecular basis of antibody diversity and what is the genetic basis for this diversity? Answers to these questions were speculative until homogeneous antibodies specific for given individual epitopes could be subjected to fine structural analysis and the methods of molecular biology applied to the genetics of antibody formation. These mechanisms of generation of diversity are described in detail in Chap. 6, on B lymphocytes, and in Chap. 5, "Generation of Diversity in the Acquired Immune Response".

Primary Structure

Requirements
Antibodies, as we have noted, consist of two types of polypeptide chains, L and H. Determination of the primary structure of antibodies requires analysis of the composition and amino acid sequence of both chains. The

methodology of peptide sequencing can only be applied meaningfully to homogeneous polypeptides. Homogeneous L and H chains became available after two discoveries: (1) Bence-Jones proteins, pathologic proteins secreted in the urine of individuals with multiple myeloma (a plasma cell malignancy where the cells may make light-chain, heavy-chain, or whole immunoglobulin molecules, which they may then secrete), were in fact L chains of immunoglobulins since they were antigenically related to L chains of antibodies of known specificity. (2) Myeloma proteins in the serum of such individuals were homogeneous monoclonal immunoglobulins derived from plasma cell tumors. Moreover, plasma cell tumors could be induced experimentally in certain strains of mice, making available a large number of homogeneous L and H chains from immunoglobulins having different binding sites for antigenic epitopes and different effector functions.

Constant and Variable Sequences
The L chain consists of 214 amino acids. The N-terminal half of the molecule, amino acids 1–107, characteristically displays variability. In contrast, the C-terminal end, amino acids 108–214, is relatively constant in its composition. Both the variable and constant portions of L have an intrachain disulfide bond between cysteine residues that influences the folding and secondary structure of the polypeptide. These links involve cysteine in positions 23 and 88 of the variable portion, and cysteine in positions 134 and 194 of the constant portion. Each of the two portions of L, as a result of its secondary structure stabilized by an intrachain disulfide bond, can best be described as a domain. The *domain*, which is approximately 110 amino acid residues in length with a central disulfide bond enclosing 60 to 70 amino acids, is the building block of immunoglobulin chains, as well as other immune molecules (Fig. 3-2). Accordingly, L comprises two domains, designed V_L and C_L.

The H chain is about twice the size of L and consists of approximately 446 amino acids. It too has an N-terminal variable

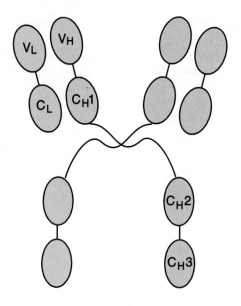

Figure 3-2 The domain, the building block of immunoglobulin chains. Both heavy and light chains consist of domain structures linked end-to-end.

region, comprising amino acids 1–107, and a C-terminal constant region, comprising amino acids 108–446. These are designated V_H and C_H, respectively. There is a single intrachain S—S bond in V_H, and three such S—S bonds in C_H, so the H chain is made up of four domains, one variable and three constant. Moving from the variable region to the C terminus the constant domains are denoted as C_H1, C_H2, and C_H3. Each of the constant domains, as does V_H, consists of about 107 amino acids. The constant domains exhibit significant homology and seem to have been conserved during evolution, perhaps being products of a replicated primordial gene (see Appendix B).

Framework and Complementarity-Determining Regions

Further scrutiny of the variability in V_L revealed hot spots of hypervariability (Fig. 3-3). These hypervariable spots occur in three regions, between amino acids 24–34, 50–56, and 89–97, associated with the epitope-bind-

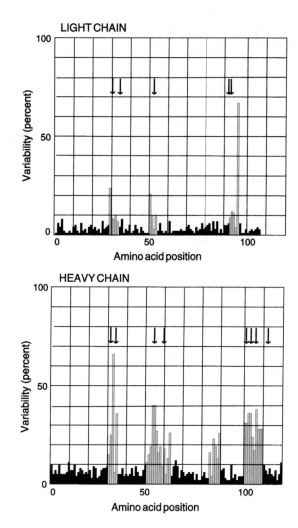

Figure 3-3 Hypervariable "hot spots" in light and heavy chains. These areas contribute to antigen-binding regions. (Used by permission of *Scientific American*.)

ing site, and are appropriately termed *complementarity-determining regions* (*CDRs*). The remaining regions of V_L provide a framework for the CDRs.

Analysis of the genes controlling L chain provided further insight into its structure. V_L is the product of two separate genes, one a minigene coding for amino acids 101–113, located just before C_L. This region serves to join the bulk of the variable domain to the constant domain and is therefore termed the *joint segment* (J_L).

The variable domain of the H chain also has regions of hypervariability associated with the epitope-binding site. There are three such CDRs; their positions correspond to the CDR of V_L. A fourth hypervariable region, between amino acids 81–85, is not involved in the formation of the epitope-binding site. The remaining amino acids provide a framework for CDRs (Fig. 3-4).

The variable domain of the H chain, like V_L, is the product of several genes, one that codes for most of the domain (the variable gene) and two minigenes, whose products serve to join the variable and constant domains and to generate diversity. The regions of amino acids coded by the minigenes are designated J_H and D_H, respectively. The joint region occurs at the end of the variable domain, and the diversity region just before it. The details of how these genes link in the development of the antibody response are discussed in Chap. 5.

Hinge Region

The H chain, unlike L, contains multiple constant domains and a hinge region between the first and second constant domains. The amino acids in this hinge region provide flexibility, thereby creating a hinge where the S—S bonds linking the H chains are located. It is this region that is susceptible to proteolytic attack by papain and pepsin, resulting in the fragmentation of immunoglobulins into Fab and F(ab')$_2$, respectively.

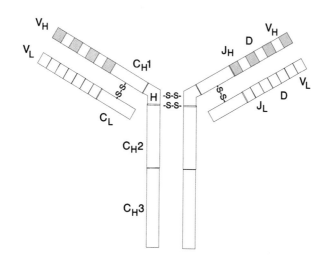

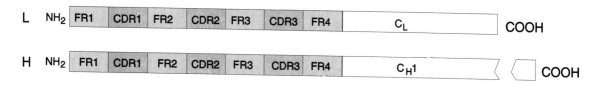

Figure 3-4 Schematic of complementarity determining regions (CDR) and framework regions (FR), which together determine the antigen-binding site of the antibody. (From Alt FW: Development of the primary antibody repertoire. *Science* 253:1679, 1987. Used with permission. Copyright 1987 by the AAAS.)

These enzymes attack different positions relative to the positions of the S—S bonds, thus explaining the difference in the valency (number of antigen-binding sites) of the fragments produced.

Carbohydrate Content

Glycosylation of immunoglobulins occurs prior to their secretion from antibody-producing plasma cells. The amount of carbohydrate, usually linked to asparagine in the H chain (C_H2), varies with the class of the immunoglobulin: 2 to 3 percent of IgG, 7 to 11 percent of IgA, about 12 percent of IgM and IgE, and 9 to 14 percent of IgD.

Classification of Immunoglobulins

The basis of classification of immunoglobulins is the antigenic specificity of the H chain, determined by species-specific immune sera induced by homogeneous H chains from plasma cell tumors. A total of five antigenically distinct H chains have been demonstrated for several species of immunoglobulins. These are designated gamma, alpha, mu, epsilon, and delta. In contrast, only two antigenically distinct L chains have been found, designated kappa and lambda. Both types of L chains are linked to each of the different H chains. Immunoglobulins are therefore classified according to the antigenicity of their H chain. They are: G, A, M, E,

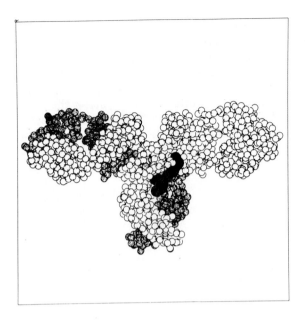

Figure 3-5   Three-dimensional structure of the combined heavy and light chains. (*From Silverton et al. Immunology. Proc Natl Acad Sci USA 74:5142, 1977, with permission.*)

and D, corresponding to the H chains gamma (γ), alpha (α), mu (μ), epsilon (ε), and delta (δ), respectively. The classes of immunoglobulins are listed in Table 3-1, using conventional nomenclature. The three-dimensional structure of the combined heavy and light chains is seen in Fig. 3-5.

TABLE 3-1   Classification of Human Immunoglobulins

Class	Subclass	H Chain	L Chain	Formula
IgG	IgG1	$\gamma1$	λ or κ	$(\gamma1)_2\lambda_2$; $(\gamma1)_2\kappa_2$
IgG	IgG2	$\gamma2$	λ or κ	$(\gamma2)_2\lambda_2$; $(\gamma2)_2\kappa x$
IgG	IgG3	$\gamma3$	λ or κ	$(\gamma3)_2\lambda_2$; $(\gamma3)_2\kappa_2$
IgG	IgG4	$\gamma4$	λ or κ	$(\gamma4)_2\lambda_2$; $(\gamma4)_2\kappa_2$
IgM	IgM1	$\mu1$	λ or κ	$[(\mu1)_2\lambda_2]5$; $[(\mu1)_2\kappa_2]5$
IgM	IgM2	$\mu2$	λ or κ	$[(\mu2)_2\lambda_2]5$; $[(\mu2)_2\kappa_2]5$
IgA	IgA1	$\alpha1$	λ or κ	$(\alpha1)_2\lambda_2$; $(\alpha1)_2\kappa_2$ =
IgA	IgA2	$\alpha2$	λ or κ	$(\alpha2)_2\lambda_2$; $(\alpha2)_2\kappa_2$
IgD		δ	λ or κ	$\delta_2\lambda_2$; $\delta_2\kappa_2$
IgE		ϵ	λ or κ	$\epsilon_2\lambda_2$; $\epsilon_2\kappa_2$

Isotypes, Idiotypes, Idiotopes, and Allotypes

An antigen elicits an immune response, producing an antibody whose paratope can bind to the antigen's epitope. There are a virtually limitless supply of antigens in nature, not to mention synthetic compounds. Antibodies can be produced to virtually all of them; the means by which such diversity can be obtained have been described in this chapter and are covered in more detail in Chap. 5. Each of these new antibodies carries antigenic markers, common to all humans, which define the heavy chain, or the class; a frequently used term synonymous with class is *isotype*. Each antibody therefore contains many areas of protein well known to the immune system. However, the antigen-binding site of the antibody, tailored specifically for the newly encountered antigen, is different from most, if not all, other antibodies and may be unique. In such a case, the new antibody represents a potential new set of epitopes, capable of inducing an immune response! This collection of new epitopes is known as the antibody's *idiotype*, with each epitope known as an *idiotope*.

The idiotype of an antibody is defined by the antigen-binding sections of the V regions of that antibody. Heavy and light chains are also antigenically diverse in their constant regions; i.e., the genes encoding the constant regions are *polymorphic*. This has nothing to do with the variable regions. The inherited differences between individuals is known as the *allotype* of the heavy chain.

Classes of Immunoglobulin

Further details of the five different isotypes of immunoglobulin are given in Table 3-2. The antigen-binding properties of the immunoglobulins are found in the Fab portions, but their biologic activities are associated with the constant domains of the H chains, also the sites of the class-determining epitopes. Therefore, it is not surprising that the classes of immunoglobulin differ in their biologic functions.

IgG

The structure of the IgG molecule is the prototypic immunoglobulin tetramer, two heavy chains and two light chains. IgG is the predominant serum immunoglobulin, although it is also found in the secretions coating the mucosal surfaces. It is the predominant *opsonin* in serum. *Opsonization* (from Greek *opsōneia,* "to buy (or prepare) victuals for a meal") is the process whereby a particle is rendered more likely to be phagocytosed. This process is accomplished by two means: (1) IgG attached to a particle can be bound to phagocytes by the interaction of the Fc portion with the receptor on the phagocyte's surface; (2) complement, fixed by IgG, can bind to specific receptors on the phagocyte's surface. (Refer back to Clinical Aside 3.1.)

TABLE 3-2 Immunoglobulin Isotype (Class)

	IgG	*IgA*	*IgM*	*IgE*	*IgD*
Serum concentration, mg/dL	1000–1500	160–300	75–175	0.03	3–5
% of total immunoglobulin	80	12	8	0.003	0.3
Molecular weight, kd	140	160	890–970	180–196	184–200
% intravascular	40–45	40–42	70–80	50	75
Serum half-life, days	23	6	5	2.8–3	1.5–2.5
Antibody valence	2	2	5 or 10	2	2
Capable of fixing complement	+	–	+	–	–
Subclasses	4	2	2	1	1
Allotypes*	About 20	2			

*Allotypic determinants reside on the designated domain of the heavy chain of that subclass; e.g., IgG1m is defined in the CH1 and CH3 domains of the G1 heavy chain, and IgA2m is defined in the CH3 domain of the A2 heavy chain.

Although IgG is the predominant immunoglobulin in serum, and most of the body's IgG is intravascular, much of it escapes to the extravascular space. There are many different molecular forms of IgG, including 4 subclasses and over 20 allotypes.

IgA

IgA is the predominant immunoglobulin in the secretions which bathe the mucosal surfaces of the upper and lower respiratory, gastrointestinal, and genitourinary tracts and in breast milk and colostrum. It is somewhat different from the serum IgA, in that the majority is polymeric, whereas in the serum over 80 percent is IgA monomer. Another difference is that most serum IgA is subclass 1, whereas the majority of secretory IgA is subclass 2. There are two IgA allotypes. When one considers the large mucosal areas covered by IgA-containing secretions, it becomes clear that on the basis of milligrams of immunoglobulin per kilogram of total body weight IgA is the predominant antibody in (or should we say, on) the body. IgA's primary role in the secretions is to bind to particles and immobilize them, thereby neutralizing viral or bacterial pathogens. IgA does not fix complement in the same way that IgG and IgM do, called the "classical pathway" (see Chap. 13). IgA can activate a second pathway that allows complement activation, called the "alternate pathway." It is interesting to note that the alternate pathway is phylogenetically much older than the classical pathway (see Appendix B).

The secretory form of IgA is a dimer bound to two other proteins. The J chain is a very elongate, highly acidic protein, of approximate molecular weight 15 kd, made by the same cells which produce the IgA. It is found in all multimeric forms of immunoglobulin, including pentameric IgM, and may be involved in the polymerization process. In the discussion of the production of immunoglobulin (Chaps. 5 and 6) and how such diverse antibodies can be generated, you will read about a J segment of immunoglobulin. The J chain discussed here and the J segment described later are not the same; however,

both accomplish the process of *joining* and the letter J is appropriately (although perhaps confusingly) used for both.

The other protein found associated with polymeric IgA in gastrointestinal secretions is called *secretory component (SC)*. It is possible that a similar or identical secretory component may be involved in the transport of polymeric IgM into secretions. Secretory component is a 70-kd protein made by the epithelial cells lining the mucosal surface. It is derived from a protein, called the *polymeric-immunoglobulin (poly-Ig) receptor*, which is found at the basolateral cell surface. The whole poly-Ig receptor includes a cytoplasmic COOH-terminal "tail," a transmembrane stretch, and an extracellular ligand-binding region. The latter consists of five repeating homologous domains of approximately 100 to 110 amino acid residues in length. Each of these are members of the immunoglobulin superfamily and are related to the immunoglobulin variable region.

After submucosal plasma cells make IgA and it has polymerized, the IgA passes to the mucosa, where the poly-Ig receptor binds covalently to the IgA Fc portion of the polymerized immunoglobulin. This complexing allows the receptor plus its ligand (the J chain plus IgA dimer) to enter the epithelial cell by endocytosis with subsequent transcellular transport in vesicles to the mucosal (or apical) surface of the cell. During this process, known as *transcytosis* (which also occurs in other cells, for other molecules, e.g., transferrin across brain capillaries), the receptor is proteolytically cleaved to yield an immunoglobulin-SC complex. This is released at the luminal surface into the secretions. Figure 3-6 shows how the IgA dimer, the J chain, and the SC all fit together. See also Chap. 11, on mucosal immunity.

Another poly-Ig receptor is found in the fetus and newborn, which mediates the transepithelial passage of maternal breast milk IgG (see Chap. 28, "The Immune Response of Normal Children"). Recent evidence suggests that a receptor for IgG (called the FcγII receptor), also found on lymphocytes and macrophages, may be part of the transport of

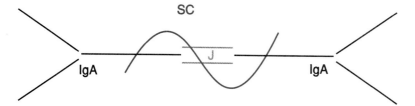

Figure 3-6 "Fit" of the IgA dimer, J chain, and secretory component (SC), which together make up dimeric secretory IgA.

IgG across the placenta. Transcytosis in neonatal rat gut makes use of a unique receptor on enterocytes, which has a different structure from the poly-Ig receptor described above. The enterocyte receptor, called the FcRn, is a heterodimer, one chain being the 14-kd protein β_2-microglobulin (about which you will hear a lot more in the next chapter, on major histocompatibility, MHC) and a larger component, called p51, which bears a strong resemblance to class I MHC molecules. β_2-microglobulin and the class I MHC molecules are also members of the immunoglobulin superfamily. These molecules, all of whose structure is based on the domain, are involved in immune recognition and cellular interactions, in a large array of settings.

IgM

IgM is a pentamer, whose monomers are linked by a J chain and intermonomer disulfide bonds. It is found predominantly in the intravascular space, predictable on the basis of its large size. There are 5 Fc portions available to fix complement, and therefore IgM is more able to start the complement cascade than is IgG. IgM is very active in the cytolytic functions of the immune response because of this efficiency in complement fixation. It also has 10 Fab portions (although in some circumstances only five sites can be used, possibly due to spatial interference or lack of flexibility of the Fab arms), so that IgM can be active in agglutination of particles or microorganisms. There are two IgM subclasses.

IgM monomer has four constant domains per μ heavy chain, rather than the three found in the γ chain. IgM is 12 percent polysaccharide by weight, the most of any class of immunoglobulin, with five oligosaccharide

chains per heavy chain. The IgM pentamer can be broken up into its five monomeric subunits by treating IgM with a mild reducing agent; 0.01 mol/L 2-mercaptoethanol is often used in experiments to eliminate IgM binding from serum.

Prior to binding to antigens, the pentamer is found with the monomers in a radial distribution, called the *star form*. Upon interaction with its target antigens, the star comes undone and IgM is found in a linear or *staple* form, bringing many Fab portions to bear on the target. The star and staple forms of IgM are shown in Fig. 3-7.

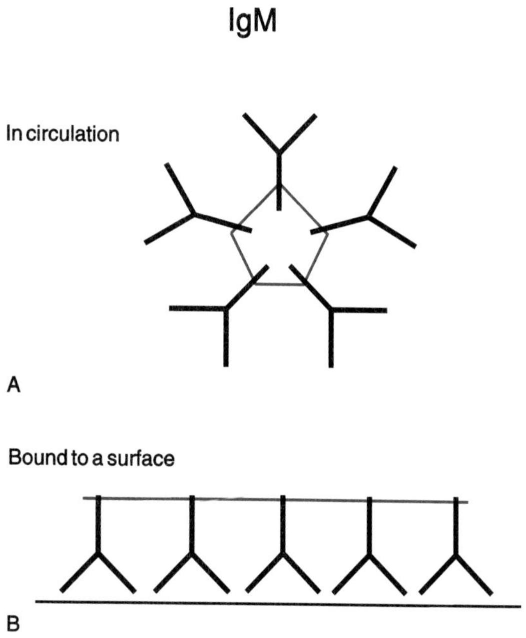

IgM

In circulation

A

Bound to a surface

B

Figure 3-7 IgM pentamer. (a) Star form, in circulation. (b) Staple form, bound to target antigen.

IgE

IgE is found primarily bound to its receptors on immune cells, including eosinophils, mast cells, and basophils. Very little IgE is found free in the circulation. In the older literature IgE was called "homocytotropic antibody," for its strong cell-binding capacity, and "reaginic antibody," for its ability to sensitize the skin in the passive transfer experiments of Prausnitz and Kustner. IgE is found only as a monomer and has no allotypic varieties or subclasses. In contrast with the other immunoglobulin classes, IgE has no hinge region.

The primary role of IgE seems related to the immune response to parasites. Once IgE binds to its appropriate target, it causes the mast cells and basophils on whose receptors it sits to liberate chemicals that increase gastrointestinal peristalsis. This increase in GI motility causes expulsion of parasites in the gut.

The ε heavy chain has four constant domains (in common with the μ heavy chain); all other heavy chains have three constant domains.

IgD

IgD is found in the serum in only trace amounts. The main residence of IgD is on the surface of B cells, where it and IgM are the predominant transmembrane immunoglobulins. Surface IgD may play a role in the maturation of B cells. Like IgE, IgD is a monomer and has no subclasses or allotypes. The δ heavy chain has a very long hinge segment.

Immunoglobulin Subclasses

IgG and IgA antibodies can be further categorized into subclasses, described in Tables 3-3 and 3-4, respectively.

IgG subclasses differ in the number and location of disulfide bonds and the size of the hinge regions. In general, the amino acid sequences of the four IgG subclasses are over 95 percent identical. IgG1 is the predominant IgG subclass. Of note is the fact that all subclasses are not equal in complement fixing ability, with IgG4 essentially incapable of that function. One major difference in the four subclasses is the size of the hinge region and the degree of flexibility of the

TABLE 3-3   Characteristics of IgG Subclasses

	IgG1	IgG2	IgG3	IgG4
Serum concentration, mg/dL	900	250–300	50–100	50–100
% of total IgG	65	23	8	4
Molecular weight, kd	146	146	170	146
% intravascular	45	45	45	45
Capable of fixing complement	2 +	1 +	3 +	0
Serum half-life, days	25	23	9	25
Hinge size (number of amino acids); flexibility of hinge region	15; very	12; little	62; very	12; >G2, <G1
Response to polysaccharide antigens	−	+	−	+
Response to protein antigens	+	−	+	−
Binding by staph protein A	+	+	−	+
Binding by rheumatoid factor	+	+	−	+

TABLE 3-4   Characteristics of IgA Subclasses

	IgA	IgA2	Secretory IgA
Serum concentration, mg/dL	300	50	5
Molecular weight, kd	160	160	385
% intravascular	42	42	Trace
Serum half-life, days	6	6	?

molecule at that site. Also of importance is the fact that polysaccharide and protein antigens elicit IgG antibody responses of different subclass types. Staphylococcal protein A binds to most IgG; this protein can be useful in experiments where purification or identification of IgG is necessary. However, staph protein A does not bind to IgG3. Rheumatoid factor is an immunoglobulin which binds to IgG, specifically the CH2 and CH3 domain of the γ heavy chain. Thus, rheumatoid factor is an auto-antibody (an antibody capable of binding to a component of self). A more detailed description of this auto-antibody is found in Chap. 31, on autoimmunity. The reason for mentioning it here is that rheumatoid factor has the same IgG subclass binding specificity as staph protein A, and, as might be suspected from these data, the binding sites for staph protein A and for rheumatoid factor are identical.

There are two IgA subclasses: IgA1 predominates in serum, and IgA2 constitutes the majority of IgA in secretions. IgA2 is more negatively charged, so that the two IgA subclasses can be separated by electrophoresis, and is slightly heavier than IgA1. The hinge region of IgA1 is more mobile than that of IgA2, so the IgA1 Fab segments are more mobile.

There are two IgA2 allotypes. IgA2m(1), the two L chains are joined by disulfide bonds, as are the two H chains; there is no H-L disulfide linkage, as there is in all other immunoglobulin molecules, including the other IgA2 allotype, IgA2m(2).

Tertiary Structure

Domains

The composition and sequence of amino acids are the determinants of the tertiary structure of proteins comprising one or more polypeptide chains. Their final three-dimensional structure in a given environment reflects the secondary interactions between amino acids to form helixes or sheets and the folding of the chains that is stabilized by S—S covalent bonds between cysteine residues at distal positions in the chain. The basic unit of immunoglobulins consists of four chains but only two types, L and H. Each is a composite of distinct segments or domains, with tertiary structures of their own. The interaction between L and H is stabilized not only by interchain S—S bonds but also by hydrophobic interactions between their corresponding domains.

Antigen-Binding Site

The tertiary structure of the variable domains of both L and H of monoclonal immunoglobulins has been determined by x-ray diffraction analysis, revealing the shape of the antigen-binding site that is formed by the interaction of the hypervariable regions of L and H.

THE PRIMARY AND SECONDARY IMMUNE RESPONSE

After exposure to a new antigen, the naive host first makes IgM antibodies. These become detectable after a short *lag* or *latent* period, usually 7 to 9 days; only in the last day or so prior to their appearance in the serum can you find cells in the secondary lymphoid structures which are making the antibodies. Thereafter a *logarithmic* or *exponential* period occurs, when there is a rise in the amount of IgM present in the serum, with subsequent leveling off, called the *plateau* or *steady-state* period. This plateau phenomenon may occur because all of the antigen is bound by the antibody and cleared from the circulation, may be due to increased catabolism of the antibody, or may be due to negative feedback mechanisms dampening synthesis. Whatever the cause, IgM levels off and IgG begins to rise. Typically, the IgM then returns to baseline levels, and IgG often remains present in very small amounts. This is called the *primary immunoglobulin (or antibody) response* (Fig. 3-8a). The bulk of the antibody made is IgM and usually of low affinity (Clinical Aside 3-2).

Clinical Aside 3-2
Use of Serologic Testing in Clinical Medicine

If a patient experiences an infection with an organism he or she has never encountered, there should be little if any serum antibody against that organism. By 10 to 20 days after exposure the primary antibody response should be well into the rising exponential phase. A comparison of serum antibody levels early in the course of the disease with levels at a later stage should reveal a significant increase, which can be used to make the specific diagnosis. Serum is drawn in the *acute phase* and compared with a sample drawn later in the *convalescent phase.* Antibody levels can be expressed as a *titer,* (i.e., the sample is tested "neat" or undiluted or at 1 : 10 and then diluted serially twofold, to 1 : 20, 1 : 40, 1 : 80, etc.); the highest or last dilution giving a "positive test" is the one reported out as the titer level. (How "positive test" is defined depends on the specific assay.) A change in titer of fourfold or greater between acute and convalescent samples is considered diagnostic of infection. Thus, if the overall antibody level is 1 : 20 in the acute phase and is 1 : 160 2 weeks later in an assay for antibodies to *Mycoplasma pneumoniae,* it can be said

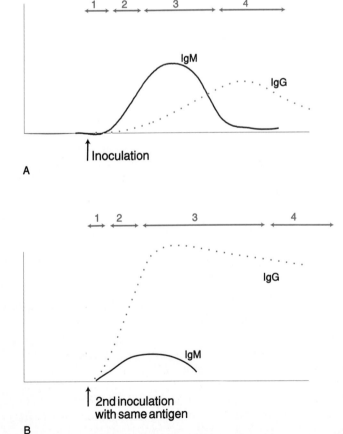

A

B

Figure 3-8 (a) Primary antibody response. Interval 1, lag or latent phase; interval 2, exponential (logarithmic, or growth) phase; interval 3, steady-state (plateau, or stationary) phase; interval 4, decline, or resolution, phase. (b) Secondary (anamnestic) antibody response. Interval 1 is about half as long as interval 1 in primary response; interval 2 reaches its peak more rapidly; interval 3 is attained sooner and lasts longer, the level of antibody reached is higher, and the antibody is more homogeneous and has higher affinity; interval 4 is longer and more shallow.

that the patient's pneumonia was due to that organism. For organisms that are difficult to culture, such serologic testing may be the only way to make a specific diagnosis.

Even better, if you can test for IgM and IgG antibodies, you can document the fact that the infection is recent. What pattern of IgM and IgG antibodies might you expect in a recent infection? In an infection of long duration?

Another useful strategy is to test the fluid obtained from the site of inflammation. Suppose you think the patient has syphilis affecting the brain. Do a spinal tap (lumbar puncture) and analyze the spinal fluid for antibodies to *Treponema pallidum*. Is Lyme disease a possible explanation for your patient's arthritis? Look at the joint fluid (synovial fluid) levels of specific antibodies and compare with the levels present in serum, in order to demonstrate relative concentration of the specific antibodies at the site of inflammation. This then allows one to make the diagnosis.

When the same individual is exposed to the *same* antigen a second time, a somewhat different response, known as the *secondary immunoglobulin* (or *antibody*) *response* (Fig. 3-8b), develops. First, the lag or latent period is shorter. Second, there is a more rapid increase in the exponential phase. The ultimate level of antibody is higher and persists longer than in the primary response. Third, there is more IgG than IgM in the antibody produced; i.e., isotype switching, which is likely T-cell dependent, has occurred. (There is an exception to this rule: T-independent antigens typically produce a smaller amplitude response in the primary response and little if any IgG, even in the secondary response). Fourth, the amount of antigen needed to elicit the secondary response is smaller than that needed for the primary response. Finally, in certain circumstances, the antibody produced has a higher mean affinity in the secondary response.

Why should the mean affinity increase in the secondary response? There are probably two mechanisms behind this fact. First, let us consider an experiment comparing a large second inoculant with a small dose. The smaller dose leads to the development of serum antibodies with a higher affinity than

does the large dose. The explanation for this is that memory cells are produced during the primary response. These cells persist for months to years after the primary exposure. They have on their surface different isotypes of antibody against the inoculant, each antibody with its own affinity for the antigen. Once the inoculant is given again and the antigen is bound to the surface immunoglobulin, these cells spring into action, making the antibody more rapidly than would naive cells. If a small second dose is given, only those cells with antibody of high affinity will bind the antigen and be stimulated to make immunoglobulin. Thus, a small dose essentially selects for the production of high-affinity antibodies. If a high dose is given, cells with lower-affinity surface immunoglobulin will also be activated. A large dose causes the production of a more heterogeneous population of antibody, but a population with a lower mean affinity.

If the second inoculation follows the initial exposure after too short a period of time, there will be a small antibody response to the second inoculation. The reasons for this are twofold. First, if there is still serum antibody present from the initial response, the second dose of antigen will be bound by free antibody and fail to reach the surface immunoglobulin on memory cells. Second, memory cells may not yet have formed. If the second inoculation is given too long after the primary exposure, the memory cells, which have a finite life-span, may have died. (See Clinical Aside 3-3.)

Clinical Aside 3-3
Inoculations and the Immune Response

Immunoglobulin can be life-saving if it can prevent an infection. Jenner identified this fact, and the science of vaccination (the Latin root *vacca*, "cow," being a permanent reminder of the cowpox Jenner used) was introduced to medicine. Inoculation with a less virulent organism or an inactivated organism can prevent a number of infections. The relevant antigen is given in an appropriate form—e.g., in alum or adjuvant, or orally—and an IgM and then an IgG response develop. In some cases, second inoculations are given with the same antigen; these so-called *booster shots* are given in order to produce higher-affinity antibodies.

It is common to inoculate elderly patients, or those with chronic diseases, for influenza every year. Every 5 to 10 years we inoculate these at risk patients with a cocktail of antigens from a number of strains of pneumococcus, one of the major causes of pneumonia. The idea is that after inoculation, the patient will develop IgG and IgA antibodies which will be very effective in opsonizing any pneumococcus that happens along; even if an infection takes place, the antibody in the serum and secretions will fight the organism and memory cells will rapidly begin to produce higher-affinity antibodies.

Finally, even if the organism which arrives is not one of those represented in the vaccine, there may be an anamnestic response because of a phenomenon now called *original antigenic sin*. Exposure to a new protein, e.g., an inoculation, often can elicit a secondary immunoglobulin response to nonidentical, but related, antigens encountered in the past. Antibodies will be produced not only to the similar epitope(s), but also to epitopes which are not found on the inoculated antigens but which are unique to the original protein. Can you think of a possible explanation for the phenomenon of original antigenic sin?

FUNCTION

Binding of Antigen

General Considerations

The binding of antigen is the essential function of all antibodies regardless of class. Antibodies have a binding site for individual antigenic epitopes, and this binding is highly specific. The molecular basis of this specificity is the complementarity in the configurations of the atoms comprising the antibody-combining site and the antigenic epitope, thus permitting a close encounter between the atoms. Close encounter is necessary because the forces of interaction are physicochemical in nature, relatively weak, and effective only at short range. Moreover, stable binding of antigen by antibody requires such interactions between a relatively

large number of corresponding atoms in close proximity to each other. The major forces of interaction are electrostatic (influenced by the pH and ionic strength of the medium), H bonds, general van der Waals forces, and interactions between hydrophobic groups. The energy of interaction between individual pairs of atoms is small, but the total sum of these weak interactions over a sufficiently large area of the antigen and antibody molecules is sufficient to ensure stable binding.

Size and Shape

Analysis of the molecular dimension of defined antigenic epitopes and their corresponding antibody-combining sites has led to a definition of the average size and shape of the antigen-binding site. Mostly it is in the form of a pocket or cleft and sometimes a superficial groove. In either case the binding site can accommodate epitopes of up to five or six monomers (amino acids, monosaccharides, and nucleotides).

Cross-Reactions

As noted, antibodies are remarkably specific in their reaction with antigenic epitopes, owing to the requirement for complementarity in the molecular configurations of the interacting atoms over a sufficiently large area of the two molecules. Nevertheless, what is required is a minimum total energy of interaction sufficient for stable binding. Thus, antibodies can bind different antigens provided their epitopes are sufficiently related structurally so as to permit a close encounter between a minimum number of corresponding atoms. Antigens that are not identical but react with the same antibodies are denoted as *cross-reacting antigens*. Such cross-reacting antigens necessarily bind antibodies with a different energy.

Affinity

The closer the molecular fit (complementarity) between the antigenic epitope and antigen-binding site of antibodies, the greater will be the energy (stability) of binding. A quantitative measure of this energy of binding is the *association constant, K*, a function of the concentrations of the free and bound antigen at equilibrium for a fixed initial concentration of antibody. This constant is appropriately called the *affinity* of the antibody-combining site for its antigenic epitope and is in essence the summation of all the attractive and repulsive forces present in the interaction between antigen-binding site and the epitope. The formula for the association constant is

$$K = [Ab - Ag]/[Ab] \times [Ag]$$

K has been determined experimentally for the reaction of antibodies with monovalent small haptens. Antigens of biologic importance are generally multivalent, which means that a single molecule of antigen can bind several molecules of antibody. The binding of one antibody to a given epitope does not alter the intrinsic affinity of a second antibody binding to its corresponding epitope. However, the binding of several antibody molecules to an antigen, and the cross-linking of antigens that results from the binding of a single antibody molecule to epitopes on different molecules of antigens, increase the stability of antigen-antibody aggregates that are formed. This apparent increase in the affinity of antibody is defined as the *avidity* of the antibody in reacting with its antigen and can be observed as a decrease in the time of formation of antigen-antibody complexes.

Immunoglobulin Receptors

Cell Surface Binding of Antibody
Antibodies can bind to circulating particles or molecules and to cells and/or tissues. As noted above, these immunoglobulin molecules can activate complement as a means of destruction of the target. The antigen-binding site of the antibody is bound to the target, but the Fc portion is exposed on the opposite end of the antibody molecule. It is through the Fc portion that the target, be it bacterium or inert protein, can interact with immune cells, because on the surface of many immune cells there are specific receptors for the Fc portion. It is important to know that antigen binding at one end of an antibody

can cause conformational changes at the other end, the Fc portion. Thus, interactions with receptors can confer *antigenic* specificity to a cellular function, which can be transmitted by the receptor to the inner workings of the cell. When the receptor is found on the surface of a *phagocyte*, this interaction may lead to uptake by the cell, known as phagocytosis. If the receptor is on the surface of a cell capable of destroying other cells, the receptor allows for specification of which target to kill. This is the crucial step in activation of a number of cells capable of accomplishing *antibody-dependent cell-mediated cytotoxicity (ADCC)*. Finally, if a receptor is internally linked to cellular activation processes, binding of immunoglobulin to that receptor may trigger proliferation or activation of that cell type in a specific fashion. Thus, these receptors are incredibly important in the function of antigen-specific immune effector function.

Different Receptors, Different Functions
Research in the past decades has defined three major types of Fc receptor for human IgG and two types for IgE (Table 3-5). IgG FcRI is probably the only Fc IgG receptor capable of binding IgG monomer; the others can bind complexed immunoglobulin only. The reason for this is the characteristic of each receptor, I being a high-affinity receptor and II and III being low-affinity receptors. Type II is the most widespread, being found on virtually all immune cells, with the exception of natural killer (NK) cells.

The three IgG Fc receptors differ in their affinity for the three subclasses of IgG (Table 3-6).

More recent work has identified three FcγII receptors, called A, B, and C, and two FcγIII receptors, A and B. The differences between IIA, IIB, and IIC are to be found in the intracellular tail amino acid sequence and glycosylation sites, as well as the cells on which they are found; neutrophils do not bear IIB receptors, B cells bear only IIB receptors, and monocytes express all three types. Type IIIB, found exclusively on neutrophils, is anchored to the outer layer of the cell's plasma

TABLE 3-5   Fc Receptors on Nonlymphoid Immune Cells

Fc Receptor	CD	PMN	Mono	Eos	Basophil/ Mast Cell	NK	Platelet	Molecular weight, kd
FcγRI	64	Some*	+	−	−	−	−	72
FcγRII	W32	+	+	+	−	−	+	40–42
FcγRIII	16	+	+†	+	+	+	+	50–80
FcεRI (high-affinity)		−	−	−	+	−	−	‡
FcεRII (low-affinity)	23	−	Some	+	−	−	+	36§

*Only PMN activated by INF-γ.
†Macrophages, not monocytes.
‡Consists of three polypeptides: 1 alpha (55 kd), 1 beta (33 kd), and 2 gamma (9 kd); interacts with the CH2 domain of IgE.
§Single polypeptide chain: amino acids 1–23, cytoplasmic tail; amino acids 24–44, hydrophobic transmembrane portion; amino acids 45–321, extracellular domain.

TABLE 3-6   Binding of IgG Subclasses to the Fcγ Receptors

	FcRI	FcRII	FcRIII
IgG1	3+	3+	2+
IgG2	+/−	1+	−
IgG3	3+	3+	2+
IgG4	1+	1+	1+

membrane by a glycosyl-phosphatidyl-inositol linkage, whereas IIIA receptors, found on macrophages, cultured monocytes, and NK cells, have the classic transmembrane insertion, with a cytoplasmic tail. Two allotypic forms of IIIB have been defined.

The function of all of these receptors has not been precisely determined yet. There is some overlap between functions, but in general terms type I seems to be involved in ADCC activities, IIA and IIC in phagocytosis and ADCC, and IIB in control of lymphocyte function. Receptor IIIA, expressed on NK cells and macrophages, is probably also involved in ADCC and phagocytosis, whereas IIIB, found only on neutrophils, may serve as a trap for circulating immune complexes and may synergize with IIA receptors in this function.

Fc Receptors for IgE   Two types of IgE Fc receptors have been identified, one of high affinity (FcεI) and one of low affinity (FcεII). The former is found on basophils and mast cells and consists of five polypeptide chains; the IgE binding site is on the α chain (Table 3-5). Aggregation of multiple receptors by multiple IgE molecules bound to antigen is needed for cell activation. Once IgE molecules are bound to receptors and in turn bind to multivalent antigen, a number of cellular events may occur, including basophil and mast cell degranulation with release of granular components and synthesis of arachidonic acid metabolites. In addition, synthesis and in certain cases release of cytokines, including IL-1, IL-3, IL-4, IL-5, IL-6, tumor necrosis factor, IFN-γ, and granulocyte-monocyte colony-stimulating factor (GM-CSF), can follow activation of these cells by means of the receptor. (Cytokines are described in more detail in Chap. 10, and basophils and mast cells are discussed in Chap. 19.)

The FcεRII, also known as CD23, is found on eosinophils, monocytes, platelets, some T cells, and B cells. The consequences of IgE binding to this receptor include the release of many inflammatory mediators from mononuclear phagocytes (including lysosomal enzymes, oxygen radicals, and arachidonic acid metabolites), release by eosinophils of platelet activating factor, oxygen metabolites, peroxidase and other eosinophil-specific cytocidal proteins, and aggregation and release of cytocidal mediators by platelets. In addition, there is evidence to suggest that when IgE molecules on the surface of eosinophils bind to target parasites, the eosinophil is capable of ADCC activity.

Comparison of Fc Receptor Structures   A comparison of the structures of the Fc receptors discussed above is seen in Fig. 3-9. Recent work has identified an IgA Fc receptor, but few details are available about the structure or function of this molecule. What is known is that it is similar to the Fc IgG receptor and the FcεRI α chain. The Fc α receptor is found on some eosinophils, where it may synergize with the IgE receptor in eosinophils resident in the gut and respiratory tracts, where secretory IgA is plentiful.

All of the Fc receptors except FcεII consist of immunoglobulin-related domains, so all of these molecules, as well as a large number of other immunologically crucial proteins, are members of what is called the *immunoglobulin superfamily.* (See Appendix B.)

Soluble Immunoglobulin Binding Proteins
In the serum and in supernatants of cultures of activated and/or cytokine-stimulated lymphocytes, one can find small amounts of soluble Fc receptors. FcγIII receptors can be proteolytically cleaved in the two external domains, to release the receptor. FcεII receptors (45-kd protein) are spontaneously cleaved from the cell surface, yielding an unstable 37-kd protein, which ultimately is modified to a 25-kd stable *immunoglobulin-binding factor (Ig-BF).* Alternative splicing of the FcγII receptor in its transmembrane exon yields a soluble form of this receptor. Ig-BF specific for IgA, IgD, and IgM have been reported, but no details are known.

The biologic functions of the well-studied Ig-BF molecules are not yet known. IgE-BF

has potent positive and negative effects on IgE synthesis, depending on the conditions of the experiment. It also may have effects on the maturation of T-cell precursors in the thymus (IgE-BF is made by thymic epithelial cells) and, in conjunction with IL-1, of granulocytes in the bone marrow. IgG-BF may have a regulatory role in immunoglobulin synthesis; recombinant soluble Fcγ receptors can suppress in vitro IgG production.

Finally, some microorganisms make proteins with functions similar to those of Fc receptors. Protein A of *Staphylococcus aureus* has already been mentioned, but others exist also. *Streptococcus* species make an IgG-binding factor, called protein G, and other isotypes may be bound by other factors. Cells infected with a number of DNA viruses, including herpes simplex, herpes zoster-varicella, and cytomegalovirus, express a virally encoded Fc receptor on their cell surfaces. Finally, a poorly characterized Fc receptor is found on the surface of schistosomula, which can bind IgG and β_2-microglobulin. These Fc receptor molecules can then bind host immunoglobulin as a means of avoiding the host immune response; this is discussed in more detail in Chap. 21, "Immunity to Microorganisms."

Host Defense
Antibodies are an integral part of the defense system of vertebrate animals. The binding of antigen by antibodies is the first essential and antigen-specific step involved in eliminating an antigen which may represent a potential noxious foreign substance. Thus, the purpose of antibodies is to effect the specific elimination or destruction of antigens, hopefully before any damage can be done to the host. IgA in respiratory and GI secretions serves this purpose. This biologic or effector function of antibodies varies with the class of antibodies and is mediated by specific functional sites on their Fc portion.

As noted in Clinical Aside 3-1, certain classes of immunoglobulin can activate another defense system, called *complement,* by activity mediated through the Fc portion.

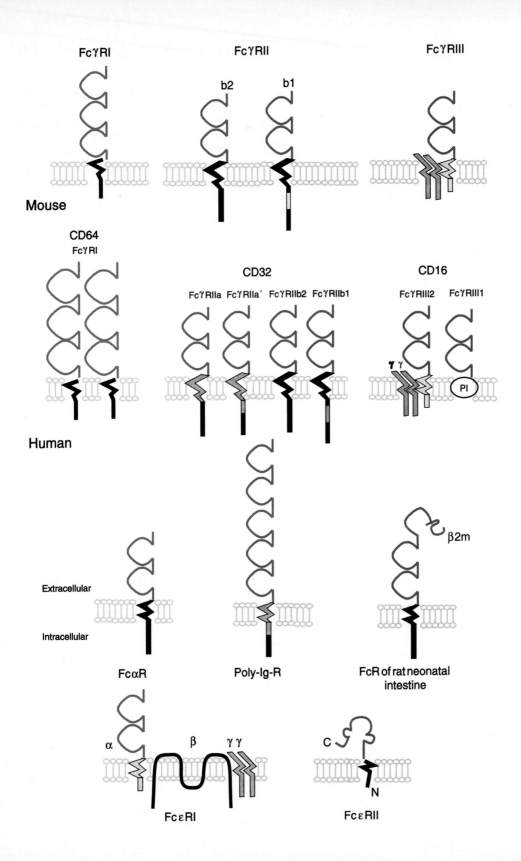

Cellular Immunity

Phagocytosis

This is an important first line of defense of the host against infectious microbes. Antibody, even in the absence of complement, can promote phagocytosis by macrophages and other phagocytic cells that have receptors for sites on the Fc portion of antibodies of a certain class. The addition of complement activation increases the ability of phagocytic cells to ingest the particle. This interaction between immunoglobulin and phagocytic cells is discussed in more detail in Chaps. 17 and 18, on polymorphonuclear cells and monocytes, respectively.

Antibody-Dependent Cell-Mediated Lysis

Antibody can sensitize target cells to lysis (killing) not only by activating the complement system but also by binding cells capable of killing the target; such antibody-dependent cytotoxicity (ADCC) has been discussed above. It is worth pointing out again that the spectrum of targets for these cells is defined by the specificity of the antibodies bound to the antigens of the target cell membrane.

IgE-Mediated Allergic Responses

Mast cells, and other such granulocytes, have receptors for sites on the Fc portion of the IgE class of antibodies and can bind such antibodies. The binding of these antibodies to the cells results in their becoming sensitized to the antigen (allergen) for which the antibody is specific. The reaction of allergen with IgE-sensitized mast cells results in degranulation, releasing vasoactive amines such as histamine, that have a profound pharmacologic effect on the vascular, contractile, and secretory systems. This is part of the allergic response. In a limited amount, these reactions are intended to benefit the host, but as is well known, severe allergic reactions of this kind can be distressful and potentially harmful. Allergic phenomena are discussed in Chap. 29, and the basophils, mast cells, and eosinophils which mediate some of these effects are discussed in Chap. 19.

T and B Lymphocytes

Certain subsets of these cells have receptors for sites on the Fc portion of antibodies that are class-specific. Antigen bound to circulating antibody can therefore be made to bind to these cells through Fc-specific receptors in addition to their direct binding to antigen-specific T-cell receptors and the transmembrane antibody on B cells. Presumably the binding of antigen, in the form of antigen-antibody complexes, to Fc-specific receptors on T and B cells provides an alternative pathway to the activation and function of the regulatory T cells and antibody-producing B cells.

SELF-TEST QUESTIONS*

Match the immunoglobulin with the correct description.

1. IgG   a. Primarily found on the surface of B cells

2. IgA   b. Active principle in allergic phenomena due to binding in Fc Rs on mast cells and basophils

3. IgM   c. Predominant serum immunoglobulin

*Answers will be found in Appendix E.

Figure 3-9 Structure of Fc receptors for IgG, IgA, and IgE. Each consists of 2, 3, or 4 extracellular domains (these are all members of the immunoglobulin superfamily) plus a transmembrane region (in all but FcγRIII1) and a cytoplasmic tail (lacking in FcγRIII1). (*From Fridman, The FASEB Journal, vol 5, Sept 1991, with permission.*)

4. IgE   d. First immunoglobulin made in the response to a new antigen
5. IgD   e. Primary antibody in the secretions on mucosal surfaces

Match the terms in 6, 7 and 8 with the correct description.
6. Isotype   a. Defined by unique features at or near the antigen-binding site
7. Allotype   b. Defined by antigenic determinants on the heavy chain
8. Idiotype   c. Defined by inherited differences between individuals at loci in the heavy chain

9. Differences between the primary and secondary immunoglobulin responses include all of the following *except*:
   a. In the secondary response, the lag or latent period is shorter.
   b. In the secondary response, the exponential phase rise in antibody levels is steeper.
   c. In the secondary response, there is more IgG than IgM produced.
   d. In the secondary response, the mean affinity of the antibody produced is higher because fewer B cells are involved.
10. The Fc segment:
    a. Binds to cell surface receptors
    b. Is where complement is bound and activated
    c. Consists of two or three (depending on the type of heavy chain) domains
    d. Contributes to the antigen-binding site of the antibody
    e. Is the part of the IgG bound by rheumatoid factor
11. The Fab segment:
    a. Has a structure consisting of components of both the heavy and light chains
    b. Contains within it the antigen-binding site and idiotypic determinants

c. Consists of CDR and FR segments in its variable region
d. Is capable of cross-linking two bound epitopes
e. Consists of hypervariable regions contributing to the antigen-binding site.

True or False
12. The effector or biologic function of antibody is mediated through the Fc fragment.
13. IgG is the predominant serum opsonin.
14. IgG and IgA are capable of activating complement by means of classic pathway; IgM activates complement through the alternate pathway.

ADDITIONAL READINGS

Alt FW, Blackwell TK, Yancopoulos GD. Development of the primary antibody repertoire. *Science.* 1987;238:1079–1087.

Apodaca G, Bomsel M, Arden J, Breitfeld PP, Tang K, Mostov KE. The polymeric immunoglobulin receptor: A model protein to study transcytosis. *J Clin Invest.* 1991;87:1877–1882.

Berzofsky JA, Berkow IJ. Immunogenicity and antigen structure. In: Paul WE, ed. *Fundamental Immunology.* 2nd ed. New York: Raven Press; 1989.

Conrad DH. Fc epsilon II/CD23: The low affinity receptor for IgE. *Annu Rev Immunol.* 1990;8:623–646.

Hasemann CA, Capra JD. Immunoglobulins: Structure and function. In: Paul WE, ed. *Fundamental Immunology.* 2nd ed. New York: Raven Press; 1989.

Ravetch JV, Kinet J-P. Fc receptors. *Annu Rev Immunol.* 1991;9:457–492.

Unkeless JC, Scigliano E, Freedman V. Structure and function of human and murine receptors for IgG. *Annu Rev Immunol.* 1988;6:251–282.

Williams AF, Barclay AN. The immunoglobulin superfamily—Domains for cell surface recognition. *Annu Rev Immunol.* 1988;5:381–405.

4

The Major Histocompatibility Complex

INTRODUCTION

The major histocompatibility complex (MHC) is one of the cornerstones of modern immunology, and the molecules of the MHC are central to the initiation of immune responses. The study of the MHC can be traced from its humble beginnings in tumor graft rejection studies, followed by research on graft rejection, through the genetics of immune responsiveness and the communication between lymphocytes. We now understand the role of the MHC molecules in T-cell activation, and this understanding has helped to shape a unified view of immune function.

In this chapter, we discuss the genes and molecules of the MHC and introduce the concepts that led eventually to our understanding of the role of the MHC in immunity. The view we have at the present time was produced by the merging of seemingly unrelated ideas and discoveries that represent a continuum of scientific thought. We'll try to recreate this continuum and the modern view, but a full appreciation of the importance of the MHC in the function of the immune system will only emerge in later chapters of this book.

THE DISCOVERY OF THE MHC

It was observed early in this century that experimental tumors could be propagated in mice only if the animals were genetically identical, and geneticists began to develop such strains. A genetic theory of tumor susceptibility emerged based on the observation that a given strain was either susceptible or resistant to the growth of a given tumor. It was reasonable to assume that the genes responsible for resistance to a tumor might encode structures important for immune responses to the tumor. In essence this assumption turned out to be right, if for the wrong reasons.

In 1933, the great geneticist J. B. S. Haldane suggested the idea that rejection in one mouse strain of a tumor from another mouse strain might be due to a response against normal tissue molecules on the surface of the cells, rather than something unique to the tumor. In testing this idea, Peter Gorer in England identified cellular antigens (cell surface molecules identified by specific antibodies) that correlated with the growth or rejection of a tumor. These antigens were found to be present on all of the tissues of mice of the same strain as that of the tumor. This led Gorer to formulate the concept of immunogenetic control of tissue transplantation.

During this time, George Snell joined the geneticist C. C. Little at the Jackson Laboratory in Bar Harbor, Maine. Taking advantage of the inbred strains of mice available at Jackson, Snell initiated a study of the formal genetics of the molecules responsible for tissue rejection. These were the *histocompatibility molecules*, and Snell called the genes that encode them the *histocompatibility genes*. Using classical genetic techniques, he bred mice that differ only in the histocompatibility genes.

THE MHC AND GRAFT REJECTION

As discussed, the original justification for studying the MHC was its role in graft rejection, and of course, this would still be sufficient reason for thorough investigation of this gene complex. As we'll see, however, the importance of the MHC in understanding the immune system goes far beyond this clinical application.

In all chordates (the phylum that includes the vertebrates) a single gene complex is primarily responsible for rapid graft rejection. Among all the vertebrates, the "rules" of graft rejection are the same, and where studied (amphibians, reptiles, birds, and mammals) the MHC is phylogenetically related. In every case, if two individuals differ at the MHC, then grafts from one will be rapidly rejected by the other. It must be noted, however, that the genes of the MHC are not the *only* genes that affect the acceptance or rejection of a graft: differences in other genes can also induce graft rejection, albeit more slowly than the genes of the MHC. These are collectively referred to as *minor histocompatibility molecules.* We now understand something of the nature of these molecules and their relationship to the MHC, a point to which we will return. For now, however, it is important to note only that the rules of vertebrate graft acceptance and rejection apply to both major and minor histocompatibility genes.

In any outbred population, the chances of finding two unrelated individuals that can exchange grafts (even if we consider only rapid rejection) are small. Below, we consider how these odds can be improved. As noted above, however, the study of histocompatibility was greatly aided by the use of genetically homozygous animals, such as inbred mice, and using such animals some rules for histocompatibility phenomena were discovered. These rules of histocompatibility are as follows:

1. Genetically identical individuals accept grafts from one another.
2. The progeny of two genetically different but genetically homozygous parents (e.g., two different strains of inbred mice) will accept grafts from either parent.
3. The parents of these progeny (in 2) will not accept grafts from the offspring.

These rules are easy to understand if we think of the MHC as a single mendelian locus with many alleles (MHC^a, MHC^b, MHC^c, etc.). The progeny of two MHC homozygous parents with different MHC alleles carry both of the parental alleles (e.g., MHC$^{a/b}$). If we consider A$\Rightarrow$B to mean that "B accepts a graft from A" and A$\not\Rightarrow$B to mean that "B rejects a graft from A," then the rules of histocompatibility become:

1. MHC$^a\Rightarrow$MHC^a
2. MHC$^a\Rightarrow$MHC$^{a/b}$
3. MHC$^{a/b}\not\Rightarrow$MHC^a

Thus, we can see that a graft will be rejected if it carries any MHC genes (and therefore molecules) that are foreign to the host.

BASIC PROPERTIES OF THE MHC

From the studies that led to these rules, several important features of the MHC became apparent. First of all, the MHC genes are *co-dominantly expressed*; i.e., the MHC genes from *both* parents are expressed in the offspring. Second, it was quickly recognized that there are several tightly linked genes in the MHC, encoding different MHC molecules. In other words, the MHC is *multigenic*. Third, each gene has many alleles in the population; i.e., the MHC is *highly polymorphic*.

For convenience, we refer to the total set of alleles for all of the MHC genes along one chromosome as the *MHC haplotype*. In describing the MHC of a human, however, one generally must describe each allele for each MHC gene (usually two per gene, one from each parent), unless one is comparing closely related individuals. This description is important for the clinical matching of tissues for organ transplantation, considered in more detail below.

The genes of the MHC are related to the genes encoding immunoglobulins and T-cell receptors (i.e., the MHC genes are members of the immunoglobulin supergene family; see also Appendix B, "The Phylogeny of the Human Immune System"). Although the genes are polymorphic from one individual to another, they are *not* variable within an individual. Unlike the genes encoding immunoglobulins and T-cell receptors (TCRs), the genes of the MHC complex do not rearrange during development.

Of course, one functional property of the MHC is the control of graft rejection. While this is of obvious clinical importance, it is

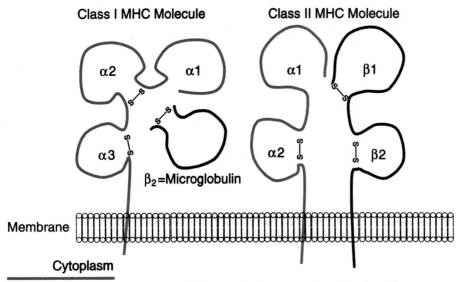

Figure 4-1. Cartoon structure of class I and class II MHC molecules. The class I molecule is shown associated with β_2-microglobulin, which is not encoded by the MHC. Also shown are the domains defined by intrachain disulfide bonds. While these models are useful for understanding the basic chain structure of MHC molecules, they are also inaccurate. A more accurate representation, based on x-ray crystal structure, is seen in Fig. 4-2.

equally obvious that the MHC did not evolve to ensure that individuals could not exchange tissues.*

DISTRIBUTION AND FUNCTION OF MHC MOLECULES

From the point of view of immunology, there are two basic classes of MHC molecules. *Class I MHC* molecules are composed of a poly-

---

*Maybe we should not be too glib in making this assertion. Most theories of the evolution of the MHC proposed before 1980 (and many proposed since then) suggest that the original function of the MHC controlled fusion and rejection reactions in colonial invertebrates. Until something is known about the genes controlling such reactions, and their relationship to vertebrate MHC genes, the validity of these theories is unknown. As we'll see, however, the MHC performs a critically important function other than that of controlling graft rejection, and it is considered likely that the genes of this complex evolved for this second function.

morphic α chain of approximately Mr 45 kd that noncovalently pairs with a nonpolymorphic molecule, called β_2-microglobulin (approximately Mr 12 kd), which is encoded outside of the MHC (see Fig. 4-1). Three regions of the molecule containing intrachain disulfide bonds are designated as domains, with the α1 domain being the furthest from the transmembrane region. The class I MHC molecules are expressed on the surface of nearly every nucleated cell in the mammalian body, although the level of expression is variable. As described later in the book, the class I MHC molecules are involved in presentation of antigenic peptides to CD8[+] T cells. For example, CD8[+] cytotoxic T cells kill their target cells following specific recognition of both a particular class I MHC molecule and its associated peptide. In addition, expression of class I MHC molecules in the thymus is required for the maturation of CD8[+] T cells.

In humans, there are three different polymorphic class I MHC molecules, called HLA-A, HLA-B, and HLA-C. In mice, the three different polymorphic class I MHC molecules are called H-2K, H-2L, and H-2D. All of these molecules are important for presentation of antigenic peptides to CD8$^+$ T cells, as mentioned above. Other, nonpolymorphic (or less polymorphic) class I MHC molecules exist in both mice and humans (although mice have many more of them); however, their function is not known. A summary of the class I molecules is given in Table 4-1.

Class II MHC molecules are each composed of two polymorphic chains, α and β of Mr 25 to 33 kd and 24 to 29 kd, respectively, both of which are encoded within the MHC (see Fig. 4-1). As with class I MHC, domains containing intrachain disulfide bonds have been designated (there are two such domains

on each chain). There is also a third, non-polymorphic chain, called the *invariant chain* (Mr 31 kd), which is involved in the transport and assembly of the class II MHC molecule with antigenic peptides. (The association of antigenic peptides with MHC molecules is discussed later in this chapter and in other chapters.) Unlike class I MHC molecules, class II MHC molecules are found only on some cells of the body. For example, macrophages and monocytes, B cells, activated T cells (in humans), dendritic cells, Langerhans cells of the skin, and some epithelial cells express class II MHC molecules, and expression is occasionally induced after exposure to certain cytokines. As discussed later in the book, class II MHC molecules are

TABLE 4-1   Some of the Alleles of the Class I and Class II HLA Loci

A	B	C	DR	DQ	DP
A1 (17.4)*	B7 (12.2)	Cw1 (2.2)	DR1 (9.5)	DQw1 (32.3)	DPw1 (4.3)
A2 (27.1)	B8 (11.9)	Cw2 (2.2)	DR2 (15.8)	DQw2 (18.1)	DPw2 (11.5)
A3 (15.5)	B13 (2.2)	Cw3 (15.1)	DR3 (12)	DQw3 (23.3)	DPw3 (4)
A11 (3.0)	B18 (6.1)	Cw4 (7.5)	DR4 (12.7)	? (26.3)	DPw4 (41.8)
A23 (4.1)	B27 (2.8)	Cw5 (7.3)	DR7 (12)		DPw5 (4.4)
A24 (10.5)	B35 (8.0)	Cw6 (7.9)	DRw8 (3)		? (40)
A25 (2.2)	B37 (1.1)	Cw7 (30.4)	DRw9 (0.8)		
A26 (2.8)	B38 (3.3)	Cw8 (5.5)	DRw10 (0.8)		
A28 (5.5)	B39 (2.8)		DRw11 (12.3)		
A29 (2.8)	B44 (13.3)		DRw12 (2)		
A30 (3.0)	B45 (0.3)		DRw13 (5.4)		
A31 (3.9)	B49 (0.8)		DRw14 (5.8)		
A32 (2.8)	B51 (4.2)		? (7.9)		
Aw33 (1.1)†	Bw31 (0.8)				
? (0.3)‡	Bw42 (0.8)				
	Bw50 (0.6)				
	Bw52 (1.4)				
	Bw53 (0.3)				
	Bw54 (0.3)				
	Bw55 (0.6)				
	Bw57 (3.3)				
	Bw58 (1.4)				
	Bw60 (5.5)				
	Bw61 (1.1)				
	Bw62 (7.8)				
	Bw63 (1.1)				
	Bw64 (1.4)				
	Bw65 (4.2)				
	? (0.6)				

*The numbers in parentheses indicate the percentage of individuals bearing that allele in a caucasoid population.
†A "w" in the designation indicates that the allele is a workshop allele, that is, that it is not confirmed as a true allele for that locus.
‡A "?" indicates unknown or uncharacterized alleles.

TABLE 4-2   Proteins Encoded in the Class III MHC

C2*
B*
C4A*
21-hydroxylase A†
C4*
21-hydroxylase B†

*Complement components.
†Gene for cytochrome p450 21-hydroxylase enzyme.

essential for presentation of antigenic peptides to CD4$^+$ T cells, such as helper T cells, and for this reason cells that bear class II MHC (and are capable of presenting antigen to such T cells) are collectively referred to as *antigen-presenting cells* (APCs). In addition, expression of class II MHC molecules in the thymus is required for the maturation of CD4$^+$ T cells.

In humans, there are three different polymorphic class II MHC molecules, called HLA-DR, HLA-DQ, and HLA-DP. In mice, there are two different polymorphic class II MHC molecules, called I-A and I-E. A summary of the class II molecules is given in Table 4-1.

Other molecules are encoded within the MHC, and these perform different functions than those of class I and class II MHC molecules. A region of the MHC called S in mice (a similar region appears in humans) is referred to as *class III MHC* and encodes a number of proteins involved in the complement pathways (Table 4-2). In addition, the genes for two cytokines, tumor necrosis factors (TNFs) α and β, are found within the MHC of rodents and humans. Other genes found within the MHC include those encoding some of the molecules probably involved in the assembly and transport of MHC molecules within the cell.

The Structure of MHC Molecules

The sketches shown in Fig. 4-1, while informative, do not reflect the actual structure of the MHC molecules. The actual structure of class I MHC molecules was determined in 1987 by Pamela Bjorkman and Donald Wiley

using x-ray crystallographic analysis. The analysis was performed on a purified molecule lacking the transmembrane and cytoplasmic regions of the protein, and the resulting structure is shown in Fig. 4-2. Note especially that the region furthest from the cell surface (the α1 and α2 domains) is in the form of a groove, bounded by two α helices on the sides and a β-pleated sheet on the bottom. This groove has been strongly implicated as the site in which processed an-

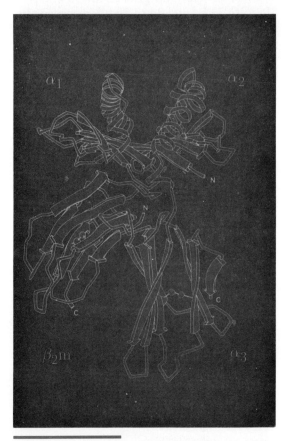

Figure 4-2.   Structure of a human class I MHC molecule. This model, based on the x-ray crystal structure of the HLA-A2 molecule, shows the antigen peptide-binding "groove" (on the top part of the figure). The part of the molecule that penetrates the cell membrane (the transmembrane region) was removed during preparation of the molecule, but would normally be found at the bottom part of the figure. (From Bjorkman, et al. *Nature.* 1987;329:506, with permission.)

tigenic peptides sit for presentation to the T-cell receptor. This and other views of the groove will appear again in this book as antigen presentation is discussed in more detail.

The structure of class II MHC molecules has not yet been determined. A model of class II MHC structure has been proposed, based on the structure of class I MHC. In this model, the α1 domain of the class II molecule takes the place of the α1 domain of the class I molecule, while the β1 domain of class II takes the place of the α2 domain of class I. Again, the model proposes a groove similar to that of class I MHC, in which antigenic peptides bind.

MHC GENES AND ASSOCIATED TRAITS

The genes encoding class I and class II (and class III) MHC molecules are found within subregions of the MHC. We will consider only the MHC of mice and humans, and the physical maps of these MHCs are shown in Fig. 4-3. The murine MHC, H-2, is found on chromosome 17 of the mouse, while the human MHC, HLA, is found on chromosome 6. H-2 is divided into the subregions, K, I, S—which encode class I, class II, and class III molecules, respectively—and D, Qa, and Tla, all three of which encode class I molecules. The maps include some genes we have not discussed, but the reader should focus on those we have considered (see Table 4-1). Three points should immediately be apparent: (1) the MHC is large, encompassing approximately 3500 kilobases (kb) in humans and 2500 kb in mice, (2) the organization of related MHC genes is different in rodents and humans, and (3) there are more genes than we expected from a consideration of MHC molecules. The implications of the latter point are not currently clear.

Long before the precise role of the MHC gene products in immune recognition was determined (discussed later in this chapter), the MHC was known to be important in the function of the immune system. In addition

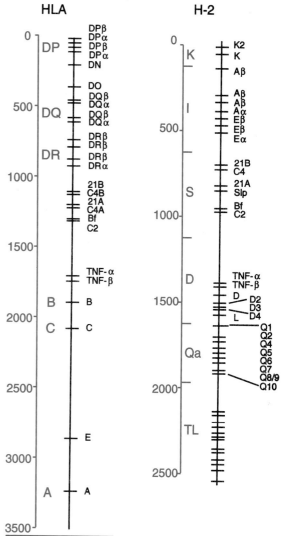

Figure 4-3. Genetic maps of the MHC in humans and mice. Genetics maps for HLA (human) and H-2 (mouse) are shown. Also included are genes found within the complex that do not encode histocompatibility molecules. The figures appearing to the left of each linear map denote the distance in kilobases.

to the studies implicating the MHC in graft rejection, specific MHC alleles were found to associate with certain diseases, most of which are clearly immunologic in nature. This association can be quantified and expressed as *relative risk*. To determine relative risk, a group of patients with a particular disease and a group of control individuals are typed for their MHC haplotypes (methods of typing are discussed below). The relative risk of acquiring the disease for individuals carrying a particular MHC allele is determined by the formula

$$\text{Relative risk} = \frac{(\text{number of patients with marker})\ (\text{number of controls without marker})}{(\text{number of patients without marker})(\text{number of controls with marker})}$$

Some examples of relative risks associated with some MHC alleles for different diseases are given in Table 4-3. A relative risk of 1 indicates that there is no increased risk of acquiring the disease which is associated with the allele. Increasing values indicate an increasing risk (if everyone with a particular allele got the disease, then the relative risk would be infinite). Most of the diseases listed in the table are known to be autoimmune in nature, and despite all that is known about the MHC and immune function, the precise reasons for these associations are not understood. It is similarly unclear why there is a general lack of association with infectious disease. Nevertheless, there is little doubt that the associations between MHC alleles and immunologic diseases are somehow a consequence of antigen fragments bound to the responsible MHC molecules (see below).

Because the MHC is large, it is not surprising that genetic recombination occurs between individual loci. This recombination, however, is not strictly random. Rodent studies have demonstrated that some recombination "hot spots," regions displaying increased recombination, exist (especially in the class II region), and studies on humans show that some MHC alleles are found to be linked with others at unexpectedly high frequencies. The latter effect is called *linkage disequilibrium*. Because of linkage disequilibrium, traits that have been attributed to a particular MHC allele may, in fact, be caused by another gene in the MHC. Thus, the relative risks given in Table 4-2 do not *necessarily* indicate that the allele directly contributes to the disease. It may, instead, indicate that another gene (for example, another MHC gene) which is in linkage disequilibrium with the allele in question is actually the major contributor to the risk of disease. For example, originally some autoimmune diseases, like Sjögrens syndrome, were thought to be linked to HLA-B8, but the primary linkage was with HLA-DR3— B8 and DR3 are "linked" to each other.

Another trait associated with MHC alleles, that of *immune response defects*, was extremely important for the elucidation of the actual function of the MHC molecules. The ability to make an immune response to

TABLE 4-3   Some Associations between HLA-DR Alleles and Autoimmune Diseases

Disease	HLA Allele	Relative Risk*
Celiac disease	DR3	10.8–54.0
Diabetes (type I)	DR3	2.9–15.3
	DR4	3.1–14.2
Goodpasture's syndrome	DR2	13.1–15.9
Grave's disease	DR3	3.3–5.5
Addison's disease	DR3	6
Juvenile rheumatoid arthritis	DR5	5.2–7.0
Multiple sclerosis	DR2	4.1–4.8
Myasthenia gravis	DR3	2.5
Pernicious anemia	DR5	5.4
	DR2	2.0–3.7
Systemic lupus erythematosus	DR3	6
Rheumatoid arthritis	DR4	2.8–13.4
Sjögren's syndrome	DR3	10
Ulcerative colitis	DR2	5.1

*Relative risk, defined in the text, may differ depending upon the reagents used in HLA typing, the definition of the autoimmune disease, and the population studied. Note that a significant relative risk of greater than 1 does not necessarily mean that the allele causes the disease; linkage disequilibrium (see text) may result in a high relative risk due to a linked allele. Alleles at other HLA loci may also be associated with autoimmune diseases (one example is the very high relative risk for ankylosing spondylitis, 87.4, associated with the B27 allele).
Source: Stastny et al. *Immunol Rev* 1982;70:113; and Svejgaard et al. *Immunol Rev* 1982;70:193.

certain antigens in mice was found to map to the class II region of the MHC. This is usually caused by a combination of effects resulting from: (1) the requirement that antigenic peptides be presented to T cells in the peptide-binding groove of an MHC molecule, and (2) preferential binding of certain peptides by different MHC molecules. Thus, one allelic form of a class II molecule may bind a particular antigenic peptide much more readily than another class II molecule, and therefore present the peptide much more efficiently. This greatly influences the response of T cells and, in turn, the immune response.

THE TCR LIGAND: A UNIFYING HYPOTHESIS

By now it should be clear that the functions we have ascribed to class I and class II MHC molecules are a consequence of the role of these molecules in antigen presentation. That is, the presentation to T cells of antigenic peptides by class I and class II MHC molecules is a major influence controlling the induction of immune responses. Because the combination of an antigenic peptide and a particular MHC molecule forms the ligand for a particular TCR, the concentration of the ligand determines whether the T cell will be triggered. And since the association of a particular peptide with different MHC molecules can vary a great deal, the "choice" of a particular peptide by the available MHC molecules restricts immune recognition (by T cells) to only a few sites on an antigen.*

Thus, it is easy to see why the MHC genes are associated with immune response defects. If there are only a few different MHC molecules available (remember that inbred mice are homozygous), then for some anti-

gens in some inbred strains of mice, the association of the MHC molecules with the antigen peptides may be too weak to generate more than a low response.† Similarly, the association between MHC alleles and autoimmune disease, while not well understood, is very likely to be due to the ability of antigenic peptides (from "self" antigens?) associated with certain MHC molecules to stimulate the T cells responsible for the disease.

The first function ascribed to MHC, that of graft acceptance or rejection, is not so easily understood in terms of our unifying hypothesis. Recent studies have shown that the response of T cells to allogeneic MHC molecules is caused by each responding T cell recognizing a combination of a foreign MHC molecule together with a peptide that appears to be derived from normal tissue (i.e., a "self" antigen). Because the antigen is associated with a "foreign" MHC molecule, the resulting ligand does not resemble self and the T cells respond. Further, a T cell that normally responds to a foreign antigenic peptide presented by a particular self MHC molecule is likely to cross-react to some foreign MHC molecule (together with an associated peptide). This cross-reaction is probably responsible for the phenomenon of the mixed lymphocyte response (see below), graft rejection, and other effects of exposing the immune system to foreign MHC molecules.

Notice that our unifying hypothesis also explains the phenomenon of minor histocompatibility loci and molecules. That is, allelic differences that result in different self peptides associated with the same MHC molecule will effectively act as minor histocompatibility loci. This is because the allelic difference in the graft has produced a new ligand that can be recognized by host T cells as foreign, even though the MHC mol-

---

*The binding of an antigenic peptide to a particular MHC molecule is not specific in the sense that antigen-antibody interactions are specific. Instead, the binding affinities for different peptides and different MHC molecules can vary extensively. *Don't* get trapped into thinking that MHC genes rearrange to generate diversity (because they don't).

†This explanation of immune response defects is called "determinant selection" based on the idea that choice of peptides (i.e., antigenic determinants) by MHC molecules is responsible. Other explanations for immune response defects might be correct for some antigens, but the majority of immune response phenomena are best explained by determinant selection.

ecules on the graft and in the host are the same. Thus, a gene or molecule that represents a minor histocompatibility difference may normally have a very different function; its role in histocompatibility is an "accidental" consequence of its polymorphism in the regions of the molecule that end up as antigenic peptides bound to MHC molecules.

Why does the TCR recognize such a complex ligand? The teleologic answer to this question is this: The recognition of a ligand composed of an antigenic peptide and a cell surface molecule (MHC) ensures that the T cell will only respond when it is in contact with another cell (e.g., an APC). When a helper T cell is triggered, it releases factors (lymphokines) that act at short range, and hence, preferentially stimulate the APC (e.g., the macrophage or B cell). Alternatively, if a cytotoxic T cell is triggered, it releases cytotoxic molecules that act at short range, and hence, preferentially kill the target cell. *It is the complex nature of the ligand for the TCR that dictates cellular interactions in the immune system.*

THE IDENTIFICATION OF MHC ALLELES

At present, the predominant clinical reason for wishing to ascertain an individual's MHC allelic profile is to determine the suitability of the individual as a graft donor or recipient (see also Chap. 26, "Transplantation Immunology"). Other possible reasons include identification of at-risk individuals in families with autoimmune disease, and even determination of paternity. From the outset, it is important to distinguish between tissue typing and tissue matching. *Tissue typing* refers to the identification of each allele at each locus of the MHC, and most of our discussion will focus on this. *Tissue matching,* on the other hand, is concerned mainly with determining whether the tissue of a donor is likely to be accepted (i.e., not rejected) by the recipient. This is done by simply mixing peripheral blood mononuclear cells from each and culturing for several days. If there is a

significant cell proliferation (determined by the incorporation of tritiated thymidine), i.e., a *mixed lymphocyte response,* the tissues are not matched.

Tissue typing is performed using different techniques employing either antibodies or molecular probes. Antibody techniques continue to be the most common, and will therefore be considered first.

Antibody-Based Methods

Antibody-based methods depend upon the use of antibodies directed to determinants on the MHC molecules that distinguish the product of one allele from another. Some of these determinants are present on several different molecules, and these are called *public specificities,* others are relatively unique to an individual MHC molcecule and are therefore called *private specificities.* By using a panel of the most specific antibodies available, a fairly accurate profile of the MHC molecules expressed on the cells of one individual can be generated. The reader should keep in mind, however, that apparently identical MHC molecules (as determined by antibody reactivity) from two unrelated individuals may have minor differences, and these differences might have major consequences.

Antibodies that are specific for MHC molecules are derived from two sources. One is sera from patients that have received multiple blood transfusions or from multiparous mothers. The second source is rodent (usually mouse) monoclonal antibodies. As more monoclonal antibodies become available, antibody-based typing systems show greater reliability.

In principle, any technique that detects the binding of antibodies to cells could be used in MHC typing; one commonly employed method is illustrated in Fig. 4-4. Cells from the individual to be typed are placed into small wells, each of which contains an antibody to a different MHC allele (this is repeated for each locus). After a period of incubation during which the appropriate antibody binds to the cells, the antibody is removed and a source of complement is added.

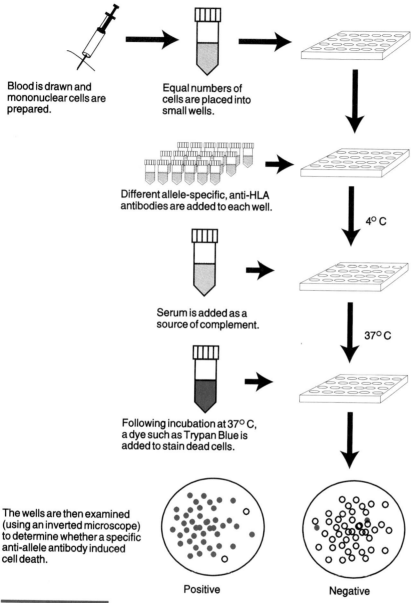

Blood is drawn and mononuclear cells are prepared.

Equal numbers of cells are placed into small wells.

Different allele-specific, anti-HLA antibodies are added to each well.

4° C

Serum is added as a source of complement.

37° C

Following incubation at 37° C, a dye such as Trypan Blue is added to stain dead cells.

The wells are then examined (using an inverted microscope) to determine whether a specific anti-allele antibody induced cell death.

Positive   Negative

Figure 4-4.   A commonly employed method for tissue typing. Peripheral blood mononuclear cells are reacted with antibodies that are known to react with defined public and private specificities. The cells are then reacted with serum that contains complement, a collection of proteins that react in an enzymatic cascade in the presence of antigen-antibody complexes. The result of the cascade is death of cells coated with antibody. This is observed by treating with dyes that stain dead but not live cells. A high proportion of stained cells indicates that the antibody reacted, i.e., that the cells bear the given determinant. By comparing the effect of a panel of antibodies, the MHC alleles expressed in the cells can be approximately determined.

The complement pathway is triggered by the presence of bound antibody, and the cells in those wells containing the appropriate antibody are killed. A dye which is actively excluded by living cells, such as Trypan blue, is then added and stains only dead cells. The wells can then be scanned quickly under a microscope for those containing mostly dead cells, indicating that the well contained antibodies that bound to the cells.

Molecular Techniques

While antibody-based assays are routine, new typing systems are currently being developed that depend upon molecular techniques. For example, DNA from the individual to be typed is treated with restriction endonucleases (yielding short pieces of DNA, or restriction fragments), electrophoresed, and blotted onto nitrocellulose. This Southern blot is then probed with labeled cDNA corresponding to different MHC genes. The positions of the various restriction fragments are then correlated with particular alleles. This method of MHC typing by *restriction fragment length polymorphism* is still being refined, but may eventually be sufficiently developed to become routine. Other methods, based on defining unique stretches of DNA corresponding to particular alleles and then identifying them by amplification with the polymerase chain reaction, are currently being developed and examined, and have the potential of surpassing the other techniques in terms of accuracy and ease.

CONCLUSION

In this chapter we have touched on a number of properties of the MHC, especially as it relates to the immune system. The central message, the key to the role of the MHC in immunity, is that an MHC molecule that is associated with an antigen peptide forms the ligand for a TCR, and it is this receptor-ligand interaction that dictates the cellular interactions that result in specific immune responses. How these interactions occur and the consequences they have are the subjects of other chapters.

SELF-TEST QUESTIONS

1. A medical scientist working with a cell line derived from a malignant tumor is accidentally exposed to the cells through an open wound. Since the original tumor was removed from her own son her colleagues are afraid that the cells will grow in her, while she remains unconcerned. Who is most likely to be right? Why?

2. During bone marrow transplantation procedures the recipient is often irradiated, which has the effect of destroying the recipient's immune system. Bone marrow cells from a donor are administered, and can under some circumstances produce a graft-versus-host disease, in which lymphocytes in the donor bone marrow react with host MHC molecules. Models of this disease are easily produced in mice for study of possible therapies. Using the homozygous parental strains A and B and their (A × B) F_1 progeny, explain why F_1 cells will not produce disease in parental recipients, while parental donor cells can produce disease in F_1 recipients, and why a (human) child's bone marrow can induce graft-versus-host disease in the child's recipient father?

3. Resting human T cells do not express class II MHC molecules, but activated T cells do. In most people, how many different MHC molecules will be found on one resting T cell? How many on an activated T cell? (Consider only the well-defined class I and class II MHC molecules.)

4. In the course of a fictitious study on narcolepsy, an investigator examined whether the individuals expressed any of three HLA molecules: DR2, DR7, and DQw1:

	DR2	DR7	DQw1
Narcoleptics	16/17	2/17	6/17
Normal	4/32	2/32	3/32

Based on these data, what are the relative risks for narcolepsy associated with each HLA allele? Which, if any, of these alleles can be said to be associated with narcolepsy? If you had a patient who appeared normal, but carried any of these alleles, would you order neurologic testing for narcolepsy based on these results? Why or why not?

5. The tissue typing facility provides you with the following data on two potential donors and your organ graft recipient, all siblings (any missing data is due to unavailability of reagents for typing):

Recipient: A2, A23, B4, B16, C2, DR3, DR6, DQw2

Donor 1: A4, A23, B4, B13, C2, DR4, DR6, DQw2

Donor 2: A2, A26, B5, B13, C2, DR3, DR7, DQ2

Mixed lymphocyte responses:
  Recipient alone: 2000 cpm
  Recipient + control stimulators (irradiated, pooled cells from multiple individuals): 120,000 cpm
  Recipient + Donor 1 (irradiated cells): 72,000 cpm
  Recipient + Donor 2 (irradiated cells): 6000 cpm

Which of the donors is the best choice based on these results? Why?

5

Generation of Diversity in the Acquired Immune Response

INTRODUCTION

The human organism confronts an unremitting and boundless assault from environmental pathogens and irritants with a varied and measured response. An encounter with protozoa, fungi, mycoplasma, bacteria, viruses, environmental allergens, parasites, vaccines, organ grafts, and even tumors elicits an immune reaction. The immune system must anticipate the potential arrival of a noxious substance or an organism without advance knowledge of the intruder. The challenge is met by the immune system with an enormous number of unique antigen receptors—T-cell receptors (TCR) expressed by T cells and immunoglobulins (Ig) expressed and secreted by B cells.

Each naive (never exposed to antigen) T and B cell displays on its surface an antigen receptor of predetermined specificity. A finite number of naive T and B cells are available in the organism to provide a primary response to a foreign antigen. T or B cells which express antigen receptors with higher affinity for a challenging antigen are selectively expanded and terminally differentiated. At the same time, some cells are triggered into the pathway of memory cell generation which provides the basis for a much more rapid and potent response upon reexposure to the same antigen.

The structures of the TCR and Ig have much in common (Fig. 5-1). Both are composed of two different polypeptides joined through disulfide linkages. The basic struc-

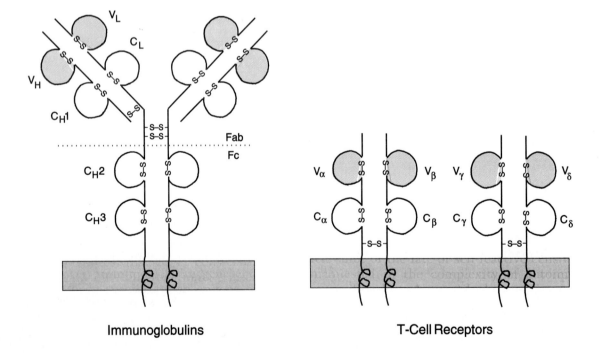

Immunoglobulins   T-Cell Receptors

Figure 5-1   Schematic representation of the immunoglobulins and the two types of T-cell receptors. The V-domain sequences (shaded) vary among different clones of lymphocytes.

ture of the Ig is a tetramer; two identical heavy chains (IgH) are joined by disulfide bonds and to each is linked, through a disulfide bond, one of two identical light chains (IgL). TCR are heterodimers. The polypeptides of both TCR and Ig are organized into domains; each domain contains a loop of about 65 amino acids formed by an internal disulfide linkage. This basic structural unit is typical of a large number of molecules collectively described as the immunoglobulin superfamily. They are thought to have a common evolutionary ancestry (see Appendix A).

IgH chains contain one variable (V) domain and three or four constant (C) domains; IgL chains contain a single V domain in addition to a single C domain. TCR polypeptides resemble the IgL chains, containing a single V and C domain. The specificity of both Ig and TCR is determined by the V domain at the amino terminus of the molecule. The V domain, as the name implies, includes regions of distinct amino acid sequences that are unique for each lymphocyte clone. The V domains of IgH and IgL, or of the TCR subunits, form the antigen-binding site, which are able to discriminate among antigens with extremely fine specificity.

Each B or T cell expresses only one antigen receptor. There is one copy of each gene on each of the two homologous chromosomes. Only one of the gene alleles for each polypeptide of the antigen receptor produces a functional protein. This phenomenon is called *allelic exclusion,* a process that permits the expression of a single antigen specificity per cell. It has been suggested that the polypeptide produced as a result of a productive rearrangement regulates the succeeding rearrangements. Thus, once an IgH μ is synthesized in a cell, further rearrangements of the IgH V domain coding gene segments are prevented in that cell.

There are two types of TCR. Each T cell expresses only one type of TCR. Both types of TCR are associated with the CD3 complex which is involved in signal transduction into the T cell after the engagement of the TCR with antigen. The dominant form of the TCR,

expressed in roughly 95 percent of thymocytes and peripheral T cells, is composed of a single-chain α subunit linked by a disulfide bond to a single-chain β subunit. This form of TCR recognizes antigen presented in the context of major histocompatibility complex (MHC) molecules rather than free soluble antigens. Many cells have the capacity to process proteins and present derivative peptide fragments on their surface in association with class I or class II MHC molecules (see Chap. 4).

A second type of TCR, composed of γ and δ subunits, is found in 1 to 15 percent of peripheral T lymphocytes. The unique function, if any, and the antigen specificity of γ/δ^+ T cells remain unknown. The abundance of these cells in the epithelium of organs such as skin, lung, intestine, vagina, etc., observed in the mouse, led to the suggestion that these molecules may serve some specific function in the immune surveillance at the epithelia (the interface of the organism and the outside environment). Nevertheless, no obvious tropism of γ/δ T cells for the epithelium is found in humans.

GENERATION OF PRIMARY DIVERSITY

Combinatorial Diversification

As shown in Fig. 5-2, a B or T lymphocyte acquires its individual specificity through gene rearrangement, combinatorial joining of disparate chromosomal segments, in somatic cells. In the process of forming an IgH in a B lymphocyte, one of a number of diversity (D) segments recombines with a single member of joining (J) segments, which in turn recombines with a V gene segment from a large cluster of V genes. In the formation of IgL, a κ or λ light-chain V gene segment combines directly with a J gene segment. There are no D segments at the light-chain gene loci. Similarly, T lymphocytes acquire their specificities by joining of V, D, and J segments of the β- or δ-TCR chain, and by joining V and J segments of the α- or γ-TCR

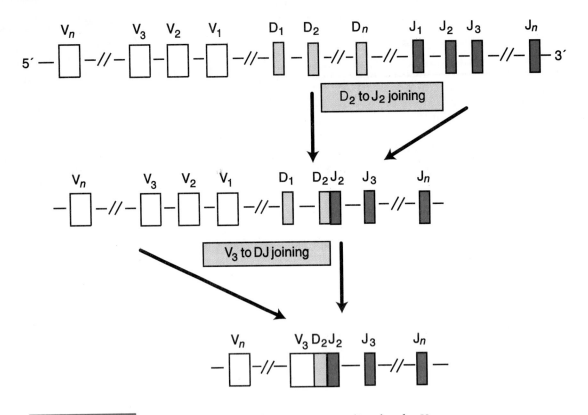

Figure 5-2   Functional immunoglobulin H-chain genes coding for the V domain are assembled by joining of a D segment to a J segment with subsequent joining of one of the V segments to the previously combined DJ segments.

chain. Combinatorial diversity of each antigen receptor can be calculated by multiplying the numbers of gene segments in each cluster of the participating loci. For example, if we estimate 200 V_H, 30 D_H, and 6 J_H in the genome, then there are $(200 \times 30 \times 6) = 3.6 \times 10^4$ rearrangements possible for IgH. With an estimated 10^3 possible rearrangements of the IgL locus, the association between IgH and IgL would generate approximately 3.6×10^7 antigen specificities. Roughly 10^6 recombinations are possible for T cells bearing the α/β heterodimer. This estimate of the potential repertoire does not take into consideration imprecise joining, addition of non-germ-line sequences at the junctions, or somatic mutation which together increase the estimated repertoire by several orders of magnitude (discussed below).

The gene segments of Ig and TCR in nonlymphoid cells or lymphoid precursor cells are in the unrearranged germ-line configuration. The rearrangement of gene segments to form the final V-domain coding sequence, with few exceptions, involves a process whereby all sequences in the germ line between the fused segments are eliminated. It is believed that joining of gene segments is mediated by recombinase enzymes, governed by recombination recognition signals (RRS) 3′ to the V, on either side of the D, and 5′ to the J segments. The RRS consists of a relatively conserved palindromic heptamer sequence separated from an AT (adenine and thymidine)-rich nonamer sequence by non-

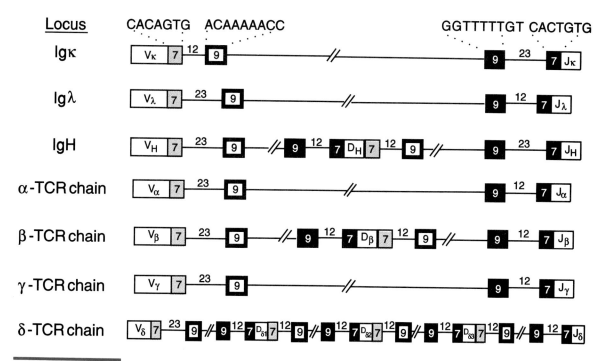

Figure 5-3 Rearrangement recognition signals (RRS) of lymphocyte antigen-receptor gene families. The numbers 7 and 9 denote the conserved heptamer and AT-rich nonamer sequences. The 12 and 23 are the lengths of nonconserved spacer between the heptamer and nonamer.

conserved 12 (± 1) or 23 (± 1) nucleotide spacers (Fig 5-3). Joining of two gene segments is possible only if their respective RRS are separated by spacers of different lengths. Thus, a gene segment followed by a 12-nucleotide spacer (corresponding to one turn of the DNA helix) can recombine only with a gene segment preceded by a 23-nucleotide spacer and vice versa. Two recombination activating genes (RAG-1 and RAG-2), transcribed only in pre-B or pre-T cells, have been isolated from both human and mouse. RAG-1 gene encodes a 119-kd protein which induces rearrangement of appropriate target sequences at low efficiency. The product of the second contiguous gene, RAG-2, is required to give high efficiency recombination.

Imprecise Joining

Each Ig V domain contains a unique amino acid sequence with the greatest variability occurring in three hypervariable regions separated by relatively invariant framework regions. The hypervariable regions define the site of antigen recognition and thus are described as *complementarity-determining regions* (CDR1, CDR2, and CDR3). X-ray crystallographic studies of Ig revealed that CDR1 and CDR2 are at the skirt of antigen-binding sites with CDR3 in the center, all contacting antigen. TCR V domains are in general more uniformly variable and less easily compartmentalized into CDR1 and CDR2 regions; CDR3 in all cases is highly variable. Based on the known Ig structure, it has been postulated that TCR recognizes antigen in the context of MHC as a result of an interaction of CDR1 and CDR2 with an MHC molecule and the highly variable CDR3 with the foreign antigen. CDR1 and CDR2 are encoded by the V gene segments; CDR3 is encoded by the D segment and sequences at the V-(D)-J junctions.

The third CDR is made much more diverse by virtue of mechanisms generating diversity at the junctions. One of these mechanisms involves a loss of coding sequences at the junctions. Imprecise joining introduces hypervariability at the junctions. This is particularly important in the case of γ- and δ-TCR-chain loci, which contain only a few germ-line V gene segments. Although imprecise joining is essential for the generation of a full immune repertoire, it is nevertheless a tightly controlled process. Defects at any point in the process of joining disparate chromosomal segments result in unsuccessful rearrangements and failure to produce functional TCR or Ig.

N Region

At the junctions of rearranging segments, nucleotides that are not present in the germ-line sequence are frequently found. Non-germ-line nucleotides can be added as another source of diversity at the V, D, and J joining junctions. These non-germ-line elements are usually referred to as *N regions*. These sequences are added by terminal deoxynucleotidyl transferase (TdT), a template-independent DNA polymerase, during the process of recombination. TdT activity can be detected in human fetal liver at 12 weeks of gestation but is not found in human fetal thymus until 21 weeks of gestation.

P Element

Although some of the added nucleotides at the junctions are strictly speaking non-germ-line elements, other nucleotides added at the junctions appear to be derived from the germ-line sequences. These are called *P elements* (P for palindrome). They are found as mono- or dinucleotides recurrent for a particular coding gene segment and only at the ends of untrimmed gene segments. P elements may be added by the following mechanism. Subsequent to DNA scission during recombination and prior to religation of disparate gene segments, a dinucleotide is excised from the exposed 5′ end of either or both of the rearranging gene segments; this dinucleotide is inverted and appended to the 3′ end of the complementary strand, generating a tetranucleotide palindrome after the single-stranded tail is converted to a duplex by DNA polymerase; this substrate is then subject to exonuclease digestion (which may remove all or part of the P element) and N-region addition.

Somatic Hypermutation

Ig diversification is further augmented by a high frequency of somatic hypermutation. Hypermutation acts on rearranged Ig V regions at a rate of 10^{-3} per base pair per generation. The majority of Ig V-region mutations are point mutations that result in amino acid replacements accumulating primarily in CDR1 and CDR2. Immunoglobulin somatic hypermutation is a T cell–dependent process triggered by antigen stimulation and occurs during the generation of memory cells. The differentiation of naive and memory B cells into antibody-secreting plasma cells is not accompanied by hypermutation. The molecular mechanism of the hypermutation remains to be uncovered.

Antibodies produced from secondary or hyperimmune responses generally have higher affinity for the challenging antigen. Somatic hypermutation plays an important role in fine-tuning the humoral immune response to maximize the affinity of an antibody to its target.

Somatic mutations do not contribute to the generation of diversity in the TCR. This makes sense: T cells are the central regulators of the immune system and do not diversify further after surviving the thymic test of restriction to self-MHC and of tolerance to self-antigens.

Gene Conversion

In chicken B cells, the λ light-chain locus contains only a single functional V_λ gene segment together with an additional 25 pseudo-V_λ genes. A gene-conversion process of unknown mechanism creates V_λ diversity by replacing a block of sequence in the rearranged V_λ region of the single functional gene with a block of sequences from different pseudo-V_λ genes. Gene conversion occurs only to the rearranged V_λ allele and exclusively in the bursa. The possibility of the same mechanism mediating human Ig loci diversification has been suggested.

THE ORGANIZATION OF IMMUNOGLOBULIN AND TCR GENES

IgH

The individual V gene segments are classified as being in the same family if they are

80 percent homologous to at least one other member of the family and less than 70 percent homologous to members of other families. (See Fig. 5-4.)

The number of V gene segments has been estimated from Southern blot analysis. As each V probe hybridizes to a group of related genes, the number of the V segments can be deduced based on the number of restriction fragments that hybridize to a panel of V probes. Such estimations are subject to error. For instance, the band detected may represent more than one gene segment, or the probe may detect related pseudogene segments. (*Pseudogenes* are defective, nonfunctional genes.)

The human IgH V locus, located on chromosome 14, includes six families. All give

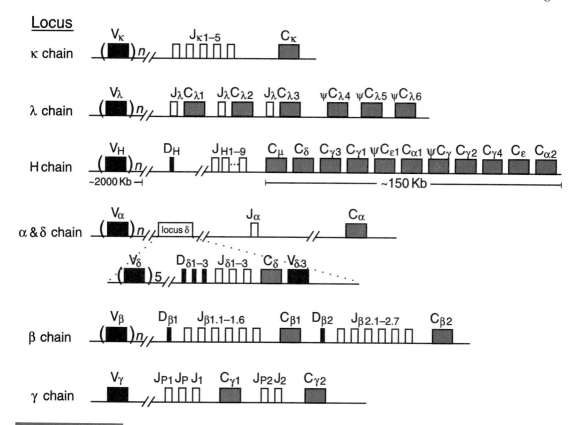

Figure 5-4   Gene organization of the human immunoglobulin H, κ, and λ loci and the human T-cell receptor α, β, γ, and δ loci. Genes with a prefix ψ are pseudogenes. This diagram shows the *overall* picture of antigen-receptor gene organizations. Map distances are not drawn to scale.

distinct and nonoverlapping patterns when used as probes for Southern blots of genomic DNA. An estimate for the minimum number of genes in each family is as follows: V_H1, 20–25; V_H2, 5–10; V_H3, 25–30; V_H4, 6–10; V_H5, 2–3; V_H6, 1. This is based on the number of distinct bands revealed by hybridization of representative members of each group to genomic DNA on Southern blots. The actual number of V_H segments is likely to be greater than 100. There are nine J_H segments, three of which are defective pseudogenes.

IgH chains have a unique feature known as *isotype switch*: a rearranged Ig can replace its C_μ region by downstream constant regions. C_μ is expressed prior to other classes of IgH constant regions. This process, influenced by antigen and T cell–derived cytokines, involves the elimination of sequences between the switch site upstream from C_μ to a switch site upstream from the new C region. The isotype switch mechanism allows clonally derived B cells to produce Ig with the same V domain linked to a different class or subclass of C domain which provides different biologic functions.

IgL

The two IgL loci are located on separate chromosomes, κ at chromosome 2 and λ at chromosome 22. Within the κ gene complex there are 75 to 80 V_κ segments, 5 functional J_κ segments, and a single C_κ segment. The human λ locus is not yet well characterized. There are six C_λ genes. By analogy with murine λ chains, each C_λ gene is likely associated with one or more J_λ segments. The proportion of the two types of light chain in the serum vary among different species. Greater than 90 percent of mouse serum light chains are κ, whereas human serum light chains are comprised of approximately 60 percent κ and 40 percent λ.

α-TCR Chain

The human α-TCR-chain gene complex, including the V, J, and C regions, spans close to 1000 kilobases (kb) of DNA on chromo-

some 14. It is estimated that the α-TCR-chain gene complex contains more than 100 V_α segments and 50 to 100 J_α gene segments. The 75 to 80 known V_α gene segments comprise approximately 20 families.

β-TCR Chain

In humans, at least 24 V_β families have been identified. The total number of V_β elements found on human chromosome 14 is estimated to be as high as 100. In addition, this gene complex consists of two very similar C_β genes. At the 5' end of each C_β region is a cluster containing a single D_β segment and either six or seven J_β segments.

There is a striking conservation of the organization of the human and murine V_β family members. Many human V_β genes have a mouse counterpart (determined by nucleotide homology) which is similarly located relative to other V_β gene segments.

γ-TCR Chain

The human γ-TCR-chain gene complex is located on human chromosome 7 and consists of 14 V_γ gene segments located 5' to five J_γ segments and two C_γ segments. Three of the J_γ segments are upstream from $C_\gamma1$; the other two are immediately upstream from $C_\gamma2$, which is separated from $C_\gamma1$ by 16 kb. Twelve of the 14 V_γ segments are categorized into four families based on relative homologies; the $V_\gamma2$, $V_\gamma3$, and $V_\gamma4$ families contain one member; the $V_\gamma1$ family contains nine members of which four are pseudogenes. The two V_γ segments not categorized are also pseudogenes.

There are no D elements present in human or mouse γ-TCR loci. However, significant variation at the V_γ-J_γ junctions has been observed; the variation is a result of imprecise joining and the addition of N regions at these junctions. Since the number of V_γ and J_γ sequences is quite limited, the diversity generated at the V-J junctions becomes the main source of diversity.

The two C_γ regions differ in their linkage with the δ-TCR chain. $C_\gamma1$ contains a cysteine residue which covalently links the γ chain to the δ chain; $C_\gamma 2$ lacks the cysteine residue and pairs with the δ chain noncovalently.

δ-TCR Chain

The human δ-TCR-chain gene complex, like the murine counterpart, is contained within the δ-TCR-bearing complex. The C_δ exons are located about 90 kb from the C_α region on chromosome 14. Three J_δ and three D_δ segments are located 5' to C_δ. Six V_δ segments have been found. One V_δ segment is located in an inverted orientation 3' of C_δ.

In spite of small numbers of V_δ gene segments, the δ-TCR chain has the potential of enormous junctional diversity. According to the 12/23 rule, the recombination recognition sequences of the δ-TCR chain allow all V-D, D-D, and D-J joinings. The δ-TCR chain is unique in that up to three D_δ segments in tandem can be found in a single δ-TCR chain polypeptide. N-region addition and imprecise joining can occur at all junctions and result in enormous diversity in the CDR3. The possible junctional diversity of the δ-TCR chain is far greater than that of the Ig or the α-TCR or β-TCR subunits. (See Clinical Aside 5-1.)

Clinical Aside 5-1 V_γ and V_δ Cells

Organ-specific V_γ and V_δ chain gene usage and pairing is probably one of the most noteworthy features of the γ/δ-TCR-bearing cell. In the mouse, the skin γ/δ cells express only one combination of the γ and δ genes utilizing a particular set of V, (D), and J gene segments. The epithelial γ/δ cells of the reproductive organs similarly express another unique combination of the γ and δ genes. No junctional diversity is found in these two locations. These T cells appear to be derived from fetal thymus during development since these two combinations of the γ and δ genes also appear in the fetal thymus in two separate waves, peaking at the 15th day of gestation and at birth, and subside after birth. The γ/δ cells of the intestinal epithelium express yet another unique γ gene sequence, in combination with highly variable δ gene sequences.

The human γ/δ cells also appear to have nonrandom V gene usage and pairing in some tissues. For example, a significant percentage of the γ/δ cells in peripheral blood express $V_\delta 2$ and $V_\gamma 9$-Jp-$C_\gamma 1$; however, they exhibit a high degree of junctional diversity. The same $V_\gamma 9$-Jp-$C_\gamma 1/V_\delta 2$ pairing is rare in postnatal thymus.

Without knowledge of the function and the antigen recognized by γ/δ cells, one can perhaps speculate that the limited V gene usage in a tissue-restricted manner reflects the interaction of the γ/δ-TCR-bearing cell with unidentified tissue-specific elements which recruit and expand the γ/δ cells expressing a particular antigen specificity.

PROCESSES THAT SELECT AND INDUCE PROLIFERATION OF LYMPHOCYTES EXPRESSING A PARTICULAR ANTIGEN RECEPTOR

The potential of primary diversity is far greater than the actual diversity found in any individual. The repertoire is not entirely random. What determines the functional V-region repertoire?

A number of considerations influence the expressed repertoire of B and T cells apart from those discussed above. For example, T cells, specifically the α/β-TCR-bearing ones, have two constraints imposed on them before they emerge from the thymus as mature circulating lymphocytes: The T cell must be made tolerant to self-antigen (negative selection), and the reactivity of the T cell is restricted by polymorphic MHC antigens present on the cells of the host. The latter is presumably a consequence of the requirement of T cells to react with processed antigen associated with MHC molecules. A T cell cannot recognize antigen presented by a cell with MHC antigens differing from that of the thymus in which it matured. There is compelling evidence that T cells are both positively selected in the thymus for recognition of either class I or class II MHC. (See Chap. 7 on the T cell.)

Despite the presence of surface Ig or TCR molecules, some B or T cells may not respond to antigen because of tolerance induced in the periphery.

SELF-TEST QUESTIONS*

1. TCR specificity of a particular T cell
   a. Is induced by interaction with antigen
   b. Is fixed after the T cell matures in the thymus
   c. May change late during the immune response via somatic point mutation
   d. May switch from one isotype to another
2. Both the B- and T-cell receptor genes are composed of V, J, and C gene segments. Which of the following also contain D gene segments?
   a. IgH
   b. IgL
   c. α-TCR chain and γ-TCR chain
   d. β-TCR chain and δ-TCR chain
3. If Mary had 100 V, 50 J, and 1 C gene segment in her α-TCR-chain gene complex and 20 V, 10 D, 10 J, and 2 C gene segment in her β-TCR chain gene complex, how many antigen specificities are possible for her α/β-TCR repertoire?
   a. Exactly 2,000
   b. Exactly 10,000,000
   c. Exactly 20,000,000
   d. More than 10,000,000
4. The immunoglobulin and T-cell receptor genes have which of the following characteristics?
   a. Allelic exclusion
   b. Diversification by rearrangement of disparate gene segments
   c. Linkage to the X chromosome
   d. Codominance
5. Which of the following statements concerning the antigen receptor is (are) incorrect?
   a. Repertoire diversity of the T cells bearing the γ/δ heterodimer is mainly achieved by imprecise joining at the V-(D)-J junctions.
   b. Clonally derived B cells can switch isotype to produce Ig with the same V domain linked to different class or subclass of C domain.
   c. The light-chain genes go through isotype switch after surface IgM is expressed.
   d. All gene rearrangement follows the 12/23 rule.
6. Mary is heterologous for IgG3 allotypes G3m(5) and G3m(21). The individual IgG3 antibodies found in her serum may have:
   a. Two H chains of allotype G3m(5)
   b. Two H chains, one of allotypes G3m(5) and one of allotype G3m(21)
   c. Two L chains of κ
   d. Two L chains, one of κ and one of λ

ADDITIONAL READINGS

Alt FW, Blackwell TK, Yancopoulos GD. Development of the primary antibody repertoire. *Science.* 1987;238: 1079.

Kronenberg M, Siu G, Hood LE, Shastri N. The molecular genetics of the T-cell antigen receptor and T-cell antigen recognition. *Ann Rev Immunol.* 1986;4: 529.

Rajewsky K, Forster I, Cumano A. Evolutionary and somatic selection of the antibody repertoire in the mouse. *Science.* 1987;238: 1088.

Raulet DH. The structure, function, and molecular genetics of the γ/δ T cell receptor. *Ann Rev Immunol.* 1987;7: 175.

*Answers will be found in Appendix E.

6

Ontogeny and Differentiation of B Lymphocytes

INTRODUCTION

B cells were originally named after the discovery in chickens of bursa-derived lymphocytes. In birds, the bursa of Fabricius is the organ in which B cells are generated and differentiate. In mammals, there is no bursa equivalent, and although B cells are produced and differentiate mainly in the bone marrow (and in fetal liver before birth), B-cell stem cells are also found and differentiate in the spleen. Hemopoiesis begins in the bone marrow where the elusive pluripotential stem cells reside. These stem cells are relatively rare, approximately 1 out of 10^5 cells in the mouse bone marrow. The definition of a pluripotential stem cell is that it is self-renewing and can give rise to multiple lineages, for example, the lymphoid, myeloid, and erythroid lineages. It is not known what induces a stem cell to differentiate to a lineage-committed stem cell. Lineage mapping studies have shown that there is a multipotential lymphoid-committed stem cell that gives rise to both T and B cells along the differentiation pathway.

Multipotent lymphoid stem cells and myeloid stem cells occur at frequencies of approximately 1 in 10^4 mouse bone marrow cells. B-cell progenitors first colonize the fetal liver in waves between days 12 and 13 of gestation in the mouse and later migrate primarily to the bone marrow. In these primary organs, B progenitors come in contact with fibroblastlike stromal cells. These stromal cells secrete cytokines and other factors, which provide important signals for lymphopoiesis. B progenitor cells remain mainly in the bone marrow and, in most rodents, also in the spleen until maturation to the stage in which they bear surface immunoglobulin (Ig). Surface-Ig-positive cells exit the bone marrow to populate the secondary lymphoid organs, the spleen and lymph nodes (Fig. 6-1).

B-cell differentiation can be divided into two phases. The first phase takes place in the primary lymphoid organ and occurs independently of antigen. The second phase occurs in the periphery and is a result of antigen-induced B-cell activation. In the first phase, the maturation process begins at the level of the stem cell, and comprises the lineage-committed B-progenitor-cell or pro-B-cell stages, and the pre-B-cell stages in which Ig gene rearrangement occurs, ending at the point of release of the virgin, surface-Ig-positive B lymphocyte into the periphery.

The second phase of B-cell differentiation occurs in response to antigenic stimulation, depending on the type of antigen. Binding of antigen to the surface Ig molecules initiates the B-cell activation pathway which leads to antibody secretion. Antibody production by B cells is in most cases dependent upon cell interaction with antigen-specific T cells, often referred to as *T-cell help*. The production of all antibody isotypes except, in some cases, for the IgM isotype, is dependent upon T-cell help. The exact nature of T-cell help is unknown, but it involves direct cell-to-cell interactions as well as the secretion of lymphokines which are involved in further B-cell activation and Ig isotype switching. Some antigens, mainly sugar polymers, cannot stimulate T cells, and elicit only the secretion of IgM antibodies by B cells. They also do not induce memory B cells. Such antigens are known as T-independent antigens. They are discussed in more detail later in the chapter.

Generally, during a primary antigen response, IgM is the first immunoglobulin isotype produced. Activated B cells in the presence of antigen can undergo immunoglobulin isotype class switching to secrete IgG, IgA, or IgE. This is accompanied by hypermutation of the variable regions in the heavy- and light-chain genes (see Chap. 5). Class switching is T-dependent and is probably induced by cytokines secreted mainly by helper T cells. It is not clear if every B cell can be induced to secrete any of the Ig isotypes by either the appropriate cytokine or a particular T-cell subset, or whether different B-cell subsets are programmed to secrete only one isotype.

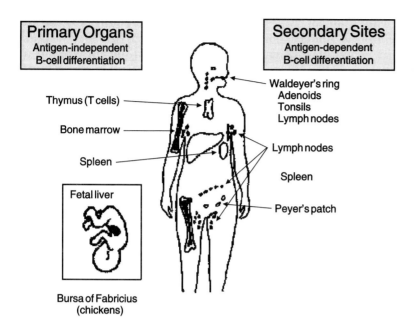

Primary Organs
Antigen-independent
B-cell differentiation

Thymus (T cells)

Bone marrow

Spleen

Fetal liver

Bursa of Fabricius
(chickens)

Secondary Sites
Antigen-dependent
B-cell differentiation

Waldeyer's ring
Adenoids
Tonsils
Lymph nodes

Lymph nodes

Spleen

Peyer's patch

Figure 6-1 Sites of lympho-poiesis.

Secondary immune responses are characterized by a much more rapid antibody response (mediated by memory B cells), and most of the antibodies produced are IgGs. Some antigens induce mainly IgA or IgE rather than IgG antibodies. Antibody-secreting B cells are called *plasma cells* and are at the end stage of the irreversible B-cell differentiation pathway.

Antigen stimulation can also induce a population of B cells to enter into a resting G_0 phase without inducing antibody secretion. These cells are memory B cells, and they comprise the bulk of the responding cells in the secondary response to most antigens. The relationship between these two B-cell subsets—those that secrete antibodies during a primary response and those that become memory cells—is a controversial issue and is dealt with in more detail later on.

CELL SURFACE MARKERS

B-cell development can be characterized by the appearance of cell surface differentiation markers throughout the maturation process. Probably the best known B-cell markers are surface immunoglobulin and MHC class II antigens, but many other markers are expressed throughout the differentiation pathway of the cell. Although many of the cell surface markers have obvious functions, e.g., lymphokine receptors, the functions of other markers remain obscure. Most of these cell surface molecules were identified by monoclonal antibodies. A numerically based *cluster of differentiation (CD)* nomenclature was developed in order to eliminate the confusion generated by different names given by different laboratories to lymphocyte surface markers. The CD nomenclature (see Appendix D) is used to describe surface molecules on all hematopoietic cells. Monoclonal antibody technology has greatly advanced research on lymphopoiesis, since it has created a tool to isolate distinct lymphocyte subpopulations, which can then be functionally characterized.

Murine B-Cell Differentiation Markers

Cells representing differentiation intermediates along the developmental pathway of the B-cell lineage can be characterized by the sequential expression of cytoplasmic and cell surface markers (Fig. 6-2). The biologic signals controlling this sequential expression have not been well defined, but certainly the microenvironment of the developing B cell plays a role. Markers unique to early pluripotential stem cells have not yet been identified; however, experimental protocols have been developed to enrich for pluripotential stem cells. Such protocols usually involve depletion of cells with various monoclonal antibodies specific for surface markers expressed on more mature cells, and complement. Although no specific stem cell marker has been identified in the mouse, most of the

cells in this enriched bone marrow subpopulation express low levels of Thy-1 and relatively high levels of the lymphocyte marker Ly-6.

The first well-characterized differentiation stage along the B-cell differentiation pathway is the pre-B cell. The pre-B-cell stage initiates with rearrangement of the heavy- and light-chain genes and ends with the appearance of Ig on the cell surface. Several genes that are expressed uniquely at the lineage-committed pre-B-cell stage, and not in mature B lymphocytes or plasma cells, have been identified in mice and in humans. These include the $\lambda 5$ and V_{pre-B} genes, which are

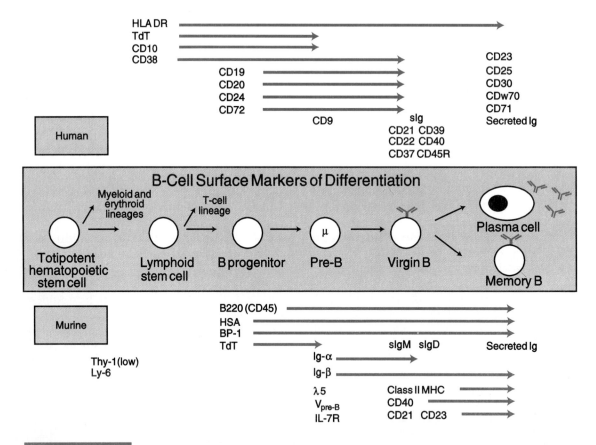

Figure 6-2   *Surface markers of B-lymphocyte differentiation.* The stages of B-cell differentiation are characterized by the appearance of surface and cytoplasmic markers. Surface markers corresponding to different stages of human B-cell development are represented on the top half of the figure. Murine differentiation markers are represented on the bottom half.

highly homologous to C_λ and V_λ, respectively. These two genes encode the ω and ι proteins, which associate with each other to form a protein resembling Ig light chain; this protein has been termed *surrogate light chain.* The surrogate light chain forms a complex with μ heavy chain on the pre-B-cell surface prior to light-chain expression. The function will be discussed in detail later on.

Other markers commonly used to characterize early stages in B-cell development are not exclusively expressed in pre-B cells but their expression starts at or before the pre-B-cell stage. Some of the most characteristic murine markers include HSA (heat-stable antigen), B220, BP-1, the interleukin-7 receptor, Ig-α, and Ig-β (Fig. 6-2). HSA, first identified by the monoclonal antibody J11d, appears very early in the B-cell differentiation pathway (as well as on myeloid cells and early T cells) and is expressed throughout B-cell development up to the memory cell stage. Recent evidence suggests that memory cells express little or no HSA. B220, a member of the common leukocyte antigen family (CD45), appears early on almost all B-lineage progenitor cells, and is commonly used to enrich for B-cell progenitors in the bone marrow. The CD45 gene is well conserved between mice and humans, and is composed of three exons, which encode up to five isoforms of the gene. Different isoforms appear on most hematopoietic cells, except for erythrocytes. The 220-kd isoform is expressed on B-lineage cells. It is a tyrosine phosphatase, which appears to play a regulatory role in antigen-specific signal transduction.

The BP-1 marker is unique to the B-cell lineage, appearing on late-stage B progenitor cells. BP-1 functions as a zinc-dependent metallopeptidase. The interleukin-7 receptor, IL-7R, is a pre-B-cell differentiation marker, also found on early thymocytes as well as on bone marrow–derived macrophages. Interleukin-7 is a pre-B-cell growth factor.

Many of the cell surface markers that appear on pre-B cells like the surrogate light chain and μ are associated with surface immunoglobulin production. Two other such molecules, Ig-α and Ig-β, are encoded by the genes *mb-1* and *B29*, respectively. Both are transmembrane glycoproteins that make up part of the surface immunoglobulin antigen receptor complex and appear to play a role in receptor signaling. Ig-α is necessary for expression of μ heavy chain on the B-cell surface. Both Ig-α and Ig-β are expressed early in pre-B cells associated with μ, which is likewise associated with the surrogate light chain. They remain associated with μ, which later associates with light chain throughout the mature B-cell stages. Ig-α is not expressed in plasma cells.

Human B-Cell Markers

Human B-cell differentiation differs from murine B-cell development most notably by the early expression of HLA-DR molecules at the lineage-committed progenitor stage. In contrast, in mice, MHC class II markers are expressed in mature B lymphocytes, and as a consequence of activation. Human lineage-committed B progenitor cells have a phenotype also defined by CD9, CD10, CD19, CD20, CD24, CD38, and CD72 (Fig. 6-2). Table 6-1 lists the characteristics of these molecules. The mature B-cell stages are characterized by surface Ig and a host of markers, some of which are expressed only on certain B-cell subsets. No markers unique to plasma cells were found; however, plasma cells express relatively high levels of CD23, the low-affinity Fc receptor for IgE, and several cryptic markers which are also expressed on activated T cells, for example, CD30, CD38, CDw70, and CD71. Many of the human markers were defined by monoclonal antibody analysis of B-lymphocytic leukemia cells. Phenotypic studies of many different leukemias have led to the concept of maturation arrest. Often, leukemic cells have a phenotype similar to normal early-stage lymphocytes, indicating that a change occurred in the cells during development which blocked further maturation but did not halt proliferation of the cells, resulting in the accumulation of immature phenotype.

CD10, otherwise known as *CALLA,* for *common acute lymphoblastic leukemia*

TABLE 6-1   Characteristics of Major Human B-Cell Surface Markers

	Cell Types	Characteristics
CD5	B-cell subset, activated B cells, B-CLL, T cells	gp 67, function unknown, controversy over lineage
CD9	Pre-B cells, early B cells, myeloid cells, thrombocytes	p24, unknown function
CD10	Pre-B cells, early B-ALL cells, PMNs, glomerular epithelium	CALLA, neutral endopeptidase
CD19	Pan B cells, follicular dendritic cells (FDCs)	Ig superfamily gp95, associated with mIg, signaling of protein kinase C pathway
CD20	Pan B cells	gp33–35, multiple transmembrane domains, cell cycle regulation
CD21	Mature B cells, FDCs	CR2, receptor for complement and Epstein-Barr virus, accessory signaling
CD22	Pan B cells: in cytoplasm—early B cells; on membrane—mature B cells	Ig superfamily gp135, accessory signaling
CD23	Mature B, monocytes, FDCs	Low-affinity receptor for IgE (FcεRII), induced by IL-4
CD24	Pan B, PMNs, epithelium	PI-linked glycoprotein, signal transduction role
CD30	Activated B and T cells, plasma cells	gp120, unknown function
CD37	Mature B cells, glial cells, epithelium, few T cells	gp40–52, multiple transmembrane domains
CD38	Pre-B cells, plasma cells, thymocytes, activated T cells	p45, unknown function
CD39	Mature B cells, FDCs, endothelium, macrophages	gp70–100, role in T-cell signaling
CD40	Pan B, FDCs, basal epithelium, carcinomas	Homology to NGF-R and TNF-α receptor, accessory signaling, coordinate expression with Ia
CD45R	Pan leukocytes	Leukocyte common antigen family, gps190–220
CD54	Mature and activated B cells, monocytes, macrophages, Kupffer cells, bone marrow	ICAM-1, ligand for CD11a on T cells, important for T-cell activation
CDw70	Mature and activated B and T cells, plasma cells	Glycoprotein 32–40 kd, unknown function
CD71	Plasma cells, activated B and T cells, macrophages	Transferrin receptor
CD72	Pan B cells, macrophages	gp43/39, lectinlike domains, homology to CD23, signal transduction role
CD73	Pan B cells, T-cell subset, FDCs, hepatocytes	PI-linked membrane ecto-5'-nucleotidase, signaling role
B7/BB1	Activated B cells, monocytes	Ig superfamily, ligand of CD28 on T cells, costimulatory for T cells

antigen, is one such marker now used to diagnose acute lymphoblastic leukemia (ALL). CD10 is normally found only on pro-B- and pre-B-cell stages; however, in ALL the proportion of cells bearing CD10 is greatly increased.

Intracellular Markers of B-Cell Development

Cytoplasmic proteins, not expressed as cell surface markers but nevertheless associated with immunoglobulin gene rearrangements, further characterize pre-B-cell development. Examples of such proteins are the enzyme terminal deoxynucleotidyl transferase (TdT), which randomly adds non-germ-line N residues to rearranging immunoglobulin genes (see Chapter 5); and the products of the *RAG-1* and *RAG-2* genes, which help activate recombination of the variable, diversity, and joining gene regions. Recently described cellular oncogenes, such as *bcl-2*, *abl*, *myc*, and *myb*, have also been shown to be differentially expressed throughout the B-cell developmental pathway. Lyn and blk are tyrosine kinases found in B cells, which are thought to noncovalently associate with the cytoplasmic domains of Ig-α and Ig-β during signal transduction through the B-cell antigen receptor.

The identification of transcriptional regulators is currently a rapidly expanding field. Several immunoglobulin gene promoter and enhancer regions have been identified that are associated with initiation and enhancement of immunoglobulin gene transcription. NF-κB is a DNA-binding protein that binds to the enhancer region of κ light-chain genes, and is actively expressed in pre-B cells during κ-chain production. The isolation of other transcriptional regulators is actively being pursued.

Markers Associated with B-Cell Activation

Differentiation markers that are expressed on virgin, immature B cells following surface expression of IgM include the MHC class II antigens (in the mouse), the complement receptor CR2 (CD21), which is also the receptor for the Epstein-Barr virus, CD22 (mainly on marginal-zone B cells), and the low-affinity Fc receptor for IgE (CD23), particularly on follicular B cells. The appearance of surface IgD, which also complexes with the Ig-α and Ig-β proteins to form the IgD receptor, is an important marker of B-cell differentiation since it defines the fully immunocompetent mature B cell.

Further stages in B-cell development are characterized by markers of activation. Expression of MHC class II molecules is drastically increased once resting B cells become activated. MHC class II molecules bind processed antigen for presentation to helper T cells. The increase in the number of class II molecules on the surface of activated B cells presumably makes antigen presentation more efficient. Expression of the CD40 molecule, a phosphorylated glycoprotein found on B cells and follicular dendritic cells which is thought to be an accessory signaling molecule, appears to be coordinately regulated with MHC class II. Signals that induce class II expression likewise induce CD40. Staining patterns with anti-CD40 and anti-MHC class II monoclonal antibodies are virtually identical in lymphoid tissues. Although its exact function is not clear, CD40 appears to have a role in promoting clonal proliferation. Expression of the B7/BB1 molecule is also induced by activation. This surface molecule is the ligand for CD28, a molecule expressed on T cells which is required for T-cell activation (see Chap. 7B).

The culmination of B-cell activation is the secretion of antibodies. This is associated with the expression of genes involved with immunoglobulin isotype switching, such as the heavy-chain constant-region genes for IgA, IgG, and IgE subclasses. Isotype switching appears to be influenced by lymphokines. For example, exogenous IL-4, when added to activated B-cell cultures, induces some of the cells to switch and secrete IgE. Immunoglobulin secretion is a result of differential mRNA splicing of the region encoding the transmembrane domain of μ heavy chain. Secreted forms of immunoglobulin are altered at the heavy-chain carboxy terminal such that the transmembrane portion is deleted making them unable to insert in the cell membrane. Secretion of IgM and IgA is associated with transcription of the gene for J chain, which is necessary for pentamerization of IgM and dimerization of IgA (see Chap. 3).

Mature B cells express many different markers that are not necessarily unique to the B-cell lineage, like receptors for lymphokines, Fc receptors, MHC class II antigens, complement receptors, and cellular adhesion molecules. Not all mature B cells express the same markers, nor must they express shared markers sequentially in the same order. The contacts that the lymphocyte has made during its lifetime with respect to helper T cells, macrophages and other accessory cells, different antigens, cytokines, etc., all influence the resultant marker phenotype of an individual lymphocyte.

THE B-CELL ANTIGEN RECEPTOR

B-cell activation is initiated through the surface immunoglobulin complex, which has recently been termed the *B-cell antigen receptor* because it is structurally analogous to the T-cell receptor. The surface B-cell antigen receptor complex is composed of immunoglobulin noncovalently complexed in the membrane to heterodimers of the transmembrane proteins Ig-α and Ig-β (Fig. 6-3). Ig-α and Ig-β are heavily glycosylated phosphoprotein subunits that mediate signal transduction through the surface immuno-globulin molecule via long cytoplasmic domains. To understand how signal transduction can occur through the surface immunoglobulin complex, it is necessary to discuss its structure in some detail.

During immunoglobulin gene rearrangement in pre-B cells, μ heavy chain is expressed first, and is inserted in the membrane only after it associates with the Ig-α/Ig-β heterodimer and the surrogate light chain. The *surrogate light chain* is composed of two polypeptides, ω and ι, which are encoded by the pre-B-cell-specific genes λ5 and V_{pre-B} and which are highly homologous to C_λ and V_λ, respectively. They associate noncovalently with each other to form an immunoglobulin

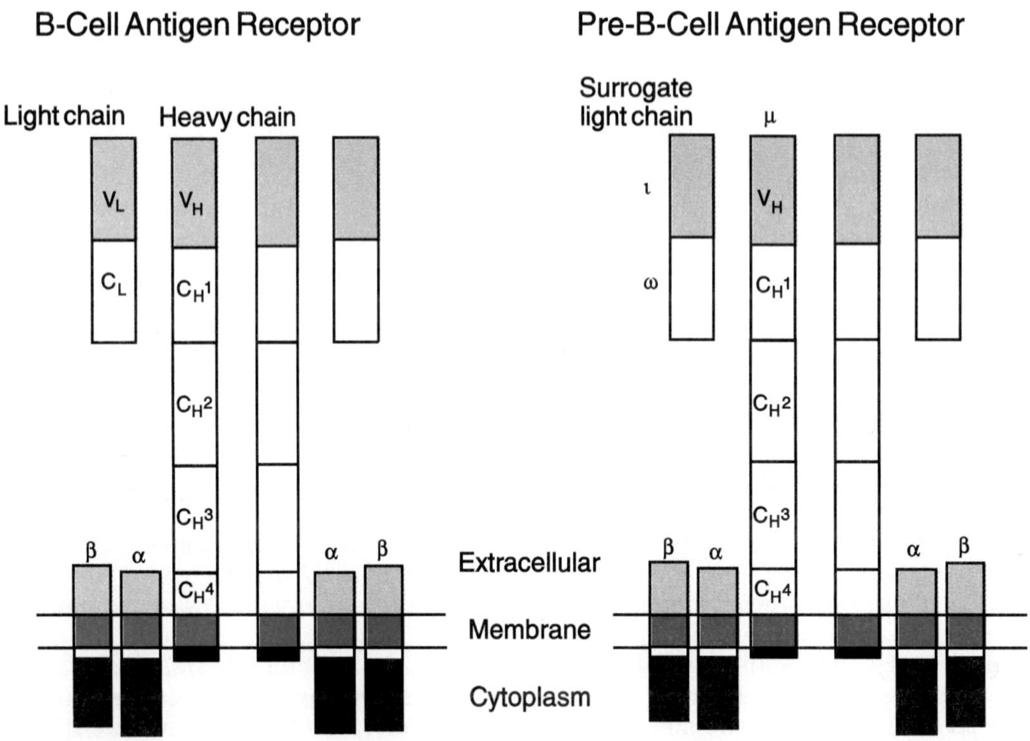

Figure 6-3   *The mature B-cell and pre-B-cell antigen receptors.* The mature B-cell antigen receptor is a dimeric molecule composed of μ or δ heavy chains and κ or λ light chains. This complex is associated with Ig-α and Ig-β. The pre-B-cell antigen receptor has a "surrogate light chain," instead of κ or λ light chains, which is bound to μ heavy chain. The surrogate light chain is composed of two noncovalently linked proteins: ι and ω. ι has some homology to V_λ and ω has homology to C_λ.

light-chain-like protein, called surrogate light chain. The surrogate light chain forms a di-sulfide-linked complex with μ heavy chain on the surface of the cell. This μ-surrogate light chain–Ig-α/Ig-β complex on the pre-B-cell surface has been termed the pre-B-cell antigen receptor. The complex appears to play a role in signal transduction and may also serve as the signal to the B cell to stop rear-ranging the heavy-chain locus. This theory is based on the fact that pre-B cells from transgenic mice that cannot express surface μ do not stop rearranging the heavy-chain locus.

The ω protein contains an N-terminal 60 amino acid sequence which bears no ho-mology to light-chain sequences. It has been proposed that this sequence protrudes from the pre-B-cell receptor and may mediate sig-nals via cross-linkage with other receptors either on the pre-B cell itself or on bone mar-row stromal cells. Its precise function is cur-rently under investigation. The surrogate light chain is replaced during differentiation by κ or λ light chain, thus defining the mature B-cell stage.

The secreted and membrane forms of the μ heavy chain, μ_s and μ_m, respectively, are generated by alternative splicing of a primary mRNA transcript. The two species differ in their carboxy-terminal regions (Fig. 6-4). The secreted form has a 22 amino acid carboxy-terminal sequence that is necessary for pen-tamerization. The membrane-bound form has

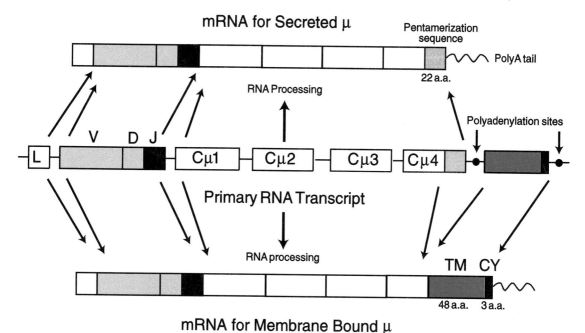

Figure 6-4   *Alternative processing of a primary μ transcript.* The secreted and the membrane forms of μ are produced by an alternative processing of the primary μ transcript. Sequences within the 3' region of the primary μ transcript determine whether μ will be secreted (pentamerization sequence) or inserted into the cell membrane (transmembrane [TM] and cytoplasmic [CY] sequences). These sequences are alternatively processed by the use of different polyadenylation signals. Utilization of the polyadenylation signal immediately 3' of the pentamerization sequence results in secretion of μ heavy chain. Utilization of the polyadenylation signal 3' of the CY sequence results in the insertion of μ protein in the membrane.

instead a 48 amino acid sequence that consists of a transmembrane domain and a very short (3 amino acid) cytoplasmic domain. The μ_m transmembrane domain is an α helix that is believed to associate with the α-helical transmembrane domain of Ig-α, which is itself complexed to the transmembrane domain of Ig-β. Since the Ig molecule is dimeric, each μ chain is associated with an Ig-α/Ig-β heterodimer (Fig. 6-3). The Ig-α and Ig-β subunits have cytoplasmic sequences that contain signaling motifs also found in the T-cell receptor ζ, γ, and δ subunits, and in the γ subunit of the IgE Fc receptor. Plasma cells do not express Ig-α, and therefore no form of membrane Ig can be expressed on the cell surface. Ig-β is expressed throughout B-cell development. Ig-β is transcribed from the B29 gene. The B29 gene product can be alternately spliced resulting in the expression of a C-terminally truncated Ig-β protein that has been termed Ig-γ. Ig-γ can also form heterodimers with Ig-α, which also appears on the surface complexed to Ig.

B-Cell Activation Through the B-Cell Antigen Receptor

Activation of the B-cell antigen receptor can occur by cross-linkage of adjacent surface immunoglobulin molecules, either by antigen or by antibody specific for immunoglobulin. It is thought that Ig-α, Ig-β, and Ig-γ are involved in signal transduction through the B-cell antigen receptor. Immediately following cross-linkage, a number of biochemical changes are induced in the B cell (Fig. 6-5). A rise in intracellular free Ca^{2+} can be measured, which is accompanied by an influx of extracellular Ca^{2+}. Protein tyrosine kinases are activated to phosphorylate a number of substrate proteins. It is believed that the intracellular domains of the Ig-α and Ig-β subunits are tyrosine-phosphorylated. Phospholipase C is activated to cleave phosphatidylinositol bisphosphate to the second messengers inositol-1,4,5-triphosphate and diacylglycerol. Diacylglycerol in turn activates protein kinase C. Within an hour of receptor cross-linkage, transcription

of the cellular proto-oncogenes c-*myc* and c-*fos* is stimulated. The expression of these proteins is associated with the cell entering the G_1 stage of the cell cycle from the resting G_0 stage. Further stimulation, either by antigen, T-cell help, or lymphokines, can at this point induce B-cell proliferation. If T-cell help is not provided at this point, cellular paralysis or clonal anergy will occur rather than activation (see the section on B-cell tolerance). The *two-signal theory*, proposed nearly two decades ago, suggested a requirement for two signals to obtain full physiologic activation of B cells. Cell surface markers of activation, such as MHC class II molecules, are expressed 12 to 24 h after receptor cross-linkage.

Polyclonal B-Cell Activation

Polyclonal B-cell activation is by definition an antigen-nonspecific activation of B cells. Many different agents qualify as polyclonal activators, and they are also called *mitogens.* The first mitogens described were polysaccharides derived mainly from various bacteria such as lipopolysaccharide (LPS) of *Escherichia coli, Staphylococcus aureus* cowan, pokeweed mitogen, purified protein derivative of tuberculin (PPD, a mitogen for murine B cells but not human B cells), and dextran sulfate. Most mitogens are only mitogenic at a relatively high dose. At lower doses most of these molecules can behave as normal antigens. For example, PPD at low doses is a potent antigen and will activate PPD-specific B cells, whereas at high doses it will activate B cells regardless of their antigenic specificity. Different mitogens can activate B cells at different stages of differentiation. PPD and dextran sulfate activate only mature B cells, whereas LPS activates immature as well as mature B cells.

B cells can also be activated polyclonally by antibodies to various cell surface markers. Cross-linking of surface Ig was the first and most studied example. Cross-linkage with anti-μ antibodies mimics specific antigen binding to the surface Ig receptor on a particular B-cell clone. Extensive cross-linking

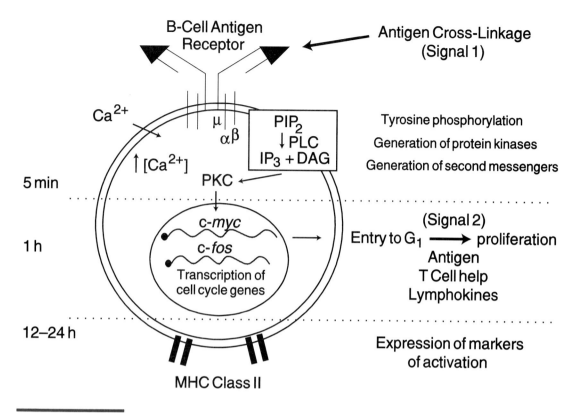

Figure 6-5 *Antigen activation of the B-cell antigen receptor.* Antigen cross-linkage of the B-cell antigen receptor induces a number of biochemical changes in the B cell, including protein tyrosine phosphorylation, activation of the protein kinase C (PKC) pathway, and increases in the level of intracellular $[Ca^{2+}]$. PKC is activated via the phospholipase C–induced (PLC-induced) cleavage of phosphatidylinositol bisphosphate (PIP_2) to diacylglycerol (DAG) and inositol triphosphate (IP_3). PKC induces transcription of the cell cycle genes c-*myc* and c-*fos*, which signal the cell to enter the G_1 phase. At this point a secondary signal to the B cell, such as T-cell help or lymphokines, will induce B-cell proliferation and expression of B-cell markers of activation.

is required to produce optimal B-cell stimulation. At suboptimal concentrations, abortive activation occurs which does not result in DNA synthesis. Anti-Ig-induced mitogenesis can be enhanced by lymphokines, mainly IL-4. In mice, antibodies to Lyb-2 (CD72), a 45-kd surface molecule expressed exclusively on B cells, will induce polyclonal B-cell activation. In humans, monoclonal antibodies to many B-cell surface differentiation markers will induce complete or partial polyclonal B-cell activation on their own or together with other costimulators such as phorbol esters and various lymphokines. These surface markers include CD20 (a Ca^{2+} channel), CD23 (FcεRII), CD21 (the complement receptor CR2), CD40 (a molecule with homologies to nerve growth factor receptor and TNF-α receptor), CD72 (Lyb-2), and CD73 (an ecto-5'-nucleotidase which catalyzes dephosphorylation of purine and pyrimidine monophosphates to nucleosides). Other B-cell surface molecules, like CD19, a member of the immunoglobulin superfamily, and CD22, a marker present on marginal-zone B cells, when similarly stimulated by monoclonal antibodies, can cause synergistic effects with either anti-Ig or with cytokines, like IL-4. The physiologic ligands for most of these molecules have not yet been identified, and it is not clear why cross-linking these surface molecules induces cell activation (Table 6-1).

B-CELL ANTIGEN PRESENTATION

Following cross-linkage by antigen binding to the surface Ig complex, the Ig molecules aggregate and form "patches," which travel to one pole of the B cell to form a "cap." This whole process is called *capping*. The antigen complex is then internalized by receptor-mediated endocytosis within an hour of antigen binding. Antigen processing ensues within the next 6 h, a process by which the antigen is digested proteolytically into short peptide sequences that are then bound intracellularly by MHC class II molecules. These processed antigen–class II complexes are transported to and presented on the B-cell surface where they are accessible to helper T cells. Antigen presentation is discussed in more detail in Chap. 7B. By a process analogous to activation of the B-cell antigen receptor, the T cell is activated to proliferate and secrete lymphokines that also effect subsequent B-cell responses to the antigen.

Although B cells are not the only cell type that can present antigen to T helper cells (e.g., macrophages and dendritic cells also present antigen, see below), B-cell antigen presentation appears to be very important in the secondary response. B cells bearing surface Ig with the highest affinity for antigen are more likely to be activated and present antigen to helper T cells during a secondary antibody response than nonspecific antigen-presenting cells (APCs).

Antigen presentation in which the B cell presents the antigen recognized by its surface Ig is the most efficient antigen-presentation process in the immune system; however, it cannot occur during primary responses. During primary responses, B cells can present antigens that are irrelevant to their surface Ig specificity, in a manner similar to the way antigen is presented by macrophages. Nonspecific antigen uptake and/or processing by B cells is not as efficient as it is by macrophages, probably because B cells have fewer lysosomes and therefore cannot degrade particulate antigens as efficiently as macrophages. In lymph nodes, B cells function as the major APC, even though they are less efficient at presenting antigen than macrophages. This was found from experiments in which lymph node T cells could not be effectively primed in B cell–depleted mice immunized subcutaneously. Only activated and not resting B cells were found to function as efficient APC. Although resting B cells can process antigen, they do not express B7/BB1, a marker of B-cell activation, which is required for T-cell activation (see Chap. 7B).

T CELL–B CELL INTERACTIONS

Although it was first thought that T cell–B cell interactions were limited to T-cell help, it has become apparent in recent years that these interactions are bidirectional. B cells function as APCs for T cells and can supply all the activation signals required for T-cell proliferation.

It was first found in the early 1960s that both T cells and B cells are required to mount an antibody response against most protein antigens. Early experiments with irradiated mice showed that an antibody response to sheep red blood cells (SRBCs) could not be generated if only B cells were adoptively transferred just prior to antigenic challenge. If, however, thymic lymphocytes were also adoptively transferred prior to challenge, an effective primary response could be generated (Fig. 6-6). This was later confirmed in in vitro experiments using purified populations of splenic B and T cells.

Other early experiments with hapten-carrier conjugate antigens further defined the

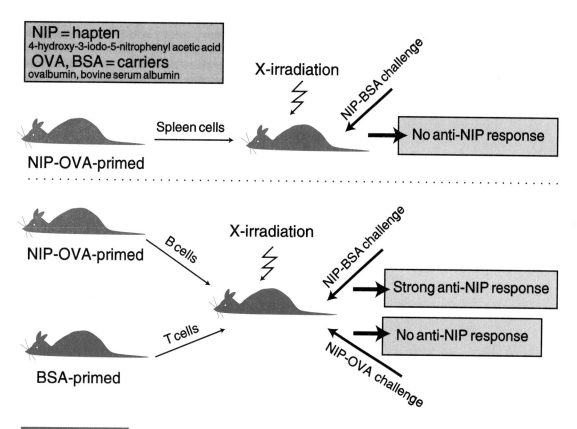

NIP = hapten
4-hydroxy-3-iodo-5-nitrophenyl acetic acid
OVA, BSA = carriers
ovalbumin, bovine serum albumin

Figure 6-6   *The hapten-carrier phenomenon.* Free haptens are not recognized by T cells and are therefore not immunogenic unless they are coupled to larger immunogenic proteins (carrier). The carrier induces T helper cells which will help hapten-specific B cells to produce antibodies provided the hapten is conjugated to the protein carrier used to prime the helper T cells. Lethally irradiated mice reconstituted with spleen from mice primed with the hapten-carrier conjugate NIP-OVA will not produce anti-NIP antibodies to a challenge with NIP-BSA. However, if T cells from mice primed with BSA are cotransferred with NIP-OVA-primed B cells, a strong antibody response will follow a NIP-BSA challenge but not a NIP-OVA challenge.

role of helper T cells in the humoral response. Haptens are small molecules (e.g., dinitrophenol [DNP]) that are not immunogenic on their own but can induce specific antibodies if they are conjugated to a protein-carrier molecule. It was found that this "carrier effect" phenomenon involves the interaction between carrier-specific T cells and hapten-specific B cells to generate hapten-specific antibody response. The response is dependent upon chemical coupling of the hapten to the carrier; i.e., the hapten and carrier cannot simply be coadministered. Furthermore, the interaction is MHC class II–restricted. (MHC restriction is described in detail in Chap. 7A.) These findings strongly suggested that antibody production is dependent on the physical interaction between T and B cells and that the antigen itself probably provides the bridge between the two cells (Fig. 6-7). The exact biochemical nature of the interaction between T and B cells that

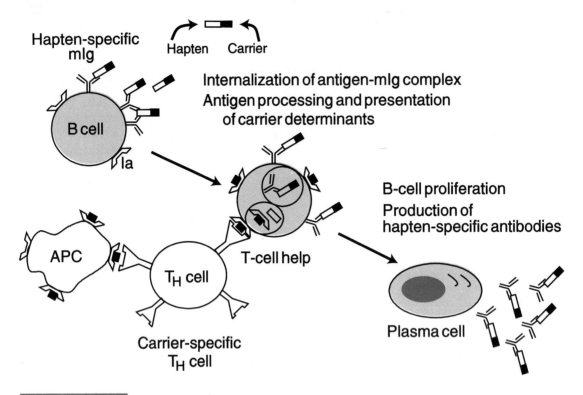

Figure 6-7   *Cellular interactions in responses to a hapten-carrier antigenic complex.* Hapten-carrier conjugates bind to the B-cell antigen receptor via the hapten portion, are internalized and processed, and carrier determinants are presented to carrier-specific T helper cells. Antigen can also be presented to T cells by other APCs, such as macrophages. T-cell help induces the production of hapten-specific antibodies.

leads to antibody production is largely unknown.

The B cell–T cell contact is additionally mediated by adhesion molecules. Adhesion molecules on both the B cell and T cell may bind ligands present on the reciprocal cell type. This can lead to activation and proliferation of either the B cell or T cell, inducing antigen-specific clonal proliferation (Fig. 6-7). Recently, it has been shown that efficient activation of T cells by antigen-presenting B cells requires adhesion of the CD11a (LFA-1) marker on T cells to the CD54 (ICAM-1) ligand present on B cells. This adhesion is likewise necessary for T cell–dependent B-cell proliferation and differentiation to the plasma cell state. A second important interaction occurs between the B-cell activation marker B7/BB1 and the CD28 T-cell signaling molecule, which appears to function as an accessory receptor in T-cell activation. Binding of CD28 on T cells that have already been activated by their T-cell receptor complex augments T-cell proliferation and stabilizes cytokine mRNAs transcribed by T cells.

Accessory signaling molecules are likewise present on B cells. For example, MHC class II molecules can also function as accessory molecules—they bind to the CD4 molecule on the surface of T cells. It has been suggested that cross-linking of MHC class II molecules during T cell–B cell interaction is by itself an activation signal for B cells. Cross-linkage of the MHC class II molecules induces the same second messengers as does cross-linking of the surface Ig molecules and also induces expression of B7/BB1 and CD40 activation markers on the cell surface.

T-INDEPENDENT ANTIGENS

Thymus-independent (TI) antigens, as the name implies, can stimulate antibody production in the absence of T-cell help. Athymic (nude) mice, which lack T cells (see Clinical Aside 3 in Chap. 7A) can therefore respond to TI antigens. TI antigens are generally polymeric sugars, usually bacterial products containing multiple identical antigenic determinants which can cross-link many adjacent Ig molecules on the surface of the B cell. This "built in" cross-linking capacity is probably the reason for their ability to stimulate specific B cells on their own. There are two types of TI antigens, TI-1 and TI-2. Perhaps the best definition of these two types came after the discovery of the CBA/N mouse, which carries the X-linked immunodeficiency gene. This mouse strain has about half the number of B cells as normal mice, and the B cells are phenotypically immature, as characterized by their high IgM/IgD ratio. These mice can mount an antibody response to some TI antigens, such as LPS at low, nonmitogenic doses, and to *Brucella abortus*, but they are completely incapable of responding to haptenated polysaccharides such as Ficoll (polysucrose) and dextran or pneumococcal polysaccharide. The former group is called TI-1 and the latter group is called TI-2. TI-2 antigens, unlike TI-1 antigens, cannot induce an antibody response in vitro if cultures are rigorously depleted of T cells.

The functional response to TI antigens is similar to a primary humoral response. Primarily, only IgM is secreted, of relatively low affinity for antigen, and there is no affinity maturation. Memory cells are rarely elicited in response to TI antigens.

It was first proposed that the responses to the two types of TI antigens are mediated by two distinct B-cell subpopulations representing two separate lineages. This theory was based on staining with a polyclonal antibody to an antigen designated Lyb-5. CBA/N mice had no detectable Lyb-5$^+$ B cells, and it was therefore suggested that the Lyb-5$^+$ B-cell subset is the only one capable of responding to TI-2 antigens. However, no one was able to produce a monoclonal antibody to Lyb-5, and thus studies of the elusive Lyb-5 marker have not been pursued. It is possible that Lyb-5 is an activation marker and Lyb-5$^+$ B cells are not found in CBA/N mice simply because the cells responding to TI-2 antigens cannot be activated in these mice.

MEMORY B CELLS

Secondary responses to most antigens are characterized by rapid production of high-affinity antibodies. They are elicited by much lower concentration of antigen and are mediated by memory (secondary) B cells. Secondary responses are dominated by high-affinity IgG and IgA antibodies. IgA is produced mainly by B cells residing in mucosal tissues such as the gut and the respiratory tract. Activation of memory B cells is also T cell–dependent and MHC-restricted.

Memory B cells and plasma cells arise in different microenviroments in secondary lymphoid organs. Most B cells are found in the B-cell areas of lymph nodes and spleen in primary follicles composed of dense colonies of resting B cells. After immunization, virgin B cells interact with T cells in the T-cell areas of the spleen and lymph nodes, and some of the B cells develop into antibody-secreting plasma cells, which then concentrate mainly in the outer periarteriolar sheaths. During the primary response to T-dependent antigens, virgin B cells responding to antigen stimulation initially proliferate in the T-dependent areas of the spleen and lymph nodes. IL-4 produced by helper T cells stimulates these activated B cells to express CD23, the low-affinity IgE Fc receptor. It has been suggested that CD23$^+$ B cells are then targeted to the follicles, where they proliferate to form a new germinal center. Targeting is likely due to CD23$^+$ B cells adhering to CD23$^+$ follicular dendritic cells.

Once antigen-antibody complexes become available, the secondary follicles containing proliferating B cells begin to form. These secondary follicles are called *germinal centers*. Germinal centers are the primary site for the formation of memory B cells; they do not contain plasma cells. They contain a unique cell type called *follicular dendritic cells (FDCs)*, which are thought to play a major role in the generation of memory B cells. FDCs are different from other macrophages and dendritic cells, which are found mainly in the T-cell area. FDC are of non-bone marrow origin; they are nonphagocytic; they express high levels of the FcγR and the complement receptors CR1 and CR2; and they have many processes which come in close contact with the surrounding B cells. Complement receptors on FDCs bind antigen-antibody complexes, and probably play a critical role in the development of memory B cells. Antigen-antibody complexes can be found bound to FDC processes for a very long time. This is thought to be responsible for the maintenance of memory B cells. Further evidence to suggest that antigen-antibody complexes are important for the maintenance of B-cell memory is the fact that cobra venom, which inactivates complement, prevents the generation of memory B cells. On the other hand, mice injected with preformed antigen-antibody complexes generate memory B cells much faster than mice immunized with antigen alone. Germinal centers are not formed in athymic mice, but it is not clear how the formation of germinal centers is dependent upon T cells.

During differentiation in germinal centers B cells acquire the memory cell phenotype which is characterized by the expression of high levels of MHC class II, CD21, and CD45 and lower IgM/IgD ratio. Some memory B cells may express other isotypes of surface Ig. They also start to express high levels of CD22, which is thought to be an accessory molecule which enhances signal transduction by the B-cell antigen receptor. Memory B cells then exit the germinal center through the marginal zone and enter the recirculating pool.

A major question in B-cell differentiation is what determines whether an antigen-primed B cell will further differentiate into an antibody-secreting plasma cell or instead enter the memory B-cell pool. Probably the most widely accepted theory is that only the microenvironment within the spleen or lymph nodes, and the presence or absence of different lymphokines, determine whether an activated B cell will become a memory cell or an antibody-secreting cell. Another theory is that memory cells and primary antibody-forming cells arise from a distinct B-cell lineage, which is programmed prior to antigenic stimulation to give rise to either memory or plasma cells. This theory is based on a few interesting experimental findings. The first is the fact that certain antigens only elicit memory cells following primary immunization. For example, in most mouse strains, phosphocholine and the Thy-1 antigen do not induce antibody responses after primary immunization; however, secondary challenge generates a normal IgG response. This indicates that memory B cells were primed during the first challenge, even though no plasma cells were induced. More recent

TABLE 6-2   Characteristics of Virgin and Memory B Cells

	Virgin B Cells	Memory B Cells
SURFACE MARKERS		
sIg Classes	IgM, IgD	IgM, IgD, IgA, IgG, IgE
mIg Level		Decreased
mIg, sIg V genes	Germ line	Mutated
J11d (HSA)	High	Low
CD21 (CR2)	Low	High
MHC class II		Increased
Affinity of Ig	Low	High
Recirculation	No	Yes
REQUIREMENTS FOR ACTIVATION		
T Dependence	High	Low
[Ag] Requirements	High	Low

experiments showed that enriched populations of B cells that differentially express high and low levels of the heat-stable antigen (HSA, defined by the monoclonal antibody J11d) had the potential to differentiate either into memory or plasma cells when adoptively transferred into SCID mice prior to antigenic challenge. Secondary responses were associated with B cells expressing low levels of surface HSA, whereas transfer of B cells expressing high levels of HSA resulted in primary antibody response but no memory induction. Cell surface markers characteristic of memory B cells are summarized in Table 6-2.

THE ROLE OF CYTOKINES IN B-CELL DEVELOPMENT AND ACTIVATION

The term *cytokines* is a general name for soluble factors that can transduce various signals to other cells bearing the appropriate receptor. They are secreted mainly (but not exclusively) by cells of hemopoietic origin. Some are growth or differentiation factors, some are chemotactic factors, and some are inhibitory factors. The nomenclature in this area is somewhat confusing, and for historical reasons the same cytokine is often referred to by different names. In this chapter we will refer to lymphokines, monokines, growth factors, interleukins, and interferons by the general name cytokines. Cytokines are discussed in more detail in Chap. 10.

B cells acquire surface receptors for different cytokines during development, and also as a consequence of activation. These cytokine receptors are typically composed of a ligand-binding domain, a signal-transducer region, an effector domain, and a regulatory unit. The majority of cytokines that activate B cells are secreted by T helper cells and macrophages. T helper cells are functionally divided into two groups in the mouse: T_H1 and T_H2; however, human T helper cells cannot always be unambiguously classified into these two groups (see Chap. 7B). T_H1 cells secrete

IL-2, IFN-γ, TNF-α, and lymphotoxin. They are typically induced in delayed-type hypersensitivity reactions. T_H2 cells secrete IL-4, IL-5, and IL-6, which are the most important cytokines in the induction of humoral immunity. An overview of the most important cytokines in B-cell signaling is presented in Fig. 6-8.

Different cytokines act at different stages along the B-cell differentiation pathway. During early B-cell development, the major cytokines known to act in lymphopoiesis are IL-3, IL-4, and IL-7. Both IL-3 and IL-4 are known to play a role in signaling early lymphoid precursors; however, the exact effects of these lymphokines are unclear. Because it is arduous to maintain early lymphoid stem cells in culture, it is difficult to study the effects of individual lymphokines on these cells. In contrast, the role of IL-7, which stimulates pre-B cells at a stage prior to surface expression of IgM, has been well studied. IL-7 is produced by bone marrow stromal cells. It was isolated from long-term in vitro cultures of mouse bone marrow after it was found that factors produced by the stromal cells which arose in these cultures supported pre-B-cell growth. IL-7 induces pre-B cells to proliferate in vitro, but there is no evidence that it can stimulate pre-B cells to differentiate. Once pre-B cells express surface Ig, they are no longer stimulated to proliferate by IL-7. IL-7 also causes early thymocytes to proliferate. The IL-7 receptor is a B-cell surface marker of differentiation. It is a transmembrane protein which forms non-covalently bound homodimers. After binding of IL-7 to the receptor, protein tyrosine phosphorylation and inositol phospholipid turnover are induced; however, the IL-7 receptor does not have intrinsic protein kinase activity. This suggests that additional proteins, which have yet to be identified, are involved in IL-7 signaling. The IL-7 receptor is also found on bone marrow stromal cells, the only cell type known to produce IL-7. There is some evidence to suggest that IL-7 acts in an autocrine fashion on these cells, stimulating its own production.

Steel factor, the ligand of the tyrosine

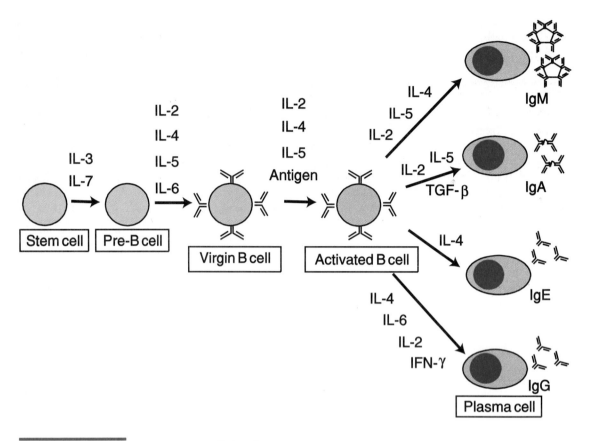

Figure 6-8   Cytokine action on B-cell development.

kinase receptor c-*kit* (which is expressed in hematopoietic stem cells), is another cytokine produced by bone marrow stromal cells. *Steel* factor appears to synergize with IL-7 at stimulating pre-B-cell growth in vitro; however, whether it actually has a role in B lymphopoiesis is not known. Long-term mouse bone marrow cultures and stromal cell lines cloned from these cultures have been instrumental in the study of pre-B cells and in the isolation of factors that act on pre-B cells.

IL-4 has many different effects on B cells, including activation, proliferation, and differentiation. It is secreted by T helper cells, particularly the T_H2 subset, and by mast cells. IL-4 can induce resting B cells to increase surface expression of MHC class II molecules and the coordinately regulated activation marker CD40, and induce expression of the adhesion molecule ICAM-1 (CD54) and the

IgE Fc receptor (CD23). IL-4 can stimulate activated B cells to proliferate and differentiate into IgM-secreting plasma cells. It is also costimulatory with low concentrations of either protein antigen or anti-immunoglobulin, inducing resting B cells to enter the G_1 phase of the cell cycle. IL-4 has also been shown to influence class switching. When added to antibody-secreting murine B cells in vitro, IL-4 induces preferential secretion of IgG1 and IgE, and suppresses secretion of IgG2b and IgG3. It is the only lymphokine capable of inducing isotype switching to IgE production, and it also induces expression of IgE Fc receptor on B cells and monocytes. IL-4 induces mast cell growth and stimulates activated mast cells to increase production of IL-4. Because of the central role that IL-4 may play in allergic responses, much research is currently being directed toward producing therapeutic regulators of IL-4 as a means of modulating allergic responses.

IL-2 and IL-5 act at the G_2 phase of the cell cycle, stimulating B cells that have already been activated to divide. IL-2 is instrumental in the induction of T-cell growth. Its role as a B-cell stimulatory agent is relatively minor; however, at high concentrations, it induces human B cells to proliferate and differentiate. IL-2 is known to synergize with IL-4 and IL-5 to promote murine B-cell growth in the response to T-dependent antigens. When added to in vitro cultures of human B cells that have been stimulated with polyclonal activators, IL-2 causes B cells to secrete high levels of antibody, particularly of the IgM and IgA isotypes, as well as low levels of IgG1.

IL-5 is another multifunctional cytokine secreted by cells of the T_H2 subset. Its main effect is the promotion of growth of activated B cells and eosinophils. IL-5 causes both B cells and T cells to up-regulate surface expression of IL-2 receptors; hence it has a key role in T-dependent antigen responses. In conjunction with IL-2, IL-5 also stimulates differentiation of cytotoxic T cells. IL-5 induces activated B cells to secrete IgM antibody, and can induce isotype switching to IgA. Because of its preferential induction of IgA class switching, it has been proposed that IL-5, along with other cytokines (e.g., TGF-β, which also induces IgA production), may be particularly important in secretory mucosal immunity.

The receptors for both IL-2 and IL-5 are heterodimeric, each being composed of an α and β subunit. The α subunits contain the primary cytokine-binding domains; the signal transduction domains are found in the β subunits, which are also necessary for high-affinity cytokine binding. The β subunit of the IL-5 receptor is also shared by the receptors for the cytokines IL-3 and GM-CSF. Each of these receptors has distinct α subunits. However, since the signaling domains are all the same, it has been proposed that crosstalk between the receptors may occur during signal transduction by one or more of the cytokines.

IL-6, or B-cell differentiation factor, is not stimulatory for resting B cells, but is known to act in the late stages of B-cell activation, inducing differentiation to the immunoglobulin-secreting plasma cell stage. Accordingly, the receptor for IL-6 is a marker of B-cell activation, not present on resting B cells. IL-6 is secreted by a wide variety of cell types, including both T and B cells, and macrophages and monocytes. It has pleiotropic action on many different cell types. It induces differentiation of macrophages and has multicolony stimulating activity on hematopoietic stem cells. IL-6 is costimulatory for both helper and cytotoxic T cells. It also induces IL-2 production by T cells. Monocytes constitutively express IL-6, and T_H2 cells secrete IL-6 upon activation in vitro. IL-6 is particularly associated with secretion of antibodies of the IgG isotype.

There have been a number of associations of IL-6 overproduction with both polyclonal B-cell abnormalities and autoimmune diseases. IL-6 was initially associated with cardiac myxoma, a benign heart tumor, which when surgically removed and cultured, produces high levels of IL-6 in vitro. Subsequently, patients with Castleman's disease, characterized by chronic hypergammaglobulinemia and lymph node hyperplasia, were shown to produce high levels of IL-6, and these patients greatly improved after surgical removal of affected lymph nodes. Cells in the germinal center of these lymph nodes constitutively overproduced IL-6. IL-6 overproduction has also been described in rheumatoid arthritis and uterine cervical carcinoma. Additionally, IL-6 has been shown to act as a growth factor for various lymphoid malignancies, including human multiple myelomas, Lennert's T lymphoma, and murine plasmacytomas.

The effects of cytokine signaling of B cells are pleiotropic (Table 6-3). Many cytokines have overlapping activities, and can act on a number of cell types. It is interesting to speculate on how different cytokines can produce similar effects, or, conversely, how a single cytokine can induce many different effects. To this end, much research is currently being

TABLE 6-3 IL-4, IL-5, IL-6, and IL-7

IL-4	IL-5	IL-6	IL-7
ACTIVITIES			
Induction of IgG$_1$ and IgE, and suppression of IgG2b in LPS blasts Induction of Ia Induces anti-μ-stimulated B cells to proliferate Induction of CD23 (FcεRII) Growth induction of early lymphoid precursors, T cells, mast cells homology to GM-CSF	Induces activated B cells to proliferate Induces Ig secretion in primed B cells Induction of IgA in LPS blasts Induction of IL-2R on B and T cells Induces eosinophil maturation Cytotoxic T-cell induction with IL-2 Homology to IL-3	Induces Ig secretion in activated B cells and B lymphoblasts Growth factor for plasmacytomas, hybridomas, human multiple myelomas Induces IL-2 production in T cells Cytotoxic T-cell induction with IL-2 Costimulatory for T-cell growth Multi-CSF activity Induces maturation of macrophages, neural cells Induction of acute-phase proteins in liver cells	Induces proliferation of large B-cell progenitors and pre-B cells Induces proliferation of early thymocytes IL-7R is a pre-B-cell differentiation marker, also present on some thymocytes, macrophages, and bone marrow stromal cells Autocrine regulation of stromal cell IL-7 production
SECRETED BY			
T cells (T$_H$2), mast cells	T cells (T$_H$2)	T and B cells, monocytes, fibroblasts, endothelial cells, keratinocytes	Bone marrow stromal cells

conducted to identify secondary binding units that act in signal transduction by different cytokine receptors. Perhaps multiple binding units are stimulated by signaling of a single receptor, each promoting different effector activities. Alternatively, signaling of different receptors may induce intracellular activation of common signal transduction pathways. Finally, it is important to keep in mind that during an immune response, an intercellular network of cytokine activity is created. Such networks exist at all times for regulation of hematopoiesis and for maintaining a homeostatic balance of the immune system.

B-CELL TOLERANCE

Immunologic tolerance is a state of specific unresponsiveness to an antigen. B-cell tolerance represents the inability to produce antibodies to a specific antigen. The mechanism by which B cells develop tolerance to self-antigens is a question first pondered by Ehrlich, in 1901, during his early experiments on the rapid lysis of erythrocytes by allogeneic and xenogeneic antisera. From these experiments, he theorized that the immune response to self is potentially more dangerous to the individual than all exogenous injuries and therefore there must be a mechanism by which lymphocytes develop tolerance to self-antigens. In this section we will deal with two types of tolerance: (1) self-tolerance and (2) induced tolerance, in the B-cell compartment, to exogenous antigens. It should be emphasized that although the mechanisms for induction of tolerance in B and T cells are different, B-cell tolerance cannot be dealt with without considering T-cell tolerance. As discussed earlier, the humoral response to most antigens is T cell–dependent, and therefore causing T cells to become tolerant to a particular antigen will also result in the lack of antibody responses to that antigen without any involvement of B-cell tolerance. T-cell tolerance is discussed in Chap. 7B.

Neonatal Tolerance

Very early on it was realized that it is relatively easy to induce tolerance to allogeneic cells at the neonatal stage. Allogeneic lymphocytes injected in large doses into newborn animals induce what is called *neonatal tolerance* to the MHC type of the donor lymphocytes. On the other hand, neonatal tolerance to exogenous proteins such as foreign serum proteins is not readily induced, and it is usually transient and incomplete. It is not clear why the neonatal stage is more receptive to induction of tolerance, but it is plausible that engagement of the Ig receptor at a very early stage of differentiation results in inactivation of the B cells. This can be mimicked by cross-linking the Ig receptor with antibodies. Indeed, mice injected continuously from birth with anti-μ antibodies mature without B cells and remain completely devoid of B cells as long as the levels of anti-μ antibodies stay above a certain threshold. It is crucial, however, to start administration of the anti-μ antibodies within 48 h of birth. Later administration does not result in depletion of B cells. Similar results have also been obtained in vitro. The addition of anti-μ antibodies to cultures containing mature B cells results in capping, internalization, and reexpression of free surface Ig. In contrast, neonatal spleen cells treated with anti-μ antibodies do not reexpress surface Ig molecules.

In the case of neonatal tolerance to allogeneic MHC antigens, the mechanism is most probably due to the establishment of partial chimerism. The allogeneic cells persist in the host, together with the host's normal lymphocytes, and both cell types are seen as self.

Induction of Tolerance in the Adult

It was first discovered three decades ago that deaggregated proteins are very potent inducers of tolerance (tolerogens) for both B and T cells. (Deaggregation of protein solutions is achieved by ultracentrifugation.) The best studied example is human γ-globulin. The aggregated form of human γ-globulin is a very strong immunogen when injected on its own or emulsified in complete Freund's adjuvant (CFA). However, even high doses of the deaggregated form induce a state of complete unresponsiveness to the immunogenic form of human γ-globulin. Tolerance is established in both B cells and T cells. This state of unresponsiveness is transient and may depend on the continuous presence of the tolerogen.

The mechanism for this type of tolerance is unknown; however, it can be readily explained by the two-signal theory discussed earlier. Since the deaggregated proteins also induce tolerance in T cells (see Chap. 7B), there is no T-cell help available for B cells. According to the two-signal theory, priming of B cells in the absence of T-cell help will result in B-cell paralysis or clonal anergy rather than activation. Memory cells, which also require T-cell help, are also susceptible to induction of unresponsiveness with deaggregated proteins, although a higher dose of the tolerogen is required.

Supportive evidence for the two-signal theory as the mechanism for induction of unresponsiveness came from experiments with TI antigens. As mentioned earlier, these antigens do not prime T cells, and only induce IgM responses without inducing memory B cells. It was found that the TI antigen DNP-pneumococcal polysaccharide will induce unresponsiveness to DNP in mice previously primed with DNP-BSA (bovine serum albumin). According to the two-signal theory, this is due to the activation of DNP-specific *memory* B cells in the absence of T-cell help, which is not induced by the TI antigen.

Acquisition of Self-Tolerance

Our current understanding of the mechanisms involved in the induction of self-tolerance have been greatly aided by recent advances in transgenic mouse technology. The frequency of a particular B-cell clone, especially in an unprimed host, is very low. Therefore, it has been very difficult to study the fate of B cells made unresponsive to a certain antigen in vivo. Transgenic mice carrying rearranged immunoglobulin transgenes were one of the first transgenic models to be developed because the transcriptional control regions for immunoglobulin genes have been well characterized, allowing for tissue-specific expression of the transgene (only in B cells). Not only was lymphoid-specific expression obtained, but as a consequence of expressing the rearranged immunoglobulin transgene in lymphocytes, it was found that endogenous immunoglobulin gene rearrangement was inhibited. This important finding was conclusive evidence in support of the theory of allelic exclusion. It effectively demonstrated that surface expression of immunoglobulin signals the B cell to halt further immunoglobulin gene rearrangement via a negative-feedback mechanism. A second application of the experiment was suggested by the fact that the majority of lymphocytes developed in these Ig-transgenic mice were of a single antigenic specificity coded for by the transgene. The question was soon posed, what happens to B cells in Ig-transgenic mice in which the rearranged Ig transgene is specific for a self-antigen?

Studies in different transgenic mouse models have so far revealed three distinct mechanisms that play a role in the establishment of self-tolerance in the B-cell compartment (Fig. 6-9):

1. Self-reactive cells may become functionally inactivated, a process termed *clonal anergy*.
2. The self-reactive cells may persist in the periphery fully immunocompetent but without causing any harm to the host, a phenomenon termed *clonal ignorance*.
3. Self-reactive B cells may be physically eliminated in the periphery, a process termed *clonal deletion* or *clonal abortion*.

The first two mechanisms were demonstrated in double transgenic mice that expressed two transgenes, one of which encoded a functionally rearranged immunoglobulin with antigen specificity for hen egg

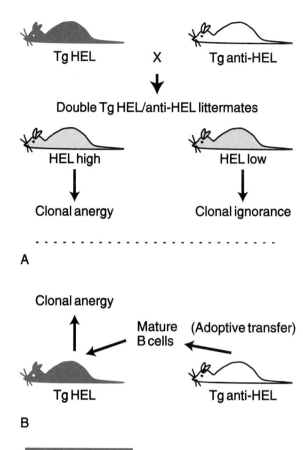

Figure 6-9 *B-cell tolerance manifested as clonal anergy and clonal ignorance.* Transgenic mice expressing hen egg lysozyme (Tg HEL) were mated to transgenic mice expressing a rearranged, HEL-specific Ig gene (Tg anti-HEL). Double transgenic mice secreting high levels of HEL exhibited clonal anergy. Double transgenic littermates that secreted lower levels of HEL exhibited clonal ignorance (*a*). Clonal anergy is also induced when mature B cells from anti-HEL Ig-transgenic mice were adoptively transferred into HEL-transgenic mice (*b*).

tibody expressed surface IgM and surface IgD specific for HEL. Several lines of HEL-transgenic mice secreting various levels of HEL were obtained. B cells in double transgenic mice secreting high levels of HEL were profoundly anergic and did not respond to immunization with HEL in the presence or absence of T-cell help. In contrast, B cells in double transgenic mice secreting low levels of HEL exhibited clonal ignorance (Fig. 6-9a). Many other examples of clonal ignorance were demonstrated when the self-antigen was present at low concentration including thyroglobulin, insulin, growth hormone, and even soluble H-2 molecules.

When clonal anergy was induced, the anergic B cells were found to express 20-fold less surface IgM than B cells in the single anti-HEL transgenic animals. Levels of surface IgD remained unchanged, but signaling through the IgD receptor with anti-IgD antibody–dextran conjugates was greatly diminished. The anergic cells failed to respond to TI antigens such as low-dose LPS, and even responses to T-dependent immunogenic conjugates of HEL in the presence of T-cell help were greatly reduced. The state of anergy was long-lasting but not irreversible. When anergic cells were transferred into nontransgenic normal mice, they recovered expression of IgM within 10 days but could not respond to an antigenic form of HEL. Moreover, in vitro stimulation of anergic cells with mitogenic doses of LPS (stimulation with LPS is independent of surface IG expression) induced proliferation to the same degree as normal B cells, but antibody secretion remained marginal for several days. If the HEL was present in the culture, antibody secretion was completely abolished. In the absence of HEL, the cells regained expression of IgM and gradually started to secrete anti-HEL antibodies.

The fact that the B cells in which tolerance has been induced can recover after a certain number of cell divisions led to speculation that a long-lived transcriptional repressor is induced by tolerance-inducing signals, and can be inactivated or diluted by mitosis. Some support for this theory came

lysozyme (HEL) and the second of which encoded a secreted form of the HEL antigen. These mice were generated by mating two transgenic parents, one carrying the transgene for HEL (Tg HEL) and the other the transgene for an antibody specific for HEL (Tg anti-HEL). Almost 90 percent of the B cells in mice transgenic for the anti-HEL an-

from experiments in which LPS-activated B cells were cultured in vitro in the presence of anti-Ig antibodies. This resulted in profound down-regulation of expression of heavy and light chains, similar to what occurs when anergy is induced in vivo. This down-regulation was dependent upon both RNA and protein synthesis, which suggests the involvement of a newly synthesized protein (repressor).

Clonal anergy was observed in a few other transgenic mouse models. For example, anti-single-stranded DNA (ssDNA) transgenic mice contain large numbers of anti-ssDNA-binding B cells, but these cells do not produce anti-ssDNA antibodies. Interestingly, no decrease in surface IgM levels was found in these mice, which suggests that anergy can be induced by mechanisms other than modulation of the surface Ig receptor.

The experimental data described above dealt with tolerance induction to a self-antigen present before the onset and during the development of the B-cell lineage. A major question remained as to whether tolerance could be induced in mature B cells in an environment where the self-antigen is expressed at high levels. This was answered in a simple experiment utilizing the same set of transgenic mice. Mature B cells from anti-HEL Ig-transgenic mice were adoptively transferred into adult HEL-transgenic animals. The transferred B cells rapidly became anergic and down-regulated the expression of surface IgM (Fig. 6-9b). This experiment elegantly demonstrated that mature B cells are also susceptible to induction of tolerance.

The third mechanism, clonal elimination or clonal deletion, was recently demonstrated in a different transgenic mouse model. Mice were made transgenic to a functionally rearranged immunoglobulin gene encoding an antibody specific for an epitope present on the MHC class I H-2K^k and H-2K^b molecules. When the transgene was expressed in H-2K^k mice, no B cells carrying the transgene could be detected in spleen, lymph nodes, or bone marrow, and the total number of peripheral B cells was markedly reduced. In contrast, when the same Ig transgene was expressed in control H-2^d mice, normal numbers of B cells were found, the majority of which expressed high levels of the transgene (Fig. 6-10).

What are the mechanisms controlling induction of clonal anergy versus clonal elimination? One possibility is the form of the tolerogen encountered by B cells. A crucial difference between the two transgenic models is that in the HEL model, the tolerance-inducing antigen is presented in a soluble form, whereas in the MHC class I model the antigen is membrane-bound. An experiment designed to test this difference used double transgenic mice expressing the anti-HEL Ig transgene and membrane-bound HEL rather than soluble HEL. In this case complete clonal elimination was observed, in contrast to the clonal anergy or clonal ignorance seen with soluble HEL.

Proposed mechanisms to account for the clonal deletion of self-reactive B cells include induction of apoptosis, or programmed cell death, by inappropriate signaling of the receptor in immature cells. Alternatively, receptor signaling of immature cells may render the cells incapable of responding to normal differentiation signals, resulting in cell death. These theories have been indirectly supported by recent evidence that demonstrates that the pre-B cell surface μ complex undergoes signal transduction by a pathway distinct from surface Ig signaling of mature B cells.

Thus the fate of autoreactive B cells appears to be dependent upon the degree and type of receptor signaling by the autoantigen, the stage of B-cell development in which signaling occurs, and the presence of costimulatory agents during signaling. The clinical relevance of the fate of self-reactive cells is manifested in the complexity of autoimmune disorders. Autoantibody secretion in different autoimmune disorders may arise by the breakdown of tolerance of anergic B-cell clones or by expansion of clones that exhibit clonal ignorance. Also, the presence of autoreactive T-cell clones may further disrupt the regulation of tolerance induction or inactivation of autoreactive B cell clones, pos-

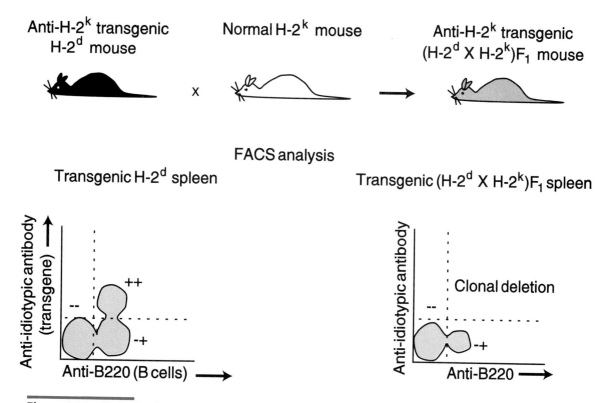

Figure 6-10   *B-Cell tolerance manifested as clonal deletion.* Transgenic mice of the H-2^d haplotype that express a rearranged Ig transgene with specificity for H-2^k were mated to normal H-2^k mice, generating H-2$^{d/k}$ mice expressing an anti-H-2^k Ig transgene. These mice exhibited clonal deletion of B cells that expressed the Ig transgene, as evidenced by fluorescence activated cell sorter (FACS) analysis of spleen cells. In control H-2^d mice carrying the transgene, about half of the B cells in the spleen were positive for the Ig transgene as illustrated by double stainings with an anti-idiotypic antibody specific for the Ig transgene, and antibodies specific for B220, a marker expressed on all B cells. In contrast, in H-2$^{d/k}$ transgenic mice, few B cells were found in the spleen, and none of these cells expressed the transgene.

sibly leading to the cycles of dysregulation seen in chronic autoimmune syndromes.

CD5 B CELLS

A small subset of B cells in both mice and humans bear the CD5 (Ly-1) cell surface marker which was first described as a T-cell marker present on most T cells. These CD5$^+$ B cells have been associated with autoanti-

body production. It was later found on an occasional human B cell tumor and on appreciable numbers of splenic B cells of the mutant autoimmune NZB mouse strain. Subsequently, CD5$^+$ B cells were found in neonatal spleen and in the adult peritoneum of normal mice. CD5 has no known function, and its presence on B cells secreting autoantibodies might very well be coincidental. It has been hypothesized that CD5$^+$ B cells are derived from a distinct lineage.

This is largely based on the fact that CD5$^+$ B cells will develop in lethally irradiated mice reconstituted with neonatal bone marrow or fetal liver, but not in mice reconstituted with adult bone marrow. This suggests that CD5$^+$ cells may arise from a distinct lineage, the precursors of which are only present in fetal bone marrow and fetal liver. Opponents of this theory suggest that CD5$^+$ B cells represent a distinct activation stage of normal B lymphocytes.

ADDITIONAL READINGS

Clark EA, Lane PJL. Regulation of human B-cell activation and adhesion. *Annu Rev Immunol.* 1991;9:97.

Desiderio SV. B cell activation. *Curr Opin Immunol.* 1992;4:252.

Goodnow CC. Transgenic mice and analysis of B cell tolerance. *Annu Rev Immunol.* 1992;10:489.

Kincade PW, et al. Cells and molecules that regulate B lymphopoiesis in bone marrow. *Annu Rev Immunol.* 1989;7:111.

Linton PJ, Klinman NR. The generation of memory B cells. *Semin Immunol.* 1992;4:3.

Osmond DG. B cell development in the bone marrow. *Semin Immunol.* 1990;2:173.

Reth M. Antigen receptors on B lymphocytes. *Annu Rev Immunol.* 1992;10:97.

Rolink A, Melchers F. Molecular and cellular origins of B lymphocyte diversity. *Cell.* 1991;66:1081.

Ontogeny and Differentiation of T Lymphocytes

A. T-Cell Development

INTRODUCTION

T lymphocytes (T cells) derive their name from the organ in which they differentiate—the thymus. T-cell progenitors develop from pluripotential stem cells in the bone marrow and enter the thymus where they undergo several steps of differentiation before they acquire immunocompetence. Mature peripheral T cells are responsible for the majority of specific cellular immune responses such as the provision of "help" signals to B cells (the production of most antibody isotypes by B cells is dependent upon T-cell help), cell-mediated cytotoxicity, delayed-type hypersensitivity, and the secretion of various lymphokines. The hallmark of T-cell reactivity is the unique pattern of antigen recognition by the T cell receptor (TCR). Unlike the antigen receptor on B cells (membrane-bound antibody), which can recognize free antigen on its own, T cells can only recognize antigen in association with major histocompatibility complex (MHC) antigens presented on the surface of cells called antigen presenting cells (APCs). Moreover, T cells in a particular individual can only recognize foreign antigens in the context of the MHC antigens they encounter in the thymus during their differentiation. This phenomenon is known as *MHC restriction*, and it implies that during T-cell differentiation in the thymus, cells undergo a process of "education" (now called positive selection), in which only T cells capable of recognizing self-MHC antigens are allowed to mature and exit the thymus. Even before the discovery of T-cell restriction, it was realized that most thymocytes never exit the thymus to the periphery. This finding suggested the existence of a negative selection process in which T cells recognizing self-antigens are deleted from the T-cell pool. Recently, using TCR transgenic mice and newly developed TCR-specific monoclonal antibodies, the positive and negative selection processes have been elegantly shown to be a part of the normal differentiation pathway of T cells in the thymus.

In this chapter, we will discuss in some detail the major events in T-cell differentiation in the thymus, T-cell restriction, acquisition of the T-cell repertoire, and T-cell selection.

T-CELL DEVELOPMENT

All blood cells, including lymphocytes, are derived from hematopoietic stem cells which themselves originate from embryonal mesenchymal cells. During embryogenesis, hematopoietic stem cells are first found in the yolk sac and then in fetal liver and spleen. After birth, stem cells in mammals are restricted to the bone marrow; in certain species, such as rodents, they are also found in the spleen. The development of lineage-specific (or committed) stem cells from pluripotential hematopoietic stem cells is still a black box. It is not clear what governs the differentiation of an early stem cell into a lineage-committed stem cell, nor is it known how many intermediate stages exist in this developmental process. It is estimated that only 0.1 percent of bone marrow cells are "T cell committed" stem cells. These cells express low amounts of the Thy-1 marker, a pan-T cell–specific marker (also expressed in the brain), but it is not known how many of these cells migrate to the thymus on a daily basis or how many are required to generate the full T-cell compartment. Interestingly, it was shown that in vitro a single stem cell can reconstitute all four subsets of thymocytes (see below) in fetal thymus organ cultures.

Anatomy of the Thymus

The thymus develops early in embryogenesis (starting at the sixth week of gestation in the human) from the third and fourth pharyngeal pouches. In the human, the thymic rudiment is formed mainly from the endoderm of the third pouch and the mesenchymal cells that surround the primitive gut. The thymic rudiment descends into the anterior mediastinum and anchors itself under the sternum. (The pharyngeal pouches are paired, and therefore the thymus develops as a bilobate organ.) T-cell precursors start to enter the human thymus via the bloodstream around week 12 of gestation (day 11–12 in the mouse) and contribute in an unknown way to the final development of the organ. In congenital diseases that affect lymphoid stem cells but not the thymus itself, the thymus remains undeveloped.

Each thymic lobe is encapsulated by a membrane that also forms inner partitions (septa) dividing the thymus into lobules. Each lobule consists of two histologically distinct regions—the peripheral cortex and the inner medulla (Fig. 7A-1). The cortex is densely populated with lymphocytes, and it therefore stains darkly with hematoxylin. In infants, the cortex comprises 80 to 90 percent of the thymic volume, but it gradually shrinks in size with age and only comprises a thin ring on the perimeter of the adult thymus. A similar histologic picture is also seen in young individuals subjected to stress or corticosteroid treatment.

The medulla contains far fewer lymphocytes; other cell types such as macrophages and dendritic cells are more apparent. The predominant cells in the medulla are epithelial cells which form a spongelike structure filled with lymphocytes; in humans, but not in mice, some of the epithelial cells also form concentric cystic structures called *Hassall's corpuscles*, the function of which, if any, is

not known. Bone marrow–derived macrophages and dendritic cells are also abundant in the corticomedullary junction, and, as will be discussed later, they play a central role in thymic selection.

T-cell precursors enter the thymic cortex via the bloodstream and move to the medulla as they mature. Mature, immunocompetent thymocytes, which are more resistant to corticosteroids and phenotypically resemble peripheral T cells (see below), reside in the medulla from where they exit the thymus.

Thymus-Dependent T-Cell Differentiation

The importance of the thymus in T-cell differentiation was discovered in the early sixties when the effects of thymectomy on the immune system were first investigated. It was clearly demonstrated that neonatal thymectomy in mice resulted in the virtual absence of T cells in all lymphoid organs. Similarly, congenital athymia (see Clinical Aside 7A-1) in various species—DiGeorge and Nezelof syndromes in humans and the *nu/nu* mutation in rodents (the "nude" phenotype)—is characterized by the absence of T cells, but not B cells, in the periphery. However, the effect of neonatal thymectomy varies between species; in humans, for example, an appreciable number of T cells exit the thymus before birth, so the effect of neonatal thymectomy is much less dramatic. (In the past, in some heart surgery operations in newborns, the thymus was removed to allow better access to the heart.) In mice, neonatal thymectomy has a more profound effect; however, some T cells do mature and enter

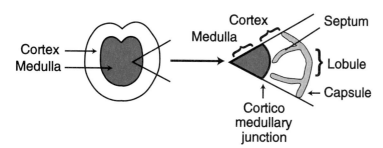

Figure 7A-1. Schematic drawing of a mammalian thymus.

the circulation before birth. Perhaps the most compelling evidence for the importance of the thymus for production of T cells came from experiments with lethally irradiated, thymectomized mice reconstituted with T cell–depleted bone marrow cells (TXBM mice). In such mice the possible entry of cells into the circulation before the removal of the thymus is overcome by the lethal irradiation which depletes the vast majority of lymphoid cells. The effect of thymectomy on mature T-cell depletion is therefore demonstrated better in TXBM mice—they are more consistently devoid of T cells.

Clinical Aside 7A-1
Immunodeficiencies due to Abnormal Development of the Thymus

Two syndromes in the human involve an underdeveloped or missing thymus (see also Chap. 22). The better-characterized one was discovered in 1965 by Angelo DiGeorge. Children with the DiGeorge syndrome usually suffer from opportunistic viral and fungal infections such as cutaneous candidiasis, severe varicella, progressive vaccinia, and *Pneumocystis carinii* pneumonia due to paucity or complete absence of T cells. This syndrome is the result of dysmorphogenesis of the third and fourth pharyngeal pouches which leads to aplasia or hypoplasia of the parathyroid glands and the thymus. It is also characterized by anomalies of other structures derived from the third and fourth pharyngeal pouches: right-sided aortic arch, congenital heart disease, esophageal atresia, bifid uvula, a short philtrum of the upper lip, an antimongoloid slant to the eyes, and low-set ears. The syndrome is not inherited and is probably the result of intrauterine damage to the region of the third and fourth pharyngeal pouches during the first 12 weeks of gestation. It is important to note that the thymic development is not uniformly affected in all cases. Some children with DiGeorge syndrome do not exhibit an obvious immunodeficiency, and in such cases the thymus is at least partially developed.

Nezelof syndrome is a rare inherited trait (an autosomal-recessive pattern was suggested in most cases and an X-linked pattern in others), and children with this syndrome have an undeveloped, embryolike thymus which is incapable of supporting normal T-cell differentiation. They also suffer from opportunistic infections much like most children with DiGeorge syndrome.

By far the best characterized congenital athymia is the recessive *nu/nu* genotype in the mouse and rat. This hairless phenotype (not to be confused with the euthymic "hairless" mouse phenotype) was discovered in 1966 in a mouse colony in Scotland. Once it was realized that this hairless phenotype was also athymic, the *nu* gene was bred into many inbred strains of mice to enable scientists to thoroughly study the role of the thymus in the immune response. Whether the same gene is responsible for both the lack of hair and the thymus is still a mystery. Although euthymic *nu/nu* mice can be found in a *nu/nu* colony, no athymic hairy mice have ever been reported, which is consistent with the presence of one gene or two unusually tightly linked genes. The *nu/nu* mouse has been the subject of many studies concerning immune surveillance, graft rejection, and other T-cell dominated immune responses. The nude mouse has also served as a model for studying the possible existence of a thymic-independent (or extrathymic) T-cell differentiation pathway. Older nude mice sometimes contain an appreciable number of T cells with a mature phenotype. How these T cells arise without a thymus is a matter of controversy. It is beyond the scope of this chapter to deal with all the arguments for and against the possible existence of an extrathymic differentiation pathway for T cells; however, it is important to note that small pockets of thymuslike tissue with dense lymphoid infiltration have been described in the anterior mediastinum of nude mice and it is possible that some T-cell maturation could take place in this tissue. It is also important to note that various studies have shown that T-cells found in nude mice are oligoclonal and that T-cell subsets are not represented in normal ratios.

Development and Classification of Thymocyte Subpopulations

For obvious reasons, most of the studies on T-cell development in the thymus were done in experimental animals, mostly in mice, but a very similar developmental pathway probably exists in humans. As mentioned earlier, T-cell progenitors (also called *prothymocytes*) in the mouse already express very low amounts of the pan-T-cell marker Thy-1 and the antigen Sca-1 (stem cell antigen 1), which is a member of the Ly6 family. (Ly-6 is discussed in Chap. 7B in the section on T-cell activation.) They also express relatively high amounts of MHC class I antigens. ("High" and "low" expression is relative to the level of expression on mature peripheral T cells.)

The first wave of T-cell progenitors enters the murine thymus on the 12th day of gestation, and these cells undergo vigorous proliferation and blast transformation. By day 14 the cells express high levels of the Thy-1 and Tla antigens (Tla, thymus leukemia antigen, is an MHC class I surface antigen expressed in some mouse strains on normal early thymocytes and on leukemia cells) and low levels of MHC class I antigens. By day 17, expression of CD8 and CD4 can first be detected, and within 1 to 2 days most cells in the thymus express both CD4 and CD8 (referred to as double-positive cells). Mature T-cell phenotypes, i.e., CD4$^+$ cells and CD8$^+$ cells (referred to as single positive cells), appear in the medulla only shortly before birth, at day 18 or 19.

In the adult, there is a constant ratio of the various thymocyte subsets for as long as the thymus remains a functional organ. Based on their sensitivity to hydrocortisone and irradiation (as defined by cell death), thymocytes were first divided into two major subpopulations. Medullary and corticomedullary cells were found to be relatively resistant, and cortical cells were found to be highly sensitive. (Human thymocytes are much less sensitive to hydrocortisone.)

The discovery of the CD4 and CD8 molecules allowed a more useful classification of thymocytes into four subsets: *double-negative* cells, which express neither molecule; *double-positive* cells, which express both molecules; and *single-positive* cells, which express either the CD4 or the CD8 molecule—CD4$^+$ cells and CD8$^+$ cells, respectively. In the adult thymus 80 percent of the cells are double-positive cells, half of which also express low levels of the CD3-TCR complex; 5 percent are double-negative cells; and 15 percent are single-positive cells, of which

about half are CD4$^+$ and half are CD8$^+$. Further subdivisions of these four subsets can be made on the basis of their reactivity to various stimuli and the expression of other surface markers defined by monoclonal antibodies (Fig. 7A-2).

One such marker is a 50-kd heat-stable antigen (HSA) found on most hematopoietic cells and originally defined by the monoclonal antibody J11d. About 50 percent of the double-positive cells and 80 to 90 percent of the double-negative cells in the thymus are HSA$^+$. HSA is not expressed on T-cell progenitors in the bone marrow. It is first expressed on T-cell precursors soon after they enter the thymus. Based on the expression of two other surface markers, Pgp-1 (CD44) and the IL-2 receptor (IL-2R), the double-negative HSA$^+$ population can be further divided into two subpopulations:

1. The Pgp-1$^+$ IL-2R$^-$ thymocytes are the less mature cells, and they have the potential to home to, and repopulate, the thymus when injected intravenously into an irradiated host.
2. The majority of double-negative HSA$^+$ cells are Pgp-1$^-$ IL-2R$^+$ thymocytes, and their ability to home to and repopulate the thymus when injected intravenously is greatly reduced. (The latter point is controversial, and is not agreed upon by some laboratories.)

The double-negative HSA$^+$ cells do not express the CD3-TCR (T-cell receptor) complex; however, some of the Pgp-1$^+$ IL-2R$^-$ and most of the Pgp-1$^-$ IL-2R$^+$ cells have already rearranged their β-TCR-chain gene. Interestingly, in some mouse strains, most of these cells express high levels of the CD3–α/β-TCR complex, predominantly of the Vβ8 family. The function of this small population of cells is unclear. It is sometimes referred to as a "dead end" population, since it does not follow the normal T-cell differentiation pathway. The rest of the double-negative HSA$^-$ thymocytes express the γ/δ TCR. The function of these cells is also poorly understood.

In contrast to the double-negative α/β-TCR$^+$ cells which accumulate with age and

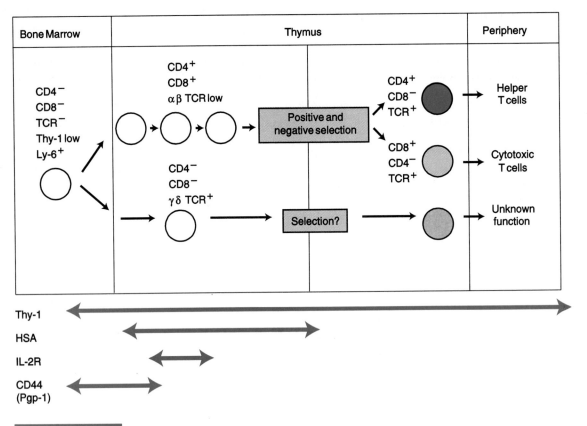

Figure 7A-2. Schematic presentation of the major steps in T-cell development in the murine thymus. T-cell maturation is characterized by the sequential expression of various cell surface markers.

are barely detectable at birth, the double-negative γ/δ-TCR$^+$ cells are first detectable in the thymus at the third week of gestation and leave the thymus as double-negative cells. In the mouse these cells accumulate in the skin and gut and they express a very restricted set of γ- and δ-TCR gene families. Their function and origin are now the subject of intense investigation. It was shown that in some cases they do not show MHC-restricted recognition of antigen (it could be argued that since they never express CD4 or CD8, they are not subjected to thymic selection and therefore cannot be MHC-restricted) and that they can only develop from precursors found in fetal liver but not in bone marrow (Fig. 7A-2).

The level of expression of the CD3-TCR complex (see Chap. 5) is also a useful tool in classification of thymocytes. The CD3–α/β-TCR complex is expressed on all four major thymocyte subsets. Single-positive cells all express these molecules at a high level, double-positive cells express low to intermediate levels, and J11d double-negative cells express low levels. During ontogeny, mRNA encoding the γ chain is the first TCR chain to appear in the cytoplasm at day 13 of gestation, followed by the β and δ chains on day 14 and the α chain on day 16. The cell surface expression of the γ/δ-chain proteins is first detected on day 14 and the expression of the α/β pair on day 16–17. The developmental pathway of the different subsets is only partially known. Most studies strongly suggest that single-positive cells arise from double-positive cells (some of the evidence is discussed later) and not directly from double-negative cells, although definitive experiments are still lacking.

Nearly three decades ago it was realized that most thymocytes are very short-lived. Experiments in which thymocytes were continuously labeled in situ with ^{3}H-thymidine (this radiolabeled thymidine analogue is incorporated into newly synthesized DNA of dividing cells and can be easily traced) showed that all cortical thymocytes were labeled within 3 days whereas medullary thymocytes lab, led much slower. These results implied that most thymocytes have a very fast turnover. Similar experiments involving in situ labeling of thymocytes mainly with fluorescein isothiocyanate showed that only a very small number of thymocytes—1 to 2 $\times$ 10^6 (1 to 2 percent of all thymocytes in a young mouse)—leave the thymus every 24 h. The vast majority of thymic emigrants are single-positive (CD4$^+$ or CD8$^+$) and they retain this phenotype in the periphery. T-cell migration will be discussed later in more detail.

ACQUISITION OF THE T-CELL REPERTOIRE

The fact that most thymocytes never leave the thymus has intrigued immunologists since the phenomenon was discovered. It laid the foundations for the hypothesis that thymocytes are subjected to a thymic selection process which allows only a handful of "qualified" T cells to exit the thymus. The factors permitting a T cell to exit the thymus were debated for quite some time. The original theory was that the main reason for cell death in the thymus was the elimination of self-reacting clones (by an unknown mechanism), which is the way the host protects itself against autoimmunity (reactivity against self). However, others believed that self-reactivity was negatively regulated extrathymically by specific suppressor cells and that the

breakdown of this regulation was the cause of autoimmunity. At that time, before the description of T-cell restriction (see below), it was also difficult to explain why 98 percent of all thymocytes were self-reactive; a biologic system in which only 2 percent of a cell population was beneficial to an individual seemed wasteful and illogical.

Direct and definitive experimental evidence for the existence of a negative selection process in which self-reactive cells are depleted in the thymus has only been obtained during the past few years. Furthermore, the existence of a positive selection process in which only cells that can recognize self-MHC antigens (self-restricted cells) are selected and allowed to leave the thymus has also been clearly demonstrated. The final T-cell repertoire of a given individual is determined by these two thymic selection processes. Before dealing with negative and positive selection in some detail, the concept of *MHC restriction* should be explained. This phenomenon was discovered long before thymic selection and conceptually paved the way for our understanding of how T cells recognize antigen and consequently how the T-cell repertoire is acquired.

MHC Restriction of T-Cell Antigen Recognition

MHC restriction of T-cell functions was first discovered in the early 1970s when it was realized that the interactions between T and B cells (T-cell help) and between T cells and *antigen-presenting cells (APCs)* could only occur when the interacting cells were of the same MHC haplotype. (These interactions will be discussed in more detail later, in the sections on T-cell activation and T-cell functions.)

A short time later, three groups discovered almost simultaneously that MHC restriction applied to antigen-specific cytotoxic T cells (CTLs) as well. These studies showed that antigen-specific CTLs could only kill target cells expressing the same MHC haplotype as the host in which the T cells were initially primed (Fig. 7A-3). More

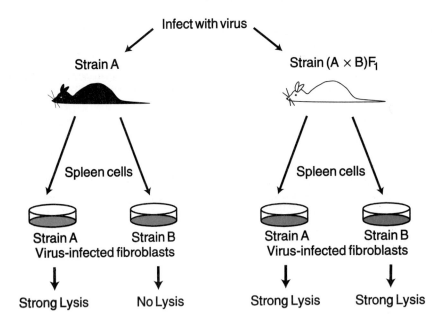

Figure 7A-3.   Demonstration of MHC restriction of CD8$^+$ cytotoxic T cells raised in vivo in virus-infected animals.

specifically, in studies initially aimed at understanding the immune response to lymphocytic choriomeningitis virus (LCMV), it was found that an LCMV-infected fibroblast cell line derived from H-2^k mice (the L fibroblast line) could only be killed with CTLs isolated from LCMV-infected H-2^k mice. CTLs isolated from infected H-2^b or H-2^d mice were ineffective in killing infected L cells. When LCMV-specific CTLs raised in H-2^k and H-2^d mice were assayed on target cells of both haplotypes, it was found that CTLs raised in H-2^k mice could only lyse H-2^k targets, whereas CTLs raised in H-2^d mice lysed only H-2^d targets.

Similar results were obtained with CTLs specific for the hapten dinitrophenyl (DNP). Such CTLs are raised in a particular mouse by immunizing it with DNP-coupled syngeneic spleen cells. As was the case for virus-infected cells, DNP-specific CTLs raised in H-2^d mice could only lyse DNP-H-2^d target cells and not DNP-H-2^k target cells. A third group showed that MHC restriction also applied to CTLs responses against tissue antigens, such as the response to the minor histocompatibility male antigen H-Y.

These experiments established two fundamental properties of antigen recognition by T cells. First, T cells do not recognize free antigen but only antigen in conjunction with MHC gene products. Second, T cells are somehow restricted to recognizing antigen only in conjunction with self- (but not allo-) MHC antigens. Using MHC recombinant mouse strains (MHC recombinant strains differ from one another only in a defined region of the MHC—see Chap. 4), it was soon realized that the restricting elements within the MHC for CD8$^+$ (then called Lyt-2) CTLs were class I genes. For example, the restricting element for the DNP hapten in H-2^b mice was found to be the class I D gene. In other words, DNP-specific CTLs raised in H-2^b mice will only kill target cells that express the H-2D^b gene product, regardless of what other MHC genes are expressed on that target cell.

The next obvious questions were where, when, and how is MHC restriction imprinted upon T cells? A great deal of experimental data from many laboratories strongly suggested that MHC restriction is imprinted in the thymus during T-cell differentiation. Thus it was shown that CTLs generated in an (A × B)F$_1$ → A irradiation bone marrow (BM) chimera (BM from an [A × B]F$_1$ is injected into a lethally irradiated A mouse— see Clinical Aside 7A-2) could only lyse A but not B targets. Furthermore, CTLs raised in a thymectomized, bone marrow–reconstituted (TXBM) (A × B)F$_1$ mouse engrafted with a type A thymus could only kill A but not B target cells. Conversely, CTLs generated in a TXBM A mouse engrafted with an A × B thymus were able to lyse both A and B target cells (Fig. 7A-4). Thus it was generally accepted that the thymus imprinted restriction, although it should be noted that

the phenomenon was "leaky." Leakiness was more prominent when short cytotoxicity assays were employed, thus raising doubts among certain investigators about the thymus being the only factor responsible for imprinting restriction.

Shortly after MHC class I restriction was demonstrated for CD8$^+$ CTLs, MHC class II restriction of CD4$^+$ T helper cells was also demonstrated experimentally. These experiments extended the finding that T cell–B cell collaboration for antibody production required MHC compatibility between the interacting cells. Using a few different experimental approaches, it was first shown that primed T cells from an (A × B)F$_1$ mouse were a mixture of A-restricted and B-restricted T cells, each of which could only interact with

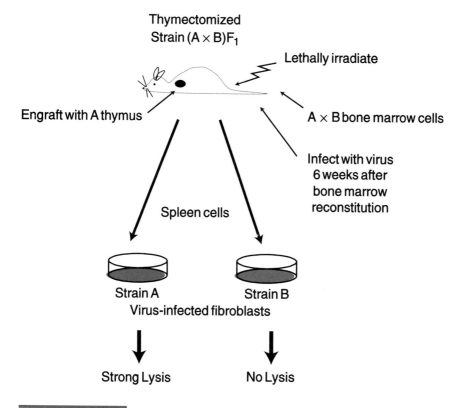

Figure 7A-4. The thymus confers MHC restriction on virus-specific cytotoxic T cells. A × B lymphocytes maturing in a lethally irradiated thymectomized A × B mouse transplanted with an A thymus and reconstituted with A × B bone marrow cells are restricted only to the A haplotype.

A- or B-type B cells, respectively. Then, using irradiation BM chimeras (Clinical Aside 7A-2), it was shown that antigen-primed T cells taken from (A × B)F$_1$ → A chimera could only collaborate with A- but not B-type B cells. Class II restriction of CD4$^+$ cells is not as leaky as class I restriction and is easily demonstrated, and was therefore less controversial (Fig. 7A-5).

Clinical Aside 7A-2
Irradiation Bone Marrow Chimeras

Hematopoietic stem cells, as well as most mature lymphocytes, are radiation-sensitive and do not survive a high dose of γ irradiation. A single dose of >8.5 gy (850 rad) is usually lethal for most mouse strains and once exposed to such a dose the mouse will die within 2 weeks *unless* protected by infusion of normal hematopoietic stem cells. Bone marrow, fetal liver, and in some spe-

cies, spleen are rich sources of stem cells. Bone marrow cells are the most commonly used source and they can be syngeneic, allogeneic, or semiallogeneic to the irradiated host. Irradiation chimeras provided a useful tool to study not only the role of the thymus in imprinting restriction and tolerance but also the role of the MHC in other cell interactions such as between T cells and APCs or between T cells and host tissues in graft-versus-host disease and in induction of experimental autoimmune diseases.

The irradiation sources most commonly used today are cobalt 65 or cesium 45. Not all species can tolerate the dose of irradiation required for elimination of stem cells and lymphocytes. The limiting factor is usually the irreversible damage to the intestinal epithelium which results in sepsis due to entry of intestinal bacteria into the bloodstream. For example, rabbits and guinea pigs cannot survive such an irradiation dose whereas mice and humans can tolerate it. Outbred strains

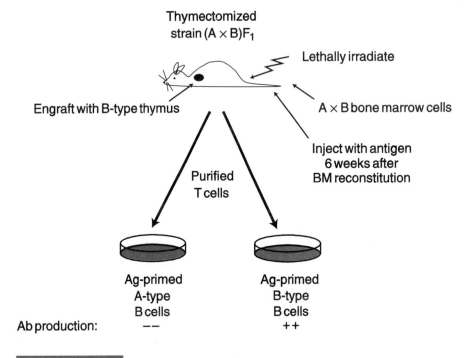

Figure 7A-5. The thymus confers MHC restriction on CD4$^+$ helper T cells. A × B lymphocytes maturing in a lethally irradiated A × B mouse transplanted with an B thymus and reconstituted with A × B bone marrow cells can only provide help to B cells from a B mouse and not to B cells from an A mouse.

of mice and most F_1 combinations of inbred strains are usually more radiation-resistant than parental inbred strains.

As stated earlier, the discovery of T-cell restriction laid the foundations for many hypotheses and experimental approaches aimed at explaining how T cells recognize antigen in association with MHC antigens. One of the fiercest arguments in immunology's rather brief history was prompted by the discovery of MHC restriction. This debate centered on the nature of antigen recognition by the then unknown T-cell receptor. Although this point is now well understood, because of its importance in the history of immunology, it is discussed in some detail in Clinical Aside 7A-3.

Clinical Aside 7A-3
Historical Perspective: The Dual-Recognition and Altered-Self Models for Antigen Recognition by the TCR

Before crystallographic data were obtained for MHC and TCR molecules, one of the most heated debates in immunology centered around two models put forward to explain the fact that the TCR recognizes both self-MHC and a foreign antigen (self + X). The dual-recognition model proposed that T cells express two highly polymorphic binding sites—one which recognizes self-MHC class I or class II antigens and the second which recognizes antigen. The two binding sites were proposed by some to be on two separate peptides and by others to be part of one receptor. This model also implied that only simultaneous binding of the two ligands to the two binding sites would result in T-cell activation.

The altered-self model proposed that there is only one polymorphic receptor, with a single binding site that recognizes a hybrid antigenic determinant composed of the MHC molecule and the foreign antigen. In this formulation, this hybrid determinant (or an altered self-determinant) is unique to any MHC-antigen combination. Many experiments were designed by many investigators specifically to rule out one or the other model.

The altered-self model has gained wide acceptance mainly due to the following experimental results: In a very elegant experiment, a T-cell hybridoma specific for antigen X + MHC^a was fused

to a T-cell hybridoma specific for antigen Y + MHC^b. The dual-recognition model would predict that the receptors for MHC and antigen should segregate (in low frequency if the two receptors are on one polypeptide) independently, resulting in some clones that would recognize antigen X + MHC^b *and* antigen Y + MHC^a. This was never the case. Antigen X was always recognized only when presented by MHC^a APCs and antigen Y was recognized only when presented by MHC^b APCs. It was, however, argued that if the two receptors are tightly linked, one should not expect to see them segregate independently.

The sequence and crystallographic data obtained in recent years clearly demonstrated that purified MHC molecules form a stable complex with processed antigenic peptides and that this complex as a whole is recognized by the TCR. Sequence analysis of TCRs predict the presence of only one binding site; however, peptide and MHC epitopes are bound by different sequences within the TCR binding site.

Negative Selection—Tolerance Induction in the Thymus

As discussed earlier, one of the mechanisms proposed for self-tolerance was the elimination of self-reactive clones during T-cell differentiation in the thymus. Several different experimental approaches have recently provided direct evidence for the existence of such an intrathymic process of negative selection.

One approach took advantage of the increasing availability of monoclonal antibodies recognizing families of TCR gene products. Such antibodies were used to screen antigen-specific T-cell hybrids to assess the usage of TCR by different clones with the same specificity. In this way, it was observed that in some cases there were strong correlations between the TCR Vβ gene used by a particular T-cell hybrid and its antigen specificity. The first such example was the usage of the Vβ17a gene family in many T cells which recognized MHC I-E molecules on the surface of B cells. Similar correlation was later found between the expression of Vβ8.1 or Vβ6 and the ability to recognize the Mls-1a antigen (minor lymphocyte stimulatory antigen locus 1^a). I-E and Mls are both self-antigens expressed in some mouse strains but not in others. (Mls is further discussed below, and I-E, an MHC class II molecular complex, is discussed in Chap. 4.) The Vβ-specific monoclonal antibodies were then used to quantify the number of peripheral T cells, as well as thymocytes, expressing Vβ17a in I-E$^+$ strains versus I-E$^-$ strains (Table 7A-1).

The key finding was that in I-E$^-$ mice approximately 10 percent of peripheral T cells were Vβ17a$^+$, whereas in I-E$^+$ mice, very few if any Vβ17a$^+$ T cells were found in the periphery. Similarly Vβ8.1- and Vβ6-positive T cells were only found in Mls ^{a}-negative mice. The conclusion drawn from these experiments was that Vβ17a-bearing T cells are deleted in I-E$^+$ mice just as Vβ8.1$^+$ and Vβ6$^+$ are deleted in Mls-1^{a+} mice because they are autoreactive. In mice that do not express I-E or Mls, these T cells are not autoreactive and are therefore not deleted. This conclusion was further tested by "forcing" T cells from a strain of mice expressing one of these Vβ-family genes to mature in the thymus of an animal which expressed the antigen recognized by this family. This was achieved by mating two such strains and also by making chimeras where the donor cells were taken from a strain positive for a particular Vβ and the recipient strain expressed the antigen recognized by that particular Vβ family. As expected, the autoreactive T cells were deleted in both cases.

Recently it was shown that the mechanism of clonal elimination by thymic negative selection could also be applied to an exogenous "superantigen" (Clinical Aside 7A-4) in the same way it applies to endogenous self-antigens. Thus, it was shown that neonatal injection of the superantigen *Staphylococcus aureus* enterotoxin (SEB) resulted in an almost complete elimination of peripheral Vβ8$^+$ and Vβ3$^+$ T cells in adult mice.

Clinical Aside 7A-4
Superantigens

Staphylococcus aureus enterotoxin (SEB) was considered for many years to be a T-cell mitogen because it induced proliferation of a large proportion of peripheral T cells. However, recent experimental evidence suggests that SEB in fact interacts mostly with T cells expressing the TCR gene families Vβ3 and Vβ8, and not with all T cells, therefore making it an antigen rather than a mitogen. (Mitogens by definition stimulate a large group of T or B cells regardless of their antigen specificity.) How do so many TCRs recognize one antigen? By mapping the exact sequence in the TCRs recognizing SEB, it was found that this antigen binds to a sequence in the β chain which is not a part of the normal antigen-binding site (Fig. 7A-A1). All members of the TCR gene families Vβ3 and Vβ8 share this sequence and therefore can be bound by SEB. By definition, a *superantigen* is an antigen that is recognized by one or more families of TCR. Encounter with a superantigen therefore causes the activation of a large number of T cells, which may have a pathologic consequence. For example, toxic shock syndrome is a result of a massive release of lymphokines by large numbers of T cells.

TABLE 7A-1   Negative Selection of Endogenous Superantigen-Reactive T Cells Expressing Particular TCR Families

Mouse Strain	I-E Expression	Mls^a Expression	Percent Peripheral T Cells Expressing Vβ17a TCR	Percent Peripheral T Cells Expressing Vβ6 TCR
SJL	−		9.4	
BALB/c	+		<0.1	
AKR		+		<0.1
B10.BR		−		9.5*/13.2†

*Vβ6 expression by CD4$^+$/CD8$^+$, lymph node cells adapted from Kappler et al., *Cell*, 1987, 49:273.
†Sprent J et al., *Science*, 1990, 248:1357.

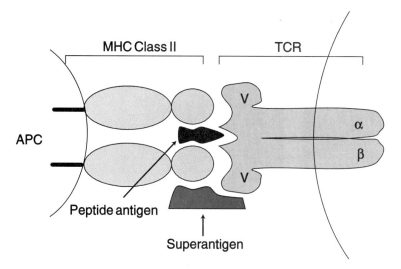

Figure 7A-A1. Binding of a superantigen to a TCR-MHC-peptide complex. Superantigens bind to determinant(s) common to a whole family of β-TCR chains and a sequence shared by many class II MHC genes.

Endogenous antigens could also be classified as superantigens if they fulfilled this definition. The best example for an endogenous superantigen is the Mls locus gene product, discovered in the early 1970s. The Mls locus gene product was defined as the protein responsible for the MHC-independent strong mixed-lymphocyte reaction observed in mixed-lymphocyte cultures made from MHC-identical strains. The identity of this gene product eluded immunologists for almost two decades, mainly because all attempts to produce Mls-specific antibodies or CTLs have failed. It was therefore defined only by its original biologic activity. Recently, it was simultaneously discovered by several laboratories that the Mls gene is in fact a murine mammary tumor virus (MMTV) gene. MMTV belongs to an endogenous group of murine retroviruses. Different MMTV genomes are highly homologous, with the exception of a gene encoded in the 3' long-terminal repeat referred to as *ORF* (open reading frame). The function of the 37-kd protein encoded by ORF is not known. Different MMTV ORF genes account for the different Mls alleles that were defined previously by mixed lymphocyte reaction. Other endogenous retrovirus genes most probably account for other endogenous superantigens.

Another approach used to study negative selection (as well as positive selection—see below) was to generate transgenic mice in which the transgene is a rearranged TCR with a known specificity. The fate of T cells expressing this TCR gene in mice that express or do not express the antigen to which the transgene is specific was then followed. It is important to remember that the introduction of rearranged TCR α and β genes into the germ line will prevent the rearrangement of most endogenous TCR genes; in other words, most of the peripheral T cells in such transgenic mice will express the transgene *unless* they were deleted in the thymus.

Two such mouse models were made around the same time by two independent groups. The first group made transgenic mice using a TCR cloned from a CD8+ H-2b CTL clone specific for the male antigen H-Y (the H-Y gene product is expressed in males but not females). The key finding concerning negative selection was that *male* mice had no CD8+ cells expressing the transgene in the periphery (some transgene positive cells expressing very *low* amounts of CD8 were found in the periphery). In contrast, most of the peripheral CD8+ cells in *females* expressed the transgene. These findings proved that T cells expressing an autoreactive TCR are eliminated in the thymus (Fig. 7A-6). In these first experiments, the results were not always clear-cut when mature lymph node cells were analyzed. An anticlonotypic antibody was not available, and some T cells not expressing the transgene or expressing a hybrid TCR were accumulating in the periphery. In later experiments, an anticlonotypic antibody to the transgene TCR was developed,

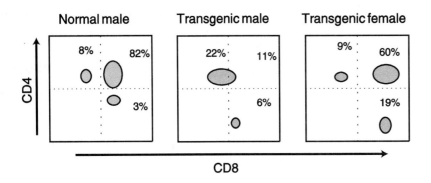

Figure 7A-6.   Effect of thymic negative selection on thymocyte subpopulations. The TCR recognizing the male H-Y antigen isolated fron a CD8+ T-cell clone was introduced as a transgene into male and female mice of the appropriate haplotype. In male mice where the transgene recognizes a self-antigen, most double-positive (CD8+/CD4+) cells are deleted. The single-positive CD8+ cells found in transgenic males did not express the transgene or expressed very low levels of CD8 (see text). The cell phenotype is analyzed on a fluorescence-activated cell sorter. Cells in the bottom right quadrant are CD8+, and cells in the top left quadrant are CD4+. Cells in the bottom left quadrant are negative for both CD4 and CD8, and cells in the top right quadrant are positive for both CD4 and CD8. (Adapted from P Kisielow et al., 1988, *Nature*, 333:742.)

and the transgene was introduced into severe combined immunodeficiency (SCID) mice which are practically devoid of endogenously rearranged TCR genes. Depletion was nearly complete in these experiments.

The second research group produced mice transgenic for a TCR cloned from a CD8+ cytotoxic T cell derived from an H-2^b mouse, specific for the MHC class I L^d gene product. In (B × D)F$_1$ transgenic mice no CD8+ T cells expressing the transgene were found in the periphery, whereas in (B × B)F$_1$ transgenic mice most of the peripheral CD8+ T cells expressed the transgene. These results demonstrated again that self-reactive T cells are deleted in the thymus during T-cell development (Fig. 7A-7).

Positive Selection in the Thymus

The discovery of the T cell–restriction phenomenon implied that somehow during the process of T-cell differentiation in the thymus, only T cells capable of recognizing self-

MHC are given the signal to exit the thymus. Experimental evidence for such a mechanism, now called *positive selection*, was first obtained from experiments using the same transgenic mice described in the previous section. First, it was found that in H-2^b H-Y-transgenic females, but not in H-2^d H-Y-transgenic females, the proportion of single-positive CD8+ thymocytes was significantly higher than in nontransgenic litter mates. It was argued that this was the result of positive selection of CD8+ cells expressing the transgene in H-2^b but in not H-2^d transgenic mice. (Remember that the H-Y-specific TCR was cloned from an H-2^b cell line.) In later experiments using SCID transgenic mice, it was clearly demonstrated again that positive selection occurred in H-2$^{d/b}$ H-Y transgenic females but not at all in H-2$^{d/d}$ transgenic females (Fig. 7A-8).

More conclusive evidence for positive selection came from experiments in which bone marrow cells from H-2^b transgenic mice were transferred into lethally irradiated mice of

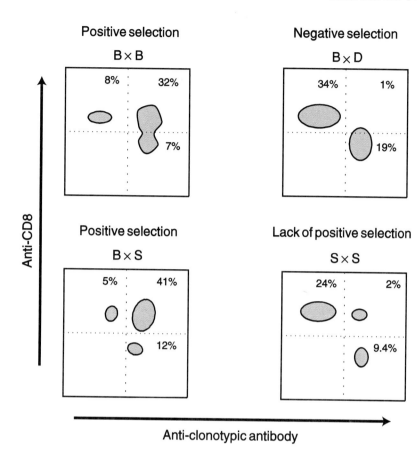

Figure 7A-7. Negative and positive selection in anti-H-2^b transgenic mice. The anti-L^d TCR gene was cloned from an H-2^b T-cell clone. Splenic T cells from transgenic H-2^b, H-2^b × H-2^d, H-2^b × H-2^s, and H-2^s × H-2^s mice were analyzed for the expression of the transgene (by an anticlonotypic antibody) and CD8. The presence of H-2^d determinants induced negative selection, the presence of H-2^b in the absence of H-2^d induced positive selection, and the absence of H-2^b resulted in the lack of positive selection. Analysis was done on a fluorescence-activated cell sorter. (Adapted from WC Sha et al., 1988, *Nature*, 336:73.

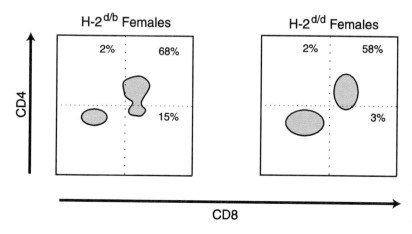

Figure 7A-8. Positive selection in H-2^b anti-H-Y transgenic SCID female mice. In H-2$^{d/b}$ transgenic females 15 percent of CD8$^+$ thymocytes expressed the transgene, whereas in H-2$^{d/d}$ transgenic females only 3 percent of CD8$^+$ cells were positive for the transgene. (Adapted from H von Bohemer, *Annu Rev Immunol*, 1990, 8:531.)

different MHC haplotypes (intra-H-2 recombinant strains were used as recipients so that the exact class I gene involved in positive selection of this particular TCR could be identified). CD8$^+$ cells expressing the transgene were only positively selected in hosts that expressed the class I D^b gene. Similar results were also obtained with the H-2^b-restricted anti-L^d TCR transgenic mice: transgene-positive CD8$^+$ T cells were only found (positively selected) in H-2^b mice and not in any other haplotype tested (Fig. 7A-7).

Positive selection was also recently demonstrated for CD4$^+$ cells in yet another transgenic mouse model. In I-E^k-positive mice transgenic for a TCR specific for pigeon cytochrome c and I-E^k, virtually all peripheral T cells expressed the transgene and were exclusively of the CD4 phenotype. Moreover, their thymuses contained an unusually high percentage of mature CD4$^+$ cells.

Recently, yet another transgenic mouse model provided an elegant proof for the existence of positive selection and its dependence on the expression of MHC gene products in the process. In this case, transgenic mice are made with embryonic stem cells in which the gene for β_2-microglobulin was "knocked out" by a process known as *homologous recombination*. In this technique, a particular gene is disrupted by an insertion of a marker gene. The new DNA is then introduced into embryonic stem cells in vitro, followed by a selection process for cells in which recombination between the altered gene and the endogenous gene has occurred. These cells are then introduced into early embryos and transplanted back into a hormonally conditioned female. In some of the progeny, one of the chromosomes will contain the disrupted gene, and when two such mice are bred again, a homozygous mouse in which both copies of the particular gene are disrupted can be identified. In this way two groups have produced mice that do not express β_2-microglobulin. As a consequence, these mice do not express any MHC class I genes. (See Chap. 4 for the structure of class I proteins.) Based on what we already know

on positive selection, one could predict that such mice would not have any CD8$^+$ cells in the periphery. This is indeed what was found by both groups of investigators.

Surface Markers and Cell Types Involved in Negative and Positive Selection

From the experiments described in the two preceding sections, a few conclusions can be drawn as to which cell surface markers on both thymocytes and thymic cells are important for negative and positive selection.

First, both positive and negative selection are dependent on the interaction of the TCR expressed on the surface of a thymocyte with MHC gene products expressed on the surface of thymic cells. If a particular TCR does not recognize the MHC molecules expressed in the thymus, neither selection process will take place. Second, it is clear that the specificity of a particular TCR for antigen in conjunction with class I or class II will determine the CD4/CD8 phenotype of the mature T cell. Recognition of class I by a particular TCR will result in the exclusive expression of CD8, whereas recognition of class II will result in the exclusive expression of CD4 on the mature T cell. Third, both CD4 and CD8 molecules are involved in the selection process itself. This last point requires some more detailed consideration. Both CD8 and CD4 molecules have been shown to bind to nonpolymorphic determinants on class I and class II molecules, respectively, and antibodies to either CD4 or CD8 have been shown to inhibit T-cell functions in vitro.

Several laboratories have examined the effects of injecting anti-CD4 or anti-CD8 antibodies in vivo on negative and positive selection. For example, injection of newborn Mls-1^a-positive mice with anti-CD4 antibodies inhibited the clonal deletion of Vβ6$^+$ cells in these mice and resulted in the appearance of Vβ6$^+$, including CD8$^+$ Vβ6$^+$ mature thymocytes. (Recall that Mls-1^a is recognized by Vβ6$^+$ T cells.)

Two important conclusions can be drawn

from these results. The first is that the interaction of CD4 with class II antigens is a necessary step for negative selection to occur. The second is that mature CD8$^+$ T cells develop from the double-positive (CD4$^+$, CD8$^+$) thymocyte population and that at least in the case of Mls, negative selection acts upon this population of cells. It should be mentioned, however, that factors other than simple blockage of the CD4 molecule could have contributed to the end result. For example, some anti-CD4 antibodies have been shown to deliver a negative signal to mature T cells and could have also effected selection in the thymus in a similar manner.

Another point to bear in mind is that although the results of the experiment described above suggest that negative selection acts upon the double-positive population, it can probably act upon single-positive cells as well. This is suggested by the fact that in different systems the degree of deletion among the various subsets of thymocytes can vary. For example, in most transgenic mouse models almost complete deletion is evident in the immature double-positive cortical population (Fig. 7A-8), whereas in normal mice, complete deletion of autoreactive clones (such as those reacting to MHC class II antigens or Mls antigens) is seen only in the mature T-cell compartment. These differences could be due to premature expression of high levels of a rearranged TCR gene on double-positive thymocytes in transgenic mice, or to differences in affinity of the TCR to the particular antigen in question. Expression of a TCR with a very high affinity for a particular antigen would lead to a more complete deletion of double-positive cells. In a double transgenic model (transgenic mice carrying two different transgenes), it was actually shown that the deletion of one set of TCR$^+$ cells occurred in the double-positive stage, whereas the other TCR$^+$ cells were only deleted at the single-positive stage.

Insufficient experimental data are currently available to suggest when during the differentiation pathway T cells are subjected to positive selection. It is, however, apparent that positive selection occurs prior to the single-positive stage. As discussed earlier, whereas in a B-haplotype host, mature, single-positive thymocytes expressing a transgenic TCR cloned from an A-haplotype-restricted clone could not be detected (due to the lack of positive selection), double-positive cells expressing the transgenic TCR were found in the thymus. This implies that positive selection occurs during the differentiation of double-positive cells into single-positive cells.

Which cells in the thymus are responsible for imparting negative and positive selection? Besides lymphocytes, the thymus contains two major cell populations: thymic epithelial cells and bone marrow–derived macrophages and dendritic cells. The fact that macrophages and dendritic cells are bone marrow–derived allows one to make irradiation bone marrow chimeras in which the thymic epithelial cells and the thymic macrophages and dendritic cells are derived from different haplotypes. One may then ask which of these cell types controls T-cell restriction (positive selection) or the induction of self-tolerance (negative selection). Most of the experimental data gathered from such chimeras strongly suggest that restriction correlates with the MHC type of the thymic epithelium rather than with the MHC type of thymic macrophages and dendritic cells, implying that positive selection is imparted mostly by thymic epithelial cells. This was corroborated by experiments with transgenic mice in which an I-E transgene was constructed such that it is expressed only in thymic epithelial cells but not in bone marrow–derived cells. In these mice, positive selection of cells with receptors recognizing antigen in conjunction with I-E was perfectly normal, implying that thymic epithelial cells are sufficient to induce positive selection.

Negative selection (induction of self-tolerance), however, is mainly governed by thymic macrophages and dendritic cells. This was first determined from experiments in which fresh thymocytes were added to organ cultures of thymuses devoid of all lymphocytes, macrophages, and dendritic cells. (Organ cultures are similar to cell cultures except that a fragment of an organ is cultured in vitro in culture medium.) Depletion of bone marrow–derived cells from a thymus can be achieved by exposing the organ in tissue culture to deoxyguanosine or high levels of oxygen. It was found that lymphocytes maturing in such thymus organ cultures can respond in a mixed-lymphocyte reaction against lymphocytes expressing the thymic haplotype.

Similar results were obtained from experiments in which T cells maturing in nude mice transplanted with deoxyguanosine-treated thymuses were tested for reactivity against the thymus and the host haplotypes. It was found that such T cells react only against the thymus haplotype, implying that the elimination of self-reactive cells in the thymus is dependent on the presence of bone marrow–derived macrophages and dendritic cells. In these experiments, however, reactivity against the thymic haplotype was not as strong as the reactivity observed in normal allogeneic responses. This suggested that although the complete elimination of self-reactive cells requires the presence of bone marrow–derived macrophages and dendritic cells, some deletion of self-reactive clones was also induced by thymic epithelial cells. The involvement of macrophages and dendritic cells in negative selection was later established in other experimental systems. A recent example is a simple experiment involving a BM chimera in which an IE$^-$ host is reconstituted with donor bone marrow cells from an I-E$^+$ strain. In this chimera, the only I-E$^+$ cells in the thymus are macrophages and dendritic cells of donor bone marrow origin, and yet no mature Vβ17a$^+$ thymocytes were found in the thymus. These results imply that macrophages and dendritic cells are sufficient to induce negative selection.

Possible Mechanisms for Negative and Positive Selection

As mentioned earlier in this chapter, around 98 percent of all thymocytes never leave the thymus, yet no signs of necrosis are ever noted in a normal thymus. Perhaps the first clue for the mechanism responsible for the elimination of thymocytes came from in vitro experiments showing that activation signals known to induce proliferation of mature T cells induce cell death when applied to immature thymocytes. For example, while anti-CD3-TCR antibodies activate mature T cells under the appropriate conditions, the same antibodies will induce cell death in immature thymocytes in tissue culture. This phenomenon has recently also been demonstrated in vivo. Injection of anti-CD3-TCR antibodies induces massive depletion of double-positive thymocytes. The dying double-negative thymocytes undergo a form of cell death known as *apoptosis*, or *programmed cell death*. This form of cell death is characteristic to developmental processes such as the cell death occurring in the resolving tail of a tadpole. Although the dying cells do not appear injured (the cell membrane remains intact), the cell's DNA is fragmented to pieces of approximately 200 bases (the size of a nucleosome) by newly synthesized cellular endonucleases. This is easily visualized by running total cellular DNA on an agarose gel.

How is apoptosis induced in thymocytes? A likely scenario is that a high-affinity interaction between the TCR expressed on immature T cells and a self-antigen results in a signal that induces apoptosis. At the same time, however, we know that cells have to recognize self-MHC in order to be positively selected, and therefore one has to assume that if a TCR does not recognize any antigen, it will also result in the induction of apoptosis. Only a "weak" interaction between a developing thymocyte and thymic epithelial cells expressing self-MHC antigens will rescue the cell from the induction of apoptosis. In other words, apoptosis is induced by high-affinity interactions of thymocytes with thymic macrophages and dendritic cells *or* by the lack of recognition of self-MHC. The exact biochemical pathway that leads to the induction of apoptosis is not known. It is worth mentioning that cell death induced by corticosteroids also involves apoptosis, and it is conceivable that other substances can also induce apoptosis in these cells.

What happens to the cells which undergo apoptosis? There is no clear answer to that question. It is obvious, however, that the thymus does not contain a large number of dead cells. The most plausible suggestion is that cells undergoing apoptosis are rapidly engulfed by thymic macrophages. These cells are abundant in the cortex and the cortico-medullary junction and have been shown to contain dense debris when examined by electron microscopy.

The Biologic Rationale for Negative and Positive Selection

The biologic sense behind negative selection is quite obvious. The organism must have a way to eliminate the majority of self-reactive cells. Thymic negative selection seems to be an adequate mechanism for that purpose. The biologic sense of positive selection is less obvious when examined at the level of an individual member of the species, but it is immediately apparent when examined at the level of the species as a whole.

As discussed earlier, the ability to mount an immune response to any antigen is dependent upon the association of the antigen with either MHC class I or class II molecules (remember that T cells only recognize antigen in conjunction with MHC molecules). Therefore, if an individual's MHC molecules cannot bind a harmful antigen, this antigen will escape the host's immune response. The more diverse the MHC molecules are within a species, the more likely it is that more members of the species will have the "right" MHC molecules that can bind the harmful antigen and mount an immune response against it. This then helps assure the survival of the species. Because T cells recognize antigen in conjunction with MHC molecules, the polymorphism of the MHC dictates that the species contain TCR combinations that can recognize all antigens with all MHC-

molecule combinations. Each individual member of the species only expresses one set of MHC molecules. Therefore there must be a mechanism to allow only cells that express TCRs which can recognize the individual's own MHC molecules to mature (TCRs that can recognize all of the other MHC molecules of the species will be useless for that particular individual). In other words, in a particular individual only a small portion of the TCR repertoire of that species will be able to recognize the individual's set of MHC antigens. This portion has to be selected in each individual. The thymic positive selection process is responsible for exactly that. Only T cells which can recognize self-MHC molecules are allowed to mature and enter the recirculating pool.

The thymic selection processes, however, are not always the perfect answer to all of the individual's "immunologic needs." Negative selection, for instance, can create "holes" in a particular individual's T-cell repertoire. It could be argued that the deletion of large families of TCRs because of their reactivity to a self-super-antigen like Mls could cause the elimination of some specificities that would be beneficial to the individual. Some examples of this have recently been reported. On the other hand, negative selection can only remove thymocytes reacting against self-antigens that are presented on thymic APCs. T cells expressing TCRs capable of recognizing tissue-specific self-antigens cannot be deleted in the thymus. This is best illustrated by the ability to induce autoimmune diseases by immunizing experimental animals with tissue-specific self-antigens like myelin basic protein or thyroglobulin. The mechanisms by which the host deals with such autoantigens will be discussed later (Chap. 31).

The positive selection process raises another fundamental question. Crystallographic studies of MHC class I antigens clearly show that class I antigens always contain a peptide bound to them. From what we know about the processing of antigen for class I presentation (discussed in Chap. 7B) this comes as no surprise. It does mean, however, that positive selection of a particular TCR is not based on the recognition of self-MHC per se, but rather on the recognition of MHC plus a particular self-peptide. How this process can select for the recognition of practically all of nature's antigens—in their absence—is still an open question.

Alloreactivity

Another issue which deserves a brief discussion is the fact that an unusually large number of T cells recognize allogeneic MHC antigens. It is estimated that the frequency of most antigen-specific T-cell clones in a mouse is 1 in 10^4 to 10^5 T cells. In contrast, from in vitro limiting dilution experiments, it was established that 1 to 2 percent of all T cells in a particular haplotype will respond in a mixed-lymphocyte reaction to a given allo MHC. In vivo experiments suggested that up to 12 percent of all T cells can recognize allo-MHC antigens. Why do so many T cells recognize allo-MHC antigens? This issue is far from being resolved, and it still presents an intellectual challenge. Three major hypotheses have been put forward.

The simplest one is that, in general, pure allo-MHC antigens "resemble" self + X antigens, and therefore many T cells recognizing different self + X determinants will also recognize a given allo-MHC determinant. Since it was discovered that MHC molecules isolated from cells always contain a bound peptide, this hypothesis actually argues that allo + Y determinants resemble self + X determinants. The finding that many T-cell clones with a known self + X specificity can also react against one or more allo-MHC antigens speaks in its favor.

The second hypothesis argues that in fact alloreactivity is mostly the response against public MHC determinants which are defined only by MHC sequences without any contribution from the bound peptide (public MHC determinants are shared by many different MHC haplotypes). According to this theory, the high number of alloreactive T-cell clones

is simply due to the very high concentration of MHC antigens (in comparison to a particular self + X antigen) which will reveal many low-affinity clones.

The third hypothesis is perhaps the most intriguing. It proposes that alloreactivity is, in fact, not a response against allo-MHC determinants per se but is actually a response against allo MHC + self. This is based on the finding that tolerance to self non-MHC antigens is also MHC-restricted. In other words, an individual develops tolerance to self-antigens (such as serum proteins) only when presented in conjunction with self-MHC, but that individual will be able to respond to the same self-antigens if they are presented on an *allo* MHC. Therefore, what we score as alloreactivity is in fact a response to many different self-antigens presented on an allo MHC. Since there are many such self-antigens, it is not surprising that such a high proportion of T cells respond to allogeneic cells. The drawback to this theory is that it does not explain how T cells can recognize self-antigen but not foreign antigens presented on allo-MHC antigens. In other words, this theory implies that positive selection somehow only restricts the recognition of foreign antigens to self-MHC but not of self-antigens. Each one of these theories is supported by some but not all experimental data.

ADDITIONAL READING

Allison JP, Harvan WL. The immunobiology of T cells with the invariant gamma/delta antigen receptor. *Annu Rev Immunol.* 1991;9:679.

Ashwell JD, Klausner RD. Genetic and mutational analysis of the T cell receptor. *Annu Rev Immunol.* 1990;8:139.

Blackman M, Kappler J, Marrack P. The role of the T cell receptor in positive and negative selection of developing T cells. *Science.* 1990;248:2355.

Herman A, Kappler J, Marrack P, Pullen AM. Superantigens: Mechanisms of T cell stimulation and role in immune responses. *Annu Rev Immunol.* 1991;9:745.

Rajewsky K, von Boehmer H, eds. Lymphocyte development. *Curr Opinion Immunol.* 1992;4:131–166.

Sha WC, Nelson CA, Newberry RD, Krantz DM, Russell JH, Lo DY. Positive and negative selection of an antigen receptor on T cells in transgenic mice. *Nature.* 1988;336:73.

Sprent J, Gao E-K, Webb SR. T cell reactivity to MHC molecules: Immunity versus tolerance. *Science.* 1990;248:1357.

von Boehmer H. Developmental biology of T cells in T cell receptor transgenic mice. *Annu Rev Immunol.* 1990;8:531.

von Boehmer H, Kisielow P. Self-nonself discrimination by T cells. *Science.* 1990;248:1369.

7

Ontogeny and Differentiation of T Lymphocytes

B. T-Cell Functions

INTRODUCTION

In this chapter we will discuss the activation pathways, the migration patterns, the immune functions, and the functional classification of mature T cells. The physiologic role of T cells is to constantly screen the body for foreign antigens so that every possible pathogen can be dealt with regardless of where it enters. As mentioned in the introduction to Chap. 7A, the hallmark of T-cell reactivity is the fact that the T-cell receptor (TCR) can only recognize antigen in conjunction with major histocompatability complex (MHC) antigens. The cardinal rule is that $CD8^+$ cells recognize antigen only in conjunction with MHC class I antigens, whereas $CD4^+$ cells recognize antigen in association with MHC class II antigens. Functional classification, however, does not correlate perfectly with the CD phenotype of T cells. Cytotoxic T lymphocytes (CTLs), for example, are mostly of the $CD8^+$ phenotype; however, $CD4^+$ cells can also be cytotoxic but they will still recognize antigen in association with MHC class II self-antigens.

T cells can exert their effector functions by direct cell-to-cell interactions, as is the case with the provision of B-cell help and lysis of a target cell, or by the secretion of a variety of lymphokines and cytokines. The biologic effects of lymphokines are discussed in Chap. 10. Certain T-cell functions are discussed in detail in other chapters. The reader should refer to Chap. 8 for detailed discussion of cytotoxic T-cell functions, including cytotoxic T lymphocytes, antibody-dependent cell-mediated cytotoxicity, and lymphokine-activated cytotoxic T cells; to Chap. 26 for discussion of the role of T cells in allograft rejection and graft-versus-host disease; to Chap. 25 for discussion of T-cell responses to tumors; to Chap. 31 for discussion of T cells in autoimmune diseases; and to Chap. 21 for discussion of T-cell responses to infections. Regulation of the immune response by suppressor T cells is discussed in Chap. 9.

Several controversial issues exist with regard to T-cell activation and function. One such issue is the general topic of T cell–T cell interactions. Many reports, mostly during the 1970s, suggested that the generation of most or all $CD8^+$ effector cells required some kind of interaction with $CD4^+$ cells. Even the generation of certain $CD4^+$ effector cells was thought to be dependent on interaction with other $CD4^+$ cells, which were termed "inducer" or "amplifier" cells. These terms are scarcely used today. Our discussion will, in general, be restricted to current classification and to current understanding of T-cell functions.

ANTIGEN PRESENTATION TO T CELLS

The biochemical pathways leading to the association of antigens with MHC molecules have been under intense investigations in recent years. We will discuss only briefly the differences between antigen presentation to class I–restricted $CD8^+$ T cells and class II–restricted $CD4^+$ T cells. As mentioned earlier, it was discovered in the early 1970s that T cells can recognize antigen only in association with MHC self-antigens on the surface of an antigen presenting cell (APC). The fundamental finding was that antigens have to be first "processed" intracellularly before they can bind MHC proteins and then be expressed on the surface of the APC as an antigen-MHC molecular complex. Antigen processing involves the proteolytic cleavage of proteins into small peptides and their subsequent association with MHC gene products. Antigen processing was first described for exogenous antigens that associated with class II gene products recognized by $CD4^+$ cells. Such antigens are phagocytosed or pynocytosed by specialized APCs that also express, or can be induced to express, MHC class II antigens. Exogenous proteins are pynocytosed into endosomes via "coated pits," and particulate antigens such as bacteria are phagocytosed into lysosomes. Inside lysosomes and endosomes, small peptides are generated by proteolytic cleavage. Drugs which can raise the pH inside cytoplasmic lysosomes (e.g., chloroquine, primaquine, and NH_4Cl) can inhibit antigen processing, suggesting that the internalized proteins are proteolytically cleaved in lysosomes and endosomes. A stable trimolecular complex composed of class II α and β chains and the invariant chain (Ii or γ chain) is assembled in the endoplasmic reticulum. This complex is transported by an unknown mechanism into lysosomes and endosomes where the invariant chain is cleaved and the α and β chains are allowed to bind short peptides generated by the proteolytic cleavage of larger proteins (Fig. 7B-1).

More recently, it was discovered that antigen processing is also required for antigen presentation in association with MHC class I antigens. The discovery stemmed from the observation that most of the cytotoxic T lymphocytes (CTLs) isolated from mice infected with the influenza virus were specific for viral nucleoproteins which are not expressed as intact proteins on the cell surface of infected cells. A plausible explanation for this finding was that all viral proteins can be processed in the cytoplasm, associate with MHC class I proteins within the cell, and then be expressed as a molecular complex on the cell surface. Shortly thereafter, it was demonstrated that any internal endogenous antigen can be processed and expressed in association with class I proteins on the cell surface. For example, a mouse cell line trans-

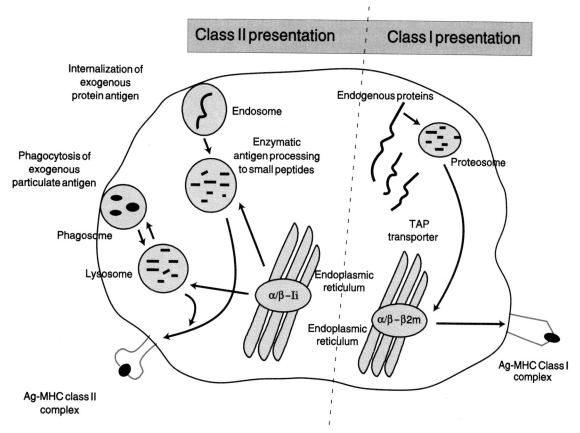

Figure 7B-1. Antigen-processing pathways for antigen presentation in association with MHC class I and class II molecules.

fected with the ovalbumin gene can present fragments of processed ovalbumin and stimulate the generation of ovalbumin-specific syngeneic CTLs.

The biochemical pathway for processing of antigens associated with MHC class I molecules is currently under intense investigation. Although we are far from understanding this complex pathway, the following picture emerges from the currently available experimental data (Fig. 7B-1). Antigen degradation of endogenous proteins produced within the cell takes place in proteosomes, which are proteolytic complexes found in the cytoplasm. These structures are related to another large proteolytic complex called the *low molecular mass polypeptide* (LMP) complex. Interestingly, at least two of the subunits that form the LMP complex are encoded by genes that map to the class II region of MHC. It is not clear what the relationship between these two structures is. One intriguing hypothesis is that once the two LMP subunits are transported into proteosomes they associate and form an LMP complex. The association of short peptides with MHC class I genes occurs in the lumen of the endoplasmic reticulum and is mediated and dependent upon a transporter protein called *TAP transporter* (TAP stands for transporter associated with antigen presentation). TAP is a heterodimer consisting of two subunits called Tap-1 and Tap-2. The Tap-1 and Tap-2 genes also map to the MHC class II region and are closely linked to the two genes coding for the two LMP subunits. TAP also resides in the endoplasmic reticulum, and it is not clear how the short peptides produced in LMP are delivered to the endoplasmic reticulum. Other chaperoninlike molecules might be involved in this process.

The α chain of MHC class I proteins and β$_2$-microglobulin also associate in the endoplasmic reticulum. In the absence of peptide, this association is unstable at physiologic temperatures, and most of this complex is degraded in the endoplasmic reticulum. In the presence of peptide, a stable complex is formed and is efficiently transported (by an unknown mechanism) to the cell surface. It

is not clear if some naked MHC class I molecules do make it to the cell surface where they can bind exogenous peptides. Some experimental evidence suggests that low levels of free α chain can also be present on the cell surface and in the presence of exogenous β$_2$-microglobulin and peptide a stable complex can be formed.

The two antigen-processing pathways leading to antigen presentation in the context of class I or class II molecules are usually well separated, although exceptions have been documented where a soluble protein can be processed by both pathways. Based on the current models for antigen processing, any protein including exogenous peptides that somehow end up in the endoplasmic reticulum could associate with class I molecules. Similarly, during the assembly of class II molecules in the endoplasmic reticulum, before the α/β dimer associates with the invariant chain (which prevents the binding of peptide), some endogenous peptides could bind to the α/β complex. It is possible that the invariant chain can bind to some of these α/β-peptide complexes, which are then transported to endosomes where the invariant chain is cleaved off and the resulting α/β–endogenous peptide complex is subsequently expressed on the cell surface.

What is the biologic significance of the fact that T cells only recognize antigen-MHC complexes? As discussed earlier, the two main functions of T cells are to kill virus-infected cells and to interact with B cells to induce antibody production. Both of these functions require cell-to-cell interactions. The fact that T cells can only recognize antigen complexed to MHC on the surface of a cell facilitates the cell-to-cell interactions required for the exertion of T cell functions. Recognition of free antigen would only distract the effector T cell from its target cell and would not make biologic sense. The biologic sense of having two separate intracellular processes for antigen presentation with MHC class I and class II molecules is obvious when one considers the different functions of CD4 and CD8 cells. It would make biologic sense for intracellular pathogens such as viruses to induce CD8-dependent responses (CTLs). On the other hand, it would not make much biologic sense for exogenous antigens and pathogens that do not enter the host's cells to induce CTL responses, but it would make sense for such antigens to induce CD4$^+$ helper T cells.

What cells can serve as APCs for T cells? For class I–restricted recognition it seems that any cell that expresses class I antigens can both stimulate CD8$^+$ cells and serve as target cells for class I–restricted CTLs. Antigen presentation for class II–restricted recognition by CD4$^+$ T cells is somewhat more complicated. As will be discussed in more detail in the section dealing with clonal anergy, antigen presentation to some CD4$^+$ T cells requires that the APC express more than just MHC class II antigens on its surface. Macrophages, dendritic cells, B cells, and various other cells expressing MHC class II molecules like astrocytes and some epithelial cells were shown to present antigen both in vitro and in vivo. Class II–transfected fibroblasts could also present antigen to most, but not all, T-cell hybridomas and T-cell clones. The ability of APCs to secrete certain lymphokines, such as IL-1, and the expression of various cell adhesion molecules were also shown to be involved in antigen presentation to class II–restricted T cells. The major adhesion molecules that were shown to play a role in T-cell interactions with APCs and B cells are listed in Table 7B-1. Some experimental data also suggest that primed

TABLE 7B-1 The Major Adhesion and Accessory Molecules for T Cells

Receptor	Other Names	Counter Receptor
LFA-1	CD11a/CD18	ICAM-1 (CD54)
	CD11b/CD18	ICAM-2
CD2	LFA-2; T11; Leu-5	LFA-3 (CD58)
CD4	Leu-3; T4; L3T4	MHC class II
CD8	Leu-2; T8; Lyt-2	MHC class I
CD44	Pgp-1; Hermes; ECMR-III	?
VLA-4	CD49d	VCAM-1

T cells might have different antigen-presenting requirements than naive T cells.

MIGRATION PATTERNS OF MATURE T CELLS

Lymphocyte migration is discussed in more detail in Chap. 12. In this section we will briefly discuss the migration patterns of T cells. As discussed earlier, the vast majority of cells emigrating from the thymus are mature CD4$^+$ or CD8$^+$ T cells. In a young mouse, $1–2 \times 10^6$ cells leave the thymus each day and enter the spleen and lymph nodes. Mature T cells are not confined to any particular lymphoid organ; they circulate among these organs and can also enter interstitial spaces throughout the body. Entry into certain organs may be limited by specific blood-organ barriers such as the blood-brain barrier.

T cells enter lymphoid organs via the bloodstream and localize in T cell–dependent areas. Entry into the spleen via the splenic artery is rapid and is independent of the expression of specific homing receptors. The splenic artery opens into the red pulp, which is not directly connected to the spleen's venous system. This forces all cells and fluids to filter through the splenic parenchyma, which is rich in APCs and lymphocytes. T cells migrate rapidly through the red pulp into the white pulp and concentrate in the T cell–dependent areas around arterioles. The T cell–dependent area is often called the *periarteriolar lymphocyte sheath* (PALS). This area is also rich in macrophages and dendritic cells and is surrounded by the B-cell area in which germinal centers are formed. T cells are also found in the outer rim of germinal centers (Chap. 6). The majority of T cells leave the spleen via the bloodstream; few exit via the efferent lymphatics. Splenic and lymph node structure was previously described in Chap. 2.

Migration to and from the lymph nodes is different. T cells enter lymph nodes via the specialized arterioles known as *high endothelial venules (HEVs)*. T cells can also enter a lymph node via the afferent lymphatics. The entry via HEV is dependent on the expression by the T cell of one or more homing receptors which recognize some surface ligand present on the endothelial cells. The HEVs are located in the paracortex, which is the T cell–dependent area of the lymph node. In order to exit the lymph nodes, T cells migrate into the medulla and leave via the efferent lymphatics. T cells that enter the lymph nodes via the afferent lymphatics do not reach the T cell–dependent areas and only pass through the lymph node. The afferent lymphatics open into the subcapsular sinus which drains directly into the efferent lymphatics. (The efferent lymphatics of a particular lymph node can drain into the afferent lymphatics of another lymph node or else directly into a lymphatic vessel.) Lymph nodes do not filter cells and foreign substances that enter through the afferent lymphatics but they do filter the lymph coming in from the bloodstream.

The recirculating pool of T cells is composed of small lymphocytes with a relatively long life span. The life span of lymphocytes is usually determined by measuring the number of cells that label with tritiated thymidine (^{3}H-TdR) after intravenous injection of the radiolabel (^{3}H-TdR only labels dividing cells). After a course of injections (8 to 10 weeks), only 40 percent of T cells become labeled. The slow turnover of T cells is also suggested by experiments utilizing adult thymectomized mice. In such animals, the number of T cells in the recirculating pool declines very slowly and reaches a plateau.

The migration pattern of activated T cells is different from that of naive T cells. Most of the primary antigenic stimulation of T cells occurs in the spleen and lymph nodes. This is characterized by blast transformation and proliferation. Activated T cells are then released into the circulation, but unlike small recirculating T cells, they can leave the bloodstream to migrate to sites of inflammation and mucosal tissues such as the breast and the lining of the gut, the upper respiratory tract, the lungs, and the brain. As an example, the cytokines released during inflammation in a joint (arthritis) can modify the endothelium of the synovium into an HEV, which then allows the influx of T cells into the inflammatory site.

T HELPER FUNCTIONS

From early experiments using neonatally thymectomized animals it became clear that the lack of T cells in these animals also correlated with drastically reduced antibody titers. It was later established that the production of antibodies to most antigens is dependent upon T-cell help. Very few antigens can stimulate B cells directly, without T-cell help, to produce IgM antibodies. (Such antigens are called *T cell–independent (TI)-antigens;* see Chaps. 2 and 6). Production of all other antibody isotypes by antigen-specific B cells requires T-cell help. Memory B cells can be induced to secrete antibodies nonspecifically even in the absence of antigen by various lymphokines, most of which are produced by T cells. T-cell help is provided by CD4$^+$ T cells. The exact nature of T-cell help is still unknown. Recent work suggests that upon activation T cells express a new 33-kd surface protein known as *T cell–induced cell-contact ligand (TICCL),* which may interact with the constitutively expressed CD40 molecule on the surface of B cells to initiate B-cell activation and proliferation. It seems that at least the initial help signal requires direct cell-to-cell interaction. As discussed earlier, the interacting T and B cells have to share the same MHC class II genes. Histoincompatible T and B cells cannot interact.

What are the antigenic requirements for effective T cell–B cell collaborations? Early studies on antigenicity of haptens suggested that the antigenic determinant for which the B cell is specific has to be on the same molecule as the antigenic determinant for which the T cell is specific. This was shown in adoptive transfer experiments in which T cells specific for keyhole limpet hemocyanin (KLH) were transferred together with trinitrophenyl-specific (TNP-specific) B cells into a syngeneic host. Help for the production of anti-TNP antibodies was provided only if the host was injected with TNP conjugated to KLH (TNP-KLH). This occurred regardless of the protein "carrier" that was used to immunize the B cells to TNP (for instance, TNP-BSA or TNP-HGG). The T cell in this case is specific for the carrier protein KLH and the B cell is specific for the hapten TNP (see Fig. 6-6).

DELAYED-TYPE HYPERSENSITIVITY AND CONTACT SENSITIVITY

Delayed-type hypersensitivity (DTH), also called type IV hypersensitivity, was the first immune system function recognized as having a cellular basis. As implied by its name, DTH is a delayed cellular reaction to a localized antigen, usually in the skin. This is in contrast to the immediate, anaphylactic type I Prausnitz-Küstner and type III Arthus' reactions, the former mediated by IgE antibodies and the latter by immune complexes. See Chap. 29 for a more detailed discussion of the four types of hypersensitivity reactions.

Perhaps the most commonly known example of DTH is the tuberculin reaction. Individuals who have been exposed to or have been immunized against tuberculosis will develop a typical erythematous indurated skin reaction when injected intradermally with a small amount of purified protein derivative of tuberculin (PPD). Individuals who have never been exposed to tuberculin will not react in this fashion even if injected locally with a much higher dose of PPD. This observation implies that DTH is a *secondary* response. The first exposure to an antigen usually does not result in a DTH reaction.

Most antigens can induce DTH reactions if they are first injected, usually intraperitoneally or subcutaneously, in complete Freund's adjuvant (CFA) or if the antigenic stimulation is the result of a persistent infection. It seems that only strong and pro-

longed immunizations will activate cells in sufficient numbers for the induction of DTH. The second introduction of the antigen must be local, not systemic, in order to observe a typical DTH reaction. Although DTH is described primarily as a skin reaction, it can occur in any tissue such as the eye or the brain. Some of the histologic features of the synovitis in rheumatoid arthritis suggest a local DTH. Such responses are sometimes referred to as "DTH-like" reactions, but conceptually they are one and the same.

The local inflammatory DTH reaction is induced by antigen-specific CD4$^+$ cells which rush to the site of entry of the antigen. The peak of the reaction occurs 48 to 72 h after local injection of the antigen; the time before the peak reaction depends on antigen dose and the level of initial sensitization. The exact sequence of events is not well characterized, but it is assumed that lymphokines secreted by the activated cells initiate the reaction. Some experimental data suggest that the initial inflammatory reaction is mediated by a distinct CD4$^+$ cell which is induced within the first 4 h of antigen injection. Inflammation is discussed in more detail in Chap. 20.

Contact sensitivity is a type of DTH in which the initial priming to the antigen also occurs through the skin, but in this case the antigen is usually much smaller in size (most often a hapten) than antigens that induce DTH. Contact sensitivity and DTH are often used interchangeably, especially in experimental animals. Some of the classical DTH models in rodents are by definition contact sensitivity reactions, since the initial sensitization is done through the skin by chemically attaching a hapten, such as dinitrophenyl (DNP), to skin cells. Although this is an artificial method of sensitization, a similar phenomenon also occurs physiologically. All the antigens that induce contact sensitivity are small molecules. Their size allows them to penetrate the skin and chemically bind to self-proteins. Most of these substances are not immunogenic on their own; they are thus typical haptens. Examples include heavy metals like mercury, nickel, and zinc or natural plant oils like uru-shiol, the contact sensitivity-inducing agent in poison ivy and poison oak. When these small molecules bind to self-proteins, how-ever, they can become highly immunogenic and can induce a potent DTH reaction.

What is the biologic importance of DTH? DTH is perhaps best viewed as an antigen-specific mechanism for the induction of in-flammation. The inflammatory reaction it-self is an important mechanism for activat-ing macrophages and thus clearing invading microorganisms and for repairing tissue damage. As a form of a specific response to a foreign antigen, however, DTH could be considered an unpleasant by-product of the immune response. Fortunately, it occurs only when a large number of antigen-specific T cells are concentrated in a small area. In fact, one might consider the massive stimulation of T cells that results from contact with such superantigens as *Staphylococcus aureus* en-terotoxin B (SEB) as a systemic analogue of DTH.

CD4$^+$ T-CELL SUBSETS

The classification of T-cell subpopulations was facilitated by the discovery of over 80 different T-cell surface markers defined by hundreds of different monoclonal antibodies and by the characterization and molecular cloning of many soluble factors, now called *lymphokines* or *interleukins*, which are pro-duced by T cells. Many laboratories have tried to correlate the expression of particular T-cell markers or the production of certain lymphokines with specific T-cell functions. Indeed, evidence has accumulated in recent years to suggest that CD4$^+$ cells can be di-vided into different functional subsets ac-cording to both cell surface markers and pat-terns of lymphokine production.

The first such subdivision of CD4$^+$ cells was recognized in murine T cells. Analysis of lymphokine production by many T-cell clones in response to antigen revealed that some CD4$^+$ clones secreted large amounts of IL-2 and IFN-γ, whereas others secreted

large amounts of IL-4. The IL-2-secreting clones were termed T$_H$1 cells and the IL-4-secreting clones were termed T$_H$2 cells. Dif-ferences in the level of secretion of other lymphokines were later also found to differ between T$_H$1 and T$_H$2 cells as well as be-tween CD4$^+$ and CD8$^+$ T cells.

More importantly, certain T-cell func-tions were also found to be preferentially as-sociated with T$_H$1 or T$_H$2 cells. DTH, for ex-ample, was found to be mediated only by T$_H$1 but not by T$_H$2 cells. The characteristics of T$_H$1 and T$_H$2 T-cell subsets are summarized in Table 7B-2. It should be emphasized, how-ever, that the subdivision of CD4$^+$ cells into T$_H$1 and T$_H$2 subsets is mostly based on prop-erties of T-cell clones grown in vitro. It is unclear whether normal resting T cells in the mouse can also be divided along the same lines. In fact, some recent studies suggest that this might not be the case. Freshly iso-lated activated T cells from immunized mice secrete IL-2, IL-4, and IFN-γ, although IL-2 is usually secreted in much larger amounts than IL-4 and IFN-γ. In addition, T-cell clones analyzed shortly after cloning could not be classified according to the T$_H$1-T$_H$2 system. It seems that the T$_H$1 and T$_H$2 phenotypes

TABLE 7B-2   Properties of Mouse CD4$^+$ T$_H$1 and T$_H$2 T Cells

	T_H1	T_H2
Lymphokine secretion		
IL-1	+ +	−
IL-3	+ +	+ +
IL-4	−	+ +
IL-5	−	+ +
IL-6	−	+ +
IFN-γ	+ +	−
TNF-α	+ +	+
TNF-β	+ +	−
GM-CSF	+ +	+
B-cell help		
IgM, IgA	+	+ +
IgG2a	+ +	+
IgE	−	+ +
DTH	+	−

Source: Adapted from TR Mossman and RL Coffman, *Annu Rev Immunol,* 1989; 7:145.

emerge only after a prolonged time in culture. Human CD4$^+$ clones can also be classified as T$_H$1 and T$_H$2, but some human T-cell clones can produce both IL-2 and IL-4. It therefore remains unclear if the classification of CD4$^+$ cells into T$_H$1 and T$_H$2 subsets is physiologically relevant. It is also unclear at what stage of differentiation this division might occur. It should be mentioned that other properties of T cells—such as life span and response to different lymphokines—were used by many investigators to classify T cells.

Another way to subdivide CD4$^+$ T cells emerged from studies on human T cells. Many laboratories discovered that human memory T cells express a different set of surface markers than naive, unprimed T cells. The best-characterized of these markers are CD45 molecules, a large family of surface molecules also known as *leukocyte common antigens (LCAs)*, present on all hemopoietic cells. Members of the CD45 family of molecules are expressed on all lymphocytes, B cells included.

Another example of subdivision of CD4$^+$ T cells (and CD8$^+$ cells in this case) into various subsets emerged from studies on human T cells. Many laboratories discovered that human memory T cells express a different set of surface markers than naive, unprimed T cells. The most characterized markers are the various isoforms of the LCA, or CD45. The different isoforms of CD45 represent splice variants of the same gene. Eight different forms are possible, but it is not known whether all forms are expressed on the cell surface. All forms of CD45 are heavily glycosylated, which might contribute further to differences in biologic functions between various forms of the molecule expressed in different cell types. All forms share the same cytoplasmic domain which is a tyrosine phosphatase. A CD45 splice isoform is called CD45R (to distinguish it from the whole, unspliced molecule CD45). Studies in humans have shown that naive T cells express high levels of the CD45RA isoform, whereas memory cell predominantly express the CD45RO isoform. CD45RA is also called

CD45^{hi}, designating a high molecular weight form of CD45 (190 to 200 kd). CD45RO is also called CD45R^{lo}, designating a low molecular weight form of CD45. In CD45RO exons 4 to 6 are spliced out, resulting in a 180-kd molecule which is the lowest molecular weight form of CD45. This isoform is recognized by the monoclonal antibody UCHL-1, and the name of the antibody is sometimes used synonymously with CD45RO. Differential expression of many other surface molecules was found to correlate with the expression of these two major forms of CD45. Table 7B-3 summarizes the major differences between naive and memory T cells. Most of the markers expressed on CD45RO$^+$ cells are characteristic of memory cells. It should be noted, however, that this division is not, at this time, accepted as complete. Several studies have shown that T cells can reverse their phenotype from CD45RO back to CD45RA, and that some of the other characteristics such as lymphokine production and expression of certain cell surface molecules can be associated, under certain conditions, with both subsets. CD45 is also discussed later on in the section dealing with T-cell activation.

TABLE 7B-3   Properties of Human CD4$^+$ Naive and Memory T Cells

	Naive	Memory
Phenotype		
CD45RA	+ + +	−
CD45RO	−	+ + +
CD29	+ +	+ + +
CD44	+ +	+ + +
CD2	+ +	+ + +
LFA-1	+ +	+ + +
LFA-3	+	+ +
ICAM-1	−	+
IL-2R	−	+
MHC class I	+ +	+ + +
MHC class II	−	+
Size	Small	Large
Life span	Long	Short
Cytokine secretion	Mostly IL-2	Various
Response to anti-CD2	+/−	+ + +

Source: Adapted from PCL Beverley, *Semin Immunol*, 1992; 4:35.

SUPPRESSOR T CELLS

The existence of a subset of lymphocytes capable of down-regulating immune responses in an antigen-specific manner was first suggested from early adoptive transfer experiments in which DTH was transferred with sensitized lymph node cells. In these experiments, transfer of DTH did not linearly correlate with the number of transferred cells. Transfer of high number of cells resulted in reduced DTH, and it was suggested that some of the transferred cells had a negative effect on DTH. In the early 1970s, experimental data first suggested that a unique subset of $CD8^+$ T cells, termed *suppressor cells*, could specifically suppress helper T cells, resulting in low or no antigen-specific antibody response. Antigen-specific suppression was under intense scrutiny during the 1970s and early 1980s, and elaborate networks of immunoregulatory circuits consisting of various inducer and effector cells and their soluble factors were proposed. (This topic is discussed in greater detail in Chap. 9.) Later on, the concept of suppression fell out of favor mainly because no reliable, reproducible protocol for cloning antigen-specific suppressor cells was ever established and because a unique marker for suppressor cells was not found. The only unique murine suppressor cell marker, called I-J, was thought to be an MHC class II gene (defined by polyclonal and monoclonal antibodies), but it was not found in the H-2 locus of the mouse when this locus was completely sequenced. It is not clear where the I-J gene is located and how its expression is linked to the expression of other H-2 genes. It should be emphasized, however, that the phenomenon of antigen-specific suppression has been well documented by many laboratories. Whether this phenomenon is mediated by a distinct T-cell subset is still an open question. It could be argued that suppression is mediated by one of the other well-characterized T-cell subsets, such as CTLs, for example. Under some conditions these cells can kill other T cells or APCs.

CLONAL ANERGY AND OTHER TYPES OF ANTIGEN-SPECIFIC UNRESPONSIVENESS

Although the immune system responds adequately to most antigens, a few general exceptions were found in different experimental systems. One example is the response to "deaggregated" proteins. (The term "deaggregated" is not well defined in physical terms; it usually means the supernatant of a protein solution spun at high speed in an ultracentrifuge.) It is well documented that the intravenous or intraperitoneal injection of deaggregated proteins results in transient, but profound, unresponsiveness to subsequent immunization with the same protein in an immunogenic form. A second example is the injection of very low amounts of an immunogenic form of an antigen like heterologous erythrocytes. Again, a profound unresponsiveness (sometimes called "low zone tolerance") is readily induced. The mechanism responsible for these types of unresponsiveness is still unknown. One hypothesis suggests that in both cases, antigen escapes processing and presentation by APCs, and for unknown reasons, this leads to unresponsiveness rather than activation.

Recently an in vitro model for induction of a different kind of unresponsiveness was established. In this model, when an antigen is presented to T_H1 T-cell clones by chemically fixed APCs, a state of unresponsiveness is induced. This unresponsiveness was termed *clonal anergy*. This term was first used to describe a state of unresponsiveness induced in B cells activated by only one of the two signals required for effective B-cell stimulation. Similarly, it was postulated that two distinct signals are required for T-cell stimulation. One is the occupation of the TCR (see below), and the other is a yet-unidentified costimulatory signal. It was found that this signal cannot be delivered by chemically fixed APCs. Stimulation of T cells by antigen bound to pure MHC molecules inserted into liposomes or by immobilized (plastic-bound) anti-TCR antibodies can also induce clonal anergy. It was therefore suggested that during normal T-cell activation the putative costimulatory factor is supplied by the normal (nonfixed) APCs, and, indeed, clonal anergy cannot be induced in the presence of normal APCs.

Interestingly, the cells providing the co-stimulatory signal do not have to be syngeneic to the T-cell clone, and it is not clear what cell types, other than conventional APCs, can provide this costimulatory signal. The induction of anergy is highly dependent on cell density. At a high cell density, clonal anergy is poorly induced and some degree of T-cell activation does occur. It is therefore possible that T cells themselves can provide low levels of the costimulatory signal, and where cell density is high, sufficient amounts of the signal are provided for activation.

The nature of the costimulatory signal is not clear. Experimental data suggest that the delivery of this signal requires direct cell-to-cell interaction between the cell providing the signal and the T cell. No soluble factor, such as IL-1 to IL-7, GM-CSF, or TGF-β, could provide the needed costimulatory signal. The costimulatory signal is not present in resting APCs, and it is not entirely clear what induces it. Recent studies on anergy induction in human T cells suggest that CD28 expressed on the surface of T cells serves as the receptor for the putative costimulatory factor. Anti-CD28 antibodies induced IL-2 production and cell proliferation by anergic human T-cell clones. The ligand for CD28 is a surface molecule called B7/BB1 which is expressed by all cells capable of presenting antigen to $CD4^+$ cells. B7/BB1 is one of the activation markers for B cells and macrophages, which is most probably the reason why resting B cells and macrophages cannot effectively present antigen.

The biochemical pathway leading to induction of clonal anergy is unclear. The initial events in TCR-mediated signal transduction seem to be normal (see below). IL-2 production, however, is almost completely shut off in anergic T-cell clones. Addition of exogenous IL-2 cannot prevent the induction of anergy, suggesting that anergy is not due simply to the absence of IL-2. The induction of clonal anergy is dependent on the synthesis of new proteins, since it can be blocked by cycloheximide. It is also dependent on a raise in intracellular calcium. Anergy induction is blocked by chelation of calcium ions, but on the other hand, calcium ionophore, a substance that induces a rapid rise in intracellular calcium, is sufficient to induce clonal anergy on its own. These findings imply that although the initial rise in intracellular calcium is a required step in the induction of anergy, it is not the only requirement.

The state of anergy, once induced, is long-lasting and usually cannot be reversed. It has been reported, however, that large amounts of IL-2 can at least partially reverse the anergic state mostly in human T cells and for murine T cells rendered anergic in vivo (see below).

In parallel with the in vitro studies described above, a state of antigen-specific unresponsiveness closely resembling clonal anergy has also been described in vivo. This state of unresponsiveness was first demonstrated in transgenic mouse models in which allogeneic MHC antigens were expressed in a tissue-specific manner in "nonconventional" APCs. The first example came from experiments (originally aimed at studying the mechanism responsible for the onset of type I diabetes) in which the I-Eα gene driven by the insulin or elastase promoters was introduced into the I-Eα-negative C57/Bl6 mouse strain. This mouse strain produces the I-Eβ chain in normal amounts, and therefore, upon introduction of the I-Eα gene it will express a complete I-E molecule on the cell surface but only in pancreatic B cells (and unexpectedly in kidney tubular epithelium) or acinar cells. Surprisingly, the cells expressing the allo class II antigen were not recognized as foreign by the host's immune system. No T-cell infiltrates were observed in the pancreas of the transgenic mice (even after priming with $I-E^+$ spleen cells), and T cells from these mice showed no reactivity to I-E in vitro.

Similar results were obtained in experiments in which the allogeneic class II I-A or class I K^b genes were expressed specifically in the pancreas and in other transgenic models in which allogeneic class I genes were expressed only in astrocytes or liver. In most cases, T cells from these transgenic mice developed tolerance to the transgene, although it is an MHC gene expressed only extrathymically, implying that an extrathymic mechanism was responsible for tolerance induction. It was suggested that MHC genes expressed on the "wrong" cell type cannot stimulate T cells. To test this hypothesis, several groups introduced normal syngeneic T cells (by direct injection, generation of bone marrow chimeras, or simply by breeding) into transgenic mice expressing a particular MHC transgene to which the introduced T cells could respond in a mixed-lymphocyte reaction.

Although the results of these experiments are by no means identical, the following general picture emerges: When mature T cells are introduced into transgenic mice expressing an allogeneic MHC gene extrathymically, the organ expressing the transgene is usually not rejected. Most of the introduced T cells expressing TCR specific for the transgene product are deleted by an unknown mechanism (constant stimulation?). In all cases, however, some of the cells (30 to 70 percent) persist in the peripheral lymphoid organs, but they become unresponsive to the transgenic antigen. This state of unresponsiveness resembles clonal anergy induced in vitro. Certain differences, however, were reported in the in vivo models. For example, the anergic cells in one model were shown to down-regulate the expression of their TCR and CD8. In other cases the anergic state could be reversed by addition of exogenous IL-2 or by stimulating the cells with anti-TCR antibodies. The similarities and differences between the in vitro and the in vivo models need to be further studied, but the concept of clonal anergy nonetheless provides a logical mechanism for tolerizing T cells extrathymically.

It is tempting to propose that anergy is induced both in vitro and in vivo when antigen is presented in the absence of the same costimulatory signal. It could be argued that this costimulatory signal is only made by "professional" APCs. If antigen is presented on cells that do not make the costimulatory signal, anergy rather than responsiveness is induced. Another appealing aspect of this theory is that it implies that T cells bearing receptors capable of recognizing tissue-specific self-antigens do not have to be deleted in the thymus. Such cells would not pose any danger to the host, since the self-antigen for which they are specific is normally expressed on cells that cannot supply the costimulatory signal needed to activate T cells. In the experimental models of unresponsiveness induced by deaggregated proteins or by very low doses of antigen, one could argue that antigen cannot be processed by normal APCs and therefore induces anergy rather than a response. Indeed it has been shown that deaggregated antigens are not pynocytosed by macrophages. Clonal anergy was also shown to occur intrathymically, so this mechanism of cell tolerance might have an even broader role in self-tolerance.

T-CELL ACTIVATION

One of the fundamental characteristics of the immune response is that the initial frequency of T (and B) cells specific for most foreign antigens is very low. Therefore, the first step in mounting an adequate response to a foreign antigen is to expand the specific T-cell clone(s) that recognize the antigen. The initial antigen recognition event is followed by a massive cell proliferation resulting in the propagation of effector cells and the generation of memory cells. The study of the biochemical and molecular events leading to this activation has become a field of intense investigation in recent years.

From experiments with T-cell mitogens

like concanavalin A (conA) and phytohem-agglutinin (PHA) it was first realized that mitogen-activated T cells both secrete and respond to the autocrine growth factor IL-2. It was subsequently shown that antigen-specific stimulation also induces the secretion of IL-2 and the expression of the IL-2 receptor (IL-2R) by the responding T cells. Upon activation, T cells can secrete other lymphokines, such as IL-4 and IFN-γ, which in turn can affect a variety of other cells (see Chap. 10).

Most of the physiologic activation signals for T cells are transduced through, or are somehow associated with, the TCR. Activation can be induced directly, by the binding of antigen to the TCR; artificially, by cross-linking the receptor with an anti-TCR antibody; or indirectly, by cross-linking other cell surface molecules that are somehow coupled to the TCR. An example of the latter case is the stimulation of T cells with conA, anti-Thy-1 or anti-Ly-6 antibodies. The Ly-6 locus encodes for at least seven distinct cell surface molecules, including the T-cell activation marker called TAP. Different Ly-6 molecules are expressed on many leukocytes, including T and B cells. The function of Ly-6 is unknown, but several studies have shown that activation of T cells via the TCR requires the presence of Ly-6 on the cell surface. In these cases, T-cell activation is considered a TCR-dependent event since it will not occur in the absence of surface expression of the TCR. The interaction between the TCR and antigen presented on the surface of the APC can be enhanced by the interaction of "accessory" molecules expressed on both cell types. The CD4 and CD8 molecules expressed on the surface of T cells interact with MHC class II and class I molecules, respectively, expressed on APCs. Although this is not their only function in signal transduction, CD4 and CD8 molecules were shown to increase the affinity of T cell–APC interactions, especially in cases of low-affinity TCR-antigen interactions. Other examples of cell surface molecules which increase the communication between cells are

the lymphocyte function antigens LFA-3–CD2 and LFA-1–ICAM-1 (intercellular adhesion molecule 1) interactions. All of these accessory molecules increase the avidity of interactions between T cells and APCs but may also be directly involved in signal transduction.

As is the case with other receptor-transduced signals (hormones and their receptors, for example), the binding of a ligand to its receptor induces conformational changes and/or internalization of the receptor-ligand complex. This induces a cascade of intracellular events culminating in the activation of transcription of new genes. TCR-mediated signal transduction is a relatively new field of research currently under intense investigation, and relatively little is known about the biochemical events that lead to cell activation. The following is a brief summary of what is known about these events.

Two major biochemical pathways were shown to be involved in signal transduction in T cells. Of the two, the better characterized is the phosphatidylinositide (PI) pathway (Fig. 7B-2). This pathway is not limited to T cells and can participate in other cell-activation models. Immediately (within minutes) after the TCR binds antigen (or after cross-linking of the TCR by any other means), the enzyme phospholipase C (PLC) is activated and hydrolyses (cleaves) phosphatidylinositol 4,5-bisphosphate (PIP_2) into 1,2-diacylglyceride (DAG) and inositol 1,4,5-triphosphate (IP_3). DAG, in turn, induces the translocation of the enzyme protein kinase C (PKC) from the cytoplasm to the cell membrane. This enzyme is a serine-threonine–specific kinase, which phosphorylates the γ and ε chains of CD3 and probably other surface molecules. c-*raf*, a cytoplasmic protein and itself a serine-threonine kinase (the substrates of which are unknown), is also phosphorylated by PKC. IP_3 activates membrane calcium channels which causes the rapid influx of Ca^{2+} ions into the cell and the release of calcium ions from intracellular pools. (Calcium influx into the cell can be easily measured by first loading the cells with a dye

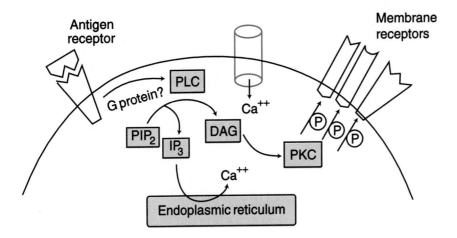

Figure 7B-2.   Activation of T and B cells via the antigen receptor. Signaling via the antigen receptor results in the activation of PLC which cleaves PIP_2 to DAG and IP_3. IP_3 induces Ca^{2+} release from the endoplasmic reticulum, and DAG activates PKC, which phosphorylates intracellular and membrane protein.

that fluoresces in the presence of Ca^{2+} ions.) The exact mechanism responsible for the activation of calcium channels is unknown, but blocking these channels prevents T-cell activation. PKC, and most probably other kinases, are Ca^{2+}-dependent. Phosphorylation of calmodulin is also dependent on Ca^{2+} influx, although it is not known whether calmodulin itself plays any role in T-cell activation.

The exact biochemical events leading from phosphorylation of cell surface proteins to cell activation is still unknown. However, it has been demonstrated that the activation of PKC is crucial for T-cell activation. Drugs which block PKC prevent T-cell activation through the TCR. Another indication that the phosphatidylinositide pathway is involved in general signal transduction comes from studies involving the pharmacologic agents phorbol myristate acetate (PMA), a phorbol diester, and calcium ionophores such as ionomycin and A23187. PMA acts as a DAG analogue and directly activates PKC, while calcium ionophores induce Ca^{2+} influx into the cell. None of these agents alone can induce cell activation, but when com-

bined they mimic at least some of the effects induced by receptor-ligand interaction and induce enough of the biochemical events to cause cell proliferation.

The coupling of the phosphatidylinositide pathway to conformational changes in the TCR is a matter still under investigation. In other systems, G proteins (GTP-binding proteins) have been shown to couple receptors to PKC, but the role of G proteins in T-cell activation remains controversial. cAMP and cGMP serve as second messengers in many other cell types, but their role in T-cell activation is also unclear. An increase in the intracellular levels of both molecules has been reported in T cells following activation, but a direct role in signal transduction has not been established.

The second major biochemical event involved in T-cell signaling is the activation of various tyrosine kinases, a common phenomenon in many receptor-ligand-induced signaling events. These enzymes are somehow associated with the receptor or can be an integral part of the receptor molecule itself. The conformational changes induced by the binding of the ligand to the receptor activates the kinase activity. This results in the phosphorylation of adjacent membrane proteins and may include the phosphorylation of the kinase molecule itself.

A few tyrosine-specific and serine-threonine-specific kinases are activated following TCR-ligand interactions. p56^{lck}, a product of the proto-oncogene *lck*, which is closely related to c-*src*, is a lymphocyte-specific membrane-associated tyrosine kinase. Most cellular p56^{lck} molecules are physically associated with the cytoplasmic domains of CD4 in CD4$^+$ cells and CD8 in CD8$^+$ cells. CD4 internalization induced either directly by anti-CD4 antibodies or indirectly by any stimulation through the TCR provokes the dissociation of p56^{lck} from CD4. Antigen stimulation of CD8$^+$ cells does not result in a similar dissociation of p56^{lck} from CD8. Aggregation of CD4 on the surface of the cell by multivalent antibodies or by binding to MHC class II stimulates the kinase activity of p56^{lck}. T-cell activation through the TCR results in the tyrosine phosphorylation of several molecules, including the CD3-associated ζ chain, and of p56^{lck} itself in positions 394 and 505. There is evidence to suggest that p56^{lck} is responsible for this activity and is therefore a part of the signal-transduction pathway in T cells. Experimental evidence supporting a pivotal role for p56^{lck} in T-cell signal transduction is accumulating rapidly.

The phosphorylation and dephosphorylation of the tyrosine residue in position 505 regulate the function of p56^{lck}. When this tyrosine is phosphorylated, the molecule loses its kinase activity. Mutation of tyrosine 505 to phenylalanine (F505), an amino acid that cannot be phosphorylated, results in constitutive activation, implying that physiologic phosphorylation of this site is down-regulating the activity of p56^{lck}. Introducing such a mutation into fibroblasts can induce transformation, suggesting that p56^{lck} might be involved in the general regulation of cell growth.

Recently, this mutant *lck* gene (F505) was introduced into transgenic mice. In F505 transgenic mice expressing low levels of the transgene, thymocytes could not be stimulated with regular TCR-mediated stimuli. Ca^{2+} influx in thymocytes from these mice was more rapid than in normal thymocytes. (A 10-fold overexpression of the *normal* p56^{lck} in other transgenic mice resulted in a similar phenotype.) An intermediate level of expression of the F505 transgene resulted in a maturational arrest; most T cells did not mature to express the CD3-TCR complex. High levels of expression resulted in T-cell tumors. (Can you think of a possible mechanism for this?) These experiments strongly suggest that p56^{lck} is also involved in signal transduction via CD4 and CD8 during thymic selection.

It could be hypothesized that the phosphorylation of p56^{lck} during early stages of T-cell development or in mature T cells in the absence of normal TCR-mediated stimulation might play a role in the induction of one form or another of unresponsiveness. This could also explain the negative effect of multivalent anti-CD4 antibodies on T-cell activation in the absence of antigen.

p56^{lck} activity is also regulated by CD45. Different forms of CD45 are expressed in different cell types. All forms are the product of one complex gene consisting of 34 exons which are alternatively spliced at the RNA level to yield up to eight different proteins. Members of the CD45 family differ in their extracellular domains but share a common cytoplasmic domain which consists of two tyrosine-specific phosphatase domains in tandem. A possible connection between CD45 and p56^{lck} was first realized when it was found that variant cell lines that do not express CD45 show increased levels of the phosphorylated form of p56^{lck}. It was also shown that CD3-mediated activation is much less effective in CD45-negative variants. These experiments suggest that CD45 can modulate signaling by keeping tyrosine residues on p56^{lck} nonphosphorylated (or in a "responsive" state). It is not yet clear if CD45 regulates the level of phosphorylation of other molecules.

Another tyrosine-specific kinase, p59^{fyn}, also a member of the *src* family of cellular proto-oncogenes, was also recently shown to be involved in TCR-mediated signaling. p59^{fyn} coprecipitates with CD3, and thymocytes from mice transgenic for this molecule are hypersensitive to CD3-mediated activation. When stimulated, these cells exhibit a very rapid increase in intracellular Ca^{2+} and tyrosine phosphorylation of a number of proteins as well as augmented IL-2 production and cell proliferation.

The number of newly discovered proteins that are phosphorylated following TCR-mediated activation is constantly growing. These proteins are being catalogued according to their molecular weight and the time at which phosphorylation occurs following T-cell activation. Correlation with cellular functions and association of a specific kinase with a particular substrate will soon follow. At the time this chapter was written, two waves of phosphorylation had been identified. Phosphorylated proteins with molecular masses of 53, 56, 59, 62, 110, and 120 kd can be detected as rapidly as 5 s after activation (with a $t_{1/2}$ of 2 min), and these phosphorylations precede Ca^{2+} mobilization and PLC activation. Some of these proteins have been identified; p59, for example, is the *fyn* protein discussed above.

A second, late ($t_{1/2}$ of 15 min) wave of phosphorylation involves the CD3γ and CD3ε chains (which are phosphorylated by PKC) and the CD3-associated ζ chain. As stated above, it is not yet known how the phosphorylation of the CD3γ and CD3ε chains is involved in signal transduction. The role of ζ-chain phosphorylation in signal transduction is under intense investigation. Recent studies with variant T-cell lines deficient in η-chain expression suggest that ζ/ζ-chain TCRs are coupled to a different stimulation pathway than TCRs containing ζ/η. The ζ/η-chain form of the TCR is coupled to the PI pathway, whereas the ζ/ζ-chain form is coupled to tyrosine phosphorylation–dependent signals. Interestingly, in T-cell hybrids, stimulation of a ζ/ζ-chain TCR induced the characteristic G_1 to S cycle block but did not induce apoptosis.

ACTIVATION OF GENE EXPRESSION

Our understanding of how all of the biochemical events discussed above culminate in gene activation is very limited. Whether the phosphatidylinositide pathway is independent of the tyrosine phosphorylation pathway or whether the two pathways converge is yet to be determined. As is the case in other signal-transduction systems, genes which are activated following stimulation can generally be categorized as *early* or *late* genes. Activation of the early genes usually does not require synthesis of new proteins. Activation of the late genes is usually regulated by the early set of genes and therefore is dependent on new protein synthesis.

Among the early genes activated following T-cell stimulation are the two proto-oncogenes c-*myc* and c-*fos*, both of which encode nucleoproteins of an as-yet-undefined function, and the gene encoding the lymphokine tumor necrosis factor α (TNF-α). c-*fos* has been shown to interact with a DNA-binding protein, AP-1, which is involved in the regulation of expression of many genes, including PKC. Both c-*myc* and c-*fos* are induced by PMA or calcium ionophore alone, implying that their activation is insufficient to induce the entire signaling pathway, since neither PKC nor calcium ionophores by themselves can induce full T-cell activation.

Lymphokine genes, some of the genes encoding their receptors, and other transcription factors such as NF-κB and NF-AT are examples of secondary or late genes activated after stimulation. So far, activation of the IL-2 gene is the most studied event. It was first thought that the activation of the PI pathway was responsible for activation of the IL-2 gene. This was based on studies that showed that IL-2 production could be elicited by PMA and ionomycin, which, as mentioned earlier, activate the PI pathway without activating tyrosine phosphorylation. It was also determined that Jurkat cells (a human T-cell line) transfected with the gene coding for the muscarinic receptor could be stimulated to produce IL-2 by the muscarinic analogue carbachol. The muscarinic receptor is coupled to the PI pathway but is normally not expressed in T cells.

Recently, however, it was found that T-cell variant lines in which the PKC-activation pathway is defective produce IL-2 when stimulated via the TCR. Tyrosine phosphorylation, including that of the ζ chain, was also unaffected in these cells. These results suggest that the IL-2 gene can be activated through both pathways. Interestingly, cyclosporine blocks IL-2 production by both pathways. It could therefore be argued that these two pathways converge somewhere down the line, although it cannot be ruled out that both pathways are independently blocked by cyclosporine. The expression of the IL-2 gene is under complex regulation. The IL-2 enhancer region contains at least four functional elements, two of which are NF-κB and NF-AT binding sequences. It seems that all four of them must be occupied in order for the enhancer to properly function. Cyclosporine was found to block the production of NF-AT.

T-cell activation also leads to the activation of genes encoding new cell surface proteins. These include nutrient receptors like the transferrin and insulin receptors and lymphokine receptors, mainly the α chain of the IL-2 receptor (IL-2R). The function of some of these gene products [for example, UCHL1, a low molecular weight form of CD45; CDw29, a member of the VLA family (see below); and the T11$_3$ epitope on the CD2 molecule] might be related to the generation of memory T cells. Some genes, like the ones encoding cell interaction molecules known as integrins, are only activated days after initial stimulation and their protein products are therefore called *very late antigens* (*VLA*). One of these genes, VLA-5, is a receptor for fibronectin, which might serve as an accessory molecule in the activation of memory cells.

The most studied gene in this category is the gene encoding the α chain of the IL-2R,

also called p55. This protein is detected by the anti-Tac (for *T* activated) monoclonal antibody and is necessary for surface expression of the high-affinity IL-2R. Three sites of transcription initiation have been found, suggesting that this gene might be activated through different pathways. Its regulation is independent of the IL-2 gene. For example, PMA is a potent inducer of the IL-2Rα gene but does not activate the IL-2 gene, whereas cyclosporine inhibits the activation of the IL-2 gene but does not inhibit the expression of the IL-2R gene. Moreover, whereas the IL-2 gene is only activated following cell stimulation, cells that were once induced to express IL-2Rα will express low levels of this receptor even in a resting state. This could provide a means for recruiting and stimulating resting memory T cells.

ADDITIONAL READINGS

Beverley PCL. Functional analysis of human T cell subsets defined by CD45 isoform expression. *Semin Immunol.* 1992;4:35.

Braciale TJ, Braciale VL. Antigen presentation: Structural themes and functional variations. *Immunol Today.* 1991;12:124.

Cambier JC. Signal transduction by T and B cell antigen receptors: Converging structures and concepts. *Curr Opin Immunol.* 1992;4:257.

Chan AC, Irving BA, Weiss A. New insights into T cell antigen receptor structure and signal transduction. *Curr Opin Immunol.* 1992;4:246.

Gerry G, Klaus B, eds. Transmembrane signalling in lymphocytes. *Semin Immunol.* 1990; vol 2.

Hemler ME. VLA proteins in the integrin family: Structure function, and their role on leukocytes. *Annu Rev Immunol.* 1990;8:365.

Janeway CA. The T cell receptor as a multicomponent signalling machine: CD4/CD8 coreceptors and CD45 in T cell activation. *Annu Rev Immunol.* 1992;10:645.

Jenkins MK, Miller RA. Memory and anergy: Challenges to traditional models of T lymphocyte differentiation. *FASEB J.* 1992;6:2430.

Kishimoto TK, Larson RS, Cobri AL, Dustin ML, Staunton DE, Springer TA. The leukocyte integrins. *Adv Immunol.* 1989;46:149.

Monaco JJ. A molecular model of MHC class I-restricted antigen processing. *Immunol Today.* 1992;13:173.

Mossman TR, Coffman RL. TH1 and TH2 cells: Different patterns of lymphokine secretion lead to different functional properties. *Annu Rev Immunol.* 1989;7:145.

Ransdell F, Fowlkes BJ. Clonal deletion versus clonal anergy—The role of the thymus in inducing self tolerance. *Science.* 1990;248:1357.

8

Specific and Nonspecific Cell-Mediated Cytotoxicity

INTRODUCTION

The essential function of cell-mediated cytotoxicity is eradication of cells responsible for sustaining an infection or other pathologic condition. Cytotoxic cells kill cells infected with virus, transformed cells, and cells infected with other intracellular pathogens. Some cytotoxic cells can also attack helminths and other parasites. Their purpose is clearance of abnormal cells, not of circulating antigen that may arise as a result of a disease process. Though humoral immunity eliminates free virus particles by means of antibody and phagocytes, it is the cytotoxic effector that destroys infected cells where virus replicates. The diverse repertoire of effector cells, consisting of cytotoxic T lymphocytes (CTLs), natural killer (NK) cells, activated macrophages, and eosinophils and other granulocytes, enables the immune system to respond to different challenges.

Cytotoxic T lymphocytes derive from the thymus; each CTL expresses a unique receptor with which to recognize antigen on target cells. Natural killer cells, on the other hand, behave as promiscuous killers, attacking broad categories of transformed cells and virally infected cells. Receptors by which NK cells distinguish targets from nontargets remain to be characterized. Whereas CTLs must be induced by antigenic challenge, i.e., viral infection, NK activity requires no prior immunization. Natural killer cells can be derived directly from the circulation or lymphoid organs of naive individuals. Natural killer cells behave as a first line of defense, ready to respond to newly arising transformed cells without induction; subsequently, antigenic stimulation gives rise to CTLs.

Macrophages are known principally as phagocytes, destroying ingested antigen with reactive oxidants and hydrolases. However, lymphokines and bacterial products, such as endotoxin, activate macrophages to a cyto-

toxic state, whereupon they kill cells independently of phagocytosis. As with NK cells, macrophages lack the fine specificity of CTLs, and the molecules mediating target recognition are not well defined. However, both macrophages and NK cells, as well as CTLs, express various Fc receptors to bind and attack antibody-coated cells by the process of antibody-dependent-cellular cytotoxicity (ADCC).

The various cytotoxic effectors employ different cytotoxic mechanisms. After recognizing a target cell, some effectors release diffusible cytokines that act not only upon the specific target cell but also upon nearby cells. Other effectors kill only the specifically recognized target by direct delivery of cytotoxic molecules. Both modes of killing are beneficial to immunity: selective killing of one cell among many healthy ones, or broad cytotoxicity within diseased tissue such as tumors. On the other hand, cytotoxic cells can damage a tissue in some autoimmune disease and can also reject transplanted tissues.

CYTOTOXIC T LYMPHOCYTES

Cytotoxic T lymphocytes (CTLs) are antigen-specific killers that recognize and lyse aberrant cells in the body (Fig. 8-1). Their principal targets consist of transformed cells and cells infected with viruses. There are reports that CTLs also act against targets infected with other nonviral intracellular pathogens, such as mycobacteria and parasites. The role of CTLs in immune responses is best exemplified in responses to viral infection. While antibody can neutralize or facilitate phagocytosis of circulating virus particles, it does not suppress production of virus in already infected cells. CTLs serve to eliminate the sites of viral replication. In in-

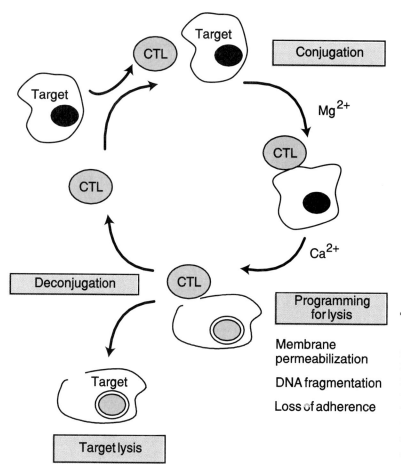

Figure 8-1 Lytic cycle of CTLs. *Conjugation:* A CTL recognizes a target cell and forms a tight conjugate with it. *Programming for lysis:* the CTL delivers toxic factors to the target cell. *Deconjugation:* The CTL and target cell dissociate; the CTL seeks other targets while the target proceeds to lyse.

stances where virus is transferred efficiently between cells without a necessary extracellular transit, effectors that attack infected cells are essential.

Antigen Recognition

The antigenic specificity of a CTL is determined by its T-cell receptor (TCR). The TCR can bind antigen only when presented on the surface of a target cell in complex with proteins encoded by the major histocompatibility complex (MHC). This receptor consists of a heterodimer of highly variable α and β chains, clonally distributed like immuno-globulin, and able to recognize a large universe of potential antigens. Functional TCR exists in complex with CD3, a pentameric protein characteristic of T lymphocytes (see Chap. 7). When a CTL encounters a target cell expressing the MHC-antigen complex recognized by its TCR, its cytotoxic potential is triggered. Thus, a CTL surveys the surface of potential targets for appropriate antigen presented on MHC.

Although TCR-CD3 imparts specificity to the discrimination of antigen, other surface molecules, such as CD4, CD8, and the lymphocyte-function-associated antigens (LFAs), cooperate in conjugation of T cells to targets

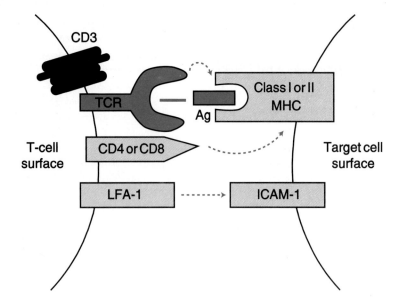

Figure 8-2 T-cell receptor interacting with MHC-antigen complex and the cooperation of accessory adhesion molecules. Antigen-specific TCR binds antigenic peptide associated with polymorphic determinants of class I or class II MHC. CD4 interacts with conserved structures of class II MHC. CD8 binds with conserved structures of class I MHC. LFA-1 interacts with ICAM-1 on target cell surface.

(Fig. 8-2). Antibody against these auxiliary molecules inhibits the cytotoxicity of CTLs and also of NK cells. Experiments with monoclonal antibodies directed to the CD4 or CD8 surface proteins demonstrate that the CD8 and CD4 proteins assist in the docking of TCR-CD3 with MHC-antigen complexes. CD4 appears to interact with nonpolymorphic determinants of class II MHC, and CD8 with class I. This interaction bolsters the low-affinity binding of TCR with the polymorphic aspects of MHC-antigen complex. There is evidence to suggest that TCRs of high avidity for MHC-antigen complex depend less on the assistance of CD4 or CD8; high-avidity clones are less easily blocked by antibody to CD4 or CD8. Other surface molecules that stabilize interactions between CTL and target cell include the lymphocyte-function-associated antigens (LFA-1) and other intracellular adhesion molecules (ICAM), interacting with specific, nonpolymorphic ligands present on most cell surfaces. Inherited deficiency in LFA, leukocyte adhesion deficiency (LAD), results in enhanced susceptibility to bacterial infections. (See Clinical Aside 8-1; also see Chap. 17.)

Clinical Aside 8-1
Lymphocyte Adhesion Deficiency

Lymphocyte-function-associated antigens (LFA) belong to the integrin family and consist of related α/β dimers. Lymphocyte adhesion deficiency (LAD) is a recessively inherited deficiency of the β_1 chain. Lymphocyte adhesion deficiency results in profound susceptibility to bacterial infection. Due to the absence of LFA-1, neutrophils of affected individuals do not adhere well to vessel walls and are deficient in ability to migrate from the circulation to sites of infection.

Although LFA-1 cooperates with the TCR in the binding of T lymphocytes to target cells, T-cell function is only mildly affected in LAD patients. Possibly, T cells with higher-avidity receptors are selected to compensate for absence of LFA-1; alternatively, an unidentified integrin may substitute for LFA-1 on T cells but not on neutrophils.

Some evidence suggests that the newly characterized T lymphocytes with receptors consisting of γ and δ chains are also cytotoxic. Epithelial tissues are enriched with γ/δ T cells. The range of variability in receptors among γ/δ cells seems much less than for α/β

CTLs. Whether γ/δ cells recognize antigen in the context of some MHC product remains unsettled. It has been suggested that these cells have evolved to recognize a set of conserved structures expressed on damaged or transformed cells arising in epithelia.

Distinct routes of antigen processing operate for presentation on class I and class II MHC molecules. Normally, fragments of endogenous protein antigens, i.e., antigens synthesized within the presenting cell, are offered on class I for T-cell recognition. Thus, antigens from virus replicating intracellularly, or neoantigens expressed in an abnormal cell, are subject to presentation on class I. However, on antigen-presenting cells, e.g., dendritic cells that express both class I and class II MHC, endogenous antigens are also presented on both classes of MHC molecules. It is likely, though not proved, that antigens from intracellular bacteria or parasites may also be presented on class I. In contrast, circulating antigens, which enter cells by phagocytosis or pinocytosis, are usually presented on cell surfaces complexed only to class II MHC. With infrequent exceptions, classical CD8 T cells (i.e., CD4$^-$, CD8$^+$) recognize antigen on class I MHC, while CD4 T cells (i.e., CD4$^+$, CD8$^-$) see antigen on class II MHC. Class I–restricted CD8 T cells induced by immunization with high doses of soluble protein have been reported, suggesting that presentation of exogenous antigen on class I MHC can occur, if only under these artificial conditions.

Studies of CTLs responding to influenza virus infections show that not only membrane proteins, but any proteins synthesized within target cells, can be processed and presented on class I MHC. In certain mice, the predominant CTL response, restricted by class I MHC, is not to the hemagglutinins, which are expressed on the cell surface, but to nucleocapsid proteins. Although nucleocapsid proteins are not themselves expressed on the membranes of infected cells, proteolytic fragments of these proteins are presented in complex with class I MHC.

It appears that CTL surveillance and an-

tigen presentation on class I MHC function as a quality control system whereby any polypeptide made within a cell is subject to immunosurveillance. It has been shown that proteins resulting from foreign genes introduced into a cell by gene transfection will be processed and presented on class I MHC in an immunogenic manner and can induce specific CTLs. In this way, the intracellular space is not "privileged," i.e., hidden from the immune system, and abnormal cellular function such as neoplastic transformation can be detected if an abnormal gene product is synthesized.

CD4 and CD8 Phenotypes of Cytotoxic T Cells

T lymphocytes can be subdivided by their expression of surface antigens CD4 and CD8. In the periphery, the expression of these antigens is mutually exclusive; thus T cells are designated CD4 or CD8 (in humans, the designations T4 and T8 are also used). It has been widely assumed that phenotypic distinction of T lymphocytes as CD4 and CD8 subsets coincides with segregation of function, that the CD4 subset consists of helper/inducer cells, and that the CD8 cells represent suppressor and cytotoxic cells. Characterization of cytotoxic CD4 cells in primates and rodents contradicts this view. When murine spleen cells are stimulated with allogeneic (histoincompatible) or virally infected targets, predominantly CD8 CTLs arise. However, protocols of in vitro stimulation with soluble protein antigen yield cytotoxic CD4 cells, along with noncytotoxic CD4 helper T cells. In humans, cytotoxic CD4 cells, as well as CD8 CTLs, arise readily from stimulation in vitro with syngeneic cells infected with Epstein-Barr virus (Fig. 8-3). Studies of the in vivo CTL response to influenza infection imply a role for both phenotypes of CTLs. It is important to note that the modes of antigen recognition by CD4 and CD8 cells do not change with function. In other words, although CD4 cells can function as CTLs, they recognize antigen only in

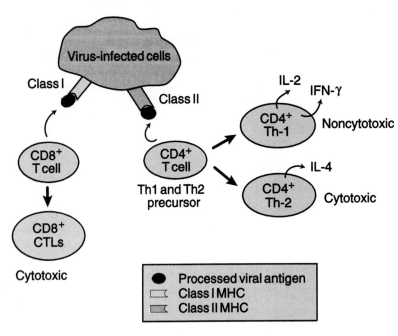

Figure 8-3 Induction of T cells by virus-infected cells. Virus-infected cells present antigen complexed to class 1 MHC, leading to induction of CD8 CTLs. The infected cells also present antigens on class II MHC, leading to activation and proliferation of Th1 and Th2 CD4 cell. Th1 cells secrete IL-2 and IFN-γ. Th2 cells secrete IL-4 and are cytotoxic. IFN-γ can induce the expression of class II MHC by many cells, thus allowing presentation to CD4 cells.

conjunction with class II MHC. Thus, the CD4/CD8 dichotomy refers to patterns of MHC restriction and antigen recognition and does not distinguish cytotoxic from noncytotoxic cells. It has yet to be determined whether CD4 and CD8 cytotoxic cells play distinct roles in immune protection.

Two subsets of CD4 cells, Th1 and Th2, are classified by their distinct secretions of lymphokines, including interleukin 2 (IL-2), interleukin 4 (IL-4), and interferon gamma (IFN-γ). Th1 cells secrete IL-2 and IFN-γ to the exclusion of IL-4, but Th2 cells secrete IL-4 with no IL-2 or IFN-γ. Other lymphokines, such as IL-3 and granulocyte-macrophage colony-stimulating factor (GM-CSF), are secreted equally by both types of CD4 cells. In their pattern of lymphokine secretion, Th1 cells more closely approach CD8 CTLs, which in some cases also secrete IL-2. Cytotoxic CD4 cells tend to belong to the Th1 subgroup. It is important to remember that IFN-γ induces many cell types that do not normally express class II MHC to do so. These cells are then capable of presenting

antigen to class II-restricted CD4 cells. Thus, CD4 CTLs can respond alongside CD8 T cells.

Activation and Induction of CTLs

Two signals are important to the development of cytotoxic T cells: antigen-presenting targets and the lymphokines IL-2 or IL-4. In vivo, IL-2 and IL-4 are secreted by helper T cells, and responding CTLs express receptors for these lymphokines. Notable differences in the function of IL-2 and IL-4 have been demonstrated. Whereas both lymphokines stimulate the antigen-dependent proliferation of CTLs, only IL-2 has been shown to generate lymphokine-activated killer (LAK) cells, noted for their promiscuous killing of tumor cells (see below).

Antigen-specific triggering of CTLs occurs when the TCR-CD3 complex interacts with antigenic peptide complexed with MHC. However, CTLs also respond to nonspecific signals. Lectins are carbohydrate-binding proteins that can be isolated from a wide variety of organisms. Certain lectins, notably concanavalin A and phytohemagglutinin, stimulate CTLs by cross-linking carbohydrate determinants on target cells with those on the CTL surfaces, including determinants on TCR-CD3. When immobilized on a solid matrix, antibody specific for TCR or CD3 can replace the need for antigen-presenting cells in stimulating proliferation of CTLs. Nonspecific stimulatory signals can be conveyed through other surface molecules, especially CD2 (the sheep erythrocyte receptor) and Thy-1 (a lipid-linked protein on T cells).

In the absence of specific antigen, the cytotoxic potential of CTLs can be activated by other means. *Lectin-dependent killing* can occur when a lectin on a target cell interacts with the TCR-CD3 on the CTL. Lectin-mediated bridging of a CTL to a target cell leads to activation of the CTL in the absence of an antigen-specific interaction. Antibodies to TCR, CD3, or CD2 can bind to and activate CTL. Target cells with Fc receptors can bind the Fc component of these antibodies and thus become targets, again in the absence of any target antigen-specific interaction. Alternatively, the Fc portion of these antibodies can be covalently attached with cross-linking reagents to the surfaces of target cells that lack the appropriate Fc receptors and thereby permit recognition by any CTL.

Events in CTL-Mediated Cytolysis

Three stages of CTL action on target cells have been defined by requirement for the divalent cations Mg^{2+} and Ca^{2+} and susceptibility to inhibition by cytochalasin B, an inhibitor of microfilament polymerization:

1. *Conjugation*, binding with a target cell strictly dependent on Mg^{2+}
2. *Programming for lysis* dependent on Ca^{2+}, when the CTL imparts a lethal signal to the target
3. The *killer cell–independent stage* requiring no divalent cation, when the target cell lyses (Fig. 8-1).

Lysis of target cells can be monitored easily by the release of entrapped radioisotopes or other cytoplasmic markers. (See Clinical Aside 8-2.) Low concentrations of cytochalasin B preferentially inhibit programing for lysis rather than conjugation; thus, conjugates form in which the targets remain viable. Recent observations that some CTL clones can kill targets, albeit less well, in very low levels of Ca^{2+} suggest that programing for lysis does not absolutely depend upon Ca^{2+}. The final phase of cell death requires no divalent cation and can occur even after the target cell is dissociated from the CTL. Death results from damage to the cell membrane and its permeability barrier. Even before membrane damage is evident, fragmentation of chromosomal DNA and loss of nuclear integrity can be detected in cells attacked by CTLs. Target cells affected by CTLs also detach from extracellular matrix. Therefore, even without cell lysis, the genetic machinery of the targeted cell is inactivated, possibly halting viral replication. CTL damage to target cells is very specific; bystander cells lacking appropriate MHC-antigen complex are spared (Clinical Aside 8-3).

Clinical Aside 8-2
Assays of Cell-Mediated Cytotoxicity

The most common quantitative assays of cell-mediated cytotoxicity rely upon the release of an intracellular marker from stricken target cells. Cells are readily labeled with the radioisotope ^{51}Cr by incubation in media containing [^{51}Cr]-sodium chromate. A fixed number of labeled target cells are incubated with varying amounts of cytotoxic cells for a standard time period. Radioactivity released into the supernatant is determined after centrifugation or filtration to remove surviving cells and debris. Data are normally presented as a plot of the percent specific release of label versus the ratio of cytotoxic effector cells to target cells (E/T). *Percent specific release* is a normalized value correct for background leakage of label in the absence of cytotoxic cells and maximum release of ^{51}Cr after lysis under hypotonic conditions or with a detergent. [Note: Percent specific release of label = 100 × (experimental release −

background release)/(maximum release − background release).] Other labels of the intracellular space besides ^{51}Cr have been employed, including cytoplasmic enzymes, such as lactate dehydrogenase, and fluorescent dyes. Other qualitative assays monitor cell death in monolayer cultures with vital stains such as crystal violet.

Activity within various cytotoxic cell preparation may be evaluated by comparing the E/T ratios at which given percent specific release is observed (e.g., at 30 percent specific release of label). Since different cytotoxic cells within a preparation may not have comparable activity, one cannot directly infer from the above comparison the number of cytotoxic cells in a preparation. Nonetheless, the activity of cytotoxic cell preparations compared in this way is useful in that those richer in cytotoxic cells must show greater specific killing at lower E/T ratios than cruder mixtures of cells. Also, the activity of cloned cytotoxic cells under different stimuli can be compared.

Clinical Aside 8-3
Cytotoxic T Cells and HIV Infection

CTLs are induced after viral infection and decline soon after eradication of the infection. In HIV-infected individuals, CTLs that recognize and lyse HIV-infected cells are readily detected. Throughout the earlier stages of infection, levels of HIV-specific CTLs remain elevated. Their levels decline in the latter stages of AIDS, as lymphokine-producing CD4 cells necessary for CTL proliferation disappear. It is thought that these CTLs may participate in the decline of HIV-infected CD4 cells. They may also lyse infected monocytes.

However, HIV-specific CTLs are unable to control the course of infection, and patients inevitably progress to AIDS. Possibly, the infection is maintained through a reservoir of infected cells that are resistant to CTL-mediated lysis.

Exocytosis and T Cell–Mediated Lysis

The discovery of perforin, a Ca^{2+}-dependent pore-forming protein located in cytoplasmic granules of CTLs and NK cells, has contrib-

uted much to current models of CTL action. In primary structure, perforin manifests some homology to the complement proteins C6, C7, C8, and C9; in its pore-forming activity, perforin behaves like C9. In the presence of Ca^{2+}, perforin rapidly inserts into membranes, forms nonspecific channels, and equilibrates ionic gradients across the membranes (Fig. 8-4). Influx of extracellular Ca^{2+} through perforin channels certainly contributes to cell death by disrupting the function of many Ca^{2+}-sensitive processes; sodium and water flow into the cell, leading to lysis by colloidal osmotic swelling.

Early studies indicated that inhibitors of trypsinlike serine hydrolases (proteases) blocked the cytotoxicity of CTLs. Serine hydrolases have been isolated from the cytoplasmic granules of both CD4 and CD8 CTLs. Their expression has been found to coincide with cytotoxicity. In the mouse, at least six distinct hydrolases, known as *granzymes*, have been purified from granules that also contain perforin. Homologous hydrolases have been characterized from human T cells. Two of these enzymes are proteolytically active. When engaging target cells, CTLs secrete the serine protease granzyme A, which is able to hydrolyze amides and esters of lysine and arginine. Presumably perforin and other contents of the granules are also released. The role of these serine hydrolases in the lytic event and their effects on target cells remain unclear. Nonetheless, inhibitors that specifically act upon the T cell–specific granzymes inhibit the cytotoxicity of CTLs.

Localization of both perforin and the serine hydrolases within secretory granules suggests that T cell–mediated lysis occurs through secretion of toxic molecules onto the membrane of target cells. CTLs themselves are highly resistant to perforin; this is essential for CTLs to survive repeated attacks on targets when their own plasma membranes are exposed to perforin secretions. However, not all aspects of CTL-mediated cytolysis can be explained by secretion of perforin. Reports of CTL-mediated

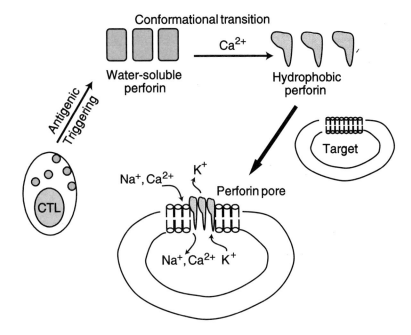

Figure 8-4 Model for the action of perforin in CTL and NK cell–mediated lysis. Soluble perforin undergoes a Ca^{2+}-dependent conformational change, leading to the exposure of hydrophobic surfaces. These hydrophobic conformers insert into membranes and associate to form pores. Ions, especially Ca^{2+} and Na^+, flow through the pore, causing activation of Ca^{2+}-dependent enzymes and lysis by colloidal osmotic swelling.

killing in media with little free Ca^{2+} argue against the secretory model and suggest the existence of alternative means of cell lysis independent of perforin, a protein requiring Ca^{2+} for membrane insertion. Remarkably, these studies find no detectable secretion of granzyme A under the "Ca^{2+}-free" conditions, despite lysis of target cells. Another limitation of the secretory, perforin-dependent model concerns the low levels of perforin in highly cytotoxic T cells derived in vivo. It remains a possibility that these cells contain relatively few, yet potent, lytic granules in comparison to CTL lines maintained in vitro.

Other cytotoxic factors are elaborated by CTLs, and these may mediate Ca^{2+}-independent lytic function (Table 8-1). Among these factors are lymphotoxin, also named *tumor necrosis factor beta* (*TNF-β*). TNF-β is homologous to the macrophage product TNF-α. Activated T cells secrete TNF-β, which has toxic activity toward a variety of tumor

lines. A form of TNF attached to the plasma membrane has received attention as a candidate molecule participating in the lethal hit. CTLs rapidly cause target cells to lose their ability to adhere to surfaces; chromosomal DNA in affected cells is also fragmented. It has not been established that loss of adherence and DNA fragmentation can

TABLE 8-1 Factors from Cytotoxic Cells

Factor	Cell Type
TNF-α	Macrophages
Lymphotoxin (TNF-β)	CTL, NK
Perforin	CTL, NK
Natural killer cytotoxic factor (NKCF)	NK
Major basic protein (MBP)	Eosinophils
Eosinophil-derived neurotoxin (EDN)	Eosinophils
Eosinophil cationic protein (ECP)	Eosinophils
Superoxide, peroxide	Eosinophils, macrophages
Hypohalites (OCl⁻, OBr⁻, OI⁻)	Eosinophils

result from the application of purified perforin on target cells.

NATURAL KILLER CELLS

CTL responses require a period of induction with antigen-presenting cells. Thus, there is need for an immediate response while antigen-specific CTLs develop. It has been observed that nonimmune cells isolated from blood, spleen, and other lymphoid organs are able to kill various tumor lines without induction or immunization. A cytotoxic response requiring no induction with antigen is termed *natural cytotoxicity*. This spontaneous cytotoxicity arises from NK cells, and serves as an initial response before the induction of antigen-specific CTLs. When activated with the proper stimuli, macrophages also acquire potent antigen-independent cytotoxicity for tumor cells and other abnormal cells. Phylogenetically, such antigen-independent cytotoxic effectors predate antigen-specific cells and may serve as the principal line of immune defense in primitive animals.

Characteristics

NK cells lyse a variety of transformed lines, designated *NK-sensitive.* Operationally, NK cells are defined by the ability to kill certain NK-sensitive target cells, including the murine lines YAC-1 and EL4 and human lines K562, U937, and MOLT4. A broader definition of NK activity is based on promiscuous killing of target cells that is neither antigen-specific nor MHC-restricted. It is not clear how NK cells recognize cells; components of NK cell and target cell membranes mediating recognition remain the subject of intense investigation.

Unlike CTLs, which are well identified by a set of surface markers (CD3, TCR, CD2, and CD8 or CD4), NK cells have thus far resisted easy categorization. NK cells express markers indicative of monocyte-gran-

ulocyte lineage (OKM1, CD16), but some fractions of NK cells also express markers normally distinguishing T lymphocytes (CD3 and CD2). Lymphokines acting on T cells also stimulate NK cells. The glycolipid asialo-GM_1 is considered a special marker of cells with NK function; however, even this molecule is expressed by some CTL lines in culture. Nonetheless, the majority of NK cells are not T cells. Athymic nude (*nu/nu*) mice lack T-cell functions, yet exhibit elevated NK function in comparison to wild-type *nu/+* mice. NK cells are heterogeneous with respect to many surface markers. Only a fraction of NK cells express CD3 or CD16, and the antibodies OKT11 and OKM1 deplete separate populations of NK cells.

The preponderance of NK activity is associated with *large granular lymphocytes* (*LGL*), filled with azurophilic granules. Although other minor populations manifest natural cytotoxicity, it may be said that LGLs are the "authentic" NK cells. LGLs seem to arise in vivo from *large agranular lymphocytes* (*LALs*); LALs can be induced in vitro to acquire LGL morphology and NK activity. The surface antigens NKH1 and asialo-GM_1 occur on most LGLs and are considered NK markers. (Recall that in Chapter 2 a marker for NK cells called HNK-1 was mentioned. NKH1 and HNK-1 are different molecules; NKH1 is the same as CD56 (also Leu-19, gp 220/135) and is an isoform of the adhesion molecule N-CAM. NKH1 is the same as CD57 (also Leu-7, gp 110). Both NKH-1 and HNK-1 refer to *h*uman *n*atural *k*iller cells.)

Mechanism of NK Cytotoxicity

In many respects, NK killing resembles CTL-mediated cytolysis (Fig. 8-4). Likewise, stages of NK killing have been distinguished by their divalent cation requirements: Mg^{2+}-dependent conjugation, Ca^{2+}-dependent programing for lysis, and a final cation-independent lysis stage proceeding after dissociation of killer from target cell. A natural killer cell cytotoxic factor (NKCF) is detected in supernatants of NK cells stimulated with NK-sensitive targets. The activity of NKCF is distinct from that of other cytotoxic factors including TNF-α, TNF-β (lymphotoxin), and perforin. A YAC-1 mutant that has become resistant to NK-mediated cytolysis manifests resistance to NKCF-containing supernatants.

LGL granules contain the cytolysin perforin as well as serine hydrolases similar to those in CTLs. The need for Ca^{2+} in programing for lysis supports an important role for perforin, which requires Ca^{2+} for membrane insertion. It has been suggested that perforin channels facilitate the entry of other cytotoxins into targets; thus, perforin might cooperate with other toxic factors produced by NK cells and CTLs.

Recognition of Targets by NK Cells

Natural killer cells attack many transformed lines and normal cell types. They show preference for killing less differentiated cells, especially in the hematopoietic lineage, and may serve to limit the expansion of these cells. It must be noted that NK cells exhibit some limited diversity with respect to target cell recognition. In one study, distinct subgroups of murine NK cells lysed YAC-1 and a methylcholanthrene-induced fibrosarcoma.

Natural killer cells seem to discriminate among targets with a receptor (or set of receptors), recognizing a ligand (or ligands) common to NK-sensitive lines. The laminin receptor has been implicated in studies that demonstrate inhibition of cytotoxicity by antibodies to the receptor and also to laminin-like structures on NK-sensitive targets. However, it is unclear whether this structure is a specific NK receptor or an accessory binding protein, like LFA-1. Other structures have been identified previously, but failed to satisfy essential criteria for an NK receptor. NK cells can also be triggered through auxiliary molecules like CD2. In CTLs, triggering through CD2 fails if the CTL surface is depleted of CD3, suggesting that CD3 is the

transmitter of signals from antigen-bound TCR and also from the auxiliary triggers. However, NK cells lacking CD3 can be triggered through the CD2 molecules. This implies that an as-yet unidentified alternative to CD3 is expressed on these cells.

Antibody-Dependent Cellular Cytotoxicity

Cytotoxic effectors expressing surface receptors for various classes of Ig can bind cells coated with Ig and kill them. Thus, even cells with no antigen-specific receptors can utilize the specificity of antibody in the process of *antibody-dependent-cellular cytotoxicity* (ADCC) (Fig. 8-5). The majority of LGLs express IgG Fc receptor (CD16) and are capable of ADCC. ADCC was once attributed to a special population of blood cells called *K cells*; it may well be that ADCC activity and NK activity reside in related, if not identical, cells. Macrophages, eosinophils, and neutrophils can also mediate ADCC through their Fc receptors. Some antigen-specific CTLs also express Fc receptor and can interact with target cells either through TCR-CD3 or through Fc.

Role of NK Cells in Immunosurveillance

Natural killer cells seem to participate in resistance to tumors and also to viral infection. For prevention of tumors, NK cells may be of greater significance than CTLs; athymic nude mice which lack T cells but which have elevated levels of NK cells are not significantly prone to neoplasia. A role of NK cells in controlling growth of primitive cells in bone marrow has been proposed. Experimental ablation of NK activity in animals with ^{89}Sr or anti-asialo-Gm₁ leads to increased susceptibility to viruses (e.g., murine hepatitis virus and cytomegalovirus), despite competent T-cell function. A notable exception, susceptibility of mice to the lymphocytic choriomeningitis virus (LCMV), is not af-

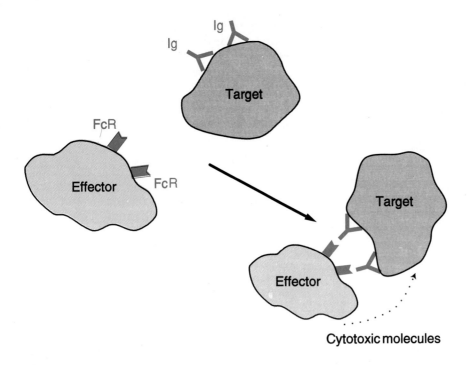

Figure 8-5   Antibody-dependent cellular cytotoxicity. Fc receptor on cytotoxic cell binds antibody associated with antigen on a target cell. Upon
conjugation of the target cell, the cytotoxic cell releases cytotoxic molecule.
Different cytotoxic effector cells release distinct toxic molecules, e.g., TNF-
α, superoxides and peroxides from macrophage, TNF-β and perforin from
CTLs and NK cells, NKCF from NK cells, and MBP, EDN, ECP, superoxides,
peroxides, and hypohalites from eosinophils.

fected by ablation of NK activity; however,
this virus does induce a potent CTL response, sufficient to curtail the infection.
Natural killer cells and CTLs may collaborate against infected cells and neoplasia. Since
they require no induction, NK cells respond
initially, while the pool of specific CTLs must
be induced and expanded as a result of antigenic challenge. Interferon alfa (IFN-α),
whose production is stimulated by virus and
poly-IC (duplexed polymers of inosine and
cytosine), augments NK activity, possibly increasing binding of target cells and release of
cytotoxic factors. Also, it has been reported

that IFN-γ enhances the cytotoxicity of NK
cells.
  Chédiak-Higashi syndrome results from a
lysosomal defect affecting NK cells and other
granular white cells. A murine model is
available in the beige (*bg/bg*) mouse. Patients
with this syndrome and other illnesses associated with defective NK function are more
prone to malignancies, especially of hematopoietic origins. This association with NK
function supports a suggested role for NK
cells in preventing overexpansion of less-dif-
ferentiated cells in bone marrow. (See Chaps.
17, "Polymorphonuclear Phagocytic Cells"

and 22, "Immunodeficiency Syndromes," for more details.)

ACTIVATED MACROPHAGES

Macrophages become activated after receiving two stimuli: first a priming stimulus and then a secondary activating signal (Fig. 8-6). In vitro, IFN-γ supplies the priming stimulus; in vivo, agents that stimulate interferon production, such as viruses and mycobacterial products, can lead to priming. Primed macrophages express class II MHC and present antigen to CD4 T cells. Activation of primed macrophages depends on the second stimulus, usually in the form of *bacterial lipopolysaccharide* (LPS), also known as *endotoxin.* It should be remembered that the immune system is continually exposed to low levels of endotoxin liberated by the bacteria normally found in the gut. It is likely that factors not of bacterial origin, including T-cell products, may activate the tumoricidal activity of macrophages in vivo. Activation leads to many biochemical and morphologic changes in macrophages, including enhanced phagocytosis and production of reactive derivatives of oxygen (Fig. 8-7). Activated macrophages are highly cytotoxic to a wide variety of tumor cells. They can also kill parasites and fungi. The lysis of tumor cells does not require phagocytosis, unlike the killing of bacteria and other small, easily phagocytosed, targets.

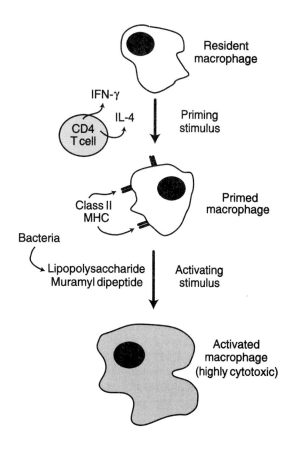

Figure 8-6 Priming and activation of macrophages. Resident macrophages or monocytes are primed by cytokines from CD4 helper cells. This stimulus consists primarily of IFN-γ; in some studies IL-4 has activity. Bacterial products, lipopolysaccharide, or muramyl dipeptide contribute activating stimuli in vitro. It remains a possibility that other factors, not bacterial in origin, may contribute the second activating stimulus.

Mechanisms of Macrophage Cytotoxicity

In response to activation, macrophages produce the potent cytokine tumor necrosis factor, TNF-α. Tumor necrosis factor has been identified as the factor known as "cachectin," which is responsible for the wasting (cachexia) associated with infections and malignancies. Secreted by macrophages, TNF-α interacts with receptors on cell surfaces, leading to death or inhibition of growth in many transformed lines. The action of TNF-α on transformed cells explains earlier observations of tumor regression in patients treated with endotoxin or suffering from coincident septic infection. Some reports claim that a form of TNF-α attached to macrophage membranes participates in killing cells directly in contact with the macro-

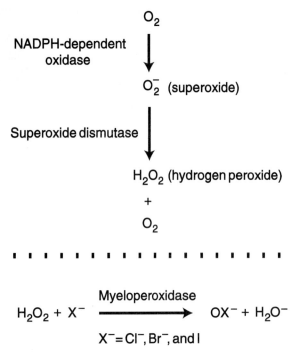

Figure 8-7 Reactive oxygen metabolites elaborated by activated macrophages and eosinophils. Hypohalite (OCl⁻, OBr⁻, and OI⁻) anions are liberated by eosinophils. Superoxide anion and hydrogen peroxide are released both by macrophages and by eosinophils.

phage. By secreting diffusible cytotoxic factors, macrophages not only affect cells in direct contact but also nearby cells sensitive to these factors. Unlike CTLs and NK cells, which focus on the target cells, macrophages can induce broad necrosis in tissues where they are activated. This can be beneficial where a solid tumor is concerned, but is detrimental in autoimmune and inflammatory diseases.

Macrophages must utilize a variety of mechanisms in killing tumors; lysis of some targets can be shown to depend on TNF-α production while lysis of other targets does not, as is shown in the ability of anti-TNF-α antibody to block lysis of certain lines but not of others. Activated macrophages also release potent oxidants, including peroxide and superoxide (Fig. 8-7). Macrophages also

direct a cytostatic effect on tumor lines. This has been shown in some studies to depend on the availability of arginine in culture medium, and is associated with profound loss of mitochondrial function due to the removal of iron from enzymes containing iron-sulfur clusters as prosthetic groups. One hypothesis proposes that macrophages derive from arginine a potent chelator that can dissociate iron from Fe-S proteins but not from heme proteins.

Target Recognition

Macrophages do not express antigen-specific receptors and, therefore, cannot specifically recognize antigens. However, macrophages, like NK cells, express Fc receptors and can utilize antibody to specifically bind targets and kill them. For example, IgG-coated schistosomes are bound via Fc receptors and lysed by ADCC. Other studies indicate that macrophages can also lyse schistosomes independently of specific antibody. Although macrophages are capable of ADCC, lysis of many tumor lines in vitro proceeds in the absence of antibody. Macrophages can select the target cells they kill; in cocultivation of tumors with bystander normal cells, tumor cells are killed preferentially while the bystanders are spared. This may result either from inability of macrophages to recognize normal cells or resistance of normal cells to soluble cytotoxic factor released by macrophages. Indeed, normal cells tend not to succumb to TNF-α.

Like NK cells, macrophages must recognize structures common to tumor cells and less differentiated cells. Little is known about the mechanism of antigen-independent target cell recognition. A stage when macrophages recognize target cells prior to target damage has been described, and killing of target cells has been shown to require intercellular contact. By killing many tumor lines not sensitive to NK activity, macrophages enhance immunosurveillance for malignancies and serve as another arm of natural immunity. For further description of macrophages, see Chap. 18.

EOSINOPHILS

Eosinophils are polymorphonuclear leukocytes with large cytoplasmic granules that stain avidly with acidic dyes. The granules contain a family of basic proteins (MBP), rich in arginine, including major basic protein, eosinophil cationic protein (ECP), and eosinophil-derived neurotoxin (EDN). Eosinophils lyse parasitic helminths in chromium release assays (see Clinical Aside 8-2), and are implicated in immune responses to schistosomes. Killing of parasites in vitro may be their most notable function. They also lyse tumor lines in vitro. Eosinophils express Fc receptor for IgE and normally depend on antibody for target cell recognition. Some reports suggest that they may also bind targets in an antibody-independent fashion.

Cationic proteins localized in secretory granules damage target cell membranes; they represent an important cytotoxic weapon of the eosinophil. Major basic protein has been shown to damage schistosomula, larvae of *Trichinella spiralis,* and tumor lines. Eosinophil cationic protein and eosinophil-derived neurotoxin are highly homologous; they are both cytotoxic to parasites and animal cells. Another cytotoxic device of the eosinophil is its peroxidase, which catalyzes oxidation of iodide and chloride to very reactive hypohalites (OI^-, OBr^-, OCl^-) (Fig. 8-7). In close contact with a cell, the eosinophil can focus high concentrations of cationic protein onto the target. Reactive oxidants, however, probably damage many other cells in the local environment (Fig. 8-8). See Chap. 19 for further details on eosinophils.

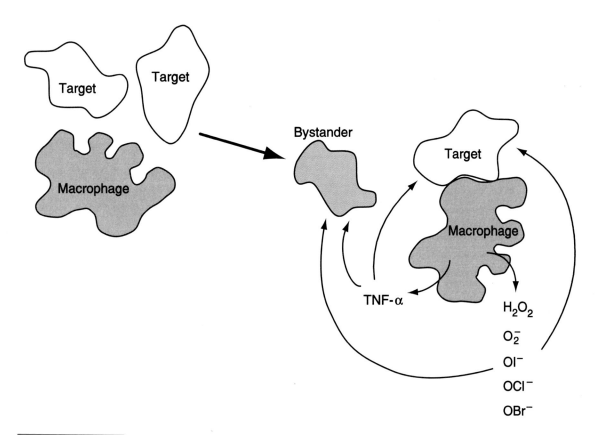

Figure 8-8 Bystander killing by macrophage (may also occur in eosinophil-mediated killing).

Neutrophils are also important in destruction of microorganisms targeted by humoral immunity. There have been reports of cellular cytotoxicity mediated by neutrophils. Although they can bind targets with Fc receptors and secrete reactive oxygen derivatives, the significance of their cytotoxicity, independent of phagocytosis, remains unclear.

TISSUE DAMAGE BY CYTOTOXIC CELLS

Damage to normal tissue does not normally accompany elimination of abnormal cells by cytotoxic T cells or NK cells, but, in some inflammatory processes, normal tissues are affected. There is much evidence to suggest that cytotoxic effectors mediate tissue damage in many autoimmune syndromes and in rejection of allografts. In tissues undergoing autoimmune reaction, CTLs have been identified by staining for granule serine hydrolases, and allospecific CTLs have been isolated from allografts. When injected into animals, allospecific CTLs, derived in vitro from mixed lymphocyte cultures, accelerate allograft rejection.

The extensive necrosis in tissues subject to autoimmune attack or allospecific rejection resembles inflammation associated with delayed-type hypersensitivity (DTH) reactions. DTH and autoimmune diseases such as multiple sclerosis have been associated with CD4 T cells, supposedly of helper phenotype. In many cases, it is not clear whether the responsible CD4 cells are themselves cytotoxic or only recruiting other cytotoxic effectors to inflammatory lesions. In animal models of autoimmune demyelinating disease, cytotoxic CD4 T cells that recognize the myelin basic protein have been demonstrated. In DTH and in allograft rejection, many cytotoxic effector cells are involved; killing of bystander cells with diffusible cytokines and oxidants is mediated mainly by macrophages, but also by eosinophils and neutrophils (Fig. 8-8).

THERAPEUTIC USES OF CYTOTOXIC CELLS

Lymphokine-Activated Killer Cells

Peripheral blood lymphocytes (PBLs) have been isolated from cancer patients and activated in culture by high levels of IL-2. When reinjected into patients, these activated cells exhibit marked cytotoxicity toward a large variety of tumor lines. Like NK cells, *lymphokine-activated killer (LAK)* cells are promiscuous killers, but the range of cells susceptible to their action far exceeds that of NK cells. Marked regression of tumors has been observed in some patients receiving LAK cells prepared from their own peripheral blood lymphocytes. Granules containing serine hydrolases and perforin have been isolated from murine LAK cells. The preponderance of LAK cells are CD3$^-$/CD16$^+$ and derive from NK cells. CTLs cultured for an extended period in the presence of IL-2 do manifest promiscuous killing; in this respect LAK cells resemble CTLs. It is possible that CTLs are activated in vivo under some circumstances to express LAK activity. It is interesting to note that IL-4, another lymphokine-supporting growth of CTLs, does not appear to induce LAK cells from CTL cultures.

Lymphokine-activated killer cells do not show much preference for autologous tumor cells in comparison to allogeneic tumors. Lymphocytes isolated directly from dissected tumors can also be stimulated to high cytotoxicity by culture with high concentrations of IL-2. These activated *tumor-infiltrating lymphocytes (TILs)* manifest more specificity toward the autologous tumor than LAK cells derived from circulating PBLs. Enrichment for tumor-specific T cells may underlie the increased therapeutic effectiveness of TILs, in contrast to LAK cells. Some evidence suggests that PBLs contain a minority of tumor-specific CD3$^+$ T cells; this subpopulation may mediate the therapeutic effect of LAK cells derived from the circulation.

Lymphokine-activated killer cell and TIL therapy have been effective for limited types of cancer, renal carcinomas, and some malignant melanoma. However, profound side effects result from the high doses of IL-2 that must be injected to support the growth and function of LAK or TIL cells. Administered IL-2 may also support proliferation of specific CTLs within tumors. The predominant side effect is increased vascular permeability causing blood pressure to decline and fluids to infiltrate tissues, especially the lungs. Modifications of IL-2 are under study to obviate its vascular side effects. Approaches that rely on combinations of lymphokines hold some promise. In order to avoid infusing patients with high levels of IL-2, some researchers are transfecting IL-2 gene constructs into PBLs in vitro for introduction into patients. The goal is that these transfected cells will secrete the lymphokine essential for proliferation and cytotoxicity.

Antibodies to CD3

Antibodies to CD3 stimulate T cells, while bypassing the antigen-specific receptor. When antibodies to CD3 are attached to the surfaces of cells, the modified cells are recognized and lysed by CTLs. Heterobifunctional antibodies have been prepared by conjugating anti-CD3 monoclonals with monoclonals specific for tumor antigens (Fig. 8-9). For tumors expressing receptors to peptide hormones, bifunctional molecules have been constructed by conjugating hormone to anti-CD3. When injected into mice, bifunctional antibodies focus CTL attack on tumor cells (Fig. 8-6). In one case, melanocyte-stimulating hormone (MSH) conjugated to anti-CD3 was used to target MSH-bearing melanomas.

The rapid clearance of foreign antibody from the circulation presents a major barrier to many promising immunotherapies. Bifunctional antibodies are rapidly cleared principally by the liver. Also, since anti-CD3 monoclonals are xenogeneic, individuals eventually mount an immune response to the monoclonals themselves. Various strategies are being explored to reduce the immunogenicity of foreign antibody and to retain them in the circulation. One promising approach attaches polyethylene glycol to antibodies to significantly enhance their longevity.

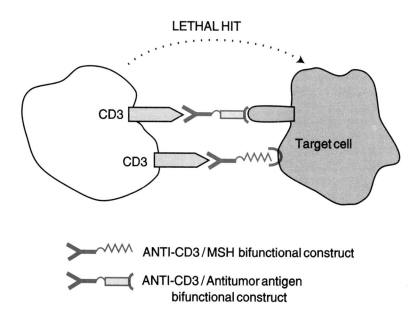

LETHAL HIT

CD3

CD3

Target cell

ANTI-CD3/MSH bifunctional construct

ANTI-CD3/Antitumor antigen bifunctional construct

Figure 8-9 Strategies for targeting CTL to tumor cells using bifunctional constructs of antibody to CD3 conjugated to peptide hormones (melanocyte stimulating hormone [MSH] in this example) which then engages the tumor receptor specific for that peptide or to antibody specific for tumor antigens.

In necrotic tumors, CD4 cells are found as well as a variety of cytotoxic cells. In many respects the situation resembles delayed-type hypersensitivity reactions, where CD4 T cells recruit cytotoxic effector cells to a site of infection. Future therapeutic applications of cytotoxic cells may depend on the use of cytokines, chemotactic factors, or tumor-specific CD4 cells in order to direct macrophages and other cytotoxic cells to solid tumors. For liquid tumors, cells derived from NK cells or from CTL may eventually prove useful. Chapter 25 describes the immune response to tumors in more detail.

SELF-TEST QUESTIONS*

For the following questions, choose the letter of the appropriate combination of correct answers.

    A. Only a, b, and c are correct.
    B. Only a and c are correct
    C. Only b and d are correct.
    D. Only d is correct.
    E. All are correct.

1. What damage to a target cell is inflicted by CTL?
    a. Inhibition of mitochondrial function
    b. Permeabilization of plasma membrane
    c. Degradation of messenger RNA
    d. Degradation of chromosomal DNA

2. How are bystander cells killed in the course of eosinophil attack on parasites?
    a. Release of hydrogen peroxide
    b. Secretion of perforin
    c. Release of hypohalite ions
    d. Random phagocytosis

3. Which of the following lymphokines induce in vitro activated killer cells for antitumor therapy?
    a. Iln-3
    b. IFN-γ
    c. ILn-4
    d. IL-2

4. Which of the following cell types can mediate ADCC?
    a. NK cells
    b. CTLs
    c. Eosinophils
    d. Dendritic cells
    e. B lymphocytes

Correctly complete the following statements:

5. Priming and activation of macrophages can be mediated by a combination of:
    a. Prostacyclins and IL-2.
    b. IFN-α and muramyl dipeptide
    c. IFN-γ and lipopolysaccharide
    d. Endotoxin and GM-CSF

6. An immune cell responsible for elimination of mature virus particles is:
    a. NK cell
    b. CTL
    c. Macrophage
    d. LAK cell

ADDITIONAL READINGS

Beutler B, Cerami A. The biology of cachectin/TNF—A primary mediator of the host response. *Ann Rev Immunol.* 1989;7:625–655.

Drapier JC, Hibbs JB Jr. Differentiation of murine macrophages to express non-specific cytotoxicity for tumor cells results in L-arginine-dependent inhibition of mitochondrial iron-sulfur enzymes in macrophage effector cells. *J Immunol.* 1988; 140:2829–2838.

Martz E, Howell DM. CTL: Virus control cells first and cytolytic second? DNA fragmentation, apoptosis and the prelytic halt hypothesis. *Immunol Today.* 1989;10:79–86.

Parmiani G. An explanation of the variable clinical response to interleukin 2 and LAK cells. *Immunol Today.* 1990;11:113–115.

Podack ER, Hentgartner H, Lichtenheld MG. A central role of perforin in cytolysis. *Ann Rev Immunol.* 1991;9:129–158.

Current topics in microbiology and immunology. In Podack ER, ed. *Cytotoxic Effector Mechanisms.* New York: Springer-Verlag; 1989.

*Answers will be found in Appendix E.

CHAPTER

9

Regulation of the Immune Response

INTRODUCTION

The immune system must be capable not only of specifically responding to and eliminating foreign antigen, but also of controlling the quality and quantity of that response should it be deleterious to the individual. Regulation of immune responses can be both nonspecific and specific, in that immunoregulatory mechanisms can exert their positive or negative effects on the immune response to all antigens (nonspecific) or only the appropriate antigen (specific). Nonspecific suppression can occur by a wide variety of mechanisms, and will be dealt with only as it relates to specific suppression. Specific regulation of immunity occurs mainly via three mechanisms: the interactive effects of cytokines produced by antigen-reactive lymphocytes (described in Chaps. 7 and 10, on T lymphocytes and cytokines, respectively), the idiotypic network, and suppressor T cells and factors. Regulation by idiotypic network interactions is accomplished by the generation of immune responses against the unique antigen-recognizing structures on the surface of either T or B cells. On the other hand, suppressor T cells appear to be a specialized group of cells whose primary purpose is to down-regulate the immune response. The generation of suppressor T-cell activity is accomplished by a series of sequential cellular interactions between suppressor/inducer T cells and suppressor/effector T cells which form a well-ordered immunologic circuit. These interactions can occur either by cell contact or by the use of cell-free factors. These factors are biologically active molecules released by suppressor cells that can functionally replace these cells in the delivery of biologic signals. Suppressor/effector T cells, once activated, are capable of inhibiting the activity of various immunologic effector cells during the course of an immune response.

A functioning, well-ordered immune system requires the capability not only of responding to the threat of pathogens, but also of controlling and fine-tuning that response in order to eliminate the pathogen most effectively, without the development of destructive or irrelevant immunity. This chapter and the chapters that follow discuss in detail the mechanisms used by the immune system to control its response to both self- and nonself-antigens, how the immune system learns to distinguish between self- and nonself-antigens, and the cells and molecules used by the immune system to both mediate and modify these responses.

Three major theories have been advanced to explain how the immune system can specifically regulate the response to self- and nonself-antigens. The first, called the *minimalist theory of immune regulation*, is based on the notion that cells which respond to antigen can either directly or indirectly affect the immune activity of other cells responding to the same antigen. This theory proposes that immune regulation is accomplished by the differential production of lymphokines by immunologic effector cells during an immune response to antigen. These lymphokines can then have differential effects on the immune system depending on the nature and immune status of their target cell. A good example of this is seen in the activities of interleukin 4 (IL-4) and interferon gamma (IFN-γ). The secretion of IL-4 by CD4$^+$ helper T cells activates B cells to express class II major histocompatibility complex (MHC) molecules, proliferate, and secrete immunoglobulin, whereas interaction of IL-4 with macrophages down-regulates class II molecules and inhibits their biologic activity. Conversely, the secretion of IFN-γ by inflammatory T cells can activate macrophages to up-regulate the expression of class II MHC molecules and to activate their biologic functions, whereas IFN-γ inhibits the expression of class II MHC molecules and the production of immunoglobulin by B cells. The synergistic and antagonistic effects of various lymphokines in immunologic responses, and how they work together in regulating immunologic responses, are covered in detail in Chap. 10.

The second theory of specific immune regulation is called the *network hypothesis*. This theory, first advanced by Neils Jerne in 1974, has had a major impact on the thinking of most immunologists on how the immune system is specifically regulated. The network theory suggests that immune regulation occurs by means of a series of interactions between antigen-recognizing structures expressed or secreted by immunocompetent cells on the one hand, and another set of cells which express or secrete receptors which are "complementary" to these antigen-recognizing structures on the other hand. This interaction can occur between antibody molecules, between antibody and lymphocytes, or even between different complementary lymphocytes, either T or B cells.

The final theory of immune regulation suggests that specialized groups of T cells function to inhibit or protect the response of antigen-specific cells during the immune response to foreign antigen. This theory, termed the *immune circuitry* theory of immune regulation, suggests the presence of distinct groups of cells, such as helper and suppressor T cells, which have a unique role in the regulation of the immune response. In this chapter, we will deal with the regulation of the immune response by idiotypic networks and immunologic circuits.

THE IDIOTYPIC NETWORK

Definition

The immune system responds to the presence of *antigen*; an antigen is simply defined as any molecule or cell capable of inducing or activating an immunologic response against it. The polymorphic structures used by the immune system to specifically recognize and respond to antigen are the immunoglobulin molecules expressed on B cells or expressed as the α/β-heterodimer (or γ/δ-heterodimer)

T-cell receptor (TCR) complex on T cells (see Chaps. 6 and 7). Regardless of the molecular nature of antigens, from small haptenic molcyte receptors recognize these antigens as small discrete units, called *determinants*, or *epitopes*. The number of epitopes on a single antigenic molecule can range from 1 to as many as 30.

Antigen-specific receptors on T and B cells possess combining sites which recognize antigenic epitopes. The antigen specificity of those receptors is determined by their unique variable regions. Thus, the variable regions on receptors which recognize different epitopes are themselves different. In fact, variable regions on receptors that recognize the same epitope may also be different, and result in differences in the affinity of binding between these two different receptors. Thus, receptors with different variable regions each possess structures that are unique to that particular receptor, and this uniqueness dictates the specificity and affinity of binding that receptor has for its corresponding epitope.

The unique antigenic structures of the variable regions of lymphocyte antigen receptors are called *idiotopes*. These idiotopes may actually be within the antigen-combining site of the receptor; these site-related idiotopes are called *paratopes*. Occupation of the receptor site by antigen blocks the binding of antiparatope antibodies to this receptor. On the other hand, idiotopes may be located outside the combining site (non-site-related idiotopes), in which case both antigen and anti-idiotopes can bind concurrently to the receptor. The totality of idiotopes (both binding-site and non-binding-site related) on an antigen-recognizing receptor determines the *idiotype* of that molecule. These concepts are detailed in Fig. 9-1.

The Autoantigenic Nature of Idiotypes

Based on the discovery of idiotypes by Kunkel et al. and by Oudin and Michel, Jerne postulated that the cells of the immune system are capable of recognizing not only

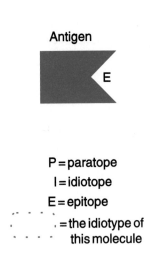

Antigen

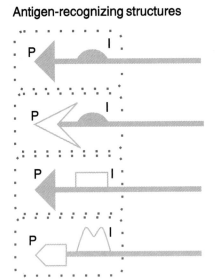

Antigen-recognizing structures

P = paratope

I = idiotope

E = epitope

= the idiotype of this molecule

Figure 9-1   Idiotypic differences on antigen-specific molecules from T and B cells. A large number of different molecules with different hypervariable regions can recognize a single antigenic determinant. The differences can be either in the site of the molecule used to bind antigen (paratope) or outside the antigen-combining site. The differences in the variable regions of these antigen-recognizing molecules are called idiotopes. A single antigen-recognizing molecule can have several idiotopes, which comprise the idiotype of this molecule.

foreign antigen, but also the unique determinants on self-receptors, or *idiotypes*, found expressed or secreted by immune cells. The first demonstration of idiotypes as self-antigens came from experiments of Rodkey, who showed that antigen-binding antibodies derived from a single rabbit could, when injected into that same rabbit a year later, elicit the production of antibodies which specifically recognized the antigen-binding antibodies used in the immunization. These antibodies were *anti-idiotypic* in that they only bound to the idiotypes expressed on the antigen-binding antibodies. These results clearly indicate that idiotypes on antigen-binding immunoglobulin molecules can elicit anti-idiotypic antibodies in an autologous system. Subsequently, investigators showed that anti-idiotypic antibodies can themselves be purified and used as immunogen in a syngeneic system to elicit the production of anti-anti-idiotypic antibodies, which can then be purified and used to elicit anti-anti-anti-idiotypic antibodies, and so on.

Network Interactions

The ability of idiotype-bearing immunoglobulin molecules to generate anti-idiotypic (and

likewise anti-anti-idiotypic) antibodies within the same individual led Jerne to formally postulate the existence of an immune network. This immune network is characterized in Fig. 9-2. After injection of antigen, the epitope binds to the paratope of the B-cell surface immunoglobulin molecule. Engagement of this paratope leads to the production of a set of antibodies reactive to that epitope, called Ab_1. This Ab_1 exhibits a number of idiotopes, which can be either binding-site or non-binding-site derived. These idiotopes on Ab_1 can themselves serve as epitopes, and bind to the paratope of "complementary" immune receptors. The engagement of the paratopes on complementary immune receptors leads to the production of a second set of antibodies, called Ab_2, which are anti-idiotypic to the Ab_1. These anti-idiotypic antibodies likewise express a set of idiotopes, either binding-site or non-binding-site derived, which can bind to the paratope of a third set of "complementary" immune receptors, leading to the production of a set of anti-anti-idiotypic antibodies termed Ab_3. This complementary induction of anti-idiotypic antibodies can continue indefinitely, with Ab_3 produced in response to Ab_2, Ab_4 produced in response to Ab_3, and so on. It was

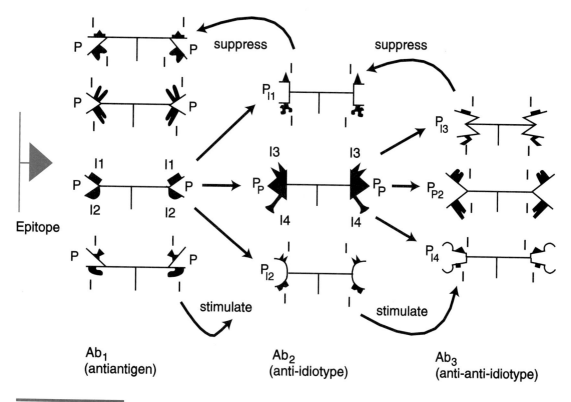

Figure 9-2   A simple network interaction. The presence of antigen induces the production of antigen-recognizing molecules. This antigen-recognizing molecule (Ab$_1$) bears a paratope (P$_1$) and an idiotope (I$_1$). These paratopes and idiotopes serve as antigen to induce the production of a second set of antibodies (Ab$_2$), which down-regulate Ab$_1$. These antibodies also bear a paratope (P$_2$) and an idiotope (I$_2$). As Ab$_1$ decreases and Ab$_2$ increases, the P$_2$ and I$_2$ now become antigenic, and induce a third set of antibodies (Ab$_3$) which down-regulates Ab$_2$. Likewise, Ab$_4$ is produced in response to Ab$_3$, and so on.

postulated that the production of anti-idiotypic antibodies was open-ended, in that the induction of complementary anti-idiotypes could go on forever. A second important feature of the network hypothesis was *directionality*. While Ab$_1$ is capable of inducing the production of Ab$_2$, Ab$_2$ is capable only of suppressing the production of Ab$_1$. Therefore, when the level of an antigen within an individual is sufficient to initiate an immune response, antibodies to that antigen (Ab$_1$) are produced (Fig. 9-3). As the level of Ab$_1$ begins to rise, two events occur: First, Ab$_1$ binds to and eliminates antigen; second, Ab$_1$ induces the production of Ab$_2$. The level of Ab$_2$ rises, and suppresses the production of Ab$_1$, so that the level of Ab$_1$ begins to decline. However, the large amount of Ab$_2$ then leads to the induction of Ab$_3$, which in turn suppresses Ab$_2$ production, but induces the production of Ab$_4$, and the cycle continues indefinitely. Thus, sequential waves of idiotypes and complementary anti-idiotypes lead to a dampening of responses to antigen, with resultant control of immunoglobulin production.

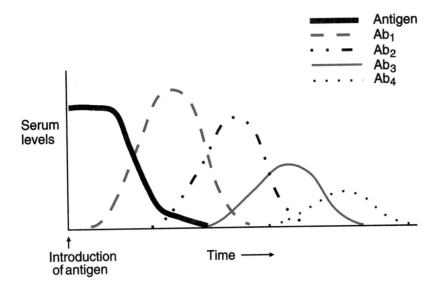

Figure 9-3 Classical network regulation. As the concentration of antigen begins to rise, antibodies to that antigen (Ab₁) are produced. As the level of Ab₁ increases, two events occur: (1) Ab₁ binds to and clears antigen, and the level of antigen begins to fall; (2) Ab₁ induces the production of Ab₂. As the level of Ab₂ rises, the Ab₂ binds to cells producing Ab₁ and inhibits further production. This leads to a drop in the amount of Ab₁ and induces the production of Ab₃. Ab₃ then inhibits Ab₂ production, leading to a drop in the amount of Ab₂, and induces the production of Ab₄, etc. This continues until the levels of anti-idiotypic antibodies produced are sufficient to eliminate idiotype-bearing antibodies, but not sufficient to induce the production of anti-anti-idiotypic antibodies, and the cascade ends.

Idiotypes as Internal Images of Antigen

As we discussed, two major types of Ab₂ can be obtained when idiotype-bearing Ab₁ is used as immunogen. The first type of anti-idiotype is directed to the binding site (paratope) of the Ab₁, while the second type is directed to non-binding-site idiotopes. Anti-idiotypic antibodies directed against the paratope of Ab₁ are referred to as *homobodies*, and represent "internal images of antigen" within the immune system. These homobodies mimic the antigen's immunogenic determinants by binding to the same region on Ab₁ as the conventional antigenic determinant. Consequently, homobodies may mimic the function of antigen in inducing immunologic responses (Fig. 9-4), or mimic the function of ligands in receptor-ligand interactions (see Chap. 31, on autoimmune disorders). In fact, homobodies to insulin, retinol-binding receptor, fMet-Leu-Phe peptide, reovirus hemagglutinin, and a host of other proteins have been described. In this sense, then, homobodies actually represent antigen; i.e., they actually induce Ab₁ production because they mimic conventional antigenic determinants and can be used in place of antigen to develop vaccines to immunogenic epitopes. Currently, homobodies are being used with significant success to develop vaccines to antigenic determinants that have proved too difficult or costly to identify and

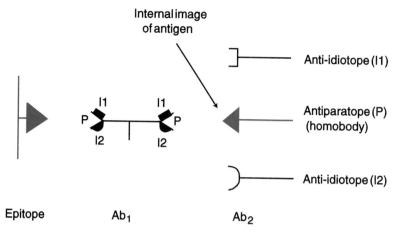

Figure 9-4 Homobodies, Ab_2 antibodies which bind to the same region of the immunoglobulin molecule as antigen (anti-paratope Ab_2). The idiotopes of homobodies are referred to as "internal images of antigen" because they can compete with antigen for binding to Ab_1 and can also mimic the function of antigen in inducing Ab_1 production.

purify, such as those found on pathogenic organisms, hormone and parasite receptors, and toxin molecules.

Parallel Sets

Since idiotypes are determined by the V-region genes of immunoglobulin or TCR molecules, it was originally postulated that antigen-recognizing receptors had a unique paratope and a unique set of idiotopes. However, it was soon found that anti-idiotypic Ab_2 could react with antibodies that did not display Ab_1, or antigen-binding activity. Thus the Ab_2 of one network could interact with the antibodies of another network. Antibodies which reacted to Ab_2, but did not react with the original immunizing antigen, i.e., did not exhibit Ab_1 activity, were termed *nonspecific parallel sets*. These parallel sets were found to occur spontaneously or after induction of immune responses by antigen, mitogen, or Ab_2. The important feature of these parallel sets is that antibodies which are stimulated by an immunizing antigen (Ab_1) induce a set of anti-idiotypic antibodies (Ab_2) which can regulate not only the production of Ab_1 but also the production of other antibodies, which have a completely different antigen recognition capability from the original Ab_1. The sole requirement is that these antibodies share idiotypic determinants with

the original Ab_1. The principle of parallel sets is demonstrated in Fig. 9-5.

Regulatory Idiotypes

Several problems with the network hypothesis as the overriding mechanism for immune regulation have been proposed. First, the network hypothesis claims that idiotype, and not antigen, is the important stimulus for all immune responses. However, studies in germ-free animals have suggested that the repertoire of immunoglobulin and T-cell receptors is shaped predominantly by antigen, and not by autostimulation of the immune system by idiotypes. Second, the network hypothesis claims that for every Ab_1, virtually unlimited numbers of Ab_2 could be produced, leading to the production of an even larger number of Ab_3, and so on. If so, then the primary function of the immune system would be to recognize idiotype and not antigen, and the degeneracy of the response to idiotype would be quite large. However, recent evidence in both rabbits and mice has suggested that the production of Ab_3 antibodies, which demonstrate anti-anti-idiotypic activity against Ab_1, are much more limited than would be predicted. The results suggest that the idiotypes expressed by Ab_1 resemble the idiotypes expressed on Ab_3, and that the idiotypes expressed on Ab_2 resemble the idiotypes on Ab_4. These results indicate

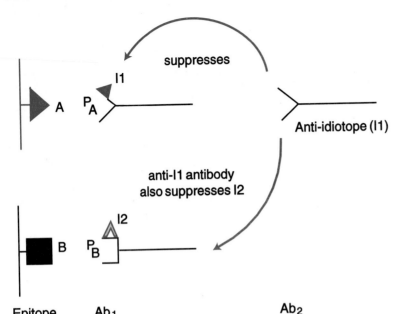

Figure 9-5 Parallel sets. Ab_1 antibodies which recognize different non-cross-reactive antigens can often bear idiotopes which are identical. Therefore, induction of Ab_2 reactive to this idiotope on one set of Ab_1 can regulate the production of the other sets of Ab_1 bearing this same idiotope.

that the network is not unidirectional, and is not as open-ended as previously thought. Rather, there seem to be two basic levels of antibodies, Ab_1 and Ab_2, which play a mutual role of coregulation.

These results have also led to the concept of regulatory idiotopes. Regulatory idiotopes are a small subset of all possible idiotopes and are highly represented on certain subsets of antigen-specific immune cells. These idiotopes may be the result of natural selection by chronic infection by endogenous pathogens, or may be germ-line-encoded and therefore expressed in high amounts prior to somatic mutation. Regulatory idiotopes are highly represented within the immunologic repertoire produced after stimulation with the appropriate antigen, and therefore reach significant levels in the periphery. This high level of expression leads to the production of anti-idiotopic Ab_2, which in turn stimulates the production of Ab_3 specifically bearing this regulatory idiotope. This in turn leads to the production of Ab_4 which is identical to Ab_2.

Network Interactions in Medicine

The network hypothesis has important implications in medicine. First, certain disease processes that directly affect patient health may arise from immune network interactions. Second, network principles are used by clinicians in the identification, diagnosis, and treatment of clinical disorders.

Diseases which may arise from immune network interactions include *insulin-resistant diabetes mellitus*. In this disease, patients who routinely take insulin develop antibodies to insulin. Continued use of insulin induces high titered antibody responses which neutralize ingested insulin. It has also been noted that in some patients anti-anti-insulin antibodies (anti-idiotypic antibodies, or Ab_2) develop, which can mimic the insulin antigen and bind to the insulin receptor. These antibodies then inhibit the binding of insulin to its receptor, thereby rendering cells unresponsive to insulin.

Other examples of anti-idiotypic antibodies in diseases are seen in Graves' disease and in cancer. Graves' disease is a type of hyperthyroidism thought to be due to the overstimulation of the thyrotropin receptor. In Graves' disease, antibodies are produced against the hormone-binding site, or idiotype, of the thyrotropin receptor. These anti-idiotypic antibodies mimic thyroid-stimulating hormone and lead to activation rather than inhibition of receptor activity. In some cancer patients, anti-idiotypic antibodies against tumor-reactive antibodies and lymphocytes develop as a result of chronic tumor stimulation. The appearance of these anti-idiotypic antibodies, which function by inhibiting the ability of tumor-reactive cells and antibodies to destroy tumor cells, has been correlated with the onset of metastasis.

Immune network interactions are also being used to identify, diagnose, and treat medical disorders. These approaches rely on the concept of antigenic mimicry, which means the production of anti-idiotypic antibodies Ab_2 which are the internal image of antigen. These internal images of antigen will then bind to the natural receptors for antigen on the appropriate cell types. Currently, these anti-idiotypic reagents are being developed to help identify a host of cell surface receptors for virus, hormones, and potentially any other protein that binds to a specific membrane receptor. In addition, anti-idiotypic vaccines are being developed which will be used to inhibit receptor-ligand interactions of parasites, viruses, or bacteria with their host entry sites, thereby limiting the pathogenicity of these infectious agents.

Another area of immediate promise is in the field of malignant myelomas and lymphomas. These cancerous cells are transformed immunocytes, each expressing a unique cell surface receptor with unique idiotypic determinants identical to the antigen-recognition structure these cells expressed prior to transformation. Because of the uniqueness of their idiotypic determinants, these cell surface receptors can serve as tumor-specific antigens (see Chap. 25, "The Immunology of Neoplasia"), thereby allowing specific targeting of the cells as treatment of the tumor, not affecting the immune response of other immunocompetent cells to the same or different antigens.

IMMUNE SUPPRESSION

Regulation by Suppressor T Cells

In addition to regulation by idiotypic network interactions, a second mechanism of regulation exists which controls and fine-tunes the immune response. This type of regulation is characterized by specialized cells within the immune system which function to down-regulate the activity of immune inducer and effector cells during an immunologic response. This activity is collectively referred to as *immune suppression*, and is generally mediated by suppressor T cells.

Suppressor T cells were first described in experimental animal systems in which it was found that inducible tolerance to certain antigens was dependent on the presence of T cells. Experimenters went on to show that cells, more specifically T cells, from tolerant animals could specifically transfer this tolerance into naive syngeneic animals (infectious immunologic tolerance), or could specifically inhibit the antibody response to antigen when added to in vitro cultures. It has now been shown that suppressor T cells play a role in the regulation of immune responses to a wide variety of antigens in a large number of different experimental systems, including immunologic tolerance, humoral immune responses, inflammatory immune responses, immune responses to tumors, hypersensitivity responses, autoimmune diseases, allotype and idiotype suppression, and in genetically low responder strains or individuals. The activity of these suppressor T cells has also been found to be either specific for the immunizing antigen or antigen-nonspecific, suggesting that several different mechanisms may exist for the generation and functional activity of suppressor T cells.

Nonspecific Suppressor T Cells

As stated above, the activity of suppressor T cells may be specific for the immunizing antigen or may exert its effects on a wide variety of immune activities. Nonspecific suppressor T cells are defined as cells which will suppress a wide variety of immunologic responses, regardless of the nature of the immune response or the antigen to which the immune system is responding. Nonspecific suppressor T cells have been found to inhibit both primary and secondary antibody responses in vivo and in vitro, the immune response of both T and B cells to mitogens in vitro, the generation of cytotoxic T cells (CTLs) in vitro, in vitro mixed lymphocyte reactions, and even macrophage-antigen presentation. These T cells are normally induced by strong, heterogenous immune responses, including graft-versus-host reactions, progressive malignant cell growth in vivo, in vitro mixed lymphocyte reactions, or mitogenic stimulation. The exact mechanism of their activity is unknown, although soluble mediators (called *soluble immune response suppressor* [*SIRS*]) have been isolated from these cells, and these mediators function in an identical fashion to nonspecifically inhibit immunologic responses.

Specific Suppressor T Cells

The majority of immune suppressive activity is mediated by specific suppressor T cells. Suppressor T cells are defined as being specific if they inhibit the immune response only to a specific antigen or immune cell, while leaving the immunologic responses to other antigenic determinants unaffected. Two major types of specific suppressor T cells exist within the immune system: antigen-specific and idiotype-specific. *Antigen-specific suppressor T cells* inhibit the immune response only to the antigen used to induce them, while not affecting the immune response to other antigens. Antigen-specific suppressor T cells have been found in virtually all immunologic responses in which they have been sought, including immune responses to both self- and nonself-antigens, as well as the response to both thymus-dependent and thymus-independent antigens. *Idiotype-specific suppressor T cells* inhibit the activity of immune cells bearing certain idiotypic determinants on their antigen-recognizing structures. Suppressor T cells can recognize idiotypic determinants on both T-cell and B-cell antigen-recognizing structures, and regulation by idiotype-specific suppressor T cells

is a functional part of the immune network detailed above.

Regulatory Circuits

The generation of most immune responses involves a sequential process of cellular interactions leading ultimately to the activation of immunologic effector cells which mediate the biologic activity. Likewise, the activation of regulatory immune mechanisms requires the stepwise passage of biologic signals through lymphoid cells resulting in a positive or negative effect on the immune response. Such a system is called an *immunologic circuit*. It differs from the immune network primarily in that it prescribes a single biologic function to a distinct cell type regardless of the idiotypic profile of the immune receptors found on that cell. Each member of the immune circuit expresses characteristic cell surface markers, and each has genetic restriction associated with both its activation and its interaction with other members of the circuit.

There are generally two cells involved in the generation of suppressor T-cell activity, a suppressor/inducer T cell (T_{SI}), which activates the immunologic circuit, and a suppressor/effector T cell (T_{SE}), which mediates the biologic activity of suppression. A simple immunologic circuit is detailed in Fig. 9-6. Cells of the circuit can be distinguished on the basis of their different functions, and their cell surface phenotypes. The T_{SI} is a CD4$^+$/CD8$^-$ T cell which is the initial cell of the immune circuit. It is identical to helper T cells with respect to its phenotype (expression of CD4 and not CD8) and to its function (inducing a second cell type to mediate an immunologic effector function, rather than carry out the effector function itself). However, T_{SI} cells differ from helper cells with regard to the target cells of their induction. The target of the T_{SI} cell is a CD4$^-$/CD8$^+$ T_{SE}, which then performs the biologic activity of suppression. Often there is a third cell type, called a suppressor/transducer T cell (T_{ST}), which accepts the signal from the T_{SI} cell,

A. Antigen-specific suppressor cell pathway

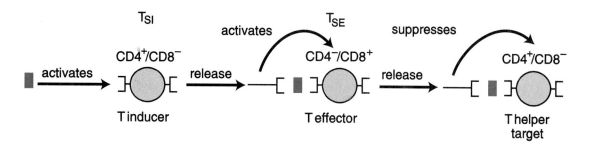

B. Idiotype-specific suppressor cell pathway

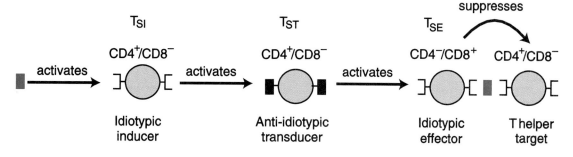

Figure 9-6 Immunologic circuits involved in the generation of suppressor T-cell activity. (*a*) Antigen-specific suppressor T-cell pathway. A CD4$^+$/CD8$^-$ T$_{SI}$ cell is activated by antigen, and this cell interacts by means of soluble mediators with a CD4$^-$/CD8$^+$ T$_{SE}$ cell of identical antigen specificity. This T$_{SE}$ cell then interacts by means of soluble mediators with susceptible target cells to deliver suppressive activity. (*b*) Idiotype-specific suppressor T-cell pathway. Antigen-activated T$_{SI}$ cells bearing idiotypic determinants interact with T$_{ST}$ cells which are anti-idiotypic. These cells in turn interact with T$_{SE}$ cells bearing idiotype.

amplifies it, and then passes the signal on to the T$_{SE}$ cell in order to increase suppressive activity. This T$_{ST}$ cell, phenotype CD4$^-$/CD8$^+$, has been described in a number of experimental animal systems, and is generally found in systems where the major mode of communication between cells of the suppressor circuit are idiotype–anti-idiotype interactions (see Fig. 9-6).

Communication between cells of the suppressor circuit has been found to parallel that found in helper circuits. First, it was found that interaction between cells is both anti-

gen-specific and genetically restricted. The interaction is antigen-specific in that the antigen specificity of the T$_{SI}$ cell must match the antigen-specificity of the T$_{SE}$ cell in order for the signal to be transduced. This form of communication requires the presence of antigen, which helps to transduce the signal from T$_{SI}$ to T$_{SE}$ cells (see Fig. 9-6). Alternatively, the specificity of the interaction between cells of the suppressor circuit could be due to idiotype–anti-idiotype interactions. In this case, the T$_{SI}$ and T$_{SE}$ cells bear the same idiotypic determinants, while a third cell, the T_{ST}, is anti-idiotypic. The idiotype-bearing T_{SI} cell interacts with the anti-idiotypic T_{ST} cell, leading to the induction of this cell. This cell then interacts with the idiotype-bearing T_{SE} cell, generating suppressive activity (see Fig. 9-6). In addition to being specific for either antigen or idiotype, the interaction between cells of the suppressor circuit is also genetically restricted. This means that both the T_{SI} and T_{SE} cells (or the T_{SI}, T_{ST}, and T_{SE} cells in the idiotype–anti-idiotype circuit) must share some genetic polymorphism in common in order for the signal to be passaged between cells. This genetic restriction has been found to map to either the HLA major histocompatibility complex (MHC) or to the immunoglobulin heavy-chain (IgH) gene locus, although the exact nature of the restriction is at present unknown.

A second way in which suppressor circuits parallel helper circuits is that communication between cells of the suppressor circuit is accomplished by soluble mediators or cytokines which convey their biologic message. These mediators are collectively called T suppressor factor (T_sF) and T_sFs produced by T_{SI} cells ($T_{SI}F$), by T_{ST} cells ($T_{ST}F$), and by T_{SE} cells ($T_{SE}F$) have been described. However, unlike cytokines produced by helper T cells, these cytokines have the following biologic properties:

1. They bind to and are specific for native antigen or idiotype.
2. They exhibit genetic restrictions in their interaction with their target cells.
3. They express determinants linked to the MHC.
4. They do not express serologic determinants found on immunoglobulin or any other known cytokine.
5. Like the cells that secrete them, they are functionally unique within the regulatory circuit, in that $T_{SI}F$ induces suppression, and $T_{SE}F$ mediates suppression, on susceptible target cells.

The structural basis of these T_sF molecules is at present relatively undefined and rather controversial, and both biochemical and mo-

lecular genetic analyses of these molecules are currently under way in many laboratories.

The Biologic Effects of Suppression

The biologic effects of suppression are as varied as their target cells. Suppressor T cells have inhibitory activities on macrophages, helper T cells, cytotoxic T cells, B cells, polymorphonuclear neutrophils and even other suppressor T cells. The effects of suppressor T-cell activity on macrophages include inhibition of interleukin 1 (IL-1) secretion, inhibition of tumoricidal activity, and even the inhibition of antigen-presentation capabilities. Suppressor T-cell effects on helper and cytotoxic T cells include inhibition of proliferation, abrogation of lymphokine secretion, and clonal anergy. Immune suppression of B cells results in the inability of these cells to produce immunoglobulin heavy chains, thereby abrogating antibody production. Effects on cell motility, homing, and even cell surface phenotype have been described. Therefore, the effects of suppression are broad and significant.

Contrasuppression

While the immune system exhibits a mechanism (suppression) by which an immune response can be inhibited when it is no longer needed or when it becomes dangerous to the individual, the immune system also requires a mechanism by which immune responses can proceed in spite of active suppression, in order to protect against premature shutdown of responses against invading pathogens or malignant cells. Such a mechanism has been described, and is called *contrasuppression*. Contrasuppression is an immunoregulatory activity which renders immunologic cells resistant to the effects of immune suppression (Fig. 9-7). Contrasuppression is similar to suppression: it is mediated by T cells, it is activated by means of a cellular circuit, and communication between cells is accomplished by soluble factors. In addition, the

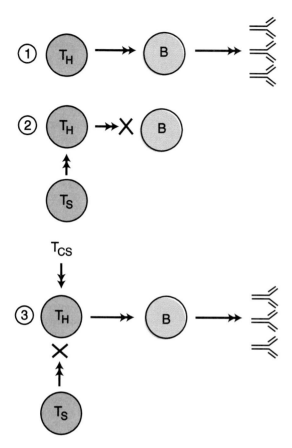

Figure 9-7   Mode of action of contrasuppression. Contrasuppression inhibits the activity of suppressor T cells and factors by interacting directly with the target helper T cell and rendering this helper T cell insensitive to suppressive signals. ① Helper T cells (T_H) interact with B cells to induce antibody production; ② Suppressor T cells (T_S) interact with T_H and inhibit their ability to help B cells; ③ Contrasuppressor T cells (T_{CS}) interact directly with T_H, rendering them resistant to T_S cell activity. Therefore, even in the presence of T_S cells, T_H cells continue to induce antibody production by B cells.

activity of contrasuppression, like suppression, is antigen-specific and genetically restricted. Contrasuppressor cells have been found in both experimental animal and human regulatory systems, and it has been suggested that contrasuppression may be im-

portant in the prevention of tolerance induction to certain harmful pathogens, as well as a factor in the ability of the immune system to generate secondary immunologic responses upon reexposure to antigen.

SELF-TEST QUESTIONS

1. What are the three major theories advanced to explain how the immune system is regulated? How are these theories interconnected?
2. What is an idiotype? What is the relationship between an idiotype and an idiotope? An idiotype and a paratope? An idiotype and an epitope?
3. Consider the relationship between Ab_0, Ab_1, Ab_2, and Ab_3. Which antibodies are likely to contain "internal images" of antigenic determinants?
4. How do network interactions play a role in disease? What diseases are believed to be due to anti-idiotypic antibodies? How can the network hypothesis be used to help the clinician identify, diagnose, and treat medical disorders?
5. How many kinds of suppressor T cells have been identified in an immunologic circuit? What are the inducers and targets of these suppressor cells?
6. What is contrasuppression? How does it differ from suppression and help? How is it the same?

ADDITIONAL READINGS

Suppression and Contrasuppression

Dorf, et al. Suppressor cells and immunoregulation. *Ann Rev Immunol.* 1984;2:127.

Flood PM, ed. Contrasuppression: A symposium. *Immunol Res.* 1988;7:1.

Green, et al. Immunoregulatory T cell circuits. *Ann Rev Immunol.* 1:439.

Ishizaka K. IgE binding factors and regulation of the IgE antibody response. *Ann Rev Immunol.* 1988;6:513.

Webb, et al. The biochemistry of antigen-specific T cell factors. *Ann Rev Immunol.* 1983;1:423.

Networks

Carson, et al. Rheumatoid factors and immune networks. *Ann Rev Immunol.* 1987;5:109.

Jerne NK. Toward a network theory of the immune response. *Ann Immunol. (Paris).* 1974;125C:373.

Periera P, et al. V-Region connectivity of T cell repertoires. *Ann Rev Immunol.* 1989;7:209.

Rajewsky, et al. Genetics, regulation, and function of idiotypes. *Ann Rev Immunol.* 1983;1:569.

10

Cytokines: Intercellular Messengers of Proliferation and Function

INTRODUCTION

The factors responsible for cellular growth, proliferation, and induction of specific functional capabilities have been the subject of intense investigation for decades. Over the last 10 years the application of the techniques of molecular biology has led to an explosion in the identification of new cytokines, substances made by specific cells which act via specific receptors on target cells to either augment or inhibit cellular proliferation or to impart new functional capabilities to the target cell. Many molecules do both; for example interleukin 2 both augments the proliferation of primed T lymphocytes and induces lymphokine-activated killer cell activity against a variety of tumors. These activities are generally part of our normal homeostatic mechanisms and work to maintain the controlled turnover of the cellular elements and to modulate immune responses. The availability of large amounts of recombinant proteins has allowed for the use of pharmacologic doses of cytokines in specific clinical problems, and several cytokines hold great promise in the therapy of hematologic, immunologic, and malignant diseases.

This chapter will describe the cytokines currently available as purified or recombinant proteins. The effects observed in vitro on target cells will be delineated, and the potential of each cytokine for the therapy of human disease will be discussed. The status of current clinical evaluations of these cytokines will also be presented.

GROWTH FACTORS

Simply stated, a *growth factor* is any substance which causes or allows a cell to proliferate. Many growth factors have been identified, with varying ranges of target cell specificity. Some, such as insulin and the insulinlike growth factors, circulate in the plasma and act on a broad range of cells. Others, notably the interleukins and hematopoietic growth factors, are produced locally and act over short distances on a restricted range of target cells. Some general characteristics of growth factors are given in Table 10-1. Growth factors work through specific receptors on the surface of target cells, and both the growth factor and the appropriate receptor are necessary for the growth factor to exert its effects. Some growth factors may act through two or more receptors on different cells; in these situations each receptor generally modulates a distinct activity of the growth factor. Like the secretion of growth factors, the expression of these receptors is dynamic and under tight control. Therefore, at least two mechanisms operate to control growth: secretion of growth factors and expression of specific receptors on target cells.

A general scheme of growth factor actions is presented in Fig. 10-1. Three models for growth factor action have been identified. Growth factors may act by one or more of these mechanisms. *Autocrine growth* is a mechanism by which a cell stimulates itself to proliferate. This is usually due to a specific stimulus, such as an encounter of a lymphocyte with the antigen for which its surface antigen receptor is specific (see Fig. 10-2). Autocrine growth may also be an important aspect of the growth of tumors whose growth has become unregulated.

Paracrine growth occurs when a growth factor produced by one cell diffuses a short distance to work on its target. An example of this is the production of several of the

TABLE 10-1   General Characteristics of Interleukins and Hematopoietic Growth Factors

Glycoproteins active at low concentration.
Act through specific receptors on target cells.
Usually active on cells of several lineages.
Active over a range of cell differentiation from stem/progenitor cells to end cells.
Often produce proliferative and differentiating effects.
Interact with other growth factors to produce synergy or, less often, inhibition.
Often active on malignant cells.
Probably act in an autocrine or paracrine manner in normal situations.

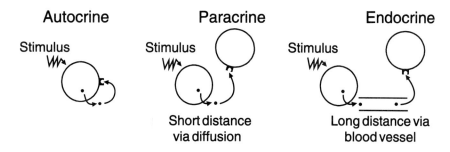

Figure 10-1 A general scheme of growth factor actions. When a factor stimulates the cell which produces it, the effect is termed *auto*crine. If the factor acts on other cells in the vicinity of the producing cell, the effect is termed *para*crine. If the factor acts on cells at long distance, often getting to the target cell by transit through blood vessels, the effect is termed *endo*crine.

hematopoietic growth factors by cells present in the stroma of the bone marrow. These act on the various precursor cells to allow for the orderly maturation of the various formed elements of the blood (Fig. 10-3).

Endocrine growth involves the secretion of a growth factor into the general circulation and is the mode of action of insulin and most hormones. The intravenous administration of therapeutic doses of recombinant interleukins or hematopoietic growth factors is another example of an endocrine mode of action.

CLINICAL TRIALS

With the availability of large amounts of pure recombinant proteins comes the potential to utilize them therapeutically. This requires a careful analysis of their toxicity and efficacy before they can be released for general use. The general strategy used to assess toxicity and efficacy follows four steps (Table 10-2).

Step 1 consists of intensive preclinical testing in animals to identify tolerable dose ranges, range and severity of toxicities, and clinical effects. From these studies an estimation is made of the toxicities to be expected in humans and a rough estimation is made of the highest tolerable dose. The first human trials (step 2), designated Phase I, are designed to treat successive cohorts of patients with increasing doses of the investigational agent to identify the maximum tolerated dose (MTD). All subjects are volunteers who have given written informed consent and who usually have cancers for which no effective treatment is available. At each dose level toxicity is closely scrutinized, and when serious toxicity occurs in an unacceptably large percentage of patients, the trial is ended. Phase II trials (step 3) then utilize the MTD determined from phase I testing to treat groups of patients with similar diseases to identify the efficacy of the drug. For instance, a single phase II trial might treat patients with myelodysplastic syndromes with G-CSF, while

TABLE 10-2 Development of Anticancer Drugs

Step 1	Preclinical trials in the laboratory involving studies of antitumor effects, biologic activity, animal toxicities.
Step 2	Phase I clinical trials: The toxicity profile in humans is established and safe doses and schedules are devised.
Step 3	Phase II clinical trials: The drug is tested for the ability to cause regression of human tumors.
Step 4	Phase III clinical trials: A new therapy is tested against standard therapy.

another might treat dialysis patients with erythropoietin. From these trials information is derived on how helpful a drug is in a particular clinical situation. Phase III trials (step 4) compare new, promising treatments with accepted standard treatments, and are often randomized to eliminate bias.

THE INTERLEUKINS

Historically, several terminologies have been applied to individual factors produced by lymphoid cells in tissue culture. Different laboratories working separately often identified an "activity" of a partially purified protein and named their factor after that activity. Others unknowingly identified a separate activity of the same protein and named their "factor" after that activity. This led to considerable confusion until purified proteins were identified as having several functional activities. The term *interleukin* was ultimately proposed to designate these lymphoid cell products and to replace previous names. The current names, previous names, and important functional characteristics of the interleukins are given in Table 10-3.

Generally speaking, interleukins have their most important effects on lymphoid target cells, although some have demonstrated effects of other hematopoietic target cells and one (IL-3) is primarily a hematopoietic growth factor. All the interleukins are single-polypeptide chains, with the single exception of IL-12, which is a heterodimer. Molecular masses range from 14 to 39 kd, and vary with the degree of glycosylation.

Interleukin 1

IL-1 is the most well investigated of the interleukins. IL-1 was initially described in the late 1960s as a protein produced by macrophages in response to infection or inflammation that induced fever. IL-1 is also produced by hepatic Kuppfer cells, alveolar macrophages, and other cells of monocyte-macrophage origin. Subsequently several additional activities have been ascribed to IL-

1, most notably the ability to induce acute-phase reactions (APRs), augment lymphocyte proliferation and lymphokine secretion, and induce the release of collagenase and prostaglandin E_2 from synovial cells. IL-1 can also induce the proliferation of fibroblasts, promote bone resorption and cartilage destruction, and participate in the activation of B cells and natural killer (NK) cells.

The clinical effects of IL-1 are well known to physicians and patients alike. It is now known that IL-1 is the same molecule as the long-studied "endogenous pyrogen." When IL-1 is given to humans or animals, its effects on the hypothalamus include the induction of rigors, chills, fever, and malaise. At high doses hypotension can result, giving rise to the picture of septic shock in the absence of infection (see Clinical Aside 10-1). IL-1 also induces the APR, resulting in leukocytosis and profound changes in plasma protein constituents. These changes include dramatic rises in C-reactive protein, SAA (serum amyloid antecedent), fibrinogen (leading to an increased ESR), haptoglobin, and α_1-proteinase inhibitor, among others. Conversely, serum iron, transferrin, and albumin fall (see Chap. 16). The APR can be induced by the administration of agents which incite inflammation or infectious agents, as well as by other lymphokines. This latter fact accounts for some of the fevers and chills seen following the administration of many recombinant proteins.

Clinical Aside 10-1
Septic Shock

An understanding of the various cytokines, why they are produced, their physiologic functions, and the interactions of the various inflammatory processes can help explain a clinical problem known as *septic shock*. This condition occurs when pathogens—often pus-forming, like streptococci or staphylococci, but also gram-negative organisms, like *Escherichia coli* and *Klebsiella*—and/or their toxins enter the blood and the tissues. Such septicemia (literally, "sepsis in the blood") has a mortality rate approaching 70 percent. About 20 percent of patients in septic shock have hemodynamic instability, with changes in peripheral

TABLE 10-3 The Interleukins

Factor	Previous Names	Biologic Activity	Therapeutic Potential
IL-1α and IL-1β	Endogenous pyrogen Lymphocyte-activating factor (LAF) Leukocyte pyrogen Leukocyte endogenous mediator (LEM)	Mediates fever in response to several inducers (endogenous pyrogen) Induces neutrophilia Chemotactic for monocytes and neutrophils Induces IL-2 production Synergizes with CSF-1, IL-3, G-CSF, and GM-CSF Induces GM-CSF production Augments B-cell responses Protects against lethal effects of radiation Induces collagenase and prostaglandins in synovial cells	
IL-2	T-cell growth factor (TCFG)	Supports proliferation of antigen- or mitogen-primed T cells Induces lymphokine-activated killer cell (LAK) activity Modulates HLA antigen expression Induces secretion of IFN-α and other lymphokines Stimulates proliferation of B cells	Used experimentally in induced LAK cells with limited antitumor effects Approved for therapy of renal cell carcinoma
IL-3	Multicolony-stimulating factor Hematopoietic growth factor	Stimulates formation of granulocytes, eosinophils, macrophages, natural killer (NK) cells, erythroid and multipotent precursors Induces acute myeloid leukemia (AML) precursors to proliferate Synergizes with GM-CSF to increase granulocyte, monocyte, and lymphocyte counts in vivo	In clinical trials (phases I and II) Potentially useful to stimulate marrow recovery from high dose chemotherapy
IL-4 (BSF-1)	B-cell stimulating factor B-cell growth factor 1 (BCGF) B-cell differentiating factor (BCDF)	Stimulates anti-μ primed B cells to proliferate Promotes IgG and IgE secretion by B lymphocytes Increases class II MHC antigen expression on B cells Enhances G-CSF-induced proliferation of granulocyte-macrophage precursors Inhibits LAK-cell induction Inhibits IL-2-induced B-cell proliferation	In limited phase I and II studies Possibly useful in therapy of humoral immunodeficiency
IL-5	Eosinophil differentiating B-cell growth factor 2 (BCGF-2) BCDF T-cell replacing factor	Promotes IgM secretion and proliferation of B-cell lines Induces hapten specific secretion of IgG by antigen-primed B cells Promotes differentiation of normal B cells to immunoglobulin secretion	Possible therapy of hypogammaglobulinemia Not yet in clinical trial
IL-6	β₂-interferon B-cell stimulating factor 2 Hepatocyte stimulating factor	Hybridoma growth factor Enhances Ig secretion by differentiation of B cells Growth factor for murine hybridomas Inhibits fibroblast growth Induces acute-phase reaction protein synthesis in hepatocytes Synergizes with other growth factors to support proliferation of blast cell colonies	Patients infected with HTLV-1 have responded to IL-6 In phase I and II clinical trials

(continued)

TABLE 10-3   *Continued*

Factor	Previous Names	Biologic Activity	Therapeutic Potential
		Induces antiviral state in fibroblasts	
		Stimulates growth of pre-B-cell colonies	
IL-7	Lymphopoietin		
IL-8	Monocyte-derived neutrophil chemotactic factor (MDNCF)	Neutrophil chemotaxis	Not yet in clinical trials
		Chemotactic for monocytes and lymphocytes	
	Monocyte-derived neutrophil-activating peptide (MONAP)	Modulates growth of hematopoietic progenitor cells	
	Lymphocyte-derived neutrophil-activating peptide (LYNAP)		
	Neutrophil-activating factor (NAF)		
	T-cell chemotactic factor		
IL-9	p40	Supports growth of T_H2 T-cell clones	Not yet in clinical trials
		Enhances proliferation effect of IL-3 on mast cells	
		Stimulates proliferation of megakaryoblastic leukemic cells	
		Stimulates erythroid colony growth	
IL-10	Cytokine synthesis inhibitory factor	Inhibits cytokine secretion of helper T cells	Not yet in clinical trials
	B cell–derived T-cell growth factor	Inhibits macrophage activity	
		Stimulates activated T cells (with IL-2 or IL-4)	
		Increases CTL numbers and activity	
		Augments B-cell proliferation	
IL-11		Increases the number of antibody-forming cells in plaque-forming assay	Not yet in clinical trials
		Supports growth of macrophages	
		Supports growth of IL-6-responsive myeloma cells	
		Augments the effect of IL-3 on megakaryocytopoiesis in murine bone marrow cells	
IL-12	Cytotoxic lymphocyte maturation factor	Stimulates antigen-primed T cells independently of IL-2	Potentially useful for adoptive immunotherapy
		Augments IL-2 induction and proliferation of CTL	
		Enhances NK-cell activity	

vascular resistance and blood pressure. About one-half of these will experience some form of end-organ damage secondary to this decreased blood flow, including renal failure, disseminated intravascular coagulation (DIC), and adult respiratory distress syndrome (ARDS).

With infection can come hypovolemia (loss of blood fluid volume), often due to diarrhea, poly-uria, insensible respiratory loss, sweating, or loss of fluid through leaky capillaries into the interstitium. Complicating this is the frequent occurrence of decreasing vascular resistance and secondary increases in cardiac output to maintain pressure. With bacteremia can come toxigenic cardiotoxicity (compounds derived from the bacteria causing heart dysfunction), in addition to the possibilities of infectious endocarditis and myocarditis. With systemic distribution of toxins comes capillary leak, fluid loss, and further vasodilatation. Some of this vasodilatation is due to the liberation of kallikrein and kinin activation by the organism. If the organism binds complement, activation of the complement cascade liberates anaphylatoxins, causes smooth muscle contraction and platelet activation, and leads to leukoagglutination, which also causes leak. As peripheral vascular resistance diminishes, cardiac output begins to fall, with attendant metabolic abnormalities (metabolic acidosis, lactic acidosis), tachypnea (attempting to "blow off" CO_2 in order to normalize the pH), renal failure, and change in mental status. With death of tissues, necrotic tissue may activate the coagulation system diffusely, with attendant "consumptive coagulopathy," another name for DIC. Local fixation of activated polymorphonuclear cells may also cause tissue damage; this is the presumed mechanism behind lung damage in ARDS.

Much of this damage can be traced back to lipopolysaccharide (LPS), a component of the cell walls of gram-negative organisms. LPS can directly activate the coagulation cascade and the kinin system, as well as act as a chemotactic factor for polymorphonuclear cells. Interleukin 1 and tumor necrosis factor (TNF) are produced by LPS-stimulated monocytes and macrophages and can be found in the circulation during sepsis. TNF is also found in the circulation after infusion of endotoxin. When volunteers are given TNF, activation of the extrinsic coagulation pathway occurs. In laboratory animals, infusion of TNF induces a full-blown septic shock syndrome, including hypotension, metabolic acidosis, tachypnea, and hemoconcentration. The animals often die of respiratory arrest. At postmortem, these mice have diffuse pulmonary hemorrhage, often with large concentrations of leukocytes in the pulmonary vasculature, acute tubular necrosis of the kidneys, adrenal hemorrhage, and ischemic and necrotic lesions of the gastrointestinal tract. Vascular leak into the gut occurs, probably due to capillary damage induced directly by TNF. Both IL-1 and TNF cause neutrophil adhesion and migration from the circulation; this effect on neutrophils may help explain capillary damage in sepsis. Animals are protected from these changes by passive immunization with anti-TNF antibodies.

But why do certain infections cause the release

of a sufficient quantity of cytokines to cause such overwhelming damage? The answer may become clearer as our understanding of certain bacterial compounds known as *superantigens* grows. (See Chap. 7, on T-cell ontogeny.) These compounds are capable of binding to many families of T-cell antigen receptors by interacting with the framework rather than the antigen-binding site. In so doing, they cause the activation of large numbers of T cells, perhaps as many as 20 percent of the total number in the body. This extreme T-cell activation causes the release of the cytokines noted above, by T cells or by other cells activated in turn by T cells, with the results noted above.

Thus, much of what is known as the septic shock syndrome may be due to inflammatory mediators, and specifically to the monokines IL-1 and TNF produced in response to the infectious agent. As our understanding of the nature of superantigens expands, the cause of septic shock and the means to prevent it may become clear.

The capacity of IL-1 to produce the protean biologic effects noted above has puzzled cellular biologists and clinicians for years. Recently, two distinct genes have been identified that code for separate proteins which possess IL-1 activity. These two proteins, designated IL-1α and IL-1β, are both 33-kd proteins; the biologically active portion of each molecule resides in the 17-kd carboxyl-terminal portion. When these proteins have been produced through molecular techniques and tested for IL-1 activity, several similarities and several differences have been observed. For instance IL-1α and IL-1β are equivalent stimulators of B-cell proliferation and antibody secretion, whereas IL-1α is a better inducer of fibroblast proliferation and IL-1β causes greater bone resorption.

These proteins are only 25 percent homologous at the amino acid level and have major structural differences, yet bind to a single cellular receptor. Much more information about their individual activities will undoubtedly be available soon.

Interleukin 2

IL-2 is perhaps the most familiar interleukin to nonscientists. Described first as T-cell growth factor (TCGF), it has since played a crucial role in the discovery of the human retroviruses HTLV-1 and HIV and has become the subject of intense study in the immunotherapy of patients with malignancies.

IL-2 was first identified as a product present in the supernatants of T-cell cultures that was able to induce proliferation of phytohemagglutinin (PHA) or antigen-stimulated T cells (Fig. 10-2). Subsequently it was shown that IL-2 was a 15-kd protein that exerts its proliferative effect through interaction with specific IL-2 receptors that appear on T-cell membranes following PHA or antigen stimulation. IL-2 receptors are not expressed on normal resting cells.

The discovery of IL-2 as a growth factor for T lymphocytes gave researchers the opportunity to grow T cells in tissue culture for prolonged periods of time. By repeatedly stimulating T cells derived from patients with

T-cell lymphomas with PHA and IL-2, researchers at the National Cancer Institute (NCI) were able to propagate long-term T-cell cultures. Eventually these cells could be weaned from their IL-2 dependency and were available for intensive study. One of these T-cell lines (HUT102) was found to produce a human retrovirus, now known as the human T-cell lymphotropic virus type 1 (HTLV-1). This was the first human retrovirus described and has been identified as the cause of epidemic lymphoma in areas where it is indigenous (notably southern Japan and the Caribbean). The clinical features of infection with HTLV-1 are protean. Some patients have only a transient T-cell lymphocytosis, while others have a chronic indolent T-cell-lymphoproliferative syndrome with peripheral blood involvement, lymphadenopathy, and hepatosplenomegaly. In the full-blown syndrome patients have a rapid downhill course

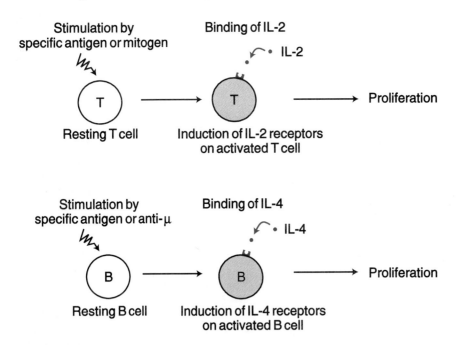

Figure 10-2   When a T cell encounters the antigen for which the T cell antigen receptor is specific, the T cell produces the IL-2 receptor and IL-2. Release of IL-2 then produces autocrine stimulation of the cell with resulting proliferation. When a B cell is stimulated appropriately, IL-4 receptor is produced by the B cell; T helper cell–derived IL-4 binds to the receptor, resulting in paracrine stimulation.

characterized by lymphadenopathy which spares the mediastinum, hypercalcemia, CNS involvement, opportunistic infections, lytic bone lesions, and skin involvement. HTLV-1 is also the cause of a progressive neurologic disorder known as HTLV-1-associated myelopathy (HAM), also called tropical spastic paraparesis (TSP). The discovery of HTLV-1 was absolutely dependent on the availability of IL-2 in order to grow the many liters of HUT102 cells required to purify sufficient virus for characterization.

In the early 1980s the acquired immunodeficiency syndrome (see Chap. 22B) began to be seen in selected populations of IV drug abusers, male homosexuals, recipients of blood transfusions, and Haitians. The cause of the syndrome was the subject of intense conjecture. Retrovirologists, however, rapidly noted the similarity to immunodeficiency diseases of cats and other animals caused by retroviral infections. Working on the assumption that the cause of human AIDS was a retrovirus, investigators adopted the technique of IL-2 propagation of PHA-stimulated lymphocytes of patient with AIDS to try to grow enough cells to isolate and characterize a virus. Initially stymied by the tendency of their cultures to die rapidly, they quickly tried adding fresh T cells to their cultures at intervals; this proved successful. The identification of the causative agent, now known as the *human immunodeficiency virus* (HIV), represents a triumph that was critically dependent on developments in cell biology and the availability of IL-2. (The HIV virus was initially called lymphadenopathy-associated virus (LAV) or HTLV-3 because of its superficial similarity to HTLV-1.)

IL-2 has several very important biologic actions. As noted above it has the capacity to induce proliferation of T cells that have been primed by exposure to the distinctive antigens for which their antigen receptors are specific. This then induces the cells to express IL-2 receptors and thus allow for the proliferation of T cells in response to antigenic challenge. This allows a precise expansion of antigen-specific T cells during the progression of an immune response. IL-2 also stimulates some lymphocytes to secrete IFN-γ, which has potent antiviral and antiproliferative effects.

IL-2 was the first interleukin to undergo clinical trials for the treatment of human disease. In 1980, workers at NCI demonstrated that the incubation of resting (i.e., unstimulated) lymphocytes with IL-2 resulted in some of the lymphocytes acquiring the capacity to mediate the lysis of tumor cells, but not normal cells. These cells, known as *lymphokine-activated killer cells* (*LAK* cells) have since been studied intensively. In animal systems (predominantly murine) they are capable of killing fresh autologous, allogeneic, or syngeneic neoplastic cell lines while sparing normal cells. LAK cells have the ability to mediate lysis of tumor cells resistant to natural killer (NK) cells.

The ability of IL-2-induced LAK cells to kill tumor cells has led to a series of studies to define how IL-2 might be clinically useful. IL-2 can be given directly to tumor-bearing animals or people resulting in the in vivo development of LAK activity in the peripheral blood. In murine studies the administration of IL-2 alone produces a dose-dependent rise in LAK activity and regression of pulmonary and hepatic metastases from sarcomas, adenocarcinomas, and melanomas.

Immunosuppression with radiation or cyclophosphamide inhibits the effects of IL-2 on micrometastases but enhances the effects on macrometastases. The reasons for this are not clear, but may involve varying mechanisms of tumor lysis. The sensitivity of macrometastases for therapy with IL-2 appears to be positively correlated with the expression of class I MHC antigens on the tumor.

IL-2 can also be used to produce LAK cells in tissue culture. These cells will proliferate and can then be reinfused into the animal with IL-2. This is often referred to as *adoptive immunotherapy*. In murine systems a dose-dependent shrinkage of metastatic tumors is seen with IL-2 and LAK-cell infusions. Both IL-2 and LAK cells are required for optimal effect. When IL-2 is infused with monoclonal antibodies with antihuman tumor specificity, the therapeutic efficacy of the antibodies is enhanced. Immunosuppression by radiation or cyclophosphamide does not prevent tumor regression from IL-2–LAK therapy.

In 1984 recombinant IL-2 became available for the first time in sufficient amounts for high-dose therapy in humans. Phase I clinical trials were quickly performed to establish the toxicity profile of IL-2 in humans and to determine the maximum amounts of IL-2 that could be administered safely with or without LAK-cell infusions. These studies were all done in patients who had advanced cancer for which no effective therapy was available or who had failed standard therapy. All patients who volunteered did so after giving informed consent, meaning that the experimental nature of the treatment with attendant risks and benefits had been explained to them. No antitumor effects were seen in these phase I studies. Phase II studies of the combination of IL-2 and LAK cells then began to identify the activity of this therapy against a variety of tumors, using the method outlined in Table 10-4. One hundred twenty-nine (129) patients with various tumors were treated at the NCI over the next 2 years. Tumor responses were seen in renal cell carcinoma, colorectal cancer, non-Hodgkin's lymphoma, and melanoma. Similarly, responses were seen in the same tumor types in patients who received IL-2 alone. Subsequently, other groups confirmed these findings.

Exciting as those tumor responses were for patients with diseases that previously could not be effectively treated, there was a significant price to pay. High-dose therapy with IL-2 was extremely toxic and most patients required intensive care for a portion of their stay. Major cardiovascular, respiratory, renal, and hepatic toxicities were observed. Much of the cardiorespiratory toxicity is due to a capillary leak leading to massive loss of fluid into the interstitium (also known as "third spacing") with resultant hypotension, edema, and organ dysfunction. This is thought to be mediated by IL-2-induced release of TNF (tumor necrosis factor) and possibly IFN-γ. Current treatment approaches attempt to limit these toxicities by treating with different doses and schedules of IL-2 that are less toxic (e.g., low-dose constant infusion seems less toxic than high-dose bolus) and by combining IL-2 with chemotherapy or monoclonal antibodies. Another approach is to utilize more appropriate effector cells as the source of LAK activity. For example, it has been reported that the lymphocytes that are often found infiltrating a tumor can be expanded in IL-2 to develop LAK activity and that these cells, known as *tumor infiltrating lymphocytes* (TILs) are 50 to 100 times more potent against homologous tumors, on a cell-per-cell basis, than LAK cells.

IL-2 may also find a role as an agent to modulate the immune response. In animals IL-2 has been shown to overcome the immune deficiency caused by prior administration of hydrocortisone or cyclophosphamide.

IL-2 has been linked to a variety of toxins (e.g., ricin or diphtheria toxin) and used to selectively poison T cells expressing the IL-2 receptor. This approach has great potential for the treatment of autoimmune disorders, graft rejection, and the therapy of HTLV-1-induced lymphomas whose T cells constitutively express the IL-2 receptor.

Interleukin 3

IL-3, formerly known as multicolony stimulating factor (multi-CSF), is one of several

---

TABLE 10-4   Adoptive Immunotherapy with IL-2 High-Dose Schedule

Day 1–5	100,00 U/kg IV tid
Day 8–12	Leukapheresis; harvested cells incubated with IL-2 to generate LAK ex vivo
Day 12–15	Reinfusion of LAK cells with IL-2, 100,000 U/kg IV tid

glycoproteins which cause proliferation of bone marrow progenitor cells. IL-3 has a broader range of target cells than do the other well-known CSFs, including GM-CSF, G-CSF, and M-CSF, which have proliferative effects restricted to granulocyte-monocyte, granulocyte, and monocyte-macrophage lineages, respectively. In contrast, IL-3 is capable of stimulating growth of erythroid, granulocyte, monocyte, eosinophil, and mixed colonies as well as megakaryocytes from human bone marrow or cord blood. IL-3 seems to work synergistically with GM-CSF and G-CSF to stimulate monocyte and granulocyte development.

IL-3 is one of several hematopoietic growth factors whose genes are located on the long arm of chromosome 5. These include IL-3, GM-CSF, M-CSF, and the gene for the M-CSF receptor which is also known as the c-*fms* oncogene. The relationship between these genes may provide insight into the development of some of the myelodysplastic disorders and cytotoxic therapy–induced acute leukemias which often have abnormalities of chromosome 5. IL-3 is currently being used in clinical trials designed to utilize its hematopoietic effects to shorten the duration of life-threatening cytopenias associated with chemotherapy. It appears to act synergistically with other cytokines, and trials using IL-3 in combination with G-CSF and GM-CSF are ongoing.

Interleukin 4

IL-4 is a product of activated T cells that was first described as a B-cell growth factor (BCGF) that stimulated antigen- or anti-μ-activated B cells to proliferate (Fig. 10-1). This allows for the selective expansion of B cells responding to a specific antigen and provides for a more effective humoral immunity. IL-4 also promotes the growth of helper T-cell lines in vitro, which may supply additional T-cell help in vivo, providing further expansion of antigen-primed B-cell clones. IL-4 also promotes the secretion of IgG and IgE; this differentiating property was initially called B-cell differentiating factor (BCDF). IL-4 serves

to inhibit LAK-cell induction in humans and also counteracts the proliferative effects of IL-2 on B-cell leukemia lines. IL-4 increases the expression of I region–associated molecules, the CD23 B-cell activation marker (which is the low-affinity receptor for IgE), and Fc receptors on B-cell lines, and stimulates the growth of mast cells.

IL-4 is of clinical interest as a possible therapy for patients with humoral immunodeficiencies and Phase I clinical trials are in progress.

Interleukin 5

IL-5 is also a product of activated T cells. Its major effects are to support proliferation of some B-cell lines, to induce some malignant B-cell lines and activated B cells to secrete IgM, and to induce eosinophil differentiation. IL-5 causes increased expression of the IL-2 receptor (Tac antigen) on activated B cells and T cells. IL-5 works synergistically with IL-4 to increase the expression of the CD23 antigen on B cells; the CD23 antigen is known to be the low-affinity receptor for IgE. IL-5 is not yet in clinical trials.

Interleukin 6

IL-6 is a multipotent molecule that has proliferative and differentiating effects on B cells and several hematopoietic progenitors. IL-6 is a product of monocytes, T cells, various carcinomas, and a wide variety of other cells. IL-6 was independently described by various groups as hepatocyte stimulating factor, hybridoma growth factor, IFN-β2 and B cell–stimulating factor 2 (BSF-2). IL-6 enhances immunoglobulin secretion by B cells and synergizes with IL-3 (and probably GM-CSF) to support proliferation of neutrophil, monocyte, eosinophil, and megakaryocyte colonies. It inhibits the growth of fibroblasts and induces class I HLA expression on their cell surfaces. IL-6 serves as a growth factor for murine plasmacytomas and hybridomas. In some systems, IL-6 can elicit the full APR of liver cells cultured in vitro, and probably serves to amplify the APR in vivo. Its effects on the APR involve a complex interaction with several other proteins, notably IL-1 and TNF. IL-6 also augments NK-cell activity. It appears to synergize with IL-1 in these last two effects. IL-6 is now in clinical trials to determine whether its ability to support neutrophil and megakaryocyte colonies will allow for higher and potentially more effective doses of chemotherapeutic agents to be given to patients with cancer.

Interleukin 7

IL-7 is a recently identified molecule produced by bone marrow and thymic stromal cells; it was first described as a B-cell growth factor. IL-7 induces the proliferation of pro- and pre-B cells but does not induce differentiation. It has a similar effect on a subpopulation of immature thymocytes and can stimulate mature T cells to proliferate in combination with suboptimal doses of IL-2. It can induce monokine secretion and induce tumoricidal activity in monocytes. IL-7 has been used in experimental models to induce and activate LAK cells in combination with IL-2 and by itself. Preliminary studies with human lymphocytes have begun recently, and if these are successful, IL-7 might be used clinically in the generation of tumor-specific effector cells in the near future. Although not in clinical trials yet, it may be helpful in therapy for various immunodeficiencies or in recovery following bone marrow ablation, for example, in bone marrow transplantation.

Interleukin 8

IL-8 is a recently described factor with a distinct receptor and no homology with previously described factors such as IL-1, TNF, the CSFs, and the IFNs. There is homology between IL-8 and platelet alpha granular peptides such as PF4 and platelet basic protein, and with CTAP-III (connective tissue activating peptide III). (See the section on chemokines below.) IL-8 is made by macrophages after stimulation by lipopolysaccharide (LPS), IL-1, TNF, IL-3, and GM-CSF, but not if the cells were treated with IL-2, IL-6, G-CSF, M-CSF, or IFN-γ. Although macrophages are the primary source of IL-8, it is also produced by fibroblasts, epithelial cells, and hepatocytes after exposure to IL-1 or TNF, and by alveolar macrophages, monocytes, and endothelial cells after stimulation with LPS.

IL-8 affects neutrophils in much the same way as the chemotactic protein C5a or the peptide fMet-Leu-Phe; IL-8 is chemotactic and induces changes in shape as well as increases in surface adhesion molecules, release of proteolytic enzymes, and production of oxygen radicals. IL-8 is more selective than C5a, fMet-Leu-Phe, PAF, and LTB$_4$, causing little if any chemoattraction for eosinophils or basophils, and has no effects on platelets or macrophages and monocytes.

IL-8 is of particular interest because it has been found in the skin of patients with psoriasis (see Clinical Aside 10-2) and could be part of the pathogenesis of the inflammation seen in the skin and in the joints of these patients. Adult respiratory distress syndrome (ARDS), idiopathic pulmonary fibrosis, and aspects of rheumatoid arthritis may all be partially explained by the local overproduction of IL-8; IL-8-like activity has been found in the bronchoalveolar lavage fluid of patients with ARDS. Thus, further study of IL-8 and other inflammatory mediators and cytokines may help explain the pathogenesis of "idiopathic" inflammatory disorders and give rise to specific methods of therapy for them.

Clinical Aside 10-2
Psoriasis

Psoriasis is a skin disease, probably first described by Hippocrates. It affects 1 to 2 percent of the population, with a peak age of onset in the second decade and a much smaller peak in the seventh decade of life. Psoriasis is usually manifested as erythematous scaling plaques, often over extensor surfaces of the elbows and knees and scalp, but it may affect the entire body surface. It can also cause nail damage, with pitting, yellowish discoloration, and onycholysis common. The lesions may be circular, drop-shaped, annular, or pustular. Patients often describe itching and flaking of the skin over a long period of time, with exacerbations and improvements. When mild, psoriasis is a nuisance. When severe, it can be devastating, both psychologically and physically. Psoriatic erythroderma, i.e., severe erythema and diffuse exfoliation, can be a life-threatening condition. About 5 to 7 percent of patients with psoriasis will have an associated arthritis. Two types of psoriasis-associated joint inflammation occur. The first type is inflammation of the spine and sacroiliac joints; over 45 percent of these patients are HLA-B27-positive. This type, known as psoriatic spondylitis, is similar to the spondylitis seen in Reiter's syndrome, where 90 percent or more of patients are HLA-B27-positive. The other kind of psoriatic joint disease affects the peripheral joints. Less than 20 percent of these patients are HLA-B27-positive. Might there be something about being HLA-B27-positive which predisposes to spinal disease?

Biopsies of affected skin reveal a thickened epidermis (up to 3 to 5 times the normal depth of epidermal cells), with more mitotic figures than in normal skin. An overlying scale of keratinized material is seen. In the dermis dilated capillaries and edema are seen, often with an epidermal neutrophilic infiltration. A lymphocytic inflammatory infiltrate, often with histiocytes, neutrophils, and mast cells, is found in the papillary dermis.

The cause of psoriasis is unclear. There is a genetic predisposition, demonstrated by the fact that one-third of patients with psoriasis have a family history of the disease. What is clear, however, is that the affected skin is metabolically very active (recall mitoses noted above) and that something is pulling inflammatory cells into the skin. The current understanding of psoriasis is that a local immunologic reaction is driving cells to produce cytokines which alter the normal skin structure and function. There is increased production of IL-1, IL-6, and IL-8 and increased expression of receptors for growth factors on skin cells. The IL-8 in the skin and in the joints of patients with psoriatic arthritis may explain the localization of neutrophils and inflammation at these sites. Arachidonic acid levels are elevated in the plaques, as are levels of 12-hydroxyeicosatetraenoic acid (12-HETE) and leukotriene B_4, both potent chemotactic factors. Activated T cells are found in the skin, and psoriatic keratinocytes express HLA-DR and ICAM molecules. Of great interest is the fact that psoriasis can be treated with immunosuppressive agents, like methotrexate and cyclosporine (see Chap. 33), suggesting that inflammation, immunologic activity, and cellular proliferation are linked in the pathogenesis of psoriasis. The common principle in all these processes is up-regulation of cytokine production and arachidonic acid metabolism.

Interleukin 9 (p40)

IL-9 (or p40) is a newly discovered lymphokine that was first identified in the mouse as a T-cell growth factor produced mainly by activated $CD4^+$ T cells. This factor could support the growth of some T_H2 type T-cell clones in the absence of IL-2 or IL-4. Like IL-2 it has no effect on resting, nonactivated T cells. IL-9 has also been found to enhance the proliferative effect of IL-3 on mast cells, to augment erythroid colony formation, and to stimulate the proliferation of megakaryoblastic leukemic cells. The human and mouse proteins are highly conserved—55 percent identity on the amino acid level. There is a perfect conservation of the nine cysteines. The genetic organization of the mouse and human genes is also highly conserved. Both consist of four introns and five exons. The exons have identical sizes in both species, and code for a 40-kd protein.

Interleukin-10

IL-10 is yet another lymphokine the gene of which was recently cloned in both mouse and human. Like IL-9, this lymphokine is a product of activated T_H2 clones (some data suggest IL-10 can be produced by B cells as well), but unlike IL-9, it is not a T-cell growth factor. IL-10 is an inhibitory factor, suppressing the production of IFN-γ by T_H1 cells; it was first called cytokine synthesis inhibitory factor (CSIF). This function of IL-10 is of potential importance in various clinical situations, since it can inhibit at least some effector functions of T_H1 cells. As discussed in detail in Chap. 7, T_H1 cells mediate delayed-type hypersensitivity (DTH) responses, whereas T_H2 cells mediate help for antibody production. IL-10 might therefore be used to specifically suppress DTH responses without affecting antibody production which could be of therapeutic value in cases of DTH reactions including some T cell–mediated autoimmune diseases. In addition, IL-10 augments IL-2- or IL-4-induced proliferation of activated T cells, increases cytotoxic T-lymphocyte (CTL) precursors and CTL activity, and stimulates B-cell proliferation.

Interestingly, IL-10 was found to have a 70 percent amino acid identity to an as-yet-uncharacterized gene in Epstein-Barr virus called BCRF-1. A protein made by this gene when expressed in COS-7 cells had the same activity as recombinant IL-10. It is tempting to speculate that the cellular gene encoding IL-10 was picked up by the virus and was conserved in evolution since it served an important biologic function for the virus, most probably by suppressing the immune response against it in an infected host.

Interleukin-11

IL-11 is a bone marrow stromal cell-derived cytokine involved in lymphopoiesis and hematopoiesis cloned from a long-term bone marrow stromal cell line derived from nonhuman primates. The human cDNA coding for IL-11 was cloned shortly thereafter. The biologic activities of IL-11 are not yet fully characterized. It was recently shown that it increases the number of antibody-forming B cells in response to an antigen in a standard plaque-forming assay. It also supports the growth of some myeloma cells which also respond to IL-6. Like IL-6, it augments the effect of IL-3 on megakaryocytopoiesis in murine bone marrow cells. The genomic organization of the IL-11 gene is not yet known.

Interleukin 12

IL-12 was the last cytokine to be given an interleukin number at the time this chapter went to print. It is a product of B-cell lines and mitogen-stimulated peripheral blood lymphocytes. IL-12 stimulates T cells in a manner very similar to that of IL-2. It acts synergistically with IL-2 to induce CTL production and proliferation. IL-12 enhances NK-cell activity and induces IFN-γ production.

CHEMOKINES

Within the past 10 years, a family of new, related cytokines has been described. They are all basic, heparin-binding polypeptides of approximately 8- to 10-kd molecular mass. They have 20 to 50 percent homology in amino acid sequence and proinflammatory and repair-oriented functions. The original term used to describe these cytokines was "macrophage inflammatory peptides" (MIPs), but this is inaccurate since some are produced by cells other than monocytes. Other workers in the field have termed them "inflammatory cytokines"; a recent review coined the term *intercrine* ("to secrete between"), but this has subsequently been replaced, by international convention, by the new term *chemokine*.

One family of chemokines, the α chemokines, is encoded on human chromosome 4(q12–21), but the murine location is unknown. The human peptides include interleukin 8 (IL-8), platelet factor 4 (PF-4), beta thromboglobulin (TG-β), IFN-γ-inducible protein (IP10), growth-related oncogene-melanoma growth-stimulating activity (GRO-MGSA), and connective tissue–activating peptide (CTAP). MIP-2 and KC are the murine analogues of GRO-MGSA, and a protein called CRG-2 is the murine analogue of IP-10. The α chemokines have 30 to 50 percent amino acid sequence homology. All of the chemokines have four cysteine residues forming two disulfide bonds. In the members of the α family the first two cysteines are separated by a single amino acid residue and so have been termed the C—X—C subfamily; members of the β subfamily have no intervening sequence and so are termed the C—C subfamily.

The β chemokines are found on human chromosome 17(q11–32) and murine chromosome 11. The members of this subfamily are 28 to 45 percent homologous with each other and 20 to 40 percent homologous with members of the α subfamily. MIP-α and MIP-β are murine members of the family. The human analogue of MIP-α is LD-78/PAT (protein activated T cell) 464/GOS19-1; the human analog of MIP-β is ACT-2/PAT 744/G26. (The other names for the human proteins are shorthand designations from the laboratory of discovery, not acronyms for a descriptive phrase.) Other human protein members of this family include I-309, RANTES (regulated upon activation, normal T expression, presumably secreted), with no known murine analogue, and macrophage chemoattractant factor (MCAF), whose murine analogue is JE.

The first chemokines identified were PF-4 and TG-β. Later it was found that IFN-γ induced monocytes to secrete certain proteins which were homologous with platelet proteins, and once IL-8 was described the chemokine family expanded rapidly. The degree of relatedness of some of these proteins is well known. When the first nine amino acids are enzymatically removed from platelet basic protein, CTAP is produced; removing four more residues produces TG-β, and with the loss of another 11 amino acids neutrophil attractant peptide II (NAP II) is formed. GRO and IL-8 bind to the same receptor, another bit of evidence suggesting the similarities of the subfamily members.

The functions of the α-subfamily peptides are better described at the time this chapter was written. Both PF-4 and IL-8 cause increased neutrophil and lymphocyte infiltration in vivo; IL-8 also causes increased vascular permeability, whereas PF-4 induces fibrosis. In vitro studies suggest that these compounds are chemoattractive and/or stimulatory for a wide array of cells, including neutrophils, basophils, T cells, and fibroblasts. PF-4 also induces endothelial cells to express more intracellular adhesion molecule 1 (ICAM-1). α Chemokines are produced by a number of cells, including monocytes and macrophages, fibroblasts, endothelial cells, and keratinocytes. T cells make IL-8, whereas platelets release both PF-4 and TG-β; synovial cells produce GRO-MGSA. Pro-

duction of the α chemokines is induced by IL-1, IL-3, TNF, IFN-γ, mitogens, and platelet activators; transforming growth factor β(TGF-β), IL-4, corticosteroids, and 1,25(OH)$_2$ vitamin D$_3$ induce the β chemokines.

Only MCAF and RANTES have been demonstrated to induce monocyte chemotaxis or superoxide release, but studies of the other β chemokines are scarce. β chemokines are produced primarily by T cells (B cells also produce LD-78 and ACT-2), but MCAF is also released by monocytes, fibroblasts, eosinophils, keratinocytes, and platelets. IL-1, TNF, and platelet-derived growth factor (PDGF) stimulate production of MCAF, and certain T-cell mitogens can increase the production of other β chemokines. Corticosteroids and cyclosporine suppress the release of certain β chemokines.

The physiologic availability of members of the chemokine family at the site of inflammatory or restorative activities suggests that they may be important players in physiologic and pathologic processes. Many more studies are necessary before their roles and importance can be documented.

HEMATOPOIETIC GROWTH FACTORS

A large number of hematopoietic growth factors have now been biologically and biochemically characterized and cloned, and are available as pure recombinant proteins. Their activities are often synergistic. They are listed in Table 10-5. Hematopoietic growth factors induce proliferation and differentiation of specific stem cells and progenitor cells. Stem cells are envisioned as giving rise to progenitor cells with restricted lineage potential, which in turn give rise to end-differentiated cells. A partial list of human stem and progenitor cells, their lineages, and active growth factors is given in Table 10-6, and their interrelationships are shown in Fig. 10-3. As can be seen, the stem cell and progenitor cells are defined by the types of colonies or smaller "bursts" to which they give rise when

TABLE 10-5   The Hematopoietic Growth Factors

Factor	Previous Names	Biologic Activity	Therapeutic Potential
EPO		Stimulates erythroid colonies to proliferate and differentiate Increases hemoglobin formation Synergizes with IL-3, GM-CSF, or IL-4 to increase erythroid colonies Stimulates erythropoiesis in vivo	Commercially available for treatment of anemia in renal failure Potentially useful for therapy of anemia in AIDS or postchemotherapy
GM-CSF	CSF Pluripoietin CSF-2	Stimulates granulocyte and monocyte colony formation in vitro and in vivo Enhances ADCC, cytotoxic, and phagocytic activity of neutrophils against bacteria, fungi, and antibody-coated tumor cells Inhibits neutrophil mobility Stimulates some AML blast progenitors to proliferate Has minimal stimulating effect on megakaryocyte colony formation and platelet production	In phase II and III clinical trials Acceleration of marrow recovery after high-dose chemotherapy Potentially useful in therapy of myelodysplasia Potentially useful in therapy of agranulocytosis or neutropenia from any cause Commercially available
G-CSF	CSF-β Differentiation factor Pluripoietin	Stimulates formation of granulocyte colonies Induces proliferation and differentiation of some but not all human AML lines Stimulates proliferation of some small cell carcinoma lines Stimulates leukocytosis in humans Synergizes with IL-3 to stimulate megakaryocytic colonies Synergizes with GM-CSF to stimulate granulocyte-macrophage colonies Enhances neutrophil migration	In phase II and III clinical trials Potentially useful in therapy of myelodysplasia Acceleration of marrow recovery after high-dose chcmotherapy Commercially available
M-CSF	CSF-1	Stimulates macrophage colony growth in vitro, with minor effect on granulocyte colonies Increases macrophage antitumor activity and secretion of O_2 reduction products Synergizes with GM-CSF in stimulation of macrophage colonies Receptor is the c-*fms* oncogene product	In phase I and II clinical trials
IL-3 (See Table 10-3)			

TABLE 10-6   Hematopoietic Growth Factors (Stem and Progenitor Cells)

Stem or Progenitor Cell	Lineage	Growth Factor(s) Active on Cell (Minor Activities in Parenthesis)
Colony-forming unit—erythroid (CFU-e)	Erythroid	Erythropoietin
Burst-forming unit—erythroid (BFU-e)	Erythroid	Erythropoietin, IL-3, GM-CSF, or IL-4
Granulocyte colony-forming cell (G-CFC)	Granulocytes	G-CSF (IL-3 and GM-CSF)
Granulocyte-macrophage colony-forming cell (GM-CFC)	Granulocytes, macrophages	GM-CSF (G-CSF, GM-CSF (CSF-2))
Colony-forming unit—granulocyte, erythroid, macrophage, megakaryocyte (CFU-GEMM)	Granulocyte, macrophages, megakaryocytes	GM-CSF and IL-3, IL-6
Macrophage colony-forming cell	Macrophages, monocytes	CSF-1 (GM-CSF, IL-3)
Burst forming unit—megakaryocyte (BFU-m)	Megakaryocytes	IL-3, GM-CSF phorbol esters, thrombopoietin activity, IL-6

cultured as single cells either in vitro or in the spleens of aplastic animals. Like their lymphoid counterparts, the interleukins, the hemopoietic growth factors often cause differentiation of specific cell types as well as provide a proliferative signal.

Erythropoietin

Erythropoietin (EPO) was the first hematopoietic growth factor to be identified. Although it was identified over 40 years ago, it was not purified until 1977. EPO was cloned in 1985 and became available for therapeutic use in 1989. EPO is a 30.4-kd single-chain heavily glycosylated polypeptide which is synthesized predominantly in the kidney, with lesser amounts made by the liver. Its secretion is governed by the kidney in response to anemia and hypoxemia. It is absolutely required for erythropoiesis, and depletion of EPO in renal failure leads to severe anemia. Serum EPO levels are depressed with infection, inflammation, or neoplasia. This contributes to the anemia seen in chronic disease but is not the sole cause. Molecular studies indicate that there is only one copy of the EPO gene, which is present on chromosome 7.

EPO is extremely specific for erythroid precursors. High-affinity EPO receptors are found only on erythroid cells. Moreover, in clinical conditions resulting in high EPO levels from endogenous sources (e.g., in chronic lung disease with hypoxemia), or in cases of exogenous administration in clinical trials, there is no effect noted on granulocytes, monocytes, or platelets. Erythropoietin exerts its action on both early and late erythroid precursors, known as burst-forming units—erythroid (BFU-e) and colony-forming units—erythroid (CFU-e), respectively.

Initial phase I and phase II clinical trials in patients with the anemia of chronic renal failure demonstrated that intravenous administration of EPO three times a week could increase the hematocrit and alleviate the symptoms of anemia. In the absence of infection or iron deficiency the hematocrit response was dose-dependent. Some patients required iron supplementation. In patients who had previously required repeated transfusion and had developed iron overload, phlebotomy could be safely performed once the anemia was corrected. The major toxicity of EPO was accelerated hypertension, which was usually easily controlled. Based on these studies EPO was approved for commercial sale and is now used extensively to treat the anemias of renal failure, AIDS, that associated with chemotherapy, and anemias seen in other diverse medical conditions.

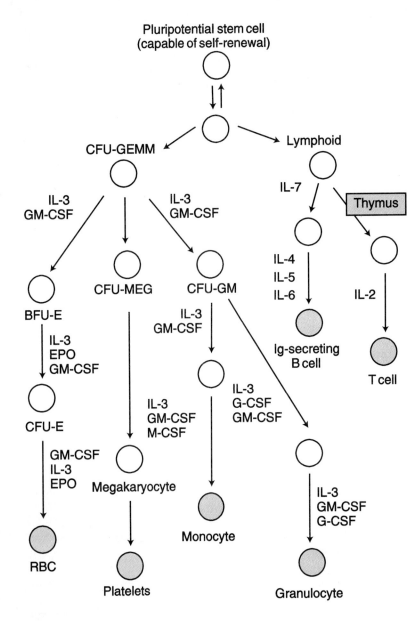

Figure 10-3   Schematic representation of the effects of various hematopoietic growth factors on precursor cells in the bone marrow. The end result of the effects of the various factors noted is the smooth differentiation and maturation of precursor cells to the end products needed. *Abbreviations*: CFU—colony forming unit; GEMM—granulocyte/erythroid/macrophage/megakaryocyte; IL—interleukin; GM—granulocyte/macrophage; CSF—colony stimulating factor; MEG—megakaryocyte; BFU—burst forming unit; E—erythroid; M—macrophage; EPO—erythropietin.

Granulocyte Colony-Stimulating Factor

Granulocyte colony-stimulating factor (G-CSF) is primarily a product of monocytes, with lesser amounts derived from endothelial and epithelial cells. It has a molecular mass of 18 kd and is encoded on the long arm of chromosome 17. G-CSF is largely granulocyte-specific and functions to promote the proliferation, differentiation, and activation of neutrophil granulocytes. G-CSF enhances the migration of neutrophils and can be detected in the serum; this is an important distinction, as GM-CSF inhibits neutrophil migration. G-CSF shortens the duration of chemotherapy-induced neutropenia and partially reverses the neutropenia of some patients with congenital neutropenia or cyclic neutropenia. G-CSF, with or without other cytokines, is clinically useful in the treatment of many patients with neutropenia, although the true magnitude of the impact it will have on the ability to cure additional cancer patients remains to be defined. It is commercially available, but its expense currently limits its use.

Granulocyte-Monocyte Colony-Stimulating Factor

Granulocyte-monocyte colony-stimulating factor (GM-CSF), like G-CSF, is a product of monocytes, but is also secreted by fibroblasts, endothelial cells, epithelial cells, and T lymphocytes. Its human gene is located on the long arm of chromosome 5. It is a glycoprotein with a molecular mass of 19 to 26 kd that stimulates the proliferation and differentiation of hematopoietic progenitor cells into mature cells of several lineages (granulocytes, macrophages, and megakaryocytes). GM-CSF induces the production of certain cytokines (e.g., IL-1 and TNF) by target cells, whereas G-CSF does not. This may be the reason for the different toxicity profiles of these two cytokines; GM-CSF treatment leads to much greater fever and IL-1-type effects in patients than does G-CSF. GM-CSF is not normally found in the serum and inhibits the migration of granulocytes; this may be of benefit when it is liberated locally in response to infection, but may be a negative characteristic when used therapeutically and administered systemically. When GM-CSF is administered to humans, a dramatic rise in circulating granulocyte and monocyte counts ensues. Toxicities include fever, myalgias, fatigue, gastrointestinal distress, bone pain, pleuritis, pericarditis, and thrombosis with pulmonary embolism. These effects are not seen with G-CSF. GM-CSF is commercially available and is used in many of the same clinical situations listed above for G-CSF.

Monocyte Colony-Stimulating Factor

Monocyte colony-stimulating factor (M-CSF) is a product of monocytes, fibroblasts, and endothelial cells. As a monocyte product and growth factor it can function as an autocrine stimulus. Its gene and the IL-3 and GM-CSF genes are present on the long arm of chromosome 5. M-CSF is capable of enhancing the proliferation and function of monocytes and is currently in clinical trials.

INTERFERONS

The interferons (IFNs) are a group of naturally occurring proteins that act as messengers between cells. They were first described in the late 1950s. At that time, it required 250,000 L of culture fluid to produce 1 mg of IFN! By 1970 high producer lines made it possible to produce 1 mg from only 25 L. Currently, unlimited quantities can be obtained by recombinant technology. There are three major types of human IFNs as distinguished antigenically; alpha (α), produced by leukocytes; beta (β), derived from fibroblasts; and gamma (γ), a product of T lymphocytes. IFN-α and IFN-β are structurally similar (45 percent homologous at the nucleotide level and 29 percent homologous at the amino acid level). Both genes are located on chromosome 9. There are at least 10 subtypes of IFN-α, but only one type of IFN-β. IFN-α and IFN-β share a common receptor and have similar functions; together they are also known as type I IFNs. IFN-γ has a distinct receptor and is functionally different from IFN-α and IFN-β; it is known as type II IFN and has only one gene. Type I IFNs are stable at pH 2; type II IFN is acid-labile.

All interferons have antiviral, immunomodulatory, and antiproliferative effects on both normal and neoplastic cells. IFN is released when various cells are stimulated by a wide variety of agents (e.g., viruses, fungal and bacterial extracts, polynucleotides, and several other cytokines).

One of the first properties of IFN to be described was its antiviral effect. When cells that are ordinarily susceptible to viral infection are first treated with IFN, they become resistant to viral infection. This is known as the *antiviral state*. IFN has been demonstrated to be of some utility in treating several viral infections, including the common cold and some types of viral hepatitis.

The immunomodulatory effects of IFN are shown in Table 10-7. IFN increases the effectiveness of immune effector cells, including cytotoxic T cells, monocytes, and NK cells. IFN can also synergize with IL-2 to augment LAK cell activity. All these effects are potential reasons to use IFN as a cancer treatment. IFN, especially IFN-γ, also has immunomodulatory effects. IFN-γ activates macrophages by increasing Fc receptor expression and superoxide generation, and augments intracellular killing of parasites and microorganisms. (In the older literature, macrophage-activating factor [MAF] was the term used to describe this activity—we now know that it is due to IFN-γ.) IFN-γ also augments the APR. All types of IFN inhibit cell growth directly in tissue culture; this antiproliferative effect forms the basis for many anticancer trials of IFN. IFN causes cells to increase the synthesis of several proteins, including HLA class I and II antigens, β₂-microglobulin, some tumor-associated antigens (e.g., carcinoembryonic antigen), and several other enzymes. IFN also causes decreased synthesis of several other enzymes and decreased expression of both the *myc* and *ras* oncogenes.

IFNs have been used extensively in attempts to treat human immunologic and malignant disease, with some notable success. IFN-α is commercially available and is used for the treatment of malignant diseases. Very respectable response rates are seen in previously untreated patients with hairy cell leukemia (> 70 percent), chronic-phase chronic myelogenous leukemia (CML) (> 70 percent), melanoma (20 percent), low-grade lymphomas (60 percent), multiple myeloma (50 percent), and renal cell carcinoma (20 percent). These antitumor effects are of significant benefit to patients; in hairy cell leukemia the need for transfusions often disappears and the incidence of neutropenic infections decreases dramatically. IFN-α can cause complete remissions in chronic-phase CML; these are often accompanied by a loss of the Philadelphia chromosome, a reciprocal translocation of the long arms of chromosomes 9 and 22, which is a clonal marker seen in 95 percent of cases of CML. Responses to IFN have also been seen in Kaposi's sarcoma and the carcinoid syndrome. In contrast to the standard cytotoxic chemotherapies where the higher the dose the greater the antitumor effect, IFN seems to exhibit maximum biologic effects at doses significantly lower than the maximum tolerated dose. The toxicities of IFN-α include a flulike syndrome, fever, myalgias, rashes, thrombocytopenia, and neutropenia.

CYTOKINES REGULATING CELL GROWTH

Transforming Growth Factor β

TGF-β is a factor produced by multiple cell types which is capable of increasing or, more often, suppressing cell growth. TGF-β was discovered as a growth inhibitor produced by monkey kidney cells which can act in an autocrine fashion. It was the first such growth

TABLE 10-7   Immunomodulatory Effects of the IFNs

Type	Effects
Type I (IFN-α, IFN-β)	Induces class I HLA on cell surfaces
	Induces antiviral state
	Induces NK-cell activity
Type II (IFN-γ)	Activates macrophages by increasing Fc receptors, superoxide generation, and intracellular killing
	Increases class II HLA expression
	Induces NK-cell activity
	Augments APR

TABLE 10-8 Cytokines Involved in Growth Regulation and Neoplastic Transformation

Growth Factor	Sources	Biologic Activity
Insulin	Pancreatic β islet	Supports growth and modulates metabolism of sugars, lipids, and amino acids
Insulinlike growth factor (IGF) I and II effects (IGF-I also called somatomedin C)	? (found in plasma)	Insulinlike Mediates hypoglycemia seen with some non-islet cell tumors (e.g., sarcoma) Mitogen for several cell types
Epidermal growth factor (EGF)	Human urine	Mitogen for epidermal cells, epithelial cells, (urogastrone), and fibroblasts
TGF-α	Transformed cells	Mitogen for transformed cells (epithelial fibroblast)
TGF-β	Platelets	Inhibits growth of many cell lines (stimulates some fibroblasts)
PDGF	Platelets	Chemotactic Immunosuppressive Stimulates growth of mesenchymal tissues
Bombesin	Small cell lung carcinoma lines	Mitogenic for carcinoma lines, respiratory and GI epithelial cells and tumors, fibroblasts Autocrine factor for small cell lung cancer

inhibitor to be biochemically identified, although such factors had long been hypothesized. TGF-β can be demonstrated to inhibit the growth of hepatocytes and prokeratinocytes but not the hepatomas or squamous cell carcinomas that are derived from them, suggesting that loss of TGF-β sensitivity might be a step in carcinogenesis. Other carcinomas have been identified which fail to secrete their own TGF-β but respond to exogenous TGF-β, providing further evidence that TGF-β may play a role in preventing neoplasia. TGF-β often blocks the proliferative signals provided by other growth factors (e.g., insulin, PDGF). It has been hypothesized that TGF-β acts to stimulate the growth of human stroma, thus promoting tumor growth. TGF-β is also capable of sustaining estrogen-dependent breast carcinoma cells in culture in the absence of estrogen, suggesting that it acts as a second messenger for estrogen.

Recent work suggests that certain leishmanial parasites can induce the production of TGF-β. In so doing, the parasite suppresses the animal host's immune response (at least in part by decreasing IFN-γ production, so that macrophages are not activated). Thus, parasites can ensure their survival by mod-

ifying the host response. This issue will be discussed in more detail in Chap. 21, "Immunity to Microorganisms."

Other Cytokines Involved in Growth Regulation

New molecules with distinct growth-modulating activities are being reported at an increasingly rapid pace due to the widespread use of molecular techniques that allow for the relatively rapid cloning and expression of large amounts of recombinant proteins. Several of these molecules have excited considerable interest, but have yet to be studied extensively. A partial listing of these molecules and their actions is given in Table 10-8.

TUMOR NECROSIS FACTOR: TNF-α AND TNF-β (LYMPHOTOXIN)

TNF-α (cachectin), a product of macrophages and monocytes, and the closely related molecule TNF-β (also known as lymphotoxin), a product of T cells, are capable of causing

TABLE 10-9 The Major Properties of TNF

Probable active factor mediating Coley's toxins
Product of macrophages and monocytes
Directly cytotoxic to many tumor lines in vitro
Probable role in cachexia (identical to cachectin)
Plays role in inflammation
Mediates pathophysiology of bacterial sepsis
Not effective in human phase I and phase II studies
(cannot achieve levels in vivo required for cytolysis in vitro

tumor necrosis in a variety of malignancies in vitro. TNF-α is also a growth factor for fibroblasts. The major properties of TNF are listed in Table 10-9. TNF activity was first detected in the serum of animals infected with BCG that were challenged with endotoxin. TNF inhibits the growth of 30 to 40 percent of human tumor lines in vitro. TNF-α secretion is stimulated by monocyte activation via infections. TNF may be the mediator of the occasional antitumor responses seen after serious bacterial infections. It is interesting to remember that nearly 100 years ago Dr. Coley administered a preparation of lysed bacteria as a cancer therapy and occasional responses were seen; these were known as "Coley's toxins" and the tumor responses may have been due to the TNF-α induced by the bacterial components. TNF-α is also a major inducer of the acute phase response. TNF-α, unfortunately, also mediates severe catabolic effects; in fact, TNF can produce all of the effects of endotoxin shock (see Clinical Aside 10-1) and infection-related cachexia. It has had limited phase I clinical trials but does not appear very promising for the treatment of human cancer. This is due to the observation that its toxicities in vivo preclude the administration of sufficient doses required to obtain blood levels high enough to cause cell death in vitro.

SUMMARY

Recent advances in cell and molecular biology have allowed for the identification and production of sufficient amounts of specific cytokines to allow for detailed in vitro investigations of their activities. Several of these molecules have dramatic influences on the growth, differentiation, and function of specific cells. These properties may explain the pathogenesis of many diseases (see Clinical Aside 10-2) and certainly hold enormous potential for the treatment of cancer either through direct biotherapy (e.g., IFN and IL-2) or as supportive measures to allow better use of chemotherapy (e.g., G-CSF). The ability to enhance specific limbs of the immune system via the interleukins holds equal promise for the therapy of certain immunodeficient states. The rapid movement of these molecules from the molecular biology laboratory to the bedside is evidence of their importance, and the potential for their use, and the use of factors that are yet to be identified, offers tremendous promise for therapy of many difficult diseases.

ADDITIONAL READINGS

Borden EC, Sandel PM. Lymphokines and cytokines as cancer treatment: immunotherapy realized. *Cancer.* 1990;65:800–814.

Quesenberry PJ. Hematopoietic stem cells, progenitor cells, and growth factors. In: Williams WJ, Beutler E, Erslev AJ, Lichtman MA eds. *Hematology.* 4th ed, New York: McGraw-Hill; 1990;129–147.

Roberts AB, Sporn MB. Principles of molecular cell biology of cancer: Growth factors related to transformation. In: De Vita VJ, Hellman S, Rosenberg SA, eds. *Cancer: Principles and Practice of Oncology.* 3rd ed, Philadelphia: Lippincott; 1989;67–82.

SELF-TEST QUESTIONS*

1. All of the following are true except:
   a. The goal of a phase I clinical trial of a new drug is to identify which tumors it has activity against.

*Answers will be found in Appendix E.

b. The goal of a phase III clinical trial is to compare a new treatment with the accepted standard.

c. All patients involved in phase I, II, or III trials must give written informed consent.

d. The maximum tolerated dose (MTD) of a drug is established in phase I testing.

2. The following general statements about growth factors are all true except:
   a. Growth factors work through specific receptors on target cells.
   b. Growth factors may have a specific or broad range of target cells.
   c. Most growth factors work through an endocrine fashion in the usual situation.
   d. Lymphocytes often demonstrate autocrine growth in response to antigenic stimulation.

3. Match the following interleukins with their major actions. Each selection may be used once, more than once, or not at all.
   a. Primary B cell growth factor
   b. Causes fever and acute phase response formerly known as endogenous pyrogen
   c. Primary growth factor for T cells
   d. Causes eosinophilia
   e. Stimulates growth of erythroid, granulocyte, and monocyte lineages in normal marrow
      1. IL-1
      2. IL-2
      3. IL-3
      4. IL-4
      5. IL-5

4. All of the following are true except:
   a. EPO is available commercially.
   b. EPO is secreted by the kidney.
   c. EPO acts specifically on erythroid precursors.
   d. EPO was discovered in 1985.
   e. EPO may cause hypertension when given to dialysis patients.

5. All of the following are true except:
   a. Type I interferons include IFN-α and IFN-β.
   b. Gamma interferon is produced by T lymphocytes.
   c. Interferons are beneficial in treatment of selected viral infections and certain malignancies.
   d. Interferons have direct antiproliferative effects.
   e. IFN-α and IFN-β have separate specific receptors.

6. All of the following are true except:
   a. TNF-α is an I-region-associated growth factor for fibroblasts.
   b. TNF-α kills 30 to 40 percent of tumor cell lines in vitro.
   c. TNF-α causes all the effects of endotoxin shock when administered to animals.
   d. TNF-α is of proven benefit for the treatment of human tumors in vivo.
   e. TNF-α causes cachexia.

INTRODUCTION

The mucosal immune system consists of lymphoid tissues associated with the lacrimal, salivary, gastrointestinal (GI), respiratory, and urogenital tracts and lactating breasts. Quantitatively, the lymphoid tissues associated with these sites, in particular with the gastrointestinal tract, contain the majority of the lymphoid tissue of the body. This fact presumably indicates the need for local immune responsiveness given the continuous assault of potential pathogens and the complex array of antigens normally present at mucosal surfaces. This is attested to by the fact that germ-free animals have a largely atrophic mucosal immune system. Most research investigation of the mucosal immune system has dealt with the GI tract, and most information regarding the mucosal immune system concerns the GI tract. There is evidence that there are considerable parallels between immunologic events which occur primarily in the GI tract and other mucosal surfaces. This is not always the case, and there are organ-specific differences. There are a number of important features of the mucosal immune system:

1. The mucosal immune system contains specialized structures, such as the Peyer's patches, where immune responses are initiated.
2. Particular subsets of lymphoid cells predominate at mucosal surfaces.
3. There is a pattern of relatively specific recirculation of lymphoid cells to the mucosa, known as mucosal homing.
4. The predominant mucosal immunoglobulin, secretory IgA, is particularly well adapted to mucosal surfaces.

These elements of the mucosal immune system function together to generate an immune response which on the one hand protects the host from harmful pathogens but on the other hand is tolerant of the ubiquitous dietary antigens and normal microbial flora of mucosal surfaces. The fact that immune responses generated in one site, such as the gastrointestinal tract, lead to generation of lymphoid cells which migrate to other mucosal sites to generate a protective immune response at all mucosae has led to the notion of a common mucosal immune system. While the major emphasis of this chapter will be the normal function of the mucosal immune system in health, it is clear that perturbations of this system occur in many diseases, and may actually underly the pathogenesis of a number of diseases including food allergies, autoimmune diseases such as systemic lupus erythematosus (see Chap. 31), and specific diseases of organ systems such as the idiopathic inflammatory bowel diseases, Crohn's disease, and ulcerative colitis (see Chap. 35). In addition, an understanding of the mechanisms of generation of protective and tolerogenic immune responses at mucosal surfaces is critical to developing immunologic strategies for immunotherapy, such as mucosally administered vaccines, recombinant lymphokines, or exogenously modified lymphoid cells.

STRUCTURAL ORGANIZATION

Peyer's Patches

The GI immune system consists of lymphoid cells in organized sites, such as Peyer's patches, mesenteric lymph nodes, and appendix, and lymphocytes that are located diffusely throughout the stromal tissue, in the lamina propria, and in the epithelial layer (intraepithelial lymphocytes). See Table 11-1. Organized tissues associated with the GI tract and pulmonary system are often referred to as *gut-associated lymphoid tissue* (*GALT*), and *bronchus-associated lymphoid*

TABLE 11-1   Essential Components of the Gastrointestinal Mucosal Immune System

Component	Function
ORGANIZED LYMPHOID STRUCTURES (PEYER'S PATCHES)	
M cells	Transport of antigens from intestinal lumen
B cells	Primarily surface IgM$^+$, but committed to IgA synthesis
T cells	
CD4	Precursors of memory T cells; isotype switching of B cells to IgA
CD8	Cytolytic T-cell precursors; T suppressors: oral tolerance
Macrophages and dendritic cells	Antigen processing and presentation; lymphokine production: IL-1, IL-6, TGF-β
NONORGANIZED LYMPHOID STRUCTURES (LAMINA PROPRIA)	
B cells and plasma cells	IgA synthesis
T cells	
CD4	Helper/effector memory cells
CD8	Cytolytic effector T cells; intraepithelial lymphocytes; ? cytolytic function
Macrophages	Nonspecific host defense—phagocytosis; production of lymphokines: IL-1, IL-6, TNF-β
Mast cells	Host defense: parasites; intestinal allergy
EPITHELIAL CELLS	
Secretory component	Receptor and transport mechanism for polymeric IgA
HLA—class II	Antigen presentation

tissue (*BALT*), respectively. It is thought that the organized sites are areas in which antigens enter the mucosal immune system and initiate immune responses, and so these sites are often referred to as the *inductive*, or *afferent*, lymphoid sites of the mucosal immune system. Lymphocytes located in the lamina propria and the intraepithelial compartments are thought to primarily carry out effector functions of the immune system, such as antibody production and cytolytic function; these sites are referred to as the *efferent*, or *effector*, compartments of the mucosal immune system. These two sites of the mucosal immune system are linked by selective migration of lymphocytes (*homing*); specifically, cells in the effector sites are derived predominantly from cells which undergo activation in the inductive sites, which ensures that the mucosal immune responses

are directed predominantly at antigens encountered in the mucosa.

The lymphoid aggregates of the GI tract, the *Peyer's patches*, are structures which are particularly well adapted to their task of induction of immune responses at mucosal surfaces. These lymphoid structures are somewhat similar to peripheral lymph nodes; however, their primary source of antigenic stimulation is by direct entry of antigens through specialized epithelial cells (M cells), rather than via afferent lymphatics. M cells are flattened epithelial cells which have poorly developed brush borders and a thin glycocalyx. They are rich in pinocytotic vesicles but are nearly devoid of the proteolytic mechanisms of mature absorptive cells. M cells take up antigens from the intestinal lumen into these pinocytotic vesicles, which are transported across the cell body and released into the subepithelial area of the Peyer's patch. This transport mechanism is capable of taking up a wide variety of materials including soluble proteins and complex particles such as intact viruses and bacteria. The uptake of materials by M cells may be in part a selective process involving specific binding of antigens to receptors on M cells. Specific antibodies against bacteria can inhibit their binding and uptake by M cells, and some organisms are able to bind to M cells while others are not. For example, binding to M cells can be conferred by transfection of specific plasmid encoded genes into *Escherichia coli*. The uptake of microorganisms by M cells can be either a positive or a negative virulence factor. Type 1 reovirus relies on the uptake by M cells to gain entry into the host, and thus is a positive virulence factor, while uptake of pathogenic *E coli* strains by M cells is the initial event in production of protective antibodies and is therefore a negative virulence factor.

Immediately below the M cells in the Peyer's patch is a dome area containing many cells bearing class II major histocompatibility complex (MHC) antigens, including macrophages, dendritic cells, and B cells in addition to T cells. It is thought that this area is particularly important in antigen processing and presentation in the initiation of mucosal immune responses. Located below the dome area are the follicular zones containing germinal centers. The proliferating B cells in this area are particularly rich in surface-IgA-positive B cells. B cells for the most part do not undergo terminal differentiation into immunoglobulin-secreting cells in this region, but instead migrate to distant sites in the lamina propria where they finally differentiate and secrete IgA.

Lymphoid cells from the Peyer's patches migrate to the draining mesenteric lymph nodes, where it is thought that mucosally derived cells undergo additional rounds of proliferation before they exit into the thoracic duct lymph and are then widely distributed to mucosal sites. For more details on lymphocyte recirculation see Chap. 12.

Intestinal Lamina Propria

The intestinal lamina propria consists of the connective tissue space between the muscularis mucosa and epithelial layer. (See Fig. 11-1.) It contains thin-walled blood vessels

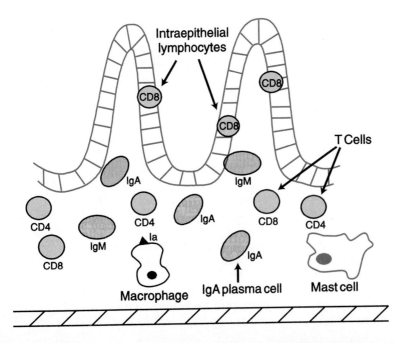

Figure 11-1 Schematic diagram of the intestinal lamina propria. Most of the B cells have differentiated into IgA-secreting plasma cells. Of the T cells, CD4 T helper/effector memory cells predominate. CD8 cytolytic effector cells are present. The T cells in the epithelial layer (intraepithelial lymphocytes) are almost exclusively CD8. Macrophages are activated.

through which lymphoid cells migrate into the connective tissue space. The lamina propria normally contains large numbers of lymphocytes, plasma cells, and macrophages. In addition, mast cells and eosinophils are normally found in this space. The epithelial layer is separated from the connective tissue layer by a basement membrane. Normally, small numbers of lymphocytes (intraepithelial lymphocytes), many of which are large and contain granules, are scattered throughout the epithelium, located between epithelial cells. As discussed below, these cells are nearly all CD8$^+$ and are thought to mediate cytolytic functions. An important feature of epithelial cells of the mucosa is the presence of the receptor for IgA on the basolateral surfaces of epithelial cells. This receptor, secretory component (SC), becomes covalently bound to dimeric IgA and is the mechanism by which IgA is transported across the epithelium and secreted at the mucosal surface. IgA and secretory component are also discussed in Chap. 3.

Nonspecific Mucosal Defenses

It should be kept in mind that there are additional nonspecific, nonimmunologic host defense mechanisms at mucosal surfaces which may equally be important as specific immunologic defenses. These mechanisms include the mucosal clearance functions (peristalsis and ciliary function) that maintain the flow of mucosal constitutents; substances such as gastric acid and intestinal bile salts that create a mucosal microenvironment unfavorable for growth of pathogens; mucus secretions that may limit penetration of microorganisms; substances such as lactoferrin, lactoperoxidase, and lysozyme that inhibit microorganisms; and, finally, the resident bacteria which inhibit growth of pathogens. All of these nonspecific mechanisms appear to be of importance, since there are clinical examples of disease states which result from disruption of any of them. Disruption of these nonspecific mucosal defenses represents a kind of immunodeficiency, as described in Chap. 22.

CELLS OF THE MUCOSAL IMMUNE SYSTEM

B Cells

As indicated above, perhaps the most characteristic feature of the mucosal immune system is the commitment of B cells to IgA secretion. Although the majority of B cells in the Peyer's patches are surface-IgM-positive, a higher proportion of B cells in this site is surface-IgA-positive than in peripheral sites. It is not clear whether surface-IgM-positive B cells that enter the Peyer's patch have already undergone the initial steps of immunoglobulin gene rearrangement which commits them to IgA secretion. This event may occur prior to entering the Peyer's patch, or it may be that the unique environment of the Peyer's patch itself contributes the factors which drive B cells to undergo switch rearrangement from IgM to IgA. There is experimental evidence that both T cells and dendritic cells of the Peyer's patches produce factors which enhance the switching of B cells to IgA-committed B cells. Thus, the mechanisms which drive IgA commitment may occur locally at the mucosal surface, rather than being the result of selective localization of B cells that are precommitted to mucosal sites. Among the soluble factors produced by T cells and macrophages which appear to be important in IgA B-cell development are the interleukins IL-1, IL-5, IL-6, and possibly transforming growth factor-beta (TGF-β). As indicated above, B cells do not undergo terminal differentiation into immunoglobulin plasma cells in the Peyer's patches; this occurs in the diffuse sites of the lamina propria, where most plasma cells secrete IgA. Smaller numbers of cells secrete IgM, which can also bind secretory component and enter secretions. Few plasma cells in the normal mucosal epithelium secrete IgG, and IgE-producing cells are rare.

T Cells

Table 11-2 gives characteristics of T cells in the GI mucosal immune system. T cells in

TABLE 11-2   Characteristics of T Cells in the Gastrointestinal Mucosal
Immune System

	Organized (Inductive) Sites	Lamina Propria Sites
Naive phenotype	+ +	−
Memory phenotype	+ +	+ + + +
Peripheral lymph node homing receptor	+ + +	−
Activation	+	+ + +
Antigen-induced proliferation	+ + +	±
Lymphokine production		
IL-2	+ +	+ + + +
IFN-γ	+ +	+ + + +
IL-4	+ + + +	+ + + +
IL-5	+ + + +	+ + + +
Helper function	+ +	+ + + +
Cytolytic T-cell function	?	+ + + +

the Peyer's patches and mesenteric lymph nodes are a mixed population, containing both CD4 and CD8 cells in similar proportions to that in peripheral blood. It is thought that CD4 cells carry out the same critical helper functions in response to antigens displayed on class II antigen-presenting cells as in the peripheral immune system. Similarly, there is evidence in animal models that CD8 cells may differentiate into cytolytic T cells in response to pathogens present in the mucosa.

There is evidence that the functional capabilities of T cells present in the intestinal lamina propria compartment have more specialized and restricted functions in comparison to T cells in the peripheral circulation. First, T cells in the lamina propria bear surface glycoproteins typical of so-called memory lymphocytes, i.e., cells that have undergone differentiation in response to antigen exposure. These include the presence of low molecular weight components of the T200 family of glycoproteins (CD45R0) and absence of the high molecular weight glycoproteins characteristic of naive lymphocytes (CD45RA). In addition, virtually all of the lymphocytes in the diffuse lamina propria compartment lack the MEL-14/Leu-8 human peripheral lymph node homing receptor, which is found on about 60 percent of circulating lymphocytes. An increased proportion of lymphocytes, both T and B cells, in the lamina propria have evidence of recent activation, as evidenced by expression of the

IL-2-receptor α chain (CD25) on about 15 percent of lamina propria lymphocytes. It has also been shown that although intestinal lamina propria lymphocytes have the capacity to proliferate in response to conventional mitogens, they show minimal or no proliferative responses to conventional protein antigens. This is not due to the absence of antigen-specific T-cell receptors on this population, since these lymphocytes have the capacity to mediate typical T-cell functions, such as providing helper activity in response to specific antigens. Although the reason for lack of proliferation is unknown, it may be analogous to the functional tolerance that is observed with T-cell clones following certain types of activation.

In healthy individuals, most of the T cells associated with the GI tract bear the α/β-heterodimer T-cell receptor. Only a minority express the γ/δ-heterodimer T-cell receptors; in contrast, in rodents the latter account for a significant proportion of T-cell receptors in the intestinal lamina propria. The role of γ/δ⁺ T cells in host defense is presently uncertain. There is experimental evidence that γ/δ⁺ T cells make up an important component of T cells responding early in particular types of immune responses. Their proportion is increased in certain disease states such as gluten-sensitive enteropathy; however, their function in these situations is still unknown (see Clinical Aside 11-1). T cells in the lamina propria have high capacity to produce lymphokines such as IL-2, IL-4, IL-5, and IFN-γ, consistent with their "memory" cell phenotype. It is likely that production of these lymphokines accounts in part for the functions of differentiated lymphocytes, including providing help for B-cell immunoglobulin production and maturation of cytolytic effector cells. These and other lymphokines may also be important in the growth and differentiation of nonlymphoid cells such as mast cells and eosinophils, both of which are normally present in large numbers in the lamina propria. Similarly, lamina propria T cells have the ability to suppress immunoglobulin production and to mediate CD3-dependent cytolytic function typical of cytolytic effector cells. There is some evidence that T cells in mucosal sites may have a selective ability to enhance IgA production by B cells. While this may be in part due to greater production of soluble factors such as IL-5 which appear to have a relatively greater enhancing effect on IgA production than other immunoglobulin isotypes, there is also evidence that T cells may express Fc receptors for IgA. One theorized role for such receptors is that they may facilitate the interaction of CD4 helper cells with the Fc portion of IgA expressed on the surface of B cells.

Clinical Aside 11-1
Gluten-Sensitive Enteropathy

Gluten-sensitive enteropathy (GSE) is a disease characterized by inflammation of the intestine caused by an immune reaction to certain components of grains (gluten) which causes villous atrophy and malabsorption. The storage proteins causing this disease are present in wheat, barley, and oats. There are two forms of the disease. One is limited to the intestine; in a second form, called *dermatitis herpetiformis*, a distinctive vesicular skin lesion predominates and intestinal lesions are mild. The intestinal inflammation is characterized by a lymphocytic infiltrate of the lamina propria. There is also lengthening of the crypts and shortening of villi due to greatly accelerated turnover of intestinal epithelial cells due to immunologic damage. The lesions of dermatitis herpetiformis are characterized by granular deposits of IgA and complement in the skin. Although high levels of antigliadin antibodies may be found in

patients, it is thought that the disease is caused by a T cell–mediated hypersensitivity reaction to gluten. The disease has a strong genetic basis, being associated with an extended HLA-B8/DR3 haplotype and having a greatly increased prevalence in particular ethnic groups, particularly individuals of Irish descent. Treatment consists of a lifelong diet free of gluten-containing foods. A late complication is an increased incidence of intestinal T-cell lymphomas which may be related to the underlying immune defect.

Although both CD4 and CD8 cells are present in the mucosa, their distribution in the lamina propria is not uniform. CD4 cells outnumber CD8 cells by a 2 : 1 to 3 : 1 ratio in the lamina propria; however, nearly all of the T cells present in the intraepithelial cell layer are CD8 cells. Although in rodents the lineage of many of the intraepithelial lymphocytes is uncertain (many are Thy-1 negative), it appears that in humans most of these cells are T cells. The increased cytoplasm/nucleus ratio and presence of granules suggest that these cells are cytolytic effector cells, for which there is some evidence in animal models. However, whether lysis of potential target cells is the only role that these cells play is presently uncertain. There is preliminary evidence that CD8+ T cells may secrete factors which are important in regulating the growth of epithelial cells; this suggests an important role of T cells in inflammatory diseases in altering epithelial cell turnover (see Clinical Aside 11-2).

Clinical Aside 11-2
Inflammatory Bowel Disease

The idiopathic inflammatory bowel diseases ulcerative colitis and Crohn's disease consist of two different but related syndromes characterized by inflammation of the intestine. Ulcerative colitis is limited to the colon, and the characteristic lesions consist of an acute and chronic inflammation of the superficial layer of the mucosa. Crohn's disease is characterized by a granulomatous inflammation involving the entire thickness of the intestinal wall, and any portion of the alimentary tract can be affected by the disease. The diseases both have a familial tendency. The etiology is unknown, but one theory of the pathogenesis of the diseases is that they represent immunologic hyperresponsiveness to ubiquitous antigens or pathogens of the gastrointestinal tract. There are numerous extraintestinal manifestations (arthritis, iritis, skin rash, fever, weight loss) and potential complications (intestinal obstruction, perforation, fistulae) of these diseases. In addition, the incidence of colon carcinoma is greatly increased in individuals with ulcerative colitis. Treatment consists of anti-inflammatory and immunosuppressive drugs and surgical management of complications.

Macrophages

Macrophages are a prominent component of the mucosal epithelium. As indicated, mast cells and specialized dendritic cells may play a critical role in the processing and presentation of antigens and in initiating immune responses in Peyer's patches. Macrophages are also prominent within the lamina propria compartment of the intestine. These cells are activated (they are larger, have more abundant enzymes), and it is likely that they play a number of different roles in host defense in this location, including processing and presentation of antigens, and production of lymphokines such as IL-1, IL-6, and tumor necrosis factor-α (TNF-α), and in nonspecific phagocytic functions. Because of their role in phagocytic functions, they may also serve as an important reservoir for pathogens in disease states, such as in viral infection with cytomegaloviruses and HIV.

Mast Cells

Mast cells are also numerous in the intestinal lamina propria. In rodents mast cells in the mucosa have atypical features which have led to the classification of mast cells into two types, connective tissue mast cells and mucosal mast cells. However, in nonhuman primates and humans these differences between mucosal and connective mast cells are less distinct. In primates mucosal mast cells contain relatively lower amounts of proteases and histamine. The role that mast cells normally play in host defense in mucosae is uncertain. Very few IgE-producing plasma cells are normally found in the intestine, and indeed it would seem undesirable for mucosal mast cells to respond to ubiquitous antigens present at mucosal surfaces. One possible clue to the importance of mast cells is that their numbers increase greatly during certain types of parasitic infections, and their major role may be in host defense against these particular pathogens. There is recent evidence that mast cells in vitro have the potential for production of numerous lymphokines, and so their functions may in part be mediated through the release of important biologic mediators. Thus, they may be able to mediate some of the same functions as T cells.

Natural Killer Cells

One cell type which is infrequent in mucosal sites is the natural killer (NK) cell. Few cells with phenotypic markers of NK cells are present either in Peyer's patches or the intestinal lamina propria. Although lymphocytes isolated from the lamina propria and from the intraepithelial compartments are capable of mediating nonspecific cytolytic function, this is probably mediated by activated cytolytic T effector cells rather than typical NK cells.

LYMPHOCYTE HOMING

One of the critical features of the mucosal immune system is the ability of cells stimulated in a particular inductive site to circulate widely and then localize in the lamina propria effector sites of the mucosa. This has the effect of focusing mucosal immune responses to mucosal tissues. There is evidence in animal models that both B and T cells are able to undergo selective migration to mucosal sites. (See Fig. 11-2.) It is currently thought that this selective migration is not due to local expansion of lymphocytes responding to antigen in mucosal sites but rather to a selective interaction of particular subsets of lymphoid cells with tissue-spe-

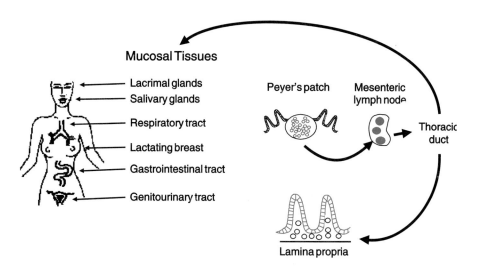

Mucosal Tissues

- Lacrimal glands
- Salivary glands
- Respiratory tract
- Lactating breast
- Gastrointestinal tract
- Genitourinary tract

Peyer's patch   Mesenteric lymph node

Thoracic duct

Lamina propria

Figure 11-2   Recirculation of lymphocytes in the mucosal immune system. Lymphocytes stimulated by encounter with antigens in organized sites, such as the Peyer's patch of the intestine, emigrate and undergo several additional rounds of proliferation in the draining mesenteric lymph nodes. Cells then emigrate to the thoracic lymph and are disseminated widely to nonorganized mucosal sites such as the intestinal lamina propria; cells originating in mucosal sites have preferential "homing" to mucosal sites.

cific receptors on vascular endothelium (which allows for lymphoid cells to enter specific tissues). At least four different lymphocyte glycoproteins are thought to play a role in lymphocyte migration through vascular endothelium. As already indicated above, the lymphocytes of the intestinal lamina propria do not express the peripheral lymph node homing receptor (MEL-14/Leu-8), a member of the *LEC-CAM* family of molecules (defined by *l*ectin domain, *E*GF domain, and *c*omplement receptor domains of *c*ellular *a*dhesion *m*olecules). Instead, lamina propria cells express markers of differentiated memory cells. Several of the molecules present on memory cells have been implicated in homing. The CD44 molecule has been suggested as a homing receptor, and it is expressed in higher amounts on memory cells and lymphoblasts. However, recent evidence indicates that this molecule plays a relative nonspecific role in adhesion to the glycocalyx. The endothelial sites that are im-

portant for homing, the so-called addressins, can be recognized by monoclonal antibody such as MECA-367, which reacts not only with the high endothelial venules present in Peyer's patches (the site where lymph node transmigration of lymphocytes is thought to occur) but also with the flat endothelium of the lamina propria. Two members of the integrin family of molecules may also be involved in homing. Antibodies against the first, LPAM-1/VLA-4, appear to selectively inhibit binding of lymphocytes to Peyer's patches; antibodies against the second, LFA-1 (lymphocyte function-associated antigen 1), also partially inhibit binding of lymphocytes to vascular endothelium; however, this does not appear to be a tissue-specific effect. Thus at present it appears that the localization of lymphoid cells in particular tissues may be the result of multiple different receptors present not only on specific subsets of lymphoid cells but also on endothelial cells of specific organs.

IgA

The central role that IgA plays in mucosal immune responses probably derives from a number of unique properties of IgA which make it especially suitable for host defense at mucosal surfaces. (See Table 11-3.) In humans IgA heavy-chain constant regions are encoded by two regions downstream of the γ and ε heavy-chain regions (Clinical Aside 11-3). The first, IgA1, encodes the predominant circulating IgA. (More than 80 percent of serum IgA is IgA1.) The second region encodes IgA2, the predominant IgA present in secretions. Circulating IgA in humans, unlike that in many other species, is mostly monomeric; in all species secreted IgA is exclusively dimeric. There are structural differences in IgA molecules: IgA1 is susceptible to cleavage in its hinge region by bacterial proteases, a potential mechanism for evasion of host defense by bacteria, but IgA2 is not susceptible to such cleavage. IgA2 exists in two allotypic forms, IgA2m(1) and IgA2m(2), which are distinguished by the absence of interchain disulfide bonds in IgA2m(2).

Clinical Aside 11-3
α-Heavy-Chain Disease

The intestine can be the site of a group of premalignant or malignant lymphoproliferative diseases classified as α-heavy-chain disease. These diseases are rare, and for the most part are found in underdeveloped countries especially in the Mediterranean and Middle East. It is thought that environmental factors may serve as a trigger for the α-heavy-chain disease because of the frequent presence of coexisting parasitic infections. In α-heavy-chain disease abnormal B cells produce aberrant α heavy chains in the absence of light chains. In early stages there is infiltration of the lamina propria with plasma cells, with associated villous flattening and malabsorption. In more advanced disease the plasma cells have a more undifferentiated appearance. The diagnosis is based on intestinal biopsy findings and the presence of circulating α heavy chains. Early forms of the disease may respond to antibiotic therapy, but in later stages the disease is malignant.

There are several important structural features of IgA which relate to its function. Like IgM, IgA has an extra cysteine residue in the C-terminal domain which permits IgA to interact with J chain to form dimers, a process that occurs within the plasma cell prior to secretion of IgA. Dimerization is probably important because dimeric IgA has an increased capacity to bind and agglutinate antigens. In addition, only the dimeric form can bind the secretory-component (SC) receptor necessary for transport of IgA to luminal surfaces. SC-bound IgA (secretory IgA) is less susceptible to digestion by proteolytic enzymes and binds more avidly to intestinal mucus than dimeric IgA, which is probably important for its survival in the intestinal lumen. The Fc portion of IgA does not react with components of either the classical or alternative complement pathway, except possibly when the IgA is highly polymerized or in the form of an immune complex. Thus

TABLE 11-3   Important Properties of IgA

IgA Subclass	Property
Monomeric IgA	Main form in serum
Polymeric IgA	Binds J chain; produced by lamina propria B cells
Secretory IgA	Covalently bound to SC; SC contributed by epithelial cell
Subclasses	
IgA1	Main form in serum
IgA2	Main form produced in lamina propria
	Resistant to proteolysis; poor activator of complement; immune exclusion: prevents absorption of intestinal antigens and pathogens

IgA does not generate inflammatory mediators as do IgM and IgG. It is thought that this is a protective adaptation in that continuous generation of such inflammatory mediators in the intestinal lumen caused by the large number of antigens normally present would be deleterious to the host. Like IgG, IgA has been shown to enhance phagocytosis and mediate antibody-dependent cellular cytotoxicity reactions (ADCC).

As noted above, the binding of dimeric IgA to SC is a critical step in rendering IgA more resistant to proteolysis and in transport of IgA to mucosal surfaces. SC, a member of the immunoglobulin superfamily of molecules, is a receptor synthesized and expressed on the basolateral surfaces of mucosal epithelium (and, in some species, hepatocytes). Dimeric IgA binds to SC and forms a covalent bond with the receptor. The complex enters epithelial cells via an endocytic vesicle and is transported to the apical surface of the cell, where a cleavage step releases the dimeric IgA and most of the covalently bound SC. Thus, the secretory IgA system is unique in that the secreted molecule is released with covalently bound receptor which is a critical component (both for transport and function) of the IgA dimer. SC is synthesized and secreted in excess of dimeric IgA, and thus free SC can be found in secretions. (See Fig. 11-3.)

SC-mediated transport occurs in the digestive tract, the salivary glands, the bronchial mucosa, and the lactating mammary glands. In addition, it occurs in the uterine epithelium, where estrogen enhances synthesis of SC by epithelial cells. Although hepatocytes transport a substantial proportion of IgA into bile in some species, such as rats, this occurs only to a minor degree in humans, and in the latter case is mediated by transport across biliary epithelium rather than hepatocytes. In humans, hepatocytes are capable of internalizing IgA; however, this appears to be mediated by asialoglycoprotein receptors, rather than SC. It has been suggested that hepatic uptake of IgA immune complexes may be one mechanism for clearance of circulating IgA immune complexes.

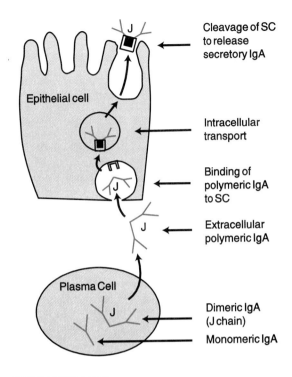

Figure 11-3 Transport of IgA into secretions. Plasma cells in the mucosal site produce monomeric IgA, which polymerizes and binds J chain intracellularly. Secreted polymeric IgA binds to the SC receptor of epithelial cells, which is then transported across the epithelial cell in intracellular vesicles to the luminal side of the epithelial cell. The bound SC-IgA complex is cleaved at the luminal side, releasing secretory IgA.

A final aspect of the protective effect of IgA involves immune exclusion, i.e., its role in preventing entry of antigens into the host. The secretion of IgA at mucosal surfaces is thought to be a mechanism which traps harmful antigens or pathogens in the mucus layer and facilitates their degradation in the intestinal lumen. That this is an important function is demonstrated by the fact that individuals with selective IgA deficiency may have high levels of circulating immune complexes containing ingested antigens (Clinical Aside 11-4). IgA may also contribute to the degradation of absorbed antigens by targeting them to the liver for degradation, as mentioned above.

Selective IgA deficiency is the most common immunodeficiency disorder, affecting as many as 1 in 500 individuals. This disorder is defined by serum IgA levels of less than 0.05 mg/mL and normal IgG and IgM levels. The cause of the disease is unknown, but since most patients have circulating IgA-bearing B cells, the defect appears to be one of failure of terminal maturation of IgA B cells. Other immunologic functions are usually normal. In many patients the deficiency is inapparent. Typical illnesses include an increased incidence of sinopulmonary infections, diarrhea, and autoimmune syndromes; when present, infections tend to be mild in nature compared to other immunodeficiency diseases. The presence of severe infections is a clue to the possible presence of other coincident immunodeficiencies; for example, patients with IgA and IgG2 subclass deficiency may have severe infections. Interestingly, many patients with selective IgA deficiency have circulating anti-IgA antibodies, and they are at risk for anaphylaxis when receiving blood products containing IgA. Treatment of the disease consists of antibiotic therapy of infectious complications and symptomatic management of autoimmune disorders. Gamma globulin treatment is not indicated unless another concomitant immunoglobulin deficiency is present. Such therapy must be instituted cautiously because of the possibility of anaphylaxis.

Other immunoglobulins in addition to IgA play a role in mucosal host defense. IgM can bind to SC and be transported in a fashion similar to the way in which IgA is transported. In fact, individuals with selective IgA deficiency are usually asymptomatic, probably because IgM can effectively substitute for IgA at mucosal surfaces, a testament to the importance of redundancy in important host defense mechanisms. IgG is normally synthesized only in small amounts in the GI tract; however, IgG is synthesized in the pulmonary tract, where it is an important component of secretions. There does not appear to be any specific transport mechanism as there is for IgA. IgE-secreting cells are normally very rare in mucosal surfaces.

ORAL TOLERANCE

A characteristic feature of the mucosal immune system is tolerance to a wide variety of common mucosal antigens. Presumably, this tolerance is critical in that it keeps the immune system from being overwhelmed by the large variety of food antigens and antigens present in normal flora of mucosal surfaces. A critical issue of current research is to determine specifically what characteristics of antigens render them immunogenic versus tolerogenic at mucosal surfaces. The mucosal immune system typically displays tolerance to a wide array of protein antigens and antigens purified from bacteria and viruses. Tolerance tends to be incomplete for thymus-independent antigens and for antigens present on living organisms, including live viruses. Certain antigens, a prime example being cholera toxin, are highly stimulatory to the mucosal immune system, possibly because of the unique binding properties of the toxin and its direct pharmacologic effects on lymphoid cells.

It is thought that several mechanisms underlie tolerance. (See Fig. 11-4.) Unresponsiveness to oral antigens involves both B cells and T cells. There is evidence in animal models that exposure to certain antigens induces potent antigen-specific suppressor T cells. This process is thought to be initiated in Peyer's patches, following which suppressor cells may be disseminated widely. The mechanisms of induction of suppressor cells in mucosal sites are not known to be different from the mechanisms at play in the peripheral immune system. It is unclear why the oral route of immunization is more likely to result in tolerance than other routes of immunization, such as in the skin, which typically result in immunogenic responses. Possible explanations include different processing of complex antigens within the GI tract, resulting in more tolerogenic fragments; more likely, the composition and functional properties of lymphoid cells in inductive sites of the intestine are significantly

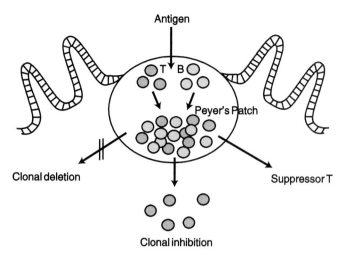

Figure 11-4 Potential mechanisms of oral tolerance. Encounter of lymphoid cells in organized structures such as the Peyer's patches has three potential outcomes which may contribute to tolerance. (1) T-cell or B-cell clones may be eliminated (clonal deletion). (2) T-cell or B-cell clones may be rendered unresponsive to further stimulation by antigen (clonal inhibition). (3) Antigen may activate a suppressor T-cell cascade resulting in antigen-specific suppressor T cells.

different from those of lymphoid cells in other sites that typically result in immunogenic responses. It has also been suggested that exposure of lymphoid cells to antigens in the mucosal environment can lead either to clonal deletion or to anergy which results in antigen-specific unresponsiveness. This unresponsiveness may be manifest in unresponsiveness of T cells, B cells, or both. The fact that tolerance can be demonstrated at a time when there is no evidence of antigen-specific suppressor T-cell activity indicates that these additional mechanisms of tolerance exist. The development of oral tolerance may be critically age-dependent. Failure to develop oral unresponsiveness may result in several different pathologic outcomes. Failure of tolerance may be an underlying mechanism in hypersensitivity to certain oral antigens, such as milk proteins. It has also been suggested that immune cross-reactivity to environmental antigens in the diet might be a contributing factor to the development of autoimmunity.

BRONCHUS-ASSOCIATED LYMPHOID TISSUE (BALT)

As indicated above, the mucosal immune system is characterized by the tendency of mucosal immune responses to result in ex-

pansion of lymphoid populations which are distributed to different mucosal sites and by the dominance of IgA immune responses. However, there are a number of differences in the structure and function of the mucosal immune system in different organ systems. The best-studied site apart from the gastrointestinal tract is the pulmonary immune system. The organized lymphoid aggregates known as BALT are associated with bronchi, particularly at the bifurcations of bronchi. Unlike the Peyer's patches, BALT contains predominantly T cells, and B cell–containing lymphoid follicles are less readily apparent. The majority of B cells in BALT bear IgM and IgG; IgA B cells are infrequent. The epithelium of BALT is similar to the respiratory epithelium of other sites, but differs from GALT in the absence of M cells. As in GALT, it is thought that lymphocytes enter BALT through a selective homing process (see below) which initially involves adhesion of lymphocytes to high endothelial venules. This selective process appears to be different in GALT and BALT in that the mucosal endothelial receptor (MECA-325) does not appear to be present on the high endothelial venules of GALT. As in the intestine, lymphocytes are also distributed diffusely thoughout the pulmonary lamina propria. However, intraepithelial lymphocytes are predominantly CD4$^+$ in BALT, whereas they are predominantly CD8$^+$ in GALT. The pulmonary immune system also functions differently from the intestine. A major component of the pulmonary immune system is the pulmonary alveolar macrophage, which is located external to the epithelium and probably plays a critical role as a first line of nonspecific defense. Finally, the major immunoglobulin in secretions in the lower respiratory tract is IgG, rather than IgA as in the upper respiratory tract.

LACTATING BREAST

The lactating breast is an important component of the mucosal immune system. The concentration of IgA in colostrum is extremely high, averaging 5 mg/mL, although the concentration falls rapidly as the volume of secreted milk increases. IgA in breast milk is derived from B cells which are thought to have originated in mucosal follicles of the digestive and respiratory tracts; IgA is transported across breast epithelium by an SC-mediated transport mechanism similar to that in the intestine. It is thought that breast milk antibodies play an important role in protecting against certain pathogens, establishing the normal intestinal flora, and preventing absorption of GI macromolecules. The beneficial role of breast milk (in comparison to formula diets) can be demonstrated in developing countries, where exposure of infants to pathogens is a greater problem. (An added problem in developing countries is the poor quality of water available to dissolve the formula. Contaminated water can spread infectious diarrhea, a major cause of infant mortality in nonindustrial nations.) Breast milk also contains cells, including macrophages, granulocytes, and small numbers of lymphocytes. Although these cells have been demonstrated to confer specific immune reactivity, their importance in normal immune physiology is uncertain.

SELF-TEST QUESTIONS*

1. Which of the following statements concerning the role of intestinal Peyer's patches in mucosal immune function is *least* correct?
   a. Specialized M cells cover the serosal surface.
   b. Antigens from the intestinal lumen can enter the patches and initiate immune responses.
   c. Lymphocytes that are activated in the patches recirculate to other mucosal surfaces.
   d. The patches are not the major site of intestinal IgA production.
   e. The patches contain a mixed population of T and B cells and macrophages.

2. Which of the following statements concerning IgA is *most* correct?
   a. IgA is comprised of four subclasses.
   b. J chain is attached to dimeric IgA by epithelial cells.
   c. Most serum IgA is monomeric.
   d. IgA in secretions is mostly of the IgA1 subclass.
   e. IgA destroys pathogens in the intestine by complement-mediated lysis.

3. Which of the following statements concerning secretory component (SC) is incorrect?
   a. SC is a cell surface receptor for dimeric IgA.
   b. SC is a member of the immunoglobulin family of molecules.
   c. Some SC is present free in secretions without IgA attached.
   d. Secretory IgA is more resistant to proteolysis than dimeric IgA.
   e. SC is attached to dimeric IgA by intestinal plasma cells.

*Answers will be found in Appendix E.

4. True or false
   a. The intestinal epithelium is characterized by a predominance of CD8 T cells in the epithelial layer.
   b. The intestinal epithelium is characterized by natural killer cells that are important as a first line of defense.
   c. The intestinal epithelium is characterized by production of immunoglobulins by plasma cells in decreasing order: IgA, IgG, IgM, IgE.
   d. The intestinal epithelium is characterized by predominance of T cells with g,d receptors in the lamina propria.
   e. The intestinal epithelium is characterized by CD4 T cells that provide helper activity.
5. True or false
   a. The bronchus associated lymphoid tissue (BALT) is characterized by a predominance of T cells.
   b. BALT is similar to intestine in producing mainly secretory IgA.
   c. BALT has M cells overlying lymphoid aggregates.
   d. BALT is characterized by selective homing of B cells.
6. True or false
   a. Oral tolerance refers to inhibition of immune responses because of exposure to an antigen by the alimentary route.
   b. Oral tolerance may be due to presence of suppressor T cells.
   c. Oral tolerance may be due to clonal elimination of B cells.
   d. Oral tolerance may be due to clonal anergy of T cells.
   e. Oral tolerance is uniformly the result of feeding of any material by mouth.

ADDITIONAL READINGS

Brown WR, Strober W. Immunological diseases of the gastrointestinal tract. In: Samter M, Talmage DW, Frank MM, Austen KF, Claman NH, eds. *Immunological Diseases.* Boston: Little, Brown; 1988:1995–2033.

Cunningham-Rundles C. Selective IgA deficiency and the gastrointestinal tract. *Immunol Allergy Clin North Am.* 1988;8:435–449.

James SP. Immunology of hepatobiliary diseases. In: Samter M, Talmage DW, Frank MM, Austen KF, Claman NH, eds. *Immunological Diseases.* Boston: Little, Brown; 1988:1945–1993.

Kagnoff MF. Celiac disease: a model of an immunologically mediated intestinal disease. *Immunol Allergy Clin North Am.* 1988;8:505–520.

Seligman M. Immunochemical, clincal and pathological features of alpha-chain disease. *Arch Intern Med.* 1975;135:78–82.

Strober W, Brown WR. The mucosal immune system. In: Samter M, Talmage DW, Frank MM, Austen KF, Claman HN, eds. *Immunological Diseases.* Boston: Little, Brown; 1988:79–139.

Strober W, James SP. The immunologic basis of inflammatory bowel disease. *J Clin Immunol.* 1986;6:415–432.

12

Mechanisms of Lymphocyte Recirculation and Homing

INTRODUCTION

If one had the luxury of being able to customize the tissues and cells of the lymphoid system with the aim of developing an efficient immune system that would allow the induction of functionally distinct immune responses in different body tissues, the customized system would likely have the following features.

First, those tissues supporting immune responses would be widely distributed throughout the body. Such a decentralized organizational structure would facilitate the rapid induction of immune responses at or near sites where immune cells are required. Localized immune responses would prove to be of value, by preventing, for example, the systemic dissemination of infectious agents from local sites of infection.

A second important feature of this customized lymphoid system would be that lymphoid cells would be highly mobile, having the ability to rapidly move both through and between different body tissues. This migratory phenotype would greatly enhance the potential of generating immune responses by allowing the full repertoire of antigen-reactive lymphocyte access to different body tissues. Lymphocyte migration through tissues would promote those cellular and subcellular interactions required for induction and regulation of immune responses. Finally, immune response potential would be further enhanced by the migration of effector and memory cells from sites of initial antigen priming to distant resting or inflamed tissues.

A third feature of this idealized lymphoid system would be that diverse lymphoid tissues would vary with respect to lymphocyte composition. As immune requirements would likely differ within anatomically distinct tissue sites (for example, mucosal versus nonmucosal), the lymphocyte types present within a given tissue would reflect tissue- or region-associated immune requirements.

A final feature of this customized lymphoid system would be that tissue-associated differences in lymphocyte composition would be maintained, at least in part, by a system allowing differential lymphocyte homing. Such a system might employ distinct molecular adhesion systems to regulate lymphocyte entry into various lymphoid and extralymphoid tissues. Such tissue-selective adhesive mechanisms would allow exquisite regulation of the tissue associations of circulating lymphocytes and would thus directly influence the character and intensity of immune responses arising in different tissues.

While we do not, at present, have the ability to custom-design lymphoid systems precisely as discussed in the previous paragraphs, it seems that evolutionary selection processes have allowed incorporation of these features into our actual immune systems. In this chapter, the process of lymphocyte recirculation through diverse body tissues will be discussed. The emphasis of the chapter is on the cellular and molecular interactions involved in the homing of blood-borne lymphocytes to lymphoid and extralymphoid tissues, including sites of inflammation.

LYMPHOCYTE RECIRCULATION

The migration or recirculation of lymphocytes between various lymphoid and extralymphoid tissues of the body is of central importance in the maintenance of a functional immune system. This continuous process of cellular shuffling allows antigen-reactive lymphocytes access to tissue sites of

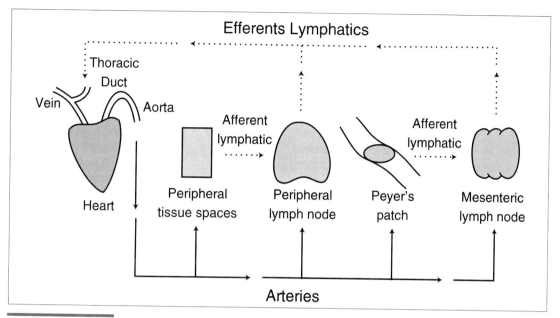

Figure 12-1   Lymphocyte recirculation. Blood-borne lymphocytes enter lymph nodes (mesenteric and peripheral) and mucosal lymphoid tissues (Peyer's patches and appendix) by first adhering to, then by passing across postcapillary HEVs. The lymphocytes then migrate through appropriate T- or B-cell domains, medullary lymphatic sinuses, and sinusoids to the lymphatics. After entry into the lymphatic system, the lymphocytes travel by way of efferent and afferent lymphatics through subsequent lymphoid tissues, and eventually these cells reenter the blood vascular compartment via the thoracic duct. Entry of lymphocytes into resting extralymphoid tissues (e.g., peripheral tissue spaces) occurs across flat-walled venules. Lymphocytes leaving these tissues migrate by way of afferent lymphatics to lymph nodes.

antigen entry and deposition, enhances cellular interactions required for the induction and regulation of immune responses, and facilitates the dispersement of locally primed effector cells to distant resting tissues and to sites of inflammation. At inflammatory sites, lymphocytes and other leukocytes participate in the elimination of tumors, the destruction of infectious agents, and the clearance of noninfectious inflammatory agents.

Lymphocytes travel between diverse tissues of the body by way of the blood and lymph vascular systems (Fig. 12-1). Blood-borne lymphocytes enter lymph nodes and mucosal lymphoid tissues (Peyer's patches and appendix) by first adhering to and then by passing across specialized postcapillary high-walled venules referred to as *high en-*

dothelial venules (HEVs) (Fig. 12-2). After moving through appropriate cortical regions in these tissues (T- and B-cell zones), lymphocytes enter the medulla and move by way of the sinusoids to the efferent lymphatics. Once in the lymphatic system, lymphocytes travel by way of afferent and efferent lymphatics through subsequent lymphoid tissues. Lymphocytes eventually reenter the blood vascular compartment by way of the thoracic duct.

The entry of blood-borne lymphocytes into sites of inflammation also requires adhesion to and passage across HEVs. These specialized venules, while not found in resting extralymphoid tissues, are readily induced as a consequence of local immune and inflammatory processes. Thus, the adhesion of

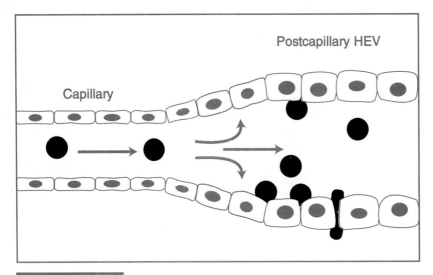

Figure 12-2   Schematic of lymphocyte entry into the extravascular compartment via postcapillary HEVs. This figure illustrates the directional movement of lymphocytes within capillaries and within and across postcapillary HEVs in organized lymphoid tissues. Lymphocytes move rapidly through capillaries in organized lymphoid tissues; their velocity is high, and few cells exit the blood via these structures. Upon entry into postcapillary HEVs, however, widening of the vessels is associated with turbulence and a reduction in lymphocyte velocity. These changes in lymphocyte flow, in combination with the presence of vascular addressins on the endothelial cells, result in high levels of lymphocyte adhesion to the vascular wall. Following adhesion, lymphocytes enter the tissue by migrating between the high endothelial cells.

blood-borne lymphocytes to specialized endothelial cells, the HEVs, in both resting and inflamed tissues is a critical controlling event in lymphocyte homing and recirculation.

TISSUE-SELECTIVE LYMPHOCYTE INTERACTIONS WITH HEVs

In leaving the blood vascular compartment, some lymphocyte subsets exhibit tissue-selective HEV-binding phenotypes. These tissue-selective interactions between lymphocytes and endothelial cells have been extensively evaluated using in vivo lymphocyte homing assays and an in vitro assay where lymphocytes bind to HEVs in frozen sections of lymphoid or inflamed extralymphoid tissues. These assay systems have allowed demonstration of distinct molecular adhesion systems that selectively control lymphocyte interactions with endothelium in peripheral lymph nodes (PLNs), mucosal lymphoid tissues, chronically inflamed skin, and chronically inflamed synovium. Tissue-selective lymphocyte localization is controlled, in part, by adhesive interactions between lymphocyte cell surface homing receptors and their endothelial cell counterparts, the vascular addressins, a functionally related group of cell surface molecules that provide tissue-position or tissue-address information to circulating lymphocytes.

The tissue-selective homing of circulating lymphocytes appears to contribute to the nonrandom distribution of lymphocyte subsets in distinct body tissues, a distribution which apparently reflects tissue- or region-associated immune requirements. Antigen-driven lymphocyte differentiation is central to the acquisition by lymphocytes of tissue-selective migratory phenotypes. Most naive B and T lymphocytes (mature lymphocytes that have not been triggered by antigen) express homing receptors for both PLNs and mucosal lymphoid tissues. B and T lymphocytes do not, however, bind equally to HEVs in these tissues: B lymphocytes preferentially bind HEVs in mucosal lymphoid tissues, while T cells exhibit preference for PLN HEVs. This tissue-selective HEV-binding potential may contribute to the predominance of B cells in Peyer's patches and T cells in PLNs. Effector lymphocyte populations differ from naive B and T cells in that they exhibit highly tissue-selective homing and HEV-binding properties. For example, IgA plasma cell precursor populations migrate al-most exclusively to mucosal sites, while IgG plasma cell precursors migrate selectively to peripheral sites, including inflamed skin.

The tissue-selective adhesion processes that direct normal lymphocyte migration into PLNs and mucosal lymphoid tissues also appear to participate in the blood-borne metastasis of lymphoid tumors. In fact, the localization of lymphoid tumors into organs containing HEVs can be accurately predicted by the HEV-binding properties of lymphoid tumors in the in vitro lymphocyte-HEV-adhesion assay. Lymphoid tumors that bind HEVs disseminate rapidly by way of the blood to spleen, bone marrow, and those organs containing HEVs (i.e., lymph nodes and mucosal Peyer's patches), yielding symmetrical lymphoid tissue involvement. Tumors that fail to bind HEVs spread by way of the blood

TABLE 12-1 Molecules Implicated in Lymphocyte Interactions with High Endothelium

Designation	Molecular Mass, kd	Function
ENDOTHELIAL CELL MOLECULES		
Mucosal vascular addressin (MAd)	58–66	Lymphocyte adhesion molecule on HEVs in resting and inflamed mucosal tissues
Peripheral lymph node addressin (PLAd)*	50 and 90	Lymphocyte adhesion molecule on HEVs in PLNs and inflamed peripheral sites
Cutaneous addressin (E-selectin)†	115	Lymphocyte adhesion molecule on HEVs in cutaneous inflammatory sites
Vascular cell adhesion molecule 1 (VCAM-1)‡	110	Lymphocyte adhesion molecule on endothelium in inflamed tissues
LYMPHOCYTE MOLECULES		
Peripheral lymph node homing receptor (L-Selectin)	70–90	PLAd-binding Ca^{2+}-dependent lectin
Mucosal homing receptor (LPAM-1)§	140 and 100	Integrin implicated in mucosal HEV binding
CD44 (Hermes)¶	85–95	Accessory molecule involved in HEV binding
Leukocyte function-related antigen (LFA-1)§	170 and 90	Accessory molecule involved in HEV binding
VLA-4§	140 and 110	Integrin implicated in synovial HEV binding

*PLAd is not a heterodimer; the 50 and 90 kd forms are distinct molecules.
†E-Selectin is also known as endothelial leukocyte adhesion molecule 1 (ELAM-1).
‡VCAM-1 is also known as inducible cell adhesion molecule 110 (INCAM-110).
§LPAM-1, LFA-1, and VLA-4 are heterodimers. The molecular masses of α and β chains are indicated.
¶Also known as H-CAM, Pgp-1, ECMRIII, and P80.

to spleen and bone marrow, but do not enter Peyer's patches or lymph nodes through HEVs. These non-HEV-binding lymphomas can, however, gain access to lymph nodes through lymphatics draining tumor-bearing tissues. As the blood-borne metastasis of lymphoid tumors can be controlled by those adhesion systems that direct normal lymphocyte homing to PLNs and mucosal tissues, it seems likely that the metastasis of lymphoid tumors may also be influenced by as-yet-undefined tissue- or inflammation-associated adhesion systems involved in lymphocyte recirculation. Functionally related adhesion systems may similarly support the metastasis of nonlymphoid tumors.

VASCULAR ADDRESSINS: TISSUE-SELECTIVE ENDOTHELIAL CELL MOLECULES THAT DIRECT LYMPHOCYTE HOMING

The tissue-selective interactions of lymphocytes with high endothelial cells clearly implied that HEVs in different tissues express distinct lymphocyte recognition elements. Such recognition elements, called *vascular addressins*, have been identified, and they function by providing tissue-position or tissue-address information to circulating lymphocytes. Three vascular addressins involved in lymphocyte recirculation are described here (Table 12-1). They include the mucosal addressin, a lymphocyte adhesion molecule present on endothelial cells in mucosa-associated lymphoid and extralymphoid tissues; the PLN addressin, a lymphocyte adhesion molecule which is expressed at high levels on PLN and tonsilar HEVs; and a putative addressin that is preferentially expressed on endothelium in inflamed skin (E-selectin).

The Mucosal Addressin

The *mucosal vascular addressin (MAd)* (Table 12-1), defined in mice with the mono-

clonal antibodies MECA-367 and MECA-89, is selectively expressed on endothelium in mucosa-associated tissues, including the Peyer's patches, the mesenteric lymph nodes, the gut lamina propria, the mammary gland, and the pancreas (Table 12-2). In mucosal-associated lymphoid tissues, the Peyer's patches, and mesenteric lymph nodes, MAd is expressed at high levels on HEVs (Fig. 12-3). In extralymphoid mucosal tissues, the gut lamina propria, the mammary gland, and the pancreas, MAd is expressed on small venules and the staining intensity is markedly reduced. The mucosal addressin is also found on sinusoidal cells of the marginal zone in spleen and on follicular dendritic cells. This addressin is not found on vessels in adult

TABLE 12-2   Tissue-Selective Distribution of MAds and PLAds in Resting and Inflamed Mouse Tissues

Tissues	Relative Expression Levels in Resting vs. Inflamed Tissues*	
	PLAd	MAd
PERIPHERAL SITES		
Peripheral lymph nodes	+ + +/+ + +	−/−
Skin†	−/+ +	−/−
Joint synovium†	−/+ +	−/−
Lacrimal gland	−/+	−/−
Salivary gland	−/+	−/−
Thyroid gland	−/+	−/−
MUCOSAL SITES		
Peyer's patches‡	+/ND	+ + +/ND
Lamina propria of the gut	−/ND	+ +/ND
Mammary gland	−/ND	+ +/ND
Stomach	−/−	+/+ +
INTERMEDIATE SITES		
Mesenteric lymph nodes	+ + +/ND	+ + +/ND
Pancreas	−/+ + +	+/+ + +

*Resting tissue/inflamed tissue.
†Expression levels reported reflect expression in human tissues.
‡ND-not determined.

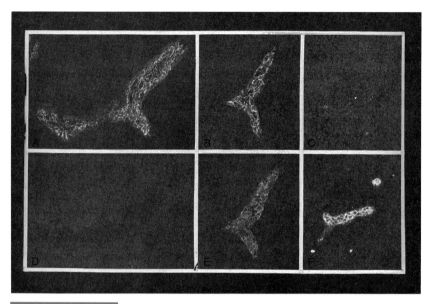

Figure 12-3   Analysis of PLAd [(a) to (c)] and MAd [(d) to (f)] on the lumenal surface of HEVs in PLNs [(a) and (d)], MLNs [(b) and (e)], and Peyer's patches [(c) and (f)]. Monoclonal antibodies MECA-79 (rat IgM) and MECA-367 (rat IgG) were administered intravenously into mice. The recipients were sacrificed 15 min later and gently perfused with HBSS to remove unbound antibody from the blood vasculature. Tissues were prepared for immunohistochemistry and serial sections were stained for lumenal PLAd versus lumenal MAd expression with peroxidase-conjugated anti-rat-IgM and anti-rat-IgG-specific reagents, respectively. PLAd was detected on HEVs in PLNs (a) and MLNs (b), but was absent or only barely detectable on Peyer's patch HEVs (c). By contrast, MAd was expressed on HEVs in Peyer's patches and MLNs and was not found on PLN HEVs. Parts a, b, and c are serial sections of d, e, and f, respectively. Bar is 50 μm. (From Streeter, et al. *J Cell Biol.* 1988;107:1853–1862, with permission.)

PLNs, thymus, or nonmucosal extralymphoid sites.

The selective expression of this endothelial cell differentiation antigen on mucosa-associated endothelium suggested that it might be involved in lymphocyte entry into anatomically separated mucosal sites. Functional studies confirmed this hypothesis. In the in vitro lymphocyte-HEV-adhesion assay, MECA-367 almost completely blocks lymphocyte adhesion to Peyer's patch. HEVs (Fig. 12-4), while having no effect on lymphocyte adhesion to HEVs in PLNs. MECA-367 exhibits an intermediate inhibitory effect on lymphocyte binding to HEV in

mesenteric lymph nodes (MLNs), an effect that is consistent with the presence of HEVs supporting lymphocyte adhesion via both mucosa- and PLN-associated adhesion systems in this tissue. The physiologic role of this molecule became apparent in short-term lymphocyte homing studies. The intravenous delivery of MECA-367 results in a dramatic decrease in lymphocyte migration to Peyer's patches, a partial reduction in trafficking to MLNs, and no significant effect on homing to PLNs (Fig. 12-5). The mucosal addressin also appears to be involved in lymphocyte homing to extralymphoid sites. However, in evaluating the ability of

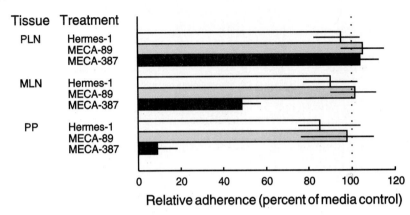

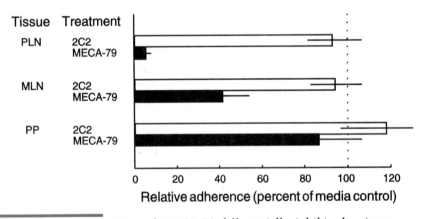

Figure 12-4 MECA-367 and MECA-79 differentially inhibit the tissue-selective adhesion of lymphocytes to HEVs in the in vitro lymphocyte-HEV-binding assay. (a) MECA-367 blocks the binding of lymphocytes to Peyer's patch (PP) and MLN HEVs without significantly influencing lymphocyte binding to PLN HEVs. Isotype-matched control antibodies (Hermes-1 and Meca-89) have no significant effect on lymphocyte binding to HEVs in any of these tissues. (b) MECA-79 inhibits lymphocyte adhesion to HEVs in PLNs and MLNs and fails to significantly inhibit lymphocyte adhesion to PP HEVs. Cell binding is not influenced by the isotype-matched control antibody, 2C2. Results in (a) and (b) are presented as a percent of the binding observed when no antibody was used in the assay (media control) (±SEM). (Part A from Streeter, et al. *Nature*. 1988;331:41–46; Part B from Streeter, et al. *J Cell Biol*. 1988;107:1853–1862, with permission.)

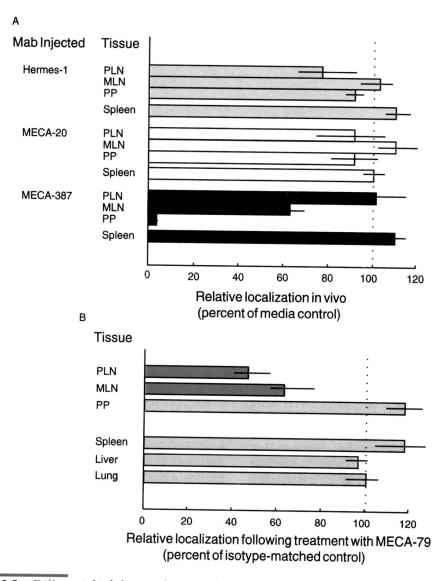

Figure 12-5 Differential inhibition of tissue-selective lymphocyte homing by MECA-367 and MECA-79. (a) MECA-367, but not isotype-matched control antibodies (Hermes-1 and MECA-20), selectively inhibits lymphocyte homing into mucosal lymphoid organs. Intravenous delivery of MECA-367 results in a substantial decrease in lymphocyte migration to Peyer's patches (PPs), a partial reduction in trafficking to MLNs, and no significant effect on homing to PLNs. Results are expressed as percent of cell localization observed in animals treated with HBSS containing no antibody (±SEM). (b) By contrast to treatment with MECA-367, the intravenous injection of MECA-79 results in the inhibition of lymphocyte homing to PLNs, it has less of an effect on lymphocyte extravasation into MLNs, and it has no significant effect on lymphocyte homing to PPs. Relative localization in MECA-79-treated recipients is expressed as a percent of that observed in recipients of an isotype-matched control antibody (±SEM). (Part *A* from Streeter, et al. *Nature.* 1988;331:41–46; Part *B* from Streeter, et al. *J Cell Biol.* 1988;107:1853–1862, with permission.)

MECA-367 to inhibit thoracic duct lymphoblast migration to such sites, this antibody only yielded a partial inhibition (roughly 50 percent), suggesting that an as-yet-undefined adhesion mechanism participates with MAd in directing lymphoblast migration into extralymphoid mucosal sites. The functional studies summarized here reveal that MAd provides a means of directing the dispersal of mucosa-associated lymphocyte populations to widely separated mucosal lymphoid and extralymphoid tissues.

The mucosal addressin, a single-chain O-glycosylated protein with a molecular mass of 58 to 66 kd, binds lymphocytes when it is immunoaffinity-purified and incorporated into artificial lipid membranes. Both normal lymphocytes and lymphomas that selectively bind mucosal HEVs bind to these membranes, while failing to bind to membranes containing control proteins. In addition, the anti-MAd specific monoclonal antibody MECA-367 inhibits the binding of these lymphocytes to MAd-containing membranes. The mucosal addressin does not, however, support the adhesion of lymphomas that selectively bind PLN HEVs. Thus, lymphocyte binding to MAd exhibits the same tissue selectivity as lymphocyte binding to HEVs in mucosal Peyer's patches.

The Peripheral Lymph Node Addressin

The *PLN vascular addressin (PLAd)* (Table 12-1), defined in both humans and mice with the monoclonal antibody MECA-79, is expressed at high levels on HEVs in both PLNs and MLNs (Table 12-2; Fig. 12-3). By contrast, expression of the MECA-79 antigen by HEVs in mucosal lymphoid tissues (i.e., Peyer's patches in mice and appendix and Peyer's patches in humans) is considerably lower than that observed in lymph nodes. Extralymphoid mucosal tissues, including the gut lamina propria and the mammary gland, are negative for the MECA-79 antigen. Indeed,

evaluation of a variety of resting nonlymphoid tissues, including skin, skeletal muscle, brain, and heart, revealed no MECA-79 antigen.

As with the mucosal addressin, the distribution of the MECA-79 antigen suggested that it might function as a vascular addressin, participating in lymphocyte homing to peripheral and mesenteric lymph nodes. Functionally, MECA-79 inhibits the binding of normal lymphocytes to PLN HEVs, while having no significant effect on lymphocyte binding to Peyer's patch HEVs (Fig. 12-4). MECA-79 also inhibits, in part, lymphocyte adhesion to MLN HEVs. As with MECA-367, the anti-MAd specific monoclonal antibody, this partial inhibition is consistent with the observation that HEVs in MLNs support lymphocyte binding by both the mucosa- and PLN-associated adhesion systems. Short-term lymphocyte homing studies yield qualitatively similar information, revealing that MECA-79 markedly reduces lymphocyte migration to PLNs, that it has a lesser effect on trafficking to MLNs, and that it has no effect on homing to mucosal Peyer's patches (Fig. 12-5). Thus, these studies confirm that the MECA-79 antigen participates in the process of lymphocyte homing and that it functions as a PLAd.

Western blot analyses indicate that MECA-79 recognizes a number of biochemically distinct species of varying molecular masses from PLNs. The predominant species are O- and N-glycosylated proteins with molecular masses of approximately 50 and 90 kd in humans and in mice. As with MAd, PLAd functions as a tissue-selective lymphocyte adhesion molecule. Immunoaffinity-isolated PLAd, when absorbed onto glass slides, binds both normal lymphocytes and lymphomas that selectively bind PLN HEVs. Furthermore, lymphocyte binding to purified PLAd is inhibited with MECA-79. Slides coated with PLAd do not support adhesion of mucosal HEV-binding lymphomas. Thus, purified PLAd supports lymphocyte adhesion in a manner that is consistent with lymphocyte adhesion to PLN HEVs.

Inflammation-Associated Endothelial Cell Molecules

Endothelial leukocyte adhesion molecule 1 (E-selectin) (see Table 12-1) is an inducible endothelial cell adhesion molecule for neutrophils, eosinophils, basophils, and lymphocytes. This molecule, a 115-kd glycoprotein, is one of three known members of the Selectin gene family, a family whose members participate in a wide variety of cellular interactions involving inflammatory cells. Additional members of this gene family include L-selectin (see Table 12-1) and P-selectin (previously GMP-140). P-Selectin is a 140-kd glycoprotein stored in α granules of platelets and Weibel-Palade bodies of endothelial cells, and is involved in neutrophil and monocyte adhesion. The three members of this family have amino-terminal sequences which are homologous to C-type or calcium-dependent lectins, a sequence homologous to an epidermal growth factor domain, and a variable number of cysteine-rich sequences that are homologous to sequences encoding complement regulatory proteins. While neutrophils have long been reported to interact with E-selectin, a putative association with lymphocyte trafficking also exists. Immunohistologically, E-selectin is selectively (although not exclusively) expressed at cutaneous sites of inflammation. In addition, E-selectin is frequently observed in association with leukocyte infiltrates that are made up principally of mononuclear cells. COS cells transfected with cDNA encoding E-selectin bind both neutrophils and a skin-associated population of memory T cells. These T cells express a cutaneous lymphocyte-associated antigen and are observed at high levels in inflamed skin and as a small T-cell subset in other tissues and in blood. Thus, inflammation-associated endothelial cell differentiation antigens, in this case E-selectin, can be expressed in a tissue-selective manner, and they may function as vascular addressins.

Vascular cell adhesion molecule 1 (VCAM-1) (Table 12-1), a member of the immunoglobulin superfamily, is a recently defined inducible adhesion molecule for lymphocytes, eosinophils, basophils, and monocytes. VCAM-1 is expressed on endothelial cells in a wide range of inflamed tissues. The physiologic role played by this molecule in recruitment of leukocytes to resting tissues or to sites of inflammation awaits further clarification. Indeed, it has recently been suggested that VCAM-1 is involved in the recruitment of T lymphocytes to inflamed joint synovium.

Inflammatory cytokines can have a profound impact on the expression of inflammation-associated endothelial cell adhesion molecules. Induction of distinct molecules on cultured endothelial cells occurs as a consequence of cytokine type, the dose of inducing cytokine, and the time following exposure to cytokine. For example, E-selectin is induced by treatment of endothelial cells with the cytokines interleukin 1 (IL-1) and tumor necrosis factor (TNF). On activated cultured endothelial cells, expression of E-selectin peaks at 4 h and is greatly reduced by 24 h. VCAM-1, by contrast, is induced on cultured endothelial cells by IL-1, IL-4, and TNF, with peak levels expressed at 6 to 24 h and some VCAM-1 remaining at 72 h. This differential induction of endothelial cell adhesion molecules may account, in part, for the changing leukocyte populations observed in acute inflammatory settings.

Lipopolysaccharide (LPS), the toxic component of bacterial endotoxin, induces production of IL-1 and TNF, and thus appears to indirectly induce E-selectin expression. The activity of LPS may be of clinical relevance; in a baboon model, exposure to LPS results in an increase in E-selectin in the postcapillary venules of the very organs most affected in septic shock—the lung, liver, kidney, and spleen.

Certain cytokines can also decrease the expression of homing molecules on endothelial cells. Transforming growth factor beta (TGF-β) decreases baseline adherence of blood cells to the endothelium and inhibits IL-1- or TNF-mediated increases in adherence for polymorphonuclear and T cells; in vitro β must be added to endothelial cells at least 9 h prior to the IL-1 or TNF in order to block the induction of homing molecules. IL-4 can stimulate VCAM, but inhibits endothelial cell expression of E-selectin; it also acts directly on monocytes to decrease their adhesiveness.

Regulation of the Expression of Vascular Addressins

While the regulatory processes controlling the tissue-selective expression of MAd and PLAd remain to be elucidated, significant evidence suggests that the expression of particular addressins is determined by regional microenvironments. In resting tissues, microenvironmental influences on expression of vascular addressin are perhaps most evident in peripheral versus mesenteric lymph nodes. High endothelial venules in adult PLNs (axillary, brachial, inguinal, popliteal, etc.) express PLAd almost exclusively, and lymphatic drainage to these tissues arrives from the periphery. By contrast, MLNs, a series of lymph nodes that drain the intestine, a mucosal site, express both MAd and PLAd. These observations suggest that afferent lymph-derived cells and/or lymph-associated factors influence expression of vascular addressins in mucosal lymphoid tissues and PLNs. This hypothesis is supported by two lines of evidence from mouse studies. In the first, the surgical disconnection of PLN afferent lymphatics results in a flattening of HEVs and a dramatic reduction in expression of PLAd. Lymph node transplantation studies, the second approach, reveal that neonatal MLNs transplanted to the popliteal fossa, a peripheral site, acquire a phenotype for expression of addressins that approaches that of PLNs (i.e., PLAd is expressed at high levels while MAd is expressed at reduced levels or is absent from most venules).

As the microenvironmental influences in mucosal versus peripheral tissues change substantially during fetal and early postnatal development, it is not surprising that the tissue associations of the mucosal and peripheral lymph node addressins differ markedly during distinct developmental stages. During late fetal development and at birth in mice, MAd is widely expressed, being found in mucosal tissues, thymus, and PLNs. PLNs and thymus at these early developmental stages differ most notably from their adult counterparts. In late fetal and neonatal PLNs, vessels express high levels of MAd, while lacking significant levels of PLAd. By 1 to 2 days after birth, vessels express PLAd, and adult levels are observed by 7 to 11 days after birth. In contrast to the increase in PLAd observed on these vessels, MAd gradually decreases over the first 3 to 4 weeks of postnatal life. Thus, the tissue-selective expression of PLAd in PLNs and MAd in mucosal sites is not achieved until mice are roughly 4 weeks of age. A similar developmental shift in expression of vascular addressin occurs in the thymus, where MAd and PLAd are sequentially observed on rare vessels. The widespread distribution of MAd in the developing immune system is suggestive of a central role for this addressin in lymphocyte seeding of both mucosal and nonmucosal tissues, and is consistent with the concept of ontogeny recapitulating phylogeny. Indeed, one can make a strong evolutionary argument for the early development of mucosa-associated adhesion systems, with requirements for alternative adhesion systems arising at later times.

There also exists an association of MAd and PLAd with inflammatory disease processes. For example, in nonobese diabetic mice (mice that develop an insulin-dependent type I diabetes), the small MAd-expressing venules associated with pancreatic islets undergo a transition to the HEV phenotype as islets become infiltrated with leukocytes. As islet infiltration proceeds, MAd expression levels on HEVs increase dramatically, and PLAd is induced and expressed at high levels. This dual expression of MAd and PLAd in chronically inflamed pancreas is consistent with expression of both of these adhesion molecules in this region of the body (i.e., the expression of vascular addressins in the inflamed pancreas is similar to that found in mesenteric lymph nodes). Functional assays confirm involvement of both MAd and PLAd in lymphocyte recruitment to chronically inflamed islets in this model. The early expression of MAd, prior to islet infiltration, is suggestive of a role for this molecule in the initial recruitment of lymphocytes to the pancreas. The later-stage expression of the peripheral addressin implies involvement of this addressin in the subsequent recruitment of lymphocytes to this tissue. This later-stage recruitment may allow effector lymphocytes access to this tissue.

Evaluation of a variety of cutaneous inflammatory conditions in humans has also led to the conclusion that while PLAd is involved in lymphocyte recruitment to chronic inflammatory sites, this molecule appears to be important in augmenting or amplifying recruitment rather than in initiating it. In cutaneous sites of inflammation, E-selectin may play the role of initiating lymphocyte recruitment. At other nonmucosal inflammatory sites, the adhesion systems responsible for initial lymphocyte recruitment remain to be defined.

In evaluating profiles of expression of vascular addressins in inflamed human and mouse tissues, it appears that expression of both MAd and PLAd on HEVs is under regional control. In peripheral sites of inflammation, including the thyroid gland, the lacrimal gland, the salivary gland, and skin (in humans), HEVs express PLAd while failing to express MAd. By contrast, in inflamed stomach, a mucosal site, HEVs exclusively express MAd. In inflamed pancreas (discussed above) both addressins are expressed. Thus, the regional expression of these molecules at inflammatory sites closely parallels the tissue-selective distribution observed in resting tissues. These data suggest that the same cellular or subcellular mechanisms control the expression of MAd and PLAd in resting and inflamed tissues. Further elucidation of the regulatory mechanisms directing the expression of vascular addressins will likely provide important insights into controlling inflammatory disease processes.

HOMING RECEPTORS: HEV-RECOGNITION ELEMENTS ON LYMPHOCYTES

The tissue-selective migration of blood-borne lymphocytes implied involvement of distinct lymphocyte cell surface molecules in the recognition of HEVs in different tissues. Such molecules, referred to as *homing receptors,* have been identified using anti-lymphocyte antibodies that inhibit tissue-selective lymphocyte interactions with endothelium (Table 12-1).

The Peripheral Lymph Node Homing Receptor

The PLN homing receptor L-selectin (Table 12-1) was originally defined in the mouse with the monoclonal antibody MEL-14. In the in vitro lymphocyte-HEV-adhesion assay, MEL-14 blocks lymphocyte adhesion to PLN HEVs, while failing to significantly alter lymphocyte adhesion to HEVs in Peyer's patches. In vivo studies confirmed involvement of this molecule in the selective homing of lymphocytes to PLNs. In humans this antigen is defined with monoclonal antibodies Leu-8, LAM-1, TQ-1, and Dreg-56. In both mouse and humans, these antibodies stain PLN HEV-binding cells and fail to stain non-HEV-binding cells.

The expression of L-selectin on lymphocyte populations is indicative of lymphocyte trafficking potential to PLNs, and supports the finding that effector and/or memory lymphocyte populations exhibit tissue-selective homing patterns. While the vast majority of naive B and T lymphocytes express L-selectin, expression of this molecule is restricted to subpopulations of memory cells. Those memory cells that preferentially migrate to the periphery express high level of L-selectin, while those that migrate to mucosal sites do not.

The PLN homing receptor, a 70- to 90-kd glycoprotein, is a member of the selectin gene family and it participates in lymphocyte-HEV interactions as a calcium-dependent mammalian lectin. As a lectin, it appears to interact with carbohydrate moieties on HEVs. Adhesion of lymphocytes to PLN HEVs in the in vitro binding assay is inhibited by treatment of lymphocytes with a variety of carbohydrates, including mannose-6-phosphate, the mannose-6-phosphate-rich yeast polyphosphomannan PPME, fructose-1-phosphate, and the fucose-rich heteropolysaccharide fucoidan, with inhibition occurring at the level of the lymphocyte. Lymphocyte adhesion to PLN HEVs is also inhibited by pretreatment of HEVs with neuraminidase, further supporting a role for carbohydrate determinants on HEVs in lymphocyte adhesion via the PLN homing receptor.

Non-HEV-binding lymphomas, when transfected with L-selectin cDNA, avidly bind to immunoaffinity-isolated PLAd. As with lymphocyte binding to PLN HEVs, the binding of these transfectants to PLAd is inhibited with anti-L-selectin antibodies, and the adhesive interaction is calcium-dependent. Furthermore, neuraminidase pretreatment of PLAd prevents transfectant binding. Thus, L-selectin appears to function as a PLN homing receptor, with PLAd as its HEV counterpart.

The Mucosal Homing Receptor

The unification of widely separated mucosal lymphoid and extralymphoid tissues into a common mucosal immune system is achieved, in part, by the tissue-selective localization of mucosa-associated lymphocyte populations. At the endothelial cell level, MAd directs the localization of lymphocytes into these widely separated mucosal sites. Functional studies suggest that a recently defined integrin, LPAM-1 (Table 12-1), may participate at the lymphocyte level in recruitment to mucosal tissues.

The integrin family of cell surface molecules has been implicated in cellular interactions with other cells, as well as cellular interactions with extracellular matrix components. Integrins generally consist of two noncovalently associated glycoprotein subunits (α and β). Multiple α and β subunits have been defined, and the differential as-

sociation of these various subunits is thought to confer distinct ligand-binding specificities. The putative mucosal homing receptor LPAM-1, described here, is a member of this gene family, and appears related to that set of integrins referred to as the *VLA antigens* (for *very late appearance* on T cells following activation). The VLA antigens are expressed on a wide range of cell types, and members of this group are composed of any of five distinct α chains associated with a common β chain. LPAM-1 consists of an α chain which is homologous to that of VLA-4 and a novel β chain which is now referred to as β_7.

The anti-LPAM-1-specific monoclonal antibody R1/2 selectively blocks the interaction of mouse lymphocytes with HEVs in Peyer's patches, while exhibiting no significant inhibitory effect on lymphocyte binding to PLN HEVs. Thus, LPAM-1 appears to function as a homing receptor for mucosal HEV. Analysis of the cellular associations (i.e., naive vs effector or memory) and cellular-distribution (i.e., tissue association) of LPAM-1-positive cells is difficult, however, since R1/2 recognizes the common α chain of both LPAM-1 and VLA-4. Antibodies to the unique β chain associated with LPAM-1 have not been described. Recent evidence suggests that LPAM-1 is a ligand for MAd.

Additional Lymphocyte Surface Molecules Implicated in Adhesion to HEVs

The lymphocyte surface antigen CD44 (Table 12-1) also appears to be involved in lymphocyte adhesion to HEVs. Rather than directing tissue-selective lymphocyte homing, however, this molecule has been implicated in lymphocyte adhesion to HEVs in a variety of tissues or regions. The monoclonal antibody Hermes-3 selectively blocks lymphocyte adhesion to HEVs in mucosal lymphoid tissues, suggesting involvement as a tissue-selective homing receptor. However, inhibition studies with a polyclonal antibody raised against the CD44 antigen reveal the involvement of this antigen in lymphocyte adhesion to HEVs in mucosal sites, PLNs, and inflamed synovium. The CD44-expression profile on naive versus memory cells is also inconsistent with this molecule functioning as a tissue-selective homing receptor. Rather than being expressed on a subset of memory cells, as is the case with L-selectin, CD44 is widely expressed on memory cells. CD44 has also recently been implicated as having a general role in cell adhesion, with fibronectin, collagen types I and IV, and hyaluronic acid as its putative ligands. These observations suggest that rather than functioning as a tissue-selective homing receptor, CD44 participates as an important accessory molecule in a variety of cell-cell and cell-substratum adhesion processes, including lymphocyte adhesion to HEVs in a variety of tissues.

The integrin VLA-4 (Table 12-1) has recently received considerable attention. This molecule, which binds both fibronectin and the inflammation-associated endothelial cell molecule VCAM-1, is thought to be involved in lymphocyte recruitment to inflammatory sites where VCAM-1 is expressed. Indeed, it has recently been suggested that VLA-4 is involved in lymphocyte recruitment to inflamed joint synovium.

The leukocyte integrin LFA-1 (Table 12-1) may also function as an accessory molecule involved in lymphocyte adhesion to HEVs. Antibodies to LFA-1 partially inhibit lymphocyte binding to HEVs in both mucosal lymphoid tissues and PLNs. However, while LFA-1 can apparently participate in this adhesion process, it is not essential. Lymphocytes from patients with leukocyte adhesion deficiency lack surface expression of LFA-1, yet they are able to home to lymphoid tissues.

THERAPEUTIC INTERVENTION IN INFLAMMATORY DISEASE PROCESSES

The recruitment of lymphocytes and other leukocytes to tissue sites, when occurring as a consequence of tissue injury, infection, or tumor metastasis, for example, is clearly an essential component of normal immune and nonimmune host defense systems. However, leukocyte infiltration of tissues is not always associated with inflammatory processes which benefit the host. Acute and chronic inflammatory diseases, as well as certain autoimmune diseases, are frequently characterized by tissue-selective leukocyte infiltrates. The continuous recruitment of inflammatory cells to these disease sites appears to both perpetuate and amplify inflammatory disease processes. Inhibition of leukocyte recruitment to inflammatory sites is theoretically achievable, using therapeutics designed to interfere directly or indirectly with those adhesion systems implicated in lymphocyte migration. It seems likely that treatment with agents that inhibit lymphocyte recruitment to inflammatory sites will have a dramatic impact on the severity and duration of inflammatory diseases.

SELF-TEST QUESTIONS*

1. Select the *true* statement(s) concerning the nature and function of vascular addressins.
   a. Vascular addressins are lymphocyte adhesion molecules expressed in a tissue-selective manner on endothelial cells.
   b. Vascular addressins are members of the selectin gene family, a family whose members have an aminoterminal lectin domain, an epidermal growth factor–like domain, and a variable number of sequences related to complement regulatory proteins.
   c. Vascular addressins can participate in lymphocyte migration to inflammatory sites.
   d. The adhesion of lymphocytes to the mucosal and peripheral vascular addressins requires the presence of accessory adhesion molecules expressed on high endothelial cells.

*Answers will be found in Appendix E.

2. Select the *correct* statement(s) regarding the process of lymphocyte recirculation.
   a. Naive lymphocytes (mature lymphocytes not triggered by antigen) enter extralymphoid sites more effectively than memory lymphocytes.
   b. The mobile nature of lymphocytes enhances their potential for participating in immune responses.
   c. Lymphocytes bind to high endothelial venules in Peyer's patches by the lymphocyte homing receptor P-selectin.
   d. Tissue-selective lymphocyte migration results in the nonrandom distribution of lymphocyte subsets in different tissues.

3. Select the *true* statement(s). Lymphocyte homing receptors and vascular addressins are involved in:
   a. The migration of lymphocytes to lymphoid tissues;
   b. The homing of lymphocytes to resting extralymphoid tissues;
   c. The migration of lymphocytes to inflamed tissues; and
   d. The blood-borne metastasis of lymphomas.

ADDITIONAL READINGS

Bevilacqua MP, Stengelin S, Gimbrone MA, Seed B. Endothelial leukocyte adhesion molecule 1: An inducible receptor for neutrophils related to complement regulatory proteins and lectins. *Science* 1989;243:1160–1165.

Butcher EC. The regulation of lymphocyte traffic. *Curr Top Microbiol Immunol.* 1986;128:85–122.

Gallatin MW, Weissman IL, Butcher EC. A cell surface molecule involved in organ-specific homing of lymphocytes. *Nature* 1983;304:30–34.

Holzmann B, McIntyre BW, Weissman IL. Identification of a murine Peyer's patch-specific lymphocyte homing receptor as an integrin molecule with an alpha chain homologous to human VLA-4 alpha. *Cell* 1989;56:37–46.

Siegelman MH, van de Rijn M, Weissman IL. Mouse lymph node homing receptor cDNA clone encodes a glycoprotein revealing tandem interaction domains. *Science* 1989;243:1165–1172.

Streeter PR, Berg EL, Rouse BN, Bargatze RF, Butcher EC. A tissue-specific endothelial cell molecule involved in lymphocyte homing. *Nature* 1988;331:41–46.

Streeter PR, Rouse BN, Butcher EC. Immunohistologic and functional characterization of a vascular addressin involved in lymphocyte homing into peripheral lymph nodes. *J Cell Biol.* 1988;107:1853–1862.

Summary of Part I: Basic Mechanisms of Immunology

In the first part of this text you have been introduced to all of the antigen-specific "players" in the immune system, how they learn to do what they are destined to accomplish, how they interact and regulate themselves, and how they do what they do. As is noted repeatedly, the full story is not yet known in all realms of immunology. Much remains to be understood, and yet what is known, if applied appropriately, provides a wealth of opportunities in the laboratory and in the clinic.

The previous twelve chapters provide the tools with which to start understanding immune mechanisms of disease (more on this later) and the means by which multi-cellular organisms can defeat pathogens, both derived from the external and the internal milieu. A description of these mechanisms from an evolutionary (phylogenetic) perspective, rather than the ontogenetic perspective used above, can be found in Appendix B. Some areas of immunology and inflammation become somewhat more understandable when viewed from this vista. All that comes now in this text and in the course you are taking is predicated upon an understanding of Part I. Much of what comes in the future as you practice medicine also will be predicated upon these principles.

PART

TWO

Basic Mechanisms of Inflammation

Learning all that is presented in Part I is not enough to fully understand how the "immune system" is capable of working its homeostatic wonders. A number of physiologic processes fall under the category of inflammation, rather than immunology (thus the title of this book). In a sense, immunology can be considered a part of inflammation, which can be described loosely as a process whereby host cells and blood proteins enter tissue injured by pathogens or by auto-aggressive behavior of the immune system (auto-immunity). In addition, may of these same cells and blood proteins can be part of a damping process, to decrease the damage and ultimately to take part in clean-up and repair of the damaged tissues.

Inflammation is discussed in Part II. Considering Immunology without inflammation is a little like studying the spinal cord with no attention to neurologic structures in the head such as the cerebral cortex and cerebellum; one without the other just does not do the job. Of most importance to medical students, considering one or the other in a vacuum gives one an artificial and incomplete picture of the medical implications of the processes described and how they magnify and help modulate each other.

Part II starts with the description of two protein cascades, the complement system (Chapter 13) and the coagulation, fibrinolytic, and kinin systems (Chapter 14). Each represents a series of enzymes which, in a step-wise fashion, activate defense and repair systems. These then interact with the mechanisms described in Part I to enhance and control the immunologic activities noted. Another prime example of immune control and function capabilities in one package is the series of compounds derived from cellular lipid compounds described in Chapter 15, "The Prostaglandins, Leukotrienes, Lipoxin, and Platelet-activating Factor."

The next four chapters in Part II describe non-antigen-specific reactivities active and/or elicited during inflammatory reactions. Upon exposure to certain cytokines (immune mediators, from Part I), the liver can produce a series of proteins which are active in defense and repair; these are discussed in Chapter 16, "The Acute Phase Response to Inflammation." The next three chapters introduce three classes of cells involved in defense, but which are not intrinsically capable of being involved in an antigen-specific fashion, i.e., they manufacture no surface receptors with antigen-specificity. The polymorphonuclear phagocytic cells (Chapter 17), mononuclear phagocytic cells (Chapter 18), basophils and mast cells (Chapter 19a), and eosinophils (Chapter 19b) are crucial participants in the wide variety of defenses called into play during infections and auto-immune damage. In the final chapter of the section many of the threads first seen in the preceding chapters are woven together to form the fabric known as the inflammatory response (Chapter 20).

13

The Complement System

INTRODUCTION

The complement system is one of the major mediators of inflammation and serves as an important part of the body's immune response. It was first discovered after observations that sera with specific antibody from immune animals lost the capability to kill bacteria after heating and that this ability was restored by the addition of small amounts of serum from nonimmune animals. This implied that lysis of bacteria requires some heat-labile serum factor that "complements" specific antibody. The complement system is composed of distinct component proteins, as well as regulators and inhibitors. It is now known that there are 21 well-defined plasma proteins which together comprise the complement system, interacting precisely to mediate the fate of antigen-antibody reactions as well as inflammation and host defense.

The complement system components are normally present in the circulation in inactive form, and are sequentially activated in a "cascading" fashion. There are two parallel pathways of activation, the classical and alternative.

The components of the *classical pathway* are designated by numbers in the order of discovery and are preceded by the letter C. Component C1 is composed of three distinct proteins, C1q, C1r, and C1s. Factors of the *alternative pathway* have been assigned names and letters: P (properdin), factor B, and factor D. Fragments of complement activation are designated by the lowercase letters a, b, c, d, and e (for example, C3a and C3b). Activated enzymes are designated by overbars (for example, $\overline{C1}$). An active form of B is designated Bb. Inhibitors are designated as factors H and I, C1INH, and C4bp (in the case of C4bp, the lowercase letters represent an abbreviation—binding protein). Note that C3 and its major fragment C3b are components of both the classical and alternative pathways.

ACTIVATION OF THE COMPLEMENT SYSTEM

The two pathways of the complement system, the classical and alternative, are distinct activation pathways which are triggered by different substances but which converge through a common set of proteins, C5 through C9, designated the terminal proteins of the complement system or *membrane attack complex (MAC)* (Fig. 13-1). The classical pathway is activated by antigen-antibody complexes and antibody-coated targets. The alternative pathway does not require the presence of antibody and may be activated by particulate activators including endotoxin and bacterial polysaccharides. Both the classical and alternative pathways require cleavage of C3.

Classical Pathway

The classical pathway is initiated when the first component of complement (C1), composed of three subcomponents C1q, C1r, C1s, binds immune complexes containing IgG or IgM antibodies (Ab) (Fig. 13-2). Activated C1 ($\overline{C1}$) has as its substrate C4 and C2, and generates $\overline{C4b2a}$, which is a C3-cleaving enzyme. $\overline{C423b}$ is formed, which then cleaves C5. C5 activation leads to assembly of C56789 (C5–C9), the membrane attack complex (the overbar is a standard way of denoting an active enzyme).

The sequence begins with antibody (immunoglobulin) interacting with antigen and with the subsequent binding of C1 through C1q subunit to the non-antigen-binding part of the antibody molecule (Fc region). The C1 complex changes configuration, activating $\overline{C1s}$, which becomes an active enzyme with C1-esterase activity.

Human immunoglobulins of subclasses IgG1, IgG2, IgG3, and IgM are capable of classical pathway activation. Immunoglobulin subclass IgG4 and classes IgA, IgD, and IgE are unable to activate the classical pathway.

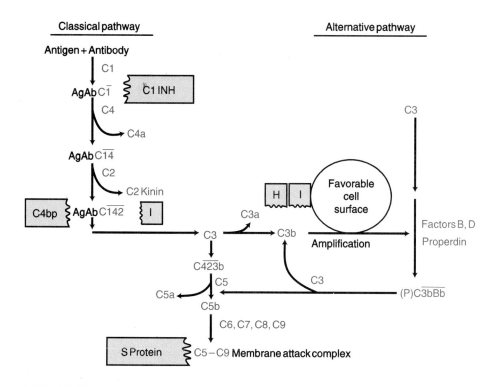

Figure 13-1   Sequence of activation of the complement components of the classical and alternative pathways. The classical pathway is initiated when the first component of complement (C1) binds to IgG or IgM antibodies (Ab) fixed to antigen (Ag). Activated $\overline{C1}$, composed of three subcomponents C1q, C1r, C1s, reacts with C4 and C2 to generate $\overline{C42}$, which is a C3-cleaving enzyme. $\overline{C423b}$ is formed, which in turn cleaves C5. A large fragment of C3 (C3b) is a powerful opsonin, and C5 activation leads to assembly of C56789 (C5–C9), known as the membrane attack complex. The alternative pathway requires C3b, which may be generated as a by-product of the classical pathway or from the alternative pathway through activity of a C3-cleaving enzyme formed from C3 and factor B ($\overline{C3bBb}$). Alternative pathway cleavage of C3 can amplify classical pathway activity. Properdin (P) can bind $\overline{C3bBb}$, stabilizing this important cleaving enzyme. The alternative pathway enzyme C3bBbC3b can cleave C5, paralleling activity of $\overline{C423b}$ of the classical pathway. Inhibitors (enclosed in notched boxes) act at several key sites: C1 inhibitor (C1INH) inhibits C1s, factor I inactivates C4b and C3b, factor H accelerates inactivation of C3b by I, and an analogous factor, C4-binding protein (C4bp), accelerates cleavage of C4b by I.

The classical pathway can also be initiated nonimmunologically through a variety of agents. *C-reactive protein (CRP)*, an acute phase reactant (see Chap. 16, "The Acute Phase Response to Inflammation") capable of binding to "C-carbohydrate" from microorganisms, may fix C1q independent of antibodies and initiate the entire sequence. Other substances which can directly activate C1 include certain RNA viruses, uric acid

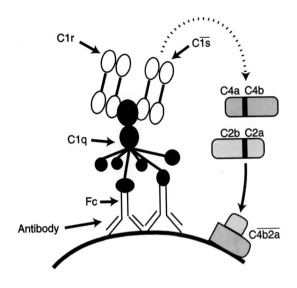

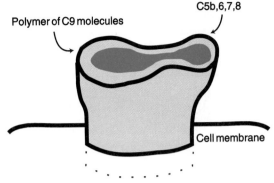

Figure 13-2 *Classical pathway activation.* C1 is composed of three components. C1q binds to the Fc region of antibody. C1r is then activated, which in turn activates C1s. Activated C1s (C1-esterase) cleaves C4 and C2. C4b and C2a form a complex (C4b2a) that attaches to the target cell and is capable of cleaving C3.

Figure 13-3 Schematic drawing of the membrane attack complex (MAC). C5b67 inserts into the lipid bilayer, and C8 and multiple molecules of C9 join to form a cylindrical structure. The outer portion of the MAC is lipophilic; the inner hydrophilic channel allows passage of water and small ions. Osmotic equilibrium is lost, resulting in cell swelling and lysis.

crystals, and membranes of intracellular organelles.

C4 and C2 are the natural substrates for activated C1. Activated C1 hydrolyses C4 and C2, generating C4b2a, the *C3 convertase* of the classical pathway. The split polypeptide fragment of C4, C4a, is a weak anaphylatoxin. The fragment released from C2, C2b, has kininlike activity which can cause increased vascular permeability.

Cleavage of C3 is crucial to the biologic effects of complement. Classical pathway C4b2a, and the C3 convertase of the alternative pathway (C3bBb), cleave C3, generating C3b and C3a. C3b acts as a binding protein for C5 and cleaves C5 by the same C4b2a enzyme that cleaves C3. Generation of C5b initiates, without further enzymatic cleavage, the assembly of the MAC (C5–C9) (Fig. 13-3). Insertion of the MAC into the cell membrane results in the formation of transmembrane channels, compromising the membrane's functional integrity and resulting in cell lysis.

C3b binds to antigen-antibody complexes permitting cells with C3b receptors, such as B lymphocytes, erythrocytes, and phagocytic cells (macrophages, neutrophils, and monocytes), to adhere to the complexes. Thus C3b is important in immune defense, leading to phagocytosis of immune complexes. (See Clinical Aside 13-1.)

The peptide C3a and the fragment product C5a have anaphylatoxin activity. C5a, as noted above, has an important chemoattractant effect on phagocytic cells.

Clinical Aside 13-1
C3 Deficiency

Individuals with C3 deficiency have a predisposition to severe pyogenic infections such as pneumococcal pneumonia and meningococcal meningitis. Without C3 to bind to most microorganisms, phagocytosis, especially by neutrophils, is greatly compromised, both in vitro and in vivo. There is also deficient killing of bacteria due to inability to produce C5a, an important chemotactic factor. C3e, another cleavage factor of C3 which normally increases the number of peripheral blood neutrophils, is diminished or absent, causing sluggish response of the neutrophil cell line to infection.

Alternative Pathway

The alternative pathway may be activated by IgA-containing immune complexes, by complex polysaccharides in pathogens, or by certain viruses in the absence of antigen-antibody interaction. Because of this direct activation by interaction with pathogens, the alternative pathway serves as part of the host's defense mechanism against microbes before specific antibody develops. C3b formation is crucial in the activation of the alternative pathway.

The initial step involves the interaction of C3 with H_2O, and the formation of a $C3H_2O$ molecule transiently capable of binding to the activating surface. $C3H_2O$ binds factor B, resulting in $\overline{C3H_2OBb}$, the initial enzyme of the alternative pathway. The attachment of factor B allows cleavage by factor D, resulting in the formation of the proteolytic enzyme $\overline{C3bBb}$ (Fig. 13-4). $\overline{C3H_2OBb}$ is an active C3-cleaving enzyme which generates C3b and initiates a positive-feedback system. This cyclic "amplification loop" is a key event in alternative pathway activation. It also serves to amplify C3 activation initiated by classical pathway activation.

The efficiency of the alternative pathway is greatly increased when C3b is bound to certain surfaces: polysaccharides from bacterial cell walls, lipopolysaccharides from endotoxin, immunoglobulin aggregates, and certain cells. When bound, C3b is protected from the action of control proteins I and H, allowing amplification of C3 activation. In the absence of this protection, C3b may be rapidly inactivated by factors H and I (Fig. 13-5). Furthermore, the activating substances favor the binding of properdin (P) to $\overline{C3bBb}$, stabilizing this important cleaving enzyme. The alternative pathway enzyme $\overline{C3bBb}$, in the presence of additional C3b, cleaves C5, paralleling activity of $\overline{C4b2a}$ of the classical pathway, leading to formation

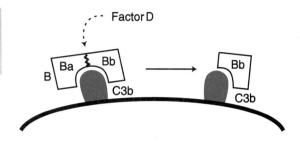

Figure 13-4 *C3b activation in the alternative pathway.* $C3H_2O$ binds factor B, which in the presence of factor D forms a complex $\overline{C3bBb}$. $\overline{C3bBb}$ is the C3-convertase of the alternative pathway.

of C5b–C9, the MAC. (See Clinical Aside 13-2.)

Clinical Aside 13-2
Alternative Pathway of Complement

The surface of rabbit red blood cells (RBCs) allows $\overline{C3bBb}$ activation by preventing inhibition by I and H. This is exploited in a clinical test of alternative pathway activity. Patient serum is mixed with rabbit RBCs and hemolysis is assayed. The erythrocytes serve both as an activating (permissive) surface and as the target of alternative pathway activity. In gram-negative sepsis, endotoxin may be released, which has the capability of altering normally "nonactivating" cell surfaces. This "disinhibition" of $\overline{C3bBb}$ may explain the activation of the alternative complement pathway seen

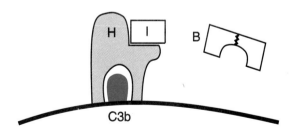

Figure 13-5 *Control proteins and C3b activation.* The control protein factor H binds to cell-bound or fluid-phase C3b, preventing C3b from binding factor B and preventing alternative pathway activation. Factor H also causes $\overline{C3bBb}$ to disassociate. Factor I may also inactivate C3b, though poorly unless in the presence of factor H.

in patients with meningococcemia and other gram-negative bacteremias.

Complement-Control Proteins

Several mechanisms constrain the complement system from unnecessary or deleterious activity or from complete consumption. Many of the active combining sites are labile, and some of the active complexes are subject to time- and temperature-dependent disassociation. In addition, there are several serum proteins which act as inhibitors and regulator proteins.

C1 has a specific inhibitor known as C1 inhibitor, or C1INH, which binds to and inhibits activity of C1r and C1s. By constraining the enzymatic activity of C1, this α-globulin inhibits cleavage of C4 and C2. Absence of C1INH is associated with a clinical syndrome known as hereditary angioedema. (See Clinical Aside 13-3.)

Clinical Aside 13-3
C1 Inhibitor Deficiency

A condition manifested by episodes of rapidly progressive cutaneous and mucous membrane edema has been associated with a deficiency of C1INH activity. This is usually an inherited disorder (hereditary angioedema), though a rare acquired form is reported, often in association with lymphoid malignancies. Patients may present with swelling of the face, larynx, or extremities, or with gastrointestinal involvement manifested by colic, nausea, vomiting, or diarrhea. This life-threatening condition may be due to failure to synthesize normal amounts of C1 inhibitor, or to synthesis of nonfunctional protein. In the acquired form it appears that either antibodies are formed to the C1 inhibitor, or, more often, the inhibitor is consumed. Without adequate C1 inhibitor, unconstrained C1 activity leads to cleavage of C4 and C2, resulting in the release of a vasoactive peptide (kinin) from C2. This kinin causes vasodilatation of the postcapillary venules, manifested as swelling and subcutaneous edema. Laryngeal edema may be fatal.

Another control protein, factor I, cleaves C4b and C3b in the presence of the cofactor

proteins C4b, binding protein, and factor H. This significantly controls both the classical and alternative pathways. Serum contains an enzyme, *anaphylatoxin inactivator*, which cleaves the carboxyterminal arginine from C3a and C5a. This greatly reduces the chemotactic effect of C5a and the anaphylatoxic effects of both C3a and C5a.

A variety of cell membrane–associated proteins interfere with complement activity and complement effects. There are a set of cellular receptors for target-bound fragments of C3, termed CR1, CR2, CR3, and CR4 (complement receptors 1, 2, 3, and 4). CR1 is the specific receptor for C3b, and is present on erythrocytes, B lymphocytes, some T lymphocytes, neutrophils, monocytes, mast cells, eosinophils, basophils, and glomerular podocytes. Binding of a C3b-coated target to CR1 is important in initiating phagocytosis. CR1 also is crucial in C3 degradation, and potently inhibits the complement cascade. CR2 is present on all B lymphocytes and epithelial cells and may be important in stimulating B-cell cycling and differentiation. CR3 is found on neutrophils, monocytes, and lymphocytes and is involved in antibody-mediated cellular cytotoxicity. When neutrophils are stimulated, CR3 present within granules is transported to the cell surface, where it promotes cellular adherence. CR4 is a similar C3-binding molecule.

Decay accelerating factor, membrane cofactor protein, and homologous restriction factor are membrane proteins that interact with activated complement proteins to preserve cell integrity and "contain" complement activity. Decay accelerating factor is present in all blood cells and endothelial cells and accelerates decay of the enzymes $C\overline{3bBb}$ and $C\overline{4b2a}$ (see the section below on paroxysmal nocturnal hemoglobinuria). Membrane control protein (also known as gp45–70), which facilitates factor I–dependent degradation of C3b, is found on a variety of blood cells, endothelial cells, epithelial cells, and fibroblasts. Homologous restriction factor is found on erythrocytes, lymphocytes, monocytes, neutrophils, and platelets. It is anchored by a phospholipid moiety into the cell membrane. By interacting with C8, it prevents C9 binding and the insertion of the MAC, protecting cells from complement-induced lysis.

Homologous restriction factor gets its name from the observation that in all species studied, this protein prevents lysis by homologous C8 and C9 but not by heterologous proteins. This may account for complement proteins being much more efficient at lysing cells of heterologous species than cells of homologous species, and may reflect a mechanism of protection of host cells from complement injury.

ACTIVITIES OF THE COMPLEMENT SYSTEM: MEDIATOR OF HOST DEFENSE

The actions of complement activities are myriad, including cellular destruction, inflammation, and immunologic effects. Complement effects are mediated through the release of vasoactive mediators and chemoattractants, neutralization of endotoxin, solubilization of immune complexes, stimulation of opsonization, and formation of lytic conduits in cell membranes (Table 13-1).

Cell Lysis

Membrane attack complexes are formed by the polymerization of C9 onto C5b678, forming cylindrical structures. When inserted into cell membranes, a channel is created with a hydrophilic center, functioning as an open channel allowing an uncontrolled influx of water into the cells, resulting in lysis. (See Fig. 13-3.) Leaky patches may also be formed by disruption of membrane lipids and phospholipids around the C5b–C9 complex. Cells susceptible to lysis include erythrocytes, lymphocytes, platelets, bacteria, viruses, virus-infected cells, tumor cells, spirochetes, and protozoa.

TABLE 13-1 Complement Peptides and Host Defense

Complement Product	Biologic Activity
C14, C1423	Viral neutralization
C3a	Suppression of antibody response
C3b	Opsonization; enhanced cell-mediated cytotoxicity; solubilization of immune complexes
C4a, C3a, C5a	Anaphylatoxin (vasoactive mediator release, increased vascular permeability)
C3 cleavage product (C3e)	Induction of granulocyes
C5a	Neutrophil, monocyte, eosinophil chemotaxis; cytokine release; enhanced antibody response
C1–C5 (? others)	Endotoxin inactivation
C1–C9	Cell lysis (viruses, virus-infected cells, bacteria, protozoa, mycoplasma, spirochetes, tumor cells, host cells)

Inflammation and Immunologic Defense

Complement activation produces peptides which mediate chemotaxis, anaphylaxis, vasodilatation, and cellular secretion of cytokines. C3a and C5a act as anaphylatoxins, causing mast cells and basophils to degranulate and release histamine and other mediators. This results in vasodilatation, redness, swelling, and other effects, including smooth muscle contraction and secretion of mucus by airway goblet cells (Fig. 13-6). C5a is a potent chemical stimulus for the migration of neutrophils, monocytes, and eosinophils into an area of inflammation. In addition, C5a bound to the surface of neutrophils stimulates neutrophil adherence, degranulation, and oxidative bursts. C5a may also induce the release of tumor necrosis factor and interleukin 1, enhancing the inflammatory response. C3b generated from C3 cleavage coats target cells (opsonization); phagocytic cells have specific C3b receptors

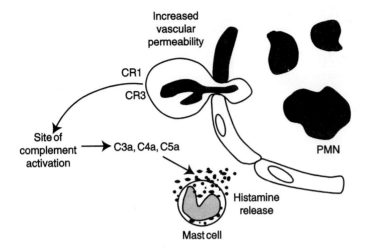

Figure 13-6 *Complement effects—anaphylatoxins and mediator release.* C3a and C5a are the biologically significant anaphylatoxins, causing release of histamines and other mediators, increasing vascular permeability. C5a promotes neutrophil migration, enhanced CR1 and CR3 expression, and adhesion. PMN stands for polymorphonuclear neutrophil.

(CR1), and can bind to opsonized cells in preparation for ingestion. C3b fixation to target cells also increases lysis by killer cells via antibody-dependent cell-mediated cytotoxicity.

The result of the interaction of these factors is the ability of a local complement-activating event to induce increased blood flow to the affected tissue, chemotaxis, activation of neutrophils and mononuclear phagocytes, secretion of cytokines, amplified complement activity, and enhanced immunologic defense.

Other effects of the complement system include its influence on both B cell–mediated and T cell-mediated immunity. In vitro, and in experimental animals, C5a enhances antibody formation, while C3a may suppress antibody formation. C3b opsonizes not only target cells, but also immune complexes. C3b coating allows cells with the C3b receptor (CR1) to bind immune complexes, and may serve to transport these complexes to the fixed macrophage system for removal. The inability to rid the circulation of immune complexes may be associated with clinical disease. (See Clinical Aside 13-4.)

Clinical Aside 13-4
SLE and Complement Receptors

Many patients with systemic lupus erythematosus (SLE), an autoimmune multisystem disease, have been shown to have reduced numbers of the C3b receptor (CR1) on red and white blood cells during active disease. The disease is partially manifested by deposition of immune complexes in multiple tissues (kidney, skin, joints, myocardium, etc). There is evidence that while in some patients the receptor deficiency may be partially genetic, receptors are depleted in active disease due to accelerated catabolism of CR1 in association with increased complement activation at the cell surface. Receptor depletion may decrease "buffering" function, permitting more immune complexes in the intravascular space and increased deposition in susceptible tissue. These unbound immune complexes may mediate tissue damage (e.g., glomerulonephritis), as well as enhance autoantibody production. (See also Chap. 31, on autoimmune disorders.)

Other Mechanisms of Host Defense and Disease

Bacteria are susceptible to direct destruction via activation of the alternative complement pathway, independent of host synthesis of specific antibody. However, some bacteria have developed resistance to this pathway through a capsular polysaccharide coat which conceals the lipopolysaccharide surface. When antibody binds to bacteria, the classical pathway is activated and can assist in killing of the organism. Neutralization of virus by antibody is enhanced by C1 and C4, assisted by C3b fixation to viral antigen-antibody complexes, through the classical or alternative pathway. Antiviral antibody may direct production, via the classical pathway, of MAC-induced "holes" in the viral surface proteins. (See Chap. 21, "Immunity to Microorganisms.")

Autoantibodies, produced after tissue damage, infection, or de novo due to poorly understood mechanisms, can bind to host tissue and activate the complement system. Deposition of immune complexes in small vessels and capillaries activates complement, a hallmark of vasculitis. There are many diseases in which immune complex deposition and complement activation contribute to tissue injury. (See Chap. 31, on autoimmune disorders.)

PRIMARY DEFICIENCIES OF THE COMPLEMENT SYSTEM

The importance of complement in immune defense is demonstrated by the susceptibility of individuals with a deficiency of complement components to a variety of infectious and other diseases. These deficiencies may be primary (inherited), or acquired.

Congenital deficiencies of all 11 of the classical complement proteins and several control proteins have been described (Tables 13-2 and 13-3). Patients with C1q, C1r, C1rC1s, C4, C2, and C3 deficiencies have a high incidence of SLE or other vasculitis syndromes. (This may be due to the fact that

TABLE 13-2 Genetic Deficiencies of Complement

Deficient Component	Clinical Findings	
	DISEASES (VASCULITIS AND AUTOIMMUNE)	INFECTIONS
C1q	SLE, discoid lupus	Bacterial, fungal meningitis
C1r	Renal disease, SLE, cutaneous vasculitis	Rare pneumonia, meningitis
C1rC1s	SLE	
C4	SLE, rare Sjögren's syndrome, Henoch-Schönlein purpura	Rare bacteremia, meningitis
C2	Arthalgia, SLE, discoid lupus, cutaneous vasculitis, rare dermatomyositis, Henoch-Schönlein purpura	Recurrent sepsis (especially pneumococcal), pneumonia, meningitis
C3	Nephritis, cutaneous vasculitis, SLE	Severe and recurrent bacterial
C5	SLE, Leiner's disease (C5 dysfunction)	Disseminated and recurrent gonococcal or meningococcal
C6	Rare SLE, rare Sjögren's, rare nephritis	Disseminated and recurrent gonococcal or meningococcal
C7	Rare SLE, rare scleroderma, rare ankylosing spondylitis, rare Raynaud's phenomenon	Disseminated and recurrent gonococcal or meningococcal
C8	Rare SLE	Disseminated and recurrent gonococcal or meningococcal
C9		Meningococcal meningitis

TABLE 13-3 Genetic Deficiencies of Control Proteins

Deficient Component	Clinical Findings
C1 inhibitor (C1INH)	Heredity angioedema, SLE
C3b inhibitor (CR1)	SLE, pyogenic infections
Factor I	Severe pyogenic infections
Factor H	Hemolytic uremic syndrome
Properdin	Meningococcal meningitis
CR3	Leukocytosis, recurrent pyogenic infections

certain of the early complement components, especially C3, increase the solubility of immune complexes. In vitro studies have shown that purified immune complexes will go into solution in normal serum, but not in serum which has been depleted of C3.) While these conditions are rare, study of patients' clinical problems has led to increased understanding of the importance of complement in the proper handling of immune complexes. Only occasionally have patients with C5, C6, C7, or C8 deficiency been found to have autoimmune diseases, but it is more common for these patients to suffer from recurrent infections. Individuals with deficiencies of the late complement components, C6, C7, C8, and C9, are at great risk for invasive disease due to meningococcus or extragenital gonococcal infection.

Neisseria meningitidis and *N. gonorrhoeae* are organisms that commonly cause severe and recurrent disease in individuals with congenital C6–C9 deficiencies. It is thought that complement-mediated bacteriolysis must be singularly important in the immune defense against these organisms. In two studies of patients with systemic meningococcal disease, 10 to 20 percent of patients had a genetic complement deficiency.

Deficiencies of control proteins include hereditary angioedema, discussed above, a manifestation of C1-inhibitor deficiency. Properdin deficiency has been shown to predispose individuals to meningococcal infections. This X-linked recessive trait has been reported only in males; there is often a fam-

ily history of male death from meningitis. Factor I deficiency has been reported to allow severe pyogenic infections, presumably due to compromised C3 function from prolonged C3 convertase activity. Partial deficiency of CR1, inherited as an autosomal recessive trait, may increase the risk of immune complex diseases such as SLE, as discussed in Clinical Aside 13-4.

SECONDARY DISORDERS OF THE COMPLEMENT SYSTEM

The secondary complement deficiencies are due to decreased synthesis, increased catabolism, or consumption of complement. Unlike the inherited complement deficiencies, secondary disorders of complement are common, displaying the importance of the complement system in disease pathogenesis (Table 13-4).

Complement Changes Associated with Activation and Consumption

Immune Complex Disease
In many autoimmune diseases circulating immune complexes play an important role in pathogenesis. Antigen-antibody complexes induce complement consumption primarily through the classical pathway, as C1 binds to antibody in the complex.

In SLE, immune complexes are deposited in multiple tissues, including the kidney, skin, joints, and myocardium. Insoluble complexes can activate both the classical and alternative complement pathways. The MAC complex C5–C9 has been seen in biopsy specimens of affected skin lesions at the dermal-epidermal junction, and in renal glomeruli. C3, C1q, and C4 may also be found. in kidney specimens by immunofluorescence assays. Complement depletion, presumably due to consumption, often parallels disease activity, and is more pronounced in patients with active renal disease. C3 and C4 levels are often used to monitor the activity

TABLE 13-4 Secondary Disorders of Complement

Disorders due primarily to activation and
  consumption
  Immune complex disease
  Serum sickness
  Infection
  Sickle cell disease
  Thermal injury
  Adult respiratory distress syndrome
  Dialysis, cardiopulmonary, and leukapheresis
    syndromes
  Nephritis, chronic hypocomplementemic nephritis
  Hypocomplementemic vasculitis syndrome
  Partial lipodystrophy
  Porphyria
  Acute pancreatitis
  Atheroembolic disease
  Reaction to radiographic contrast media
  C1-inhibitor deficiency with B-cell
    lymphoproliferative disorder or autoantibody to
    the inhibitor
Disorders due primarily to increased catabolism
  and/or loss
  Increased C1q catabolism associated with
    hypogammaglobulinemia
  Nephrotic syndrome
Disorders due primarily to decreased synthesis
  Neonatal period
  Malnutrition and anorexia nervosa
  Cirrhosis and hepatic failure
  Reye syndrome
Disorders secondary to deficiency of noncomplement
  serum or membrane protein
  Paroxysmal nocturnal hemoglobinuria
  Decreased alternative pathway function associated
    with hypogammaglobulinemia, β-thalassemia
    major, or splenectomy

of lupus glomerulonephritis. Reduced numbers of CR1 (the C3b receptor) are seen with active SLE, as discussed previously.

Immune complex formation and hypocomplementemia have also been seen with rheumatoid arthritis, serum sickness (see Clinical Aside 13-5), subacute bacterial endocarditis, infectious mononucleosis, hepatitis B, malaria, Felty's syndrome, leprosy, and dermatitis herpetiformis.

Complement effects in immune complex disease are not limited to tissue damage and injury. The complement system also participates in the normal processing of immune complexes. C3b opsonization and C3b receptors on erythrocytes and monocytes are

particularly important. Antigen-antibody complexes may be "opsonized" by C3b. C3b-bound complexes bind to C3b receptors (CR1) on the surface of cells such as erythrocytes, neutrophils, mononuclear cells, B lymphocytes, and glomerular podocytes.

Clinical Aside 13-5
Serum Sickness

Serum sickness is a prototype for immune complex disease. Patients receiving antithymocyte globulin (ATG), a preparation derived from horse serum, for treatment of aplastic anemia, develop antibodies to the foreign serum proteins. Classic manifestations of serum sickness include fever, arthralgias, adenopathy, proteinuria or frank glomerulonephritis, and a distinctive erythematous petechial eruption on the sides of the hands and feet. These findings are all due to deposition of immune complexes. Complement is activated as shown by a decrease in C3, C4, and CH_{50} (see "Measurement of the Complement System and Clinical Applications," below), and increased levels of activation products such as the anaphylatoxin C3a.

Infections

Infections may activate the complement system in several ways. Antimicrobial antibody may bind microbes, forming immune complexes which can activate early complement components. Bacteria and endotoxin directly activate the alternative pathway with consumption of C3. Alternative pathway activity and complement depletion have been seen with pneumococcal pneumonia, typhoid fever, dengue fever, cryptococcal sepsis, and several viral infections. Malarial paroxysms have been associated with decreases in C1, C4, and C2.

Sickle Cell Disease

Children and adults with sickle cell disease have an increased susceptibility to pyogenic infections, especially to pneumococci, *Haemophilus influenzae*, and *Salmonella* species. In addition to poor splenic function secondary to recurrent splenic infarction from sickling, there is compromised ability to opsonize pneumococci, and defective opsonization and bacteriolysis of salmonellae by the alternative complement pathway. Complement deficiency associated with sickle cell disease may be due to activation of complement in the circulation or tissues by free hemoglobin or red cell stroma.

Burns and Adult Respiratory Distress Syndrome (ARDS)

Thermal injury can induce massive complement activation. C3a and C5a are rapidly produced, stimulating neutrophil aggregation and sequestering in lung parenchyma. ARDS is a condition of respiratory failure due to increased permeability of the alveolar-capillary membrane with interstitial and alveolar edema. ARDS can develop as a complication of burns, shock, or severe trauma. Clinical and experimental studies have correlated complement activation with development of ARDS as well as with granulocyte "entrapment" in pulmonary parenchyma. It is likely that generation of vasoactive amines, histamine, and leukotrienes may mediate the increased pulmonary vasculature permeability. Burn-damaged tissue can directly activate the alternative pathway. Complement by-product C5a depresses neutrophil chemotaxis and degranulation, and together with complement deficiency contributes to predilection for infection in patients with significant burns.

Dialysis, Cardiopulmonary Bypass, and Leukapheresis Syndromes

Renal dialysis, leukapheresis, and cardiopulmonary bypass are occasionally complicated by hemolysis, leukopenia, and a "postperfusion syndrome" of fever, shock, and multisystem dysfunction. The exchange membranes can activate complement, generating factors C3a and C5a, the anaphylatoxins.

The membrane attack complex C5b–C9 is found on erythrocytes and granulocytes during cardiopulmonary bypass. Hemolysis occurs in all patients, and the MAC has been demonstrated on "ghost" RBCs. The MAC "pore former" is a cylinder with a lipophilic outer layer that allows it to intercalate into the lipid of the cell membrane. The hydro-

philic inner layer of the MAC permits free passage of water and small ions through the channel, and the cell swells and lyses. Interestingly, studies have shown that the MAC is seen on membranes of lysed red blood cells, but not on intact cells.

Renal Disease, Partial Lipodystrophy, and Hypocomplementemic Vasculitis

Many types of nephritis are associated with diminished levels of complement in the serum and deposition of complement in renal tissue as demonstrated by immunofluorescence. In acute poststreptococcal nephritis, complement levels return to normal over time. In some types of chronic membranoproliferative glomerulonephritis, low complement levels persist. It has been found that some patients with chronic hypocomplementemic nephritis have factors in their serum (C3b nephritic factor and C4b nephritic factor) that cause rapid consumption of C3. C3 nephritic factor (C3NeF) has also been found in patients with partial lipodystrophy, with or without nephritis. These factors are IgG autoantibodies to either the classical or alternative pathway C3 convertase, which suppress the decay-accelerating activity of C4bp and factor H. The stabilized C3 convertase permits unchecked consumption of C3, resulting in low serum C3 levels. There is also a syndrome of recurrent urticaria, angioedema, and vasculitis in children and adults that is associated with depression of C1 through C5 (especially C1q). The pathogenesis of this *hypocomplementemic vasculitis syndrome* is unknown, although deposition of immunoglobulin and complement is seen in vessel walls, and one-half of patients have mild glomerulonephritis.

Porphyria

Patients with porphyria cutanea tarda (PCT) or erythropoietic protoporphyria have enzymatic defects of heme synthesis, creating buildup of porphyrins in the body. Patients are photosensitive, and develop blisters on hands, forearms, and face when exposed to certain wavelengths of light. When these patients are experimentally exposed to these wavelengths, complement is activated, levels of serum C3 and C5 are decreased, and chemotaxis-inducing C5 byproducts are produced. When blood is taken from patients with PCT, the serum, independent of the patient, consumes complement and generates chemotactic factors when irradiated with light. Porphyrins added to normal serum will similarly cause complement consumption when the serum is exposed to the correct wavelengths of light. Blistering may be due to porphyrins in skin absorbing light energy, forming oxygen radicals, and allowing tissue oxidation and complement activation.

Complement Changes Associated with Increased Catabolism

Factor B deficiency has been associated with nephrotic syndrome in children, as well as occasional slight decreases in C3, C4, and properdin. Factor B deficiency has been correlated with defective bacterial opsonization, and may contribute to the increased risk of serious infection in these children. There is also an inconsistent decrease in serum C1q in patients with hypogammaglobulinemia. IgG normally protects C1q from catabolism, and this protection is absent in hypogammaglobulinemia. Treatment of these patients with IgG corrects the complement deficiency.

Complement Changes Secondary to Decreased Synthesis

Newborns are complement deficient, with hemolytic complement values approximately 75 percent of normal adults (see also Chap. 28). All individual components of both the classical and alternative pathway are mildly or moderately decreased. Term infants have compromised opsonization as well. It is likely that suboptimal complement function contributes to neonates' increased susceptibility to infection. Patients with malnutrition and patients with chronic cirrhosis of the liver may have significant depletion of complement due both to decreased synthesis and to consumption.

Complement Changes Secondary to Deficiency of Noncomplement Serum or Membrane Proteins

Paroxysmal Nocturnal Hemoglobinuria

Paroxysmal nocturnal hemoglobinuria (PNH) is a rare disorder in which RBCs are abnormally sensitive to complement-induced lysis. Abnormal cells have an inherited deficiency of the membrane control protein called *decay accelerating factor (DAF)*, as well as *homologous restriction protein (HRF)*, also known as C8-binding protein. DAF inhibits assembly of C3-cleaving enzymes, blocking amplification of both the classical and alternative pathways. PNH cells, without DAF present, are vulnerable to increased C3b deposited on the cell surface. The absence of HRF allows the generation of MAC (C5b–C9) and cell lysis. The Ham test involves acidification of serum, allowing spontaneous activation of the alternative pathway and lysis of PNH cells. Normal erythrocytes are resistant to lysis by the MAC or human complement; thus a positive Ham test is diagnostic of PNH.

MEASUREMENT OF THE COMPLEMENT SYSTEM AND CLINICAL APPLICATIONS

Serum levels of complement components reflect a balance between synthesis and catabolism. The most useful test for screening for most of the diseases of the complement system is the assay for total hemolytic complement, known as the CH_{50}. Antibody-coated sheep erythrocytes are mixed with various dilutions of patient serum. If the serum contains functional classical pathway components, lysis occurs. The dilution of serum that lyses 50 percent of the cells is the CH_{50} (usually recorded as the reciprocal of the dilution). Inherited deficiencies of factors C1 to C8 cause CH_{50} values of 0; the CH_{50} in C9 deficiency will be approximately half of normal. The CH_{50} will not reflect deficiencies in the alternative pathway components B, D, or properdin. Testing for individual complement components may be done through a variation of the hemolytic assay, with all components present in excess other than the one being assessed. If the test serum has an adequate concentration of the component in question, lysis occurs. There are also specific antisera available which may be used in immunochemical assays, such as radial immunodiffusion, to measure the total levels of complement component present. Alternative pathway activity can be measured with a hemolytic assay using unsensitized rabbit erythrocytes, which directly activate the pathway and serve as its target.

The presence or absence of complement in tissue specimens as determined by immunofluorescence is commonly used to aid in diagnosis, especially in organ-specific autoimmune diseases and immune complex–mediated diseases. For example, the intraepidermal blistering skin disease pemphigus vulgaris is characterized by deposition of C4, C3, and C5b–C9 (MAC) as well as IgG on direct immunofluorescent studies of lesional skin.

Complement components are also used as reagents in several widely used tests. Complement-fixation tests are commonly used to detect specific antibodies and antigen in serum or other body fluids. Tests for measuring circulating immune complexes use specific qualities of complement binding and activation to detect the presence of antigen-antibody complexes (For example, the C1q-binding assay measures radiolabeled C1q binding to complexes in the serum sample, and the Raji cell assay measures binding complexes to the C3 receptor on the B-cell tumor-line Raji cell.)

SELF-TEST QUESTIONS

1. How are the classical and alternative pathways of the complement system activated, and by what agents?
2. Where do the classical and alternative pathways converge and what proteins comprise the terminal portion of the complement sequence?
3. How does C3b allow "amplification" of the alternative complement response?
4. What are the complement control proteins and how do they mediate the system?
5. How do complement activation by-products mediate inflammation? What is the membrane attack complex?
6. How does complement mediate the pathogenesis of immune complex disease?

ADDITIONAL READINGS

Berger M, Frank MM. The complement system. In: Steihm ER, ed. *Immunologic Disorders in Infants and Children.* 3rd ed. Philadelphia: WB Saunders; 1989.

Eichenfield LF, Johnston RB, Jr. Secondary disorders of the complement system *Am J Dis Child.* 1989;143:595.

Frank MM. Complement in the pathophysiology of human disease. *N Engl J Med.* 1987;316:1525.

Johnston RB, Jr. Disorders of the complement system. In: Steihm ER, ed. *Immunologic Disorders in Infants and Children.* 3rd ed. Philadelphia: WB Saunders; 1989.

Muller-Eberhard HJ. Molecular organization and function of the complement system. *Annu Rev Biochem.* 1988;57:321.

14

The Contact Activation System:

Proteases Mediating Inflammation, Tissue Damage, and Healing

Key to the symbols used in the art for Chapter 14

Activating Surface

Neutrophil

Zymogen

⟶ Translocation

⟶ Activation

▽ Active Enzyme

➡ Conversion

▭ Cofactor

▶▶▶ Cascade

List of Abbreviations Used in the Art for Chapter 14

BK	Bradykinin	HMWKa	High molecular weight kininogen–activated
C1	Complement component 1	HMWKi	High molecular weight kininogen–inactivated
C$\bar{\text{I}}$	Complement component 1—activated	Kal	Kallikrein
C$\bar{\text{I}}$-INH	C$\bar{\text{I}}$-inhibitor	Kal-C$\bar{\text{I}}$-INH	Kallikrein–C$\bar{\text{I}}$ inhibitor complex
C2	Complement component 2	PK	Prekallikrein
C2b	Complement component 2—fragment	Plgn	Plasminogen
		Pln	Plasmin
C3a	Complement component 3—fragment	ProUk	Prourokinase
		TF	Tissue Factor
C3b	Complement component 3—fragment	Thr	Thrombin
		Uk	Urokinase
C4	Complement component 4	VII	Factor VII
		VIIa	Factor VI–activated
C5a	Complement component 5—fragment	IX	Factor IX
		IXa	Factor IX–activated
C5b	Complement component 5—fragment	Xa	Factor X–activated
		XI	Factor XI
DIC	Disseminated intravascular coagulation	XIa	Factor XI–activated
		XII	Factor XII
		XIIa	Factor XII–activated
FDPs	Fibrinogen degradation products	XIIa-C$\bar{\text{I}}$-INH	Factor XIIa–C$\bar{\text{I}}$ inhibitor complex
HMWK	High molecular weight kininogen	XIIf	Factor XII fragments
		XIII	Factor XIII
		XIIIa	Factor XIII–activated

INTRODUCTION

The inflammatory response is the primary process by which the body defends itself against infectious agents and toxic substances and the principal mechanism by which the body repairs tissue damage resulting from acute or chronic diseases. Both cells and humoral agents are involved in the complex process of inflammation, which is initiated and propagated by components of the coagulation, kinin, fibrinolytic, and complement systems (Fig. 14-1). These complex networks are intricately interconnected and may be activated by exposure to a foreign surface such as an injured blood vessel or artificial organ. In this chapter each of the first three systems will be outlined, its components defined, and its role in inflammation examined, and some of the disease states in which there are significant alterations of the

systems will be discussed. The complement system is dealt with in Chap. 13.

The fundamental histologic characteristic of acute inflammation is the infiltration of neutrophils into tissues. In response to various agonists, neutrophils release proteolytic enzymes, primarily neutrophil elastase, cathepsin G, and myeloperoxidase (which, together with oxygen free radicals, is involved in forming the toxic oxygen compound hypochlorous acid). Stimulated neutrophils also synthesize arachidonic acid metabolites (including leukotrienes) and platelet activating factor (PAF), which further enhance the inflammatory response (congenital absence of the inhibitor is dealt with in Chap. 16.)

Human neutrophil elastase degrades elastin, and both elastase and cathepsin G proteolytically modify collagen, rendering it susceptible to digestion by collagenase. In addition to directly damaging tissue, human

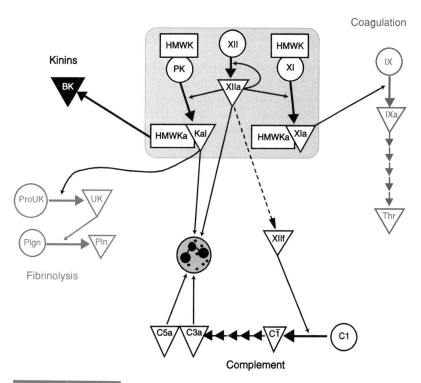

Figure 14-1 Overview of plasma mediators of inflammation.

neutrophil elastase inactivates IgG, IgM, and the third component of complement, thereby reducing opsonin activity, impairing phagocytosis of microorganisms, and possibly leading to persistence of infection.

α_1-Protease inhibitor, the major inhibitor of both elastase and cathepsin G, is necessary to protect against degradation of connective tissue and plasma proteins by these enzymes. Inactivation of this inhibitor by either proteolytic (plasmin) or oxidative mechanisms (promoted by neutrophil myeloperoxidase) enhances tissue injury.

THE CONTACT SYSTEM

The contact pathway of intrinsic coagulation consists of four major proteins: factor XII (Hageman factor), prekallikrein (Fletcher factor), factor XI (plasma thromboplastin antecedent), and high molecular weight kininogen (Williams-Fitzgerald-Flaujeac factor). The system's name refers to the fact that activation of these proteins occurs upon exposure to (*contact* with) artificial negatively charged surfaces (glass, kaolin, talc, diatomaceous earth, celite, supercel, barium carbonate, cellulose sulfate, silicon dioxide, dextran sulfate, carrageenan, ellagic acid) and naturally occurring substances (including sodium urate crystals, calcium pyrophosphate crystals, cholesterol sulfate, and L-homocysteine). Additionally, circulating immune complexes and bacterial lipopolysaccharides have been associated with activation of these proteins.

Human plasma factor XII (Hageman factor) deficiency was first identified by Ratnoff in 1955 in a patient who had a markedly prolonged partial thromboplastin time (PTT). This laboratory test is a commonly used method of screening for abnormalities in the intrinsic coagulation pathway. Factor XII deficiency is an autosomal-recessive trait with no apparent clinical bleeding disorder. The single-polypeptide chain of factor XII (80 kd), a β-globulin, occurs in plasma at a concentration of 30 μg/mL. Factor XII, as the initiator of the contact pathway of intrinsic coagulation, undergoes conformational changes upon binding to a negatively charged surface. Conversion of the zymogen to an active enzyme in this manner is referred to as solid-phase activation. Additionally, autoactivation of factor XII provides a small quantity of activated factor XII, which then converts prekallikrein to kallikrein. This kallikrein then further activates factor XII in the presence of high molecular weight kininogen. In the absence of a surface, activation of factor XII by kallikrein may also occur in the fluid phase, although the rate is much slower. Factor XII may also be activated by factor XI or plasmin, but these activators are only one-tenth as potent as kallikrein.

There are two major forms of activated factor XII: factor XIIa, a molecule (80 kd) consisting of two disulfide-linked polypeptide chains (52 kd and 28 kd), and factor XII fragments (28 kd), both of which are derived from the native molecule (Fig. 14-2). Factor XIIa, which initiates the intrinsic coagulation cascade, results from the single cleavage of an Arg-Val peptide bond in zymogen factor XII. This cleavage results in expression of coagulant activity by exposure of the active site, which hydrolyzes Arg substrates. Factor XII fragments, known to activate prekallikrein (see below), result from further proteolysis of the factor XIIa molecule and contain mainly the catalytic light chain and a tiny fragment of the heavy chain. The surface binding property of factor XIIa resides in its heavy chain (52 kd), whose amino acid sequence contains putative collagen-binding domains, growth-factor regions, and a single kringlelike structure (a highly folded peptide loop with multiple disulfide loops). Substrates of activated factor XII include prekallikrein, factor XI, the first component of complement, high molecular weight kininogen, and factor VII. Factor XII fragments are responsible for the nonimmunologic activation of the classical complement pathway (Fig. 14-3). C1 inhibitor accounts for 90 percent of the inhibition of both factor XIIa and factor XII fragments, while antithrombin III is responsible for inhibition of the remainder of the activity. In conditions where C1 inhibitor is either absent or decreased, e.g., hereditary angioedema, antithrombin III

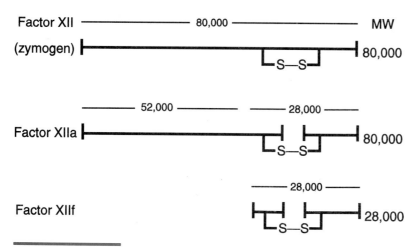

Figure 14-2 Structure of factors XII, XIIa, and XIIf.

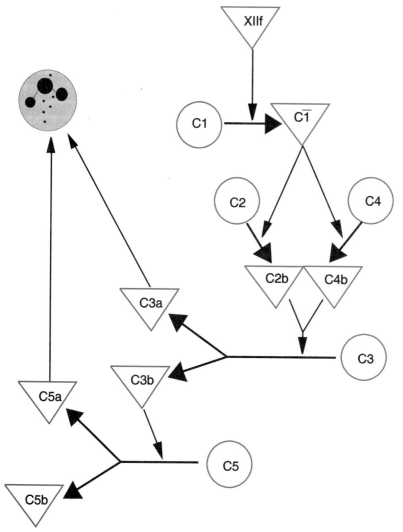

Figure 14-3 Nonimmunologic activation of the classical complement pathway.

becomes the major inhibitor of both factor XIIa and factor XII fragments, but it is much less potent.

Factor XII is routinely assayed by a modified partial thromboplastin time, utilizing factor XII–deficient plasma. Substrates containing the peptide sequence Pro-Phe-Arg or Ile-Glu-Gly-Arg may be used to measure the functional activity of factor XIIa or factor XII fragments. Radioimmunoassays and enzyme-linked immunosorbent assays have been developed that measure generation of factor XIIa–C1 inhibitor complexes. Both polyclonal and monoclonal antibodies against factor XII have been raised in a variety of animals, and these may be used to determine antigenic levels directly.

Human plasma prekallikrein (Fletcher factor) deficiency was first identified by Hathaway in 1965 in a patient who had a markedly increased partial thromboplastin time which corrected after prolonged incubation with a surface (i.e., the rate of contact activation seemed to be impaired). Prekallikrein deficiency, like factor XII deficiency, is an autosomal recessive trait with no apparent clinical bleeding disorder. Prekallikrein is a γ-globulin with two components (88 kd and 85 kd), occurring in plasma at a concentration of 35 to 50 μg/mL. Approximately 75 percent of the zymogen prekallikrein circulates in plasma in a complex with high molecular weight kininogen, while 25 percent circulates in a free form. Kallikrein, the active enzyme, is formed as a consequence of the cleavage of prekallikrein by either factor XIIa or factor XII fragments. This cleavage results in the formation of one heavy chain (55 kd) with four large amino acid sequence repeats, and one light chain (36 kd or 33 kd) linked by disulfide bridges (Fig. 4). Kallikrein also forms a complex with high molecular weight kininogen, which can protect it from its inhibitors. Substrates of kallikrein include factor XII, high molecular weight kininogen, low molecular weight kininogen, plasminogen, and prorenin.

C1 inhibitor is the major inhibitor of kallikrein, with which it combines to form an inactive complex. α2-Macroglobulin, the other major inhibitor, also combines with kallikrein to form a complex, suppressing 75 percent of its functional activity against small substrates. Antithrombin III is a minor inhibitor of kallikrein. Heparin is a catalytic cofactor that markedly accelerates the action of antithrombin III to inactivate factor Xa and thrombin. Heparin contains a specific sulfated carbohydrate sequence that facilitates its binding to antithrombin III, resulting in a conformational change in the structure of the inhibitor to form a more efficient enzyme inactivator. However, heparin does not appreciably accelerate the inhibition of kallikrein by antithrombin III.

Prekallikrein can be assayed by a modified partial thromboplastin time, utilizing prekallikrein-deficient plasma, but recently developed chromogenic assays using Pro-Phe-Arg substrates to measure the functional activity associated with kallikrein are more accurate. Radioimmunoassays and

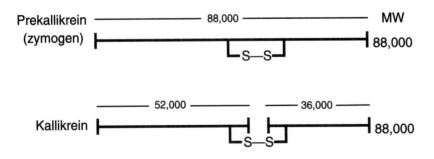

Figure 14-4   Structure of prekallikrein and kallikrein.

enzyme-linked immunosorbent assays have been developed that measure the generation of kallikrein–CĪ inhibitor complexes and kallikrein–α_2-macroglobulin complexes. Both polyclonal and monoclonal antibodies against prekallikrein have been raised in a variety of animals, and these may be used to determine antigenic levels directly.

Human plasma factor XI (plasma thromboplastin antecedent) deficiency, first described in 1953 as a new hemophiliac syndrome, is distinct from other intrinsic coagulation deficiencies in that it results in bleeding in about 50 percent of patients. Spontaneous bleeding, however, is uncommon, and the decrease or absence of factor XI may present solely as an abnormal partial thromboplastin time during preoperative screening. Factor XI deficiency is an autosomal-dominant trait found mostly in Ashkenazi Jews. Factor XI (160 kd), a γ-globulin, is composed of two identical polypeptide chains (80 kd) linked by disulfide bridges, occurring in plasma at a concentration of only 5 μg/mL. The protein exhibits 60 percent homology with prekallikrein, suggesting a common ancestral gene. Factor XI is acti-

vated to factor XIa upon cleavage by factor XIIa. This results in two heavy chains (50 kd) and two light chains (30 kd) (Fig. 14-5). The binding region of factor XI is found on the heavy chains, while the active site is located on the light chains. Substrates of factor XIa include high molecular weight kininogen, plasminogen, and factor IX. Virtually all of factor XI forms a complex with high molecular weight kininogen, protecting it from its inhibitors. α_1-Protease inhibitor is the major inhibitor of factor XI. Antithrombin III has also been shown to inhibit the active form of factor XI in purified systems, but it is not a significant inhibitor in plasma even in the presence of pharmacologic levels of heparin.

Factor XI is routinely assayed by a modified partial thromboplastin time, utilizing factor XI–deficient plasma. Substrates containing the peptide sequence pyro-Glu-Pro-Arg may be used to measure the functional activity of factor XIa in a more accurate manner. Both polyclonal and monoclonal antibodies have been raised in a variety of animals against factor XI, and these may be used to determine antigenic levels directly by radioimmunoassay.

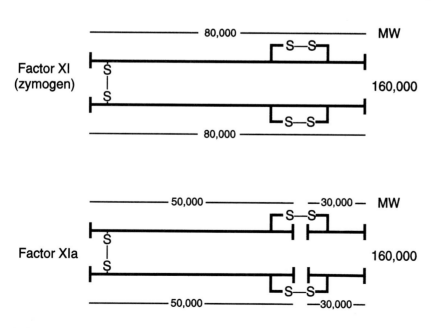

Figure 14-5 Structure of factors XI and XIIa.

Human plasma high molecular weight kininogen (Williams-Fitzgerald-Flaujeac factor) deficiency was identified in this laboratory in 1975 in a patient who had a markedly prolonged partial thromboplastin time and no kinin formation. In the same year, two other laboratories reported similar patients deficient in high molecular weight kininogen. High molecular weight kininogen is required for contact activation, and is therefore referred to as the *contact-activation cofactor*. High molecular weight kininogen deficiency is also an autosomal-recessive trait with no associated clinical bleeding disorder. Two different kininogens are present in human plasma: a high molecular weight form (molecular mass of 120 kd) that is rapidly cleaved by human plasma kallikrein (Fig. 14-6), and a low molecular weight form (molecular mass of 67 kd) that is more readily proteolyzed by the tissue kallikreins. The two proteins are produced by differential splicing of mRNA transcribed from a single copy gene, and they both contain the identical heavy-chain region (D1–D3) and bradykinin (D4). High molecular weight kininogen, a γ-globulin, exists in plasma at a concentration of 80 μg/mL and contains a unique light chain (56 kd) (D5–D6) which accounts for its coagulant activity. Low molecular weight kininogen occurs in plasma at a concentration of 160 μg/mL and contains

a different light chain (5 kd) of unknown function. High molecular weight kininogen is synthesized in the liver, and is present in human platelets, neutrophils, and endothelial cells, which also express it on their surfaces after activation.

High molecular weight kininogen is routinely assayed by a modified partial thromboplastin time, utilizing high molecular weight kininogen–deficient plasma as its substrate. Radioimmunoassays and enzyme-linked immunosorbent assays have been developed that measure high molecular weight kininogen. Both polyclonal and monoclonal antibodies against high molecular weight kininogen have been raised in a variety of animals, and these may be used to determine antigenic levels directly.

High molecular weight kininogen directly enhances the surface-mediated formation and function of factor XII, prekallikrein, and factor XI, so that activation proceeds optimally. Domain D5 contains positive charges (histidine and lysine) that facilitate interaction with anionic surfaces. Domain D6 has specific amino acid sequences that bind either prekallikrein or factor XI, thus bringing these zymogens to the surface for cleavage by factor XIIa. High molecular weight kininogen is a procofactor which does not bind appreciably to activating surfaces in plasma until it has been cleaved by human plasma kalli-

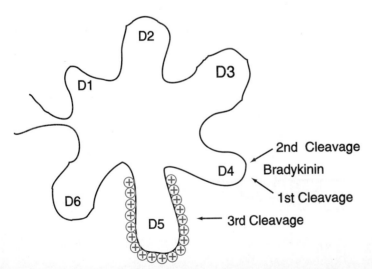

Figure 14-6 Structure of high molecular weight kininogen.

krein. The cofactor is destroyed when factor XI or plasmin proteolyzes the light chain of high molecular weight kininogen. Human plasma kallikrein cleaves high molecular weight kininogen in a three-step sequential pattern. The first cleavage produces a "nicked" kininogen composed of two disulfide-linked chains (64 kd and 56 kd). The second cleavage yields bradykinin (which mediates vasodilatation, pain, and increased capillary permeability), an intermediate kinin-free protein of the same molecular weight as "nicked" kininogen. The third cleavage results in a stable kinin-free protein composed of two disulfide-linked chains (64 kd and 45 kd) and an additional peptide (10 kd) (Fig. 14-6). Both high and low molecular weight kininogen, which contain the same amino acid sequence in their heavy chain (D1–D3), are immunochemically and structurally identi-

cal to the two plasma α-cysteine protease inhibitors. α-Cysteine protease inhibitor is the major plasma protease inhibitor of a group of tissue-derived neutral calcium-activated proteases (calpains) which play a role in intracellular proteolysis of cytoskeletal proteins and processing of proteins on the external plasma membrane of cells.

INTERACTIONS BETWEEN THE CONTACT SYSTEM AND NEUTROPHILS

Since the neutrophil plays a significant role in inflammation, the interaction of the contact pathway proteins and neutrophils must be considered (Fig. 14-7). Human plasma

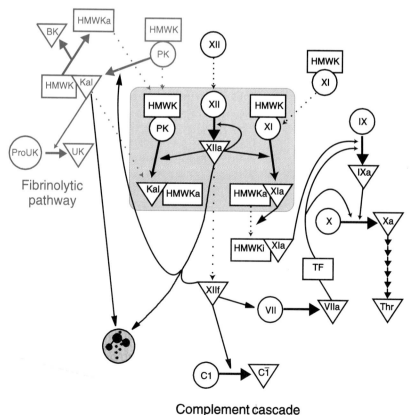

Complement cascade

Figure 14-7   Overview of intrinsic coagulation.

factor XIIa stimulates neutrophil aggregation and degranulation. Human plasma kallikrein (the active species), but not prekallikrein (the zymogen), is chemotactic for neutrophils. Exposure of neutrophils to chemotactic levels of human plasma kallikrein results in a significant increase in aerobic glycolysis and activity of the hexose-monophosphate shunt. Neutrophils, in the presence of divalent cations (calcium and magnesium), aggregate in response to human plasma kallikrein. This interaction is associated with a stimulation of the respiratory burst in neutrophils, as indicated by an increase in oxygen uptake. Human plasma kallikrein also induces neutrophils to release human neutrophil elastase from their azurophilic granules. In the test tube, this reaction requires that the neutrophils first be primed with cytochalasin B, a substance which causes the membranes of the azurophilic granules to fuse with the cellular membrane, thus facilitating release of elastase granules. In an in vitro plasma system, human neutrophils release elastase during blood coagulation in the absence of cytochalasin B, but neutrophils resuspended in either prekallikrein- or factor XII–deficient plasma release less than one-third of the amount released in normal human plasma. This suggests that both kallikrein and factor XIIa stimulate the release of elastase from neutrophils. In addition, in an in vitro nonplasma system, kallikrein causes the release of neutrophil elastase in a concentration-dependent fashion that requires the presence of both the active site of kallikrein (on its light chain) and an intact heavy chain. Furthermore, the formation of either kallikrein or activated factor XII in circulating blood in an in vitro model of cardiopulmonary bypass is associated with a marked rise in release of human neutrophil elastase. High molecular weight kininogen binds to neutrophils in a specific, reversible, and saturable manner, and is required for kallikrein to optimally stimulate neutrophils. Factor XIIa down-regulates one of the immunoglobulin receptors on monocytes.

THE KININ SYSTEM

Bradykinin was first described by Rocha E. Silva in 1949 when he incubated blood in the presence of trypsin or snake venoms and found that a potent stimulator of smooth muscle was generated. *Bradykinin* is slow in its ability to stimulate smooth muscle, and the name is derived from the Greek *bradys* ("slow") and *kinein* ("to move"). Bradykinin is generated from high molecular weight kininogen upon cleavage by kallikrein. It is a nonapeptide with an amino acid sequence of Arg-Pro-Pro-Gly-Phe-Ser-Pro-Phe-Arg. Immunoassays have been developed that measure bradykinin directly. Specific receptors for bradykinin exist on both smooth muscle and endothelial cells. Bradykinin stimulates the latter to synthesize prostacyclin (PGI_2) and release tissue plasminogen activator. Bradykinin is a potent vasoactive peptide which has a number of effects, many of which contribute to the inflammatory reaction. These include smooth muscle contraction, increased vascular permeability, venular dilatation, electrolyte secretion, ion transport, cell proliferation, and activation of phospholipase A_2. The end results of the liberation of bradykinin by the kallikrein-kinin system include constriction of uterine and gastrointestinal smooth muscle, constriction of coronary and pulmonary vasculature, mucosal inflammation, bronchoconstriction, edema, hypotension, flushing, pain, and rhinitis.

CLINICAL DISORDERS ASSOCIATED WITH THE CONTACT AND KININ SYSTEMS

Neither the intrinsic coagulation cascade (the contact pathway) nor bradykinin, a by-product of contact activation, significantly contribute to physiologic hemostasis. Patients deficient in either factor XII, prekallikrein, or high molecular weight kininogen display no overt bleeding diathesis, and spontaneous bleeding is rare in patients deficient in factor XI. However, activation of the contact system and generation of bradykinin occur in a variety of pathophysiologic conditions in which the inflammatory response has been implicated.

Because of its ability to lower blood pressure in normal humans and animals, bradykinin has been implicated in the pathogenesis of septic shock. The early peripheral vascular changes accompanying gram-negative bacteremia and endotoxic shock are similar to those of bradykinin infusion, including arteriolar dilatation and venular constriction. Infusion of *Escherichia coli* endotoxin in normal volunteers, as well as naturally occurring sepsis, leads to a decrease in plasma levels of factor XII, prekallikrein, and high molecular weight kininogen. Levels of kallikrein–α_2-macroglobulin complexes and cleaved $\overline{C1}$ inhibitor are also increased. Activation of the kallikrein-kinin system in septic shock is probably mediated by factor XIIa or factor XII fragments. The mechanism of in vitro activation of factor XII by endotoxin is not clear but might be due to tumor necrosis factor (TNF). The sequence of events of kinin production in human septic shock includes several stages. First, factor XII is activated by the lipid A component of endotoxin, with a resultant decrease in its plasma level and formation of factor XIIa and factor XII fragments. These enzymes then activate prekallikrein with a resultant decrease in its plasma level. Kallikrein then cleaves kininogen to release kinins into the circulation, coincident with depletion of plasma kininogen. The measurement of plasma kininogen in patients with septic shock may have prognostic value. In young victims of traumatic injuries complicated by sepsis, a good correlation was found between kininogen level and survival. A drop in the kininogen level to near zero usually indicated a lethal outcome of the shock in hospitalized patients, while kininogen levels rose toward

normal in those shock patients who survived.

In patients with disseminated intravascular coagulation associated with septicemia due to bacteria, viruses, fungi, or parasites, decreased plasma levels of factor XII, prekallikrein, and high molecular weight kininogen are seen, indicating contact-system activation. These changes are probably mediated by endotoxin and other products of infecting organisms acting through monokines, i.e., TNF, which perturb endothelial cells and/or expose components of the basement membrane, potentially activating factor XII. These changes are not seen in patients with disseminated intravascular coagulation associated with leukemia, carcinoma, or abortion, where endothelial alterations are not a primary mechanism.

There is abundant evidence implicating kinins in the manifestations of the carcinoid syndrome, a disorder consisting of episodic cutaneous flushing, abdominal cramps, diarrhea, and right-sided valvular heart disease. The syndrome is usually caused by metastatic intestinal carcinoid tumors that secrete excessive amounts of vasoactive substances. In normal persons, infusion of bradykinin mimics carcinoid flushes. Additionally, approximately half of patients with the carcinoid syndrome have a significant increase in kinin concentration in hepatic venous blood during catecholamine-induced flushes. An anionic tissue kallikrein which releases bradykinin from human kininogen has been identified in carcinoid tumor tissue.

Bradykinin is generated in patients with allergic rhinitis following challenge with ragweed pollen, leading to vasodilatation, edema, increased mucus secretion and cellular recruitment, and increased capillary and mucosal permeability. Plasma levels of high molecular weight kininogen are decreased during acute allergic reactions as a result of anaphylaxis after a wasp sting or after administration of radiologic contrast media.

The clinical features of the postgastrectomy (dumping) syndrome include nausea, vomiting, epigastric fullness, diarrhea, and vasomotor phenomena such as flushing, diaphoresis, palpitations, tachycardia, and hypotension. Postulated mechanisms include proximal small bowel distension from a food bolus, rapid fluid influx into the small bowel in response to the presence of hyperosmolar small bowel contents, and the release of vasoactive substances such as bradykinin. Elevated bradykinin and decreased plasma prekallikrein concentrations are found in patients with dumping syndrome after administration of hypertonic glucose by mouth, presumably secondary to the presence of hyperosmolar small bowel contents.

A deficiency of $C\bar{1}$ inhibitor, the single most important plasma protease inhibitor of contact system proteases, results in the severe clinical disease known as *hereditary angioedema*. This is an autosomal-dominant disorder, which can first appear in infancy up through the fourth decade. Prominent symptoms include recurrent episodes of edema of the gastrointestinal tract, manifested by abdominal pain or vomiting, and edema of the skin and subcutaneous tissues. In one-third of the cases, the disorder terminates in fatal edema of the larynx and upper respiratory tract. During acute episodes, decreased functional activity and antigenic levels of prekallikrein are noted, as well as a decrease in high molecular weight kininogen. Blisters resulting from these acute episodes contain high levels of kallikrein, which lead to subsequent bradykinin generation. Prophylactic therapy for hereditary angioedema may include anabolic steroids (which increase the functional level of $C\bar{1}$ inhibitor protein), ε-aminocaproic acid (an inhibitor of $C\bar{1}$, plasmin, and plasminogen), or fresh frozen plasma infusion prior to surgical procedures.

Plasma levels of factor XII, factor XI, and prekallikrein are significantly decreased in patients with the nephrotic syndrome, not due to urinary losses of the proteins as first thought, but as a result of activation of the contact system. Patients with polycythemia vera have chronically decreased levels of factor XII and prekallikrein.

Prekallikrein and $C\bar{1}$ inhibitor are depleted, and kallikrein–$C\bar{1}$ inhibitor complexes are detectable in patients with typhoid fever. Factor XII and prekallikrein are depleted in patients with renal allograft rejection. Patients with Rocky Mountain spotted fever have decreased prekallikrein levels with increased kallikrein–$C\bar{1}$ inhibitor complexes. In a model of simulated extracorporeal circulation, levels of kallikrein–$C\bar{1}$ inhibitor complexes are markedly increased. Factor XII, prekallikrein, and high molecular weight kininogen are depleted in patients with cirrhosis. Levels of factor XII and prekallikrein are decreased in patients with hyperlipidemia.

The presence of kallikrein in the synovial fluid of patients with rheumatoid arthritis suggests a role for the contact system in this disease. Chondroitin sulfate, articular cartilage components, and microcrystals found in joint fluids all may serve as negatively charged surfaces to activate the contact system. Uric acid in gout, calcium pyrophosphate crystals in pseudogout, as well as L-homocysteine crystals in homocystinuria may act as pathologic surfaces for activation of the contact pathway of intrinsic coagulation.

The adult respiratory distress syndrome is a clinical complex of noncardiogenic pulmonary edema with refractory hypoxemia and decreased pulmonary compliance which may occur following a variety of insults, and results from an abnormally permeable alveolar-capillary membrane. Activation of proteins of the contact system may play a significant role in the pathogenesis of this disorder by stimulating neutrophils to synthesize and release substances which can cause endothelial and epithelial injury and enhance the inflammatory response. Patients with the adult respiratory distress syndrome have significantly reduced plasma levels of factor XII, prekallikrein, and high molecular weight kininogen activity, increased levels of $C\bar{1}$-inhibitor antigen, and decreased levels of $C\bar{1}$-inhibitor activity.

THE FIBRINOLYTIC SYSTEM

The fibrinolytic system regulates the deposition of fibrin in vessels and tissues. Following the formation of a hemostatic plug or thrombus, a localized response is initiated to dissolve the fibrin deposit. This reaction sequence involves the activation of the precursor plasminogen by plasminogen activators, i.e., urokinase and tissue plasminogen activator, generating plasmin, whose basic physiologic function in the circulation is to digest fibrin clots and thrombi (Fig. 14-8).

Earlier in the chapter, when we described the actions of the key members of the contact pathway of intrinsic coagulation, plasminogen was listed among the substrates of factor XIIa, factor XII fragments, kallikrein, and factor XIa. Plasminogen is activated to form plasmin, and thus the fibrinolytic system might be initiated via the contact pathway of intrinsic coagulation (Fig. 14-8). We will therefore discuss the contact pathway–related aspects of fibrinolysis in the remaining paragraphs.

The finding that fibrinolytic activity was much greater if plasma was exposed to a negatively charged surface was observed by Niewiarowski et al. in 1959. However, this effect could not be demonstrated if the plasma was deficient in any of the contact factors of intrinsic coagulation. One of the ways in which plasminogen is converted to plasmin to initiate fibrinolysis is by the action of the plasminogen activator urokinase. Subsequent studies have shown that prourokinase is converted to urokinase by kallikrein, explaining the findings of Niewiarowski et al. and elucidating the initiating role of the contact pathway of intrinsic coagulation in fibrinolysis. Thus, the same mechanisms which initiate coagulation also start fibrinolysis.

The key component of the fibrinolytic pathway is the single-chain polypeptide, plasminogen (80 kd), occurring in plasma at a concentration of 210 μg/mL. Plasminogen is activated to plasmin following cleavage by urokinase, tissue plasminogen activator, or

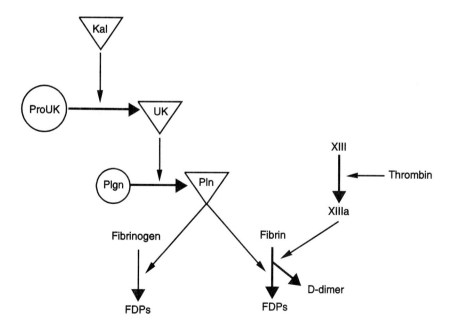

Figure 14-8 Overview of fibrinolysis.

streptokinase. This results in the formation of a serine protease with trypsinlike activity. Substrates of plasmin include fibrin, fibrinogen, factor XIIa, factor V, factor VIII, prothrombin, C$\bar{1}$ inhibitor, the first, third and fifth components of complement (C1, C3, C5), proaccelerin, antihemophilic factor, ACTH, glucagon, and γ-globulin. Plasmin also degrades fibronectin to produce fibronectin degradation products which stimulate neutrophils. Plasmin cleaves its substrates at Lys and Arg bonds. α$_2$-Plasmin inhibitor is the major inhibitor of plasmin. Minor inhibitors of plasmin include α$_1$-protease inhibitor, α$_2$-macroglobulin, and antithrombin III. Plasmin is routinely assayed by measuring amidolysis of Val-Leu-Lys with substrates containing the peptide sequence.

Fibrinolysis may also be initiated by a neutrophil-dependent mechanism. Proteases liberated from the neutrophil, upon migration to the site of inflammation, degrade fibrinogen. Neutrophils bind specifically to fibrin and fibrinogen and may be involved in the dissolution of clots.

Neuroimmunologic disease is associated with the release of biologically active peptides cleaved from fibrin which open the blood-brain barrier, setting the stage for the inflammatory response in experimental allergic encephalomyelitis. Patients with renal allograft rejection have increased fibrin(ogen) products and shortened euglobulin lysis. Levels of fibrin(ogen) derivatives are elevated in patients with hyperlipidemia.

SELF-TEST QUESTIONS*

Matching (*use one or more*)

1. Factor XII
2. Prekallikrein
3. Factor XI
4. High molecular weight kininogen
5. Low molecular weight kininogen

a. Nonenzymatic cofactor for contact activation
b. Responsible for clinical hemorrhagic disorder
c. Cysteine protease inhibitor
d. When activated, causes neutrophil aggregation
e. Decreases in sepsis or endotoxin infusion
f. Adsorbs directly to anionic surfaces
g. When activated, initiates classical complement pathway
h. When activated, initiates fibrinolysis

ADDITIONAL READINGS

Carvalho AC, DeMarinis S, Scott CF, Silver LD, Schmaier AH, Colman RW. Activation of the contact system of plasma proteolysis in the adult respiratory distress syndrome. *J Lab Clin Med.* 1988;112:270–277.

Colman RW. Contact systems in infectious disease. *Rev Infect Dis.* 1989;11(Suppl 4):S689–S699.

Colman RW. The role of plasma proteases in septic shock. *N Engl J Med.* 1989;320:1207–1209.

Colman RW, Scott CF, Schmaier AH, Wachtfogel YT, Pixley RA, Edmunds LH, Jr. Initiation of blood coagulation at artificial surfaces. *Ann NY Acad Sci.* 1987;516:253–267.

Gustafson EJ, Colman RW. Interaction of polymorphonuclear cells with contact activation factors. *Semin Thromb Hemost.* 1987;13:95–104.

Schapira M, DeAgostini A, Schifferli JA, Colman RW. Biochemistry and pathophysiology of human C1 inhibitor: Current issues. *Complement.* 1985;2:111–126.

Schmaier AH, Silverberg M, Kaplan AP, Colman RW. Contact activation and its abnormalities. In: *Hemostasis and Thrombosis: Basic Principles and Clinical Practice.* 2nd ed. Philadelphia: Lippincott; 1987:18–38.

*Answers will be found in Appendix E.

15

The Prostaglandins, Leukotrienes, Lipoxins, and Platelet-Activating Factor

INTRODUCTION

Acute inflammation is characterized by pain, redness, swelling, heat, and eventual loss of function of the affected area. There is an expanding body of evidence to suggest that these events are mediated in part by lipid-derived mediators such as the eicosanoids and platelet-activating factor (PAF), which are synthesized de novo from membrane lipids of inflammatory cells. Eicosanoids are 20-carbon oxygenation products derived from arachidonic acid and are generated, in part, by

the actions of three major classes of intracellular enzymes: cyclooxygenases (prostaglandins), lipoxygenases (leukotrienes, lipoxins, and hydroxyeicosatetraenoic acids), and epoxygenases (epoxyeicosatrienoic acids) (Fig. 15-1). Since our understanding of the role of epoxygenase-derived products in the pathogenesis of inflammation is still evolving, this chapter will focus on the biosynthesis and actions of cyclooxygenase- and lipoxygenase-derived products. Table 15-1 summarizes some of the proinflammatory actions of the major series of eicosanoids and PAF

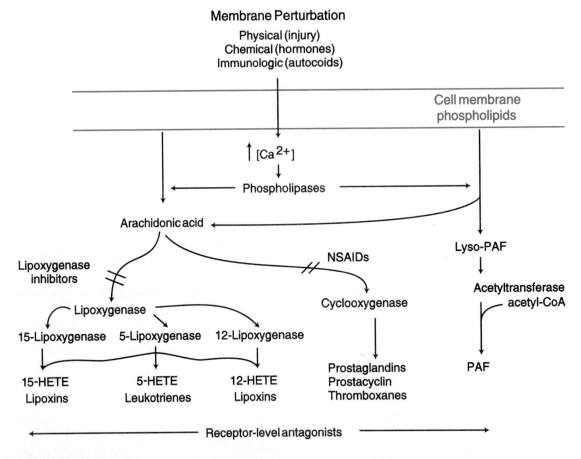

Figure 15-1   Lipid mediators of inflammation—overview of eicosanoid and PAF biosynthesis and sites of action of anti-inflammatory drugs. [NSAIDs = nonsteroidal anti-inflammatory drugs (e.g., aspirin, indomethacin); 15-HETE = 15-hydroxyeicosatetraenoic acid.]

TABLE 15-1 Proinflammatory Actions of Lipid-Derived Molecules (Eicosanoids and PAF)

Cardinal Sign	Lipid Mediator
Pain and hyperalgesia	PGE_2, LTB_4, PAF
Redness (vasodilation)	PGE_2, PGI_2, LTB_4, LXA_4, PAF
Heat (local and systemic fever)	PGE_2, PGI_2, LXA_4, PAF
Edema	PGE_2, LTB_4, LTC_4, LTD_4, LTE_4, PAF

in various experimental models. It is evident that many of these compounds can mimic the cardinal signs of inflammation (pain, heat, redness, and swelling) and thus have the potential to serve as inflammatory mediators in vivo.

SIGNALS FOR THE RELEASE AND FORMATION OF LIPID MEDIATORS

Lipid-derived mediators are not stored by inflammatory cells but rather their biosynthesis from cellular precursors is triggered by various stimuli. Arachidonic acid is derived from dietary sources or is synthesized in the body from the essential fatty acid linoleic acid. It is stored in lipid bilayers of cell membranes and is esterified predominantly to phospholipids such as phosphatidylcholine, phosphatidylethanolamine, and phosphatidylinositol. Thus, a rate-limiting step in eicosanoid biosynthesis is the release or deacylation of arachidonic acid from esterified sources (i.e., membrane storage sites) by specific phospholipases. One such enzyme is phospholipase A_2. This particular phospholipase cleaves the ester bond joining arachidonate to the glycerol backbone of the phospholipid precursor. In many cell types, phospholipase A_2 is a membrane-associated Ca^{2+}-dependent enzyme which is activated by increments in intracellular calcium concentration. Thus eicosanoid biosynthesis can be initiated by a wide variety of stimuli which increase the level of intracellular calcium. This may occur through specific receptor-

mediated signal-transduction mechanisms (e.g., hormones and autocoids) or through disruption of cell membrane integrity (physical, chemical, or immunologic trauma), events which will lead to phospholipase activation. For example, thrombin, a potent platelet agonist, stimulates thromboxane A_2 formation by platelets through its interaction with a membrane-bound cell surface receptor. Receptor binding, through activation of a GTP-binding protein, initiates a cascade of cellular events which culminates in a rise in intracellular calcium concentration, activation of phospholipase A_2, and release of arachidonic acid, followed by biosynthesis and release of eicosanoids to surrounding tissues. Less elegant stimuli such as abrasion or burning of epithelial surfaces, or shear stress to endothelial cells, also cause an increase in intracellular calcium which can lead to a similar result, namely eicosanoid biosynthesis.

TRANSFORMATION OF ARACHIDONIC ACID

The fate of unesterified arachidonic acid, once released from membrane phospholipid storage sites, is cell-specific and depends initially on the presence or absence of arachidonic acid–converting enzymes, such as cyclooxygenases or lipoxygenases, and then on the presence of specific synthetases which convert lipoxygenase and cyclooxygenase products to biologically active eicosanoids. Arachidonic acid is converted to prostaglandins by the initial action of cyclooxygenases, while leukotrienes and lipoxins are formed from arachidonic acid by the initial action of lipoxygenases (Fig. 15-1). Other fatty acids, such as C18:2 and eicosadienoic acid (EDA), are also substrates for these enzymes. However, arachidonic acid appears to be the preferred substrate in most mammalian cell types. PAF is also formed de novo from precursors found in membrane phospholipids. Again phospholipase A_2 plays a critical role in this biosynthetic scheme. Phospholipase A_2 causes the release of a precursor molecule, termed lyso-PAF, from alkylacylglycerophosphoryl-choline in cell membranes (Fig. 15-1).

Because of the complexity of this lipid mediator network, the pathways of biosynthesis and biologic actions of each class of lipid mediator will be introduced separately.

PROSTAGLANDINS

Pathways of Biosynthesis and Cell Sources of Prostaglandins

The basic structure of a prostaglandin molecule (PG) is a 20-carbon carboxylic acid containing a cyclopentane ring between carbons 9, 10, 11, and 12 and a hydroxyl group at carbon 15. This basic structure has been termed *prostanoic acid* or, in more recent literature, *prostanoid*. Prostaglandins are divided into series that differ in the oxygen substitution in the cyclopentane ring as coded by a letter (PGD, PGE, PGF, PGG, PGH). The subscript numeral in prostaglandin nomenclature indicates the number of double bonds present in the compound. In general, prostaglandins in the 1 series are derived from the precursor linoleic acid, while compounds in the 2 series are derived from arachidonic acid. Prostaglandins are formed from arachidonic acid by the initial action of cyclooxygenase (prostaglandin endoperoxide G\H synthase) (Fig. 15-2). Cyclooxygenase is a heme-containing enzyme which is most abundant in the endoplasmic reticulum and catalyzes two distinct reactions: (1) cyclization of arachidonic acid to form PGG_2 and (2) hydroperoxidation of PGG_2 to yield PGH_2. The latter is a relatively unstable compound which has a half-life of seconds and is a common intermediate that is converted to biologically active products, including thromboxane (TXA_2), prostacyclin (PGI_2), PGD_2, PGE_2, and $PGF_{1\alpha}$, in a cell-specific manner. Thus, cells which generate TXA_2 from PGH_2 do not usually generate appreciable quantities of PGI_2.

Figure 15-2 depicts the pathways for prostaglandin biosynthesis and the major cell sources of the individual compounds. PGH_2 is converted to PGE_2 by an enzyme termed PGE_2 isomerase. This enzyme is expressed by a wide range of cell types, including phagocytic cells such as neutrophils and macrophages. PGD_2 isomerase, an enzyme which is particularly abundant in the brain and certain inflammatory cells such as mast cells, converts PGH_2 to PGD_2. PGF reductase converts PGH_2 to $PGF_{2\alpha}$. This enzyme is abundant, for example, in uterine tissue. Prostacyclin synthetase and thromboxane synthetase convert PGH_2 to prostacyclin and thromboxane, respectively. Prostacyclin is the main arachidonic acid product generated by endothelial cells, while thromboxane is formed by platelets and macrophages. These two compounds have a critical role in hemostasis as well as inflammation.

Biologic Actions of Prostaglandins

The major biologic actions of prostaglandins are summarized in Fig. 15-2. Prostaglandins act locally (autocoids) and are unstable or metabolized rapidly in the circulation. PGE_2 is a potent vasodilator, while $PGF_{1\alpha}$, in contrast, causes vasoconstriction. PGD_2 inhibits platelet aggregation and causes contraction of smooth muscle. Prostacyclin and thromboxane have opposing actions on vascular tone and platelet aggregability. Prostacyclin is a potent vasodilator which also inhibits platelet aggregation. Thromboxane A_2 causes vasoconstriction and promotes platelet aggregation. Thus, the balance between these opposing forces may be critical in the control of vascular tone and blood coagulability in health and disease. (See Clinical Aside 15-1.)

Clinical Aside 15-1 PGI_2 and TXA_2 in cardio- and cerebrovascular disease

A TXA_2-PGI_2 imbalance has been implicated as an early event in thrombus formation in coronary and cerebral blood vessels and may be a pivotal event in the pathogenesis of myocardial infarction and stroke. Atheromatous change in blood vessel walls leads to endothelial damage and reduced prostacyclin generation. The unopposed actions of thromboxane on platelets (aggregation) and vascular smooth muscle (contraction) favor vasoconstriction and platelet aggregation and

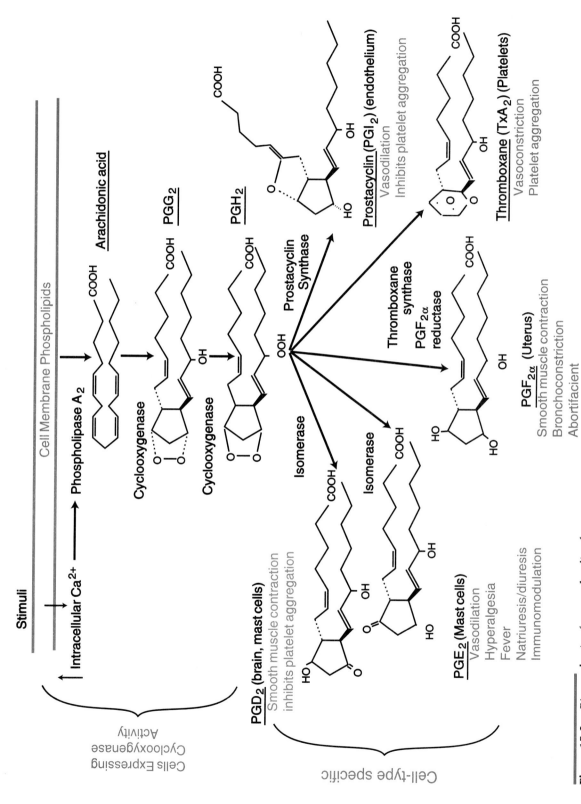

Figure 15-2 Biosynthesis of prostaglandins from membrane phospholipids, cell sources, and major biologic actions.

275

thrombus formation. Daily low-dose aspirin therapy reduces the incidence of myocardial infarction and stroke in these patients by irreversibly inhibiting platelet cyclooxygenase activity and thromboxane generation. Although aspirin inhibits endothelial cell cyclooxygenase also, and thus inhibits prostacyclin generation, this enzyme is constitutively regenerated while the platelet enzyme is inactivated for the life span of the cell (approximately 10 days).

Role of Prostaglandins in Inflammation

There are several lines of evidence to support the notion that cyclooxygenase-derived products are important mediators of inflammation: (1) prostaglandin synthesis is increased at sites of inflammation, (2) prostaglandin administration, e.g., intradermal injection, causes pathologic changes almost identical to those seen in inflammation, and (3) aspirin and other nonsteroidal anti-inflammatory drugs, molecules of differing chemical structures, share as a common action the ability to inhibit cyclooxygenase, the enzyme involved in prostaglandin synthesis. Increased synthesis of prostaglandin is an almost invariable consequence of tissue injury, whether physically, chemically, or immunologically induced. This is not surprising, perhaps, given that significant cell injury virtually always results in a rise in intracellular calcium concentration.

In humans a variety of inflammatory arthritides (e.g., rheumatoid arthritis, gout) are associated with increased levels of PGE_2 in the synovial fluid. Aspirin, one of the original and most effective treatments for arthritis, is a potent inhibitor of cyclooxygenase activity; aspirin successfully relieves the symptoms and signs of inflammation and causes a parallel fall in PGE_2 levels. Similar findings have been reported with various animal models of inflammation and arthritis. Local administration of PGE_2 causes many of the cardinal signs of inflammation. Injection of PGE_2 into human skin, for example, causes arteriolar dilatation and, as a result, redness and increased skin temperature. PGE_2

causes fever when administered into the subarachnoid space and is one of the most pyretic substances known. PGE_2 by itself does not produce pain or changes in vascular permeability and swelling, but does potentiate the effects of other autocoids such as histamine and serotonin. To date, the precise role of other cyclooxygenase products in mediating acute inflammation in humans is less clear, although prostacyclin, thromboxane, PGD_2, and $PGF_{1\alpha}$ have all been detected in significant concentrations at sites of inflammation. Prostacyclin, like PGE_2, causes marked vasodilatation and hyperalgesia. Whether the other prostaglandins contribute to the inflammatory response or are merely generated in response to tissue injury has yet to be demonstrated.

The actions of prostaglandins on the acquired immune response are less well defined. PGE_2 has been reported to inhibit the function of T and B lymphocytes and natural killer cell activity in vitro (Table 15-2). It remains to be determined whether prostaglandins are important modulators of cellular or humoral immunity in vivo.

LEUKOTRIENES

Pathways of Biosynthesis and Cell Sources of Leukotrienes

The *leukotrienes* were discovered in the mid-1970s and were so-named because they were originally isolated from leukocytes and contain a conjugated triene structure (three conjugated double bonds). The subscript numeral in leukotriene nomenclature refers to the number of double bonds in the precursor molecule. Thus, leukotrienes of the 4 series are derived from arachidonic acid (eicosatetranoic acid), which has four double bonds, while leukotrienes of the 5 series are generated from eicosapentanoic acid, which contains five double bonds. Leukotrienes are formed from arachidonic acid by the initial action of the enzyme 5-lipoxygenase (Fig. 15-3). This enzyme catalyzes two sequential reactions: (1) the insertion of molecular ox-

TABLE 15-2 Major Immunomodulatory Effects of Lipoxygenase and
Cyclooxygenase Products

Product	Immunomodulatory Effect
LTB_4	Inhibition of immunoglobulin synthesis
	Inhibition of mixed lymphocyte response—inhibition of helper cell (CD4) proliferation; induction of suppressor cell (CD8) proliferation
	Enhancement of NK-cell activity
	Enhancement of monocyte cytokine production
LTC_4, LTD_4, LTE_4	Inhibition of mitogen-induced lymphocyte proliferation
LXA_4, LXB_4	Inhibition of NK-cell activity
PGE_2	Inhibition of T- and B-lymphocyte activation
	Inhibition of NK-cell activity

ygen at the carbon-5 position of arachidonic acid (counting from the carboxylic acid end as 1) to form 5-hydroperoxyeicosatetraenoic acid (5-HPETE) and (2) the subsequent transformation of 5-HPETE to an epoxide denoted LTA_4. LTA_4 is also a relatively unstable molecule (with a half-life of seconds) which is rapidly transformed in a cell-specific manner, a situation analogous to the transformation of PGH_2 in prostaglandin synthesis. The epoxide LTA_4 can be hydrated enzymatically to LTB_4 by LTA_4 hydrolase (e.g., in neutrophils) or conjugated with glutathione to form LTC_4 (e.g., in mast cells and eosinophils) by LTC_4 synthetase, a glutathione-S-transferase. LTC_4 can be converted in turn to LTD_4 and LTE_4 by the successive elimination of glutamyl and glycine residues. Transformation in this manner is associated with relative loss of biologic activity. The mixture of peptido-containing leukotrienes (LTC_4, LTD_4, and LTE_4) was formerly known as slow-reacting substance of anaphylaxis (SRS-A) (see Chap. 29). Together these substances are generated by mast cells following antigenic challenge and IgE-receptor-mediated signal transduction.

Biologic Actions of Leukotrienes

Figure 15-3 lists the major biologic actions of leukotrienes relevant to the immune response. LTB_4 is a potent activator of human neutrophils (vide infra), while LTC_4, LTD_4,

and LTE_4 display strikingly different biologic actions, causing, for example, smooth muscle contraction in a variety of tissues. These compounds are potent constrictors of bronchial smooth muscle. This effect is rapid in onset and lasts for hours. Inhalation of LTC_4 or LTD_4 by normal volunteers results in prolonged bronchoconstriction. In addition, both LTC_4 and LTD_4 are vasoconstrictors. Despite this effect, systemic administration of LTC_4, LTD_4, and LTE_4 causes hypotension due to (1) reduced myocardial contractility and coronary blood flow and (2) loss of plasma to the extravascular space as a consequence of increased vascular permeability. Since these compounds are released along with histamine following antigenic challenge of mast cells, eosinophils, or basophils, it is likely that they represent major inflammatory mediators derived from these cells.

Role of Leukotrienes in Inflammation

There is strong evidence supporting the role of leukotrienes as important mediators of acute inflammation, including acute hypersensitivity. LTB_4 is a potent activator of neutrophil functional responses (i.e., generation of oxygen free radicals and release of lysosomal enzymes), and is an important early signal which mediates the migration of neutrophils to sites of inflammation (neutrophil chemotaxis). In health approximately 50

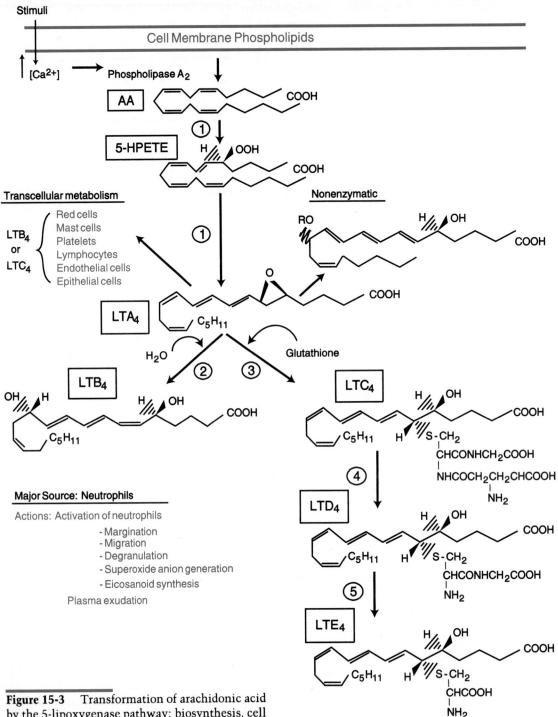

Figure 15-3 Transformation of arachidonic acid by the 5-lipoxygenase pathway: biosynthesis, cell sources, and major biologic actions of leukotrienes. The enzymes involved in leukotriene biosynthesis are depicted by encircled numerals and are ① 5-lipoxygenase, ② LTA₄ hydrolase, ③ LTC₄ synthetase, ④ γ-glutamyl transpeptidase, and ⑤ dipeptidase.

percent of neutrophils circulate freely in blood, while 50 percent crawl (stick and roll) along the endothelial surface lining of blood vessel walls. In inflammatory states, circulating neutrophils adhere to the endothelial cell layer, pass through the cells of the vessel wall (diapedesis), and migrate to the site of inflammation where they attack and ingest foreign antigen. This latter process of phagocytosis results in the formation of a phagosome which fuses with neutrophil lysosomes to form phagolysosomes. Ingested particles are then destroyed within this organelle by proteases, hydrolases, and reactive oxygen species, with relative protection of host tissues. In addition, activated neutrophils synthesize and release more eicosanoids. LTB_4, through its interaction with a neutrophil cell surface receptor, is a stimulus for all of these events (i.e., neutrophil adhesion, diapedesis, migration, the generation of reactive oxygen species, and lysosomal enzyme release). For more details on the function of neutrophil phagocytosis see Chap. 17, "Polymorphonuclear Phagocytic Cells."

Administration of LTB_4 to experimental animals in vivo is associated with increased neutrophil margination along vessel walls and migration to the extracellular space. LTB_4 is not believed to affect vascular tone directly, and is considered a weak inducer of plasma exudation. However, combined exposure to LTB_4 and PGE_2, another weak inducer of plasma exudation, results in a profound increase in vascular permeability. Thus, under some circumstances prostaglandins and leukotrienes may act synergistically to promote inflammation. LTB_4 does not induce pain directly but lowers the threshold for other stimuli. (See Clinical Aside 15-2).

Clinical Aside 15-2   The role of LTB_4 in inflammation

LTB_4 has been identified in inflammatory exudates in arthritis and cystic fibrosis and in the epidermis of patients with psoriasis. Several inhibitors of LTA_4 hydrolase have been developed, but are, as yet, only available for experimental use. These agents will help define the role of LTB_4 as a mediator of inflammation in these diseases and promise to be potent and pathway-specific anti-inflammatory drugs.

The peptido-containing leukotrienes (LTC_4, LTD_4, and LTE_4) have also been identified in several experimental models of inflammation, and may be particularly important in the pathogenesis of hypersensitivity disorders such as asthma. (See Chap. 29.) Asthmatic subjects appear to be hypersensitive to these compounds. In addition to their effects on vascular tone, LTC_4 and LTD_4 increase vascular permeability and increase the leakage of plasma and macromolecules from the intravascular space. Unlike LTB_4 these compounds do not affect neutrophil functional responses and do not appear to alter the pain threshold after topical administration.

Recent evidence suggests that leukotrienes may also be important regulators of both cellular and humoral immunity. Table 15-2 summarizes some of the major effects of these compounds on the immune system. It should be noted, however, that the majority of these actions have been described in vitro and their relevance to the immune response in vivo remains a subject of intense research interest.

LIPOXINS

Pathways of Biosynthesis and Cell Sources of Lipoxins

Whereas the biosynthesis of leukotrienes is initiated by the insertion of molecular oxygen at the carbon-5 position of arachidonic acid by 5-lipoxygenase, the sequential oxygenation of arachidonic acid at the carbon-15 and then carbon-5 position by 15- and 5-lipoxygenase, respectively, results in the formation of *lipoxins* (*lipox*ygenase *in*teraction products). These compounds are the most recent addition to the family of bioactive products generated from arachidonic acid. These novel eicosanoids differ markedly from the leukotrienes in both their structure and biologic actions (Fig. 15-4). Dual oxygenation produces an epoxide intermediate denoted as 5,6-epoxytetraene, which is

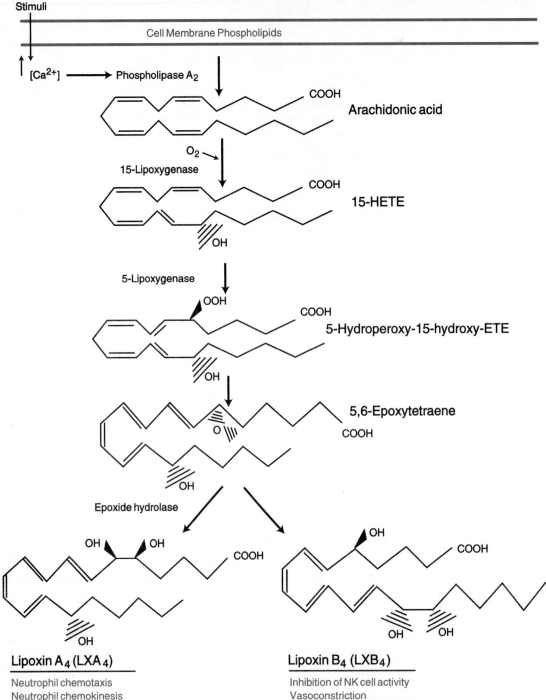

Stimuli

Cell Membrane Phospholipids

$[Ca^{2+}]$ ⟶ Phospholipase A_2

COOH
Arachidonic acid

O_2 ⟶
15-Lipoxygenase

COOH
15-HETE
OH

5-Lipoxygenase

OOH
COOH
5-Hydroperoxy-15-hydroxy-ETE
OH

5,6-Epoxytetraene
O
COOH
OH

Epoxide hydrolase

OH   OH
COOH
Lipoxin A$_4$ (LXA$_4$)
OH

OH
COOH
Lipoxin B$_4$ (LXB$_4$)
OH   OH

Lipoxin A$_4$ (LXA$_4$)

Neutrophil chemotaxis
Neutrophil chemokinesis
Inhibits NK cell activity
Arteriolar dilatation
Leukotriene antagonist
Release of TxA$_2$, PGI$_2$
Bronchial smooth muscle contraction
Activates PMN
Stimulates PG formation

Lipoxin B$_4$ (LXB$_4$)

Inhibition of NK cell activity
Vasoconstriction
Bronchial smooth muscle contraction

Figure 15-4   Biosynthesis and major biologic actions of lipoxins. [15-HETE = 15-hydroxyeicosatetraenoic acid; 5-hydroperoxy-15-hydroxy-ETE = 5-hydroperoxy-15-hydroxyeicosatetraenoic acid.]

280

rapidly converted to either lipoxin A_4 or B_4 by epoxide hydrolases. More recently, it has been demonstrated that lipoxin formation may be achieved by oxygenation of leuko-cyte-derived LTA_4 by platelet lipoxygenase through cell-cell interaction (vide infra). Li-poxins are characterized structurally by the presence of four conjugated double bonds. These confer a characteristic appearance on ultraviolet spectroscopy, which is the hall-mark of the compounds in this series and different from that seen with leukotrienes. Interestingly, there appears to be an inverse relationship between the amount of lipoxin and leukotriene formed in vitro, which sug-gests the potential for counterregulatory in-teractions between these two series of lipox-ygenase products. The nature of this control mechanism remains to be determined.

Biologic Actions of Lipoxins

Although the lipoxins were identified rela-tively recently, it is already apparent that these compounds have important effects on a number of inflammatory cells. Lipoxin A_4 causes neutrophil chemotaxis, but not neu-trophil aggregation or adhesion in vitro. Un-like LTB_4, the administration of lipoxins in vivo does not provoke neutrophil adhesion to endothelial cells or neutrophil migration to the extracellular space. Instead, lipoxin A_4 may inhibit LTB_4-induced neutrophil migra-tion. Thus, there exists the exciting possi-bility that these compounds may have an "anti-inflammatory" or counterregulatory role(s). In addition to their actions on human neutrophils, both LXA_4 and LXB_4 inhibit nat-ural killer (NK) cell cytotoxic activity in vi-tro, suggesting that they may regulate other facets of the immune response.

Lipoxins also have profound effects on va-somotor tone when administered to labora-tory animals. LXA_4 stimulates vasodilation, while LXB_4 causes vasoconstriction. The va-sodilation caused by LXA_4 appears to be a secondary effect in certain tissues due to the generation of prostaglandins, probably pros-tacyclin and/or PGE_2, as LXA_4 causes vaso-constriction in the presence of a cyclooxy-genase inhibitor. Thus, lipoxins can also regulate the production of other eicosanoids by stimulating prostaglandin biosynthesis. Lipoxins also cause contraction of other smooth muscle cells such as renal glomer-ular mesangial cells and bronchial smooth muscle. These actions of lipoxins appear to be due to a partial agonist action of lipoxins on the vascular smooth muscle LTD_4 recep-tor. Along these lines, LXA_4 has been shown to attenuate the actions of LTC_4 and LTD_4 on bronchial smooth muscle and the renal microcirculation, suggesting that these com-pounds may serve as nature's endogenous leukotriene antagonists as well as act at their own recognition sites.

Role of Lipoxins in Inflammation

There is compelling evidence to suggest that the lipoxins may be important lipoxygenase-derived lipid mediators involved in both acute inflammation and the control of cellular im-munity. Lipoxins have, indeed, been identi-fied already in bronchoalveolar lavage sam-ples from patients with sarcoidosis and pneumonia. Their exact role in this context remains to be defined, although the possi-bility that lipoxins represent endogenous modulators of leukotriene responses in in-flammation is exciting and an area of active research.

PLATELET-ACTIVATING FACTOR (PAF)

Pathways of Biosynthesis and Cell Sources of PAF

The name *platelet-activating factor* was coined in the early 1970s to describe an ac-tivity or substance(s) which, when released from basophils during IgE-induced anaphy-laxis, activated platelets. Subsequently, this bioactive substance was isolated and its structure was elucidated as a group of mol-ecules characterized by the common struc-ture 1-*O*-alkyl-2-acyl-*sn*-glycero-3-phospho-choline. Individual compounds differ only within the number of carbon atoms in the alkyl group (Fig. 15-5). PAF, like the eicosanoids, is derived from membrane phospholipids by the action of phospholipase A_2. Upon activation of a cell, phospholipase A_2 effects deacylation of 1-O-alkyl-2-acyl-glycero-3-phosphocholine in the cell membrane, yielding lyso-PAF and free fatty acid. Lyso-PAF is then acetylated by acetyl-coenzyme A (acetyl-CoA) transferase, yielding PAF. It is noteworthy that up to 40 percent of the fatty acid released from the 2 position during PAF synthesis by human neutrophils is arachidonic acid. As a result, increased PAF biosynthesis by activated inflammatory cells is often accompanied by the generation of prostaglandins and lipoxygenase products.

PAF production has been documented with a number of different cell types, including leukocytes (neutrophils, basophils, and eosinophils), macrophages, mast cells, and platelets. It is intriguing that the biosynthesis of PAF can also occur in various non-inflammatory cells, such as endothelial and epithelial cells. This suggests that PAF may serve as an important physiologic regulator of cellular function in addition to its role as a mediator of acute inflammation. A second pathway of PAF synthesis has been documented with renal cells. In this case choline transferase catalyzes the formation of PAF from 1-O-alkyl-2-acetylglycerol (Fig. 15-5). The importance of this pathway as a source of PAF in inflammatory cells has yet to be determined.

A variety of stimuli trigger PAF synthesis

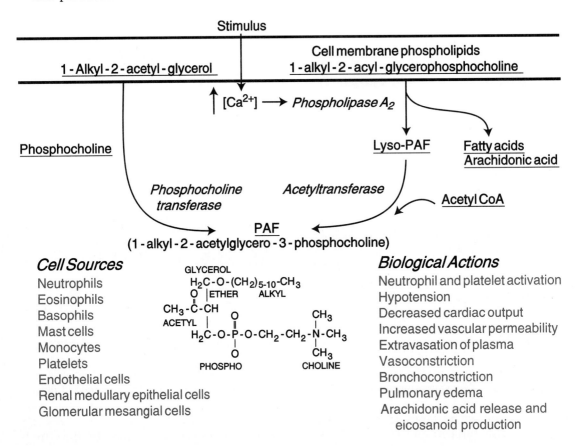

Figure 15-5   Biosynthesis, cell sources, and major biologic actions of PAF.

in inflammatory cells. PAF synthesis by neutrophils is stimulated by phagocytosis of serum-treated zymosan, C5a fraction of complement, formylmethionylleucylphenyl-alanine (a synthetic peptide which mimics the action of the formylated peptides contained in bacterial cell walls), and the calcium ionophore A23187. All of these stimuli increase the level of intracellular calcium and activate phospholipase A_2. The stimuli for PAF biosynthesis are, however, cell-specific. For example, thrombin, angiotensin II, and vasopressin do not trigger the generation of PAF in inflammatory cells, but stimulate PAF formation in vascular endothelial cells.

Biologic Actions and Role in Inflammation of PAF

PAF has been implicated in the pathogenesis of both acute inflammation and hypersensitivity disorders. In addition, PAF may be an important inflammatory mediator in a variety of other conditions, including endotoxic shock, vasculitis, and arterial thrombosis. PAF is a potent activator of human neutrophils in vitro and stimulates neutrophil adhesion, lysosomal enzyme release, and the generation of reactive oxygen species and eicosanoids. PAF causes rapid margination of neutrophils onto endothelial cell walls in vivo, and promotes neutrophil migration to the extracellular space. As the name implies, PAF causes platelet activation and aggregation. In keeping with these observations, local administration of PAF by intradermal injection in laboratory animals or human subjects is associated with neutrophil margination and intravascular thrombosis. There is an associated increase in vascular permeability and edema and in hyperalgesia. Thus PAF causes many of the cardinal features of inflammation.

Intravenous injection of PAF has profound effects on bronchial smooth muscle tone and the cardiovascular function of laboratory animals. Indeed, intravenous PAF causes a syndrome which is very similar to that of acute anaphylaxis (i.e., severe acute hypersensitivity reaction). PAF induces contraction of bronchial and vascular smooth muscle, including coronary artery smooth muscle. In addition, there is a marked increase in vascular permeability and exudation of plasma into the extravascular space, including the lungs (pulmonary edema). As a result, the animals develop respiratory insufficiency, decreased cardiac output, and hypotension.

PAF may also be a regulator of lymphocyte function, either directly or indirectly, through the generation of prostaglandins and leukotrienes. PAF has been shown to inhibit lymphocyte proliferation in response to various mitogens. Furthermore, lymphocytes generate PAF upon stimulation by agents which increase intracellular calcium. The significance of these findings is currently being investigated.

CELL-CELL INTERACTION AND EICOSANOID BIOSYNTHESIS

Acute inflammation is characterized by the local accumulation of inflammatory cells at the site of injury where they function in juxtaposition with, and often while adherent to, resident endothelial, epithelial, mesenchymal, and other inflammatory cells. It has become apparent in recent years that arachidonic acid and arachidonate-derived lipoxygenase products may pass from one cell type to another and that different cell types may cooperate with each other (i.e., pool their enzymatic machinery) to generate eicosanoids. In this way, cell types that on their own may not be able to generate a particular class of eicosanoid (for example, cells which lack a lipoxygenase) can generate eicosanoids from intermediates generated in other cells if they have the enzymes to convert the intermediate to a biologically active product. Figure 15-6 illustrates this phenomenon. In this example, neither neutrophils alone nor platelets alone can generate LTC_4, because

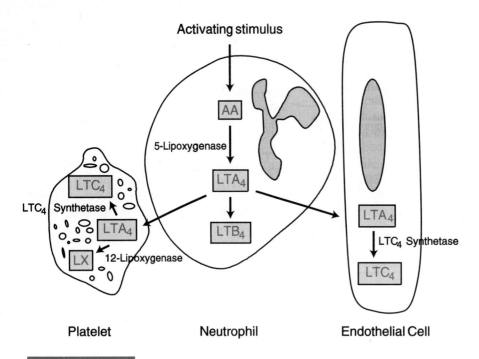

Figure 15-6   Biosynthesis of leukotrienes and lipoxins by cell-cell interaction. Activated neutrophils generate LTB_4 from arachidonic acid–derived LTA_4 by the action of 5-lipoxygenase, but do not possess LTC_4-synthetase activity and so do not generate LTC_4. However, platelets and endothelial cells, which themselves do not form LTC_4 from endogenous substrates, can generate LTC_4 in abundance from neutrophil-derived LTA_4. Platelets can also generate lipoxins from neutrophil-derived LTA_4. Thus, cell-cell interaction greatly enhances the quantities of eicosanoids generated at sites of inflammation and the variety of cells which can form these compounds.

neutrophils do not have LTC_4 synthetase and platelets do not possess a 5-lipoxygenase activity. Nevertheless, when these different cell types interact, LTC_4 is formed in abundance since platelets can convert neutrophil-derived LTA_4 to LTC_4. Similarly, LTC_4 can be generated by endothelial cells from neutrophil-derived LTA_4. Lipoxins are also formed during platelet-neutrophil interaction. Platelets alone do not generate lipoxins. However, when platelets and neutrophils interact, platelets can form lipoxins from neutrophil-derived intermediates. Thus, the phenomenon of cell-cell interaction not only expands the array of eicosanoids that can be generated at sites of inflammation but may also amplify the quantity of eicosanoids produced.

TARGETS FOR ANTI-INFLAMMATORY THERAPY

As can be seen from Figs. 15-1 to 15-4, there are many sites or targets along eicosanoid and PAF biosynthetic pathways at which to direct anti-inflammatory therapy. Clearly, a potent inhibitor of phospholipase activity would have the advantage of inhibiting the formation of prostaglandins, leukotrienes, lipoxins, and PAF. Corticosteroids are potent anti-inflammatory compounds which are effective in the treatment of a wide variety of inflammatory and hypersensitivity states (see Chap. 33A). Corticosteroids can, under certain conditions, block phospholipase A_2 activity in vitro and inhibit eicosanoid synthesis. Whether the anti-inflammatory actions of corticosteroids are related to their ability to block phospholipase A_2 activity in vivo remains unclear, since corticosteroids can also inhibit a range of other functional responses by immune cells including lymphocytes, monocytes, and natural killer cells.

On the other hand, there are a large number of relatively specific and potent inhibitors of cyclooxygenase activity available (e.g., aspirin, indomethacin, and ibuprofen). Their efficacy as anti-inflammatory agents has been well demonstrated, and the resolution of inflammation is paralleled by a fall in tissue prostaglandin levels. It should be remembered, however, that prostaglandins are intimately involved in many physiologic functions such as fluid and electrolyte homeostasis and the control of vascular tone and tissue perfusion. For example, PGE_2 has natriuretic and diuretic properties, while PGE_2 and PGI_2 are vasodilators which appear to play an important role in the preservation of renal blood flow during renal ischemia. In addition, PGE_2 appears to have a cytoprotective role in the upper gastrointestinal tract. Thus, cyclooxygenase inhibitors, while being effective anti-inflammatory drugs, may also interfere with these homeostatic mechanisms and cause salt and water retention or gastrointestinal ulceration, exacerbate renal ischemia, and precipitate acute renal failure. To date there are no specific or selective inhibitors of lipoxygenases available for clinical or experimental purposes, and this is an area of intense research. Similarly, research is currently ongoing to synthesize drugs which selectively inhibit the various synthetase enzymes which are involved in the generation of eicosanoids or which antagonize the actions of specific eicosanoids with cells by blocking their interaction with cell surface receptors on target tissues. The development of such agents will not only allow more specific, and hopefully more effective, anti-inflammatory drug regimens to be designed, but will also enable a complete dissection of the roles of individual eicosanoids in the pathophysiology of acute inflammation and hypersensitivity. A recent approach to the manipulation of inflammation has been to modify the intake and content of dietary lipids, using fish oils. The biochemical basis for this approach lies in the finding that in many settings leukotrienes derived from eicosapentanoic acid (the 5 series) are less potent than those derived from arachidonic acid (the 4 series). The replacement of arachidonic acid at membrane storage sites in phospholipid by dietary fish oil–derived eicosapentanoic acid results in a decrease in the agonist-induced formation of series 4 leukotrienes and shifts product formation to the less active series 5 leukotrienes. This dietary approach has had reported success in the treatment of arthritis and SLE and is an important area of active research.

SELF-TEST QUESTIONS*

For the following incomplete statements, choose the letter of the appropriate combination of correct completions.

1. Cardinal signs of inflammation are:
   a. Headache   A. a
   b. Swelling   B. a, b, c
   c. Pain   C. b, c
   d. Tremor   D. All are correct.
2. Enzymes involved in prostaglandin biosynthesis include:
   a. 12-Lipoxygenase   A. d
   b. Cyclooxygenase   B. b, c
   c. Phospholipase A_2 C. a, d
   d. Carboxypeptidase   D. a, c, e
   e. 12-HETE   E. b, c, d, e
3. Actions of prostacyclin include:
   a. Vasoconstriction   A. b
   b. Vasodilatation   B. a, c
   c. Platelet aggregation   C. a, c, d
   d. Bronchoconstriction   D. a, c, d, e
   e. Neutrophil activation
4. Actions of leukotriene C_4 include:
   a. Neutrophil activation   A. a, e
   b. Vasoconstriction   B. b, c
   c. Bronchoconstriction   C. b, d

*Answers will be found in Appendix E.

d. Platelet aggregation   D. a, b, c, d
e. Vasodilatation   E. b, c, d, e

5. Enzymes involved in lipoxin biosynthesis include:
   a. LTA_4 hydrolase   A. a
   b. 12-Lipoxygenase   B. a, c, d
   c. 5-Lipoxygenase   C. b, c, d
   d. 15-Lipoxygenase   D. b, c, d, e
   e. Phospholipase A_2 E. All are correct.

6. Actions of lipoxin A_4 include:
   a. Vasodilatation   A. a
   b. Platelet aggregation   B. a, c
       C. a, c, d
   c. Inhibition of NK-cell activity   D. a, d, e
       E. All are correct.
   d. Stimulation of prostacyclin biosynthesis
   e. Pyrogenic action

7. Eicosanoids generated by cell-cell interaction include:
   a. Prostacyclin   A. c
   b. Lipoxins   B. b, d
   c. Leukotriene A_4 C. a, e
   d. Leukotriene C_4 D. a, b, d
   e. Arachidonic acid   E. b, c, d

8. Potential treatments for acute inflammation include:
   a. Platelet-activating factor   A. a
       B. b, c
   b. Azathioprine   C. a, e
   c. Corticosteroids   D. c, d, e
   d. Fish oils   E. All are correct.
   e. Aspirin

ADDITIONAL READINGS

Braquet P, Toqui L, Shen TY, Vargaftig BB. Perspectives in platelet-activating factor research. *Pharmacol Rev.* 1987;39:98–133.

Rola-Pleszczynski M. Immunoregulation by leukotrienes and other lipoxygenase metabolites. *Immunol Today.* 1985;6:302–307.

Samuelsson B, Dahlen S-E, Lindgren JA, Rouzer CA, Serhan CN. Leukotrienes and lipoxins: Structures, biosynthesis, and biological effects. *Science.* 1987;237:1171–1176.

Smith WM. The eicosanoids and their biochemical mechanisms of action. *Biochem J.* 1989;259:315–324.

Williams KI and Higgs GA. Eicosanoids and inflammation. *J Pathol.* 1988;156:101–110.

16

The Acute Phase Response to Inflammation

INTRODUCTION

The primary goal of any organism is to survive. Therefore, after significant tissue damage, be it ischemic, traumatic, or infectious, there must be an effective means of restoring homeostatic balance. The systemic mechanisms called into play must be able to focus the energies of the organism on the new problem, even at the expense of routine metabolic processes. They must start quickly after the onset of damage, and provide an effective means of disposing of dead tissue and debris after the response is completed. The damaged tissue must be repaired. Finally, all these changes must be reversed once the conditions return to the *status quo ante bellum.* These responses, both local and systemic, must be integrated with each other and tailored to the individual problem, but must retain the ability to cope with a wide variety of new assaults.

If the damage has been caused by an infectious agent, it is important to expose the damaged area to the full immune potential of the organism and enhance that immune capacity. Once infection is controlled, the response must be dampened before it can do harm to undamaged tissues. If some way of depriving the invading pathogen of vital nutrients could occur, this would also help. All of these functions are served by what is known as the acute phase response.

The *acute phase response (APR)*, also known as the *acute phase reaction*, represents a complex, nonspecific, rapid response to many types of tissue damage. It represents local and systemic modifications of normal

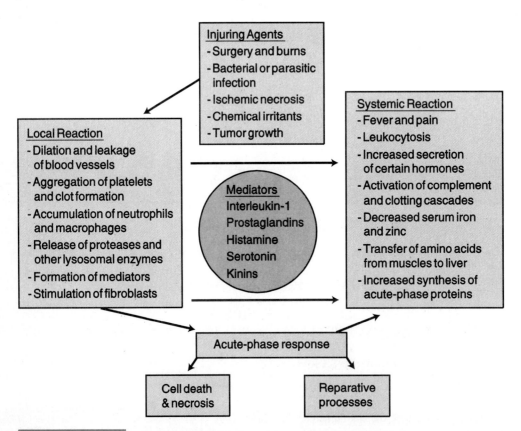

Figure 16-1 Development and effects of the APR.

physiology, all of which serve to control damage, clean up debris, and start repair. These functions are accomplished by alterations in hepatic protein synthesis which accompany inflammation (Fig. 16-1). Those proteins which are up-regulated during inflammation are called *positive acute phase reactants;* those whose synthesis is diminished are termed *negative acute phase reactants.*

At the site of inflammation, a great number of local changes occur; these and the inflow of cells which take part in the inflammatory reaction are described in Chap. 20, "The Inflammatory Response."

THE APR IN EARLY INFLAMMATION

In the very early phases of inflammation tissue macrophages and recruited blood monocytes begin to produce monokines (please review these compounds, which are described in Chap. 10). The monokines most clearly implicated in the APR are interleukin-1 (IL-1), tumor necrosis factor (TNF; also known as cachectin), and IL-6, also known as hepatocyte stimulating factor(s) (HSF). [Other names for HSF include B-cell differentiation factor (BCDF), B-cell stimulatory factor (BSF), hybridoma-plasmacytoma growth factor (HPGF), and beta$_2$ interferon. (This proliferation of names is a result of the fact that different laboratories define functions for undefined factors, often in unprocessed conditioned media, realizing only after molecular cloning that the stuff they have been calling Ronnie is just the same as the stuff other labs have been calling George.)]

Early in inflammation, serum cortisol levels increase, peaking at about 6 h. The circulating white blood cell count begins to increase and peaks at about 10 h. Large numbers of white blood cells are loosely associated with the endothelial cells which line the blood vessels; these white blood cells are released into the circulation during inflammation in a process known as *demargination.* In ad-

dition to these cortisol effects, another cause of leukocytosis is the release of neutrophils from the bone marrow, caused by IL-1. Other effects of IL-1 and TNF on hypothalamus, muscle, and adipose tissue are described in Chaps. 18 and 10, on monocytes and cytokines, respectively.

ALTERATION OF HEPATIC FUNCTION IN THE APR

Monokines also alter hepatic function. There is a change in fat metabolism, with an increase in the synthesis of very low density lipoproteins (VLDL) and a decrease of high density lipoprotein (HDL). Amino acids which have been liberated from muscle are taken up by hepatocytes. Hepatocyte synthesis of an intracellular zinc-binding protein, metalothienein, increases with subsequent uptake of serum zinc and decrease in serum zinc levels. (Increased metalothienein synthesis during inflammation is not represented in the serum, an intracellular APR of sorts.) Increased levels of ferritin (storage protein for iron) have also been found. The synthesis of other nonsecreted proteins is also modified. There is a decrease in the levels of enzymes involved in gluconeogenesis, e.g., phosphoenol pyruvate carboxykinase and glucose-6-phosphatase, and an increase in the enzymes providing fuel and in those involved in protein glycosylation.

Among the secreted proteins, there is a mild increase in the levels of ceruloplasmin and complement components C3, C4, and B. These are termed group I APR proteins, defined as proteins whose serum levels increase by about 50 percent (Table 16-1; also Fig. 16-3). [The prefixes α_1 or α_2 refer to the mobility of serum proteins when subjected to gel electrophoresis (Fig. 16-2; also Appendix C).] A two- to fourfold increase in serum levels of α_1-acid glycoprotein (AGP), haptoglobin, fibrinogen, α_1-protease inhibitor (α_1-PI) (formerly called α_1-antitrypsin before its broader range of inhibition was appreciated), and α_1-antichymotrypsin defines these as group II APR proteins.

TABLE 16-1   APR Proteins

APR	Serum Level Change
Positive APR	
Group I	↑ 50%: ceruloplasmin, C3, C4, B, C1-esterase inhibitor
	Rat: CRP, prekallikrein, kininogen
Group II	↑ 2 to 4×: α_1-acid glycoprotein, haptoglobin; fibrinogen,
	α_1-protease inhibitor, α_1-chymotrypsin inhibitor
	Mouse: SAP
Group III	↑ 100 to 1000 ×: CRP, SAA
	Rat: α_2-macroglobulin
Negative APR	↓: albumin, transferrin, transthyretin

Group III includes the most spectacular APR proteins, where 100- to 1000-fold increases are not uncommon. These include C-reactive protein (CRP) and serum amyloid A (SAA) component, which increase within 8 h of the onset of inflammation and peak at about 48 h (Fig. 16-3). The group III proteins, with the most rapid increase and the highest peak levels, are the only positive APR proteins which are not glycosylated. AGP, haptoglobin, and the protease inhibitors begin to increase by about 12 h, but peak at different times; fibrinogen typically peaks late. Serum levels of AGP and haptoglobin are diminished for the first 6 to 8 h of the APR and then begin to rise.

Other proteins have a prolonged diminution in serum level, persisting for as long as the inflammation. The negative APR proteins (Table 16-1; also Fig. 16-3) include albumen, transferrin, and transthyretin. (Transthyretin is involved in transport of thyroid hormone and, in association with a small molecule known as retinol-binding protein, in the transport of vitamin A.)

There is some controversy as to whether the following serum proteins also change as APR in humans: complement components C2 and C9, kininogen, kininogenase, angiotensinogen, and fibronectin. Some of these are APR proteins in other species; the APR varies greatly from species to species.

VARIATIONS IN THE APR

There is evidence that the APR may be different in various types of inflammation. The change in rate of synthesis of the APR proteins and the type of protein glycosylation vary with different pathologic processes. Different molecular forms of SAA have been found in individuals, and there is heterogeneity of glycosylation of AGP. For example, the forms of AGP in the blood in infection are different from those in systemic lupus erythematosus (SLE), a systemic inflammatory "autoimmune" disease. There may be a *local* APR, as well, in which production of APR proteins by macrophages occurs at the site of inflammation.

THE FUNCTION OF THE APR

A reasonable approach to the question "What is the function of the APR?" is to look at the

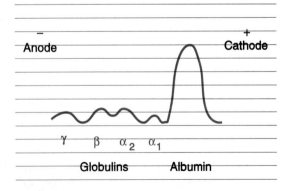

Figure 16-2   Normal serum protein electrophoresis pattern.

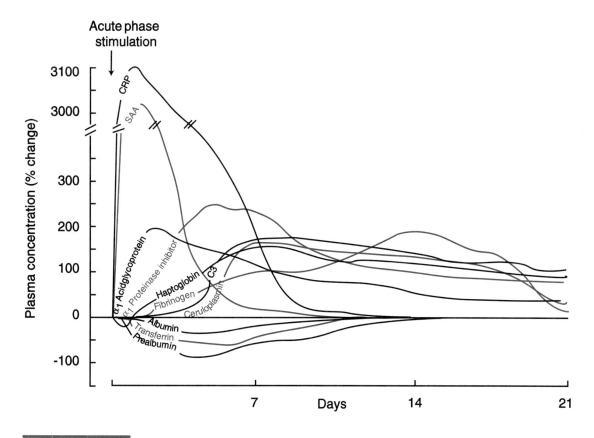

Figure 16-3 Typical plasma concentrations of APR proteins following tissue injury or infection.

function of each protein. Knowing the role of the protein should make the purpose of the change during the APR clearer.

The Negative APR

Albumin binds many drugs, bilirubin, amino acids, and some lipids, and transports about 65 percent of serum zinc. Aside from providing about 75 percent of the oncotic pressure of serum, albumin serves no defined, unique function. Some people have essentially no circulating albumin. These individuals, and a rat strain which is analbuminemic, are healthy, save for dependent edema. This lack of a specific function has led some researchers to suggest that albumin is a "metabolic adaptor," which keeps protein synthetic processes active, but whose rate of synthesis can decrease when the need for other proteins is increased. This reciprocal change then maintains the overall rate of protein synthesis at a relatively constant level. A decrease of albumin, the transport protein for zinc, in concert with increased levels of metalothienein, decreases serum zinc levels; perhaps decreased serum zinc is advantageous during inflammation. One last note about albumin as a negative APR: What do you think is the value of using the serum concentration of albumin as an indicator of nutritional status in patients with infection, parasitic infestation, or malignancy, or without any inflammatory process?

Transferrin (a β-globulin), another negative APR, is the major iron transport protein. Iron is a requirement for growth of mammalian cells *and* for bacteria. The concomitant decrease in circulating transferrin and increase in intrahepatic ferritin decreases available iron at the site of infection. Transferrin levels return to normal 7 to 10 days after onset of the APR.

Transthyretin (formerly known as prealbumin) is a carrier protein for thyroid hormone (the major carrier is thyroid-binding globulin, an α_1-globulin), and also transports retinols and progesterone. It may be helpful to lower the level of thyroid hormone in the periphery, perhaps modifying metabolism during inflammation. Patients with chronic inflammation may have alterations in thyroid hormone levels with normal thyroxine but diminished triiodothyronine concentrations, the so-called sick euthyroid state. Whether changes in the peripheral conversion of thyroxine to triiodothyronine or changes in transthyretin levels are the primary cause in such alterations is not known.

The Positive APR

The proteins which make up the positive APR can be broadly grouped into six overlapping functions (Table 16-2). A note of caution: We know these molecules by what they do in a test tube or by in vitro bioassays. There is no guarantee that these lab tests are a true indication of their in vivo physiologic roles.

Group I

Ceruloplasmin (an α_2-globulin) is the major copper transport protein. It also may have the ability to scavenge oxygen radicals in a noncatalytic, stoichiometric fashion and/or may have superoxide-dismutase activity, thus possibly preventing tissue damage. Ceruloplasmin may have a role in iron metabolism. It has ferroxidase activity, changing ferrous (Fe^{2+}) to ferric (Fe^{3+}) ions; ferrous iron is released from hemoglobin and ferric iron is the form bound by transferrin. Thus ceruloplasmin may play a role in the removal of iron derived from hemoglobin released from red blood cells at the site of an inflammatory process. Efficient removal would deny the iron to pathogens.

Also in group I are the complement components B, C3, and C4 (all β-globulins). The function of complement is described in Chap. 5; this is a good time to review these functions from your new perspective of the integrated APR. It is clear that the opsonic, chemotactic, vasodilatory, and cytolytic activities of the protein fragments produced in the complement cascade are all of importance in inflammation and immune responsiveness.

Group II

AGP, previously known as orosomucoid, is the plasma protein with the highest carbohydrate content, about 50 percent by weight. AGP accounts for about 30 percent of the total α_1-serum fraction. It is likely that the polysaccharide chains of AGP account for some of its physiologic functions, e.g., its

---

TABLE 16-2   Functions of Positive APR Proteins

Function	APR Proteins Engaged
Inhibition of proteases	Macroglobulins, α_1-PI, α_1-antichymotrypsin, haptoglobin
Blood clotting and fibrinolysis	Fibrinogen, C1-esterase inhibitor, AGP, SAP, CRP
Removal of foreign materials	CRP, SAA, SAP, C3, fibrinogen
Modulation of immune response	Protease inhibitors, CRP, C3, AGP, fibrinogen, haptoglobin
Anti-inflammatory properties	Protease inhibitors, haptoglobin, ceruloplasmin, fibrinopeptides
Binding and transport of metals and biologically active compounds	Haptoglobin, transferrin, albumin, transthyretin, ceruloplasmin, AGP, macrogobulin

ability to interact with a variety of cellular membranes. AGP blocks the interaction of malaria parasites (*Plasmodium* species) with red blood cells. AGP may inhibit platelet aggregation. Other possible functions include activity as an antiprotease (e.g., inhibition of thromboplastin, part of the coagulation cascade; see Chap. 14), and binding to and inactivating heparin.

There is in vitro evidence to suggest that AGP may be immunosuppressive. When added to cultures, AGP decreases T-cell mitogen responses, cell-mediated cytolysis, and mixed lymphocyte reactions, diminishes monocyte chemotaxis and phagocytosis, and decreases antibody responses to sheep red blood cells. No effect on natural killer (NK) cell activity has been found. Which, if any, of these is of physiologic relevance is not known. (It is clear that the proteases on the surface of some immune cells have a role in normal function. In general, if a compound has antiprotease activity, in vitro immunomodulatory effects are likely.)

Haptoglobin, which accounts for about 25 percent of the total α_2 fraction, binds hemoglobin and functions in the disposal of free hemoglobin at sites of inflammation (recall the function of ceruloplasmin in iron removal). Haptoglobin may also have antiprotease activity, and there are reports that it may modify prostaglandin production. (Chapter 15 discusses the role of prostaglandins in modifying immune reactivity.) Haptoglobin also may have natural bacteriostatic activity. The specific immune response is not instantaneous; it may be a few days until antigen-specific T cells and antibodies are available to defeat an invading organism. In the meantime, a variety of nonspecific responses must suffice. These nonspecific aspects of the immune response include interferon and the APR, as well as other "defenses" described in Chap. 22, on immunodeficiency.

Haptoglobin may also be immunomodulatory; it can suppress lymphocyte blastogenesis and monocyte chemotaxis, in vitro. Recent studies suggest that haptoglobin may play a role in bone resorption.

Fibrinogen, a β-globulin, is well known as a key protein in coagulation (see Chap. 14), but also may act as an opsonin by enhancing the clumping of certain microorganisms, including staphylococci and streptococci. Proteolytic fragments of fibrinogen, known as fibrinopeptides A and B, may have anti-inflammatory activity. Fibrinogen itself has been reported to block T-cell mitogen reactivity and macrophage chemotaxis.

α_1-PI is the major protease inhibitor in human plasma, providing about 70 percent of the inhibition of serine proteases in the coagulation, fibrinolytic, kinin, and complement systems. Table 16-3 lists the serine proteases inhibited. It is the major α_1-protein, accounting for nearly 70 percent of that serum fraction. α_1-PI is involved in modulation of serine proteases, as well as in control of tissue damage. About 55 percent of α-PI is extravascular, in keeping with its major role in tissue protease control. The crucial nature of this role is well demonstrated by the problems found in people with

TABLE 16-3   Serine Proteases Inhibited by α_1-PI

Most Activity	Moderate Activity	Some Activity
Chymotrypsin	Plasminogen activator	Kallikrein
Trypsin	Renin	Plasmin
Cathepsin	Sperm acrosin	Thrombin
Leukocyte elastase	Hyaluronidase	Hageman factor
Collagenase		
Urokinase		
Leukocyte neutral protease		
Complement proteases		

a congenital absence of α_1-PI, where the tissue damage is likely due to the uncontrolled activity of leukocyte-derived elastase. (See Clinical Aside 16-1.) This is one example of the many inborn errors of metabolism which may lead to tissue damage.

Clinical Aside 16-1
α_1-Protease Inhibitor (α_1-PI) Deficiency

A number of years ago a group of patients who had the onset of a type of lung damage known as emphysema in the third to fourth decade were identified; these patients were often dead by age 50. They were found to have deficient serum α_1-PI activity. This problem often ran in families and was often accompanied by liver disease or frank cirrhosis, which could occur in the neonatal period. On liver biopsy, the hepatocytes were often full of globules that stained positively with the periodic acid-Schiff reagent; this material turned out to be unsecreted α_1-PI. On acid-starch gel electrophoresis analysis some of these people had an abnormal inhibitor which migrated either slower (S type) or much slower (Z type) than normal (called M for medium speed migration). The S type had diminished activity, so that a heterozygote with half M and half S had only 75 percent of normal inhibitory activity. MZ heterozygotes had 57 percent activity, and SZ had 37 percent; individuals with only Z (who could be a ZZ homozygote or have one Z gene and one null allele) had only 16 percent activity. Replacement therapy with intravenous purified α-PI has been successful. Currently recombinant inhibitor, delivered directly by aerosol into the lung, is being tested.

Thus the absence of a protease inhibitor predisposes to the development of disease in the liver and lung, both places where leukocyte elastase might mediate tissue damage.

α_1-PI binds to secretory and serum IgA and protects them from the IgA proteases of *Neisseria gonorrhoeae* (the agent which causes gonorrhea), *N meningitidis* (a common cause of meningitis), *Haemophilus influenzae* (a leading cause of infection in young children until an effective vaccine became available), and *Streptococcus pneumoniae* (a common cause of pneumonia and of sepsis in older patients).

α_1-PI also has immunosuppressive effects. Both B-cell responses to antigens and T-cell responses to mitogens have been suppressed by α_1-PI. Decreased NK cell activity, antibody-dependent cytotoxicity, and polymorphonuclear cell and macrophage chemiluminescence have been found. Alteration of cell surface proteases by α_1-PI may be the explanation for the decreased IL-1 production or binding induced by α_1-PI.

The parsimony of nature dictates that when a molecular structure is efficient it is often reused in different settings. There are many "superfamilies," where a shared molecular motif is reused in different proteins. Antithrombin III (coagulation control protein), α_1-PI, α_1-antichymotrypsin, and angiotensinogen are all part of such a superfamily. (For other examples of superfamilies and their evolution, see Appendix A.)

Another superfamily includes complement components C3 and C4, α_2-macroglobulin, and a recently defined protein called *PZP* (for *pregnancy zone protein*, also called α_2-pregnancy-associated glycoprotein). The common structure in each is an internal reactive β-cysteinyl-γ-glutamyl thiol ester. Normally present in trace quantities (10 to 30 mg/L in women, less than 10 mg/L in men), PZP levels increase rapidly in the first trimester of pregnancy; by the end of pregnancy PZP levels reach 1000 mg/L. It is found in fluids of the reproductive organs and has been isolated from placenta.

PZP can covalently bind proteases, with two potential outcomes. PZP inhibits the activity of urokinase and of plasmin, and inhibits complement-induced cytolysis. By binding to enzymes PZP can also prevent binding of α_1-PI and preserve protease activity. PZP may have immunosuppressive activity; in vitro PZP suppresses mixed lymphocyte reaction, T-cell mitogen response reactivity, and macrophage mobility; intravenous PZP increases survival of murine heart transplants. PZP is found on the surface of a subpopulation of about 25 percent of peripheral blood T cells and on some macrophages, but not on B cells.

What is the presumed function of PZP? Recall that the fetus is a foreign graft on the mother. (See Chap. 27, "Pregnancy and the Fetal-Maternal Relationship" for a more detailed discussion of the issues involved in maintenance of the graft.) It is possible that PZP has a role in the maintenance of pregnancy, perhaps by modulating surface proteases, perhaps as an immunomodulatory substance.

α_1-Antichymotrypsin is another protease inhibitor of more limited spectrum, affecting collagenase, cathepsin, chymase, and leukocyte elastase. It also has immunosuppressive effects on both NK and antibody-dependent cytotoxic cell activity.

Group III

SAA-related protein levels increase 100- to 1000-fold during inflammation. SAA is found in association with the high density lipoprotein HDL_3, leading to the theory that SAA may help in eliminating microorganism-derived lipids or toxins complexed to lipoproteins. In describing the previous APR proteins, it has been implicit that there is no heterogeneity of structure, with the stated exception of α_1-PI. However, microheterogeneity of the SAA molecule has been found in comparisons of individuals and over time in a given individual. This may help explain the occurrence of amyloidosis, a disease seen in some people with chronic inflammatory conditions, including rheumatoid arthritis, chronic osteomyelitis, and Still's disease (systemic childhood chronic arthritis). See Clinical Aside 16-2.

Clinical Aside 16-2
Amyloidosis

Amyloidosis is the buildup of a waxy, eosinophilic material which causes dysfunction of various organs. The material was thought to be a starch, or celluloselike material; hence it was called *amyloidosis*, which has the same root as *amylase*, the enzyme which degrades starch. The deposits are actually a packed mass of fibrillar proteins, which assume a beta pleated sheet structure. A number of proteins can assume this structure and can theoretically form amyloid deposits, often after proteolytic digestion of a normal serum protein precursor. A characteristic of amyloid deposits is staining with the dye Congo red.

The unanswered question: Is amyloidosis due to (1) abnormal proteolytic modification of a normal protein, (2) an enzymatic defect which makes it impossible to remove a normal protein, or (3) production of a protein whose amino acid sequence is slightly different from the usual? There is good evidence in support of the last model. Microheterogeneity of SAA has been described, and at least four discrete amino acid substitutions have been described in transthyretin in the different hereditary polyneuropathic amyloidoses; refer to a general medical text.

Amyloidosis is not a single disease (a triumph of "splitters" over "lumpers"); it can be: (1) primary, associated with an underlying myeloma, (2) secondary to an underlying chronic inflammatory state, (3) hereditary, and (4) localized (a grab bag of different phenomena); see Table 16A-1.

C-Reactive protein (CRP) is the other spectacular human APR. First described and named for its ability to precipitate the C polysaccharide of the organism *S. pneumoniae*, CRP can bind to a large number of organisms and to a range of molecules including polysaccharides, phospholipids, and polycations. CRP has a peculiar structure, with five platelike molecules in a pentagon. It is also the structure of serum amyloid P component and rat female serum protein, all of which are called *pentaxins* or *pentraxins*. This structure is phylogenetically highly conserved; pentaxinlike compounds are found as early in evolution as the horseshoe crab, *Limulus polyphemus*. The persistence of the pentaxin motif, coupled with the impressive acute phase increase in CRP, suggests that CRP may have an important role in human defenses.

The end result of the binding of CRP to bacteria is capsular swelling, precipitation, and agglutination of the microorganism. CRP bound to microorganisms, phospholipids, or polycations fixes complement, increasing opsonization and clearance of the bound

TABLE 16A-1   Types of Amyloidosis

Name	Underlying Condition	Precursor Protein	Amyloid Type
Primary	Myeloma	Ig V_L	AL (L = light)
Secondary	Inflammatory conditions*	SAA	AA (A = amyloid A)
Hereditary familial polyneuropathies	None	Transthyretin	AF (F = familial)
Familial Mediterranean fever	None	SAA	AA
Localized			
Endocrine-related			
Thyroid	Medullary cancer of the thyroid	Calcitonin	AE_T (Endocrine, thyroid)
Pancreatic islet	None	Insulin	AE_P (Endocrine, pancreas)
Senile cardiac	None	?Transthyretin	AS_C (Senile cardiac)
Carpal tunnel and osteoarticular	Long-term hemodialysis	β_2-microglobulin	$AM\beta_{2m}$
Cerebral amyloid angiopathy†*	None	γ trace protein (cystatin)	—

*The major causes in 1991 were poorly controlled rheumatoid arthritis and chronic osteomyelitis; years ago the number 1 cause was tuberculosis.
†May be inherited as an autosomal dominant trait. This entity is not to be confused with Alzheimer's disease, where examination of the brain shows neuritic plaques and neurofibrillary tangles; transthyretin may be a major component of these structures.

particle and causing the generation of chemotactic factors. CRP binds to necrotic tissue and may help speed phagocytic removal. By binding to a wide variety of self-antigens, especially chromatin, CRP may protect the immune system from exposure to autoantigens and help avoid autoimmune reactions. CRP can bind to other biologic molecules, and may be part of the pathogenesis of two entities not usually associated with the APR: fat embolization and gout (see Clinical Aside 16-3).

Clinical Aside 16-3
CRP and the Pathogenesis of Disease

Purified CRP or acute phase serum can agglutinate very low density lipoproteins (VLDL) and the fats found in intravenous dietary supplements. It has been suggested that this may be relevant to a relatively rare complication of surgery, known as *fat embolus*, which occurs about 2 days after trauma or surgery. It is theorized that the increasing levels of CRP present 2 days after surgery or trauma (both of which engender an APR, right?) complex with circulating VLDL. Complement fixation by this complex causes the vascular collapse seen in the fat embolization syndrome.

Monosodium urate crystals can bind CRP. Such coated crystals fix complement, causing local inflammation; this may be the pathogenesis of attacks of the gout often seen after surgery. (Please refer to a medical text for a full discussion of both of these clinical entities.)

CRP binds to immune cells, especially to antigen-activated, rather than mitogen-activated, T cells, and to NK cells and macrophages. CRP can alter NK-cell activity and B-cell responses, and can cause platelet aggregation. CRP given to animals increases survival from infection and decreases the growth of tumors. Thus, there is reason to suspect that CRP may have an ancient and important role in survival.

CRP has a role in the evaluation of inflammatory disease. The rapid rise of CRP levels makes it a good lab marker of recent acute inflammation. Neonates normally make CRP by day 3 of life, due to umbilical cord necrosis. (Neonates also make AGP, but not haptoglobin or α_1-PI, in what seems to be an "immature" APR.) Checking CRP levels may be valuable in determining whether an infant is infected.

Other inflammatory diseases are associated with elevated serum concentrations of CRP. Patients with severe rheumatoid arthritis have elevated CRP levels (why?). Disease progression and severity correlate with the levels of CRP, and fall during remission. Patients with vasculitis, ankylosing spondylitis, and childhood chronic arthritis also have elevated CRP levels. In contrast, some studies of patients with other autoimmune diseases, including SLE, progressive systemic sclerosis, and dermatomyositis, have found normal serum CRP (see Chap. 31, on autoimmunity). Patients with SLE may develop fever and other clinical manifestations compatible with either a flare of SLE or with an intercurrent infection; in such a setting an elevated CRP may be the first clue to the presence of a problem not related to a lupus flare, although this is of unproven clinical value.

Thus, a discussion of CRP is in many ways a good summary of the APR proteins. CRP has many in vitro activities, although the in vivo significance of these is unclear. It may assist the immune system by participating in control of infection before the emergence of a true immune response to the pathogen. CRP may modulate a variety of immune mechanisms and has activities which suggest the ability to speed the clean-up of debris and repair of damaged tissue. (Some studies suggest that APR proteins may actually *interfere* with the immune response to malignancy and/or help tumors grow. Recall that the APR is a response to necrosis. The furtherance of tissue repair and growth is seemingly one of the APR's main functions. Can you see how the APR proteins might favor tumor growth?) Finally, CRP is not uniformly elevated in all forms of inflammation.

Induction of the APR

After the onset of inflammation there is a rapid change in the pattern of hepatic protein synthesis. But how is this complicated change orchestrated? Before you read the next section, please review the chapters on cytokines and monocytes, for it is the cytokines which are at the root of the APR.

Rat liver cells, in sections of whole organ, suspensions of cells, or cultures of hepatoma lines, can make an APR in vitro. Stimulation with the crude supernatant from a culture of rat macrophages (containing IL-1, TNF, and other monokines) causes the in vitro elaboration of a typical rat APR. Exposure of the cells to IL-1, TNF, or IL-6 (formerly known as beta$_2$ interferon) alone causes an incomplete APR. Thus, the complete APR seems to be induced by the combined effects of multiple cytokines.

Hormonal influences on the APR, e.g., synergy of cytokines with dexamethasone, was shown in rat hepatocyte cultures. Hormones like thyroxine, epinephrine, estrogens, and testosterone, and peptide hormones like glucagon, insulin, and growth hormone, have a variety of effects on the spectrum of APR proteins.

Of major clinical relevance is the influence of the steroid sex hormones, most notably estrogen, on levels of APR proteins. Estrogen increases the synthesis of PZP, a member of the α_2-macroglobulin superfamily. Pregnancy and oral contraceptives cause an increase in ceruloplasmin, α_1-PI, fibrinogen, C3, and C4. The increase in fibrinogen induced by the estrogens in oral contraceptives is one of the causes of a major side effect of their use: thrombosis, strokes, and pulmonary emboli.

C3 and C4 levels increase in pregnancy. We often measure C3 and C4 levels in lupus; lowered levels are a relatively early indication of consumption of complement in the inflammatory lesion of the kidney, glomerulonephritis. Would this knowledge of changes in complement levels affect your interpretation of C3 and C4 levels in your pregnant lupus patient?

There is an optimal concentration of particular hormones for the maximal synthesis of each APR protein, with glucocorticoids probably permissive for most. It is known that glucocorticoids decrease inflammation and therefore dampen the APR. There is another negative-feedback loop: IL-6 and IL-1 both induce the production of adrenocorticotrophic hormone (ACTH) in the pituitary, which then stimulates the production of glucocorticoids in the adrenal cortex. Dexamethasone directly blocks the production of IL-6 by monocytes (such feedback systems interlocking the immune, endocrine, and neurologic systems are discussed in more detail in Chap. 23, "Psychoneuroimmunology").

Products of the APR themselves influence the APR. The digestion of fibrinogen by plasmin releases two fragments, fibrinopeptides D and E. These both suppress IL-6 production by monocytes; native fibrinogen has no such effect.

So, the APR is regulated by hormones, cytokines, and interactions with other physiologic systems. As is so often the case, the diagram which summarizes the known influences on the APR is a complex array of crisscrossing lines (Fig. 16-4). But what ultimately happens within hepatocytes? It is worthwhile reviewing the steps involved in protein synthesis. The control of the APR may occur at multiple levels, including transcription, translation, and posttranslational processes.

In the negative APR, decreases in transcription precede any decrease in the level of APR protein mRNA, suggesting rapid turnoff of transcription. In the positive APR, an absolute increase in mRNA levels occurs, followed a few hours later by increased serum

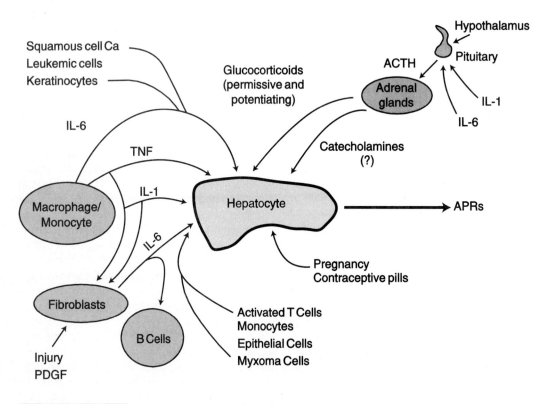

Figure 16-4 Mechanisms active in the control of the APR.

levels of the APR proteins. The increase in mRNA levels is due to decreased degradation and/or increased stability of the mRNA for some proteins and a combination of increased stability and transcription rate in others. Rates of protein secretion may also be increased, each molecule's residence within the cell being shorter. Glycosylation of proteins and changes in the patterns of glycosylation occur independently of changes in cellular mRNA or serum protein levels.

Each hepatocyte can produce multiple APR proteins, as well as increase the amount of protein produced. The coordinately increased expression of multiple proteins may be due to common regulatory sequences; the 5' untranslated region of α_1-PI, AGP, and haptoglobin share consensus sequences, with possible regulatory significance.

The pattern of sequential recruitment of new hepatocytes supports the belief that blood-borne messengers signal the liver to start the APR. Early in inflammation, only hepatocytes in the periportal region (nearest the blood vessels) synthesize APR proteins. Later, cells further from the portal tracts, in the midlobule and then the center of the hepatic lobule, begin.

APR proteins can also be produced outside of the liver. α_1-PI is made by monocytes and neutrophils, and monocytes probably produce C3, C4, factor B, and other complement components. Transthyretin and transferrin are produced in the placenta, the yolk sac, and the choroid plexus; there is evidence that a peptide derived from transthyretin may form the plaques seen in Alzheimers disease (see Table 16A-1).

ERYTHROCYTE SEDIMENTATION RATE

The most commonly used measure of the APR is called the *erythrocyte sedimentation rate* (*ESR*, or "sed rate"). Centuries ago, Galen was the first to note that the red blood cells (RBCs) of people with disease sedimented rapidly. In the eighteenth century physicians first tried to measure and explain the phenomenon, and since 1921 physicians have been using the ESR clinically.

Two techniques have been widely used. The Wintrobe ESR uses undiluted blood, anticoagulated with sodium oxalate and placed in a 100-mm-long small-bore tube. Due to packing of the RBCs at the bottom of the tube, ESRs of over 60 mm/h cannot be measured, and this technique is very sensitive to anemia. The Wintrobe ESR has been supplanted by the Westergren ESR, which uses a 200-mm tube and blood diluted 4 : 1 with an anticoagulant, either sodium citrate or EDTA. The advantage of the Westergren ESR is its lower normal range, less sensitivity to anemia, better reproducibility, and, due to the longer tube used, greater accuracy at higher ESR values. [For males normal is age/2; for females normal is (age + 10)/2. Why do you think there is a change in normal values with age?]

RBCs have sialic acid residues on their surface, whose negative charge causes the cells to repel. Serum proteins with a positive charge could neutralize the sialic acid charges; were this to happen, the cells would come together more easily. The more positive the charge and the more asymmetric the positively charged molecule the more the neutralization. Once the charge is neutralized, the RBC can pack more closely and sedimentation results. Fibrinogen is a positively charged molecule and is the most asymmetric of plasma proteins. Anything which increases fibrinogen levels would therefore be expected to increase sedimentation. Since fibrinogen is an APR protein, it stands to reason that the ESR would increase in inflammatory conditions. Other proteins, including α_2-, β-, and γ-globulins, contribute as well, but fibrinogen is the major cause of the increased ESR in inflammation. (Given the influence of estrogens and pregnancy on fibrinogen levels, what would you predict would happen to the ESR during pregnancy?) Patients with certain kinds of plasma cell malignancies produce large quantities of very positively charged immunoglobulin (γ-globulin)—as you would predict, these patients have very accelerated ESRs.

Sedimentation depends on the ability of cells to aggregate in a rouleau, the RBCs stacking like pennies in a wrapper. Normal serum causes a slight increase in rouleaux formation; with an increase in the concentration of either RBC or aggregating substances, there is an increase in the speed and stability of rouleaux formation. Any abnormality of the RBC shape which interferes with stacking and rouleaux formation will depress the ESR. Thus, patients with sickle cell anemia or abnormalities of RBC like spherocytosis, acanthocytosis, or anisocytosis may not increase their ESR even during severe infection.

In the presence of extremely elevated WBC counts (e.g., leukemia) RBCs may have trouble forming rouleaux and the ESR may be falsely low. Any form of anemia will tend to increase the ESR (less frictional forces to keep the RBCs suspended). Any form of polycythemia (increased number of RBCs per milliliter of blood) will decrease the ESR; thus patients with the myelodysplastic syndrome polycythemia rubra vera (literally, "truly increased number of RBCs") and infants, who have very high hemoglobin and hematocrit for the first few weeks of life, will have artifactually low ESR, making interpretation difficult. In all these cases the ESR, which can be a very useful test when appreciated in the clinical context, may be misleading. In the case of a newborn infant thought to be septic, a good pediatrician would not wait for the ESR or the CRP results—he or she would evaluate the infant, culture appropriately, and treat aggressively, pending results of the cultures. In certain circumstances, tests may be of little value; a too-often-ignored message in medical practice is *treat the patient, not the lab test!*

Drugs and physiologic compounds may also affect the ESR. Extremely elevated serum bile salt levels or therapy with the antiseizure medication valproic acid can decrease the ESR, whereas extreme elevations of cholesterol levels and therapy with heparin may increase the ESR. Both hyper- and hypothyroidism have been associated with elevated ESR, as has chronic renal failure; such patients have a normal CRP and an accelerated ESR. (How might this be valuable knowledge to the clinician?)

What would you predict the ESR to be in patients with the congenital inability to make fibrinogen (congenital hypofibrinogenemia)? In sepsis, where the coagulation system is activated and much of the fibrinogen is consumed (called *consumption coagulopathy* or *disseminated intravascular coagulation—DIC* for short)? In a hyperviscosity syndrome, where abnormal serum proteins increase the plasma viscosity?

So, the ESR can be altered by a lot more than the APR. When properly used, the ESR serves as a confirmation of a diagnosis suggested by historical and physical findings. An abnormal ESR itself does not make a diagnosis. The ESR can be elevated in perfectly healthy people and it can be normal in patients with active inflammatory diseases. An elevated ESR may also be transitory.

An extremely accelerated ESR (over 100 mm/h), however, is a very powerful predictor of the presence of disease. In one study, only 2 percent of patients with such an elevated ESR did not have disease, and 95 percent of the patients had infection, malignancy, or a connective tissue disease. Such an extremely accelerated ESR is rarely the only clue to illness; a complete history and physical examination are the best way to make a diagnosis.

Despite the above caveat, the ESR and the CRP can be very useful tests in the management of certain inflammatory diseases. It may be that the CRP is a better test in assessing response to therapy, since the CRP begins to fall before the ESR (why?); CRP also correlates better than ESR with disease activity in rheumatoid arthritis. However, when used properly, these tests, which directly measure APR proteins, are useful as confirmation of clinical impressions. The ESR and the CRP and all the other tests available are merely tools, valuable only when used by a thoughtful clinician in conjunction with, and subservient to, clinical judgement.

SELF-TEST QUESTIONS*

Identify each of the following as a positive (+) or a negative (−) APR:
1. Ceruloplasmin
2. Transthyretin
3. Haptoglobin
4. Albumin
5. Fibrinogen
6. C-reactive protein
7. Transferrin
8. All of the following are descriptions of major functions of APR proteins *except:*
   a. Inhibition of proteases
   b. Binding and transport of metals
   c. Suppression of endothelial procoagulant activity
   d. Removal of foreign proteins
9. Which of the following cytokines has not been implicated in the control of the APR
   a. IL-6
   b. IL-1
   c. TNF
   d. IFN-γ
10. Clinical conditions known to be associated with an artifactually decreased erythrocyte sedimentation rate include all of the following *except:*
   a. Pregnancy
   b. Sickle cell anemia
   c. Normal infants
   d. Polycythemia

ADDITIONAL READINGS

Fey GH, Fuller GM. Regulation of acute phase gene expression by inflammatory mediators. *Mol Biol Med.* 1987;4:323–338.

Fleck A. Acute phase response: Implications for nutrition and recovery. *Nutrition.* 1989;4:109–117.

Kushner I, Volanakis JE, Gewurz G, eds. C-reactive protein and the plasma protein response to tissue injury. *Ann NY Acad Sci.* 1982;389.

Sehgal PB, Grieninger G, Tosato G, eds. Regulation of the acute phase and immune responses: Interleukin-6. *Ann NY Acad Sci.* 1989;557.

*Answers will be found in Appendix E.

17

Polymorphonuclear Phagocytic Cells

INTRODUCTION

Human neutrophils, or polymorphonuclear leukocytes (PMN), comprise 60 to 70 percent of the total leukocyte count in the peripheral blood of the adult. The neutrophil life cycle can be divided into a bone marrow, blood, and tissue phase. An ancestral stem cell in the bone marrow undergoes a series of cell divisions, then maturation through myeloblast, promyelocyte, myelocyte, metamyelocyte, band, and finally mature neutrophil. Granulocyte colony-stimulating factor (G-CSF) is elaborated by activated monocytes and drives neutrophil production and differentiation. Distinct classes of granules appear with cell maturation, classically referred to as primary, secondary, and tertiary granules. However, recent evidence suggests a more complex heterogeneity of these granules.

Neutrophils are phagocytic cells whose major function is to seek out and destroy microorganisms. Chemotaxins generated by bacteria or the inflammatory process bind to specific neutrophil receptors and initiate chemotaxis toward offending agents. Phagocytosis and degranulation initiate a respiratory burst which enzymatically generates oxidants that participate in killing microorganisms. The granules also release a number of components which facilitate bacterial killing or digestions by anaerobic mechanisms. Disorders of neutrophil function arise from aberrations of their normal physiology. This can result in clinical manifestations and profound consequences from recurrent life-threatening bacterial infections.

NEUTROPHIL GRANULOCYTE

Neutrophil Life Cycle

The life cycle of the neutrophil encompasses residence within the bone marrow and blood and final arrival in the tissues. Within the bone marrow there is a mitotic compartment

and a nonmitotic storage compartment consisting of relatively mature cells. Transit time through the marrow compartment is approximately 14 days, with 6 of those days being spent in the mitotic compartment. The bone marrow produces approximately 60 to 400 $\times$ 10^7 neutrophils per day. The bone marrow storage compartment in adults contains approximately 8.8×10^9 cells, whereas the circulating granulocyte pool and the marginating granulocyte pool, composed of blood neutrophils, contain 0.7×10^9 cells. Thus, most of the neutrophils in the body reside in the bone marrow, and peripheral blood counts directly measure less than 10 percent of total body neutrophils.

Peripheral blood neutrophil counts vary significantly with age. During the first few days of life there is a leukocytosis with generally over 10,000 neutrophils per mm^3 of blood. This rapidly falls to an average of approximately 3000 to 4000 neutrophils per mm^3, which is maintained throughout life. Up to 2 years of age lymphocytes generally outnumber neutrophils; after that, neutrophils comprise more than 50 percent of peripheral blood leukocytes. Absolute neutrophil counts can fall to as low as 1000 cells per mm^3 during the first year of life; however, after that neutrophil counts are generally greater than 1500 cells per mm.[3]

Granulocytes from the bone marrow are released as a result of complex interactions between the mature leukocyte membrane and the endothelial lining and basement membrane of bone marrow capillaries and sinusoids and a number of stimulating or releasing factors. Once released into the blood the neutrophils have a half-life of 6 to 9 h and reversibly move from circulating to marginating (attached to endothelial cells) pools. The granulocytes leave the blood by penetrating endothelial cells which are modified by inflammatory reactions or as a result of neutrophil attachment. Once in the tissues the major functions of the neutrophils are performed which generally involve utilization of granules through phagocytosis and secretory activities related to clearance of foreign material or unwanted debris.

Neutrophil Development

Stem Cells and Myeloblasts

Neutrophilic leukocytes and other granulocytes are derived from undifferentiated blasts and myeloblasts which comprise up to 3 percent of bone marrow cells. The earliest cell committed to a multipotent differentiation pathway has been termed CFU-GEMM (colony-forming unit—granulocyte, erythrocyte, monocyte, megakaryocyte), which forms as a result of GM-CSF (granulocyte-monocyte colony-stimulating factor) action on the stem cell. This in turn differentiates to CFU-GM, which is driven toward myeloid differentiation by the hematopoietic hormone G-CSF. Both GM-CSF and G-CSF are elaborated by a variety of marrow cells including endothelial cells and activated monocytes.

Myeloblasts represent the earliest stage of the mitotic myeloid compartment, with a transit time of approximately 18 h. Myeloblasts often lack morphologic features that predict their differentiation into one of the granulocytic lines and vary from 10 to 15 μm in diameter. The single round nucleus contains abundant dispersed chromatin and one to four distinct nucleoli averaging 1.5 μm in diameter. The cytoplasm appears gray-blue in Wright-stained preparations and circumferentially surrounds the nucleus. Numerous polyribosomes and some segments of endoplasmic reticulum are present (Fig. 17-1). There is a variably prominent Golgi region from which the formation of the first cytoplasmic granules allows definitive identification of differentiation of myeloblasts into neutrophilic leukocytes. Peroxidase can frequently be identified in these granules or in the Golgi complex and endoplasmic reticulum. The appearance of myeloperoxidase in the granule marks the transition of a myeloblast to a promyelocyte in the course of granulocytic differentiation. Myeloperoxidase is a central component of the myeloperoxidase–hydrogen peroxide–halide microbicidal system of the phagocyte and, therefore,

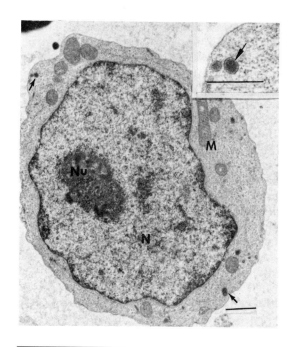

Figure 17-1 This typical myeloblast contains a single nucleus (N) with dispersed nuclear chromatin and a large nucleolus (Nu). The cytoplasm is less prominent with sparse endoplasmic reticulum, large mitochondria (M), and occasional identifying small primary granules (arrows and enlarged in inset). Human bone marrow, stained with uranyl acetate and lead citrate. Bar = 1 μm, inset bar = 0.5 μm.

is an important element of the body's host defenses. The human myeloperoxidase gene has recently been cloned by several laboratories and localized to human chromosome 17q22-24.

Promyelocytes and Azurophilic Granules

Early neutrophilic leukocytes or promyelocytes comprise approximately 2 to 4 percent of marrow cells and include a morphologic spectrum of cells involved in synthesis of lysosomal granules termed primary or azurophilic granules. This cell is in the mid stage of the mitotic compartment, with a transit time of approximately 24 h. In Wright-stained smears, the cells average 13 to 18 μm in diameter, with a single round nucleus that contains predominantly dispersed nuclear chromatin and one to two nucleoli. The cytoplasm is abundant and contains numerous segments of dilated rough endoplasmic reticulum and polyribosomes accounting for the basophilia seen in light microscopic preparations. The Golgi apparatus is prominent and appears as a clear perinuclear zone in light microscopic preparations (Fig. 17-2). Numerous vesicles can be observed budding from the Golgi apparatus and coalescing to form condensing vacuoles or granule precursors. Variable numbers of primary granules in different stages of maturation and/or con-

densation can be observed throughout the cytoplasm. Secondary or specific granules are not observed at the promyelocyte stage of development.

Primary granules vary from deeply azurophilic to neutral in Wright-stained preparations with the most intense staining observed in the immature granules (Fig. 17-2). At least some of this staining appears to represent glycosaminoglycans, including chondroitin sulfate. Primary granules, as seen in ultrastructural preparations, vary from 0.2 to 0.4 μm in diameter. Ultrastructural cyto-

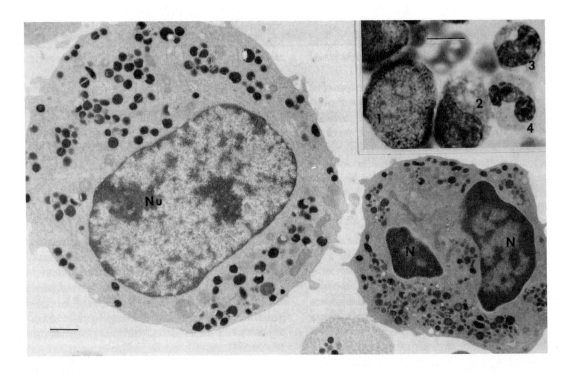

Figure 17-2 A promyelocyte with a moderate number of cytoplasmic primary or azurophilic granules and endoplasmic reticulum. The large, round nucleus contains dispersed nuclear chromatin and prominent nucleoli (Nu). The smaller segmented neutrophil at the right contains numerous pleomorphic cytoplasmic granules but otherwise sparse cytoplasmic organelles; and two nuclear lobes (N) with condensed chromatin. Electron micrograph from human bone marrow stained with uranyl acetate and lead citrate. Bar = 1 μm. The inset compares a similar Wright's stained promyelocyte (1) with numerous azurophil granules; a myelocyte (2); metamyelocyte (3); and segmented neutrophil (4, right). Neutrophils contain numerous secondary or specific granules which lack affinity for cationic dyes and primary granules are less prominent. Bar = 10 μm.

chemistry and biochemical studies have localized peroxidase (Fig. 17-3), acid phosphate, β-glucuronidase, aryl sulfatase, elastase, and proteases in endoplasmic reticulum, Golgi vesicles, and primary granules of promyelocytes and/or isolated primary granules.

Myelocytes and Specific Granules

Neutrophilic myelocytes vary from 10 to 15 μm in diameter and comprise approximately 13 percent of marrow nucleated cells. Myelocytes represent the last stage of the mitotic compartment, with a transit time of 104 h, which presumably represents three to four cell divisions. The cells contain a slightly indented nucleus with predominantly dispersed nuclear chromatin and one or two small nucleoli. The abundant cytoplasm contains numerous cytoplasmic granules, some of which lack azurophilia and represent specific or secondary granules not found in promyelocytes. The cytoplasm is less basophilic than promyelocytes and corresponds ultrastructurally to the presence of less dilated rough endoplasmic reticulum and fewer polyribosomes. The Golgi apparatus of neutrophilic myelocytes is rather prominent, corresponding to a clear zone in light microscopic preparations, and to an area with distinct lamellae and budding vesicles forming secondary granules in ultrastructural preparations.

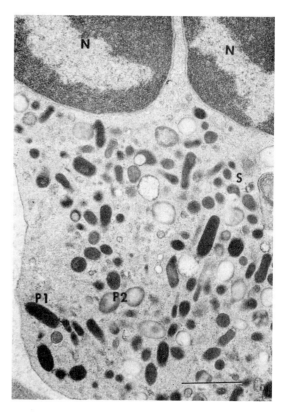

Figure 17-4 This electron micrograph enlarges a portion of human neutrophil cytoplasm demonstrating a variety of cytoplasmic granules. In general, primary granules are larger and tend to have a uniformly dense (P1) or rim density (P2) type of staining. Presumed secondary granules (S) tend to be smaller and are moderately dense, often overlapping in size with primary granules. N = nuclei. Peripheral blood stained with uranyl acetate and lead citrate. Bar = 1 μm.

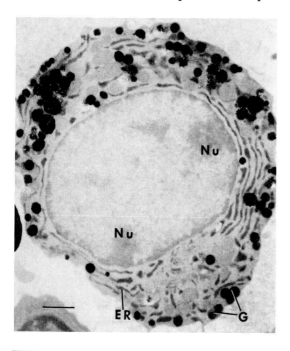

Figure 17-3 Diaminobenzidine stains myeloperoxidase in the endoplasmic reticulum (ER) and cytoplasmic granules (G) of this human bone marrow promyelocyte. The cell contains a single round nucleus with two nucleoli (Nu). Thin section not counterstained. Bar = 1 μm.

The onset of secondary granule genesis appears to be the most consistent morphologic feature which identifies neutrophilic myelocytes. Ultrastructurally, human secondary granules vary from 0.1 to 0.3 μm in diameter, are moderately dense, and may be elongated in appearance (Fig. 17-4). Although in humans the granules overlap in size with primary granules, they appear to have less osmiophilia and less affinity for metal counterstains in ultrastructural preparations. In most species, secondary granules outnumber primary granules by a ratio of 3:1 in late myeloid cells.

Secondary granules contain glycoproteins, lactoferrin, vitamin B_{12}–binding protein, NADPH oxidase, and cytochrome B. Lacto-

ferrin is an iron-binding protein with antimicrobial properties that is present in mature neutrophils but not in the immature blasts or early promyelocytes. Ultrastructural studies have identified intense matrix staining for glycoprotein in secondary granules (Fig. 17-5), which is not found in mature primary granules. Lysozyme has been reported in both primary and/or secondary granules by various investigators. Secondary granules lack peroxidase (Fig. 17-6), acid phosphatase, elastase, acidic glycoconju-

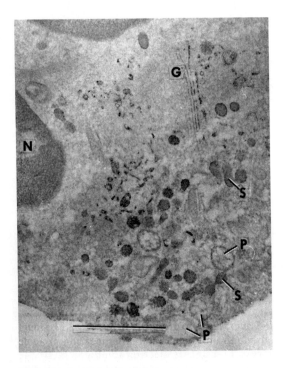

Figure 17-5   After amylase or distase digestion, glycogen staining (with periodate-thiocarbohydrazide silver proteinate) is removed from this human segmented neutrophil. Staining of glycoprotein persists in Golgi lamellae (G) and numerous secondary granules (S). Less vicinal glycol containing glycoconjugate staining is evident in the larger primary granules (P). Bar = 1 μm.

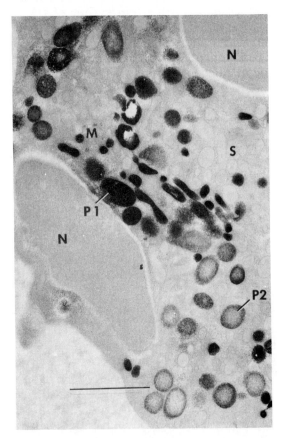

Figure 17-6   Intense diaminobenzidine staining of myeloperoxidase is evident in primary granules, whereas more numerous secondary (S) granules lack staining in this human blood neutrophil. Peroxidase may be found in a microgranule population (M) as well as in larger, uniformly stained (P1) and rim-stained (P2) granules. Portions of two nuclear lobes (N) are evident. Bar = 1 μm.

gates (i.e., sulfated glycosaminoglycans), and basic proteins and peptides found in primary granules.

Late Neutrophils

Metamyelocytes, band neutrophils, and segmented neutrophils represent nondividing cells in which a progressive condensation of nuclear chromatin occurs. Nucleoli are indistinct. In fully developed cells, an average of three nuclear lobes with fully condensed nuclear chromatin may be identified (Figs. 17-2 and 17-4). In females distinct drumstick appendages corresponding to inactivated X chromosomes may be seen, although these may be confused with less distinct clublike appendages seen in both males and females. The Golgi apparatus is much less prominent than that in early and mid myeloid cells, and the cytoplasm contains very little endoplasmic reticulum. There are sparse, small mitochondria and no large increase in granules in segmented neutrophils compared to metamyelocytes. Glycogen is prominent and may be stained using the PAS method at the light microscope level (Fig. 17-7).

Tertiary granules are found in late neutrophils where they appear to be actively synthesized. These granules are smaller than most primary and secondary granules, varying from 0.1 to 0.2 μm in diameter in humans. Ultrastructurally, they are moderately electron-dense and stain for acid phosphatase, aryl sulfatase, and sulfated glycosaminoglycans but not for peroxidase. Biochemical studies have also suggested that gelatinase and some membrane receptor proteins reside in this granule.

Although at least three types of granules (primary, secondary, and tertiary) have been generally identified in neutrophils, significant heterogeneity and overlap can be demonstrated. Recent data indicate that size, density distribution, and biochemical, cytochemical, and functional properties are not entirely consistent with a simple two- or three-granule model. While some if not all of this heterogeneity appears related to maturation and continued programmed or environmental modification of preformed gran-

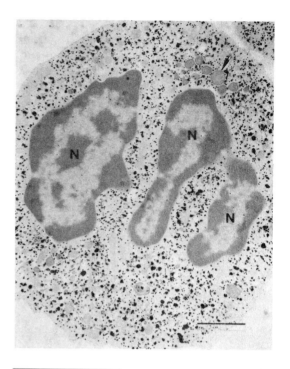

Figure 17-7 Intense staining of particulate glycogen is scattered throughout the cytoplasm of this segmented neutrophil and corresponds to the intense PAS staining seen in neutrophils at the light microscope level. Finer staining of glycoprotein is evident in cytoplasmic granules (arrow). N = nuclei. This section is stained with periodate-thiocarbohydrazide silver proteinate. Bar = 1 μm.

ules, further studies are required to determine if more than three de novo granule types are produced by neutrophils.

In addition to cytoplasmic granules, a variety of vesicles are present in late neutrophils. Some of these contain hydrolases being transported from the Golgi region to form tertiary granules. Some vesicles appear derived from the plasmalemma and may contain endocytosed material and/or NADH oxidase. Other vesicles appear to contain elastaselike enzymes. Alkaline phosphatase, which strongly stains late neutrophils, is confined to vesicles in human neutrophils but can be localized in secondary granules of rabbit heterophils. A centriole is usually located near the Golgi apparatus, and microtubules can be identified radiating from this structure in appropriately fixed tissues. Microfilaments are located throughout the cytoplasm and often in a subplasmalemmal distribution. Microtubules and microfilaments play significant roles in endocytosis, secretion of lysosomes, and determining neutrophil shape. Circulating neutrophils have a spherical appearance, with microvillus projections and surface ruffles (Fig. 17-8); however the shape can change dramatically with attachment, migration, and phagocytosis.

Neutrophil Physiology

Neutrophils are phagocytic cells whose major function is to seek out and destroy mi-

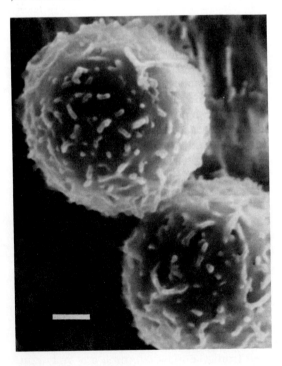

Figure 17-8   Portions of two neutrophils are evident in this scanning electron micrograph. The isolated neutrophils were fixed in suspension, resulting in a spherical shape as seen for circulating neutrophils. The surface contains numerous cytoplasmic projections and occasional ruffles. Bar = 1 μm.

croorganisms, particularly bacteria. This requires both an ability to migrate to the location of the invading organism and, once there, to participate in the destruction and removal of the organism.

Chemotaxins and Chemotaxis

Chemotaxis is the movement of neutrophils toward the site of infection or injury in response to a positive chemical gradient of chemotaxin (or chemoattractant) produced at that site. Chemotaxins are produced or released by bacteria, other inflammatory cells, or damaged tissues involved in the inflammatory reaction. Specific examples of chemotaxins include bacterial formylmethionyl peptides; components of the activated complement system such as C3a, C5a; and metabolites from lipooxygenation of arachidonic acid such as leukotriene B_4 (LTB$_4$). Human neutrophils have been found to possess a variety of specific surface receptors for chemotactic formyl peptides such as *N*-formylmethionylleucylphenylalanine (*N*-fMet-Leu-Phe, or fMLP). These receptors exist in low- and high-affinity forms, resulting in a dose-dependent chemotactic response. Receptors for complement-derived factors or anaphylatoxins such as C5a have not been well defined. LTB$_4$ similarly binds to a distinct subset of surface receptors eliciting chemotaxis in low concentrations, whereas high concentrations of LTB$_4$ result in lysosomal degranulation.

Chemotaxin-Receptor Interaction, Signal Transduction, and Adherence

After chemotaxins bind to distinct neutrophil surface sites, a number of reactions are initiated, including an increase in free intracellular calcium and alterations of membrane phospholipids with activation of a G protein (with binding of GTP), phospholipase C, protein kinase C, and cAMP-dependent protein kinase pathways. These events lead to a decrease in the net negative charge in the neutrophil membrane and promote cell attachment or increased adhesion to cell surfaces and tissue matrixes. Attachment is further facilitated by neutrophil receptors for the extracellular matrix components laminin and fibronectin and a receptor for the complement fragment 3b. The latter receptor appears to be the site detected by monoclonal antibodies Mo1 or Mac-1. Another closely related receptor with neutrophil adherence functions is LFA-1. Signal transduction also results in release of some secondary and tertiary granules and primes the oxidative burst.

Neutrophil Orientation, Microtubules, and Microfilaments

The first morphologic changes observed in vitro as the neutrophil prepares to move toward a higher concentration of chemotaxins involves polarization or orientation. Granules become located in the front of the neutrophil, and the nucleus is found at the rear of the cell. Pseudopodia are prominent at the leading edge and appear to facilitate cell movement. Ultrastructurally, actin filaments are prominent just beneath the surface of the leading edge. Cytochemical studies suggest that cations, particularly Ca^{2+}, accumulate in submembranous areas at the leading edge where they can presumably be utilized by ATPase in actin interactions necessary for movement. Microtubules radiating from a centriole maintain a skeletal framework responsible for cell shape. The actual movement of the cells can be observed with a light microscope using a Boyden chamber, in which neutrophils in a glass chamber accumulate on a filter as they migrate toward a chemotaxin released on the other side of that filter. Agents that inhibit the formation of microtubules, such as colchicine, result in rounding of cells and impaired pseudopod formation, thereby inhibiting neutrophil movement. Disruption of microfilaments by cytochalasin B also inhibits neutrophil migration.

In vivo neutrophil migration begins with margination from the circulation or attachment to the luminal surface of an endothelial cell. The neutrophils become firmly anchored on the endothelial surface and begin movement through endothelial junctions. The basement membrane becomes the next ob-

stacle through which the neutrophil passes. This is facilitated by release of enzymes from the neutrophil which create an opening in the basement membrane. The neutrophil then migrates through the tissue to the site of inflammation. Once the neutrophil has migrated out of the blood, it cannot return to the circulation. It remains in tissues for several hours; it then dies and is subsequently cleared by macrophages.

Phagocytosis and Degranulation

After arrival at the site of inflammation, the neutrophil must attach to the microorganism and phagocytose it. Often this is facilitated by neutrophil surface receptors for C3bi and the Fc portion of immunoglobulin molecules which are opsonins coating the bacteria. Once attachment occurs, pseudopodia extend around the microorganism and completely engulf it in a phagosome (Fig. 17-9).

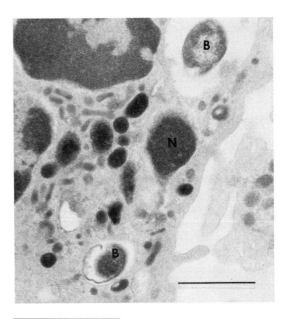

Figure 17-9 Two phagocyte vacuoles containing variably digested *Pseudomonas* bacteria (B) are evident in this human segmented neutrophil. Several cytoplasmic granules are still intact, although degranulated material is evident in the vacuoles containing the bacteria. Specimen stained with uranyl acetate and lead citrate. N = nuclear lobe. Bar = 1 μm.

After engulfment, neutrophil lysosomes fuse with phagosomes to form phagolysosomes. A drop in pH is observed soon afterward. This appears to correspond with sequential fusion of granule constituents.

Degranulation into the extracellular space may occur in vivo and in vitro and may be induced by fMLP and other agents such as phorbol esters. Both ultrastructural and biochemical studies indicate sequential degranulation with release of secondary granules followed by primary granules. The release of the granular contents, called by some *phagocytic regurgitation*, can then cause extensive tissue damage. This mechanism is thought to be a cause of the tissue damage seen in rheumatoid arthritis.

Metabolic Burst and Microbicidal Activity

During phagocytosis a respiratory burst occurs that generates oxidants which participate in bacterial killing. Initially a membrane oxidase oxidizes NADPH or NADH to form an O_2^- radical and NADP or NAD through the following reaction:

$$2O_2 + NADPH \xrightarrow[\text{oxidase}]{\text{respiratory burst}} 2O_2^- + NADP^+ + H^+$$

The superoxide (O_2^-) reacts with hydrogen ions spontaneously or with superoxide dismutase to form hydrogen peroxide. NADP and H_2O_2 further stimulate the hexose monophosphate (HMP) shunt, which makes more NADPH available. Glucose utilization and lactate production are increased. Detoxification is accomplished by the following reactions involving the sulfhydryl-containing tripeptide-reduced glutathione (GSH) and oxidized glutathione (GSSG):

$$2GSH + H_2O_2 \xrightarrow[\text{peroxidase}]{\text{glutathione}} GSSG + H_2O$$

$$GSSG + NADPH \xrightarrow[\text{reductase}]{\text{glutathione}} 2GSH + NADP^+$$

Catalase may also contribute to detoxification by catalyzing divalent reduction of H_2O_2 to water and oxygen. Oxygen-dependent killing occurs when myeloperoxidase catalyzes the formation of additional highly reactive oxidizing radicals from H_2O_2 and a halide such as chloride. Similarly, superoxide radicals can contribute to formation of hydroxyl or iron hydroxide radicals which are active in bacterial killing. These metabolic pathways are summarized in Fig. 17-10. The ability to generate superoxide anion and subsequently H_2O_2 can be evaluated at the light microscope level in viable neutrophils by observing a calorimetric change with reduction of nitroblue tetrazolium (NBT).

Bacterial killing may also occur as a result of oxygen-independent or anaerobic mechanisms. Lysozyme, a cationic enzyme, destroys muramic acid in bacterial cell walls. Cathepsin G, a serine protease with chymotrypsin-like activity, is located in primary granules and has antibacterial and antifungal properties. A number of cationic proteins and lactoferrin, a component of specific granules which binds iron avidly, may also contribute to killing. Another protein, called *bactericidal permeability-increasing (BPI)* factor, has antimicrobial activity against gram-negative bacteria. Similarly, a family of small cationic polypeptides of about 30 amino acids termed *defensins* appears to have a significant role in killing certain microorganisms, including bacteria, fungi, and viruses. In addition, many of the enzymes within the phagocytic vacuole contribute primarily in completing digestion of dead microorganisms.

NEUTROPHIL DISORDERS

Phagocytic dysfunctions represent a group of quantitative or qualitative disorders of phagocytic cells (neutrophils, monocytes, and macrophages) which present with recurrent bacterial infections (skin, gastrointestinal tract, and bone) resulting in chronic abscess formation. Specific disorders and their cellular defects are presented in Table 17-1.

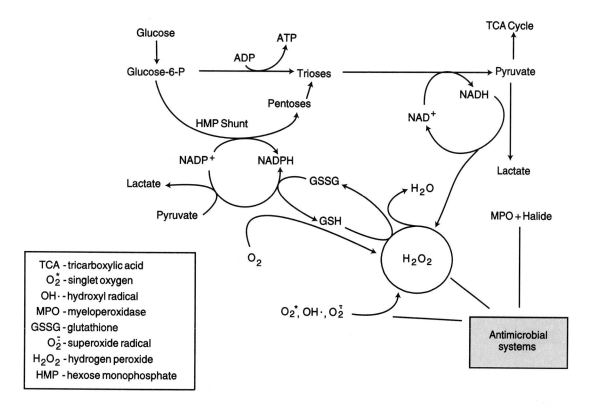

Figure 17-10   Metabolic pathways in human neutrophils.

TABLE 17-1   Disorders of Phagocytic Cell Functions Which Present As Recurrent Infections

Disease	Cellular Defect(s)
Neutropenias (cyclic, drug-induced, malignancy, etc.)	No cellular defect (too few white cells)
Complement deficiency (e.g., C_3 deficency)	Chemotaxis, phagocytosis
Agammaglobulinemia, hypogammaglobulinemia	Chemotaxis, phagocytosis
Chédiak-Higashi syndrome	Chemotaxis, microbicidal activity
Neutrophil actin dysfunction	Chemotaxis, phagocytosis
Job-Buckley syndrome	Chemotaxis
Wiskott-Aldrich syndrome	Chemotaxis
Chronic granulomatous disease	Microbicidal activity
Myeloperoxidase deficiency	Microbicidal activity
"Lazy leukocyte" syndrome	Chemotaxis
Adherence glycoprotein deficiency	Adherence

Quantitative Neutrophil Defects

Neutropenia refers to a reduction in the number of circulating neutrophils. Patients are at greatest risk for infection when the absolute neutrophil count falls below 0.5×10^9 per liter. Neutropenia can be induced by chemotherapeutic agents which cause bone marrow suppression (Clinical Aside 17-1). *Cyclic neutropenia* is a rare disorder characterized by periodic variations in the number of absolute neutrophils from normal to neutropenic levels. These patients are variably symptomatic, and this disorder has been associated with various types of immunologic dysfunctions. Severe neutropenia also occurs as a congenital disease (Kostman's syndrome) which is associated with severe life-threatening infections. Recent studies indicate that the neutropenia in this disorder can be corrected with administration of G-CSF.

Clinical Aside 17-1
Clinical Problems Associated with Neutropenia

Anything that damages the bone marrow granulocyte stem cells can decrease the number of granulocytes produced. An important example of this in clinical practice is the effect that myelosuppressive agents, such as cyclophosphamide, azathioprine, chlorambucil, and methotrexate, have in decreasing neutrophil counts in patients treated for malignancies. When the number of circulating neutrophils is decreased below 1×10^9 per liter there is an increased incidence of infection, which is even more marked when the level goes below 0.5×10^9 per liter. In parallel with this increased risk of infection is a decrease in the clinical manifestations of infection. After all, what causes the symptoms of an infection is the inflammation induced by that infection. If there are very few cells to cause the inflammation, it stands to reason that the signs and symptoms of that infection might be minimal. This is in fact the case.

In a large review at the Baltimore Cancer Center of the National Cancer Institute, the most common infections noted in their neutropenic patients were pharyngitis; skin, anorectal, and urinary tract infections; and pneumonia. The patients were divided into three groups: those with an absolute granulocyte count of over 10^9 per liter,

those with counts between 0.1 and 1.0×10^9 per liter, and those with a count less than 0.1×10^9 per liter. Signs like warmth, swelling, fluctuance, and ulceration were significantly less frequent in the patients with lowest counts. Cough and sputum production were less common in those with pneumonia and a lower cell count, as were pyuria, urinary frequency, and dysuria in those with urinary tract infections and the lowest counts. Bacteremia is, on the contrary, more common in the patients with the lowest counts.

What is the take-home message from these findings? The criteria you use to diagnose an immunocompetent patient as having an infection do not work in the very patients where you are most concerned about infection. The answer? Eternal vigilance, with attention to even the most minimal complaints and physical findings.

Disorders of Degranulation and Chemotaxis

Chédiak-Higashi syndrome is characterized by partial oculocutaneous albinism, neurologic abnormalities, a high incidence of lymphoreticular malignancies, and recurrent infections. The underlying abnormality in Chédiak-Higashi syndrome is not known. The giant primary granules that are characteristic of the disorder fuse with each other to form huge lysosomes (Fig. 17-11). Inconsistent delivery of hydrolytic enzymes from the giant granules into the phagosome results in impaired killing. In the "lazy leukocyte" syndrome there is an unknown intrinsic defect in neutrophil random mobility and inability to mobilize leukocytes to endotoxin stimulation. The ability to engulf and kill bacteria appears to be normal. Isolated cases with abnormal actin have been described. Patients with Job-Buckley syndrome have markedly elevated levels of IgE with eczema and ineffective neutrophil chemotaxis. Wiskott-Aldrich syndrome is an X-linked disorder characterized by thrombocytopenia, eczema, and immunodeficiency with recurrent infections. Neutrophil adherence and/or chemotaxis are decreased in these patients. Recent studies have identified isolated deficiencies

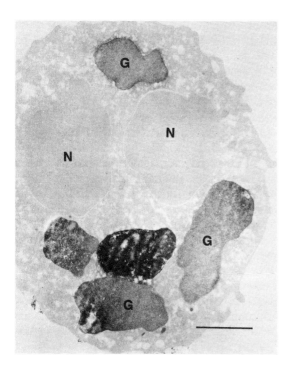

Figure 17-11 Giant lysosomes (G), stained with peroxidase, are characteristic of neutrophils from this patient with Chédiak-Higashi syndrome. Few normal-sized azurophilic or primary (peroxidase positive) granules remain (compare with Fig. 17-6). N = nuclei. Bar = 1 μm.

of adherence protein (detected by Mo1 and Mac-1) which result in increased problems with infection (Clinical Aside 17-2).

Clinical Aside 17-2
Integrins

Cell-cell interactions are crucial in a large number of physiologic functions. The ability of leukocytes to adhere to other cells is determined, in large measure, by the presence of surface molecules, designated as CD11/CD18, or *integrins*. This family of heterodimeric molecules, all having the same β chain, but different α chains, includes Mac-1 (CD11b/CD18), LFA-1 (lymphocyte function related antigen 1; CD11a/CD18), and p150,95 (CD11c/CD18). The Mac-1 molecule is the receptor for the complement degradation compo-

nent C3bi (CR3) and is found on monocytes, neutrophils, and natural killer (NK) cells; the absence of CR3 activity decreases polymorphonuclear cell adherence, spreading, aggregation, and chemotaxis. LFA-1 is found on all human leukocytes; its adhesion-promoting function facilitates helper T-cell function, cytolytic T cell–mediated killing, and NK-cell binding to targets. LFA-1 binds to intercellular adhesion molecule 1 (ICAM-1), a member of the immunoglobulin superfamily, on the surface of target cells. p150,95, which has recently been identified as the complement receptor 4 (CR4), is found on monocytes and neutrophils, where it promotes cellular adhesion.

In the absence of production of the normal β chain, there is no assembly or transport of the heterodimers to the cell surface. The result is profound cellular dysfunction. Neutrophils are unable to migrate to sites of inflammation, not because they are unable to detect or react to chemotactic signals, but because they are unable to adhere to surfaces, the first step in migration across these surfaces into the inflammatory site. Once at the site of inflammation, these cells cannot recognize and bind articles or organisms opsonized by C3bi. The steps triggered by such recognition, like degranulation and a burst in oxidative metabolism, are therefore blunted.

The clinical features of defective integrin expression include recurrent soft tissue infection, with necrosis and even gangrenous changes. Bacterial (often *Staphylococcus aureus*, *Pseudomonas*, and other gram-negative bacilli) and fungal (usually *Candida*) infections predominate; periodontal infection is virtually universal in patients who survive infancy. As one might predict, examination of the infected tissues (or of implanted skin windows) reveals few neutrophils. Delayed wound healing is common, often first noted as delayed umbilical cord separation.

The defect in cell surface expression of these proteins is inherited in an autosomal recessive fashion (in one family a pattern compatible with X linkage was described); unaffected carriers of the defect have 50 percent of normal levels of Mac-1 on their cells' surfaces. Some affected individuals have less deficiency of surface expression and less severe infections, with a better prognosis. Supportive therapy includes antibiotic treatment of infections and prophylaxis. Successful bone marrow transplantation of this frequently fatal disorder has been reported.

Disorders of Phagocytosis

When the neutrophil reaches the site of pathogen invasion, it must prepare to ingest the offending agent. If the microbe is adequately opsonized with antibody and complement, phagocytosis proceeds normally. Phagocytosis is defective when antibodies or complement components are not available for opsonization. Thus, disorders of phagocytic ingestion can result from defects in components of the complement system such as C3 and C5. (For more details about the function of complement and about complement deficiencies, see Chap. 13.) Likewise, deficiency of specific antibodies found in patients with defects of humoral immunity or after splenectomy can cause defective phagocytosis. Intrinsic defects of neutrophil ingestion are rare but have been reported in patients whose neutrophils have defective actin polymerization resulting in inability to engulf foreign particles.

Disorders of Microbicidal Activity

Chronic granulomatous disease (CGD) is an X-linked disorder where the underlying defect is impaired generation of H_2O_2 and oxygen metabolism resulting from a defect of NADHP oxidase. An autosomal recessive form of the disease has also been described. The inability to reduce O_2 to the bactericidal product H_2O_2 predisposes these patients to life-threatening infections with catalase-positive bacteria such as *Staphylococcus aureus*, *Klebsiella*, and *Escherichia coli*. (Why specifically catalase positive bacteria?) Recently, absence of a component of the NADPH-oxidase system, cytochrome b, has been defined as the molecular basis of the X-linked type of CGD. The gene for the X-linked form of CGD has also been identified and localized to chromosome Xp2.13. This gene is expressed in phagocytes but is absent or structurally abnormal in some patients with the disorder. A disease resembling CGD is seen in patients with less than 1 percent glucose-6-phosphate dehydrogenase (G-6P-D) activity in their leukocytes. Defective mi-crobicidal function has also been described in patients with myeloperoxidase deficiency. The disorder is inherited as an autosomal recessive trait and the patients are typically asymptomatic.

SELF-TEST QUESTIONS*

1. Chronic granulomatous disease is a disorder which results from:
   a. Abnormality in antibody production
   b. Impairment in cell-mediated immunity
   c. Abnormality in complement-dependent chemotaxis
   d. Defective microbicidal activity in neutrophils
2. Neutrophils are attracted to the site of infection of injury by all of the following *except*:
   a. Complement components such as C3a, C5a, and C567
   b. Leukotriene B_4
   c. Secretory products of lymphocytes
   d. Protein kinase C
3. The phagocytic process induces several metabolic perturbations in phagocytes which are oxidative in nature and are collectively termed the *metabolic burst*. These changes consist of all of the following *except*:
   a. Increase in oxygen consumption
   b. Activation of phospholipase C
   c. Increase in glucose utilization and lactate production
   d. Increase in glucose metabolism through the hexose monophosphate shunt
   e. Generation of H_2O_2 and several activated forms of oxygen
4. Most of the neutrophils in the body may be found in the:
   a. Bone marrow
   b. Blood

*Answers will be found in Appendix E.

  c. Spleen
  d. Extravascular space
5. Primary granules are produced in:
  a. Promyelocytes
  b. Myelocytes
  c. Segmented neutrophils
  d. All of the above
6. Secondary granules contain:
  a. Peroxidase
  b. Vitamin B_{12}–binding protein
  c. Acid phosphatase
  d. None of the above
7. Division of myeloid cells occurs at:
  a. The myeloblast stage only
  b. The promyelocyte, metamyelocyte, and myelocyte stages
  c. The myeloblast, promyelocyte, and myelocyte stages
  d. The myelocyte and metamyelocyte stages
8. Chemotaxin-receptor interaction and signal transduction in neutrophils result in:
  a. Decrease in free intracellular calcium
  b. Inactivation of protein kinase C
  c. Decrease in net surface membrane charge
  d. Release of LTB_4

ADDITIONAL READINGS

Hurst JK. Barrette WC Jr. Leukocytic oxygen activation and microbicidal oxidative toxins. *Crit Rev Biochem Mol Biol.* 1989;24:271.

Lehrer RI, Ganz T, Selsted ME, et al. Neutrophils and host defense. *Ann Intern Med.* 1988;15:127.

Marmont AM, Damasio E, Zucker-Franklin D. Neutrophils. In: Zucker-Franklin D, Greaves MF, Grossi CE, Marmont AM, eds. *Atlas of Blood Cells.* Philadelphia: Lea & Febiger; 1988:157.

Sawyer DW, Donowitz GR, Mandell GL. Polymorphonuclear neutrophils: An effective antimicrobial force. *Rev Infect Dis.* 1989;11(suppl 7):S1532.

Yang KD, Hill HR. Neutrophil function disorders: Pathophysiology, prevention and therapy. *J Pediatr.* 1991; 119:343.

18

Mononuclear Phagocytic Cells

INTRODUCTION

Monocytes and macrophages were discovered 100 years ago by Eli Metchnikoff, who first identified this cell type as a major component of the host defense. Monocytes and macrophages are essential elements of the *mononuclear phagocytic system* (*MPS*), a multiorgan collection of cells whose common functional capacity is phagocytosis. Since the time of Metchnikoff our understanding of the the role of monocytes and macrophages has evolved. We know now that monocytes and macrophages are more than cells primarily utilizing their phagocytic ability; rather they are multifunctional cells intimately involved in many aspects of the the immune response. *Monocytes* constitute the blood-borne constituent of the MPS, while *macrophages* reside in specific tissue locations, including the liver (Kupffer cells), lungs (alveolar macrophages), spleen, lymph nodes, bone marrow, uterus, and brain (microglia). Monocytes mature into macrophages when they enter the tissue compartment. During maturation, these cells acquire many functions, some relating to phagocytic capacity, including (1) host defense against microorganisms, particularly intracellular parasites, (2) the ability to initiate immune responses through stimulation of and/or antigen presentation to immunocompetent T cells, (3) secretion of various mediators which regulate the proliferation and production of factors by lymphocytes and other nonmesenchymal cells, and (4) control of tumor growth.

ORIGIN AND TRAFFIC OF MONOCYTES AND MACROPHAGES

Cells of the monocyte and macrophage lineage originate from precursors in the bone marrow called *monoblasts*. In the bone marrow, monoblasts divide and differentiate into *promonocytes*, which eventually become monocytes. Monocytes remain in the bone marrow for only a short time after which they enter the circulation for 8 to 10 h. This process is illustrated in Fig. 18-1. Monocytes represent 3 to 5 percent of the total circulating white blood cells and are produced at a rate of 1×10^8 cells per kilogram of body weight per day to maintain normal circulating populations. Peripheral blood monocytes vary in size between 20 to 25 μm; they have a large, oval, indented nucleus which can be either horseshoe- or kidney-shaped. They are characterized by abundant cytoplasm with a fine granular texture owing to a large lysosomal content as well as the presence of mitrochondria. This is illustrated in Fig. 18-2a. Monocytes may exit the circulation and migrate into the tissues where they differentiate into macrophages. The circulating population of monocytes is extremely heterogeneous, and individual monocyte subpopulations are programmed to populate specific tissues. However, local regulatory influences can alter monocyte differentiation and trafficking. Monocytes are attracted to sites of inflammation by a number of chemotactic factors, the most potent of which are derived from lymphocytes (lymphokines). Other nonlymphokine factors possess chemotactic activity for monocytes, including the complement fragment C5a, fMet peptides, and endotoxin (a lipopolysaccharide derived from the bacterial cell wall of gram-negative bacteria). When the monocyte enters into tissue, a metamorphosis ensues. The maturation process is associated with a rapid increase in protein synthesis, lysosomal content, and cell size; the appearance of dendritic processes and granular cytoplasm; and a wrinkled appearance. The mature macrophages are terminally differentiated cells which do not divide. They have a half-life of 3 months, after which they die and are cleared

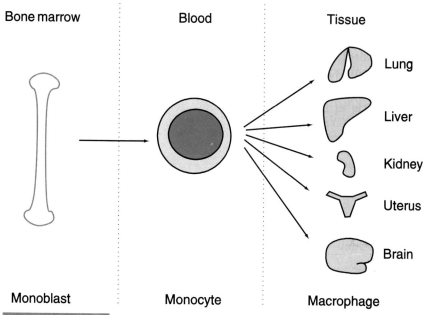

Figure 18-1 Monocytic cells exist in different forms in three separate tissue compartments: bone marrow precursors, peripheral blood monocytes, and tissue macrophages. The proliferation and differentiation are influenced by a series of factors, particularly monocyte-macrophage colony-stimulating factors (M-CSF), which act directly on bone marrow precursors. Monocytes are released into the peripheral blood where they circulate until they are attracted to sites of inflammation by inflammatory mediators. At local sites further differentiation into macrophages takes place.

from the body. Some evidence indicates that a small percentage of tissue macrophages (2 to 3 percent) are capable of limited division and that this population is not dependent on the blood-borne monocyte. Typical macrophage morphology is illustrated in Fig. 18-2b.

CHARACTERISTICS OF MONOCYTES AND MACROPHAGES

The maturation of monocytes and macrophages is characterized by the sequential expression of a series of surface membrane proteins, intracytoplasmic enzymes, and receptors, and the acquisition of functional capabilities (Table 18-1). One of the most re-liable features used to identify monocytes is the presence of intracytoplasmic enzymes, i.e., nonspecific esterase, lysozyme, and per-oxidase, that can be identified biochemi-cally. Esterase is identified by its ability to metabolize α-naphthyl butyrate or acetate with subsequent change in color of the sub-strate, so that when these substrates are in-cubated with monocytes, diffuse cytoplas-mic staining results. All monocytes and macrophages are positive for nonspecific es-terase, although the intensity of the reaction may differ with developmental stage and functional state. Another intracellular en-zyme, lysozyme, can be visualized using ly-sozyme-specific fluorescein-labeled anti-bodies. A third enzymatic marker, perox-idase, is used to identify monocytic cells and to a limited extent define the various stages of monocyte differentiation. Immature

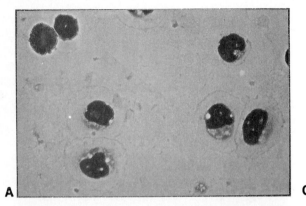

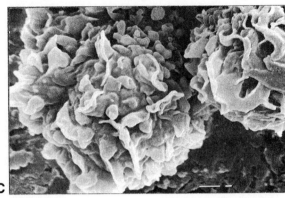

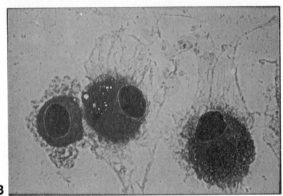

Figure 18-2   (*a*) High-power magnification (×400) of peripheral blood monocytes showing typical morphology with indented oval-shaped nucleus. (*b*) High-power magnification (×400) of normal macrophages. During the maturation process, dramatic changes in monocyte morphology occur. As is illustrated in this figure, monocytes acquire dendritic processes, increase greatly in size, develop abundant lysosomal enzymes, and take on a wrinkled appearance. Both the monocytes and macrophages were stained with Pappenhein stain. (*c*) Scanning electron micrograph (×2000) of mature macrophages demonstrates the numerous dendritic processes. (Courtesy Dr. J. Bauer, Freiburg University, Germany.)

monocytic cells (monoblasts, promonocytes and monocytes), contain large amounts of peroxidase; macrophages do not contain this enzyme. All of these enzymatic markers appear to be relatively specific to monocytes and macrophages, although other cell types, including granulocytes and natural killer (NK) cells, have limited amounts of peroxidase.

Although intracytoplasmic enzymes can

TABLE 18-1   Cell Surface Characteristics of Monocytes

huFcRI
huFcRII
huFcRIII
C3b receptor
Lymphokine receptor (IL-1 and IL-6)
CD14
Fibronectin
HDL receptor
Lactoferrin receptor
Insulin receptor
Class II molecules
fMLP receptors

be useful in identifying monocytes and macrophages, specific surface markers are not as well defined as are those for B cells or T cells. The presence of receptors for the Fc fragment of IgG and for complement fragment C3b are, in addition to phagocytic abilities, the criteria most widely accepted for definition of monocytes and macrophages. Over the past several years, however, a series of monoclonal antibodies have been generated against both monocytes and macrophages; the most useful of the monocyte-specific antigens is CD14 (cluster of designation 14, identified by a series of murine monoclonal antibodies including Leu-M3, P9, S1, and S39), which identifies a protein present on both monocytes and macrophages but not on immature monocytic cells. None of the currently available antibodies is absolutely reliable; the developmental state of the cells as well as their state of activation must be taken into account. Immature cells may not express certain surface characteristics of monocytes; alternatively, activated cells may lose antigens which distinguish their lineage.

Monocyte characteristics can change when cells are attracted to sites of inflammation. (See also Chap. 20, "The Inflammatory Response.") At these sites monocytes may differentiate into macrophages or epithelioid cells, or fuse with other macrophages to become multinucleated giant cells. *Epithelioid cells* resemble epithelial cells morphologically but have many monocyte characteristics, including Fc and C3b receptors. Epithelioid cells can persist for long periods of time in tissue as components of granulomas. *Multinucleated giant cells* are formed by fusion of macrophages in the absence of cytoplasmic division. There are two general types: (1) *Langhans type*, with relatively few nuclei arranged peripherally in the cytoplasm and (2) *foreign-body type*, with multiple nuclei dispersed in the cytoplasm. Multinucleated giant cells are generally less phagocytic than macrophages and, like epithelioid cells, are long-lived in tissue. Epithelioid cells and multinucleated giant cells are essential for the formation of *granulomas* (a collection of modified inflammatory cells made in response to a poorly degraded antigen), which wall off infected areas of tissue. Granulomas are formed, for example, in response to tuberculosis. It is unclear how macrophages, multinucleated giant cells, and epithelioid cells disappear when the inflammatory response subsides.

Kupffer cells, originating from peripheral blood monocytes, are the resident macrophages of the liver and represent a special type of tissue macrophage. Kupffer cells are situated between the venous return from the GI tract and the systemic circulation, making these cells the first members of the mononuclear phagocytic system to encounter the wide variety of immunogens absorbed from the intestine. Their primary function appears to be ingestion and degradation of soluble and particulate material from portal blood. They therefore play an essential role in clearing a large number of harmful agents, including bacteria and other microorganisms, as well as immune complexes from the

circulation. In order to perform this function, Kupffer cells have very well-developed lysosomes.

A specific type of nonphagocytic cell, the *dendritic cell*, represents a special category of cells of uncertain lineage. Unusual features of dendritic cells include their unique morphology; abundant spherical, dense mitochondria; irregularly shaped nuclei; and numerous long cytoplasmic prolongations. Cells of this type include the Langerhans cells of the skin, veiled cells in the afferent lymphatics, and the interdigitating reticulum cells of the lymph node. These three cells may represent different stages of differentiation of the same nonmonocytic cell type; veiled cells and interdigitating reticulum cells are the more immature types, while Langerhans cells are thought to represent a more differentiated state.

Although sharing many other properties with monocytes, the dendritic cell is incapable of phagocytosis. These cells differ from monocytes in that they lack peroxidase and nonspecific esterase. Bierbec granules, rod-shaped granules present in the cytoplasm, are a unique morphologic feature of dendritic cells. Dendritic cells are highly efficient in antigen presentation and express abundant class II MHC (major histocompatibility complex) antigens on their surfaces. It is estimated by some investigators that these cells are 10- to 100-fold more efficient than monocytes in presenting antigens and perhaps antigen fragments processed by other cells adherent to their surface antigens. Thus, dendritic cells are thought to play a very important role in the stimulation of cellular immune responses. They are commonly found in the skin but are rarely present in peripheral blood.

Veiled cells, which are mononuclear cells with long cytoplasmic veils, are found in lymph; *interdigitating reticulum cells* reside in the thymus-dependent inner portion of the periarteriolar sheaths of the spleen and in the paracortical areas of the lymph nodes. Aside from different tissue locations, the two cell types are similar. They bear class II antigens, and are both reported to be very efficient in antigen presentation. Interdigitating cells may

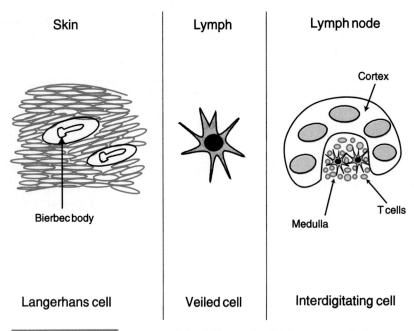

Skin	Lymph	Lymph node

Figure 18-3   Characteristics of the different dendritic cell populations present in skin (Langerhans cells), lymph (veiled cells), and lymph nodes (interdigitating cells). These cells have high levels of class II molecules on their surface and are highly efficient in presenting antigen to surrounding T helper cells.

increase in number after antigenic stimulation, and a rapid increase is noted in the dermal lymphatics from draining sites of a contact hypersensitivity reaction. The major characteristics of these three types of dendritic cells—Langerhans cells, veiled cells, and interdigitating cells—are illustrated in Fig. 18-3.

MONOCYTES AS PHAGOCYTIC CELLS

One of the most important functions of monocytes and macrophages is their ability to ingest foreign material. This process is called *phagocytosis* (from the Greek *phagein*, "to eat"), and is defined as the mechanism of engulfment of corpuscular particles by macrophages and white blood cells. Phagocytosis is often enhanced by interaction of the phagocyte with *opsonins* (from the Greek *opsonein*, "to purchase food for eating"). *Pino-*

cytosis (from the Greek *pinein*, "to drink") is the mechanism of uptake of colloidal or soluble macromolecules. These processes are combined under the general term *endocytosis*, which can be nonspecific or can be greatly enhanced in a receptor-mediated manner, either by specific antibody (via the Fc receptor) or by a complement-mediated mechanism (via the C3b fragment). The endocytosis process occurs in several stages: (1) chemotaxis, (2) attachment, (3) engulfment, and (4) intracellular events.

Chemotaxis is unidirectional movement of phagocytic cells across a concentration gradient of substances which attract them. It is distinct from *chemokinesis*, which is increased activity due to the presence of a chemical substance. Chemotaxis-inducing substances include soluble bacterial factors, plasmin-treated fresh serum, immune complexes, T-cell lymphokines, and cationic proteins (e.g., histones and protamines). Chemotactic activity can be demonstrated in vitro using specialized culture conditions and a Boyden chamber, consisting of two compartments separated by a 10-micron filter. The cell suspension is placed in the upper chamber and the substance to be assayed for chemotactic activity in the lower chamber. Monocytes and macrophages will migrate through the pores from the upper to the lower chamber if a chemotactic substance is present in the lower chamber.

Attachment is the binding of a particle to the monocytic membrane. This process initiates the internalization of particles into the cytoplasm. The particle is then engulfed by the macrophage cytoplasm, and a vacuole, called a *phagosome,* is formed. Intracellular events involving interaction between lysosomes and phagosomes then occur. *Lysosomes* are minute bodies in the cell cytoplasm which contain various hydrolytic enzymes. Initially, the phagosomes are found near the cell membrane, but in time they migrate toward the perinuclear area where they fuse with lysosomes to form *phagolysosomes.* This fusion process discharges lysosomal contents, including lysosomal enzymes (e.g., acid hydrolases and peptidase), into the phagolysosomes. The lysosomal enzymes are subsequently activated by the low pH (produced by proton pumps located in the phagosome) and can digest the engulfed substances, either storing them as "dense bodies" or eliminating them by exocytosis. Some phagosomes, or *endosomes,* are recycled to the cell surface. This recycling process is important. As will be seen later, antigen processing, which can occur in the absence of lysosomal enzymes, takes place in the endosome. The entire phagocytic process is illustrated in Fig. 18-4.

Fc-Mediated Antigen Uptake

Fc receptors are a group of surface membrane molecules that specifically recognize and bind the Fc portion of the immunoglobulin molecule and then presumably mediate biologic function. Human phagocytic cells have at least three separate protein receptors for IgG on their surface: huFcRI, huFcRII, and hu-FcRIII. These receptors are members of the immunoglobulin superfamily. (See also Chap. 3, "Antibodies: Structure and Function.")

huFcRI

huFcRI is found on monocytes and macrophages and binds IgG with great avidity. Three of the four subclasses of IgG—IgG1, IgG3, and IgG4—bind to huFcRI, whereas IgG2 does not. This receptor is a glycoprotein with a molecular mass of 70 kd and a valency of 1 (binds only one IgG at a time). huFcRI is thought to be involved in antibody-dependent cellular cytotoxicity (ADCC) (see Chap. 8). This allows the monocyte or macrophage to increase its phagocytic ability 1000-fold allowing clearance of a wide variety of opsonized (antibody-coated) invading microorganisms as well as eliminating immune complexes. Several factors can influence surface expression of huFcRI. Gamma interferon (INF-γ) can increase surface expression by 10-fold, suggesting that this agent may play a role in enhancing macrophage effector function. Conversely, dexamethasone, a corticosteroid widely used in a variety of inflammatory diseases, can decrease huFcRI expression; this may explain, at least in part, some of the anti-inflammatory action of dexamethasone.

huFcRII

A second Fc receptor, with a molecular mass of 40 kd, has been described recently. In addition to being expressed on monocytes, huFcRII is also found on platelets and neutrophils. huFcRII, in contrast to huFcRI, has a relatively low affinity for IgG.

huFcRIII

A third Fc receptor, which is present on macrophages but not on monocytes, has also been discovered recently. Unlike huFcRI and huFcRII, huFcRIII is a receptor of low avidity that binds immune complexes but not monomeric IgG. This receptor probably plays an important role in clearing immune complexes. Several animal studies utilizing antibodies that block this receptor have demonstrated that subsequent clearance of

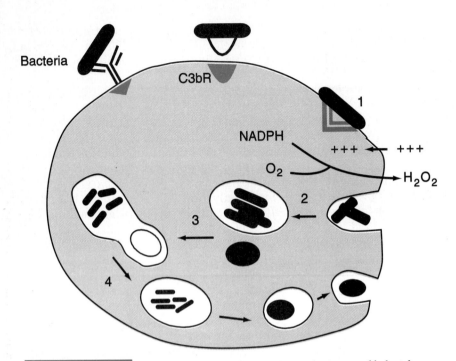

Figure 18-4   The normal phagocytic process. Antigen is engulfed either nonspecifically or via Fc or C3b receptors (1). A phagosome is formed which contains the ingested foreign material. During the ingestion there is cation influx and the hexose monophosphate shunt is activated (2). Oxygen, which is consumed during this process, undergoes enzyme catalytic univalent reduction to form superoxide anion O_2^-. Two O_2^- molecules, one of which may be in the form of HO_2^-, interact with each other to form the anion of hydrogen peroxide (O_2^-) and oxygen. Superoxide anion and H_2O_2 interact with each other to form the hydroxyl radical ($\cdot OH$). The hydroxyl radical is critical in killing a wide variety of microorganisms. The phagosome fuses (3) with lysosomes produced in the Golgi apparatus. Lysosomal enzymes are activated after the fusion process, and the foreign material is digested. The digested material is then removed by exocytosis (4).

immune complexes can be decreased 20-fold. huFcRIII is important in phagocytosis and is also thought to mediate ADCC.

Fc-Receptor Expression in Autoimmune Disorders

Several studies have documented a decreased rate of immune complex clearance in autoimmune diseases such as systemic lupus erythematosus (SLE), Sjögren's syndrome, and dermatitis herpetiformis. Additionally, it has been reported that there is decreased Fc-me-diated phagocytosis by normal individuals with the HLA haplotypes DR2 and DR3, which are associated with autoimmune disease. The severity of disease in SLE correlates with a depression in clearance of immune complexes, while remission is associated with a normalization of the clearance rate. In Sjögren's syndrome, prolonged clearance time of immune complexes is associated with diffuse tissue damage. The change in activity of Fc-mediated clearance in these diseases is undoubtedly complex. Moreover, most studies involve measurement of huFcRI and not huFcRIII. The decrease in clearance of immune complexes could be either the primary event leading to accumulation of circulating immune complexes or a secondary phenomena with the system being overloaded with excess of complexes because of overproduction.

Autoimmune thrombocytopenic purpura (ATP), formerly called idiopathic thrombocytopenic purpura (ITP), is an autoimmune disease associated with circulating levels of antiplatelet antibodies. These antibodies cause opsonization of the platelets and phagocytosis by monocytes and macrophages, which leads to a decrease in platelet levels (thrombocytopenia) and bleeding. Clinical management of ATP includes administration of steroids, which can inhibit expression of huFcRI, and intravenous γ-globulin, which competes with the opsonized platelets for Fc receptors on monocytes and macrophages. Splenectomy is occasionally necessary; removing the spleen surgically eliminates the site where Ig-coated platelets are removed from the circulation. It has been demonstrated that antibodies to huFcRIII can block immune complex clearance in chimpanzees. It has also been shown that in selected patients with refractory ATP, treatment with anti-huFcRIII antibodies can elevate platelet levels. The therapeutic efficacy of anti-Fc antibodies in ATP and other autoimmune diseases is currently under investigation. ATP and other hematologic diseases caused by autoimmune mechanisms are described in more detail in Chap. 30, "Immunohematology."

Antigen Processing, Antigen Presentation, and MHC Restriction

Antigen processing comprises the initial events leading to antigen recognition and specific stimulation of CD4 and CD8 T lymphocytes. It is a critical event in the generation of an immune response because intact antigens cannot be recognized either by helper T cells or by cytotoxic T cells and must be processed and presented together with MHC

antigens. Monocytes and macrophages phagocytose bulky antigens and "process" them within the endosome with subsequent reexpression of an immunogenic peptide fragment on the cell surface in association with class II molecules. CD4 cells recognize foreign antigens only when they are associated with class II molecules. When T cells bind to the antigen-MHC complex, they become activated; they proliferate and secrete a variety of mediators, including INF-γ, which serves as a stimulatory factor for monocytes. Stimulation of the monocyte results in further secretion of monokines by the monocyte, including IL-1, which in turn stimulates antigen-activated T cells to express IL-2R and to produce IL-2, which then serves as the principal T-cell growth factor. IL-2 in turn expands the number of antigen-activated T cells (Fig. 18-5). Helper T cells traffic through tissues until they encounter the appropriate antigen recognized by the specific T-cell antigen.

Nonmonocytic cells capable of antigen presentation include B cells themselves, endothelial cells, intestinal epithelium, and microglial cells in the brain. All these cell types express class II molecules. A model that shows monocytes and macrophages directly interacting with both helper T cells and B cells and functioning as an intermediary between the two provides a very efficient means for the transfer of T-cell signals to specific B cells. This can be seen in Fig. 18-5, where antigen-stimulated T cells provide the factors required by B cells, B-cell growth factor (IL-4) and B-cell differentiation factor (IL-6).

At this point it would be useful to briefly review class II structure. (The structure of class II molecules is described in more detail in Chap. 4.) Human HLA class II antigens are composed of three alleles—DR, DQ, and DP—which are located on the short arm of chromosome 6 centromeric to the class I genes. The whole region is roughly 1100 to 1500 kb (kilobases) and is composed of several well-defined and several less-well-defined subregions. Class II molecules are composed of two chains, a 34-kd α heavy chain and a 29-kd β light chain. Each chain consists of

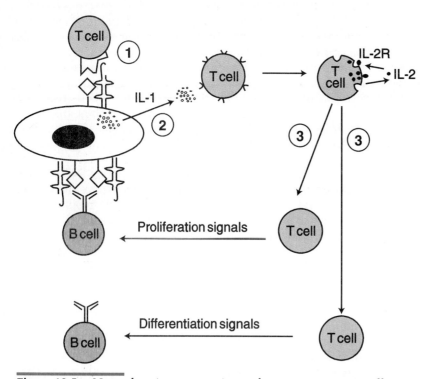

Figure 18-5   Normal antigen processing and presentation to T cells. Antigen is phagocytosed and reexpressed on the cell surface in association with class II molecules (1). T cells and B cells traffic through tissues until they encounter the antigen, recognized either by the T-cell receptor (T cells) or by immunoglobulin (B cells). T cells recognize antigen, become activated, and produce soluble factors such as interferon (IFN) which stimulates monocytes and macrophages to produce IL-1, which acts as a coactivator for T cells (2). The activation also induces IL-2 production (the T-cell growth factor), which binds to its receptor on the T cell (IL-2R), causing further T-cell proliferation. Proliferating T cells secrete factors BCGF and BCDF, which influence B-cell growth and differentiation (3). B cells may also recognize antigen processed by monocytes and macrophages, but this is not an absolute requirement.

external domains, a transmembrane domain, and a cytoplasmic tail. Each of the external domains (except the distal α chain) has two cysteine residues which form a disulfide loop. The chains are noncovalently linked; however, the exact three-dimensional arrangement of these molecules is still unknown. The distal external domains show marked diversity, accounting for these serologic specificities and alternatively peptide binding, while the proximal external domains as well as the transmembrane and intracyto-

plasmic portions are well conserved. Activation of human monocytes and macrophages with IFN-γ up-regulates the expression of class II molecules.

The DR subregion is composed of one DR α gene and three DR β genes. Genetic polymorphism is confined to the β genes and accounts for the distinct specificities of the gene products (DR haplotypes). The DQ subregion has extremely polymorphic α and β chains. The DP gene also exhibits extreme polymorphism but is incompletely studied. The class II DR, DQ, and DP antigens, as products of the immunoglobulin supergene family, demonstrate significant homology with different domains of class I molecules and the immunoglobulin heavy and light chains. The class II molecules are structurally related to immunoglobulins, and their organization into the polymorphic (first) and conserved (second) domains is similar to the variable and constant regions of immunoglobulin molecules.

How do antigen fragments and HLA-D molecules become associated in monocytes? As noted above, the surface of the monocyte is rich in class II molecules. A portion of the monocyte surface becomes part of the cavity which forms during endocytosis. The internalized antigen is contained within an endosome which contains proteases. The proteases and the proton pump are present in the endosomes and are not found at the cell surface. It is unclear how both the proteases and the proton pump become part of the endosome in this process. The proteases are activated to partially degrade and "unfold" the antigen through a proton pump which lowers pH in the endosome. Small peptide residues of from 8 to 12 amino acids are produced, which interact with class II molecules. The endocytic vacuole is then recycled to the cell surface with the antigen fragment and the class II molecule displayed together on the cell surface where they can be recognized by T cells. This is shown in Fig. 18-6. Protein antigens are usually of high molecular weight with complex structure, and it has become apparent that a given peptide may give rise to more than one antigenic determinant. The class II molecules present an interesting peptide transport system, since by binding to the partially degraded peptides they create antigenic determinants recognized by T lymphocytes while at the same time rescuing the peptide from further intracellular proteolysis. Compounds that either block acidification of the endosome (e.g., chloroquine, a drug used to treat malaria and certain autoimmune disorders) or inhibit the proteases (e.g., leupeptin, an inhibitor of endosomal enzymes) will impair antigen pro-

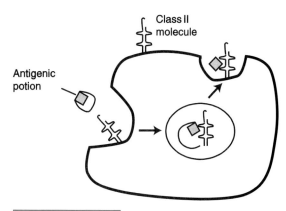

Figure 18-6   The interaction of antigen with class II molecules in monocytes. As the antigen is phagocytosed, it interacts with class II molecules which are present in the phagosome. The antigen is "unfolded" and linked to the class II molecule which is recycled to the cell surface. (The nonimmunogenic peptides are cleaved away.) The immunogenic portion of the antigen, now coupled with a class II molecule on the cell surface, can now be recognized by a helper T cell.

cessing. Some investigators have reported antigen processing at the cell surface without internalization.

As mentioned previously, there are three separate class II molecules expressed on the cell surface which can each form a complex with the processed antigen. The type of immune response to a particular antigen depends not only on its antigenicity but may also depend on the type of class II molecule to which it is complexed. It has been observed by several investigators that DR and DQ have opposite functions (i.e., they are *epistatic*), and in at least one case (with *Schistosoma*), antigens complexed with DR generate greater T-cell proliferative response, than the same antigens complexed with DQ, which generate a suppressor T-cell response.

Antigens can be processed by another route as well, of importance in processing viral antigens. In this system, which is not restricted to monocytes and macrophages, predominantly viral antigens are synthesized by host cell ribosomes. The peptides that are generated bind to class I antigens (see Chap 4) and are expressed on the cell surface. All nucleated cells produce HLA class I molecules and are capable of antigen processing by this route. The cells which express these antigens complexed to class I molecules serve as targets for cytotoxic T cells. In contrast to helper T cells, which recognize the class II antigen complex, cytotoxic T cells recognize antigen only in the context of class I molecules. In vivo, this process eliminates virally infected cells as well as selected tumor cells.

MONOCYTES AND MACROPHAGE EFFECTOR CELLS

Monokines

In addition to antigen processing and expression of class II molecules, monocytes produce soluble mediators which can have broad biologic activities. The regulation of monokine production is generally under T-cell control. Although there are a myriad of substances produced by monocytes, we will concentrate on four of the most important: interleukin 1 (IL-1), colony-stimulating factors, interleukin 6 (IL-6), and tumor necrosis factor (TNF). A consideration of these four should demonstrate the crucial role of monocytes in the organization of immune responses and host reactions to tissue damage. These and other cytokines are described in more detail in Chap. 10.

Interleukin 1

IL-1 not only activates T cells but affects other cells as well. There are two different molecules with IL-1 activity, an α form and a β form. The two differ considerably in molecular mass and amino acid sequence. IL-1α has a molecular mass of 17.5 kd, and IL-1β has a molecular mass of 25 kd. There is 30 percent sequence homology between the two. IL-1β is predominantly membrane-bound, and IL-1α is not. Both are synthesized by monocytes in response to activation signals. IL-1

acts on T cells as a comitogenic signal, i.e., IL-1 plus mitogen (e.g., phytohemagglutinin) will cause T-cell proliferation. Additionally it causes neutrophil release from the bone marrow and accumulation of neutrophils in tissues. It induces increased fibroblast proliferation as well as increased prostaglandin PGE$_2$ and collagenase production by fibroblasts. IL-1 is an endogenous pyrogen causing fever by increases of PGE$_2$ in the hypothalmus. IL-1 can induce the production of acute phase reactants by hepatocytes although IL-6 is a necessary cofactor. Thus it is clear that IL-1 is a critical inflammatory cytokine important in regulating acute responses and repair processes. Please see Chap. 16, on acute phase reactants.

Colony-Stimulating Factors

Monocytes and macrophages synthesize factors which enhance hematopoiesis of certain white blood precursors including granulocytes and monocytes. These substances specifically stimulate precursors of defined lineages: *granulocyte colony-stimulating factor (G-CSF)* stimulates granulocyte colonies, while *monocyte-macrophage colony-stimulating factor (M-CSF)* stimulates only monoblasts. G-CSF has a molecular mass of 20 kd, and M-CSF has a molecular mass of 40 kd. There is 60 percent sequence homology between these two cytokines. M-CSF and G-CSF are not constitutively expressed, and are secreted only after stimulation with a variety of agents, including bacterial endotoxin, interferon, or phorbol esters. The lack of secretion of these cytokines in unstimulated cells leaves open the question of the role of G-CSF and M-CSF in normal hematopoiesis. However, the lack of constitutive expression supports the concept that infections which stimulate monocytes cause increases in both granulocytes and monocytes through the direct stimulation of bone marrow precursors by these secreted factors. In this way, infection or other processes which activate monocytes can be eradicated through direct stimulation of the bone marrow.

Interleukin 6

This remarkable lymphokine was first isolated from an HTLV-I–infected T-cell clone as well as from an atrial myxoma in 1986. Although IL-6 was initially isolated from T cells and certain tumors, it has been shown that monocytes are the main source of this cytokine. IL-6 (previously called hepatocyte-stimulating factor, B-cell differentiation factor, and IFN-β_2) has a molecular mass of 19, 21, or 32 kd, depending on the presence or absence of added sulphate, phosphate, or polysaccharide side chains. IL-6 has many biologic properties, including stimulation of B-cell differentiation, myeloma growth, and hepatic protein synthesis (acute phase response, see Chap. 16); it also exhibits hematopoietic activity, and induces differentiation similar to that induced by nerve growth factor (NGF). IL-6 drives activated B cells to mature and secrete immunoglobulin, but IL-6 has no B-cell growth activity. In recent studies, growth of both plasmacytomas (a focal neoplasm of plasma cells) and multiple myeloma (a malignancy of antibody-producing plasma cells) were shown to be dependent on the presence of IL-6, whereas antibody to IL-6 could inhibit growth. These studies indicate that IL-6 is intimately involved in B-cell differentiation; disorders in its regulation may have far-reaching consequences.

Although IL-6 has some activity on B cells, its main biologic activity is on hepatocytes. IL-6 causes hepatocytes to release a wide variety of proteins collectively known as *acute phase reactants (APRs)*, which are produced in response to tissue injury or inflammation. Although, as previously mentioned, IL-1 can stimulate the release of all acute reactants from normal human hepatocytes, this cannot occur in the absence of IL-6. HSF activity can also be neutralized by anti-IL-6 antibody but not by anti-IL-1 antibody.

IL-6 can stimulate differentiation of malignant glioblastomas into neuronal cells. IL-6 supports the proliferation of multipotent bone marrow precursors.

Several tumors, including atrial myxomas, bladder carcinomas, and cervical carcinomas, produce large amounts of IL-6. Patients with these tumors can show autoimmune phenomena which might be related to uncontrolled IL-6 stimulation of B-cell function. Other autoimmune disorders are associated with elevated levels of IL-6 from stimulated monocytes. Synovial (joint) fluid from patients with acute rheumatoid arthritis shows markedly elevated levels of IL-6. Unregulated production of IL-6 may cause plasma cell infiltration in synovial tissue and support autoantibody production.

TUMOR NECROSIS FACTOR

The macrophage product called *tumor necrosis factor (TNF)*, or cachectin, was first described in the late 1800s when William Colley observed hemorrhagic necrosis of tumors in patients with concurrent bacterial infections, especially with gram-negative organisms. In 1985 Carwell isolated a factor in mice that was capable of inducing necrosis of a sarcoma. This factor was subsequently found to be produced by a variety of human malignant tumor lines. It was purified and found to be a single pleiotrophic protein with a molecular mass of 17 kd. There are two distinct molecules called TNF, TNF-α, which is produced by monocytes, and TNF-β, which is produced by lymphocytes and is also called *lymphotoxin*. Although these two molecules have the same name and bind to the same receptor, they have only 46 percent sequence homology. The discussion here is confined to TNF-α.

The regulation of TNF-α synthesis is incompletely understood, but agents like lipopolysaccharide (LPS) can dramatically increase its synthesis. TNF-α possesses many biologic activities; one of the most important is its ability to cause chronic wasting (hence the name *cachectin*). TNF-α has been shown to induce a catabolic state by suppressing key lipogenic enzymes, including lypoprotein lipase, acetyl-CoA, carboxylase and fatty acid synthetase. By inhibiting these enzymes, TNF prevents accumulation of lipids within adipocytes and causes mature lipid-containing adipocytes to lose stored tri-glycerides. TNF-α also causes a marked stimulation of glycogenolysis which causes glycogen storage depletion with increased lactate production. Therefore, along with stimulation of lipolysis, necessary mobilization of peripheral energy reserves can take place for the acute metabolic demands of inflammatory responses. These mechanisms may also contribute to the cachexia associated with many chronic diseases. Animal models support a role for TNF-α in cachexia. It has been demonstrated that metabolic changes with weight loss, depletion of whole-body protein and lipid stores, and anemia can be reproduced with injection of TNF-α.

TNF-α has other effects aside from altering host metabolism. It enhances neutrophil phagocytosis, and has been shown to increase antibody-dependent cytotoxicity and up-regulate the expression of class II molecules. TNF-α causes fibroblast proliferation along with release of lymphokines, including IL-1 and IL-6, from hepatocytes, leading to fever and other systemic symptoms. Additionally, it induces osteoclast-mediated bone resorption.

MACROPHAGE ACTIVATION

Another aspect of the role of macrophages in an immune response to infectious agents or neoplastic cells involves the development of an "activated" state. The term *activated macrophage* refers to enhanced microbicidal ability primarily due to its production of superoxide anion (O_2^-) and H_2O_2. This activation is produced by interaction of monocytes with the products of stimulated T cells. Thus, in the interaction of antigen and the immune system, the macrophage is necessary to present antigen to T cells, which in turn produce products which activate the macrophage to eliminate the antigen. The monocyte then serves a dual function, first as a scavenger cell and second as a recruiter and stimulator of T lymphocytes.

MACROPHAGES AS SECRETORY CELLS

Macrophages produce many secretory enzymes, some of which are listed in Table 18-2, which play important roles in a variety of diseases. The secretory repertoire of the macrophage rivals that of the hepatocyte. Because the number of products is so extensive, we will concentrate on a few of the most important enzymes and the complement proteins.

Among the most important products are plasminogen activator, collagenase, elastase, and proteases active at neutral pH. Plasminogen activator is a monocyte-macrophage product that is responsible for the formation of plasmin from plasminogen, a circulating plasma protein (see also Chap. 14, "Coagulation, Fibrinolytic, and Kinin Systems"). Plasmin is a thrombolytic agent that actively cleaves fibrogen polymers (which constitute blood clots) which form in damaged vessel walls. It resembles trypsin and splits lysine and arginine bonds. This monocyte-macro-

TABLE 18-2   Secretory Products of Monocytes and Macrophages

Enzymes
Lysozyme
Neutral proteases
Plasminogn activator
Collagenase
Elastase
Angiotensin convertase
Acid hydrolases
Lipases
Ribonucleases
Glycosidases
Vitamin D
Arachidonic acid metabolites
Complement components
C1, C4, C2, C3, C5
Factor B
Factor D
Properdin
C3b inactivator (C3bINH)
Binding proteins
Transferrin
Transcobalimin II
Fibronectin

phage enzyme is essential for resolution of thrombi which form throughout the body. Collagenase and elastase are two neutral proteases secreted by activated macrophages which can degrade vessel walls (which contain elastin), perivascular tissue, and articular surfaces (which contain collagen). These enzymes are important in degrading and resolving sites of inflammation throughout the body. However, in certain autoimmune diseases like rheumatoid arthritis, activation of these enzymes can lead to joint destruction. Products of collagen (produced by collagenase) are chemotactic for macrophages, so accumulation of more macrophages at sites of collagen degradation can occur, potentially causing more inflammation. Additionally, collagen degraded by collagenase is susceptible to further degradation by less specific proteases. The secretion of the neutral proteases is inducible by a variety of agents including endotoxin and immune complexes, whereas other enzymes which are usually intracellular, like lysosomal hydrolases, can be secreted (usually associated with a low pH) into extracellular fluid where they degrade collagen, basement membrane, and other connective tissue components. These enzymes can cause extensive destruction of joints in a variety of arthritides. In fact, macrophages may be a crucial cellular component in chronic inflammatory joint disease. Macrophages also secrete products which inhibit these catalytic enzymes. These include α_2-macroglobulin, which inhibits plasmin, collagenase, and elastase. The regulation of production of both neutral proteases and α_2-macroglobulin is incompletely understood.

Macrophages also synthesize and secrete a number of complement components, including C1, C4, C2, C3, C5, factor B, factor D, and properdin (Table 18-2) and generate the active fragments C3a, C5a, and Bb through the action of macrophage proteases. Macrophage migration can be influenced by complement. Fragments C3a and C5a stimulate macrophage migration; fragment Bb suppresses migration. As discussed in Chap. 13, complement proteins are essential components of the immune system. Macrophages,

along with hepatocytes, constitute the principal source for complement protein synthesis.

Macrophages also produce significant quantities of fibronectin, a large molecular mass protein dimer (450 kd) that has been implicated in cellular adhesion and locomotion. Macrophages also make a considerable quantity of biologically active lipids, including PGE_2, TXA_2, leukotrienes B and C, and a variety of eicosatetraenoic acids such as 5-HETE and 15-HETE. Macrophages are more active than neutrophils in the production of PGE_2, TXA_2, and leukotrienes. PGE_2, in fact, may directly mediate many of the in vitro actions of macrophages, particularly those involving suppression. Macrophage-derived PGE_2 has been reported to decrease neutrophil cytotoxicity and NK-cell activity, as well as lymphocyte-mediated cytotoxicity. In addition to its effect on other cells, PGE_2 acts on endogenous regulation of protein synthesis, affecting the formation of CSFs and interferon.

A characteristic enzyme made by activated macrophages is angiotensin-coverting enzyme (ACE), which converts angiotensin I to angiotensin II. ACE is important in the regulation of normal arterial blood pressure, since angiotensin II is the most potent pressor compound made by the body having a direct action on arterial smooth muscle. ACE is normally present in serum, but levels are markedly increased in a variety of granulomatous diseases including sarcoidosis, a multisystem disorder primarily involving the lung. (See Clinical Aside 18-1). However, an elevated ACE is not a specific diagnostic test for sarcoidosis.

Clinical Aside 18-1
Sarcoidosis

Sarcoidosis is a multisystem granulomatous disease of unclear etiology affecting predominantly black and Scandinavian populations. Females are slightly more affected than males. Two-thirds of patients are under 40 years of age at the onset of disease. Granuloma formation occurs in response to an as-yet-unidentified antigen. The organ most affected is the lung, and both the parenchyma and the intrathoracic lymph nodes are involved. Hilar adenopathy can usually be seen on chest x-ray with or without interstitial parenchymal infiltrates. Although the disease spontaneously remits in the majority of cases, if the granulomas are present in the alveolar septa and in the walls of bronchi, lung function can be altered, which can progress to respiratory insufficiency and death. There is a systemic granuloma formation involving other organs as well, including the central nervous system, muscles, skin, liver, eyes, bones, joints, and heart. The most characteristic histologic feature of this disease is the presence of epithelioid cell granulomas consisting of tightly packed central follicles of epithelioid cells derived from peripheral blood monocytes, as well as multinucleated giant cells of the Langerhans type.

The diagnosis of sarcoidosis is made on clinical history, the histologic finding of noncaseating granulomas, and the exclusion of other diseases which can produce a similar histologic and clinical picture. However, one can make a diagnosis of sarcoidosis utilizing the Kveim reaction. This test consists of intracutaneous injection of heat-sterilized extracts from either a lymph node or a spleen obtained from sarcoid patients and presumably containing the sarcoid antigen. If the patient injected with this material has sarcoidosis, a nodular lesion usually occurs 4 to 6 weeks later which when biopsied contains the characteristic epithelioid granuloma. Other characteristic laboratory features of sarcoidosis include elevated levels of all classes of immunoglobulin, failure to respond to recall antigens (anergy), elevated levels of ACE, which is produced by macrophages and epithelioid cells, and hypercalcemia. The hypercalcemia is caused by increased circulating levels of vitamin D, derived from the activated macrophages found in patients with sarcoidosis.

Monocytes also possess a low level of procoagulant activity, which increases considerably in the presence of stimulated lymphocytes. A variety of stimuli, including immune complexes, complement fragments, and lipopolysaccharide, can greatly increase procoagulant activity. Deposition of fibrin is a characteristic feature of delayed-type hypersensitivity reactions in the skin, as well as inflammation in other sites such as the kidney in proliferative glomerulonephritis. Macrophages contain receptors for fibrin and

fibrinogen degradation products which underlies the association between the coagulation cascade and monocytes.

MACROPHAGES IN CLINICAL MEDICINE

Macrophages serve as effector cells with potent antibacterial and antitumor activity. The resistance to infection with many intracellular bacteria (e.g., *Salmonella, Brucella, Listeria, Mycobacteria*), fungi, or other protozoal parasites revolves around the activation of macrophages in order to eradicate the infection. The functional expression of macrophage activation in vivo is a complex phenomenon that occurs at the site of inflammation. Activated macrophages have enhanced microbicidal activity, but activation is not specific to a particular pathogen;

TABLE 18-3   Secondary Causes of Monocyte Dysfunction

Affected Activity	Cause
Adherence	Drugs: ethanol, steroids, aspirin, tetracycline
Phagocytosis	Cigarette smoke (alveolar macrophages)
	Sepsis
Chemotaxis	Drugs: adrenergic agents, lipid emulsions, colchicine, penicillamine, amphotericin B
	Diabetes mellitus
	Down's syndrome
	Infections: sepsis, measles
	Severe allergic disorders
	Sickle cell crisis
	Thermal injury
	Surgical trauma
	Cancer
	Cirrhosis
	Kwashiorkor
Killing	Adrenergic agents
	Radiation therapy
	Down's syndrome
	Sepsis
	Cancer
	Vitamin B_{12} deficiency, iron deficiency

TABLE 18-4 Causes of Monocytosis

Infectious
   Tuberculosis, brucellosis, bacterial endocarditis,
     malaria, kala azar, trypanosomiasis, typhus
Inflammatory
   Sarcoidosis, ulcerative colitis, Crohn's disease,
     rheumatoid arthritis, SLE
Neoplastic
   Hodgkin's disease, acute myelocytic leukemia,
     myelodysplastic anemia, chronic myelomonocytic
     leukemia

macrophages activated by one organism are capable of killing others.

Diseases associated with macrophage dysfunction may be associated with other diseases or may be idiopathic. Defects in macrophage functions can lead to increased infections with bacterial organisms. Several rare conditions have been described in which macrophage defects predominate. *Malakoplakia*, an acquired granulomatous disease usually involving the ureters and characterized by the presence in tissue specimens of a collection of large mononuclear cells called *Hansmann macrophages*, is thought to result from a defect in macrophage phagocytosis. *Hydradenitis suppurativa* is a chronic staphylococcal infection of lymph nodes, particularly axillary, in which monocyte defects in phagocytosis and intracytoplasmic killing predominate. Secondary defects of monocyte function are listed in Table 18-3. *Monocytosis*, increased numbers of circulating monocytes, is seen in a number of disease states, including chronic infections, inflammatory disease, and malignancy (see Table 18-4).

Recent studies have described the important role of the monocyte in HIV-1 infection. Experimental evidence suggests that the peripheral blood monocyte serves as a reservoir for HIV-1. The virus is related to a family of lentiviruses which causes immunodeficiency in animals. A key feature of these infections is the role that the monocyte plays as the vehicle of transmission into the central nervous system. As the virus-infected monocyte matures into a macrophage, the HIV-1 viral genome is activated and production of intact virus occurs. This may have a direct deleterious effect on neighboring cells, including neurons. Studies of brains from patients with AIDS dementia complex have revealed HIV-1 infection of mononuclear cells but not neurons. It has been observed that HIV-1 grown in monocytes will preferentially infect other monocytes and not T cells. This pattern of HIV-1 replication may explain the latency period occurring between the actual viral infection and the development of opportunistic infections. If monocytes and not T cells were infected, the number of T cells might not decrease to the critical level associated with opportunistic infections for many years. Thus, HIV-1 infection may be a disease of monocytes as well as helper T cells.

CONCLUSION

Monocytes, when first described by Metchnikoff 100 years ago, were thought of only as scavenger cells with the ability to protect the host by engulfing and destroying invading bacteria. New experimental work has documented the importance of monocytes and macrophages in all phases of both humoral and cell-mediated immune responses. In preserving immune homeostasis, monocytes serve a key role in antigen processing and in the production of soluble factors which modulate or regulate the function of other immune cells.

SELF-TEST QUESTIONS*

1. Antigen processing is a function of all of the following cells *except*:
   a. Intestinal epithelial cells
   b. Monocytes
   c. Microglial cells
   d. Red blood cells
   e. Endothelial cells

*Answers will be found in Appendix E.

2. All of the following are produced by monocytes and macrophages *except*:
   a. IL-6
   b. IL-3
   c. IL-1
   d. IL-2
   e. Vitamin D
3. Monocytes enter into sites of inflammation in response to which of the following stimuli:
   a. Endotoxin
   b. *f*Met peptides
   c. Lymphokines
   e. All of the above
4. All of the following are necessary for antigen processing by monocytes *except*:

   a. Class II molecules
   b. Antigen internalization
   c. Endosomes
   d. Proton pumps

ADDITIONAL READINGS

Nathan CF, Secretory products of macrophages. *J Clin Invest.* 1987;79:319.

Unanue ER, Cerottini JC. Antigen presentation. *FASEB J.* 1989;3:2496–2502.

Unkeless JC, Scigliano E, Freedman VH. Structure and function of human and murine receptors for Fc. *Ann Rev Immunol.* 1988;8:251.

19

Basophils, Mast Cells, and Eosinophils

A. Mast Cells and Basophils

INTRODUCTION

Mast cells and basophils are a morphologically distinct population of cells, characterized by numerous granules which appear metachromatic (i.e., display a shift in color) if appropriately stained. These cells are derived from precursor cells residing in the bone marrow. The basophil develops along a granulocytic pathway, and eventually the mature cell enters and normally remains in the circulation. In contrast, mast cell differentiation stems from mononuclear cells and appears to be under separate control. The mast cell eventually resides fixed in connective tissue, usually in proximity to microvasculature, or in mucosal tissue. Not all mast cells assume an identical appearance or contain an identical array of secretory products, but precisely what influences the development of a particular subset of mast cells remains unclear. Experimental evidence derived from studies using rodents indicates that mast cells residing in mucosal tissue can multiply in response to interleukin 3 (IL-3) elaborated by T lymphocytes and have a unique phenotype, in contrast to mast cells found in connective tissue. A similar subset of mast cells likely exists in humans, although conclusive evidence for this is lacking.

The role played by these cells in mounting an allergic reaction in humans is of major importance in clinical medicine. Thus the pathologic events which occur in an individual with atopic dermatitis, bronchial asthma, allergic rhinitis, conjuctivitis, contact dermatitis, or anaphylaxis all serve to highlight the capacity of mast cells to mediate diverse inflammatory disorders. In each case the manner in which these cells are recruited and activated may be variable, but the result is the secretion of substances which have considerable effect on the vasculature and the surrounding tissue. This chapter describes the events surrounding mediator release and reviews some of the major secretory products.

MORPHOLOGIC CHARACTERISTICS

Mast cells are relatively large cells with a mean diameter of approximately 12 μm, although the size and shape of these cells may be quite variable. At times they resemble fibroblasts with an elongated narrow shape; at other times they assume the appearance of a rounded cell. However, certain characteristic features of mast cells are especially notable under the electron microscope. In fact, lacking these identifying features, it may be virtually impossible for even the most experienced histopathologist to label a particular cell as a mast cell. In 1879, Paul Ehrlich used basic aniline dyes and described the striking purple-violet staining and prominent appearance of the cytoplasmic granules characteristic of mast cells. This is the property of *metachromasia:* when cells are exposed to light of a certain wavelength, there is a shift in the wavelength emitted as visualized by light microscopy. This phenomenon results from interactions of the dye with the dense electron cloud imparted by the highly negatively charged proteoglycan within the granules. Basophils share this notable staining feature, and indeed at times it is difficult to differentiate basophils from mast cells in tissue specimens (normally basophils are circulating cells and rarely enter tissues in the absence of inflammation). Nonetheless, differences do exist. As you read through this chapter, it is important to bear in mind both the differences and the similarities of basophils and mast cells. Clearly, when one considers the common features, including the biochemical events initiated by aggregating

338

IgE, the array of potent chemical mediators released from the granules, and the similarities in appearance, it becomes evident why these cells are often grouped together in discussions of allergic responses.

Ultrastructural analysis of mast cells and basophils has led to advances in our ability to conceptualize the events which occur during activation and release of secretory products (Fig. 19A-1). In the resting state, basophils contain numerous electron-dense granules which range from 0.2 to 0.4 μm in

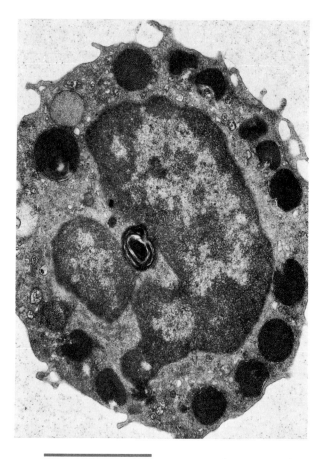

Figure 19A-1. Ultrastructure of a mature basophil. Note segmented nucleus and abundant electron-dense heterochromatin. ×18,000 (Reproduced from Lichtman MA: Basophilopenia, basophilia, and mastocytosis, in Williams WJ et al (eds): *Hematology*, 4/e. New York, McGraw-Hill, 1990, with permission.)

diameter. Mature human basophils are similar in overall size to other granulocytes (5 to 7 μm) and likewise contain a segmented nucleus. Within this nucleus, the chromatin tends to be heavily condensed (see Fig. 19A-1). The cytoplasm contains many dense particles (i.e., the granules) along with glycogen particles and aggregates. In general, the rough endoplasmic reticulum and the Golgi apparatus are inconspicuous. Overall, these cells appear round, with surface projections that are short, blunted, and irregularly distributed.

Human mast cells are quite pleomorphic ultrastructurally, in contrast to basophils. The nucleus of the mast cell is not segmented and tends to assume an eccentric location. The granules are more numerous and variable, and generally smaller. The granules themselves occasionally take on a highly ordered internal structure, consisting of scrolls, particles, and/or crystals (see Fig. 19A-2). The cytoplasm also lacks glycogen particles, but contains numerous oval lipid bodies which appear electron-dense and are usually larger than the granules. The surface of mast cells is covered with multiple thin projections, and the plasma membrane often has prominent folds. The morphologic changes observed following anaphylactic degranulation are dramatic and extensive. These are described in greater detail below, in the section depicting the biochemical events leading to degranulation.

Progress in recognizing mast cells within tissue sections has extended well beyond the routine usage of metachromatic dyes. The cytoplasmic granules can be visualized following reactions with compounds such as avidin or berberine, the latter requiring fluorescent microscopy. Technical advances in immunohistologic techniques employing monoclonal antibodies which react to specific membrane markers on mast cells (e.g., surface-bound IgE) or specific granule constituents (e.g., enzymes unique to mast cells) have led to a growing ability to identify these cells in tissue specimens. (See Clinical Aside 19A-1.)

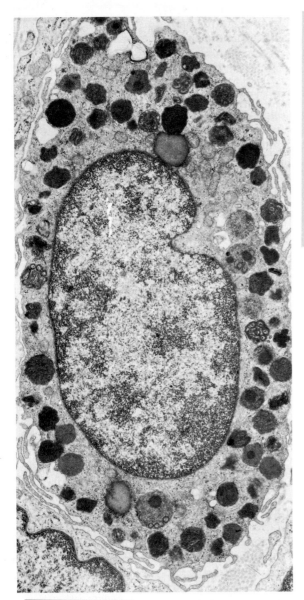

Figure 19A-2   Ultrastructure of a mast cell. Nucleus is not segmented and has more finely dispersed chromatin than the basophil. ×14,000. (Reproduced from Lichtman MA: Basophilopenia, basophilia, and mastocytosis, in Williams WJ et al (eds): *Hematology*, 4/e. New York, McGraw-Hill, 1990, with permission.)

Clinical Aside 19A-1
Mast Cells and Rheumatoid Arthritis

With better ability to recognize mast cells, there has been a growing realization that the number of mast cells may increase manyfold in a variety of disease states. An example of such an unexpected finding is seen in rheumatoid arthritis. It has been known for some time that in rheumatoid arthritis the synovial membrane lining the joint cavity becomes inflamed (synovitis), with a predominantly mononuclear cell infiltrate. However, newer techniques have revealed clusters of mast cells in this tissue, which often grow and invade the underlying cartilage and bone (see Fig. 19A-A1). The role of the mast cell in this setting

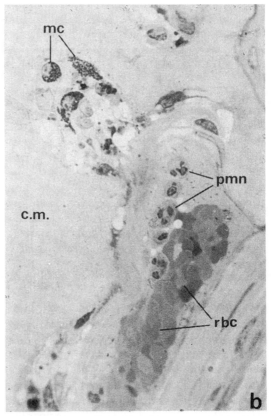

Figure 19A-A1   Cluster of mast cells seen at the junction of invading synovial tissue and cartilage in a rheumatoid joint. Seen nearby is a blood vessel. ×825. (From Bromley M, Fisher WD, Woolley DE. *Ann Rheum Dis.* 1984;43:76–79, with permission.)

and its contribution to the disease process is not yet clear. As you proceed through this chapter and become familiar with the more classical assignments for mast cells in allergic disorders, try to formulate your own hypothesis as to how mast cell secretory products might contribute to the pathologic process of inflammatory arthritis.

ORIGIN AND DISTRIBUTION

Accumulated evidence indicates that basophils stem from a precursor within the monocyte-granulocyte lineage. These cells mature in the bone marrow and then enter the circulation, representing approximately 0.5 percent of the total granulocyte pool. In general, the kinetics of basophil turnover are very similar to those of eosinophils, which is perhaps not surprising, since both cells are involved in allergic responses and may evolve from a common precursor. Like eosinophils, basophils can be recruited into the tissue following the appropriate signals during an inflammatory or immunologic response. An example of this is seen in the skin in contact dermatitis. The precise function of the basophil in this setting is unknown.

It is believed that basophils, like eosinophils, express immunity against certain parasitic infestations (ectoparasites). Strong support for this exists in rabbits and guinea pigs, where immunity to ticks is, in large part, a function of basophils. Occasionally, basophilia is an indication of an underlying neoplastic hematologic process. For example, basophilia is seen in chronic myelogenous leukemia, where basophils often enter the circulation in large numbers as part of the neoplastic process.

In contrast to basophils mast cells are not found in the circulation but rather comprise a ubiquitous portion of the fixed connective tissue cells. Virtually every organ contains mast cells. They are particularly abundant within mucosal tissues, lungs, and skin; they are found throughout the gastrointestinal system, and are often situated around blood

vessels, lymphatics, and nerves, or in close proximity with fibroblasts (see Fig. 19A-3). The density of mast cells in normal human skin is approximately 10,000/mm³. The origin of mast cells is also assumed to be the bone marrow, but considerably less is known about the proliferation, maturation, and recruitment of these cells (especially in humans). In rodents, mast cells can be derived from bone marrow cells placed in culture for several weeks in the presence of growth factors, notably IL-3. Furthermore, certain mice strains which are genetically deficient in mast cells can be reconstituted by bone marrow transplantation. Hence mast cell precursors likely reside in the bone marrow, albeit the proof in humans awaits identification of the appropriate growth factors and the critical microenvironment in which these cells can be grown from bone marrow. Furthermore, the stimuli which lead to mast cell

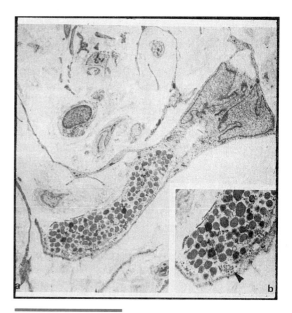

Figure 19A-3 (a) Two perineurial fibroblasts investing a mast cell, ×3000. (b) High-power view of the intimate association between the mast cell and the cytoplasmic process of the fibroblast. Note the presence of numerous vesiclelike strictures in the intracellular space (arrowhead). ×7600. (From Kirkpatrick CJ, Curry A. *Pathol Res Pract.* 1988;183:453, with permission.)

hyperplasia in disease states remain elusive at present. The recent finding that mast cells can synthesize and secrete specific lymphokines and monokines (as these substances are normally recognized as products of lymphocytes and monocytes) strongly supports the mononuclear cell origin of these cells, and suggests immunoregulatory functions for these cells. Indeed, in response to the appropriate signals (e.g., INF-γ), mast cells can express major histocompatibility complex (MHC) class II antigens.

MAST CELL HETEROGENEITY

In rodents, it is generally accepted that at least two distinct and different phenotypic populations of mast cells exist. This is readily apparent as one compares the mast cells which reside in connective tissue to those found in the superficial layers of mucosal tissue. A number of terms have been applied to differentiate these cells, including "typical" versus "atypical," "connective tissue" versus "mucosal," and "lymphocyte-dependent" versus "lymphocyte-independent." The scientific basis for the concept that not all mast cells are created equal (or, at least, do not mature along identical pathways) was confirmed with the discovery that the growth of mucosal mast cells, but not connective tissue mast cells, is dependent on IL-3, which is elaborated by T lymphocytes. Prior to this finding, the heterogeneity was based on slight differences in size, fixative requirements, response to specific secretagogues and antagonists, and staining properties. A complete description of these differences is beyond the scope of this textbook. The biochemical basis for many of the morphologic differences lies in the proportion of heparin versus chondroitin sulfate which the particular mast cell packages into its granules.

Mast cell–deficient mice have afforded researchers further insight in this area. If these mice are injected with competent mast cell precursors, the phenotype of the cell will be largely determined by its site of residence (i.e., connective tissue or mucosal). This sug-

gests that factors within the local environment control the mast cell phenotype found in that particular tissue. Indeed, recent data indicate that direct contact with fibroblasts may influence the development of mast cells toward a connective tissue phenotype.

These observations have proved difficult to extrapolate to humans. The problem in applying these findings stems largely from our inability to isolate lymphocyte-dependent mast cells in humans. An alternative classification system has recently been devised which is based on differences noted in the protease content of human mast cell granules. Two of the major granule-associated enzymes of mast cells are tryptase and chymase. Mast cells located in connective tissue contain both of these enzymes. Mast cells in mucosal tissue have been found to be deficient in chymase (hence the current proposed nomenclature involves use of the terms T mast cells and TC mast cells). Interestingly, in settings of T-lymphocyte deficiencies [such as AIDS and severe combined immunodeficiency disease (SCID)], biopsies of mucosal tissues show a paucity of T mast cells. (Caution: the use of T for both lymphocytes and mast cells can be confusing.) These data suggest that certain human mast cells are lymphocyte-dependent and these may be identified by their protease content.

The exact relevance and importance of cellular heterogeneity within a population of mast cells are difficult to determine at this time. However, for precisely this reason, one must be aware of the possibility that in the future we may be able to assign different functions to these subsets of mast cells with different implications in normal physiology and disease states (much in the way the biology of lymphocytes has evolved).

ACTIVATION AND THE DEGRANULATION PROCESS

Both basophils and mast cells are uniquely linked to the allergic response through their capacity to bind IgE. This is accomplished with great efficiency, as these cells are equipped with over 200,000 receptors per cell which have a very high affinity for the Fc portion of the IgE molecule (affinity constant greater than 10^{-9} mol/L). IgE may also bind with a much lower affinity to receptors on a variety of cells, including lymphocytes, neutrophils, platelets, monocytes, eosinophils, and dendritic cells. The function of these low-affinity receptors is not entirely clear. The high-affinity receptor (found only on basophils and mast cells) generates the signal, initiated by an allergen reacting with reagin (IgE), which is then transmitted internally to activate these cells to mount an allergic response. The presence and specificity of the pool of IgE molecules in an individual determine the potential for an allergic response to a particular substance. On the other hand, the mast cell (and basophil) allow for the expression of the allergic response. (See also Chap. 29, "Allergy.")

The allergic response is mediated by a complex set of reactions which begins at the cell membrane. This set of reactions can be initiated by IgE, as a minimum of two molecules on the membrane are brought into proximity by bound antigen at the cell surface. This in turn brings together two receptors in the cell membrane, an interaction which is then transmitted to the cytoplasmic component of the receptors, initiating a cascade of biochemical reactions. In fact, one can bypass the need for IgE by using antisera directed to the membrane receptors themselves. It should be emphasized that the classical IgE pathway is not the only means of activating these cells. Basophils degranulate in response to a number of cytokines, including IL-1, IL-3, and IL-8, granulocyte colony-stimulating factors, and other products released from monocytes, platelets, and neutrophils which are currently undergoing characterization. In addition, basophils respond to products generated during an inflammatory response, e.g., cleavage fragments of complement components generated during complement activation (C3a, C4a, and C5a all represent anaphylatoxins), neuropeptides, and proteases. Certain chemicals can

also induce basophil degranulation, such as morphine, several antibiotics (polymixin B, vancomycin), calcium ionophores, and specific polysaccharides or polymers (concanavalin A and compound 48/80), as well as hyperosmotic stimuli. The ways in which these substances lead to degranulation are poorly understood and controversial, especially in comparison to the well-studied antigen-IgE-coupled cell activation.

The biochemical events leading to the actual degranulation process are poorly understood, and a number of previous notions have become controversial. Although many textbooks describe a series of enzymatic reactions involving methyltransferases acting on phospholipids along the plasma membrane, disagreement about the presence and role of these pathways has recently arisen. Certainly, phospholipids are involved, and their metabolism generates a number of important secreted products as well as intracellular factors which promote granule fusion and exocytosis. However, the details of these reactions require further exploration. Regardless, electron microscopy reveals gross morphologic changes when these cells are exposed to a potent stimulus in vitro (such as crosslinking by anti-IgE antibodies). In mast cells derived from human lung specimens, the changes occur within minutes, and consist of swelling of individual granules, reduction of electron density of the granule matrix, and eventually fusion of several granules. These fused granules grow progressively larger, and the matrix becomes more fibrillar in appearance. Within approximately 10 min, the giant altered granules contact the plasma membrane and, through a pore, extrude their granule contents. At this point they appear as empty channels in the cytoplasm (see Fig. 19A-4). These ultrastructural characteristics are somewhat in contrast to what is observed when studying human basophils. Stimulation of basophils results in fusion of individual granule membranes with the plasma membrane (see Fig. 19A-4). The contents of the granules are released through multiple narrow communications to the exterior surface. Again, as the mediators are released, the granules appear hypodense. It is likely that

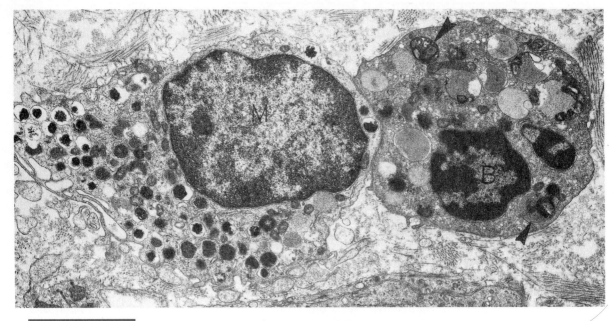

Figure 19A-4.   Mast cell (M) and basophil (B) in the ileal submucosa of a patient with Crohn disease. The mast cell is a larger, mononuclear cell with a more complex plasma membrane surface, and cytoplasmic granules that are smaller and more numerous than those of the basophil. In this section plane, the basophil exhibits two nuclear lobes. Several basophil cytoplasmic granules contain whorls of membranes (arrowheads). Osmium collidine uranyl en bloc processing. ×7650. (Reproduced from Galli SJ et al: Morphology, biochemistry, and function of basophils and mast cells, in Williams WJ et al (eds): *Hematology*, 4/e. New York, McGraw-Hill, 1990.)

exocytosis is induced when certain substances which comprise the backbone of the granule matrix undergo solubilization upon exposure to the exterior environment, leading to changes in electron microscopic appearance.

The aggregation of the IgE receptors sets into motion a number of biochemical events which act both to induce degranulation and to counter the activation process. The latter are known collectively as *desensitization*, and desensitization has been observed with a variety of stimuli. Obviously, considerable attention has been given to the details of this process, since pharmacologic intervention mimicking desensitization may allow better control of allergic conditions. It is known that this phenomenon involves enzymatic

pathways, as protease inhibitors tend to enhance histamine release and prevent desensitization. It is also known that release of mediators follows an increase in intracellular calcium, although this may not be required of all stimuli (phorbol esters, for example).

Despite the disagreement as to the precise role of membrane phospholipid metabolism in mediator release, it is likely that many cell types share certain common mechanisms in signal transduction. These involve release of inositol phosphates, calcium mobilization, and activation of protein kinase C via metabolites of the phospholipids (i.e., diglycerides). This in turn leads to assembly of microtubule-associated proteins. During this process, a number of proteins become phosphorylated, and these have been analyzed in considerable detail with the hope of designing or understanding effective drug therapy for allergic symptoms.

In addition to the events mentioned above, cross-linkage of IgE receptors induces the release of the membrane-associated unsaturated fatty acid, arachidonic acid. Metabolism of arachidonic acid then leads to the formation of products of the cyclooxygenase (prostaglandins) and lipoxygenase (leukotrienes) pathways; the potent platelet-activating factor (PAF) is also released (see Chap. 15 for a more detailed discussion of these inflammatory mediators). As discussed below, these mast cell products are formed in the process of cell activation and not stored in the granules. The activation process generates arachidonic acid by stimulating phospholipase A_2 to act on membrane phospholipids and at the same time stimulating the enzymes which metabolize this fatty acid.

CELL-DERIVED INFLAMMATORY MEDIATORS

Mast cells and basophils are replete with substances which have the capacity to regulate the microcirculation, leading to changes in vascular permeability. In addition, mast cell products influence cell traffic in and out of tissues, potentiate neural pathways, and may severely constrict the smooth muscles of airways. Thus massive release of mast cell and basophil products can mediate a violent immediate-type hypersensitivity reaction that can lead to death within a brief period. This type of response is known as *anaphylaxis*. (See Clinical Aside 19A-2.)

Clinical Aside 19A-2
Anaphylaxis

Each year, a number of deaths occur as a result of anaphylaxis. Insect stings and drug reactions comprise the most common inciting events. Among the insects, hornets, wasps, bees, and yellow jackets are each capable of inducing a systemic, even fatal, reaction in the sensitive individual. The reaction occurs within minutes of the sting, although we now recognize that even if the immediate reaction is brought under control, a more sustained reaction may appear several hours later. An appreciation that a late reaction can occur, heralded in some fashion by the initial reaction, dictates that the prudent physician continue to observe affected individuals in a hospital setting for up to 24 h. At some later date, the allergist can confirm the existence of antivenom IgE antibodies by skin testing using commercially available highly purified venom preparations. If the sensitivity is confirmed, the allergist may decide to gradually desensitize the individual by administering minute amounts of the venom (usually provoking a local reaction at the site of injection but hopefully not a systemic reaction). The amount of the venom is gradually increased on a weekly basis until a state of tolerance is reached. Monthly maintenance therapy is then required.

For convenience, mast cell mediators are often classified into three categories: preformed and easily eluted, preformed and granule-associated, and newly generated (see Table 19A-1). Although many biologic

TABLE 19A-1   Human Mast Cell Mediators

Preformed and eluted
  Histamine
  Eosinophil chemotactic factors
  Neutrophil chemotactic factors
  Superoxide
  Arylsulfatase A
  Elastase
  Hexosaminidase
  Glucosonidase
  Galactosidase
  Kallikrein-like enzyme
  Interleukins 3, 4, 5, 6, and 8
  Interferon-γ, TNF-α
Preformed and granule associated
  Heparin-chondroitin sulfate E
  Tryptase
  Chymotrypsin-like protease (chymase)
  Carboxypeptidase
  Superoxide dismutase, catalase (rodents)
  Arylsulfatase B
Newly generated
  Leukotrienes (LTC$_4$, LTD$_4$, LTE$_4$)
  PAF
  Prostaglandins (PGD$_2$)

TABLE 19A-2   Biologic Activities of Mast Cell Products

Selected Mediators	Actions
Histamine	Triple response of Lewis (vasodilatation, endothelial cell contraction, and increased vascular permeability, axon reflex) (H_1), pruritus (H_1), gastric acid secretion (H_2), lymphocyte suppression (H_2), chondrocyte activation (H_2), regulation of microcirculation (H_2), chemoattraction (eosinophils)
Heparin	Anticoagulation, anticomplementary (C1q binding, C4, C2, C3 activation, C3bBb convertase), stimulation of angiogenesis, enhancement of elastase activity, modulation of parathyroid hormone to induce osteoporosis, stimulation of collagenase synthesis, inhibition of activated collagenase, stabilization of tryptase, potentiation of fibronectin binding to collagen, inhibition of smooth muscle cell proliferation
Tryptase	Cleavage of trypsin substrates, inactivation of fibrinogen and high molecular weight kininogen, activation of latent metalloproteinases
Chymotrypsin-like protease (chymase)	Cleavage of chymotrypsin substrates, cleavage of fibronectin, laminin, and type IV collagen, conversion of angiotensin I to II, cleavage of dermal-epidermal junction
Prostaglandins (PGD_2)	Bronchoconstriction, chemoattraction, inhibition of platelet aggregation, vasodilatation, potentiation of LTC_4 on vasculature
Leukotrienes (LTC_4, LTD_4, LTE_4)	SRS-A, sustained smooth muscle contraction, vasodilatation, airway mucus secretion
PAF	Activation of neutrophils and platelets, smooth muscle contraction, vasopermeability, chemotaxis for eosinophils and neutrophils
Kallikrein-like enzyme	Generation of bradykinin

activities resulting from these substances have been well documented, the in vivo function of some of them still must be elucidated. Furthermore, among the many activities of each product, it is difficult to determine the most prominent during an immune response. Often these mediators are released during the inflammatory response, when numerous cell types are present, and this results in a very complex reaction. Therefore, the precise contributions of mast cells may be difficult to define, although experiments with mast cell–deficient mice indicate that these cells do, in fact, augment the inflammatory response within a tissue.

The bulk of our knowledge concerning the actions of mast cell products comes from the arduous task of isolating the substance, purifying to homogeneity, and administering to experimental animals or human subjects for observation purposes. A summary of these mediators and their activities is found in Table 19A-2.

What follows is a brief discussion of several major products secreted by these cells. In no way is this meant to be complete, and

Histamine

The granule-associated amine which has attracted great attention for its role in the allergic response is histamine. It is formed through the action of the cytoplasmic enzyme histidine decarboxylase on the amino acid histidine. Mast cells and basophils contain approximately 1 to 5 μg of histamine per million cells. This comprises between 5 and 10 percent of the weight of granules. Within the granules, histamine is bound to the core proteoglycan (see below). Almost all of the histamine in the human body is contained or released from mast cells or basophils. Normally a small amount is detectable in the circulation (less than 500 pg/mL). About 3 percent is excreted unchanged in the urine; the remainder is metabolized either by diamine oxidase or histamine methyltransferase. The excreted products in that case are methylhistamine and imidazole acetic acid.

The biologic activities of histamine are mediated predominantly by two major receptors, termed H_1 and H_2, and the ratio of these two receptors in any given tissue determines the effect of histamine. Histamine binding to H_1 receptors leads to bronchial and smooth muscle contraction, increased vascular permeability, pulmonary vasoconstriction, increased intracellular cyclic GMP (cGMP) levels, and increased nasal mucus production, and it also directs eosinophils and neutrophils to migrate against a gradient (chemotaxis). Most of these effects are blocked with antihistamines. Histamine occupying the H_2 receptors leads to increased airway mucus production, gastric acid release, and intracellular cAMP levels; stimulates a subset of suppressor lymphocytes; inhibits lymphocytotoxicity; decreases histamine release from basophils and some mast cells (which may represent feedback regulation); and leads to bronchodilatation. These effects can be blocked by H_2 antagonists, which have become a mainstay in the treatment of peptic ulcer disease. Stimulation of both receptors induces pruritus, vasodilatation, and cardiac irritability. Clinically, the local release of histamine in skin causes edema, flushing, and pruritus, collectively referred to as the *wheal-and-flare reaction,* or *triple response of Lewis.* At least a portion of this response is due to the simultaneous release of the neuropeptide, substance P. In the gut, local histamine release leads to diarrhea, cramping, acid release, and mucus production; in the lung, bronchoconstriction and mucus production are observed. If histamine is infused in the circulation, cardiac arrhythmias, profound hypotension, and fluid shifts (so-called third spacing) occur.

Platelet-Activating Factor (PAF)

As mentioned earlier, several subtances are formed as a result of the membrane events associated with IgE-antigen-coupled activation. The extremely potent spasmogen PAF, which is released by metabolism of membrane-associated phospholipids, is such a compound. Removal of an acetate group from the PAF molecule produces lyso-PAF, an inactive substance. Several cell types appear capable of releasing PAF, including macrophages, neutrophils, eosinophils, and mast cells. It is not certain that human basophils are capable of synthesizing PAF.

Originally described by its ability to aggregate platelets following IgE-mediated basophil release, this molecule possesses extraordinary potent biologic activities at concentrations below 10^{-10} mol/L. In addition to being the most effective platelet aggregator known, it also aggregates neutrophils and monocytes. Neutrophils are particularly sensitive to the actions of PAF through a specific receptor and will respond with directed migration, an oxidative burst, and the production of lipoxygenase products. Injected into skin, PAF causes a wheal-and-flare response which can be associated with leukocyte infiltration. It also can induce spasm of ileal smooth muscle, lung strips, and can lead to dramatic hypotension and cardiovascular collapse when given intravenously. Compliance changes in the lungs are reflected by pulmonary artery hypertension, edema formation, and a prolonged increase in total pulmonary resistance. It is no wonder that this substance has created so much excitement among researchers studying mediators of allergic reactions. (See also Chap. 15, on the lipid mediators of inflammation.)

Arachidonic Acid Metabolites

The prostaglandins and the sulfidopeptide leukotrienes represent a large family of compounds, at least one of which virtually every cell is capable of generating. The specific products that human mast cells release following stimulation (alas, another example of a secreted product not stored by these cells) deserve mention. The major cyclooxygenase pathway in human lung mast cells leads to synthesis of large amounts of prostaglandin D_2 (PGD_2). When injected intracutaneously PGD_2 produces an asymptomatic wheal and flare, followed by progressive dermal edema lasting over 2 h. Accompanying this, a biphasic perivenular infiltrate of neutrophils is apparent at 30 min and then at 6 h. Some evidence suggests that the flushing and hypotension that occur in people with mastocytosis (see below) is a result of circulating PGD_2.

The lipoxygenase pathway in mast cells is rich in enzymes which generate hydroperoxy products of the 5-HPETE (5-hydroxyperoxyeicosatetraenoic acid) group, which are rapidly metabolized to 5-HETE (5-hydroxyeicosatetraenoic acid). Alternatively, the 5-HPETE is transformed into the leukotrienes LTB_4, LTC_4, LTD_4, and LTE_4. It is not clear that human mast cells are a source of LTB_4, but the latter three compounds comprise a group of mast cell products previously called *slow-reacting substances of anaphylaxis (SRS-A)*. This term reflects the biologic activities of these substances. Injection into the skin generates a burning, erythematous wheal-and-flare response which persists for 4 h. Microscopically, one finds dermal edema, dilatation of venules and capillaries, and endothelial cell activation (as reflected by alterations in morphology). Inhalation studies using LTD_4 have demonstrated reversible constriction of peripheral airways, with a potency 100- to 1000-fold that of histamine. In general, the sulfidopeptides have activities similar to those of histamine; however, they are much more potent on a mole per mole basis and are longer-lasting. (See also Chap. 15.)

Chemotactic Factors

A number of mast cell products have been identified which mediate migration of granulocytes and mononuclear cells. *Neutrophil chemotactic factors (NCFs)* (e.g., high molecular weight NCF, or HMW-NCF) are released in the circulation shortly after mast cell activation. The release of HMW-NCF can be demonstrated in asthmatic patients in response to antigen challenge and is accompanied by transient leukocytosis. As mentioned above, the arachidonic acid metabolites (particularly LTB_4), PAF, and histamine are chemotactic for human neutrophils.

In the low molecular weight region of mast cell supernatants, an eosinophilic chemotactic factor has been identified following antigen challenge. This factor, termed *eosinophil chemotactic factor of anaphylaxis (ECF-A)*, may explain the often-observed eosinophilic infiltrates or eosinophilia associated with allergic responses. Some of this activity is attributed to two synthetic tetrapeptides, Val-Gly-Ser-Glu and Ala-Gly-Ser-Glu. Clearly, the most potent eosinophilic factor yet described is PAF.

Other factors have been identified which affect T and B lymphocytes; some of these inhibit and others promote directed migration. In addition, numerous effects have been demonstrated in vitro by leukotrienes, prostanoids, and biogenic amines on mononuclear cells.

Enzymes

The most prominent enzyme found in human mast cells is tryptase, a tryptic protease that comprises approximately 25 percent of the dry weight of mast cells. It is stabilized in an active form with a molecular mass of 134 kd by forming a tight complex with heparin. Human basophils contain a minute amount of tryptase; no other human cell appears capable of synthesizing this enzyme. For this reason, immunolocalization of tryptase serves as a convenient way of highlighting mast cells in tissue specimens. Furthermore, the detection of elevated levels of tryptase in the circulation reflects mast cell activation. (See Clinical Aside 19A-3.)

Clinical Aside 19A-3
Chest Pain after Bee Stings:
Measuring Serum Tryptase Levels

The following situation attests to the clinical utility of measuring circulating tryptase levels. A middle-aged man presents to the emergency ward clutching his chest with pain. He is hypotensive and states that he was stung by a bee while working in his garden. Shortly thereafter he began to sweat, became dizzy, and developed chest pain. The electrocardiogram identified changes consistent with myocardial ischemia. The question at hand is, Did the bee sting lead to an anaphylactic reaction inducing hypotension with subsequent coronary insufficiency or is this clinical situation due to garden-variety effort-related angina? (Why is this differentiation important to you as a clinician and to the patient's future?) A serum sample was submitted for tryptase level, which was subsequently determined to be elevated. Hopefully, the reader can continue the evaluation from this point.

Tryptase is an endopeptidase at neutral pH which can be quantified by hydrolysis of the synthetic substrate, tosyl-L-arginine methyl ester (TAMe), or by immunoassays. Unique to tryptase is the fact that the normal mechanisms which exist to inhibit active proteases through circulating or tissue-bound inhibitors appear not to have activity against this enzyme. Although tryptase has been shown to destroy high molecular weight kininogen, the major substrate in vivo for this protease remains unknown. In concert with the finding of mast cells in areas of collagen degradation, recent in vitro experiments indicate that tryptase can activate the latent metalloproteinases, which in turn dissolve matrix. In this manner, mast cells may play a role in connective tissue homeostasis or pathology.

Chymase, which is characterized as a monomer with a molecular mass of 28 kd, has been purified from human dermal mast cells. This enzyme converts angiotensin I to angiotensin II in vitro and degrades certain matrix components of basement membranes, including substrates such as laminin and type IV collagen. Some of these activities may explain an apparent dermal-epidermal separation that is observed when fragments of human skin are incubated with chymase.

Other enzymes described in mast cells include a unique carboxypeptidase, acid hydrolases, β-hexosaminidase, β-glucuronidase, β-D-galactosidase, and arylsulfatases. In addition, oxidative enzymes such as superoxide dismutase and peroxidase are ubiquitous among respiring cells. Peroxidases are capable of destroying the activities of sulfidopeptide leukotrienes.

Proteoglycans

The core of the granules of both mast cells and basophils is composed of proteoglycan molecules. The metachromatic staining of these cells is due to the presence of the highly sulfated proteoglycans. The predominant proteoglycan in human mast cells is heparin, the most acidic molecule in the entire body. Bone marrow–derived mouse mast cells and human basophils apparently contain mostly chondroitin sulfate. The difference in structure between these proteoglycans is found in their glycosaminoglycan side chains: heparin consists of uronic acids linked to glucosamine and chondroitin sulfate is composed of uronic acid linked to galactosamine. These molecules are relatively resistant to proteases mainly because of the dense distribution of the glycosaminoglycan side chains.

Proteoglycans, as they exist in the granules, have many functions, one of which is to stabilize other stored active substances such as the proteases. In addition, both secreted heparin and the commercial product isolated from porcine gut have diverse biologic activities. A clinically useful activity is the inhibition of blood coagulation by potentiating the activity of antithrombin III. Other miscellaneous effects of heparin include increasing the enzymatic activity of elastase, promoting the release of plasminogen activator from endothelial cells, and enhancing collagen binding to fibronectin. Heparin also appears to potentiate endothelial cell–derived growth factors by inducing their release, prolonging their half-life by binding, protecting them from protease degradation, and enhancing their effects on other cells. Heparin inhibits the proliferation of smooth muscle cells through the modulation of oncogene expression. Certain protooncogenes, such as c-*myc* and c-*fos*, are requisite for cells to enter the growth cycle, and heparin appears to inhibit their expression following mitogenic stimuli (such as phorbol esters). Heparin also inhibits multiple steps within the complement cascade, including C1q binding to immune complexes, C1s activation of C4 and C2, the amplification of convertase C3bBb, and zymosan-dependent activation of C3. On the other hand, C1-inhibitor activity appears to be enhanced in the presence of heparin. It has also been shown that heparin has the ability to induce osteoporosis when administered as an anticoagulant for prolonged periods of time. This may be the result of a synergistic effect of parathormone and heparin on bone matrix. (See Clinical Aside 19A-4.)

Clinical Aside 19A-4
Mastocytosis

Much can be learned about the biologic effects of mast cell products by studying the rare individual in whom mast cells accumulate to pathologic levels. A spectrum of clinical manifestations is found in the patient with this condition, known as *mastocytosis*. Often presenting in childhood, mastocytosis can be as benign as a pruritic skin eruption (known as *urticaria pigmentosa*) or as serious and devastating as the life-threatening condition, *systemic mastocytosis*, where generalized mast cell infiltration occurs. The latter may be manifested by flushing, hypotension, disorientation, head-aches, or abdominal cramps and diarrhea. Mast cell infiltration may enlarge the liver, spleen, and lymph nodes. Bones are frequently involved, resulting in areas of osteoporosis adjacent to bony sclerosis. Many of the clinical manifestations are a result of circulating vasoactive compounds, whereas some occur as a consequence of the effects of mast cell products on neighboring cells.

Other Mediators

Recently, investigators in the field have discovered that mast cells are a rich source of cytokines, once believed to be solely in the parlance of mononuclear cells. The mRNA encoding interleukins 3, 4, 5, 6, and 8, GM-CSF, and IFN-γ has been detected in bone marrow–derived mouse mast cells following cross-linkage of IgE, using probes currently available. In addition, human endothelial cells in situ can be activated (as demonstrated by the expression of receptors which promote adhesion to neutrophils) within 2 h after mast cells are stimulated; this phenomenon can be inhibited by the addition of monoclonal antibodies to tumor necrosis factor alpha (TNF-α). This exciting information allows further speculation concerning the role of mast cells in a number of cell-mediated immune responses, as well as their contribution to hematopoiesis and general inflammation.

CONCLUSION

Mast cells and basophils have high-affinity receptors for IgE which allow these cells to respond by secreting numerous potent products in an allergic response. Differences exist between these cells and probably between different subpopulations of mast cells themselves. The extent to which these cells are harmful or beneficial to an individual probably depends on a host of factors, including the quantity of cells infiltrating a tissue, the presence of effective stimuli, the processing and degradation of secreted products, and perhaps on the particular subset of mast cell.

Detailed histologic studies of normal physiologic processes such as wound healing, bone fracture repair, and neovascularization reveal the presence of numerous mast cells. This has suggested that these cells are actively involved in the homeostasis of connective tissue metabolism. Supporting this hypothesis is the finding of mast cell hyperplasia in diseased states characterized by excessive fibrosis or turnover of tissue. A role for mast cells has been proposed in diseases which are characterized by excessive scarring such as scleroderma (where numerous organs including the skin are crowded out by excessive collagen deposits), keloidosis, pulmonary fibrosis, and rheumatoid arthritis (the latter being an example of excessive breakdown of tissue). Therefore, mast cell mediators when acutely released may provoke anaphylaxis, hives, or bronchospasm, but over an extended period of time may alter mesenchymal tissue in ways which are incompletely understood. On the other hand, basophils and mast cells may be critical for defense against ticks and helminths (the latter in part due to the ability of mast cell mediators to mobilize eosinophils).

ADDITIONAL READINGS

Galli SJ, Lichtenstein LM. Biology of mast cells and basophils. In Middleton E, Jr, ed. *Allergy and Practice.* 3rd ed. St. Louis, Mo: Mosby; 1988;106–134.

Mast cell activation and mediator release. In: Ishizaka K, ed. *Progress in Allergy.* S. Karger AG; 1984.

Metcalfe DD, Corta JJ, Burd PR. Mast cells and basophils. In: Gallin JI, Goldstein IM, Snyderman R, eds. *Inflammation: Basic Principles and Clinical Correlates.* 2nd ed. New York: Raven Press; 1992.

Metcalfe DD, Kaliner M, Donlon MA. The mast cell. *Crit Rev Immunol* 1981;3:23.

Wasserman SI. Mediators of immediate hypersensitivity. *J Allergy Clin Immunol.* 1983;72:107–117.

19

Basophils, Mast Cells, and Eosinophils

B. Eosinophils

INTRODUCTION

Eosinophils are formed in the bone marrow, from precursors which are themselves derived from a stem cell common to neutrophils and possibly basophils. Eosinophils mature in about 2 to 6 days; they then enter the circulation, with a half-life of only 6 to 12 h. Blood eosinophils are easily recognized by their distinct features in stained preparations of peripheral blood (bilobed nucleus and many granules), but these blood-borne cells represent a tiny percentage of the total body store of eosinophils. It has been estimated that there are 300 tissue-resident eosinophils for each circulating cell in the rat. In humans there may be as many as 200 eosinophils in the bone marrow and 500 in the loose submucosal tissues for each eosinophil in the blood. Thus, these cells are primarily tissue-dwelling, with the majority of eosinophils found in the same sites as mast cells, often in those tissues whose epithelial surfaces are in contact with the outside world. Eosinophils, basophils, mast cells, and IgE are all components of immunity at body surfaces. Eosinophils have much in common with basophils and mast cells, although there are clear differences, which will be discussed later.

SURFACE COMPONENTS

The surface of the eosinophil contains Fc receptors for IgE, IgA, IgG, and perhaps IgM. There are also receptors for the complement components C3b and C4; the number of receptors increases after exposure of the cell to two basophil-derived inflammatory mediators, histamine and eosinophil chemotactic factor of anaphylaxis (ECF-A). All of these binding activities are of great relevance to the physiologic and pathologic functions of eosinophils.

The surface membrane of the eosinophil also contains lysophospholipase. When large numbers of eosinophils are involved in an immune response and die, the liberated lysophospholipase may coalesce into particles known as *Charcot-Leyden crystals.* These are elongate bipyramidal crystals occasionally seen in clinical specimens, e.g., the sputum of patients with asthma. This Charcot-Leyden protein was long thought to be unique to eosinophils, but it is now known that this protein is also found in basophils.

GRANULE COMPONENTS

The granules of the eosinophil gave rise to the cell's name; the same Paul Ehrlich who identified the basophil found another blood cell, one whose granules bound the rose-colored dye eosin very strongly. And it is the granules of the eosinophil which are among its most fascinating features (Fig. 19B-1). There are about 200 granules in each cell, of three types. The small granule, present only in mature eosinophils, contains acid phosphatase and arylsulfatase; arylsulfatase is capable of modulating slow reacting substance of analyphylaxis (SRS-A), now known to be leukotrienes. The primary granule is round and electron-dense and prominent in the eosinophilic promyelocyte. The third type of granule, called the *secondary granule*, provides most of the "punch" of the eosinophil.

The secondary granule consists of an electron-dense core made up of a crystal of the protein known as *major basic protein* (MBP). The name is a good description of the protein—*protein*, because it is chemically a protein; *basic*, because of the very high isoelectric point (pH 11.6), which is due to the fact that about 16 percent of the amino acid residues are arginine; and *major*, because it makes up 55 percent of the granule protein and about 25 percent of the total cellular protein in the rat eosinophil.

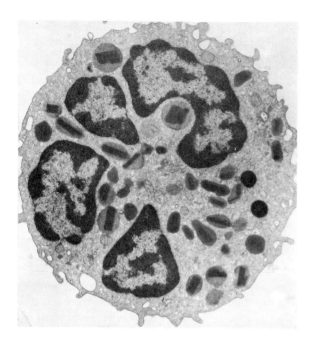

Figure 19B-1 Electron photomicrograph of a mature eosinophil. Granules have a central electron-dense core, or crystalloid, surrounded by matrix, which is less dense. ×16,500. (From Zucker-Franklin D: Eosinophils: Morphology, production, chemistry, and function, in Williams WJ et al (eds): *Hematology*, 4/e. New York, McGraw-Hill, 1990, used with permission.)

MBP causes the release of histamine from basophils and mast cells and binds to and neutralizes heparin anticoagulant activity. Initially, MBP was thought to be a protein unique to the eosinophil. However, just as with the Charcot-Leyden crystal protein, MBP was also found in basophils, but at only a fraction of the amount found in eosinophils. One study found nearly 5000 ng of MBP per 1 million eosinophils and only 140 ng per 1 million basophils, a ratio of about 35:1. MBP is also taken up by mast cells, perhaps as a means of neutralizing MBP at sites of inflammation.

MBP plays a major role in the eosinophil's ability to destroy parasites, the best studied example being *Schistosoma.* This killing is accomplished in two steps. The surface Fc receptor of the eosinophil binds immunoglobulin already bound to the parasite, which brings the target and effector cell into close proximity in an antigen-specific fashion. Following this, irreversible binding of the eosinophil to the parasite takes place, with degranulation of the cells. MBP in the liberated material then binds to the surface of the parasite, causing both damage to the surface membrane and diminution in mobility of the membrane and sluggish movement of the organism.

MBP may be implicated in other, pathologic, effects of eosinophils. Mammalian cells, both neoplastic and normal, can be damaged by MBP. MBP has a direct toxic effect on respiratory epithelium, with slowing of ciliary beating in studies on tracheal explants. This may be a crucial contribution to the respiratory epithelial damage found in asthma; large amounts of MBP are found in the sputum of patients with asthma.

Also within the secondary granules are other very basic proteins which constitute the matrix, as opposed to the core. These include eosinophil cationic protein (ECP), eosinophil-derived neurotoxin (EDN) [also known as eosinophil protein X (EPX)], and eosinophil peroxidase (EPO).

ECP is a potent neurotoxin and helminthotoxin. As a helminthotoxin, ECP may be a very potent agent; in killing *Schistosoma mansoni*, ECP is 8 to 10 times more potent on a mole per mole basis than MBP. ECP has no intrinsic antibacterial activity. In addition, ECP has been shown to alter coagulation and fibrinolytic function by enhancing factor XII–dependent reactions. ECP also binds to heparin and neutralizes the latter's anticoagulant activity. (What cell, intimately involved with the function of eosinophils, is very rich in heparin?). Finally, ECP inhibits in vitro proliferation of peripheral blood mononuclear cells in cultures.

EDN bears strong N-terminal-sequence homology with ECP; both of these compounds are structurally closely related to human pancreatic ribonuclease and both have

RNase activity (EDN more than ECP). EDN, like ECP, is toxic to helminths and can inhibit peripheral blood mononuclear cell cultures, but is named for its ability to induce damage to myelinated neurons in experimental animals. Between 3 and 11 days after intrathecal injection of EDN, the animal develops stiffness, followed by incoordination and ataxia. Finally, severe wasting and weakness occur, occasionally associated with nystagmus and repetitive, jerky head motions. On light microscopy, there is extensive spongiform degeneration of white matter, with no change in gray matter; disappearance of the Purkinje cells of the cerebellum is a classic finding. This syndrome due to EDN (also caused by ECP injection, a final note of parallelism of ECP and EDN) is called the *Gordon phenomenon.*

EPO, another basic matrix granule protein, is very active in killing microorganisms (including bacteria, mycoplasma, viruses, fungi, helminths, and other parasites, as well as other cells like neoplastic and mast cells). This occurs when EPO, hydrogen peroxide, and iodide interact to iodinate and kill the cell; part of the increased killing may be mediated by mononuclear phagocytes. Surface-bound EPO on tumor cells increases their sensitivity to lysis by hydrogen peroxide, and spontaneous cytolysis of tumor cells by macrophages is increased if the tumor cells are EPO-coated. In addition, EPO and hydrogen peroxide can oxidize other molecules; an example of this is the inactivation of leukotrienes.

Mast cell degranulation can be stimulated by EPO. The peroxidase can bind to the surface of mast cells and, at levels of EPO which are not toxic to the mast cell, is more efficient in inducing degranulation and release of histamine.

OTHER BIOCHEMICAL ACTIVITIES OF EOSINOPHILS

Eosinophils contain other, often less well described, enzymatic activities, including col-lagenase, acetylcholinesterase, acid glycerophosphatase, ATPase, β-glucuronidase, cathepsin, acid and alkaline phosphatase, histaminase, and phospholipase D. Arachidonic acid metabolism by the eosinophil yields such products of the lipoxygenase pathway as leukotrienes C_4 and D_4, and 5-hydroxyeicosatetraenoic acid (5-HETE). The production of LTC_4 and LTD_4 by eosinophils is in contrast to the production of LTB_4 by neutrophils; LTC_4 production is increased when the EPO–hydrogen peroxide–halide system is inhibited. Of note is the fact that eosinophils stimulated by allergens or anti-IgE antibodies (which cross-link the surface IgE receptors) produce prostaglandins PGE_1 and PGE_2, potent inhibitors of histamine release from leukocytes. The Charcot-Leyden crystal protein lysophospholipase may have a regulatory function also; lysophospholipases can inactivate the toxic lysophosphates liberated by the action of phospholipase A_2. Enzymes found in the eosinophil can neutralize other mediators of anaphylaxis, including histamine, platelet-activating factor, and SRS-A.

Thus, this recent evidence suggests another role for eosinophils. Eosinophils are capable of inactivating certain mediators of inflammation produced by mast cells. This provides a means of decreasing the severity of IGE-mediated phenomena, which includes responses to parasites, as well as allergic reactions and anaphylaxis. (See Chap. 29, "Allergy".)

Eosinophils play a key role in the response to parasites, although there is incomplete understanding of how eosinophils help defeat the invader. Elevated levels of eosinophils in the blood (eosinophilia) can be seen in patients with a number of types of disorders (Table 19B-1). It is clear that eosinophils have a role in the pathogenesis of hypersensitivity phenomena, like asthma, hay fever, atopic dermatitis, and anaphylaxis (see Chap. 29, "Allergy"). Cardiac localization of MBP in acute necrotizing myocarditis and the correlation, in asthmatics, of the amount of ECP in bronchoalveolar lavage with the severity of the asthma would seem to con-

TABLE 19B-1   Some Causes of Eosinophilia

Allergic phenomena
  Hay fever, asthma
  Drug reactions, e.g., to iodides, sulfonamides, β-lactam antibiotics (penicillins and
    cephalosporins)
Parasitic disease
  Tissue forms—*Trichinella, Strongyloides, Echinococcus,* cysticercosis, filariasis,
    schistosomiasis
  Intestinal forms—Roundworm: *Ascaria*
  Hookworm: *Ancylostoma duodenale, Ancylostoma ceylanicum, Necator americanus*
Malignancy
  Hodgkin's disease, chronic myelogenous leukemia and myelodysplastic syndromes,
    carcinomas (ovary, stomach, and lung, among others)
Autoimmune and collagen vascular disease
  Rheumatoid arthritis, dermatomyositis, polyarteritis nodosa
Hypereosinophilic syndrome

firm this role of eosinophilic inflammation in these diseases. Eosinophils may also be involved in the pathogenesis of other non-allergic diseases, including chronic eosinophilic pneumonia and the hypereosinophilic syndrome (see Clinical Aside 19B-1).

Clinical Aside 19B-1
The Hypereosinophilic Syndrome

This is a term which describes a spectrum of clinical disorders all of which include an elevation in peripheral blood eosinophil levels; the eosinophil count may be as high as 100,000/μL and may comprise 30 to 80 percent of the total peripheral blood cell count. The bone marrow is hypercellular, containing many eosinophils and eosinophil precursors. Anemia may be present as well. Eosinophilic infiltration of different organs occurs, with damage probably mediated by the mechanisms described in this chapter. There may be fibroplastic endocardial growth and/or fibrosis, pulmonary infiltrates and/or pleural effusions, and splenomegaly and hepatomegaly. Due to left-sided endocardial damage there may be local thrombus formation; if pieces of this mural thrombus break off, damage may be done elsewhere due to occlusion of systemic blood vessels. Neurologic damage may occur caused by ischemic central nervous system, possibly due to embolization; polyneuropathy or encephalopathy may occur, possibly caused by the direct toxic effects of granule contents of the eosinophil, like MBP and ECP.

There is an interesting heterogeneity in eosinophil populations. Most eosinophils are of approximate density 1.088, but a light-density (or hypodense) population (density 1.075 to 1.077) is also found. These cells are preferentially represented in eosinophilic pleural effusions. The hypodense population has a greater percentage of cells with receptors for IgG, and cells in this population exhibit greater oxygen consumption, produce more LTC_4, have fewer granules, and are more cytotoxic. This population may represent preactivated cells, cells which have already been partially degranulated, or may be released from the bone marrow as a separate functional class of cell.

EOSINOPHIL CHEMOTACTIC FACTORS

A number of molecules have the potential to induce eosinophil chemotaxis or modification of eosinophil function. T cells produce growth factors which enhance differentiation of eosinophils from bone marrow stem cells and chemotactic factors which cause infiltration of eosinophils into tissues; the net effect is increased production and delivery of these cells. As well, factors in T-cell culture supernatants, including an activity called *eosinophil stimulator promoter,* induce increased efficiency of eosinophil killing of pathogens. Mast cells produce ECF-A, a tetrapeptide, and histamine; both ECF-A and histamine are very active in attracting eosinophils and enhancing killing (as well as increasing the expression of cell surface receptors for C4 and C3b, as noted above). A variety of colony-stimulating factors, including T cell–derived granulocyte-macrophage colony-stimulating factor and eosinophil differentiation factor (IL-4) have an effect on eosinophil activation as well as eosinophil maturation. Monocyte-derived eosinophil-cytotoxicity-enhancing factor (M-ECEF), which may be identical to TNF, also enhances eosinophil killing. LTB$_4$ also increases eosinophil cytotoxicity. Immune complexes and complement fragment C5a are also chemotactic for eosinophils and neutrophils; eosinophils can phagocytose immune complexes, as well. The ability of eosinophils to devour immune complexes may be the explanation for the finding of large numbers of eosinophils in long-standing pleural and synovial effusions occasionally seen in inflammatory diseases, like rheumatoid arthritis and systemic lupus erythematosus. Finally, molecules derived from the parasite targets of eosinophils serve as eosinophil chemotactic factors, beckoning these effector cells to the very site where they are needed.

SIMILARITIES OF EOSINOPHILS, MAST CELLS, AND BASOPHILS

As noted above, eosinophils, mast cells, and basophils are linked in function and often share molecular characteristics. Basophils and mast cells have high-affinity receptors for IgE and histamine, and basophils contain Charcot-Leyden crystal proteins and MBP. There is a single combined congenital deficiency of basophils and eosinophils, and there are patients who lack both populations of cells. Finally, colony formation studies have shown

the coexistence of basophils and mast cells in eosinophil colonies and mixed eosinophil-basophil colonies.

ANOTHER ROLE FOR MBP?

We will end this section on a speculative note. The uterus of rats in estrus is infiltrated with eosinophils, although no eosinophils are found in the gravid uterus of rats or humans. However, all pregnant human females in one study had elevated serum levels of MBP, without eosinophilia or elevated levels of ECP or EDN. This increase started at about 4 weeks of gestation, increased until about 20 weeks, and then plateaued until about 33 weeks. A further increase was noted 2 to 3 weeks prior to labor. After delivery, MBP levels rapidly fell to normal. Elevation of MBP is not seen in women with prolonged gestation who do not have spontaneous labor, and MBP levels do not rise during induced labor. Elevations are found during premature labor and correlate with the onset of spontaneous labor. Although no eosinophils were found in the uterus, MBP was isolated in certain populations of placental cells, found at the junction between maternal and placental tissues. These findings taken together suggest that MBP may have a role in the induction or progression of labor. MBP may alter the contractility of uterine muscle or might have a role in the release of the placenta from the uterine wall. If these findings are correct, this may represent yet another example of the parsimony of nature: how a single molecule can be used in different physiologic systems.

ADDITIONAL READINGS

Gleich GJ. Current understanding of eosinophil function. *Hosp Pract.* March 15, 1988;97–119.

Gleich GJ, Adolphson CR. The eosinophil leukocyte: Structure and function. *Adv Immunol.* 1986;39:177–210.

INTRODUCTION

The development of an inflammatory response is an important mechanism by which an organism defends itself against pathogenic agents and initiates both structural and functional repair of damaged tissues. It represents a complex interaction between pathogenic agents, parenchymal cell and tissue components, the vasculature, and both plasma and cellular components of blood. Traditionally, the evolution of the inflammatory response has been viewed as a continuum from the early stages of acute inflammation to a more chronic inflammatory reaction followed by wound healing and repair. The initial stages of the classical inflammatory response to tissue injury are characterized by the release of vasoactive mediators from tissue mast cells (e.g., histamine, leukotrienes), platelets, and plasma components (e.g., bradykinin), resulting in vasodilation and edema formation. This is followed by the activation of the coagulation and complement systems and the generation of plasma- (e.g., C5a) and cell-derived [e.g., interleukin 8 (IL-8)] chemotactic factors for neutrophils and other inflammatory cells. The chemotactic factors function to recruit inflammatory cells to sites of inflammation and promote their migration into tissues. Once present in tissues, inflammatory cells (e.g., neutrophils) may be stimulated to release bactericidal and degranulation products including reactive oxygen metabolites and proteases, as well as biologically active lipid mediators such as leukotriene B_4 and platelet-activating factor (PAF). In addition, depending on the nature of the pathogenic insult, mononuclear phagocytic cells may be stimulated by immune and nonimmune (e.g., bacterial endotoxin) pathways to generate products of arachidonic acid metabolism and potent cytokines that further modulate the evolution of the inflammatory response. Recently, it has become evident that the vascular endothelial cell is an important active participant in the modulation of the inflammatory response secondary to its ability to express on its surface and secrete potent mediators that regulate not only vascular tone and permeability, but also the activation of the coagulation and fibrinolytic pathways and inflammatory cell function.

The morphologic hallmarks of acute inflammation are edema formation, fibrin deposition, and the presence of neutrophils within the injured tissue. Depending on the nature of the pathogenic insult and/or extent of injury, the number of neutrophils at the site of injury may decrease with development of a chronic inflammatory response. Chronic inflammation is characterized by an increase in the number of macrophages, lymphocytes, plasma cells, and eosinophils. At this point several outcomes are possible. First, there may be elimination of the pathogenic agent and injured tissue with repair and return to normal tissue structure and function. Second, there may be persistence of the pathogenic insult with or without activation of immune mechanisms leading to the development of granulomatous inflammation. Third, there may be irreversible injury of tissue, resulting in an active proliferation of capillaries, fibroblasts, and mesenchymal elements leading to scar formation and loss of tissue function. The evolution of the inflammatory response is dictated by the nature of the pathogenic insult, extent of tissue injury, and the degree of immune activation that occurs. For instance, gram-positive bacterial infections are characterized by a prominent acute inflammatory response that frequently resolves without irreversible tissue injury, while *Mycobacterium tuberculosis* and certain fungal infections are typified by activated cell-mediated immune mechanisms and a granulomatous inflammatory response. In contrast, viral infections are characterized by lymphocyte and macrophage immune-dependent reactions, and parasitic infection and allergic reactions frequently have a prominent eosinophil infiltrate. Also, it is important to remember that a large number of plasma- and cell-derived mediators regulate the function of inflammatory and parenchymal cells and direct the course of the inflammatory response. These include a variety of cytokines, plasma- and cell-derived growth factors, lipid mediators, and proteases. Current laboratory research is intensely focused on defining the role of the plasma- and cell-derived mediators in specific inflammatory conditions and the mechanisms by which their activity is regulated.

OVERVIEW

Inflammation is characterized by the movement of fluid, plasma proteins, and leukocytes into tissues in response to injury, microbial invasion, foreign material, or antigens. The purpose of this response is to contain or destroy the pathogenic insult and to remove the tissue debris resulting from this response. Consider the following clinical situation.

Mr. H. stepped on a nail at work which penetrated his foot to a depth of 2 cm. Because the wound stopped bleeding immediately, no medical attention was sought. Over the first 6 h, the skin immediately surrounding the wound was red and swollen, but by the next morning (12 to 16 h) a surrounding area 5 cm in diameter had become red, swollen, hard, and painful. Because of these changes, Mr. H. went to his family doctor. On examination, redness and swelling were noted, as well as a white discharge (pus) from the wound and a fever of 40°C. Laboratory studies showed an increased peripheral blood neutrophil count of 10,000 neutrophils per μL (normal $\leq$ 5000/μL). Due to the obvious signs of infection, Mr. H. was admitted to the hospital, bacterial cultures were taken, and appropriate antibiotics were started. After 2 to 3 days, the pain, swelling, and redness lessened and Mr. H. was discharged home on oral antibiotics. Follow-up examination 2 weeks later showed a healed wound with minimal scarring.

This case history illustrates the typical phases of the inflammatory response. The four cardinal signs of inflammation—redness, swelling, heat, and pain—are indicative of the acute phase of the inflammatory response where local release of mediators results in an increase in capillary blood flow, leakage of plasma into the tissue, and pain. Subsequent activation of the complement and coagulation systems as well as circulating inflammatory and endothelial cells lead to the generation of additional soluble inflammatory mediators and biologically active compounds. These mediators also have systemic effects which result in fever, neutrophilia (an increase in the blood neutrophil content), and, potentially, an acute phase response (APR) (see Chap. 16). At the site of injury, neutrophils accumulate in the capillaries and postcapillary venules, cross the endothelial cell lining into the tissue, and move toward the source of the inflammatory mediators. At the heart of the wound, neutrophils phagocytose (ingest) foreign materials and altered tissue components, releasing digestive enzymes, bactericidal proteins, and powerful oxidants. In Mr. H.'s case, the net result is the destruction of the invading bacteria (with the aid of antibiotics). Following the initial acute phase there is a recruitment of monocytes, macrophages, and lymphocytes to the site of injury. The macrophages and monocytes ingest and/or kill any infectious agents or foreign materials resistant to the action of the neutrophil. Further, these cells digest and clear any damaged tissue that has not survived the inflammatory response. Final resolution of the injury occurs when viable cells at the site and adjacent to the site of injury proliferate in an attempt to restore normal tissue architecture and function. Depending on the extent of injury and the nature of the pathogenic insult, this may result in (1) the return to normal tissue structure and function, (2) scar formation with altered tissue function, (3) the creation of an abscess, or (4) persistence of a chronic inflammatory process.

At this point, it is important to remember that for the large proportion of the world's population that is infected by parasites eosinophils are important cellular components of the inflammatory response. In response to parasitic infections, eosinophils are recruited to the inflammatory site in much the same manner as neutrophils.

The inflammatory response is designed to clear injured tissue, facilitate the repair process, and protect the host from microbial invasion or tumorous cell growth. Yet in autoimmune diseases where antibodies or antibody-antigen complexes are deposited in host tissues, or cell-mediated immune reactions are activated, these inflammatory cells may show little restraint and injure host cells and damage tissue components. Similarly, the activation of neutrophils results in the release of considerable amounts of toxic products which are cytotoxic not only to their intended targets, but also to "innocent bystanders" in the area (e.g., endothelial cells, smooth muscle cells). Thus, the inflammatory response serves to protect the host from invasion, but, at times, this protection is achieved at considerable cost.

INITIATION OF THE INFLAMMATORY RESPONSE

Initiation of the inflammatory response is a dynamic process involving the interaction of tissue-derived soluble mediators with the vascular wall, inflammatory cells, and plasma components. Of the four cardinal signs of inflammation, redness and heat are due to a redistribution and an increase in blood flow to the site of inflammation. Following tissue injury, there is a release of potent vasoactive mediators from tissue mast cells and components of the vascular wall causing a brief episode of vasoconstriction (3 to 5 s) followed by dilation of precapillary arterioles and increased blood flow to the capillary beds. The clinical manifestation of this pathophysiologic response is redness. This is accompanied by an increase in permeability in the postcapillary venule due to retraction of endothelial cells and gap formation at the endothelial cell–endothelial cell junctions. The increase in permeability allows proteins and

TABLE 20-1   Vasoactive Mediators

Mediator	Source
VASOCONSTRICTION	
Neurogenic	Nerves
LTC_4, LTD_4, LTE_4	Mast cells, basophils
VASODILATION	
PGI_2	Endothelial cells
PGE_2, PGD_2	Monocytes, macrophages, mast cells
Histamine	Mast cells, basophils
Serotonin	Platelets
Bradykinin	Contact activation system (plasma)
NO·	Endothelial cells
INCREASED VASCULAR PERMEABILITY	
Histamine	Mast cells, basophils
Serotonin	Platelets
C3a, C5a	Plasma via histamine release
Bradykinin	Contact activation system (plasma)
LTC_4, LTD_4, LTE_4	Eosinophils, mast cells, monocytes
PAF	Mast cells, basophils, monocytes, macrophages, neutrophils, eosinophils, platelets, endothelial cells

fluid to leak from the intravascular space, resulting in edema and swelling. This process also causes a relative concentration of blood cells within the vasculature with sludging and the slowing of blood flow in venules. This slowing facilitates margination of leukocytes and encourages the adherence of leukocytes to the endothelium. The redistribution of blood by the precapillary arterioles and edema formation are also affected by neurogenic mediators released at sites of injury (Table 20-1).

Capillary blood flow is an important component of the inflammatory response. Leukocytes have the ability to move under their own power through the extravascular tissues, but this movement is practically limited to only a few millimeters. Thus, cells rely heavily upon capillaries to deliver them to a region adjacent to the site of inflammation from which they can migrate. This point is of clinical importance in dealing with infections involving large areas of tissue death associated with a loss of local blood supply. Under these circumstances, neutrophils cannot adequately permeate the tissue and the infection can continue unchecked. Thus to adequately deal with an abscess (large avascular collections of neutrophils, necrotic tissue, and proteinaceous fluid) or a gangrenous limb (avascular tissue), surgery may be required. The surgeon may have to drain or remove (debride) the avascular tissue if the body is to cope successfully with the infection.

THE ROLE OF PLASMA FACTORS IN THE INFLAMMATORY RESPONSE

Plasma contains factors which augment the role of inflammatory cells, including immunoglobulins, complement, and the coagulation, fibrinolytic, and contact-activating systems. Since each of these systems is dealt with in detail elsewhere (Chaps. 3, 13, and 14), this discussion will only briefly touch on these topics in the general context of the inflammatory response.

Immunoglobulins (see Chap. 3) bind to specific epitopes on target antigens via the Fab portion of the immunoglobulin molecule, leaving the Fc portion directed away from the target surface. This Fc portion is responsible for complement activation and binding to inflammatory cells through class-specific receptors (Table 20-2). While immunoglobulins are generally directed against invading pathogens (nonself-antigens), the response described below can be equally applied to antibodies directed against self-antigens (autoantibodies) or to antibody-antigen complexes deposited in tissues. In the latter two cases, these autoantibodies or immune complexes can result in major tissue injury and are an important cause of autoimmune disease (Chap. 31).

TABLE 20-2 Inflammatory Cells with FcγR (Fc Receptors for IgG Heavy Chain) and FCεR (Fc Receptors for IgE Heavy Chain)

	Fcγ	*Fcε*
Neutrophils	+	
Macrophages	+	
Eosinophils	+	+
Platelets	+	+
NK cells	+	

Complement activation (see Chap. 13) via the classical or alternative pathways (Table 20-3) can result in direct plasma-mediated cytotoxicity. Surface-bound immunoglobulins (IgG, IgM) or other factors act through the classical pathway of the complement cascade by binding C1q to the plasma membrane. The alternative pathway is triggered by polysaccharide, fungi, bacteria, or viruses through direct activation of C3. Activation of either pathway leads to the generation of C3a and C5a, as well as the formation of the membrane attack complex (MAC) (C6–C9).

Complement activation is one of the first responses to bacterial invasion (via contact with surface polysaccharides, endotoxin, or surface-bound immunoglobulins). This pathway can act as the first cytotoxic response to invasion while also initiating recruitment of leukocytes and vascular changes. Complement fragments C3a, C4a (generated during activation of the classical pathway only), and C5a are collectively referred to as *anaphylatoxins*. C3a and C4a share a common receptor (and the same spectrum of activity),

TABLE 20-3 Activators of the Complement System

Classical Pathway	*Alternative Pathway*
Immune complexes (IgG, IgM)	Zymosan (yeast cell wall)
	Cobra venom factor
Aggregated antibodies	Endotoxin
Proteases	Polysaccharides
Urate crystals	X-ray contrast material
Polyanions (polynucleotides)	Dialysis membrane
	Parasites, fungi, viruses

but C3a appears to be the more important of the two. C5a has an entirely separate receptor and has biologic effects that are slightly different from those of C3a. C3a and C5a both cause histamine release from mast cells and increased vascular permeability. C5a, in addition, is the most important chemotactic factor generated from plasma for neutrophils, monocytes, eosinophils, and basophils.

The MAC is an assembling of the terminal complement components (C6–C9). The most recognized function of these proteins is the formation of cytotoxic ion channels in both microbial pathogens and host cells upon which complement has been deposited. There is also experimental evidence indicating that the MAC or parts of it can aggregate platelets, prime leukocytes, or act as chemotactic factors.

The coating of particles with antibody or complement (C3b, C4b, C3bi) is referred to as *opsonization*, and is one of the most im-

portant roles that immunoglobulins and complement play in combating bacterial infections. Opsonized particles are more readily recognized by neutrophils, monocytes, macrophages, and, to a lesser extent, eosinophils. These cells have specific receptors for the C3b, C3bi, and the Fc portion of specific classes of Ig which are used in recognition and phagocytosis of these particles. In addition, aggregate IgG is a stimulus for the production of toxic oxygen products and lysosomal enzyme release. Thus, opsonization of pathogens provides an efficient system for recognition, uptake, and destruction by phagocytes.

The contact-activation system plays an important role in the inflammatory response mainly through the generation of bradykinin and activation of the coagulation system. To initiate this pathway, factor XII (Hageman factor), bound to a negatively charged surface, is activated spontaneously or via proteolytic cleavage by kallikrein (Fig. 20-1). The

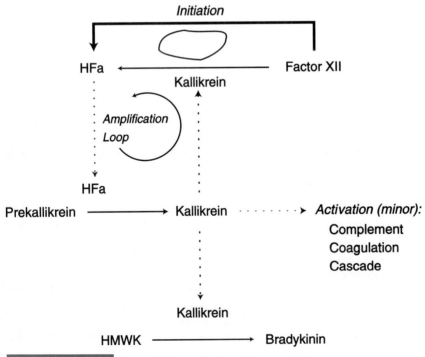

Figure 20-1 Factor XII and the contact activating system.

resulting activated factor (XIIa) cleaves pre-kallikrein to kallikrein, thereby establishing an amplification loop. Kallikrein is active in a number of reactions, including activation of factor XI, plasminogen, and C1q of the complement cascade. Perhaps, however, its most important proinflammatory role is the cleavage of high molecular weight kininogen (HMWK) to bradykinin (with the aid of aminopeptidases). Bradykinin increases vascular permeability, decreases arterial resistance, and causes smooth contraction and, in combination with prostaglandins, is the major source of mediator-induced pain associated with the inflammatory response.

In addition, activation of the coagulation cascade may be initiated secondary to either factor XII activation or the generation of procoagulant factors such as "tissue factor" by endothelial cells, smooth muscle cells, fibroblasts, or mononuclear phagocytic cells (e.g., monocytes). The generation of thrombin at inflammatory sites functions to promote platelet aggregation and the secretion of additional inflammatory mediators by platelets and endothelial cells. Formation of a fibrin thrombus would decrease blood flow to the inflammatory site, leading to tissue ischemia. Fortunately, the coagulation pathway is highly regulated and coupled to enzymatic pathways of fibrinolysis (see Chap. 14).

What is the role of these plasma factors in the inflammatory response? Patients with genetic defects in these pathways give us some clues. X-linked congenital hypogammaglobulinema (agammaglobulinemia of Bruton) and common variable immunodeficiency are both associated with severe or complete deficiency of IgG. These patients have persistent and recurrent bacterial infections mainly due to encapsulated organisms at sites of heavy bacterial colonization—conjunctiva, throat, ear, lung, and skin. Infections by viruses and mycobacteria are handled relatively well in the absence of IgG. Patients with complement deficiencies have problems mainly associated with deficiency in the ability to opsonize bacteria. Those patients deficient in the early components of either the classical

pathway (C1 to C3) or the alternative pathway (factor D) have recurrent pyogenic bacterial infections, as well as particular susceptibility to meningococcal infections. In contrast, patients with deficiencies of C5 or the components of the MAC (C6–C9) are relatively normal with the exception of an increased susceptibility to *Neisseria meningitidis* infections. Thus, the opsonization of bacteria by C3 appears to be necessary for the handling of bacterial infection successfully, while C5 and the MAC are apparently less important. Patients with factor XII deficiency show abnormal laboratory findings (prolongation of the partial thromboplastin time) but do not show increased susceptibility to infection or problems with the inflammatory response. Thus, it is evident that there exist multiple interacting plasma components that play an important role in host defense mechanisms and the initiation of the inflammatory response. However, it is apparent that there is some duplication of function between the various components of the inflammatory response, since deficiencies of a single component do not necessarily result in a general defect in the ability of the host to mount an effective inflammatory response.

MOBILIZATION OF INFLAMMATORY CELLS

One of the essential events for the development of the inflammatory response is the recruitment of circulating inflammatory cells to sites of tissue injury. This phase involves the release of the mobile effector cells (neutrophils, monocytes, eosinophils) from storage sites and the modulation of their response by extracellular matrix, plasma, and cellular factors with the ultimate goal of delivering the effector cells to the capillaries and postcapillary venules adjacent to the inflammatory site.

Neutrophils, monocytes, and eosinophils are all produced in the bone marrow, stored there for a short time, and then released into the bloodstream. Macrophages are mainly derived from circulating monocytes but also have a limited ability to undergo mitotic division in tissue. In appreciating the role of the neutrophils, eosinophils, and mononuclear phagocytes, it is important to realize that these cells are relatively short-lived (Table 20-4) and to maintain their number at an inflammatory site requires constant influx of new cells.

With acute inflammation the peripheral blood neutrophil content rises from 5000/μL to as high as 30,000/μL. This increase is due to the movement of neutrophils into the circulating blood from two storage sites—a marginating intravascular pool of cells and bone marrow stores. Increased production of new neutrophils in bone marrow from precursor cells plays only a very small role in the immediate inflammatory response. The *marginating pool* represents a population of neutrophils within blood vessels which has adhered temporarily to the vessel wall and so has been taken out of the main circulating stream. Margination occurs in relatively slow-moving blood where the dynamics of axial blood flow force the red blood cells to occupy the central stream of blood, displacing the leukocytes to the periphery in contact with the endothelium of the vessel wall. These leukocytes adhere to the endothelial wall and are "removed" from the circulating population to join the marginating pool. Of the total neutrophil population within the intravascular space, 45 percent are circulating and 55 percent are marginated. This pool can be rapidly mobilized and accounts for the immediate increase in neutrophils in the periph-

eral blood associated with strenuous exercise or with steroid use. The bone marrow pool is composed of cells which are mature or in the last stages of differentiation and which are normally held in the bone marrow for a short time prior to being released into the peripheral blood. This bone marrow pool represents a neutrophil population 20 times larger than that in circulation. In response to inflammatory mediators such as tumor necrosis factor (TNF), IL-1, and endotoxin, these cells move from the bone marrow pool into the bloodstream. The contribution of the bone marrow pool can be seen by examining the peripheral blood microscopically. Under normal conditions immature neutrophils (band or stab cells) which lack the characteristic lobulation of the nuclei represent only 20 percent of the total neutrophil count. However, with acute inflammation, these immature cells are released from the bone marrow and may become the predominant cell type (> 70 percent of the total neutrophil count). Indeed, if the inflammatory insult is overwhelming, there may be the release of large numbers of very immature granulocytes; this condition resembles chronic myelogenous leukemia and is referred to as a *leukemoid reaction.*

Monocytes, in contrast to neutrophils, have a small bone marrow storage pool, and mobilization of monocytes from the marrow requires division of monocytic stem cells to repopulate the bone marrow and to meet the peripheral demand. This replenishment of the bone marrow pool is brought about by an increase in precursor cells (promonocytes) and by a decrease in the time that the stem cells spend between mitotic divisions. Examination of the peripheral blood seldom shows monocytosis (increase in absolute monocyte count) to the same degree as seen with neutrophils. Unlike neutrophils, cells of the monocytic cell line have a prominent resident population in tissues under normal noninflammatory states. These resident tissue macrophages compose the reticuloendothelial system (Table 20-5). In addition to their inflammatory role, these cells provide the

TABLE 20-4 Life Span of Neutrophils, Eosinophils, and Monocytes and Macrophages

	Blood	Tissue
Neutrophil	10 h	1–2 days
Eosinophil	2 days	4–10 days
Monocytes and macrophages	1 day	4–12 days

TABLE 20-5 Components of the Reticuloendothelial System

Cell	Site
Monoblast, promonocyte	Bone marrow
Monocyte	Blood
Macrophage	Pleural and peritoneal space, spleen, lymph nodes, bone marrow
Kupffer cell	Liver sinusoids
Alveolar macrophage	Lung, alveolar space
Microglial cell	Central nervous system
Osteoblast	Bone
Histiocyte	Connective tissue
Langerhans cell (disputed)*	Skin
Dendritic cell (disputed)*	Lymphoid tissue

*"Disputed" means there is lack of agreement as to what criteria (antigenic phenotype, functional responses, and stem cell of origin) define the cells of the reticuloendothelial system.

day-to-day removal of cellular debris resulting from natural cell turnover.

Eosinophils also have both bone marrow and marginating pools. Like monocytic cells, eosinophils have a prominent tissue component, most notably in the connective tissues below epithelium-lined surfaces (e.g., beneath bronchial mucosa).

Figure 20-2 is a section through a capillary adjacent to a site of inflammation. This figure shows the intravascular localization of the inflammatory effector cells—neutrophils, monocytes, and eosinophils. One key point to note is that within this capillary, each cell is in intimate contact with several cell types, serum proteins, and proteins of the extracellular matrix that potentially influence the leukocytes and modulate their function.

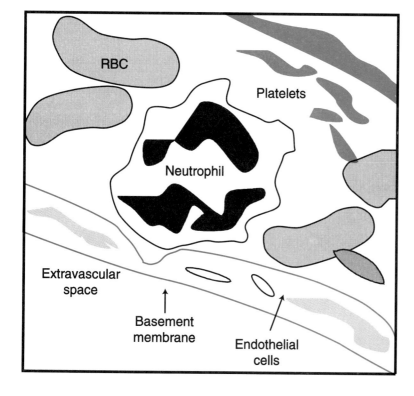

Figure 20-2 Cartoon based on an electron micrograph of a pulmonary capillary at the center of an inflammatory focus. The extravascular space shows considerable fluid accumulation due to capillary leakage. The endothelial cells show degenerative changes due to the neutrophil-mediated injury.

ENDOTHELIAL CELLS

Endothelial cells (ECs) provide an interface between the blood and the extravascular space. Much of inflammation involves the movement of cells and plasma into the extravascular space in response to injury or infection. Under normal conditions, ECs provide a "nonstick" surface that prevents coagulation, cellular adhesion, and leakage of fluid from the intravascular space. In addition, the endothelial cell plays an important role in regulating vascular tone and tissue perfusion due to the selective release of vasodilatory compounds [e.g., prostacyclin (PGI_2)], adenosine, and endothelial cell–derived relaxing factor (EDRF, an activity now known to be due to nitric oxide—see below) and vasoconstrictor compounds (e.g., endothelin).

If endothelial cell function is altered or the integration of the vascular lining is disrupted, the anticoagulant properties are lost and the basement membrane is exposed, allowing or initiating the aggregation of platelets and leukocytes. Further, the altered production of mediators such as endothelin and PGI_2 would have potentially profound effects on tissue perfusion. Recently, it has also been shown that endothelial cell function is modified in response to the inflammatory mediators (e.g., TNF, IL-1, and endotoxin) and the endothelial cells become active participants in the inflammatory response. This is in contrast to the previously held view that endothelial cells have a primarily passive anti-inflammatory role.

Leukocytes normally have only a small propensity to adhere to ECs, but with the appropriate inflammatory stimuli the adherence between leukocytes and ECs is markedly increased. The adhesive interactions between leukocytes and endothelial cells are regulated by the expression on cell surfaces of two families of adhesion molecules (selectins and integrins) and their respective counterreceptors. The initial interaction between circulating leukocytes and endothelial cells is the result of binding between selectins expressed on the leukocyte (L-selectin) and endothelial cell (P-selectin and E-selectin) and their respective carbohydrate-based counterreceptor. These interactions are responsible for the initial localization and "rolling" of leukocytes along the vasculature at inflammatory sites. Increases in chemoattractant concentrations induce expression of β_2 integrins on the leukocyte surfaces, which further promotes leukocyte adhesion and spreading along the vasculature. The subsequent interactions between leukocyte β_2-integrin molecules and extracellular matrix protein (e.g., collagen, fibronectin, laminin) play an important role in chemotaxis of the cells to the inflammatory nidus.

Our understanding of the mechanism involved in the regulation of leukocyte and endothelial cell adhesive interactions has increased greatly in recent years and has revealed important interactions between soluble inflammatory mediators and adhesion molecule expression. For instance, E-selectin (also referred to as ELAM-1, endothelial-leukocyte adhesion molecule) is not normally present on ECs but is expressed following exposure to TNF, IL-1, or endotoxin. ICAM-1 (intercellular adhesion molecule), present on normal ECs although at relatively low concentrations, is similarly up-regulated with exposure to cytokines.

The β_2-integrin family of leukocyte adhesion molecules participates not only in cell chemotactic responses but also in phagocytic and cytotoxic processes of leukocytes. This family of proteins includes lymphocyte function-associated antigen (LFA-1), Mo1, and Leu-M5. These molecules all share a common β subunit (designated CD18) but have antigenically unique α subunits (designated CD11a, CD11b, and CD11c for LFA-1, Mo1, and Leu-M5, respectively). CD11a/CD18 (LFA-1) is expressed on phagocytes and lymphocytes and promotes cytotoxic T-cell, NK-cell (natural-killer-cell), and tumorolytic macrophage adhesion to their respective targets. CD11c/CD18 (Leu-M5) is also expressed on phagocytic cells and has been shown to play an important role in phagocytic cell adhesion to cellular and extracellular matrix components. CD11b/CD18 (Mo1) is perhaps the best characterized of this family of leukocyte adherence proteins. It is present on monocytes, macrophages, and neutrophils and is, in part, responsible for adhesion of these cells to their targets. This molecule has complement receptor activity for the C3 degradation product C3bi, also referred to as CR3 (complement receptor 3). The C3bi receptor, as its name suggests, is responsible for the binding of C3bi-coated particles (e.g., bacteria, cells). However, Mo1 also mediates the adherence to other surfaces (yeast, bacteria, and ECs) in the absence of complement. ICAM-1 has been shown to be a ligand for CD11b/CD18. Whether additional ligands exist for CD11b/CD18 is unclear. As was the case for ELAM-1 on ECs,

circulating neutrophils show a low level of expression of CD11b/CD18 but increase the number of surface CD11b/CD18 molecules upon stimulation by a wide range of stimuli including C5a, LTB$_4$, PAF, and TNF-α. This increased expression is associated with increased neutrophil adherence to ECs.

Acute inflammation associated with mediator release results in an increase in adhesion molecules on both inflammatory effector cells (e.g., neutrophils and monocytes) and on ECs. This increased "stickiness," in conjunction with the local changes in blood flow and margination, fixes the leukocyte to the EC near the site of inflammation. It is from here that neutrophils, monocytes, and eosinophils migrate in response to chemotactic factors toward the heart of the inflammatory focus. In addition, the adherence of

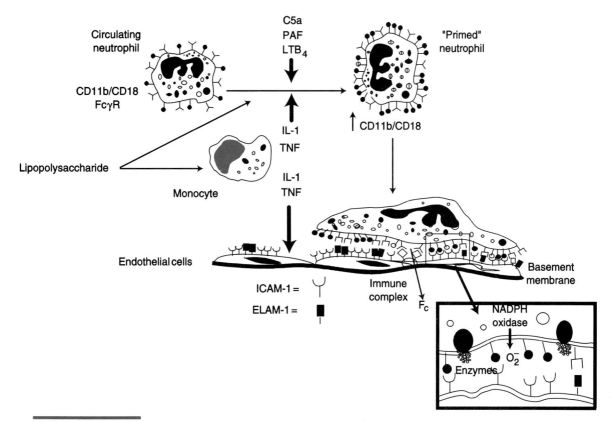

Figure 20-3 Adhesive interaction between neutrophils and endothelial cells.

neutrophils to a target results in an heightened respiratory burst following stimulation, focuses degranulation and production of reactive oxygen species along the adherent surface, and excludes scavengers of reactive oxygen species and antiproteases, present in extracellular fluids, from the site of interactions between neutrophil and target. Thus, it enhances the toxic action of the neutrophil on its target (Fig. 20-3).

The importance of leukocyte adhesion in the evolution of the inflammatory response and cell cytotoxicity is demonstrated in a small number of patients who are deficient in the expression of LFA-1, Mo1, and Leu-M5 glycoproteins. These patients present in infancy with severe recurrent bacterial and fungal infections that eventually prove to be fatal. The clinical syndrome is associated with an impaired inflammatory response with persistent leukocytosis (an increase in leukocyte content in blood) and defective adherence-dependent leukocyte functions. The result of this abnormality is that the patient's neutrophils have a marked inability to localize to sites of infection and function in the clearance of pathogens. Similar deficiencies of other adherence-promoting glycoproteins (e.g., ICAM and ELAM) have yet to be described, and so the precise role of these molecules is unknown.

Endothelial cells stimulated by bacterial endotoxin and specific cytokines (e.g., IL-1, TNF-α) have also been shown to express and secrete low molecular weight peptides that are chemotactic for leukocytes. The production of a neutrophil chemotactic factor, interleukin-8 (IL-8), by endothelial cells has been implicated as an important mechanism for the activation of neutrophils at sites of bacterial infection and during sepsis. Similarly, a monocyte-specific chemotactic peptide (MCP-1) has also been shown to be secreted by cytokine-stimulated endothelial cells and is thought to play an important role in the selected recruitment of circulating monocytes to sites of tissue injury. These cytokines are discussed in more detail in Chap. 10. This further underscores the important

role that endothelial cells play as active participants in the inflammatory response.

PLATELETS

Traditionally, the major role of platelets is that of hemostasis by acting as a plug where the integrity of the blood vessel wall has been breached. This view is substantiated clinically, since a profound lack of platelets is associated with life-threatening bleeding. However, the role of platelets in inflammation should not be overlooked. Platelets are the second most numerous circulating cell (after the red blood cells), and there are 20 to 50 platelets for every leukocyte in circulation. Many of the conditions which result in leukocyte activation are also associated with platelet aggregation. Aggregates containing platelets and neutrophils have been found in such conditions as septic shock, adult respiratory distress syndrome, bacterial endocarditis, and some acute autoimmune diseases. Thus, during the inflammatory response, platelets and leukocytes are brought in intimate contact with one another and so greatly enhance the potential for exchange of mediators between them.

The role of platelets can be divided into four major areas: (1) hemostasis; (2) modulation of the inflammatory response; (3) direct cytotoxicity as an effector cell; (4) repair.

Platelet aggregation and the coagulation pathway play a key role in the response to injury by providing hemostasis (Fig. 20-4). In general, it is best to think of the coagulation cascade and platelet aggregation as two arms of the same process, since stimulation of one results in activation of the other. Platelet aggregation is initiated primarily by: (1) exposure to extracellular matrix following a breach in the endothelial lining, (2) exposure to thrombin of the coagulation cascade, and (3) exposure to ADP and the arachidonic acid metabolite thromboxane A_2 (TXA$_2$) released from other platelets (Table 20-6). Coagulation is triggered by platelet aggregation, by the procoagulant surfaces of the ECs and

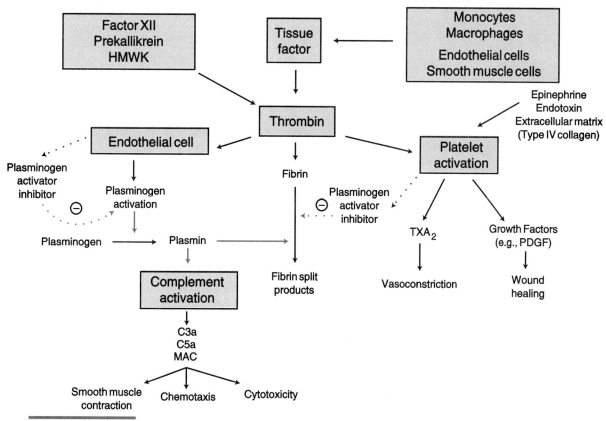

Figure 20-4   Interaction between the complement system and inflammatory cells.

monocytes, and by the release of tissue factors associated with injury. These two processes ultimately result in the production of a polymerized fibrin meshwork and platelet plug whose purpose is to occlude affected vessels.

Aggregation of platelets brings them in direct contact with other cells in the vicinity, allowing platelets to modulate endothelial and inflammatory cell function. As was the case for endothelial cells and leukocytes, platelets have specific adhesion molecules on their surface which promote intercellular contact. Glycoprotein 1b, in combination with factor vWF (formerly von Willebrand factor), is responsible for platelet adhesion to the subendothelial surface. Platelets bind to monocytes via the interaction of thrombo-

spondin present on their surface and thrombospondin receptors of the monocytes. Activated platelets also show similar binding to the neutrophils, but the exact nature of this adhesion is unknown. The aggregation of platelets exposes endothelial cells, vascular smooth muscle cells, and leukocytes to relatively high concentrations of products released from platelet granules or produced de novo. These products have predominantly proinflammatory effects and include metabolites of arachidonic acid, proteases, ADP, and growth factors (Table 20-7). Platelets are capable of modulating the neutrophil in all phases of the neutrophil's response to inflammation. Platelets, by inducing adherence, aggregation, and chemotaxis, recruit neutrophils to sites of injury. In addition,

TABLE 20-6   Platelet-Aggregating Agents

Agent	Source
ADP, TXA2	Released by platelets resulting in further aggregation
Collagen	Basement membrane, extracellular matrix
Thrombin	Produced by coagulation pathway; increased production associated with blood stasis, infection, or alteration of the surface of endothelial cells
PAF	Released by a variety of cells during the inflammatory response
Bacteria, viruses, IgG-coated parasites, aggregated IgG and surface-bound IgG	Part of the immune response to infection or associated with autoimmune disease and immune complexes
C-reactive protein	Acute phase reactant

platelet products initiate or potentiate the toxic responses of neutrophils for their targets. Platelets may have much the same effect on monocytes and eosinophils.

The third function of platelets is as effector cells in parasitic infections. Platelets appear ill equipped for this role since they lack the toxic granular proteins or an active mechanism for superoxide anion production as is found in neutrophils and eosinophils. However, platelets from patients infected with schistosomes or filariae are cytotoxic to these parasites both in vivo and in vitro, although the precise mechanism of their cytotoxic activity is not known.

Platelets fulfill their fourth function by promoting the cellular responses associated with repair. Platelet-derived growth factor and transforming growth factor β (TGF-β) are potent stimuli for the migration, proliferation, and stimulation of fibroblasts and smooth muscle and play an important role in wound healing and the development of fibrotic reactions and scar formation. These growth factors have also been implicated as important mediators in the pathogenesis of a number of disease states, including atherosclerosis.

The relative role of platelets in the modulation of inflammatory reaction is difficult to ascertain since hemostasis overshadows all other platelet functions. In experimental animal models, platelet depletion results in about 50 percent reduction in the acute inflammatory response and an increased susceptibility to parasitic infections. If these animal studies can be applied to humans, it would appear that platelets play an important proinflammatory role.

EXTRAVASCULAR EVENTS

The preceding discussion has dealt with the egress of leukocytes from bone marrow and marginating pools and the localization to the vascular bed adjacent to the inflammatory site with the aid of ECs, platelets, serum factors, and changes in blood flow. The next part of this discussion will focus more upon the leukocyte itself and those processes by which the cell leaves the vascular space, moves specifically toward the inflammatory stimuli, and delivers its toxic metabolites.

Chemotaxis

Leukocytes share with bacteria and some eukaryotic cells the ability to orient and move along a gradient of increasing concentrations of chemical attractant—a process referred to as *chemotaxis*. Under most circumstances inflammation and infection are located outside the vascular space, and chemotaxis provides the mechanism by which leukocytes can leave the intravascular space and traverse through the extracellular matrix to the site of injury or infection. Neutrophils in response to chemoattractants orient toward the stimulus by forming a knoblike protru-

TABLE 20-7   Platelet Mediators of Inflammation

Content	Function
	DENSE GRANULE FRACTION
Serotonin	Increases vascular permeability, increases neutrophil adhesion, increases neutrophil phagocytosis
ADP	Aggregates platelets, degrades to adenosine (a neutrophil inhibitor)
ATP	Primes neutrophils, increases neutrophil adherence, degrades to adenosine (a neutrophil inhibitor)
Histamine (minor component)	Increases vascular permeability
	α GRANULE FRACTION
Fibrinogen	Aggregates platelets, coagulation factor
Factor Va	Coagulation factor
Cationic proteins	Antibacterial (?)
Factor VII	Coagulation factor
Platelet factor 4	Chemoattractant for neutrophils, enhances neutrophil elastase activity, antagonizes histamine, stimulates histamine release from basophils
Platelet-derived growth factor	Chemotactic for neutrophils, monocytes, smooth muscles, and fibroblasts; induces proliferation of fibroblasts and vascular smooth muscle, stimulates fibroblast collagenase production
Thrombospondin	Platelet-monocyte adhesion molecule
vWF	Adhesion molecule for platelets to subendothelium
Glycoprotein IIB, IIa	Platelet adhesion protein
Glycoprotein Ib	vWF receptor
TGF-β	Stimulates collagen formation by fibroblasts, induces vessel proliferation
B-Lysin	Antibacterial
	LYSOSOMAL AND VESICULAR FRACTION
Protease (neutral)	Cleaves C5 to C5a
Cathepsin A, collagenase, elastase, galactosyltransferase	Digestion of extracellular matrix
	NONPREFORMED PRODUCTS
12-hydroxyeicosatetraenoic acid	Enhances endothelial production of PGI_2 (decreased neutrophil adherence), stimulates oxidative burst of neutrophils, increases neutrophil adherence, enhances monocyte expression of tissue factor (procoagulant); chemotactic for neutrophils, monocytes, and eosinophils
12-hydroperoxyeicosatetraenoic acid	Stimulates neutrophil LTB_4 production, converted to 12,20-DiHETE (12,20-dihydroxyeicosatetraenoic acid) by neutrophil (which is chemotatic to neutrophils)
PAF	Chemotactic for neutrophils; stimulates respiratory burst and/or primes neutrophils and monocytes, aggregates neutrophils and platelets, increases vascular permeability
TXA_2	Aggregates platelets, increases neutrophil adhesion
Reactive oxygen products	Antiparasitic

sion anteriorly (toward the stimulus) and a trailing tail (uropod). Associated with this polarization is migration of chemoattractant receptors to the anterior surface. This redistribution is thought to play an important role in the ability of the leukocyte to "sense" concentration gradients. The physical movement of the cells is brought about by fixing a region of plasma membrane to the extracellular matrix through binding of specific

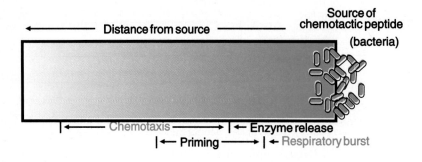

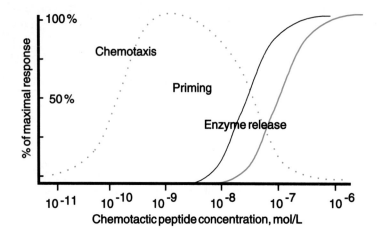

Figure 20-5 Relation of neutrophil responses to chemotactic peptide concentration and distance from inflammatory focus.

receptors to matrix components. Selective solubilization and repolymerization of the cytosolic actin-myosin matrix propels the cell in the direction of the increasing chemotactic factor gradient.

Leukocytes detect the presence of inflammatory mediators using surface receptors that are specific for each compound to which they respond. Chemotactic factors may be either plasma- or cell-derived and include products of complement activation, metabolites of arachidonic acid metabolism, and low molecular weight peptides derived from host cells and bacteria. Unlike classical neurotransmitter receptors which have an all-or-none response, leukocyte chemotactic receptors have gradations of their responses. At low concentrations of chemoattractant, a chemotactic response is initiated, while at high concentrations (such as occurs at the site of injury) leukocyte degranulation and a respiratory burst occur associated with enhanced

phospholipid metabolism and release of granular proteins, arachidonic acid metabolites, PAF, and reactive oxygen products. This is outlined graphically in Fig. 20-5. The division of the responses prevents the premature release of granule or reactive oxygen products that would cause unnecessary damage to the surrounding tissues and would lessen the ability of the leukocyte to respond where it is most needed.

Phagocytosis

When neutrophils, monocytes, macrophages, or eosinophils come into direct apposition with the inflammatory target (bacteria, parasite, foreign body, etc.), they can engulf the target by surrounding it with plasma membrane by a process referred to as *phagocytosis*. As the plasma membrane comes in contact with itself, it fuses and separates the newly formed phagosome (phagocytic vesicle) from the surface membrane. The phagosome can then fuse with intracellular lysosomal granules (resulting in a phagolysosome) and expose the target to the granular proteins or reactive oxygen products. Thus, phagocytosis effectively sequesters pathogens within the cell, exposes them to high concentrations of bactericidal products, and minimizes the damage to the surrounding tissues.

Recognition of the particulate matter for phagocytosis occurs by both specific and nonspecific mechanisms. As mentioned previously, opsonization (binding of immunoglobulin or complement to the surface) allows direct interaction between these particles and complement and immunoglobulin (Fc) receptors on the phagocyte. Nonopsonized particles also undergo phagocytosis without the benefit of specific surface receptors, although less efficiently.

Obviously, there are limits to the size of particles that can be taken up into phagosomes. In response to the large surfaces that cannot be surrounded, leukocytes react in much the same manner as with simple phagocytosis. Specific and nonspecific recognition bring the plasma membrane in direct, tight contact with the target surface. Into this region, lysosomal granules and reactive oxygen products are released with much the same results as would have been seen in phagolysosomes.

Phagocytosis is a process common to neutrophils, eosinophils, and monocytic phagocytes. Eosinophils are less adept at phagocytosis than are neutrophils. This is not surprising, since their natural targets (parasites) are often many times larger than the eosinophil and the eosinophil relies more upon bringing its membrane in apposition with its target. Macrophages of the reticuloendothelial system use phagocytosis extensively to resorb cellular debris in both inflammatory and noninflammatory states. Macrophages also use phagocytosis to isolate certain organisms resistant to killing, such as *M tuberculosis,* and so prevent the dissemination of these organisms. The sequestration of specific pathogens and particulate

materials within the macrophages underlies granuloma formation (see below).

Priming

Priming is the process by which preexposure of leukocytes to a stimulus (Fig. 20-6) alters the cell such that a subsequent exposure to a second stimulus results in an increased or exaggerated response when compared to the response of unprimed cells. (See Clinical Aside 20-1.) These responses include cell aggregation, superoxide production, degranulation, and arachidonic acid metabolite formation. As indicated, many priming agents can also act as direct stimulants. Priming occurs at concentrations lower than that necessary for stimulation.

Clinical Aside 20-1
Clinical Consequences of Priming Leukocytes

Mrs. Y. has a renal stone which has obstructed the collecting system of the kidney, resulting in bacterial pyelonephritis (infection and inflammation of the collecting system of the kidney). As a result of her infection, Mrs. Y. develops bacteremia (bacteria in the bloodstream) associated with the systemic release of low molecular weight bacterial proteins (e.g., formylated bacterial peptides), endotoxin, and a variety of inflammatory mediators, including TNF and IL-1. Her symptoms include low back pain, fever, and dysuria and laboratory tests show neutrophilia and elevation of specific plasma proteins.

In this situation, the presence of specific circulating inflammatory mediators will prime marginated and circulating neutrophils. When these primed neutrophils are recruited to Mrs. Y.'s kidney, they will be more effective in their bactericidal activity since they can release greater amounts of toxic products.

Priming may be a common event in the inflammatory response, even in the absence of systemic release of priming factors. As shown in Fig. 20-5, leukocyte chemotaxis involves movement of leukocytes through a range of mediator concentrations. Thus, as neutrophils approach the heart of the inflammatory site, these cells in fact are primed as they pass along the chemotactic factor

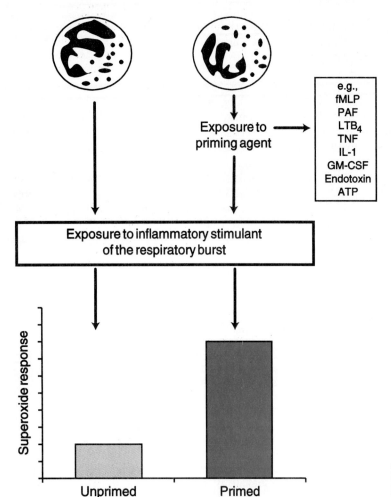

Exposure to priming agent →

e.g.,
fMLP
PAF
LTB$_4$
TNF
IL-1
GM-CSF
Endotoxin
ATP

Exposure to inflammatory stimulant
of the respiratory burst

Superoxide response

Unprimed   Primed

Figure 20-6 Priming of leukocyte responses.

concentration gradient prior to their final activation by the phagocytic stimulus.

The exact role that priming plays in the inflammatory response is difficult to judge. However, the relative production of reactive oxygen products and extent of degranulation that occur upon stimulation of "primed" cells suggest that leukocyte priming represents a major component in the inflammatory response since it markedly increases leukocyte bactericidal efficiency.

Cytotoxic Mechanisms

The key effector role of mononuclear phagocytes, neutrophils, and eosinophils is to de-

liver cytotoxic products to specific targets (bacteria, viruses, parasites, and tumor cells). The cytotoxic mechanism of phagocytic leukocytes can be divided into two major groups: (1) reactive oxygen products and (2) granule proteins.

Clinical Aside 20-2
Chronic Granulomatous Disease of Childhood

A 1-year-old male presented to the hospital with fever, chills, shortness of breath, and wheezing. He had been discharged from the hospital one month earlier, having been treated for viral pneumonia complicated by a secondary *Staphylococcus aureus* lung infection. Physical examination on this admission showed generalized lymphadenopathy (increased lymph node size), hepatosplenomegaly (increased size of liver and spleen), and a very localized area of wheezing over the right lung fields. Laboratory studies showed a high normal neutrophil count, normal lymphocyte count (total, T cells, and B cells), and elevated serum IgG and IgM. A sweat chloride test (for cystic fibrosis) was normal. X-Ray examination revealed multiple lung masses with a large mass compressing the right main bronchus (accounting for wheezing). A biopsy of this mass showed granulomatous inflammation (giant cells, epithelioid macrophages, and lymphocytes) and fungal hyphae. Because of the clinical history, neutrophils were evaluated for their ability to reduce nitroblue tetrazolium. This and subsequent tests demonstrated a defect in the production of the reactive oxygen products O_2^- and H_2O_2.

The key role that reactive oxygen products play in the host's response to infection is seen in patients, such as the one described above, with chronic granulomatous disease (CGD) of childhood. CGD represents a heterogenous group of individuals with genetic defects in phagocytic cell NADPH oxidase associated with an inability to produce O_2^- and other related oxygen products. These patients present in infancy with recurrent and persistent bacterial and fungal infections that often prove fatal within the first two decades, in spite of antibiotic support. The reason for the granulomatous response that is so characteristic of this disease is not entirely understood. The general inability to eradicate infections may result in persistent chronic inflammation with an associated granulomatous response. In contrast to O_2^- and H_2O_2, the roles of hypochlorous acid (HOCl) and the peroxidases myeloperoxidase (MPO) and eosinophil peroxidase (EPO) are less important in combating infection. With the advent of the use of automated flow cytochemical systems which use an MPO staining reaction as a parameter to differentiate cell types, it was discovered that MPO deficiency is a relatively common disorder (1 in 2000 individuals). These individuals have few clinical problems unless they have underlying immunodeficiency (e.g., poorly controlled diabetes). In the latter cases, there is an increased risk of disseminated infection by *Candida albicans*. It is interesting to note that patients with CGD are able to cope with bacteria that produce their own H_2O_2. This suggests that bacterial production of

H_2O_2 and the patient's MPO are sufficient to combat such infections. The role that EPO plays in eosinophil-mediated oxygen-dependent killing appears to be relatively minor. In fact, the eosinophils of lions, tigers, and domestic cats function without any EPO.

Reactive Oxygen Products and Respiratory Burst

Reactive oxygen products are a major component of the armamentarium of neutrophils, monocytes and macrophages, and eosinophils. (See Clinical Aside 20-2.) All of these products are related to one another, with the superoxide anion (O_2^-) and hydrogen peroxide (H_2O_2) being central to their production (Fig. 20-7). O_2^- is produced by an NADPH-dependent oxidase which utilizes NADPH as an electron donor to reduce molecular oxygen (O_2), generating O_2^-. This reaction which briefly increases O_2 consumption of these cells is referred to as the *respiratory burst*. Similar to the mitochondrial electron transport chain, this reduction involves a flavin adenine dinucleotide (FAD), and a specific b cytochrome. O_2^- is produced predominantly on the plasma membrane or the membrane of the phagosome (invaginated segment of the plasma membrane) and released into the extracellular medium or the interior of the phagosome. H_2O_2 is formed predominantly from the spontaneous dismutation of O_2^- and serves as a branching point in the production of the hydroxyl radical OH• and hypochlorous acid, HOCl.

The biologic production of OH• proceeds through reduction of H_2O_2 with aid of O_2^-. The production of OH• from H_2O_2 requires a reduced transition metal such as Fe^{2+} (ferrous) ion to act as reductant, with O_2^- perpetuating the reaction by recycling the Fe^{3+} back to Fe^{2+} (Fig. 20-7). The potential role of iron in these reactions emphasizes the importance of tight biologic control of free iron.

HOCl is a strong oxidant derived from H_2O_2 with the aid of leukocyte-derived peroxidases. Two main peroxidases exist in phagocytes: (1) myeloperoxidase (MPO) in neutrophils and monocytes, and (2) eosinophil

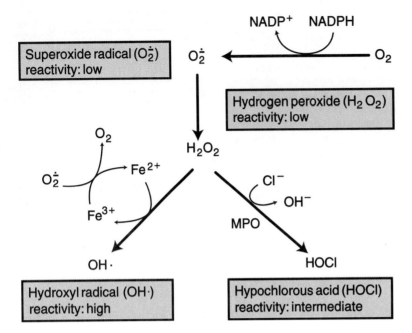

Figure 20-7   Reactive oxygen metabolite formation by phagocytic cell NADPH oxidase.

peroxidase (EPO). MPO is found in the azurophilic granules of neutrophils and represents 2 to 5 percent of the dry weight of the cell. Monocytes contain only about one-third of the MPO activity of neutrophils, and as these monocytes differentiate into macrophages, their granular peroxidase is lost. However, macrophages may take advantage of the MPO released from other cells at inflammatory sites to convert H_2O_2 to HOCl. EPO is unique to the eosinophil, and although it is functionally related to MPO, it is antigenically distinct. Both peroxidases are highly cationic (positively charged) and when released into the extracellular medium tend to adhere tightly to the adjacent membrane of the target organism or basement membrane. In this way, EPO and MPO can be localized to the desired site of action.

O_2^- and H_2O_2 are much less reactive than OH• and HOCl and probably do not have a major direct role as an oxidant in the biologic systems. The highly reactive products OH• and HOCl are short-lived in vitro and are consumed in the immediate vicinity of their production. The less reactive products are capable of diffusing away from their site of

production and cross plasma membranes (H_2O_2) or pass through anion channels (O_2^-) before their conversion to the more reactive products. Thus, phagocytic cells can effect oxidant-dependent injury of not only target cell plasma membranes but also susceptible intracellular sites, thereby altering cell function.

In recent years an additional reactive oxygen species has been shown to play an important role in macrophage cytotoxic reactions and tissue injury. Nitric oxide (NO•) is synthesized from L-arginine by nitric oxide synthase. This enzyme exists in at least two forms: a constitutively expressed isozyme expressed in endothelial cells and an inducible isozyme expressed in macrophages. Endothelial cell–derived NO• has been identified as the biologically active molecule originally referred to as endothelium-derived relaxing factor (EDRF). Thus NO• plays an important effector role both as a modulator of vascular tone and tissue perfusion as well as in macrophage-dependent cytotoxicity.

The reactive oxygen products discussed are capable of reacting with a wide variety of biologic molecules, including both cellular and extracellular proteins (especially those containing sulfur groups), DNA, lipids, and glycosaminoglycans. These products are also able to modulate the inflammatory response by inactivation of inflammatory mediators (C5a, chemotactic peptides, prostaglandins, and LTC_4) or by stimulation of the release of mediators from platelets and mast cells.

The disadvantage of the reactive oxygen products in the extracellular medium is that they cannot discriminate between friend and foe. Thus, cytotoxic activity can also be directed against leukocytes, endothelial cells, and surrounding tissue. Both bacteria and host cells possess antioxidant systems (glutathione-glutathione peroxidase, superoxide dismutase, catalase, and vitamin E) which react with these oxygen products and protect against their toxic effects. Thus a critical balance exists between pro- and antioxidant reactions that determines the extent of cell injury.

Granule Proteins

The granule-associated proteins of phagocytes are necessary for the killing of microbes as well as for digestion of the extracellular matrix and debris. In all phagocytes, these proteins are partitioned into discrete lysosomal granules which are subclassified based upon their morphologic appearance or enzyme content. With the appropriate stimulus, lysosomal granules can fuse with phagosomes or the plasma membrane. The granular proteins have a wide spectrum of enzymatic activity for biologic molecules (proteases, lipases, and deoxyribonucleases) and can directly promote cell and tissue injury. The protease content of the phagocytic cell granules is diverse and includes both serine proteases (e.g., neutrophil elastase) and metalloproteases (e.g., collagenase) which have potent biologic activity toward extracellular matrix proteins and basement membrane. The metalloproteases are secreted as latent enzymes that can be activated by both serine proteases and reactive oxygen species. The activity of these proteases is regulated by both plasma-derived (e.g., α_1-antiprotease, α_2-macroglobulin) and cell-derived (e.g., tissue inhibitor of metalloproteases, TIMP-1, -2) protease inhibitors. The regulated secretion and activity of these enzymes play key roles in phagocytic cell chemotaxis, tissue injury, and repair. An additional class of granular proteins are cationic proteins with intrinsic antimicrobial action independent of any enzymatic activity. These include bacterial-permeability increasing protein (BPI), defensin proteins, myelin basic protein (MBP), and eosinophilic cationic protein (ECP). Cationic proteins are highly positively charged at physiologic pH and readily adhere to biologic membranes which carry a negative charge. The exact mechanism of the toxic effects of these proteins is not precisely known. BPI is found in neutrophils and is selectively active against gram-negative bacteria. ECP and MPB are released by eosinophils and have little or no effect on bacteria, but are toxic to parasites. Thus the granules of different granuloycte-lineage cells have different contents, which help determine their disparate functions.

MPO and EPO are also present within lysosomal granules; as mentioned above, their main action is through the conversion of H_2O_2 to the highly reactive species HOCl.

CHRONIC INFLAMMATION AND GRANULOMATOUS INFLAMMATION

Following the development of the immediate (acute) response to an inflammatory insult, there is a subsequent influx of monocytes, eosinophils, and lymphocytes (Fig. 20-8). As the initial insult is controlled, diminished, or contained, neutrophils are no longer recruited, the neutrophils already present degenerate, and mononuclear cells accumulate. At this point, where monocytes and macrophages, lymphocytes, and plasma cells predominate, the site takes on the histologic appearance of chronic inflammation.

In reference to chronic inflammation, it is appropriate to point out that monocytes and macrophages have two major roles in the

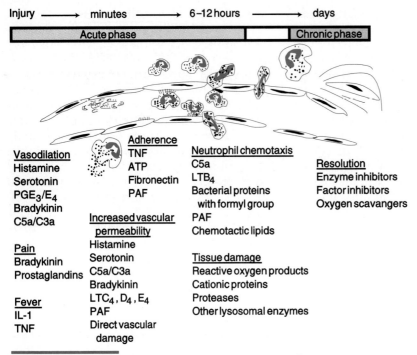

Injury ⟶ minutes ⟶ 6–12 hours ⟶ days

| Acute phase | | Chronic phase |

Vasodilation
Histamine
Serotonin
PGE_3/E_4
Bradykinin
C5a/C3a

Pain
Bradykinin
Prostaglandins

Fever
IL-1
TNF

Adherence
TNF
ATP
Fibronectin
PAF

Increased vascular permeability
Histamine
Serotonin
C5a/C3a
Bradykinin
LTC_4, D_4, E_4
PAF
Direct vascular damage

Neutrophil chemotaxis
C5a
LTB_4
Bacterial proteins with formyl group
PAF
Chemotactic lipids

Tissue damage
Reactive oxygen products
Cationic proteins
Proteases
Other lysosomal enzymes

Resolution
Enzyme inhibitors
Factor inhibitors
Oxygen scavangers

Figure 20-8   The acute and chronic phases of the inflammatory response.

immune response. The first, as previously discussed, is that of a phagocytic cell capable of ingesting and degrading microbes, cellular debris, and degenerating neutrophils. The second function (Chap. 18) is the modulation of the immune response and T-cell function through antigen presentation and the secretion of specific cytokines. Further, monocytes and macrophages have the potential to modulate the process of wound healing and repair secondary to the secretion of cytokines that affect both parenchymal and inflammatory cell function. As the inflammatory response enters the chronic stage, the monocytes and macrophages continue to phagocytose cellular debris and material that has not been adequately cleared by neutrophils. Depending on the extent of tissue injury, this can result in return to normal structure and function of the tissue or an active repair reaction with fibrosis and altered tissue structure and function. Alternatively, if there is persistence of the remaining pathogen, macrophages can also aid

in switching the response to a delayed-type hypersensitivity reaction involving the full spectrum of responses of lymphocytes (Chap. 7). Thus, chronic inflammation can be thought of as a turning point in the inflammatory response and the monocyte or macrophage as the pivotal cell in directing the course of the response.

One morphologically unique response that may be associated with chronic inflammation is the formation of granulomas (granulomatous inflammation). A *granuloma* is recognized histologically as an organized aggregate of mononuclear phagocytes surrounded by lymphocytes and plasma cells (Fig. 20-9). The phagocytes involved are derived mainly from recently recruited monocytes with a small contribution from resident tissue macrophages. The cells of the granuloma typically take on an epithelioid appearance (that is, they resemble epithelial cells, with pale nuclei and abundant cytoplasm) and lose much of their phagocytic activity. Occasionally, there is also fusion of macrophages in

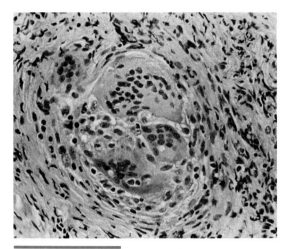

Figure 20-9 Morphologic features of granulomatous inflammation with multinucleated giant cells.

the granuloma to form distinctive multinucleated cells (giant cells). Granulomas are typically seen in association with poorly digestible material (e.g., suture, glass, talc) and/or initiators of cellular hypersensitivity (*M tuberculosis, M lepra, Histoplasma capsulatum*). Granuloma formation isolates the persistent inflammatory focus and limits its dissemination, and allows the mononuclear phagocytes to present antigens to the surrounding lymphocytes.

CYTOKINES AND ENDOTOXIN

With the advent of molecular biology, much attention has been directed at the characterization of peptides which mediate inflammation and have marked local and systemic effects. These factors were first referred to as *monokines* and *lymphokines* (i.e., immunoregulatory peptides produced by monocytes and macrophages or lymphocytes, respectively). Current terminology identifies these biologically active peptides as *cytokines*, since they are elaborated by a wide variety of inflammatory cells (monocytes,

macrophages, lymphocytes, and endothelial cells) as well as noninflammatory cells (keratinocytes, astrocytes, fibroblasts, and smooth muscle cells). (See also Chap. 10.)

TNF-α and IL-1 are two cytokines which play a key role in the inflammatory response. Intravenous infusion of either TNF-α or IL-1 reproduces many of the systemic signs and symptoms of infection and inflammation. While the systemic response (Table 20-8) is virtually identical for IL-1 and TNF-α, they are structurally different and each has separate receptors.

TNF-α and IL-1 play a major role in the localization of leukocytes to inflammatory sites. Both of these cytokines can cause an increased release of neutrophils from the bone marrow and so increase the number of circulating neutrophils (neutrophilia). IL-1 and TNF-α directly affect ECs, increasing the production of vasodilating prostaglandins (PGI_2 and PGE_2) and chemotactic factors for inflammatory cells (e.g., IL-8), and also increasing the procoagulant activity on the EC surface. In addition, they can increase the expression of adhesion molecules on both neutrophils and endothelial cells and promote leukocyte–endothelial cell adhesion. These cytokines are also able to prime the

TABLE 20-8 Biologic Properties of IL-1 and TNF-α

Biological Property	IL-1	TNF-α
Fever (endogenous pyrogen)	+	+
Slow-wave sleep	+	+
Hemodynamic shock	+	+
Increased hepatic acute phase protein synthesis	+	+
Decreased albumin synthesis	+	+
Activation of endothelium	+	+
Priming of neutrophils	+	+
Priming of macrophages	+	+
Chemotactic for neutrophils	±	±
Decreased plasma levels of iron and zinc	+	+
Increased fibroblast proliferation	+	+
Increased synovial cell collagenase and PGE_2 levels	+	+
T- and B-cell activation	+	−

respiratory burst of monocytes and macrophages and neutrophils, thereby increasing the cytotoxic responses of these cells.

TNF-α and IL-1 may have a role in modulating the response of resident cells at a variety of anatomic sites. For example, synoviocytes (cells which line joint cavities and produce synovial fluid) can release collagenase in response to IL-1 and contribute to tissue destruction in inflammatory diseases of the joint (e.g., arthritis). Similarly, resorption of bone at sites of injury (fracture) or infection (osteomyelitis) is, in part, mediated by IL-1 (which was once referred to as osteoclast activating factor.)

At this point, it is appropriate to introduce the bacterial product endotoxin, since this is intimately linked to IL-1 and TNF-α production. *Endotoxin,* also referred to as *lipopolysaccharide,* is a component of the cell walls of gram-negative bacteria, and can be shed by viable bacteria or released following cell death. Infusion of endotoxin produces physiologic responses similar to those outlined previously for TNF-α and IL-1. This is not surprising, since endotoxin is one of the most potent agents inducing production of IL-1 and TNF-α in monocytes and macrophages. Endotoxin is relatively heat-stable, and so the commonly used methods of sterilization (autoclaving, filtration, etc.) that kill bacteria do not remove already present endotoxin. This is one reason why pharmaceutical companies go to such great lengths to avoid bacterial contamination at all stages of production of drugs, since sterilization of the end product cannot eliminate endotoxin. It should be realized that in spite of even elaborate precautions trace amounts of endotoxin are present in virtually all solutions and chemical preparations, although at levels below a threshold concentration necessary to produce systemic effects.

TNF-α, IL-1, and endotoxin release are a mixed blessing for the host. Low concentrations of these agents are proinflammatory, enhancing the bactericidal activity of phagocytes. As the systemic concentration increases, the effects noted in Table 20-8 are seen. While some are beneficial to the host in combating infection or tumors, others contribute to the debility associated with chronic disease (e.g., anorexia and wasting). In addition, the induction of high levels of IL-1, TNF-α, and (IL-6) have marked effects on hepatocyte function and are thought to be the primary mediators of the acute phase response associated with inflammatory conditions (Chap. 16). IL-1, through its ability to stimulate arachidonic acid metabolism in the hypothalmus, has also been shown to be an important mediator for the fever response associated with inflammatory conditions. Inhibition of cyclooxygenase (e.g., by aspirin) blocks the fever response by inhibiting IL-1-dependent PGE_2 synthesis in the hypothalmus. At the extreme, very high concentrations of endotoxin (as seen with overwhelming sepsis) are associated with profound hypotension and death. This response appears to be in part mediated by endotoxin-dependent production of TNF-α and PAF.

VIRAL INFECTIONS

Viruses are obligate intracellular organisms which require the use of DNA, RNA, or protein synthesis of host cells to reproduce. Viral infections involve intracellular reproduction of virus within host cells followed by release of virions secondary to host cell lysis or budding from the plasma membrane. Released virus particles can reinfect tissue locally or spread to distant tissues by circulation of free virus or in parasitized host cells. To combat these infections, the immune response must recognize these free virions or identify foreign viral proteins on the plasma membrane of infected cells.

As anyone with a cold sore (herpes simplex) can attest, early viral infections provoke the cardinal signs associated with acute inflammation (redness, swelling, heat, and pain). In general, viral infections initiate all of the early inflammatory responses discussed above. Sites of infection release cytokines (TNF-α) and chemotactic factors (C3a, C5a) that mobilize and recruit first neutrophils, then lymphocytes and macrophages. Neutrophils are not as effective in defeating infection by intracellular organisms such as viruses as they are with extracellular bacteria. However, opsonization of free virus or deposition of immune globulins and complement on plasma membrane of infected cells promotes neutrophil participation in the acute response to viral infections. Opsonization of free circulating viruses also provides an effective means by which the reticuloendothelial system can remove and inactivate particles. This is one mechanism by which immunity to viral infection is induced by vaccines.

The resolution of viral infection relies heavily upon macrophages and lymphocytes—the cells of chronic inflammation. Cytotoxic T cells recognize the presence of foreign viral antigens on HLA-identical host cells and specifically kill these infected host cells, thus limiting the spread of virus. T cells, in addition, release interferon-γ which primes macrophages and limits viral replication in newly infected cells. NK cells also contribute to the cytotoxicity of antibody-coated infected host cells.

The relative role of the components of the acute and chronic inflammatory response in viral infections can be inferred from patients with immunodeficiencies. Patients with defects in neutrophil-mediated killing (chronic granulomatous disease), complement, or antibody production (X-linked congenital hypogammaglobulinemia) can generally cope well with viral infections. However, patients with T-cell defects (e.g., DiGeorge syndrome, AIDS) are often unable to eradicate viral infections. Thus, viral infections elicit the full spectrum of acute and chronic inflammatory response (see Clinical Aside 20-3) and are associated with delayed-type hypersensitivity response.

Clinical Aside 20-3
Viral Meningitis

G.B., a 22-year-old female, presented at the emergency room with a 1-day history of malaise, sore throat, rash, severe headaches, and photophobia. Physical examination revealed no abnormality other than the rash and a slight exacerbation of her headache with movement. No nuchal rigidity (resistance to flexion of the neck suggestive of meningeal inflammation) was found. Blood work showed a mild neutrophilia and mild lymphocytosis (a lymphocyte count higher than normal) with a few atypical lymphocytes ("activated" lymphocytes). Because of the headache and photophobia, a spinal tap was performed to obtain cerebral spinal fluid (CSF). Examination of this fluid showed protein: 20 mg/dL (normal, 14 to 45 mg/dL); glucose: 50 mg/dL (normal, 44 to 100 mg/dL); cells: 30 neutrophils per μL and 10 lymphocytes per μL (normal < 5 lymphocytes per μL, no neutrophils). No bacteria were found on Gram's stain. The presence of neutrophils in the CSF is generally a good indication of the presence of bacterial meningitis (bacterial infection of the meninges covering the spinal cord and brain).

In spite of the CSF results, the clinical impression was that the signs and symptoms were due to a virus-associated meningitis, and so antibiotics were not given and G.B. was admitted to the hospital. Repeat blood work, the next day, showed a marked lymphocytosis with numerous atypical lymphocytes (very characteristic of viral infections). A second spinal tap 8 h later showed protein: 22 mg/dL; glucose: 55 mg/dL; cells: 2 neutrophils per mL and 400 lymphocytes per μL.

This case demonstrates the two phases of the inflammatory response to viral infections. Mononuclear infiltrates (lymphocytes and monocytes) are characteristic of viral infections; however, on rare occasions, an acute neutrophilic response may be seen in samples of tissue or fluid, as in G.B.'s case.

SELF-TEST QUESTIONS

1. The underlying tissue process that is most directly associated with redness (erythema), a clinical sign of acute inflammation, is:
   a. Vasoconstriction
   b. Vasodilation
   c. Fibrin deposition in tissues
   d. Increased vascular permeability
   e. Leukocyte margination
   f. Vessel thrombosis

2. The underlying tissue process that is most directly associated with swelling, a clinical sign of acute inflammation, is:
   a. Vasoconstriction
   b. Vasodilation
   c. Fibrin deposition in tissues
   d. Increased vascular permeability
   e. Leukocyte margination
   f. Vessel thrombosis

3. The most important plasma-derived chemotactic factor for neutrophils is:
   a. Bradykinin
   b. Thrombin
   c. C5a
   d. Leukotriene B_4
   e. Thromboxane A_2

4. Pain associated with acute inflammation is most closely associated with which of the following mediators?
   a. Fibrin
   b. Leukotriene B_4
   c. IL-1
   d. Bradykinin
   e. Thromboxane A_2

5. Cell surface glycoproteins directly implicated in mediating neutrophil adherence to endothelial cells include all of the following *except*:
   a. Mo1 (CD11b/CD18)
   b. ELAM-1
   c. IL-1
   d. ICAM-1
   e. Leu-M5 (CD11c/CD18)

6. The most important inflammatory mediator responsible for edema formation in the early phase of acute inflammation is:
   a. IL-1
   b. C5a
   c. Histamine
   d. Factor XII
   e. Myeloperoxidase

7. The *characteristic* cell associated with parasitic infections is the:
   a. Neutrophil
   b. Eosinophil
   c. Monocyte
   d. Lymphocyte
   e. Mast cell

8. A biopsy of lesion in the skin of a 47-year-old woman shows aggregates of monocytes surrounded by lymphocytes with multinucleated giant cells and fibroblasts. This is characteristic of:
   a. Acute inflammation
   b. Granulomatous inflammation
   c. Thrombus formation
   d. Wound healing

9. The inflammatory cell most closely associated with virus infection is the:
   a. Neutrophil
   b. Eosinophil
   c. Platelet
   d. Lymphocyte
   e. Basophil

10. All of the following functions of endothelial cells contribute to the evolution of the inflammatory response *except*:
    a. Regulate vascular tone
    b. A source of tissue factor
    c. A source of plasminogen activator
    d. Express the adherence glycoprotein Mo1
    e. A source of neutrophil chemotactic factor (IL-8)

11. The reactive oxygen metabolite produced by myeloperoxidase is:
    a. O_2^-
    b. H_2O_2
    c. HOCl
    d. OH•
    e. $^1O_2$

12. Reaction of reduced transition metals such as Fe^{2+} with H_2O_2 promotes the formation of:
    a. O_2^-
    b. OH•
    c. HOCl
    d. $^1O_2$
    e. O_3

13. Secretory products of activated monocytes/macrophages include all of the following *except*:
    a. O_2^-
    b. TNF
    c. IL-1
    d. Tissue factor
    e. Histamine

14. The primary role of opsonization of pathogens is to:
    a. Promote phagocytosis and clearance of the pathogen
    b. Activate coagulation pathways
    c. Prevent complement system activation
    d. Facilitate pathogen localization to the vasculature
    d. Prevent platelet activation

15. The primary effect of phagocytic cell priming is to:

a. Block cell activation
b. Cause cell desensitization to a specific stimulus
c. Enhance the functional responses of the cell to a second stimulus
d. Inhibit cell adherence to endothelium

ADDITIONAL READINGS

General

Gallin JI, Goldstein IM, Snyderman R, eds. *Inflammation: Basic Principles and Clinical Correlates.* 2nd ed. New York: Raven Press; 1992.

Adhesion

Bevilacqua MP. Endothelial-leukocyte adhesion molecules. *Annu Rev Immunol.* 1993; 11:767–804.

Eosinophils

Weller PF. The immunobiology of eosinophils. *N Engl J Med.* 1991;324:1110–1118.

Platelets

Capron A, Ameison JC, Joseph M, Auriault C, Tonnel AB, Caen J. New functions for platelets and their pathological implications. *Int Arch Allergy Appl Immunol.* 1985;77:107–114.

Weksler BB. Roles for human platelets in inflammation in platelet membrane receptors: In: Jamieson GA, ed. *Molecular Biology, Immunology, Biochemistry, and Pathology.* New York: Liss; 1988;611–638.

Chemotaxis and Phagocytosis

Cochrane CG, Gimbrone MA (eds). *Cellular and Molecular Mechanisms of Inflammation. Receptors of Inflammatory Cells: Structure Function Relationships.* Orlando, Fla.: Academic Press; 1990.

Granulomatous Inflammation

Hunninghake GW et al. Pathogenesis of granulomatous lung diseases. *Am Rev Respir Dis.* 1984;130:476–496.

Remick DG, Scales WE, Chensue SW, Kunkel SL. The pathophysiology of interleukins and tumor necrosis factor. In: Sayeed MH, ed. *Cellular Pathophysiology.* Boca Raton, Fla.: CRC Press; 1989.

Summary of Part II: Basic Mechanisms of Inflammation

So, here we are at the end of Part II of "Immunology and Inflammation: Basic Mechanisms and Clinical Consequences", a bit over half way through the book. But where are we really?

You have read about antigen-specific and non-antigen-specific responses to pathogens and the internal invader, neoplasia. You have read about how the endless array of antigen-specific immune receptors is created and how their elaboration is modulated and focused by many different supervisory systems. You have read how the various cells and molecules that are part of immunology and inflammation interact in a constantly shifting pattern of cooperation and control.

Hopefully you now appreciate how immunology and inflammation, rather than being independent systems, are actually complementary and mutually supportive in many of their effector functions. Perhaps another look at Appendix B ("The Phylogeny of the Humane Immune System") might be helpful in appreciating the ancient needs that called forth these responses and how, despite epochs of developmental time, the original structures and functions are still represented. Even more interesting is the realization that obscured by the genetic shuffling, duplication, and mutation that have occurred during that time, widely differing functions of multi-cellular organisms, e.g., digestion and inflammation, can be traced back to a common underlying functional principle.

This text now shifts gears a bit, now delving into the practical importance of all that has been presented. Part III describes the ways all of these mechanisms of immunology and inflammation are of importance in disease and health.

PART

THREE

Clinical Consequences

Parts I and II provided all that you need in order to understand the immunopathogenesis and immune responses seen in human disease and health. Part III will help you to apply these principles in ways that seem quite logical and straightforward. However, there are circumstances in which immune mechanisms seem to be active in physiologic activities which are totally unrelated to what seems like an "immune" function (recall the nonimmune activities of certain of the cytokines you learned about in Chapter 10?). By considering these disparate areas of immune activity, we hope that you will appreciate the broad activity of the molecules and cells you have learned about.

We begin by considering how immune mechanisms help defeat infectious agents in Chapter 21 ("Immunity to Micro-organisms") and then look at the clinical ramifications of a defective or absent immune response (Chapter 22, "Immunodeficiency Syndromes," made up of 22a, "Primary, Secondary, and Congenital Syndromes" and 22b, "AIDS"). Next come two somewhat less traditional topics: how the immune system is functionally linked with neurologic, psychologic, and endocrine function (Chapter 23, "Psychoneuroimmunology") and how aging and nutrition can be responsible for modification of immune function (Chapter 24a, "Aging and the Immune System" and Chapter 24b, "Nutrition and the Immune System").

Two "pathologic" conditions are next discussed: how the immune system deals with malignancy (Chapter 25, "The Immunology of Neoplasia") and how we can manipulate the concept of "tolerance" to allow patients with end organ failure to successfully receive new replacement organs (Chapter 26, "Transplantation Immunology").

The miracle of the development of normal children has an immunologic aspect which is described in the following chapters. If the baby has paternal antigens on its cell, why is it not rejected? This and the possibility that just such a mismatch is important in the survival of the fertilized ovum are discussed in Chapter 27, "Pregnancy and the Feto-maternal Relationship." Chapter 28 then deals with the development of the immune response of normal children.

A key to the normal immune response is control, the prevention of a response which can be damaging to self. The next three chapters describe situations in which autoregulation is defective. Allergic phenomena are discussed in Chapter 29, auto-aggressive behavior directed at blood cells in Chapter 30, and a more general discussion of auto-immunity is provided in Chapter 31 ("Systemic and Organ-Specific Auto-Immune Disorders").

Exogenous materials, be they man-made or artificial, can interact with the immune system, producing salubrious or pernicious effects. Immunotoxicity (Chapter 32) is the study of how environmental and man-made materials can damage the immune system. Immunomodulatory therapy, altering the immune system for clinical advantage, is described in Chapter 33a, "Immunopharmacology", Chapter 33b, "Transfer Factor", and Chapter 34, "Clinical Use of Intravenous Gammaglobulin."

The final chapter of the book is a collection of four disease states where immune mechanisms are clearly part of the pathogenesis of the disease. Each is written by clinicians who see patients with that disease so that you will be able to apply the material contained in the preceding chapters to a specific disease process. By analogy, we hope that you will be able to apply the contents of this book to the clinical problems you encounter on the clinical services on which you will serve, in medical school and beyond.

21

Immunity to Microorganisms

INTRODUCTION

Infection occurs when a microorganism successfully enters the host, having evaded mucosal barriers and the host immune defense mechanisms. Once this happens, a coordinated immune response to the invading organism occurs. T-cell immune responses give rise to cytotoxic cells and activate cells which coordinate humoral responses. Macrophage activation is triggered by a T-cell product, INF-γ. Macrophages present antigens to T cells, and, as the name implies, these cells can ingest and kill pathogens. The humoral immune response produces circulating and cell-surface-bound immunoglobulin. Circulating immunoglobulin binds to invaders, increasing clearance by phagocytic cells, and, by activating the complement system, leads directly to further increases in phagocytosis and to the destruction of the invaders. Cell-surface-bound immunoglobulin allows the B cells to recognize the invader. In most types of infections, there is a coordinated immune response which involves T cells, antibodies, macrophages, and polymorphonuclear cells, as well as complement and other nonspecific defense mechanisms. Antibody production is the primary adaptive immune response. Immunity on mucosal surfaces is often IgA-dependent and may not correlate with the systemic response.

In most cases microorganisms are destroyed in a phagocytic cell, complement and antibodies serving as opsonins. Antibody-dependent cytotoxic cells are capable of destroying infected cells. Only infected host cells are killed by cytotoxic T cells.

The point of the preceding paragraphs is that many of the immune mechanisms detailed in this text are active in the fight against infections, collaborating in an integrated immune response. If the invading organism overcomes innate mechanisms of defense, a specific immune response will occur. The specific cellular and humoral responses enhance and amplify the innate mechanisms by providing specificity and by recruiting other cells and defenses. One or more of the many forms of immune response may be the primary defense active against a particular infection. The desired end result is the uptake and destruction of the invader. Recall that immunology is a direct outgrowth of the study of the host response to infections. It is therefore fitting that the first topic in Part III of this text, on clinical immunology, is the host response to infection.

In order to proceed with a discussion of immune responses to microorganisms, it is important to define the terms used. Before proceeding, check the glossary at the end of this chapter to make sure you know the terms and concepts important for a precise understanding of the material in this chapter.

You have learned about the inducible immune mechanisms which protect us from infection. These include:

B-cell responses: immunoglobulin, local (IgA) and systemic (IgM, IgG, IgA, IgE)

T-cell responses: cytotoxic, helper, and delayed-type hypersensitivity cells

Macrophages: none intrinsically antigen-specific

Natural killer (NK) cells: specificity conferred by antibodies

Complement: produced by B cells

These defense mechanisms are not all equally active in the response to each and every infection. As an example, the response to viruses does not involve a large contribution from polymorphonuclear cells (PMNs), and the effect of antibody is only to eliminate extracellular virus and decrease the likelihood of reinfection. In general, the type of defense most active in infections with a given type of organism is as follows:

Bacteria:	T cells, monocytes, complement, B cells, PMNs
Mycobacteria:	T cells, monocytes, PMNs
Viruses:	T cells, monocytes, complement

390

Parasites: T cells, monocytes,
Fungi: T cells

There are, in addition, numerous nonspecific barriers which can prevent entry of microorganisms and help to eliminate them while specific immune mechanisms are developing. In some circumstances, these forms of nonspecific defenses are sufficient to avoid infection. Even when infection does develop, these mechanisms are active in minimizing the severity of infection.

Intact Integument
Intact integument is a physical barrier to entry of microorganisms.

Normal desquamation and shedding of skin also sheds attached microorganisms.

Hostile Environments
Sweat (lactic acid), fatty acids on skin surface, and acid pH in stomach and vagina are important nonspecific hostile environments.

Lysozyme (small cationic enzyme) present in tears, nasal secretions, and saliva acts on the mucopeptides of bacterial cell walls.

Seminal plasma spermine and other compounds in prostatic secretions inhibit certain bacteria.

Salivary glycolipids decrease bacterial adhesion.

Local Mechanisms
Cilia and mucus "sweep" surfaces clean.

Air passes over nasal turbinates with adhesion and clearance of particles.

Urinary system and gastrointestinal tract flush out invading microorganisms.

Competition
Commensual organisms in and on the body already fill the microbiologic niche; some produce fatty acids or deconjugate bile salts to produce toxic compounds while others may produce antibiotics.

Innate Immunity
"Natural antibodies," probably made in response to intestinal bacteria, have low affinity but broad specificity.

Complement fixes directly to cell walls (by the phylogenetically older alternative pathway) and acts as an opsonin. (Once specific antibodies are formed, complement can be fixed by IgM and IgG bound to the organism's cell surface by means of the classical pathway.)

Another serum protein, unrelated to the complement proteins, is C-reactive protein, which can bind nonspecifically to organisms and decreases alternative pathway deposition but markedly increases classical pathway activation.

Complement degradation products act as chemotactic factors, increase degranulation and aggregation of PMNs, and increase production of superoxides and lactoferrin, which inhibit growth of bacteria.

Phagocytes, both macrophages and PMNs, may kill the organism and release lactoferrin.

Tissue injury may trigger the coagulation cascade, with fibrin deposition inhibiting the spread of the organism.

Coagulation cascade also initiates bradykinin production, with subsequent vasodilatation, increased permeability of blood vessels, and local prostaglandin production; bradykinin also produces the sensation of pain.

Platelets contain β-lysin, a cationic protein which is bactericidal for many organisms.

Host damage from infection occurs because the invading organism has been able to successfully

Invade

Attach

Proliferate

Avoid destruction and/or digestion by defense mechanisms

Damage the host by
    Elaboration of toxins
    Direct tissue invasion
    Action of the immune response (see Clinical Aside 21-1)

Clinical Aside 21-1
Heat Shock Proteins in the Initial Immune Response to Infection

Any time a cell is stressed, be it from exposure to heat, oxidants, heavy metals, or cytokines, it begins to make a group of proteins called *heat shock proteins* (HSPs), which help protect it from that stress. This is the case for every cell yet studied; bacteria, yeasts, and mammals all make a "heat shock response." The structure of these proteins is remarkably conserved throughout evolution, so that the HSPs made by bacteria are quite similar to those made by humans.

Some of these proteins help to refold denatured proteins into their native conformation; some unfold proteins to allow transport into organelles, e.g., chloroplast, mitochondria, nucleus; other related proteins (chaperonins) are part of the protein folding, assembly, and processing functions of normal cells; yet other proteins serve to maintain unliganded glucocorticoid, androgen, and progesterone receptors and certain cellular kinases in their nonactivated state. Recent evidence suggests that one member of an HSP superfamily may be involved in transport of the T cell–immunomodulatory molecule FK-506.

HSPs are often immunodominant proteins, which means that a large part of the specific B- or T-cell response to a microbe is directed against the HSP, e.g., 20 percent of the murine T cells reacting with *Mycobacterium tuberculosis* after mouse inoculation recognize a single protein, hsp65. Normal people have anti-HSP antibodies and anti-HSP T cells. The universality of this immunodominance suggests that this reactivity has survival value to the host. This then raises two interrelated questions: (1) What is the role of the immune reactivity with HSPs? (2) Can the high degree of conservation of these molecules lead to problems, i.e., autoimmunity?

As you have learned, it takes a few days for an antigen-specific immune response to develop. A number of innate or natural, immune mechanisms exist to contain infection (e.g., lysozyme, isohemagglutinins, IFN-γ) before the antigen-specific response can be mounted. We can probably add HSPs to this list; bacteria subjected to changes in environment, oxygen radicals, and proteolytic enzymes make HSPs which are displayed on their surfaces. Antibodies and T cells preformed to these HSPs can then bind to the cells and destroy them.

Many transformed cells and cells infected with DNA viruses (as well as infected with other intracellular pathogens) express HSPs on their surface. Thus, it is possible that anti-HSP immune reactivity may play a role in defense against intracellular infections and malignancies.

IFN-γ induces macrophages to make HSPs and express them on the cell surface. One theory suggests that HSP production in activated macrophages may help protect the macrophage from its own oxygen radicals and enzymes.

HSPs may be present on the surface of normal cells and are released by cells during immune reactivity. As discussed in the "Molecular Mimicry" section of Chapt. 31 on autoimmunity, anti-HSP reactivity has been implicated in the pathogenesis of adjuvant-induced arthritis (AA). AA is a model of rheumatoid arthritis in the rat in which adjuvant that contains mycobacterial proteins, notably hsp65, induces arthritis in susceptible animals. The arthritis can be transferred to naive animals by hsp65-reactive cells. Anti-hsp65 T cells are noted in the synovial fluid of patients with rheumatoid arthritis. In normal people there are T-cell-idiotype networks that keep anti-HSP T-cell reactivity under tight control. It may be that these controls fail after certain occult or minor infections, and the unfettered anti-HSP reactivity may be involved in the production of persisting inflammation, e.g., rheumatoid arthritis. Although in 1993 this is merely speculation, such mechanisms may be involved in the chronic phases of inflammation, long after the initiating infection has disappeared.

BACTERIAL INFECTION

Bacteria adhere to, and may enter, cells by means of surface structures on the invader and host cell. Receptors on the surface of mammalian cells are often polysaccharides, and may be normal mammalian cell surface structures, such as the P blood group antigens, fibronectin, CD4 molecule, and, perhaps, HLA markers including β_2-microglobulin. These molecules are recognized by lectins on bacteria; pili and fimbriae on certain bacteria mediate adhesion. IgA in mucosal surface secretions is often directed at these bacterial surface structures and blocks attachment to the target.

It is not surprising that bacteria have evolved means by which to avoid immune defenses. The multiplicity and complexity of the mechanisms used by bacteria (and by other pathogens, most notably parasites) is quite amazing:

Microbial mobility may overcome the defensive qualities of mucus.

Organisms can shed their surface molecules in mucus; these will then bind immunoglobulin and complement and so deplete the stores of molecules available to bind the infectious particle.

By attaching to the epithelial lining of the respiratory, digestive, or genitourinary tracts, organisms can avoid being flushed away by local mucus plus ciliary action.

Certain organisms have the ability to survive the hostile acid environment of the stomach (including *Salmonella typhosa*).

Certain polysaccharides in the capsule of organisms (including *Streptococcus pneumoniae*, *Haemophilus influenzae*, *Neisseria meningitidis*, and *Staphylococcus aureus*) interfere with phagocytosis; antibodies to these molecules may increase uptake. Coagulase, an enzyme produced by certain staphylococci, may activate the coagulation system and envelope the organism in a protective coat of fibrin.

Pili (*N meningitidis*) and fimbriae (*Staphylococcus aureus*) on the surface of organisms also interfere with phagocytosis. Antibodies to these organisms lead to increased phagocytosis.

By means of genetic recombination, some organisms (e.g., *Borrelia*) can alter their surface proteins, so that antibodies do not bind as well.

Certain strains of *N meningitidis* are resistant to IgM-mediated complement fixation.

Some strains of *N meningitidis* cleave IgA on mucosal surfaces.

Proteins like the protein A made by *S aureus* can bind to IgG and block its opsonizing effects.

Inhibition of phagolysosomal fusion occurs in infection with *S aureus*, *Chlamydia psittaci* and *Chlamydia trachomatis*, and *Mycobacterium tuberculosis*. The organism may produce enzymes which interfere with intraleukocytic killing (catalase by staphylococci and *Escherichia coli*, among others).

Rickettsia and *Mycobacterium leprae* can escape from the phagosome into the phagocyte's cytoplasm.

Legionella pneumatophila blocks the gravitation of cellular organelles to the phagosome. Other organisms can survive the effect of the digestive enzymes in phagolysosomes and grow within macrophages (certain rickettsiae, mycobacteria, and *Brucella*; *Listeria monocytogenes*; *Legionella pneumophila*; and cryptococci).

However many means of evading the human immune response there may be, most people avoid infections most of the time. In the absence of clear breaches in our defenses, the immune response is very effective.

Immunoglobulin is one of the primary immune defenses against bacteria, and antibodies can block many of the mechanisms used by microorganisms listed above. The mucosal IgA response is often the crucial first step in frustrating infection; e.g., mucosal IgA can block adherence of bacteria to respiratory or gut mucosa. External secretions, including saliva, tears, and bile and nasal, tracheobronchial, intestinal, and cervical fluids, contain much more IgA than IgG or IgM; internal secretions, like the aqueous humor and cerebrospinal, synovial, pleural, and peritoneal fluids, contain more IgG than IgA, and even less IgM. (Topologically speaking, the human body is essentially a torus or doughnut, with the skin, gut, and respiratory tracts on the surface, thus, intestinal fluid and bile are truly external secretions.) Local production of IgA may correlate with systemic production of IgA, but may be independent of immunoglobulin production in the rest of the body. The unique qualities of IgA and the mucosal immune response are discussed in Chap. 11.

The humoral response at nonmucosal locations is induced at regional lymph nodes, where bacteria arrive, either free or within macrophages (Fig. 21-1) Early in an infection, polyclonal B-cell activation, stimulated by bacterial molecules like lipopolysaccharide and staphylococcal protein A, may cause the production of mostly low-affinity, nonspecific IgM, which is very effective in fixing complement. This requires little cellular collaboration and provides efficient opsonization, more efficient phagolysosomal fusion, bacteriolysis, and toxin neutralization until high-affinity specific immunoglobulin and T-cell mechanisms evolve.

Specific IgG can fix complement and lead to either increased efficiency of phagocytosis (opsonization) or to lysis (Fig. 21-2). IgG may bind to and block the surface molecules which help the organism enter host cells and can bind and neutralize toxins and enzymes produced by the invader which promote tissue damage and spread of the organism.

The diseases tetanus, diphtheria, and botulism are caused by toxins elaborated by *Clostridium tetani, Corynebacterium diphtheriae,* and *Clostridium botulinum,* respectively. In these three diseases passive treatment with immunoglobulin antitoxin may be life-saving. In other, non-toxin-producing infections, serotherapy may help opsonize virulent encapsulated organisms (e.g., *N meningitidis* and *S pneumoniae*) and decrease the severity of infection. Such passive treatment may also be valuable in certain forms of bacterial sepsis and cases in which the host is unable to mount a specific humoral response.

Once chemotactic factors—e.g., complement degradation components, certain arachidonic acid metabolites, and bacteria-derived molecules—are elaborated, the professional phagocytes arrive. PMNs and monocytes have receptors for C3b, IgG1, and IgG3 on their surface, each of which increases the efficiency of phagocytosis by interacting with specific compounds already bound to the organism. PMNs destroy microorganisms that rely upon evasion of phagocytosis for their survival. Monocytes are often important in controlling chronic infections with microbes capable of intracellular survival. Acting as antigen-presenting cells, monocytes can sensitize T cells and T cell–derived lympho-

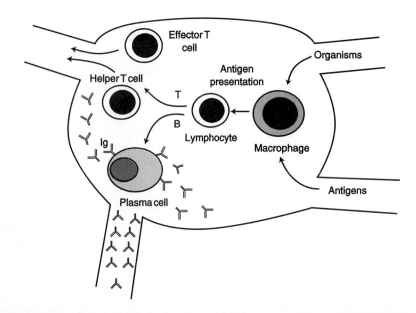

Figure 21-1 Humoral response of regional lymph nodes. With arrival of organisms or discrete antigens, a local immune response takes place in the germinal center(s) of the regional lymph node.

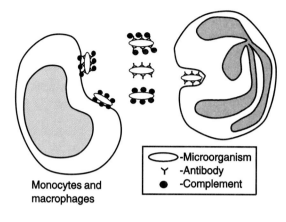

Figure 21-2 Complement fixing by specific IgG leads to increased efficiency of phagocytosis or to lysis. Phagocytic cells are more able to bind and ingest organisms/particles that are coated with complement (binding to complement receptors) and immunoglobulin (binding to Fc receptors).

kines such as INF-γ, increase monocyte activity, and mediate other immune functions.

During ingestion of the organism, PMNs undergo a respiratory burst of metabolism. This occurs with any perturbation of the cell membrane, even without ingestion, and gives rise to oxygen radicals, superoxide, hydrogen peroxide, and products of the hexose-monophosphate shunt. Myeloperoxidase can act on hydrogen peroxide in the presence of a halide ion to produce bactericidal activity within phagocytic vacuoles. Superoxides which escape from the vacuoles are metabolized by superoxide dismutase into hydrogen peroxide. The latter is then detoxified by catalase or glutathione peroxidase–glutathione reductase (Fig. 21-3). If the oxygen radicals are not confined to the phagolysosome, as is seen when phagocytes attempt to ingest very large and/or nondigestible particles, there may be leakage of the radicals and other intracellular components; when this occurs, tissue death rather than the death of the microorganism may result.

PMN granules contain a number of compounds with antibacterial activity (see Chap. 17). Nuclear histones and cytoplasmic proteases also help kill ingested organisms, as does the very low pH of the phagolysosome (recall that the low pHs of the stomach and vagina are natural defenses). Thus, PMNs can kill microorganisms by both oxygen-dependent and oxygen-independent mechanisms.

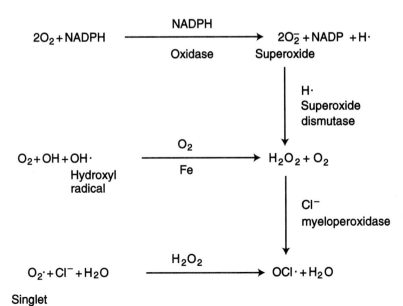

Figure 21-3 Generation of hydrogen peroxide, oxygen radicals, and hypochlorite. Hydrogen peroxide can be detoxified by catalase or glutathione peroxidase–glutathione reductase.

Monocytes are the other major phagocytic population. (Recall that other cell types, including endothelial and epithelial cells and fibroblasts, are capable of phagocytosis, but with much less efficiency, in part due to the lack of surface receptors for Ig and C3b.) The mononuclear phagocytes exit the bloodstream and enter organs, where they may proliferate, unlike PMNs, which are already terminally differentiated. Approximately 75 percent of monocytes exist in a marginal, noncirculating pool and can be mobilized as needs dictate. Monocytes phagocytose less rapidly and with less efficiency than PMNs, but are an important response when PMNs are unable to kill and degrade the organism. Monocyte granules are different from those of PMNs, in that they do not contain lactoferrin or cationic proteins, but do have neutral proteases and lysozyme. Monocytes are circulating biochemical factories, capable of making prostaglandins, leukotrienes, and complement components, as well as the arylsulfatases and acid phosphatases in their granules. Both types of phagocytic cells are made more efficient by opsonins.

Monocytes also produce IL-1 and tumor necrosis factor (TNF) (Chap. 10). As is so often the case in immunology, the names of these two compounds are far too restrictive; IL-1 acts on lymphoid cells, as first described, but it also causes fever (it is the "endogenous pyrogen"), fatigue (IL-1 is one of the reasons why an infection makes you tired), anorexia (perhaps the origin of the saying "feed a cold and starve a fever"), and myalgias. (In order to mobilize amino acids for use in production of proteins essential in the immune response, there is muscle breakdown—thus the aches and pains often felt during viral infections.) TNF has actions having nothing to do with response to tumor. It induces wasting in animals and probably humans (thus its original name, *cachectin*), and, in common with IL-1, is also a pyrogen and a growth factor for osteoclasts and fibroblasts and has antiviral activity by inducing INF-β. Both compounds also induce the cell surface expression of a variety of markers on endo-

thelial cells. Plasminogen activator, which promotes local thrombosis, may help to isolate infection; however, uncontrolled coagulation may be the cause of the disseminated intravascular coagulation (DIC) that may complicate infection with endotoxin-containing organisms and may be the cause of hemorrhagic necrosis of tumors.

IL-1 and TNF also induce a marked increase in the "stickiness" of endothelial cells for PMNs, monocytes, and lymphocytes. The adherence of circulating cells to the endothelium at the site of ongoing inflammation then allows a more efficient egress of cells where they are needed and makes the inflammatory response more effective.

One other major advantage of the monocyte phagocytic system is its ability to interact with T cells. Activated T cells produce lymphokines which are chemotactic for monocytes and increase the efficiency of the endocytic and microbicidal activity of monocytes and the macrophages.

T cell–mediated responses include three subsets of T cells, helper, cytotoxic, and delayed-type hypersensitivity (DTH).

Certain bacterial antigens, especially large polysaccharides with a repeating structure, can elicit an immunoglobulin response without the action of helper T cells; these are called *T-independent antigens*. Immunoglobulin response to other antigens, often proteins, requires T-cell assistance, and these are classified as *T-dependent antigens*. Helper cells are also involved in expanding other cellular responses. (See Chap. 7, "Ontogeny and Differentiation of T Lymphocytes.")

Cytotoxic cells are involved in killing virus-infected cells (see below) but are probably not very active in resistance to bacterial infections. NK cells, however, do react against *N meningitidis*, and antibody-dependent cellular cytotoxicity (ADCC) may be vital, especially where there is little complement or antibody, e.g., the cerebrospinal fluid or mucosal surfaces.

DTH T cells are often active where monocytes have been infected. Monocytes, as antigen-presenting cells, can activate T cells, which then secrete factors which attract, immobilize, and activate monocytes. These lymphokine-activated monocytes then produce more reactive oxygen metabolites and become more efficient phagocytes; the net result is a more microbicidal cell.

DTH activity, measured by skin testing, correlates directly with the potential magnitude of the granulomatous reaction to the organism. The most commonly used skin test is PPD (purified protein derivative of *Mycobacterium tuberculosis*), used to test for prior exposure to TB. (One reason for non-response to PPD is the absence of a previous exposure. What might be another explanation for lack of response and how might this be tested?) PPD (or an antigen from any other organism to be tested) is injected intradermally. The antigen is then picked up by resident antigen-presenting cells. In a previously exposed individual the site of the skin test is infiltrated with PMNs and then with lymphocytes. The antigen specificity of the reaction is defined by the influx of specific T cells and the subsequent inflow of monocytes. The presence of antigen decreases the exit of cells from the draining lymph nodes of that region, at least in part due to the local production of migration inhibition factor(s) keeping the cells from leaving. DTH is called "delayed" because it takes about 48 h for this process to occur and cause the erythema and induration we as clinicians can then measure as a positive skin test.

The inability of an individual to mount a DTH reaction to any antigens previously encountered is called *anergy*. It is very important not to adjudge someone anergic too quickly, however. An important part of skin testing is the use of positive controls, antigens derived from ubiquitous microbes, to which exposure would be expected. Commonly used controls are dermatophytes, including *Trichophyton, Candida,* and mumps. The absence of any response to multiple controls on two occasions can be said to indicate anergy, which must then be evaluated.

Some of the same processes are at work in the tissues of patients with TB. The same

factors and macrophage-fusion inducing substance(s) cause the production of giant cells and granulomata at sites of chronic inflammation in disease. There is selective recruitment of antigen-sensitized, primed memory T cells into the area, and such cells can be found in these granulomata. Some antigen-specific T cells do escape the region of infection and, through recirculation, disseminate immune memory to the rest of the body.

Humoral and cellular immune responses cooperate in a combined and balanced response to infection. One or the other may predominate, depending on the type of invader; if the former is the major response, there may be a *purulent* reaction. Especially where organisms parasitize monocytes, a primarily cellular response may lead to a *granulomatous* reaction. In either case the response is focused on the organism, and is designed to eliminate the invader with minimal damage to the host.

When an organism makes toxins or enzymes which are released into the environment, host tissue destruction may result. There are, however, examples of disease (tissue damage) being caused not by the organism but by the type of inflammatory response elicited. The degree of DTH correlates with tissue damage in TB, and the organism which causes syphilis, *Treponema pallidum,* is itself not harmful to host tissues. Thus the immune response, not the infecting organism, may cause tissue damage. As PMNs respond to a local infection, they may regurgitate their lysosomal enzymes into the tissue, with damage to the host. Immunoglobulin may bind to bacterial antigens and the immune complexes formed may cause tissue damage, e.g., glomerulonephritis in subacute bacterial endocarditis.

It is known that the individual's genotype at least in part determines the immune response to an organism [recall major histocompatibility complex (MHC) linkage of immune responses, Chap. 4]. The type of immune response can determine the presence (or absence) of tissue damage in infection. The best described example of this is leprosy, caused by infection with *M leprae*. The "proper" immune response to exposure would be to have no disease, because the defense system has successfully dealt with the infection; the end result would be the development of clones of T cells which can recognize the organism, manifested only by a positive skin test when using lepromin, a protein derived from the organism.

If, on the other hand, the immune response is insufficient, the organism may survive, especially within immune cells, and extensive disease may occur. This is what happens in lepromatous leprosy—many organisms are seen and there is widespread disease, with an inefficient granulomatous reaction. The skin test for specific DTH using lepromin is weak or negative.

The other end of the spectrum is an overly strong response. In tuberculoid leprosy there are very few organisms seen, but the immune response produces an aggressive infiltration with lymphocytes and epithelioid cells, which mediate local damage. The lepromin-induced skin test is usually positive. It has been shown that antigen-induced suppressor cells are very active in lepromatous leprosy, are nearly absent in tuberculoid leprosy, and are present at an intermediate level in the "proper" response alluded to above. Whether this immunoregulatory dysfunction is a consequence of the ongoing disease or represents a premorbid immune abnormality is not clear (Table 21-1).

VIRAL INFECTION

Viruses are obligate intracellular parasites capable of causing a wide spectrum of disease. The illness may be acute (with or without lifetime immunity), subclinical, recurrent, chronic, or latent. The specific immune response includes both humoral and cell-mediated mechanisms, but it is important to remember that those responses which can be demonstrated in vitro may not be the critical in vivo events.

Viruses must enter host cells in order to replicate. The specific site of entry on the target cell is not known for most viruses; where known, the portal of entry is a cell surface protein, e.g., the T-cell marker CD4 (HIV), the acetylcholine receptor (rabies), the complement CR2 receptor [Epstein-Barr virus (EBV)], and the HLA molecules (Sindbis virus and others). (Recall that interferon, which is produced in response to viral infection, induces the expression of HLA markers on the surface of a number of cells; over the course of the evolution viruses have been able to bend a part of the immune response to their own needs!) The type of illness, if any, is dictated by a variety of factors related to the virus and the host. Depending on local conditions, the tropism of the virus, and the status of the immune system of the host, viral infections may abort, may be local, or may be widespread.

TABLE 21-1   Features of Tuberculoid and Lepromatous Leprosy

Feature	Tuberculoid Leprosy	Lepromatous Leprosy
Lesions	Localized	Disseminated
Organisms	Rare	Many, in macrophages
Lymphocytes	Many	Few
Granulomata	Many	Absent
Skin test	Positive	Negative
In vitro tests		
Lymphocyte proliferation	Positive	Negative
MIF production*	Positive	Negative
Cause of tissue damage	Immune response to organism	Organism

*Migration inhibition factor production upon exposure of peripheral blood mononuclear cells to *M leprae* antigens.

After penetration, the virion uncoats and may then replicate. Budding of daughter virus particles or lysis of the host cell may occur. The virus may become dormant, perhaps to be activated at a later date. Finally, the virus's genetic material may insert into the host's genome, with virus production or subsequent neoplastic transformation the result.

From the initial site of invasion virus may spread via the extracellular (hematogenous or contiguous) route, the intracellular (delivery of circulating cells to remote sites) route, or the intercellular (parent to progeny, or vertical) route. Viruses may lie dormant within host cells, only to reemerge clinically at a later date. For example, varicella, the virus which causes chickenpox, can chronically and subclinically infect nerve cells and upon reactivation cause shingles many years after the initial infection (Fig. 21-4).

Viruses which do not produce an acute infection, elaborate no viral antigens on the surface of infected cells, cause little or no tissue destruction, or infect only immunologically privileged sites may elicit a minimal immune response and so evade host defenses. Slow viruses, like those which cause Creutzfeldt-Jakob disease, kuru, and subacute sclerosing panencephalitis (SSPE—a rare

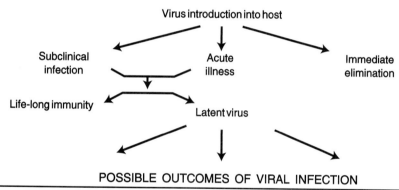

Carrier state	Neoplastic transformation of affected cells		Chronic illness		Later acute illness	
EBV	EBV	⟶ Burkitt's lymphoma	Measles (prior acute illness)	⟶ Subacute sclerosing panencephalitis (SSPE)	Varicella-zoster (prior acute illness)	⟶ Shingles
Hepatitis B virus	Human papilloma virus	⟶ Genital squamous cell carcinoma			Herpes simplex (oral or genital) (prior acute illness)	⟶ Herpes simplex
Varicella-zoster virus						
Human papilloma virus						
Herpes simplex virus	Hepatitis B virus	⟶ Hepatocellular carcinoma				

Figure 21-4 Viral activity in the host. Depending on the prior and present immune status of a host, viral infection can result in many different clinical outcomes.

manifestation of infection with the virus that causes measles) cause chronic diseases which avoid detection and elimination by these means.

Evasion of the immune response remains the most effective way for viruses to survive. Certain viral surface markers are poorly immunogenic and so the virus is unscathed by immune attack. When an antibody is formed to a nonneutralizing antigen, the antibody may not inhibit the virus; instead it may form circulating immune complexes which can themselves mediate tissue destruction. Rapid changes in surface antigens and multiple variants of the same virus with little cross-reactivity help the virus survive.

Influenza A virus is quite adept at avoiding the immune response. The virus has two major classes of proteins on its surface, neuraminidase and hemagglutinin (Fig. 21-5). Influenza virus antigens can undergo two general types of antigenic changes, known as *drift* (point mutations in a given subtype; a subtype is defined by viruses having neuraminidase and hemagglutinin surface proteins which cross-react) and *shift* (major alterations in antigenic characteristics leading to a change in subtype, perhaps by genetic recombination between human and animal viruses). Epidemics and pandemics of influenza are associated with shift and drift of these surface proteins; if the antigenic change is great enough, antibodies produced from previous exposure to influenza will not help in the current experience. Antibody to the hemagglutinin is the most important component preventing reinfection with the same subtype, whereas antibody to the neuraminidase molecule interferes with release of the virus from infected cells.

Herpesviruses, as well as other viruses, make a compound resembling Fc receptor which, when elaborated on the surface of infected cells, binds immunoglobulin, thus eliminating the bound immunoglobulin molecules from the hunt. Recent studies suggest that myxoma virus–infected cells secrete a viral protein with significant sequence similarity to human and murine IFN-γ receptor. The viral protein (called M-T7) binds IFN-γ. Virulence factors in other viruses include complement-binding proteins, as well as proteins with serine protease inhibitor. In addition, viruses can adopt a camouflage of sorts; they may carry along host membrane molecules as they bud from infected cells. The host will in general not make an immune response against self, so that the viral particle escapes notice and can proceed to infect another cell.

Despite their advantage in speed of genetic turnover and alteration, viruses are generally well controlled by the intact immune system. Antibodies produced during a prior exposure to the same or closely related viruses may still be present in the circulation

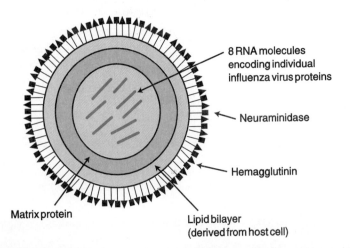

Figure 21-5 The structure of influenza virus A.

and neutralize the virus particles. The alternative complement pathway may directly bind to virus particles, with subsequent lysis or phagocytosis; this occurs *before* the specific immune response has had a chance to begin. During the same early, "preimmune" period of infection, the elaboration of interferon by infected cells induces viral resistance and antiviral immunity (Fig. 21-6; also see Chap. 10). The side effects of interferon (when given as therapy) include fever, malaise, fatigue, and anorexia. (Note that these are the very symptoms of a cold, and closely resemble the systemic effects of IL-1. Fever as an effect of both of these mediators suggests that elevated temperature may have a purpose in fighting infection. And in fact there is evidence that T cells and phagocytes work better at higher temperatures.)

Once specific antibodies are made, they can fix complement and aid in the clearance of virus. IgA on mucosal surfaces can neutralize viruses, and may prevent systemic spread. Neutralizing antibodies prevent the virus from binding to the target cell, may block certain surface enzymatic activities needed for penetration, or may prevent virus

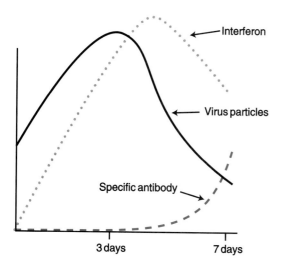

from uncoating, once already in the cell. Neutralization is never quite complete, however, and a fraction of the virus particles remain at liberty for further infection.

As stated above, if a virus-infected cell does not manifest either viral or some sort of never-before-elaborated antigens on its surface, the host's immune response will ignore the cell. However, the presence of either type of unusual antigen can lead to lysis of the cell, mediated by specific immunoglobulin plus complement or by any of three types of lymphoid cells. Cytotoxic T cells are capable of killing cells with these new antigens, expressed in the context of HLA class I antigens (see Chap. 8). It is important to note that this killing is not always virus-strain-specific (viral strains are defined by serologic, not cell-mediated determinants, and these may be different). For example, HLA-restricted cytotoxic responses can develop against cells infected with several different strains of influenza A after immunization with one strain. NK cells and antibody-dependent cytotoxic cells are also capable of killing infected cells. The latter are not directed at any particular type of cell or virus and, you will recall, are not MHC-restricted in their activity. Such cells have Fc receptors on their surfaces. The antibody-dependent cytotoxic cell's target (its specificity) is dictated by its interaction with the Fc segment of a specific immunoglobulin bound to the infected cell. Thus, MHC-restricted and MHC-nonrestricted cytotoxicity may be active in the response to viral infection, in addition to humoral responses, depending on the type of viral infection (see Fig. 21-7).

In all of these interactions, genetically determined host restrictions are active. Thus, part of the severity of disease, or of "intrinsic" resistance to infection, may be due to inborn factors. The type of immune response can, in part, determine the manifestations of viral infection. A good example of this is EBV, which is a herpesvirus. Most of the adult population has serum antibodies to EBV (is *seropositive*), but many seropositive individuals have never had any clinical manifestations of infection. In lower socioeconomic

Figure 21-6 Elaboration of interferon before the specific immune response emerges allows for rapid clearance of virus before specific antibodies are available.

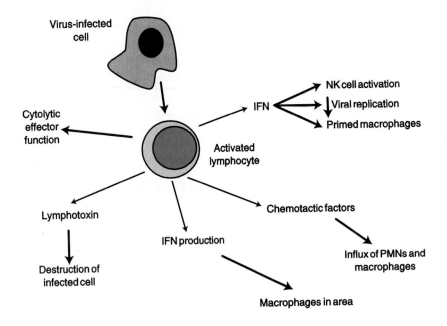

Figure 21-7   Lymphocyte-mediated mechanisms capable of causing destruction of virus-infected cells. By MHC-restricted and nonrestricted means, lymphocytes can kill cells expressing unique cellular or viral antigens on their surfaces. In addition to natural killer (NK) cells, cytotoxic T cells, and antibody-dependent cytotoxic cells, macrophages and polymorphonuclear (PMN) cells can be enlisted. The direct effects of cytokines like lymphotoxins and interferon (IFN) are also active participants in this response.

groups and especially in nonindustrialized parts of the world, infection occurs early in life and is usually asymptomatic; in the United States and other industrialized parts of the world, approximately 50 percent of people will get infected with EBV later in life and may experience the syndrome known as infectious mononucleosis.

EBV is acquired via the oropharynx and enters epithelial cells on its way to infecting B cells (or it may infect B cells directly). Once in circulating B cells, the virus disseminates. Latent infection remains throughout life. During the acute phase of infection, a cytotoxic T-cell response is made; some of these cells are MHC-restricted, some are not. The large number of atypical cells in the blood of a patient with "mononucleosis" are actually activated CD8$^+$ T cells with suppressor/cytotoxic activity. The elevated suppressor and cytotoxic activity seen in the peripheral blood of patients decreases toward normal with convalescence. These cells and certain neutralizing antibodies may prevent the latent infection from becoming symptomatic.

The ability of EBV to infect B cells has made it useful to research immunologists, since these B cells will continue to divide and grow in tissue culture (known as becoming "immortal"). In vivo, the absence of a T-cell response to control this phenomenon translates into malignant growth of the cells which are infected with EBV, nasal epithelial cells (nasopharyngeal cancer), or B cells (Burkitt's lymphoma). Recently a nonmalignant, chronic infection with EBV has been recognized, as well. An individual's ability to mount an immune response to EBV probably determines what the ultimate outcome of infection will be (Fig. 21-8).

The immune response to viruses may also cause host damage. Specific cytolysis and secondary metabolic changes at the site of inflammation may cause direct tissue damage. Local buildup of antibody and complement, immune complexes, and activated cells may cause the destruction of healthy tissues.

Circulating immune complexes formed by the combination of antigens shed by the virus and the specific antibodies produced during the immune response may cause systemic inflammation; the preicteric (before jaundice) phase of hepatitis B virus infection may be associated with dermatitis, arthritis, or damage to blood vessels (vasculitis) caused by such immune complexes. The systemic damage caused by deposition of immune complexes can cause a syndrome virtually identical to the systemic necrotizing vasculitis known as *polyarteritis nodosa*. This phenomenon is seen especially in chronic viral infections, with long-term antigenemia. The organs involved include the kidneys, lung, joints, and choroid plexus. Despite the fact that there is no firm evidence that such a

virus-induced mechanism is the cause of systemic lupus erythematosus (SLE), this is one of the abiding theories of the immunopathogenesis of SLE, an (at least partially) immune complex–mediated "autoimmune" illness.

Viral antigens may resemble those of host tissues. When this is the case, an immune response to the virus may also bind to and damage host tissue, a circumstance known as *molecular mimicry* (see below).

If viruses enter target cells by binding to surface cellular molecules, it seems reasonable that, as part of the idiotype–anti-idiotype network, there might be an antibody produced which resembles the internal structure of the binding site. Were this antibody to be capable of fixing complement, or of activating antibody-dependent cytotoxic cells, there could be destruction of the cellular target of the virus, i.e., host tissues. This mechanism has been noted as another way that a virus could cause "autoimmune" disease (Fig. 21-9).

In 1911 Von Pirquet, the father of the study of allergy, noted that in the first days after the onset of the rash of measles, skin reactivity to PPD diminished. Over the years this

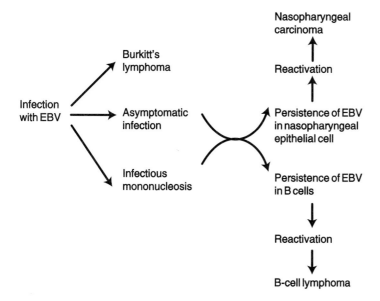

Figure 21-8 The immune response to EBV. A single virus can produce a number of clinical outcomes.

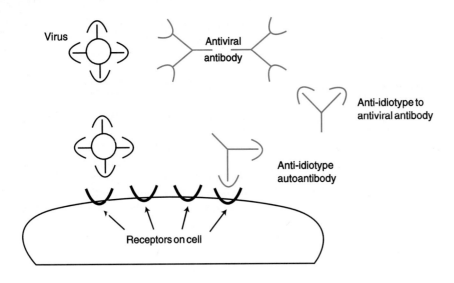

Figure 21-9   Proposed mechanism by which a virus may cause "autoimmune" disease.

and other examples of virus-induced immunosuppression have been documented. As a result of Von Pirquet's observation, for many years a negative PPD skin test was required before giving the attenuated live measles vaccine; occasionally, a child being inoculated for measles would experience a sudden flare of his or her previously inactive tuberculosis.

The coincidence of defective suppressor cell activity, the stimulation of polyclonal B- and T-cell activation, and the release of previously sequestered self-antigens provides an excellent opportunity to mount an autoimmune reaction. These and other possible mechanisms will be explored in greater detail in Chap. 31, on autoimmunity.

PARASITIC INFECTION

Although usually not a major problem in the United States, parasitic disease, both human and animal, is *the* major health problem in the world. They are usually chronic and persistent infestations which do not kill their hosts. [This last point is a good one to remember: it is a foolish (and suicidal!) parasite which kills its host.] In general the host-parasite interaction has evolved to the point where neither the host nor the parasite dies; both species survive and reproduce. The ultimate outcome is determined by the balance of the parasite's ability to evade the immune response and the ability of the host to efficiently recognize and dispose of the parasite. However, even an effective response will simply decrease the total parasitic burden, not totally eliminate the invader.

Parasites are more complicated organisms than bacteria or viruses and have developed highly effective means of evading the host's immune response:

Many parasites can inhibit fusion of lysosomes to phagosomes (*Toxoplasma gondii*), escape from the phagosome into the cytoplasm (*Trypanosoma cruzi*), or are resistant to the enzymes of the phagolysosome (*Leishmania*).

Many parasites, such as *T cruzi*, *T gondii*, and *Leishmania*, can hide within host cells, without expressing parasite-derived antigens on the host cell surface. *Plasmodium* and *Babesia* species hide within red blood cells. These organisms are then inaccessible to the immune reactivity of the host.

Parasites often exist in the gut, without tissue invasion—without invasion, there can be no inflammatory response in tissue.

Parasites may form cysts, which are resistant to immune functions.

Parasites may frequently change their coat proteins probably by genetic recombination; by the time host antibodies recognize the parasite's surface markers, the organism has changed its surface antigens. Examples of this include African trypanosomiasis and some diseases caused by *Plasmodium* species.

During their normal life cycle, parasites shed large quantities of their coat proteins. These molecules in tissue and the circulation bind the parasite-specific antibodies, which are thus unable to attach to the parasite, and immune complex–mediated tissue damage occasionally occurs.

Schistosomes can add host cell surface antigens to their own outer coat, thus appearing to be a part of "self."

Leishmania species and schistosomes elaborate compounds which induce suppressor cells, thus dampening the host's immune response.

Plasmodium species induce polyclonal B-cell activation. The large amounts of immunoglobulin (especially IgM) produced, termed "garbage antibodies," are not functional. Tropical splenomegaly syndrome, including enlargement of the spleen and increases in serum IgM, may be caused by *Plasmodium* species.

The T-cell response is critical in defense against parasites, directly contributing to control of the parasites and survival of the host. Stimulated T cells produce INF-γ, which activates macrophages. Certain organisms can survive within nonactivated macrophages, but once activated, the macrophages can destroy organisms like *T cruzi, T gondii, Leishmania,* schistosomes, and *Plasmodium*. INF-γ also has a direct suppressive effect on the growth of some parasites. T cells from helminth-infected patients provide help for the production of IgE, possibly by the production of IL-4 by TH2 helper T cells. Cytotoxic T

cells usually play only a minor role (how might cytotoxic T cells be involved?). In the immune response to *Theileria parvum* and *T cruzi*, cytotoxic T cells are able to kill infected host cells.

As macrophages accumulate and release monokines, a granulomatous reaction may develop. This occurs when the host is incapable of eliminating the parasite. Walling off the invader minimizes damage to the host. Typically the continuing presence of the organism elicits a chronic cell-mediated immune response. The presence of this cellular reactivity can be measured by skin testing with organism-specific antigens. (When a chronic parasitic or fungal infection is suggested clinically, skin tests and tests for antibody levels may be important diagnostic tests. It is crucial to obtain blood for the serologic tests first—Why?)

Eosinophils play a key role in the response to parasites, although there is an incomplete understanding of how eosinophils help defeat the invader (Chap. 19B). These white blood cells contain compounds known as major basic protein, eosinophil cationic protein, and eosinophil protein-X (also known as eosinophil-derived neurotoxin) which may help kill parasites as well as mediating host tissue damage. In addition, eosinophils use the peroxidase-halide system to produce activated oxygen and related compounds which are cytotoxic. There is evidence that eosinophils are antibody-dependent cytotoxic cells, active in the destruction of *T cruzi* and schistosomes (Fig. 21-10). T cells produce a factor known as IL-6, which causes infiltration of eosinophils into tissues and may increase the bone marrow's production of these cells. Mast cells produce eosinophil chemotactic factor of anaphylaxis (ECF-A), a tetrapeptide very active in attracting eosinophils. PMNs are less potent than eosinophils in killing parasites, but they too may have a role in the integrated immune response to parasites.

Specific antibodies of a number of isotypes are produced during parasitic infestation. IgE, IgG, and IgM, either by their own action or with the assistance of complement, can kill some blood-borne parasites. Antibodies can

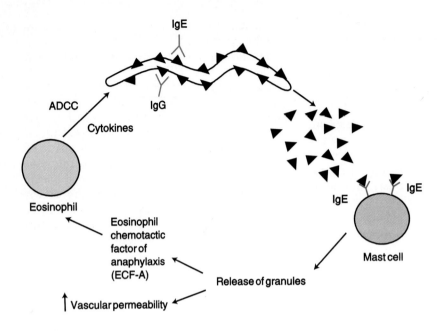

Figure 21-10   Antibody-dependent cellular cytotoxicity (ADCC) action by eosinophils in the response to a helminth.

bind to the receptors on the surface of parasites and block their ability to enter target cells. Both of these mechanisms are active in the defense against *Plasmodium* species, where antibodies to the 175-kd erythrocyte-binding protein or to the 85-kd antigen of *T cruzi* may have a protective role. Opsonization of parasites due to bound immunoglobulin (via Fc receptors) and/or complement (via C3b receptors) is effective in the phagocytosis of *Plasmodium* species and *T brucei*. As stated above, immunoglobulin may allow the cytotoxic potential of eosinophils to be activated, and there is evidence that IgE can activate macrophages directly, as well.

IgE is very important in the response to a variety of parasites, especially helminths, but the exact mechanism is unclear. IgE may act as an opsonin for macrophages and eosinophils and may activate mast cells via an interaction with IgE-specific Fc receptors. Release of mast cell contents may induce vasodilatation and allow other defensive mechanisms better access to the parasite. When released in the bowel wall, mast cell

contents can induce peristaltic contraction of the muscles, which can speed elimination of the parasite. Mast cells may be able to engage in an ADCC response. In addition, as noted above, mast cell–derived ECF-A is a powerful chemoattractant for eosinophils.

Platelets may provide another important defense against parasites and may represent another role for IgE. Platelets bear a surface IgE receptor, termed Fcε RII, related to the IgE surface receptors on eosinophils, basophils, macrophages, and lymphocytes. (Obviously if there is a type II receptor, there must be a type I receptor; it is found on basophils and mast cells.) About 20 percent of platelets from naive individuals can bind IgE, but this proportion increases to 50 percent of the platelets of patients with parasites or asthma. Cross-linking this surface-bound IgE leads to platelet aggregation and release of granular contents, some of which can be directly toxic to parasites in vivo. IgE from infected animals can imbue the platelets of naive animals with the ability to provide protection from subsequent challenge with parasites. Thus, platelets may mediate an ADCC-like response in parasitic infestation and may be more active than merely ensuring hemostatic integrity in human immune responses to parasites.

FUNGAL INFECTION

With the emergence of immunodeficiency due to the use of chemotherapy for malignancies and other diseases and the AIDS epidemic, fungal infections have become a major clinical problem. Fungi may cause acute inflammation, in which case antifungal medicines and the immune response combine to eliminate the organism. However, chronic infection, where large numbers of live but quiescent organisms persist, may not be eradicated, especially where the immune response of the host is defective.

Some fungi, like viruses, have specific tissue targets. Some fungi affect the skin, hair, or nails, causing dermatomycoses, and rarely affect internal organs. Others gain access to the body through breaks in skin or mucosa or via the respiratory tract. Opportunistic infection may occur in the setting of previous broad-spectrum antibiotic therapy (e.g., after oral or vaginal thrush, an infection with fungi of the genus *Candida*, has been treated by ampicillin or tetracycline therapy, which has eliminated the usual local flora), or immunodeficiency. This immunodeficiency may be of the global type seen in AIDS, may be the neutropenia seen in chemotherapy patients, or may be the T-cell defect isolated to the response to *Candida* known as chronic mucocutaneous candidiasis, which is discussed in Chap. 22, on immunodeficiency.

The primary immune responders to fungal infection are T cells which, once activated, secrete lymphokines that activate macrophages and make them better able to destroy fungi. The combination of macrophages and T cell–mediated cellular response often produces a granulomatous response, as noted above. PMNs are also active in phagocytosis of fungi; fungal infection is a serious problem in neutropenic patients. The alternative

pathway of complement may be activated. As is the case with parasites, the immune system may never totally eradicate fungi, but is able to control them. In general macrophages are not very effective in controlling superficial fungal infections.

Antibodies may be important in controlling cutaneous fungi and may prevent blood-borne spread, but are not effective in containing systemic fungal infection. The measurement of complement-fixing antibodies is often a valuable tool in diagnosing fungal infections.

People with seemingly normal immune systems can get fungal infections. Environmental factors are sometimes invoked: e.g., the hot, dry air of the southwest desert plus a high exposure rate predisposes people in Arizona and California to *Coccidioides* infection (coccidioidomycosis, also known as San Joaquin Valley fever). The higher incidence of severe coccidioidomycosis in exposed Filipinos and blacks suggests that a genetic factor may, to some degree, determine the status of immunity.

Serum from patients with fungal infections may contain factors which suppress lymphocyte function; these antigen-specific factors may be antibodies or circulating immune complexes. The role of immune complexes in fungal disease is not well understood; they may cause adverse effects as they are deposited through the body, or the immunosuppression they produce may represent an appropriate control of the immune response. It is known that certain polysaccharide antigens found in *Candida* can induce immunosuppression directly, by activating adherent cells to produce prostaglandins.

Hypersensitivity reactions to certain fungi may occur. An IgE-mediated asthmatic reaction (Gell and Coombs type I) may occur. In patients with "farmer's lung," IgG binds to fungal antigens and produces immune complex–mediated (Gell and Coombs type III) tissue damage. Systemic granulomatous reactions (Gell and Coombs type IV) can also occur.

Fungus need not invade host tissues to

cause tissue damage. *Aspergillus* is a common fungus which can cause extensive invasive disease of the lungs of immunocompromised patients. Alternatively, it can grow into a fungus ball (a mycetoma) in the airways of normal individuals without tissue invasion; occasionally a mycetoma can be seen as a radiopaque ball in a pulmonary cavity, with no active disease clinically apparent. Finally, *Aspergillus* can cause an entity called allergic bronchopulmonary aspergillosis (ABPA); see Clinical Aside 21-2.

Clinical Aside 21-2
Allergic Bronchopulmonary Aspergillosis

Allergic bronchopulmonary aspergillosis usually affects patients with chronic lung diseases, e.g., chronic obstructive pulmonary disease, asthma, or cystic fibrosis. Episodic exacerbations of wheezing occur in association with shifting areas of pulmonary infiltration on chest x-ray. Peripheral blood eosinophilia is common. On bronchoscopic examination, there is no tissue invasion in the bronchial tree; rather, spores of the *Aspergillus* (usually *A fumigatus*) are found in the mucus secretions. It is thought that the immune response to the fungus, in the form of IgE and eosinophils, causes a local hypersensitivity reaction, with liberation of bronchoconstrictive substances like histamine and leukotrienes.

The diagnosis of ABPA can be made, in the appropriate clinical setting (see above), by finding serum precipitins (antibodies) for *Aspergillus*, elevated serum levels of anti-*Aspergillus* IgE antibodies, skin-test reactivity to *Aspergillus* antigens, and occasionally *Aspergillus* on sputum examination or culture. Early treatment with oral corticosteroids can prevent worsening of lung disease and progression to pulmonary fibrosis. Thus, an astute clinician who suspects this entity and makes the correct diagnosis is practicing the best kind of medicine—prevention.

MOLECULAR MIMICRY

Certain pathogens contain antigens which resemble constituents of human cells. Infection with these organisms can elicit an immune response which can recognize and damage the host, a process known as *molec-*

ular mimicry. This is thought to be the mechanism behind certain features of at least two diseases in which the immune response, rather than the organism itself, causes the tissue damage. These are rheumatic fever (due to infection with *Streptococcus*) and Chagas' disease (caused by infection with *T cruzi*). Current research suggests that molecular mimicry may be part of the immunopathogenesis of Reiter's syndrome (*Chlamydia* and certain enterobacteria) and Lyme disease (*Borrelia burgdorferi*). This also may be the mechanism behind Coxsackie virus–induced myositis; the amino acid identity between certain viruses and human cell surface markers is a possible immunologic cause of other poorly understood "autoimmune" diseases. Such similarity of microbial and host structures may be the reason that patients with *Mycoplasma* pneumonia infections make antibodies to I antigens on red blood cells and that syphilitics often have antibodies to P antigens on red cells. In sufficient quantities, these antibodies, produced because the pathogen and the host red blood cell have components which resemble each other, can cause hemolysis.

In addition, as described above, the idiotype network may help explain how certain infections cause autoantibodies and perhaps autoimmune diseases. If an invading microorganism uses a host cell surface receptor as an entry site, the immune response to that microbe might recognize the site of attachment. An anti-idiotype to this antibody might then resemble the microbe's ligand and could interact with the receptor. If the antibody fixes complement or a cell capable of ADCC interacts with the Fc of the anti-idiotype on the receptor, tissue damage might ensue. Thus, the immune response to a microbe might induce tissue-specific autoimmunity.

Recall that some viruses, including herpes simplex, contain Fc receptors on their surfaces. Antibodies to this receptorlike molecule will elicit anti-idiotype antibodies, in kind. (How might this ultimately lead to the production of rheumatoid factor, an IgM which binds to the Fc region of normal IgG? *Hint:* What if the antireceptor antibody were to represent an internal image of the receptor?)

The investigation of molecular mimicry is one of the most active areas in clinical immunology today. As the amino acid sequence and tertiary structures of microbial structures are defined and compared to mammalian proteins, there is a long list of potential cross-reactivities which might prove to be of clinical relevance.

SELF-TEST QUESTIONS*

1. In order to cause an infection, the potential invading organism must do all of the following *except:*
   a. Invade
   b. Attach
   c. Proliferate
   d. Immunosuppress

   For the following mechanisms of antimicrobial activity choose the letter of the component which is active in that mechanism.

2. Blocks attach-   a. Granules of PMNs
   ment   b. Cytotoxic T cells
3. Fever   c. IgA in secretions
4. Proteases   d. IL-1
   destroy
   organism
5. Cytolysis of
   infected cells

True or false

6. A primarily cellular immune response to a pathogen may result in a granulomatous rather than purulent reaction.
7. The production of immunoglobulin represents one of the primary responses to bacteria.
8. There is no intrinsic antigen specificity within the macrophage-associated part of the immune response.
9. The term *T-independent antigen* refers to an antigen that can induce a cytotoxic effect on the organism without the intervention of an effector T cell.

*Answers will be found in Appendix E.

ADDITIONAL READINGS

Dannanberg AM, Jr. Delayed-type hypersensitivity and cell-mediated immunity in the pathogenesis of tuberculosis. *Immunol Today.* 1991;12:228–233.

Immunol Today. 1991; 12:(Special issue 3). (Special issue on immunoparasitology).

McChesney MB, Oldstone MBA. Viruses perturb lymphocyte function: Selected principles characterizing virus-induced immunosuppression. *Ann Rev Immunol* 1987;5:279–304.

Seifert HS, So M. Genetic mechanisms of bacterial antigenic variation. *Microbiol Rev.* 1988;52:327–336.

Tyler KL. Host and viral factors that influence viral neurotropism. *Trends Neurosci.* 1987;10:455–460, 492–497.

GLOSSARY

Abscess—localized collection of pus in a cavity formed by the disintegration of tissues.

Acute infection—highly productive infection, with clear-cut signs and symptoms.

Adjuvanticity—ability of certain components of microorganisms to induce a broad spectrum of responses, including polyclonal B-cell and T-cell activation, and occasionally the ability to activate macrophages and complement directly; these occur before the host has had sufficient time to produce antigen-specific responses.

Anaerobic organism—microorganism that lives and grows only on the complete or almost complete absence of molecular oxygen.

Arthropoda—multicellular organisms with jointed appendages; includes Crustacea (crabs, shrimps, crayfish), Chilopoda (centipedes), Arachnida [scorpions, spiders, ticks, mites (*Sarcoptes scabiei*, the "itch mite," causes scabies)], and Insecta [lice (*Pthirus pubis* causes "crabs"), beetles, bedbugs, reduviids, ants, wasps, bees, fleas, flies, gnats, mosquitoes]. Crustacea may be a reservoir for infectious diseases such as paragonimiasis. The bite of arachnidae and insects can spread a variety of disease, including Rocky Mountain spotted fever (Rickettsia), Lyme disease (*Borrelia*), Colorado tick fever (virus), Chagas' disease (*Trypanosoma*), malaria (*Plasmodium*), African sleeping sickness (*Trypanosoma*).

Carrier state—special case of inapparent infection in which a pathogenic organism is still excreted by the host after recovering from the infection (e.g., hepatitis B virus)

Chronic infection—the capacity of certain organisms to evade immune defense mechanisms, often by residing in an intracellular location.

Commensalism—(literally "eating at the same table") symbiosis which is beneficial to one of the pair and at least not detrimental to the other.

Communicability—ease with which an infection is transmitted from one individual to another.

Endotoxin—bacterial toxin (often a lipopolysaccharide) not freely liberated into the surrounding medium, in contrast to an *exotoxin*.

Exotoxin—extracellular protein elaborated by an organism which can then diffuse into surrounding tissues.

Facultative intracellular organism—an organism that is readily taken up by a phagocyte and is relatively resistant to subsequent digestion.

Facultative parasite—an organism which can exist in a free-living, commensal, or parasitic state.

Gram stain—a staining protocol using Gram's stain (crystal violet and iodine), which divides bacteria into gram-positive and gram-negative organisms, depending on certain features of the cell wall. Bacterial cell walls include an inner layer, known as the *murein layer* (polymer of *N*-acetylglucosamine and *N*-acetylmuramic acid, linked to tetrapeptide side chains), and a set of peptide linking chains. Most gram-positive organisms have teichoic acids in their cell wall, and some may contain polysaccharides. The cell walls of gram-negative organisms contain three polymers outside of the murein layer, including lipoproteins, an outer membrane of phospholipids, and lipopolysaccharide (which consists of a complex lipid, known as lipid A, attached to a polysaccharide core).

Inapparent (subclinical) infection—infection not sufficiently active to cause signs and symptoms.

Infection—colonization by organism in or on a host.

Infectious disease—pathologic condition, with signs and symptoms, associated with frank clinical illness, resulting from infection of a tissue normally free of significant numbers of organisms.

Latent infection—persistent, inapparent infection where the presence of the microbe cannot readily be detected.

Metazoa—parasitic worms; includes nematodes and platyhelminths.

Mutualism—mutually beneficial symbiosis.

Nematodes—multicellular roundworms, with well-defined digestive tracts and a variety of surface structures at their anterior and posterior ends; includes *Ascaris*, *Ancylostoma* (old World hookworm), *Necator* (new World hookworm); *Strongyloides*, filariae, *Trichinella spiralis*.

Nonpathogenic organisms—organisms usually incapable of causing illness; often incapable of penetrating natural defenses.

Obligate intracellular organism—an organism which resides within a cell requiring the use of certain cellular mechanisms in order to reproduce.

Obligate parasite—an organism which cannot survive unless it is parasitizing a host.

Opportunistic infections—infections caused by organisms not usually considered pathogenic or virulent, but which may cause disease when the host's defenses are compromised.

Parasitism—a symbiotic relationship in which the host is, at least to some degree, injured through the actions of the other animal, the parasite.

Pathogenic organisms—organisms capable of overwhelming defenses and producing disease.

Platyhelminths—multicellular flatworms (flukes), usually hermaphroditic; includes trematodes (*Fasciolopsis, Schistosoma, Paragonimus*) and cestodes (*Diphyllobothrium, Sparganum, Taenia, Cysticercus, Echinococcus, Hymenolepsis*).

Protozoa—eukaryotic unicellular organisms, with organelles; includes *Entamoebae, Giardia lamblia, Trichomonas vaginalis, Toxoplasma gondii, Plasmodium* (malaria), *Trypanosoma, Leishmania, Pneumocystis carinii.*

Pus—liquid inflammatory product, consisting of white blood cells, microorganisms, dead tissue, and a thin liquid called *liquor puris.*

Pyogenic infection—infection with an organism which elicits pus formation.

Symbiosis—(literally "living together") the association of individuals from two species, which depend on each other for food gathering or mutual protection; they are dependent upon each other for survival.

Toxigenic infection—infection the manifestations of which are due to the elaboration by the microbe of toxic compounds which cause tissue destruction, rather than tissue damage being due to direct invasion by the pathogen.

Tropism—selectivity by an organism for specific host tissue(s).

Vector—an invertebrate animal (e.g., tick, flea, fly, mosquito, snail) capable of transmitting an infectious agent among vertebrates.

Virulent organisms—organisms so highly pathogenic that whenever they infect a host they are capable of producing disease.

22

Immunodeficiency Syndromes

A. Primary and Secondary Immunodeficiencies

INTRODUCTION

The role of the immune system in response to infection is to produce a functional response at a protective level at the site of inflammation; anything short of this, for any reason, represents relative immunodeficiency. When responses are too vigorous or uncontrolled, they may cause tissue destruction, even after the infection is controlled. On the other hand, if the immune system is defective or down-regulated and unable to defeat an invading organism, increased numbers and severity of infection may occur, which we call *immunodeficiency*. Relative immunodeficiency often contributes to the morbidity and mortality of nonimmune disease, though the immunodeficiency may be masked by the other manifestations of disease. There is a good correlation between the type of defect and the type of infection(s). Therefore, it is possible to predict the kind of infection to be expected in most of the immunodeficiency syndromes. Likewise, obtaining a complete history from a patient with a suspected immunodeficiency can go a long way toward making a proper diagnosis of the type of immune deficit.

Specific immune responses are mediated by two principal cell types, B cells and T cells. These two types have different lineages, arise from different microenvironments, and cope with foreign antigens in different ways. T cells recognize antigen in the context of "self," as defined by markers of the major histocompatibility complex (MHC). The end results of this recognition process are the activation of helper and suppressor T cells, which provide a balanced yin and yang of influences, and of cytotoxic cells, as well as the liberation of lymphokines. Even without an intact humoral response, T-cell and natural killer (NK) cell responses, in conjunction with macrophages, control most viral and fungal infections, reject foreign grafts, and mediate delayed-type hypersensitivity reactions. B cells, often requiring T-cell help, become plasma cells, which secrete immunoglobulin. Antibodies can eliminate bacteria, neutralize bacterial toxins and virulence factors, neutralize extracellular viral particles and prevent reinfection, and mediate immediate allergic reactions. Both cell types can produce soluble products (lymphokines) which can recruit and/or make other cell types more efficient, including polymorphonuclear cells, macrophages and monocytes, eosinophils, basophils, mast cells, NK cells, and antibody-dependent cytotoxic cells.

T cells arise from pluripotent stem cells originating in the fetal liver and then enter the microenvironment of the thymus. The thymus, located in the anterior mediastinum, is derived from tissues of the third and fourth pharyngeal pouches; other tissues from these embryologic sources contribute to the structures of the face, the aortic arch, and the parathyroid glands. The thymic epithelium attracts precursor stem cells from the circulation and alters them by their interaction with the thymic epithelial cell.

Events in the thymus are poorly understood. What is known is that nearly 99 percent of all prospective T cells never escape the thymus (What do you think the reason for this remarkable death rate might be? In general, the body is not "inefficient" without reason.)

Once mature, the surviving T cells leave the thymus and populate the peripheral lymphoid organs, filling the T-cell compartments of the spleen, lymph nodes, and Peyer's patches. Specific markers on the surface of T cells and target organs allow different types of T cells to home in on their intended destination. Once a T cell has partaken of the local immunologic environment, it can recirculate repeatedly; this allows for the dissemination of information learned locally. Interruption of this recirculation can result in local lymphoid depletion and compromised immunity. The development of T cells is described in more detail in Chap. 7.

Beginning in the eighth to ninth week of gestation, B-lineage cells are found in the fetal liver, with a shift to the bone marrow later. B cells also circulate, leaving the fetal liver or bone marrow to fill the specialized areas of the spleen, lymph nodes, and Peyer's patches. It has been suggested that suppression of B-cell development may occur as self-antigens are presented to fetal B cells, with subsequent deletion of autoreactive clones. Were such deletion to become too extensive, a global suppression of B-cell development might lead to an immunodeficiency. Any interference with the development of pre-B cells in fetal liver or bone marrow would also seriously compromise the future humoral system. The development of B cells is described in more detail in Chap. 6.

The first important clinical question to ask is "*When* should an immunodeficiency be suspected?" In general, the clinician should suspect that the immune system is not working properly in the following situations:

A patient has experienced frequent, protracted, or recurrent severe infections.

A patient has an infection caused by an organism of usually low virulence.

There has been incomplete clearance of infection or incomplete response to treatment, despite appropriate antibiotic therapy.

Unexpected complications occur.

The Clinical Asides briefly describe rather typical presentations of very different immunodeficiency syndromes.

Clinical Aside 22A-1

A 12-month-old boy is referred for evaluation of multiple infections over the last 6 months. He has had three episodes of otitis media, each responding poorly to appropriate antibiotic therapy, bronchitis (*Streptococcus pneumoniae*) at age 8 months, and meningitis (*Haemophilus influenzae*) at age 11 months. He had a normal case of chickenpox at age 7 months, and is now at the 4th percentile for both height and weight, having "fallen off his curves" at about 7 months of age. Physical examination is remarkable for bilaterally scarred tympanic membranes (eardrums), mild conjunctivitis, and an eczematoid skin rash over the lower extremities. No splenomegaly (enlarged spleen) or lymphadenopathy (enlargement of the lymph nodes) is noted.

Clinical Aside 22A-2

A 19-month-old boy is referred for evaluation of multiple infections over the last 10 months. He had pneumonia at age 13 months; he has had chronic diarrhea, ulcers of the mucus membranes of the mouth, osteomyelitis of the left humerus due to *Staphylococcus aureus* with a draining sinus, and recently has had drainage from a left axillary lymph node. His growth began to slow at about age 12 months, and he is now at the 5th percentile in both height and weight. Physical examination reveals cervical, axillary, and inguinal lymphadenopathy, hepatosplenomegaly, and two chronic draining sinuses.

Clinical Aside 22A-3

A 23-year-old male presents with weight loss and fatigue. He has had one episode of gonorrhea and one episode of syphilis; he recently had *Entamoeba histolytica* enteritis. He notes a nonproductive cough. Recently he has felt a burning sensation in his throat upon drinking orange juice at breakfast. Examination reveals blood pressure, 120/80; heart rate, 84; temperature, 37.7°C orally; white plaques on his hard palate which can be dislodged by a cotton swab; clear lungs; internal and external hemorrhoids; brown, guaiac-positive stool. (A positive guaiac reaction indicates that there may be blood in the stool specimen tested.)

SECONDARY IMMUNODEFICIENCIES

Recall that the body's defenses against infection include more than specific T- and B-cell responses. Any breaching of the innate defense mechanisms, including the mucocutaneous barrier and its antimicrobial products, should be classified as an immunodeficiency. Such breachings, which include surgical wounds, extensive burns, infections, and a host of other influences and which occur in an individual with a previously healthy immune system, are classified as *secondary immunodeficiencies*. Table 22A-1 lists the major types of secondary immunodeficiencies.

TABLE 22A-1 Secondary Immunodeficiencies

Epithelial Defect
  Chemotherapy-induced decreased cell turnover
  Wound
  Surgery
  Decreased tears, saliva, or secretions
  Defective ciliary function
  Loss of acid in stomach
Decreased Production of Active Principles
  Chemotherapy-induced: lymphoid cells, PMNs
  Radiotherapy-induced: lymphoid cells, PMNs
  Malnutrition
  Infection-induced suppression: HIV, EBV, CMV, protozoans, *Mycobacterium leprae*
  Malignancy-associated suppression: multiple myeloma, Hodgkin's disease
  Splenectomy
  Thymectomy
Increased Loss of Active Principles
  GI tract: Protein-losing enteropathy, intestinal lymphangiectasia
  Renal: proteinuria, nephrotic syndrome
  Burns: serous fluid drainage
Diseases or Factors Suppressing the Function of Lymphoid Cells
  Diabetes mellitus: hyperglycemia
  Renal failure: molecules in uremic serum
  Burns: defective PMN and T-cell function, suppressive factors or increased suppressor
    T cells
  Drugs: corticosteroids, depressing lymphoid, PMN, and macrophage function

---

The loss of functioning lymphoid tissue, due to surgical removal or disruption of the lymphatic-venular circulation, may compromise the host. After splenectomy there is an increased incidence and severity of infections with encapsulated organisms. (*Streptococcus pneumoniae* and *Haemophilus influenzae* are frequent pathogens; a new addition to this list of organisms of concern is *Babesia microti*, an intraerythrocytic parasite spread by the bite of infected *Ixodes dammini* ticks.) In splenectomized patients these infections may cause circulatory collapse, the syndrome of overwhelming sepsis, and death, all because of a diminution in circulating opsonins, including immunoglobulin, which would have been produced in the absent splenic tissue. "Autosplenectomy" occurs when splenic tissue is destroyed by an endogenous process. A good example of this is sickle cell anemia, where sickled red blood cells obliterate small blood vessels in the spleen and ultimately cause splenic tissue to die; sickle cell patients, with low levels of opsonins, often have difficulty clearing

infections with these encapsulated organisms. Patients with sickle cell anemia are also susceptible to *Salmonella typhimurium* osteomyelitis. This frequent association should be kept in mind, since patients with sickle cell disease can present with painful "sickle crisis," including bone and joint pain, which can obscure the underlying infectious bone problem.

Other disorders may predispose an individual to infection. Any time a tube is obstructed, be it ureter, urethra, gut, bronchus, or eustachian tube, there is a disruption of local antimicrobial mechanisms and an increased risk of infection. Any time a foreign body is introduced into the body, be it central venous catheter, artificial heart valve, ventricular shunt, or urinary catheter, there is a focus which can provide an attachment site for a microbe. Any irregularity of circulation, be it decreased circulation in an elderly patient with peripheral vascular disease, turbulent flow over a congenital heart lesion, or a diseased heart valve, may provide a location for a microbe. Alteration of the clearance systems of the reticuloendothelial system, as in hepatic cirrhosis or splenectomy, or an increase in blood flow and filtering elsewhere, as in inflammatory joint disease or after trauma, may allow an organism to escape into tissues whose defenses against the invader have been rendered ineffective. (In devitalized tissue, for example, a focus of necrosed bone after trauma, there is an increase in local circulation due to the local inflammation that is part of the healing process.)

There is some debate as to the status of the senescent immune system: Is aging a form of immune deficiency? This, as well as the effects of malnourishment and stress, will be discussed in later chapters (Chaps. 24B and 23, respectively.)

The secondary immunodeficiency which has gotten the most attention in both the medical and lay press is, of course, the *acquired immunodeficiency syndrome—AIDS.* AIDS first occurred in the United States in 1980 and was described in 1981 in male homosexuals. In addition to male homosexuals, others affected have included unfortunate individuals who received "tainted" blood transfusions and clotting factor transfusions for hemophiliacs, intravenous drug users, prostitutes, and the children of infected women. The causative agent was originally named HTLV-III (human T lymphotropic virus type III), the third human T-cell retrovirus discovered. The current name is *HIV* (human immunodeficiency virus). HIV has a tropism for human cells which carry the CD4 (OKT4) antigen, including those T cells which interact with class II antigens (also known as helper cells), and probably certain macrophages and brain cells. Infected blood cells are free to circulate around the victim's body and spread the infection throughout. The virus is most easily able to infect activated CD4-positive cells, which explains, in part, the remarkably increased susceptibility of gay men and drug abusers: both groups are exposed to an incredible antigenic burden. Gays, especially those in the "fast lane," are exposed to various venereal infectious agents, different semens, and the

various drugs used to heighten the sexual experience, like amyl nitrite. Drug users inject not only their chosen substances for abuse, but also the material which is used to "cut" the drugs, to say nothing of microbes injected inadvertently due to the absence of sterile technique. Both groups then make immune responses to many of these antigens and therefore have many activated T cells.

CD4-positive cells are destroyed, although the exact mechanism is not known. (With what you know of the control mechanisms of T- and B-cell responses, and how these responses are elicited, can you think of ways an infected T4 cell might be destroyed?) As fewer and fewer CD4 cells are available to provide help for immune responses, there is a gradual diminution in overall T-cell function. Patients with AIDS may not make antibody to infectious agents, so that serologic testing may be ineffective as a diagnostic tool. Paradoxically, excess activity of B cells occurs, with elevated serum IgA and IgG and increased spontaneous in vitro production of immunoglobulin by the peripheral blood cells of these patients.

On analysis of peripheral blood, there is a drop in T-cell reactivity to antigens and mitogens, a drop in the ratio of CD4/CD8 cells (from about 1.7 to 2.0; this is the "helper/suppressor ratio" quoted in the literature) and then a drop in the total number of T cells (from a normal of over 1200/μL, the count may drop to 10). Skin tests for delayed-type hypersensitivity (Gell and Coombs type IV) become negative. The end result is a propensity to infections with low-virulence organisms (opportunistic infections) and/or neoplasms (Table 22A-2).

The exact incubation time for AIDS is not known, but is probably in excess of 2 years. The number of cases has doubled every 6 months since statistics first became available, and there are now over 250,000 cases in the United States. By comparison the polio outbreaks of the 1950s never exceeded 21,000 cases. The AIDS mortality rate is essentially 100 percent for those with the full-blown syndrome; by way of comparison, the bubonic plague (now treatable with

---

TABLE 22A-2   Common Infections in AIDS

Protozoal
  Pneumocystis carinii pneumonia
  Toxoplasmosis of the lung or central nervous system
  Cryptosporidium of the gut
  Strongyloidosis of the lung, central nervous system, or disseminated
Fungal
  Candidiasis of the esophagus
  Cryptococcosis of the lung, central nervous system, or disseminated
  Aspergillosis of the central nervous system or disseminated
Viral
  Cytomegalovirus of the lung, gut, or retina or central nervous system
  Herpes simplex, mucocutaneous or disseminated
  Progressive multifocal leukoencephalopathy (presumed due to papovavirus)
Bacterial
  Atypical (*Mycobacterium*, especially *M. avium-intracellulare*, of the gut and lung, or
    disseminated

---

tetracycline, a drug which was unfortunately not available in Europe in the Middle Ages) had a mortality rate of about 40 percent.

There is hope, however. First, recent figures from the U.S. armed forces screening studies suggest that fewer of their candidates are seropositive than they had predicted in their projections. Second, testing of blood used for transfusions and for the preparation of coagulation factor supplements makes these less of a risk. Many patients are electing to give blood in advance of elective surgical procedures, eliminating exposure to donated blood products. Third, there has been a change in life-styles in certain groups at risk, "fast lane" gays and straights, alike. Many HIV-positive individuals have become "monogamous;" others have decreased the number of their sexual partners and started using condoms and practicing "safe sex". These changes help to decrease the spread of HIV and decrease the frequency with which any individual might be re-exposed. Fourth, a few forms of therapy seem promising. Drugs which reduce or eliminate the virus have been tested and have shown clinical effect; the problem is that upon discontinuation of therapy, the virus reappears. Drugs which interfere with the ability of the virus to bind to the CD4 molecule can block the entry of the virus into its target cell, and such compounds are being tested. A major focus of research is the development of a vaccine

against HIV. Glycoproteins derived from the virus have been evaluated for immunogenicity, and two, gp120 and gp41, are potential candidates for this use. Immunization has not been attempted, but this will doubtless be an area of ongoing study. Recent studies suggest that inoculation of patients with early HIV infection with a vaccine derived from the gp160 HIV envelope protein molecule may actually retard progressive CD4 cell loss. Fifth, the mere presence of antibodies to HIV in the blood does not necessarily mean progression to AIDS. AIDS-related complex (ARC), which includes seropositivity, lymphadenopathy, malaise, but no opportunistic infections or neoplasias, may be a self-limited process in the proper setting. It was especially in ARC patients that a change in life-style made a difference in the natural history of disease. It is possible that those with antibodies may remain seropositive and never progress to any clinical manifestations. Only time (and research) will tell.

AIDS is discussed in more detail in Chapter 22B.

PRIMARY IMMUNODEFICIENCIES

AIDS is a *secondary, acquired* defect of T cells. *Primary* defects are much less common

TABLE 22A-3   Prevalence of Some Primary Immunodeficiency Syndromes

Deficiency	Prevalence
Isolated IgA deficiency	1:328 to 1:3000
Myeloperoxidase deficiency	1:3000
C2 deficiency	1:10,000 to 1:40,000
Common variable immunodeficiency	1:70,000
Severe combined immunodeficiency	1:100,000
Adenosine deaminase deficiency	<1:200,000
X-linked hypogammaglobulinemia	1:200,000

than secondary defects. Primary defects are often congenital or inherited, are typically manifest at birth or shortly thereafter, and often have associated, extraimmunologic manifestations. These can include:

1. Manifestations of the immune defect, e.g., skin rash or destruction of lung tissue.
2. Other congenital anomalies which occur in conjunction with the immune defect. (Recall the ontogeny of the thymus. Absence of the thymus is associated with abnormalities of the other structures which originate from the branchial pouches.)

Primary immunodeficiencies are usually classified in one of four main groups, depending on which immune effector mechanism is defective: T cell, B cell, polymorphonuclear leukocyte, or complement. The coexistence of defects in T- and B-cell function is not unusual, especially in congenital primary deficiencies. This is really predictable; any defect which arises at the stem cell or lymphoid precursor stage might cause a defect in more than one lineage. Cellular defects occurring after commitment to T- and B-cell lineages would affect solely T or B cells, although T cells must help B cells in order to produce certain responses; thus, a T-cell defect might cause a defect in B-cell function.

The most common form of primary deficiency is a selective IgA deficiency, which is often asymptomatic. This defect occurs in approximately 1 individual in 400 to 500 in the population; this frequency is compared with those of some of the other syndromes in Table 22A-3. Table 22A-4 shows the four

general types of immune defects and the contribution of each to the prevalence of immunodeficiency syndromes.

As described in Chap. 21, the different components of the immune system cooperate in defeating microbial invaders. However, each of the four immunologic response mechanisms contributes to the response to various pathogens differently. It is possible to predict the kind of infections most likely to affect a patient with a given deficiency type (Table 22A-5). Conversely, once one has identified the pathogens affecting an individual, one can make an educated guess as to which kind of immunodeficiency the patient is suffering.

Many primary immunodeficiencies are hereditary, and are often congenital, and so these problems often occur in the pediatric population. The X-linked genetics of congenital deficiencies, including X-linked hypogammaglobulinemia, severe combined immunodeficiency, immunodeficiency with hyper-IgM, Wiskott-Aldrich syndrome, and

TABLE 22A-4   Distribution of Types of Defects in All Patients with Primary Immunodeficiency Syndromes

Type of Deficiency	Percent of Total
B cell	~50
T cell	30–40
With antibody deficiency	20–30
Isolated cellular defect	~10
Phagocyte	6–18
Isolated mononuclear cell	~1
Complement	2–4

TABLE 22A-5   Type of Infection Correlated with Type of Immunodeficiency

Type of Immunodeficiency	Agent	Infection
T-cell deficiency	Viruses	CMV, herpes, measles, varicella-zoster
	Protozoans	P carinii, T gondii
	Fungi	Candida, Aspergillus
	Bacteria	Mycobacterium
Immunoglobulin deficiency	Bacteria	S pneumoniae, H influenzae
	Intestinal parasites	Giardia lamblia
Complement deficiency	Bacteria	Neisseria meningitides, N gonorrhoeae
PMN deficiency	Bacteria	Pseudomonas, S aureus, E coli
	Fungi	Candida

chronic granulomatous disease, are such that better than 70 percent of all primary immunodeficiencies occur in males.

Antibody (B-Cell) Immunodeficiency Syndromes

Deficiencies of All Immunoglobulin Isotypes

X-Linked Congenital Agammaglobulinemia
X-linked congenital agammaglobulinemia was also known as Bruton's agammaglobulinemia. However, this term has fallen from favor because there is a trend away from eponyms.

This was the first clinically described and laboratory-documented immunodeficiency syndrome; a 4½-year old boy with recurrent infections was referred to Dr. Bruton at the Walter Reed Army Hospital, who then used serum electrophoresis to analyze the boy's serum. The absence of gamma globulin in the serum defined the problem. Of note is the fact that this young man had normal varicella at age $3^{10}/_{12}$ years, but had multiple, severe infections, often with Streptococcus pneumoniae. In the first and subsequent cases, no IgG, IgA, IgM, IgD, or IgE could be demonstrated in the serum.

As the name implies, only males are affected, although rare cases of a similar syndrome have been described in females. In these little girls the syndrome is called autosomal recessive agammaglobulinemia, and is, by clinical and laboratory measures, identical to the X-linked form except for the sex of the patient and the occasional presence of both male and female affected family members.

Babies with X-linked hypogammaglobulinemia are usually clinically normal until about 6 months of age (what protects them until that age?), when they begin to experience recurrent pyogenic infections, including bacterial otitis media, bronchitis, pneumonia, meningitis, and dermatitis. The most common causes of infection are S pneumoniae and H influenzae. (Both of these are encapsulated organisms—can you explain this?) Occasionally the babies respond well to appropriate antibiotic therapy, which may delay diagnosing the immunodeficiency. More often they will not respond promptly, one of the hallmarks of immunodeficiency syndromes.

The cell-mediated immune response is intact, as are the complement and phagocytic systems. Thus, measles, mumps, and varicella infections are unremarkable, but poliomyelitis (wild-type or from live vaccines) and echoviruses may produce fatal illnesses (paralysis in the former and encephalitis in the latter). This is an indication of the difficulty patients without antibodies have clearing some viruses from their circulation.

A disease resembling rheumatoid arthritis has been reported in patients with X-linked hypogammaglobulinemia; in those patients developing chronic echovirus infection an illness resembling dermatomyositis may develop. This is the first example of a recurring theme in the study of immunodeficiency syndromes: the absence of an intact immune system seems to predispose patients to *autoimmune* diseases as well as to malignancies.

Some children do not become symptomatic until later in childhood, presenting with chronic conjunctivitis, severe dental caries, or malabsorption (sometimes due to bowel infection with *Giardia lamblia*). About 20 percent of children with Bruton's (we will go against the trend and have a bit of respect for Dr. Bruton) have affected male maternal relatives (why male *maternal* relatives?) and some of these relatives have a different expression of what is presumably the same genetic defect.

The defect seems to be in B-cell maturation. Since there is an intact T-cell system in these children, the defense cannot be proximal to the point where the stem cells become committed to T-cell versus B-cell growth. Deficiency of all isotypes makes it unlikely that there is an abnormality occurring after B-cell commitment to the various isotypes. Very few plasma cells and B cells are present in the circulation. There are usually a normal number of pre-B cells in the bone marrow, although in one recent study normal infant bone marrow had 18 to 36 percent cells with a pre-B cell phenotype, whereas Bruton's marrows contained only 12 to 18 percent such cells. The same study found that 95 percent of the cells in normal marrow contained V_H protein, whereas only 5 percent of cells in the marrow of the Bruton's patients were positive. The defect may thus be at the level of maturation from pre-B to B cell, with absent or abnormal translocation of V_H genes during B-cell ontogeny. Recent studies have shown a short cytoplasmic μ chain, confirming that the block occurs at the level of the pre-B cell. The defect appears to be in a recently identified tyrosine kinase

needed to attach V to DJ segments. Other theories include premature death of immature B cells or even an abnormality of the bursa equivalent, with subsequent defective B-cell maturation. Different X-chromosomal abnormalities have been found (this may be a heterogeneous syndrome), with many occurring at Xq21.3-Xq22.

Routine laboratory evaluation reveals a marked deficiency or absence of all five immunoglobulin isotypes. Affected babies who have had immunizations will have no demonstrable antibodies to these organisms, and will have no isohemagglutinins. (Natural exposure to the environment, probably in the form of colonic flora, leads to the elaboration of IgM antibodies which can agglutinate red blood cells with the type A or type B antigens on their surfaces. Normal babies have low titers of these antibodies, usually about 1:4, by 1 year of age.) A baby suspected of having this immunodeficiency should *never* be immunized with live attenuated virus vaccines.

Older references suggest the need for lymph node biopsy to make the diagnosis, but this is usually unnecessary. (What might such a biopsy, or a biopsy of the intestine, show?) The diagnosis should be suspected on clinical grounds and made by quantitative immunoelectrophoresis. In contrast to B cells, there are normal or elevated numbers of T cells, and tests of T-cell function are normal.

Therapy of this entity has been made practical by the introduction of a form of immunoglobulin which can be given by vein (see Chap. 34). Optimal doses are determined on an individual basis. Some patients with chronic echovirus infections have improved after intravenous gamma globulin therapy. The ability of such therapy to prevent severe tissue damage due to chronic infections has not yet been demonstrated. Many of these patients must receive continuous antibiotics and postural drainage for bronchiectasis or chronic lung disease; a high degree of concern over even the most trivial infection is indicated, even if the patient is on appropriate gamma globulin replacement therapy.

Many patients succumb to chronic lung disease, due to scarring from recurrent pyogenic infections; to central nervous system infections with echovirus; and, occasionally, to leukemia or lymphoma (up to 6 percent of cases in one recent report).

Thus, X-linked hypogammaglobulinemia has many of the features common to immunodeficiency syndromes: variable presentation and manifestations, predictable types of infections with predictable types of organisms, increased risk of autoimmune and neoplastic complications, severe tissue damage developing due to recurrent infection, and frequent poor outcome.

Transient Hypogammaglobulinemia of the Newborn At about 6 months of age, the baby's serum level of maternal IgG has decreased to the point where humoral immunocompetence increasingly depends on the child's synthetic capability (see Chap. 28). If the infant does not begin to produce immunoglobulin, transient hypogammaglobulinemia may develop and recurrent infections may occur. Usually this entity can be differentiated from X-linked hypogammaglobulinemia by the presence of normal levels of IgM and IgA, but some infants with transient hypogammaglobulinemia may also lack these isotypes. In these cases, biopsy of lymph node or intestine demonstrates plasma cells and peripheral blood samples contain B cells, which suggests the diagnosis of hypogammaglobulinemia of the transient, rather than the permanent, X-linked, variety. Also, lateral x-rays of the nasopharynx may demonstrate lymphoid tissue in transient hypogammaglobulinemia; these lymphoid organs are hypoplastic in the X-linked disorder. However, if the baby is not suffering from infections, it is best to "temporize." Don't subject the infant to invasive tests; merely follow the patient clinically and repeat the immunoglobulin levels in 3 to 6 months. Levels of immunoglobulin must be compared to normal levels *for that age* in order to know if there is a deficiency. If the serum levels increase, the diagnosis of transient hypogammaglobulinemia is made.

This "transient" entity may persist for up to 2 years. If there is a problem with infections, intravenous gamma globulin therapy can be given. Immunizations should wait until the child has demonstrated his or her ability to make immunoglobulin.

Common Variable Immunodeficiency (CVI) A clinical syndrome superficially resembling X-linked hypogammaglobulinemia, CVI occurs in an older population in both males and females, at a similar incidence. This syndrome is probably the result of a heterogeneous group of cellular defects: increased suppressor T-cell activity (up to 10 percent of all CVI patients in one series), decreased helper T-cell activity (in 5 to 7 percent of all CVI, in the same series), intrinsic B-cell abnormalities of maturation, defective antigen-presenting (dendritic) cell function, defective glycosylation of the heavy chain of IgG, or autoantibodies to T or B cells.

Recent work has suggested that up to *80 percent* of all CVI may, in fact, be due to T-cell abnormalities. Clinical abnormalities of cell-mediated immunity may be seen in up to 30 percent of carefully studied patients, with many of them having diminution in T-cell responses to mitogens. Some patients with CVI experience a deterioration of T-cell function with time. One intriguing study showed that the addition of B-cell differentiating factors can boost in vitro immunoglobulin production from cells of patients with CVI. This may mean that the problem lies in cytokine production or recognition, with the B cells "stuck" at the maturational level of a nonsecreting germinal center B cell. Elevated serum interleukin 6 (IL-6) levels were found in another study, with normal levels of IL-6 surface receptor on B cells; this suggests that an abnormality of transmission of IL-6 signal may be a cause of some cases of CVI. In certain familial cases, an autosomal-recessive inheritance pattern has been demonstrated. In most cases, however, no genetic abnormality can be documented.

Recurrent sinopulmonary infections are usually the clinical problem which brings CVI patients to the immunologist. These are typically chronic and recurrent, rather than overwhelming, infections, with incomplete response to appropriate therapy. On occasion, neutropenia or lymphopenia can complicate CVI.

CVI can occur in the pediatric population and is generally a less severe problem than X-linked hypogammaglobulinemia. Echovirus and poliovirus infections are not a major problem. Also, in contrast to X-linked hypogammaglobulinemia , there may be significant lymphadenopathy and/or splenomegaly in CVI. Nodular lymphoid hyperplasia of the intestine may occur and is often associated with malabsorption, often due to infection with *Giardia lamblia.* A granulomatous disease of the liver and spleen has been described, as have a few cases of inflammatory bowel disease.

In up to 20 percent of patients with CVI, autoimmune problems may develop, including a syndrome resembling rheumatoid arthritis, a syndrome resembling systemic lupus erythematosus (SLE), idiopathic thrombocytopenic purpura, hemolytic anemia, Graves' disease, hypothyroidism, and pernicious anemia. (Two to four percent of patients with hypogammaglobulinemia have or will develop pernicious anemia, compared to 0.17 percent of the total population.) Occasionally, CVI will be found in the presence of complement component C4 deficiency, suggesting a genetic linkage. There is a 2:1 ratio of females to males in this autoimmune group, as is seen in "idiopathic" autoimmune maladies. This seemingly bewildering array of endocrine and systemic disorders are all due to the attack of the immune system on components of self, with subsequent damage. Thus, autoimmunity can occur in the absence of normal humoral immune responses, and autoantibodies can be found in patients with barely detectable levels of immunoglobulin. It may be that chronic, low levels of infection predispose to autoimmune reactivity. (Could it be that the absence of normal immunoglobulin synthesis precludes a normal immunomodulatory function of the idiotype–anti-idiotype net-

work?) These complications of CVI may make therapy of the underlying disease more difficult.

As was true of X-linked hypogammaglobulinemia, CVI is associated with an increased incidence of malignancy. About 7 percent of CVI patients will develop lymphoma or leukemia. Gastric carcinoma and thymoma are found in CVI at a higher than expected incidence, as well. Recent studies suggest that CVI patients have a 438 percent excess of lymphoma when compared to the general population.

Laboratory testing reveals hypogammaglobulinemia, but often with higher levels of IgG than found in the X-linked disorder. Antibodies to previous immunizing antigens are usually absent, even after a booster immunization (*not* with a live virus vaccine); it is the failure to respond to such a booster which establishes the diagnosis.

Peripheral blood samples contain B cells, again a contrast to X-linked hypogammaglobulinemia. Biopsy of lymphoid structures may reveal B cells, but no plasma cells are found. Intestinal tissue samples may reveal blunted villi, as seen in nontropical sprue, or nodular aggregates of mononuclear cells.

Differentiation of CVI from X-linked hypogammaglobulinemia is usually not difficult. When the presenting problem is the autoimmune manifestations noted above, the true underlying diagnosis may be overlooked. Malabsorption in some patients may be severe enough to suggest that the major problem is actually a protein-losing enteropathy (itself a secondary immune deficiency, see above).

Treatment of the immune deficiency in CVI is intravenous gamma globulin, just as it is for the X-linked syndrome. Malabsorption may require treatment of an underlying *Giardia* infection or may respond to dietary manipulation. In those patients whose T-cell function begins to decay, the kinds of infections seen in T-cell deficiencies may develop and must be treated. Certain of the autoimmune phenomena seen in CVI can be treated with replacement, e.g., thyroid hormone or vitamin B_{12}. The development of these phenomena, especially hormonal deficiencies, should be considered at all times in the longitudinal care of these patients, as they are often late features of the syndrome, occurring after years of autoimmune damage. Splenectomy may be required for the control of hemolytic anemia or thrombocytopenia (but splenectomy is a secondary immune deficiency in itself!), and steroids, often used for the treatment of SLE, should be used only with great caution in CVI patients.

Infection is a major concern. Diagnostic evaluation should be aggressive. (One recent paper suggests that computed tomography or magnetic resonance imaging is more accurate in diagnosing sinusitis or pulmonary infections than is routine X-ray.) Chronic lung disease is a cause of significant morbidity and mortality in these patients, despite appropriate therapy. The malignancies, the endocrine and other autoimmune disorders, and the possible T-cell deficiencies noted above are all serious problems, but a significant number of patients with CVI survive into the seventh and eighth decades.

Transcobalamin II Deficiency   Rarely, the specific biochemical lesion which causes an immune deficiency is known; such is the case for transcobalamin II deficiency. This β-globulin is required for vitamin B_{12} to enter cells, including B cells. In the absence of this protein B cells are unable to undergo terminal differentiation into plasma cells; the resultant hypogammaglobulinemia is usually manifested by failure to thrive and chronic diarrhea in childhood. Associated decreases in total lymphocyte, polymorphonuclear cell, and platelet counts occur.

Treatment is high doses of intramuscular vitamin B_{12} which enters the cells by diffusion down a concentration gradient. Before therapy, childhood immunizations result in no antibody production. However, after vitamin B_{12} therapy immunoglobulin is produced to the very antigens inoculated previously. Priming with these antigens had already occurred, and all that remained was to overcome the block in terminal differentiation into plasma cells.

Deficiencies of Individual Immunoglobulin Isotypes or Subclasses

The B-cell abnormalities noted above prevent the production of all isotypes of immunoglobulin. Recall that the first antibody response to a new antigen is IgM, followed by the other isotypes. Isotype switching is a T cell–dependent event. It could be predicted that immunodeficiencies might occur in which one or more isotype is absent and that in some of these, T-cell abnormalities might be the cause. It is also reasonable to predict that one or more subclasses of IgG might be absent in a given individual.

Immunodeficiency with Hyper-IgM   Rarely, patients with severe recurrent pyogenic infections are found to have elevated levels of IgM (and occasionally IgD), but are deficient in IgG and IgA. The first cases seen were young boys, and in several families the inheritance pattern suggested an X-linked inheritance. Subsequently females with the same clinical disorder have been described, as have several examples of acquired forms of this syndrome (some occurring after rubella infections). There are circulating plasmacytoid cells capable of secreting IgM spontaneously, and cellular immunity is intact. The defect(s) seem to be in isotype switching, from the initial IgM response to IgG and IgA secretion. Studies have demonstrated disparate abnormalities: intrinsic B-cell inability to switch from IgM to IgG synthesis (inability to respond to the T cell–derived signal), deficient "T switch" cell activity, and increased suppressor T-cell activity. Recent work has suggested that a deletion in a T cell surface protein (gp38, the ligand for the CD40 molecule on the B cell surface) may be at the root of the defective isotype switching.

Recurrent otitis media, pneumonia, and sepsis with pyogenic organisms occur. Neutropenia, lymphopenia, thrombocytopenia, and hemolytic and aplastic anemia have been described, often associated with IgM autoantibodies. Hyperplasia of mucosa-associated lymphoid tissues, pseudo-lymphomatous adenopathy and true lymphoid malignancy of IgM-containing cells may occur.

Laboratory evaluation reveals elevated IgM levels, with absent IgG and IgA. Isohemagglutinins are present, and IgM responses to immunization are normal. No IgG is made, as would be expected in a normal response to such immunization.

Therapy is similar to therapy for the other hypogammaglobulinemic syndromes: intravenous gamma globulin. In some cases, this has resulted in a decrease in the IgM levels and occasionally the lymphoid hyperplasia has diminished. It has been suggested that these phenomena represent feedback inhibition of IgM production by the infused IgG.

Selective IgA Deficiency The role of IgA in human immunology is still not clear, some 30 years after IgA was first described. It is the major immunoglobulin on mucosal surfaces and probably plays a major role in local immune responses. The fact that IgA is unable to fix complement by the classical pathway and is a poor opsonin may actually be an advantage, as a local inflammatory reaction in the mucosal secretions could injure the major local barrier to invasion, the mucosal surface. It seems likely that IgA is active in neutralizing toxins and preventing microorganisms from adhering to the mucosa. The nonadherent organism can then be flushed away by ciliary or peristaltic mechanisms.

But IgA is also found in the serum, comprising between 6 and 15 percent of the total serum immunoglobulin. In the circulation IgA may serve the role of a housekeeper, helping to remove antigens which have entered the body through defects in mucosal surfaces; in favor of this is the high incidence of antimilk protein IgG and IgM antibodies in IgA-deficient individuals.

Total serum IgA and secretory IgA are different. There are two distinct subclasses of IgA in humans, IgA1 and IgA2; these can exist as monomers or polymers. In secre-

tions, the two subclasses are about equal, 40 to 50 percent IgA1 and 50 to 60 percent IgA2 and about 95 percent polymeric. In serum, about 90 percent is IgA1; about 80 percent of serum IgA is monomeric. Of note, plasma cells producing IgA1 predominate in bone marrow, tonsils, spleen, and some lymph nodes, whereas IgA2-producing cells are in the majority in most areas of the gut, with the exclusion of the large intestine. The structural difference between the two IgA subtype heavy chains resides primarily in the hinge region. The functional differences between the two IgA subtypes are not clear.

Absence of IgA in the serum is the most common immunodeficiency described, occurring in as many as 1 of 400 individuals. (Some studies suggest incidence figures as low as 1 of 1000.) In most of these cases there is a concomitant decrease in secretory IgA, as well. (Four cases of isolated serum IgA deficiency and one case of isolated secretory IgA absence have been reported.) The majority of these individuals are entirely asymptomatic. Symptomatic IgA deficiency, including recurrent infections of the gastrointestinal, respiratory, and genitourinary tracts, accounts for 10 to 15 percent of cases of clinical immunodeficiency.

Why some individuals with little or no IgA are asymptomatic and others have infections may be explained by recent studies showing that IgG or IgM may take the place of IgA in the mucosal defenses of IgA-deficient individuals—some of the symptomatic IgA-deficient patients have a coexisting IgG2 deficiency. Many IgA-deficient patients without a predisposition to infection have normal or elevated IgG4 levels, suggesting that it may adequately substitute for IgA. Like IgA, IgG4 is a secretory immunoglobulin. Colostrum contains four times the concentration of IgG4 that serum does, suggesting local production of IgG4 in breast tissue, not simple serum transudation.

The incidence of autoimmune disorders, including SLE, rheumatoid arthritis, dermatomyositis, Coombs-positive hemolytic anemia, pernicious anemia, and autoimmune thyroid and liver disease, may be increased in IgA deficiency. Like CVI, isolated IgA deficiency may occur in patients who are also C4-deficient. There is an increased incidence of atopic disease and of celiac disease in IgA-deficient persons. This may be due to the inability to clear antigens before they can enter the circulation from the gastrointestinal tract and cause a systemic immune response. Selective IgA deficiency has also been associated with an increased risk of malignancies.

The cause of IgA deficiency is usually unknown. Examples of IgA deficiency in patients taking phenytoin (an antiseizure medicine) have been reported as due to the induction of suppressor T cells; cases of sulfasalazine- and penicillamine-induced IgA deficiency have also been reported. IgA deficiency has been related to preceding rubella in utero infection. Some IgA-deficient individuals have family members with CVI, suggesting a genetic predisposition to B-cell dysfunction with different expression or manifestations.

There are normal numbers of IgA-containing B cells in the peripheral blood of patients with selective IgA deficiency. Normal serum levels of the other immunoglobulins are usually found, suggesting that this is a selective abnormality of isotype switching. There are, however, patients with coexisting IgG2 deficiency; IgG4 and IgE deficiencies have also been found in patients lacking IgA, suggesting that there may be a more generalized defect in isotype switching. Occasionally suppressor T cells have been found which interfere with IgA production. Routine in vivo and in vitro T-cell tests are usually normal.

There is no treatment for IgA deficiency. If coexisting IgG subclass deficiency exists, treatment with intravenous gamma globulin can be tried, but only with IgA-deficient preparations. As commercially available preparations of gamma globulin contain small amounts of IgA, the IgA-deficient recipient can make an immune response to this (seemingly) new, "foreign" protein and experience anaphylaxis. The same kind of reaction can follow blood transfusions, as there is a small amount of IgA in even packed red blood cells;

all transfusions should be with packed *washed* red blood cells or with blood donated from another IgA-deficient individual. In any event, intravenous administration of immunoglobulin is a very inefficient way to get the antibodies to the mucosal surfaces (bronchi, upper respiratory tract, and gut), where they would be needed.

As stated previously, most IgA-deficient patients never become symptomatic; many are fine until given a transfusion which causes unexpected anaphylaxis. If an increased rate of infection is going to occur, symptoms usually occur within the first decade of life. Management includes prompt therapy of infections and regular follow-up in order to detect autoimmune and neoplastic complications.

Selective Deficiency of Other Isotypes Deficiencies of IgM have been reported; this is somewhat difficult to explain given the current understanding of isotype switching from an initial IgM response. These patients have no IgM in their serum, despite normal numbers of IgM-containing B cells. Most have normal levels of IgG and IgA, although some patients are unable to make antibodies upon antigenic challenge. Some studies of these patients have shown suppressor T cells in the peripheral blood which can block isotype switching.

Patients may develop severe infections with encapsulated organisms, including pneumococci and *H influenzae*. Meningococcemia has also been associated with isolated IgM deficiency. Some of these patients have developed autoimmune disease.

One of the hottest topics in immunodeficiency today is the selective absence of certain IgG subclasses. It is known that the different subclasses differ in structure and function. Subclasses 1 and 3 activate complement better than does subclass 2, and subclass 4 does not activate complement at all. Subclasses 1 and 3 bind well to Fc receptors, whereas subclass 3 binds very poorly to staphylococcal protein A. IgG4 competes with IgE for the specific Fc receptor on mast cells and basophils. (Allergy shots, which consist of the specific antigen which elicits the allergic symptoms, probably work by causing the production of "blocking" IgG4 antibodies, which compete with IgE and thereby block antigen from activating mast cells, etc. IgG4 may be naturally elevated in patients with atopic disease and/or eczema.) IgG against polysaccharide antigens is predominantly IgG2, whereas antitetanus toxoid (a protein antigen) is mostly IgG1 and IgG3. One recently studied adult with recurrent sinopulmonary infections was unable to produce IgG2 in response to polysaccharide antigens.

In certain patients there is an isolated deficiency of one or more of the IgG subclasses. Total IgG is often normal. In one group levels of total immunoglobulin and total IgG were normal, as was the number of CD4 and CD8 cells found in the blood, but the number of B cells was markedly diminished. These patients often suffer from recurrent sinopulmonary infections. In individuals who lack IgG2, infections are due to those organisms which have polysaccharide capsules (see above).

Therapy of individuals with symptomatic IgG subclass deficiency is intravenous gamma globulin. Commercial gamma globulin for intravenous use is only 2 percent IgG4 (normal serum is 10 to 12 percent IgG4), so replacement therapy is very difficult in IgG4 deficiency.

Antibody Deficiency with Normal Immunoglobulin Levels   The mere presence of normal IgG levels does not guarantee immunity, as is seen in the subclass deficiencies described above. To further complicate matters, there are patients who prove that the words "immunoglobulin" and "antibody" are not synonymous. There are patients who have normal levels of serum immunoglobulin isotypes and subclasses, but when immunized do not make antibodies which bind to the inoculating antigen(s). They have normal numbers of B cells and T cells, but few have been studied in enough detail to elucidate the underlying mechanism.

**Summary: Isolated B Cell
Immunodeficiencies**
The primary humoral immunodeficiencies

may be due to intrinsic B-cell defects; defective antigen processing or defective presentation by accessory cells; abnormalities of T-cell help, suppression, or cytokine production; autoantibodies or other serum inhibitory factors. The clinical ramifications of the defects depend on the specific type of immunoglobulin missing and the severity of the defect. As noted earlier, B-cell defects are often associated with T-cell defects; in these combined deficiency syndromes manifestations may be a combination of the clinical problems of each deficiency. A recurring theme in studying the antibody deficiencies is the increased incidence of autoimmune phenomena and malignancy, especially of the lymphoreticular system.

Therapy with intravenous gamma globulin is often effective. This topic is described in much greater detail in Chap. 34.

Cellular (T-Cell) Immunodeficiency Syndromes

In certain individuals there may be a selective defect in T-cell function. As described above, isolated T-cell deficiencies are rare, but may occur in the setting of other, stereotyped, nonimmune findings, which may be discernible as syndromes.

**Congenital Thymic Aplasia (DiGeorge
Syndrome, Third and Fourth Pharyngeal
Pouch Syndrome, Immunodeficiency
with Hypoparathyroidism)**
The proper development of T cells requires an intact thymus, which is formed from the invagination of the endoderm of the third and fourth pharyngeal pouches starting at about the sixth week of gestation. The parathyroid glands and parts of the aortic arch are also derived from the same tissues, as are structures of the lip, outer ear, and mandible. DiGeorge syndrome probably develops from a problem with normal embryologic developments at about 12 weeks of gestation, when the thymus should be migrating caudally and the other structures noted should be differentiating. Recent work suggests that the

underlying abnormality may not be in the pouches. Neural crest mesenchymal cells must interact with the pharyngeal epithelium in order for the structures noted above to develop; in the absence of cooperation the anomalies of DiGeorge may develop.

There is a spectrum of abnormalities, from total thymic aplasia with profound hypocalcemia and cardiac and facial abnormalities, to a small thymus at birth and subsequent hypertrophy leading to normal immune responsiveness. Affected infants often present within the first day of life with hypocalcemic tetany. The additional findings of congenital heart disease, including right-sided aortic arch, tetralogy of Fallot, interrupted aortic arch, patent ductus arteriosus, septal defects, and truncus arteriosus, and the typical facies of low-set ears, midline facial clefts, hypomandibular abnormalities, and hypertelorism, suggest that third and fourth pharyngeal pouch structures may be maldeveloped.

In addition to hypocalcemia with low or absent parathyroid hormone levels, T-cell counts and function may be very low, or may be normal or high initially, with later deterioration in function. Alternatively, as noted above, there may be spontaneous resolution of T-cell abnormalities, suggesting that thymic hypoplasia rather than thymic aplasia was the lesion. Skin tests for delayed-type hypersensitivity are usually negative in infants and so are not valuable in evaluating the competence of their T cells. Specific immunoglobulin synthesis may be abnormal in patients with DiGeorge syndrome (why should this be the case?), but IgG levels are normal in infancy (what is the source of the IgG in a DiGeorge baby's serum at birth?). NK-cell activity is normal.

The clinical manifestations of the T-cell defect include infections with viral, protozoal, fungal, and bacterial pathogens; mucus membrane infections with *Candida* (see below); pneumonia; diarrhea; failure to thrive.

In the normal nonstressed newborn, a lateral or anteroposterior x-ray view of the chest should reveal a thymus in the anterior mediastinum; infants with DiGeorge syndrome do not have a thymic shadow on these films.

The best way to make the diagnosis of DiGeorge syndrome is to suspect it in any infant with any of the features of pharyngeal pouch maldevelopment. Transient hypocalcemia may occur in infants with congenital heart anomalies, but is not a typical feature of neonatal sepsis or stress; the hypocalcemia of DiGeorge syndrome is usually permanent. (Two cases of DiGeorge syndrome where parathyroid function normalized have been reported.) Even in the absence of T-cell abnormalities DiGeorge syndrome should be considered, and it is prudent to continue evaluating T-cell function for at least 1 year. Most infants with the DiGeorge phenotype will have normal immune function. A recent study suggests that low CD4-cell count and a low phytohemagglutinin mitogen response of peripheral blood mononuclear cells may define those with an immune deficit.

The features of DiGeorge syndrome are sufficiently distinct as to be differentiable from other immunodeficiencies of the newborn. There are features of DiGeorge syndrome which overlap with features of other congenital-anomaly syndromes, e.g., the fetal alcohol and monosomy 22 syndromes, and features of isoretinoin embryopathy. The key point is to recall that these are *syndromes*, with a constellation of findings, and there may be more than superficial similarity between them.

Hypocalcemia and congenital heart disease are often acutely life-threatening problems in infants with DiGeorge syndrome, and the immune abnormalities may be overlooked as the physicians try to stabilize a critically ill infant. These infants may require blood transfusion, especially if heart surgery is necessary; if DiGeorge syndrome is suspected, it is vital that the transfused blood be irradiated to prevent the small number of viable donor lymphocytes found in packed red blood cells from mounting a graft-versus-host (GVH) reaction.

Treatment of the T-cell defect has been possible with fetal thymus transplants, resulting in normal immune function in some cases. The fetal thymic epithelium is the crucial tissue, as recipient precursor cells are available to colonize the transplant. Donor tissue of less than 14 weeks of gestational age is used, as older thymuses contain immunocompetent T cells which can produce a GVH reaction. Reconstitution with matched sibling bone marrow has also been reported as effective, suggesting there may have been a small thymic remnant or undescended small thymus in these patients.

Chronic Mucocutaneous Candidiasis

In this syndrome there is a selective T-cell deficiency, with an inability to control *Candida*; the result is chronic infection of the skin and mucus membranes, as is described in the name of the syndrome. B-cell function is normal and antibodies to *Candida* are present. (The section on immune responses to infection suggested that antibodies may have a role in control of cutaneous fungal infections, but such antibodies are clearly not sufficient to control infection in all sites.)

Some of these patients (up to 20 percent in some series) may develop autoimmune endocrinopathies with circulating autoantibodies specific for endocrine glands. These glandular deficiencies may occur 10 to 15 years after the onset of the chronic *Candida* infections. Hypoparathyroidism is the most common endocrine abnormality, but the adrenal, thyroid, pancreas, or ovary may be affected; pernicious anemia, interstitial pulmonary fibrosis, chronic liver disease (with occasional cirrhosis), and Sjögren's syndrome may occur, as well. *Candida* infection or the endocrinopathy may be the initial manifestation of the syndrome.

Mucocutaneous candidiasis has been classified into four groups: I, early onset; II, late onset; III, familial; IV, familial juvenile with polyendocrinopathy.

Immunologic testing reveals a selective abnormality of T-cell responses to *Candida* antigens. There are normal delayed-type hypersensitivity skin tests, T-cell proliferative responses, and production of macrophage migration inhibitory factor in response to other fungal antigens. The T cells have normal responses to mitogens, like phytohemagglutinin (PHA), and to allogeneic cells (the mixed lymphocyte reaction, or MLR).

It is of course critical to evaluate the immune system of these children in order to differentiate chronic mucocutaneous candidiasis from other immunodeficiency syndromes.

There is no treatment for the endocrinopathies aside from replacement therapy. The long delay in the onset of endocrine deficiencies makes vigilant long-term follow-up a crucial part of the ongoing care of these individuals; the leading causes of death are adrenal failure (Addison's disease), which may develop suddenly, and hepatic failure. The *Candida* infections are typically difficult to control with topical therapy, but usually do not become systemic.

Some forms of immunologic therapy have been successful. *Transfer factor* is a dialyzable extract of leukocytes taken from normal individuals whose lymphocytes can respond to *Candida* antigens (See Chap. 33B). Transfer factor, either alone or in combination with the antifungal compound amphotericin B, has been effective in relief of infection.

A subpopulation of these patients have circulating antigen-specific suppressor T cells. One study found that resolution of mucocutaneous infections resulted after treatment with oral cimetidine (an inhibitor of histamine, which binds to and blocks the H_2 receptors on the surface of the suppressor cells). Fetal thymus transplantation and thymic hormones have also been reported as effective in small series of patients.

Other examples of seemingly isolated antigen-specific reversible defects have been described. There are individuals who are susceptible to recurrent herpes simplex I infections, but are otherwise immunologically intact. (In dealing with such an individual it is crucial to evaluate other aspects of the cellular and humoral immune response in order to assure that the rest of the immune system is, in fact, in proper order.) Antigen-specific transfer factor has been effective in some patients.

An intriguing example of an antigen-specific defect has been reported in a few patients with manic-depressive disorders.

These patients, with recurrent herpes simplex I infections, had complete resolution of infection, with no recurrences, after treatment of their psychiatric disorder with lithium chloride. The interpretation of these findings is problematic. Is this merely a coincidence? Can a major psychiatric disorder negatively affect the immune system and does resolution remove this deleterious influence? Or do the psychiatric disorder and the impaired immune system represent two manifestations of the same defect, both of which are then modified by lithium chloride? The reader is left to her or his own thoughts. Suffice it to say that such peculiar deficits, or blind spots, in the immune response are probably more common than heretofore appreciated. Take-home message: think of the possible immune mechanisms of disease and you may find a previously unknown immune deficit.

X-Linked Lymphoproliferative Syndrome (Duncan's Syndrome)

In 1969 an 8-year-old boy died with infectious mononucleosis (IM), an infection with the Epstein-Barr virus (EBV). At autopsy, systemic B-cell proliferation was found, although there was depletion of T cells in the thymus, lymph node, and spleen. Five other maternally related males of this family (the Duncans) had also died of either hypogammaglobulinemia or malignant lymphoma following IM due to EBV. It seemed that an X-linked trait determined an abnormal response to infection with EBV. (An infection can cause very different clinical manifestations, depending on the type and quality of the immune response an individual mounts. This may be genetically determined.)

EBV infection can cause a minimally symptomatic infection with seroconversion, "classic" IM, fatal IM with severe liver disease as the cause of death, fatal IM with lymphoma, fatal IM with bone marrow aplasia, or fatal IM with immunodeficiency. In the fatal cases of IM, there was no evidence of immune abnormality prior to the infection with EBV. After infection, there was evidence of profound immunoregulatory abnor-

mality, presumably due to a suppressor T-cell imbalance. EBV specifically infects B cells, and the proliferation of these infected B cells is normally under the control of suppressor T cells. Too little suppressor T-cell activity may lead to the development of B-cell lymphoma; too much activity may lead to aplasia or hypogammaglobulinemia. Progressive destruction of the thymus following EBV infection leads to further immunoregulatory deterioration.

The susceptibility to EBV has also been found in females, suggesting that this syndrome may be caused by other genetic defects or that the X-linked defect may not be the only problem.

Patients usually make an incomplete EBV-specific antibody response and have impaired isotype switching. As in mucocutaneous candidiasis, the T-cell defect is isolated to the response to one organism; in both entities, the nature of the defect is still unknown, although the locus for the abnormality in X-linked lymphoproliferative syndrome has been identified as Xq26-q27.

Miscellaneous T-Cell Defects of Interest

Individual cases of immunodeficiency, where some of the biochemistry or molecular biology has been described, appear in the literature frequently. Cases of children with T-cell abnormalities due to defective response to secreted IL-1 or due to defective IL-2 production have been described.

A 9-year-old whose mother took azathioprine and prednisone during the pregnancy in order to control renal allograft rejection was described who had Hodgkin's disease and chronic infections. The child made no antibody and had absent delayed-type hypersensitivity and abnormal mitogen-induced T-cell proliferation in vitro. The defect in his T cells was found to be an inability for cell surface receptors to deliver their signal to the cell, due to an uncoupling of a guanosine nucleotide–binding protein.

Two siblings whose T cells lacked surface CD3 TCR have been reported. The abnormality was identified as the inability to make normal amounts of one of the proteins in the five-molecule CD3 complex. The CD3-TCR complex was present on only 2 to 12 percent of their T cells and then only at very low levels. Most intriguing is that one sib died of recurrent infections and autoimmune hemolytic anemia at age 3, but the other sib with the same defect was alive with no immune deficit at age 6.

A defect where lymphocytes lack class I molecules, class II molecules, or both is known as the *bare lymphocyte syndrome.* T- and B-cell deficits have been noted; a primary B-cell defect has been described where the B cells lack the C3d-EBV receptor and are unable to respond to membrane activation. The precise molecular defect in cases where class II markers are absent has been identified: the cells lack the molecule RF-X, the specific DNA-binding molecule that binds to and activates the class II promoter in lymphocytes.

Summary of Isolated T-Cell Immunodeficiencies

A full understanding of the mechanisms underlying T-cell activation and of all the steps that go into the maturation of T cells suggests that there are a great number of steps at which the process can go wrong. Until the advent of molecular-biologic and cell-cloning techniques, the explanation for the many T-cell deficiencies were unknown. As these techniques are applied, new subtle defects and ways to repair the more serious defects will emerge.

Combined T-Cell and B-Cell Immunodeficiency Syndromes

In certain forms of immunodeficiency there are both T- and B-cell abnormalities. These may occur because of stem cell defects, or because B-cell maturation is T cell–dependent; the absolute absence of T-cell influences precludes the normal development of normal immunoglobulin-secreting cells.

Severe Combined Immunodeficiency (SCID)

Severe combined immunodeficiency (SCID) is a fatal form of immune defect, resulting in the onset of recurrent or chronic infections and failure to thrive in the first 6 months

of life; death usually occurs by 1 year of age. The onset of infections may be delayed until about 6 months of age in some patients due to the presence of maternal antibodies. The persistence of transplacentally transfused maternal lymphocytes in the infant may result in a GVH reaction manifested by a chronic morbilliform rash.

There are two patterns of familial SCID: an X-linked recessive form (the most frequent form of SCID—75 percent of SCID patients are male) and an autosomal-recessive form (previously known as *Swiss-type agammaglobulinemia with lymphopenia*). In many cases there is no family history, which makes the early diagnosis of SCID difficult. The absence of a family history may reflect the rapidity with which many of these infants die or may indicate that spontaneous mutations are the cause of SCID, as is thought to be the case in one-third to one-half of all males with SCID and no family history.

The defect is unknown, but is thought to be an abnormality of stem cells. Alternative theories include failure of normal development of the thymus or thymus and bursa-equivalent organs, with improper T- and B-cell maturation. Cases where histocompatible bone marrow transplantation has led to immunologic reconstitution suggest that a stem cell abnormality is the basic defect.

Infections with viruses, fungi, protozoa, and bacteria cause chronic and recurrent infections, including oral candidiasis, otitis media, pneumonia, diarrhea, and sepsis. There is a notable susceptibility to the large DNA viruses, notably cytomegalovirus, varicella, and herpes. Live viral vaccines, including smallpox and poliomyelitis, have led to progressive and fatal infections. Maternal antibodies may protect these children from bacterial infections for the first 6 months of life, but ultimately gram-positive and -negative infections develop.

In the absence of T cell–mediated immunity, there is a risk of a GVH reaction from maternal lymphocytes (see above) and from viable lymphocytes in transfusions. As in DiGeorge syndrome, all transfused blood must be irradiated prior to infusion in order to prevent GVH reactions. The presence of a GVH reaction can confuse the clinical picture and delay the diagnosis. For example, SCID patients do not have lymphoid tissue or hepatosplenomegaly—in the presence of a GVH reaction, these may develop and suggest immunodeficiency syndromes other than SCID.

The T-cell defect in SCID is usually apparent in the first days of life, with low numbers of circulating T cells. There may be circulating early or late thymocytes in the circulation of these infants; mature T cells present in the infant are usually maternal in origin. B cells may be absent or remarkably diminished in number at birth.

Biopsy of lymphoid tissues (if they can be found) is usually not necessary, but when done demonstrates severe lymphoid depletion with no follicles in lymph nodes. Gastrointestinal lymphoid tissue contains no plasma cells. The histology of the thymus is virtually pathognomonic, with no Hassall's corpuscles or lymphoid cells present; nests of endodermal cells are found.

An aggressive diagnostic workup, with equally aggressive treatment of infections, is required if these infants are to survive. Intravenous gamma globulin may be used to support the child until definitive therapy—transplant of bone marrow, containing stem cells, from a histocompatible donor (usually a sibling)—can be accomplished. When an appropriate bone marrow donor is not available, fetal liver (less than 8 weeks gestational age) and thymus transplants have also been used, but neither is as effective as bone marrow transplantation.

Adenosine Deaminase Deficiency

Half of the autosomal-recessive SCID cases apparently result from a deficiency of the enzyme adenosine deaminase (ADA). ADA is found in all cells of the body, but no organ other than the thymus is affected by ADA deficiency. ADA and purine nucleoside phosphorylase (PNP, to be discussed below) are critical enzymes involved in the purine salvage pathway. Less than 1 percent of all cells which enter the thymus survive to become T cells. The sheer volume of cell death in the thymus liberates a large amount of RNA and DNA metabolites. ADA catalyzes the conversion of adenosine and deoxyadenosine to inosine and deoxyinosine, and PNP helps in the conversion of inosine, deoxyinosine, guanosine, and deoxyguanosine to hypoxanthine and xanthine (Fig. 22A-1). In the absence of ADA, there is buildup of adenosine which may increase intracellular cyclic AMP and inhibit lymphocyte function. Adenosine is also directly toxic to lymphocytes, at least in part because adenosine inhibits the generation of S-adenosylmethionine, the molecule which donates methyl groups in the methylation of DNA. Deoxyadenosine is incorporated in deoxyadenosine triphosphate, which is also toxic, as it inhibits ribonucleotide reductase and depletes deoxyribonucleoside triphosphates. Thus, by this explanation, T-cell deficiency is a bystander effect!

The end result is even more and inappropriate cell death in the thymus. If enough cell death occurs in utero, the newborn will be immunodeficient. Damage to the immune system continues after birth, as well. Immunodeficiency may present as early as the tenth day of life, or cell-mediated immunity may be normal for up to 2 years before deterioration. The degree of the immune defect is variable, ranging from complete B- and T-cell deficiency to milder abnormalities of function. Diminished ADA or PNP activity can be demonstrated in individuals who are heterozygous carriers of the defect. Even low levels of ADA activity are compatible with immunocompetence. ADA deficiency seems to be a spectrum of abnormalities.

Treatment is similar to that for SCID; without treatment ADA deficiency is fatal within the first 2 years of life, usually at between 4 and 6 months. Bone marrow transplantation has been successful in returning normal immune function. Red blood cells contain ADA *and* have receptors which help in removing adenosine and deoxyadenosine from the plasma. A reduction of the elevated levels of these compounds then allows de-

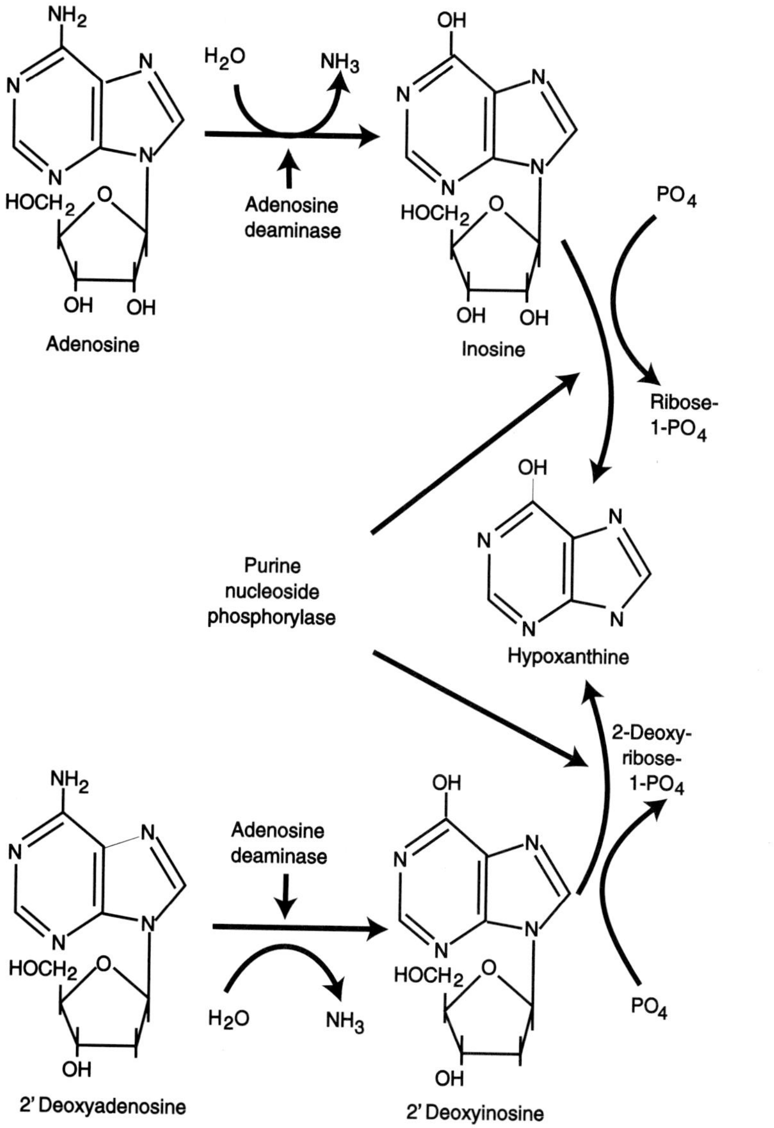

Figure 22A-1 The role of ADA and PNP in the conversion of inosine, deoxyadenosine, guanosine, and deoxyguanosine to hypoxanthine and xanthine.

oxyadenosine to leave lymphocytes, down a concentration gradient. In the absence of an appropriate bone marrow donor, irradiated red blood cells (why irradiate the red cells?) have been used to provide ADA activity, with variable results. More recently bovine ADA, modified by conjugation with polyethylene glycol, has been tried, with reversal of the biochemical abnormalities and improvement of T-cell function.

Of great potential importance is a genetic engineering approach—the introduction of

the ADA gene into target cells with the subsequent expression of enzymatic activity. The ADA gene is packaged in a replication-deficient retroviral vector. Bone marrow cells of the patient are grown in culture and infected with the defective virus containing the ADA gene, and then these transfected cells are used for autologous bone marrow transplant. This approach might also work with fibroblasts, with implantation in the peritoneum or liver, or even as a skin patch graft. These last two techniques offer the opportunity to treat ADA deficiency and other metabolic diseases where accumulation of normal metabolites leads to poisoning of the cell by long-term or possibly permanent repair of the metabolic defect— in essence, a permanent implantation of a "depot" of the enzyme needed.

PNP Deficiency

Deficiency of PNP leads to severe immunodeficiency. Affected infants have very low numbers of T cells, but normal numbers of B cells, with relatively normal antibody-forming ability. This may be due to the fact that the CD8-positive cells (suppressor/cytotoxic subset) are more severely affected than the CD4-positive cells (helper/inducer subset), although the reason for this is not well understood. With absent or defective CD8-positive cells one might expect that viral infections and unsuppressed immune function might be a problem. In fact, fatal varicella is frequent and some patients have been reported to have serum autoantibodies.

In this enzymatic deficiency, the toxic compound implicated is deoxyguanosine triphosphate, which inhibits ribonucleotide reductase and inhibits cell division. Infusion of irradiated red blood cells has reversed the measured metabolic abnormalities, but has not been successful in repairing the immune defect.

Nezelof Syndrome: Cellular Immunodeficiency with Abnormal Immunoglobulin Synthesis

In DiGeorge syndrome, there is near total absence of thymus. In Nezelof syndrome, the thymus is present but is not well differentiated and is incapable of allowing for normal T-cell development. T-cell deficiency can be moderate to quite severe and is often associated with B-cell abnormalities, perhaps secondary to T-cell defects. Patients are susceptible to viral, protozoal, fungal, and bacterial infections, as predicted by the nature of the immune defect; the infectious complications are similar to those seen in other combined deficiencies. One distinctive feature of Nezelof syndrome is that patients may

have lymphadenopathy and hepatosplenomegaly, which is absent in SCID and X-linked hypogammaglobulinemia. The syndrome is not well defined and diagnosis rests heavily on excluding other combined deficiency syndromes, like SCID, ataxia-telangiectasia, and Wiskott-Aldrich syndrome. See Chap. 7 for more details on the thymus and T cells in Nezelof syndrome.

T cells are usually diminished in number. B cells are usually found in the peripheral blood, although phenotypic markers on the B cells may be abnormal. Levels of immunoglobulin may be decreased or normal, but there is a markedly diminished ability to make specific antibodies after inoculation.

Aggressive evaluation and therapy for infections are crucial in the management of patients with Nezelof syndrome. Intravenous gamma globulin therapy is effective in supporting these patients. Thymus transplant, thymus-derived factors, and bone marrow transplant have been used with varying success to reconstitute B- and T-cell compartments.

Hyperimmunoglobulin E (Hyper-IgE) Syndrome with Recurrent Infections— Job's Syndrome

In the Bible, Job was said to be afflicted with "sore boils from the sole of his feet unto his crown." This condition was recalled by the physicians who described two red-haired little girls with recurrent "cold" (pus, but no inflammation), large subcutaneous staphylococcal abscesses and a history of eczema with onset shortly after birth. Furunculosis, cellulitis, otitis, and sinusitis were also noted. Eosinophilia and increased levels of serum IgE were noted; much of the IgE was found to have anti-*Staphylococcus aureus* or anti-*Candida albicans* activity. Later, deficits in salivary IgA secretion, impaired antibody responses to both protein and polysaccharide antigens, abnormalities of T-cell number and function, and a neutrophil chemotactic defect were described, establishing the hyper-IgE syndrome as being more than just a problem with regulation of IgE synthesis. Deficient suppressor cell activity and increased in vitro synthesis of IgE by peripheral blood mononuclear cells suggest an element of immunodysregulation. And, the syndrome has been described in African-Americans and others without red hair.

Treatment for the recurrent staphylococcal infections is crucial, and prophylactic therapy is often necessary, despite the risk of fungal overgrowth. There have been reports of successful therapy with vitamin C for the neutrophil defect and levamisole directed at the T-cell abnormalities.

Reticular Dysgenesis

A small number of children have been reported who have a syndrome resembling SCID *and* have no polymorphonuclear cells. The defect is presumably an even earlier stem cell defect than in SCID. Infections are present within the first days of life, and none of these infants has survived beyond 3 months. The severity of the immunodeficiency is such that none of these infants has survived long enough to be considered for bone marrow transplant, which theoretically might provide the missing stem cells.

Immunodeficiency Associated with Nonimmune Defects

Congenital Thymic Aplasia (DiGeorge Syndrome, Third and Fourth Pharyngeal Pouch Syndrome, Immunodeficiency with Hypoparathyroidism)

See discussion above, under Cellular (T-Cell) Immunodeficiency Syndromes

Wiskott-Aldrich Syndrome

In approximately 4 of every 1 million male births the combination of severe eczema, thrombocytopenia, and increased incidence of infection occurs; this is called the *Wiskott-Aldrich syndrome (WAS)*. Hypercatabolism of immunoglobulin and an inability to make antibodies to polysaccharide antigens are usually present within the first year of life, but infections do not become a problem until after the first 6 months. The child usually becomes symptomatic early in life

because of bleeding due to thrombocytopenia, often presenting with bloody diarrhea. Eczema usually occurs within the first year of life, and the lesions often become secondarily infected. In a study of 301 patients, the median survival was 5.7 years, with 59 percent dying of infections, 27 percent from hemorrhage, and 5 percent of tumors (leukemia or Hodgkin's disease). Of note, myelogenous leukemia occurs more frequently than in the other immunodeficiency syndromes.

Recurrent infections with the types of organisms seen in the hypogammaglobulinemias occur, causing meningitis, otitis, and pneumonia. T-cell function may be normal at first, but often deteriorates with time. Lymphopenia and depletion of the T-cell areas of lymphoid organs often develop after 6 months of age.

Affected boys have normal IgG, elevated IgA and IgE, and decreased IgM levels. There are normal numbers of B cells, and there is normal follicle production in both lymph nodes and gastrointestinal tracts. The inability to make antibodies to polysaccharide antigens is first manifested by absent isohemagglutinins in the child's serum. Paraproteins may be present, otherwise very rare in the pediatric population. Coombs-positive hemolytic anemia may develop, and autoantibodies may be found in the serum. Hypercatabolism of all immunoglobulin isotypes has been attributed to reticuloendothelial hyperplasia.

There are features of "incomplete" WAS which resemble other pediatric diseases. For example, idiopathic thrombocytopenia in a male child could be a forme fruste of WAS, as could eczema and elevated IgE in an atopic child. However, in the former, isohemagglutinins and antibody responses to polysaccharide antigens are normal. The platelets look different in WAS: they are typically small, whereas in idiopathic thrombocytopenia the young platelets remaining in the circulation are usually large. In addition, there is decreased thrombopoiesis in the bone marrow in WAS, whereas the opposite is the case in idiopathic thrombocytopenia. In the patient with eczema, a normal platelet count should be found, and there is often a family history of atopic disease.

Recent experiments have found the T cell of patients with WAS are lacking a specific surface glycoprotein known as *sialophorin* or CD43. CD43, related to the gpIB protein in platelets, interacts with ICAM molecule and therefore probably plays a role in cell-cell interactions. This protein, encoded on chromosome 16, may be involved in an alternative T-cell activation pathway. It is also found on the surface membranes of mononuclear phagocytes, neutrophils, some B cells, NK cells, and platelets.

WAS patients' circulating platelets are small, as are the lymphocytes. By scanning electron microscopy the lymphocytes are also abnormally smooth. All of this suggests that a membrane abnormality may be present. Studies of the actin filaments in WAS lymphocytes show a lack of normal bundling of these filaments, with rapid destruction of the unbundled filaments.

Treatment of infections and bleeding is vital. Corticosteroids, used in idiopathic thrombocytopenia, should not be used in WAS. Splenectomy, although resulting in an increase in platelet counts, has often been associated with subsequent fatal infection. Attenuated viral vaccines and nonirradiated blood products are also dangerous in these patients (recall the other examples of immunodeficiency syndromes where these are contraindicated). Intravenous gamma globulin is useful as replacement therapy.

Bone marrow transplantation is probably the treatment of choice. In early disease, total body irradiation or chemical ablation of host bone marrow is required, but in late disease, with lymphoid depletion, rejection is less often a problem. When there is "a take" of the transplant, the eczema disappears and B- and T-cell function normalize, but thrombocytopenia persists.

Ataxia-Telangiectasia

Ataxia-telangiectasia was originally described as a neurologic defect, with cerebellar ataxia developing in the first 2 years of life. As time passes, other neurologic impairments develop, including choreoathetoid movements, pyramidal tract and posterior column findings, and dysconjugate gaze. Telangiectasia usually develops by the second year, but may be absent until age 6.

The early clinical finding that these patients are unusually sensitive to x-rays, confirmed by the laboratory finding of defective DNA repair in fibroblasts and lymphocytes, may explain the immunodeficiency often seen. Numerous chromosomal breaks have been reported in both normal and malignant cells taken from these patients. In many cases the breakpoints in chromosomes 7 and 14 match with the areas encoding the T-cell antigen receptor and immunoglobulin heavy chain, respectively. The defect in such patients is probably due to multiple different genetic abnormalities, as fusion of the fibroblasts of different patients may cross-correct the DNA repair defect. There is a fivefold increase in the incidence of malignancy in the immunologically and neurologically normal relatives of patients with ataxia-telangiectasia.

Recurrent sinopulmonary infections and increased susceptibility to both viral and bacterial infections may develop early in life or may be delayed 10 years or more. (In most of these syndromes the clinical pattern is quite varied, with individual components occasionally very delayed or never appearing—incomplete clinical patterns abound.) Endocrine and hepatic abnormalities have been reported in these patients, as well. Increased levels of alpha-fetoprotein and carcinoembryonic antigen (CEA) are the rule; this suggests a more widespread aberrancy in control of genetic expression.

The immune defect varies, as well. Of patients with ataxia-telangiectasia, 40 percent have a defect in IgA, 50 percent have low IgG, and 75 percent have low IgE levels. IgA2, IgG2, and IgG4 subclass deficiencies have been reported, as have responses to specific antigens. As in IgA deficiency, patients with deficiencies of both IgA and IgG2 appear to be at increased risk of infection; there may be autoantibodies to IgA in the serum of these patients. Autoantibodies to other tissues, including brain and thymus, may occur. Helper T activity may be defective, although suppressor T activity is normal. T-cell response to mitogen and skin testing may be defective or normal, but often diminishes with age. An increase in T cells bearing the γ/δ TCR markers, with a decrease in α/β T cells has been described, perhaps indicating a defect in T-cell ontogeny.

If the immune abnormality occurs before the neurologic and skin components of this syndrome, there may be difficulty in making the diagnosis. The physician may have to wait several years until the rest of the syndrome develops. Recall that IgA is the most frequent primary immune deficiency known and is often totally asymptomatic. The finding of IgA deficiency may therefore be little more than a laboratory finding or may be the first sign of ataxia-telangiectasia; an elevated alpha-fetoprotein and/or CEA may help differentiate between the two.

Treatment of ataxia-telangiectasia consists primarily of controlling infections. Intravenous gamma globulin has been useful in those patients with deficiency of antibody production. Transfer factor and bone marrow transplants have been unsuccessful. Fetal thymus transplantation and thymic factor therapy have been used with some effect. Attenuated viral vaccines and nonirradiated blood products should not be used.

Survival into the fifth decade has been documented, with increasing morbidity secondary to chronic lung disease and mental retardation or physical disability. Death is due to overwhelming infection or lymphoreticular or epithelial malignancy.

Immunodeficiency with Thymoma

Thymomas are often associated with immunologic and hematopoietic abnormalities. Recurrent infections, diarrhea, dermatitis, and sepsis may occur due to hypogammaglobulinemia. All patients with acquired hypogammaglobulinemia should be followed for the development of a thymoma, which can usually be detected on chest x-rays.

In some cases, T-cell abnormalities have been described. Autoimmune phenomena associated with thymoma include pure red cell aplasia, thrombocytopenia, granulocytopenia, myasthenia gravis, diabetes, chronic hepatitis, and circulating autoantibodies. The removal of the thymoma may result in the amelioration of the autoimmune disease, but does not reverse the immunodeficiency. In 75 percent of cases the thymoma is of the spindle cell type, and occasionally the thymoma may be malignant.

Treatment of the hypogammaglobulinemia with intravenous gamma globulin may be effective in controlling the infections. Death secondary to infections or the manifestations of the hematologic disease or myasthenia is common.

NK-Cell Deficiencies

Not much is known about isolated NK-cell deficiency in humans. Individual cases of such an immunodeficiency have been described in which the patient was normal for a number of years, suggesting that the defect is an acquired phenomenon (or that it might somehow be related to changes of levels of sex hormones at puberty). One such case was in good health until age 13, having received live virus vaccines with no difficulty, only to experience severe, life-threatening viral infections with CMV, herpes simplex, and varicella.

Animal models of NK deficiency may help in understanding the role of these cells in normal immune function. The beige mouse is NK-deficient. These mice cannot reject allogeneic bone marrow grafts, and have an increased susceptibility to viral infection and metastatic spread of tumors. Beige mice given NK cells can reject bone marrow grafts and control melanoma metastases like normal mice. Thus, it is possible that the NK defect seen in Chédiak-Higashi syndrome and in X-linked lymphoproliferative syndrome may contribute to the increased risk of malignancy in those syndromes.

Complement Deficiency Syndromes

These syndromes are discussed in Chap. 13, on complement. See Tables 22A-4 and 22A-5 in this chapter.

Polymorphonuclear Cell Abnormalities

These syndromes are discussed in Chap. 17, on polymorphonuclear cells. See Tables 22A-4 and 22A-5 in this chapter.

LABORATORY EVALUATION OF POSSIBLE IMMUNODEFICIENCY SYNDROMES

Once a physician suspects an immunodeficiency, it is important to use laboratory tests prudently. First, in the infected patient there may be little time available for testing; this is especially true for the newborn. Second, some of these tests are not easily available,

often requiring transportation of the patient or specimens to another medical center or laboratory. Third, some tests are modified by infection and so should be done only in intercritical periods. The possibility of infection should be sought, and treatment completed prior to doing many of the more sophisticated assays. Finally, most of the tests noted here are quite expensive; often tests ordered incorrectly are a waste of money and time. With a good understanding of the types of immunodeficiencies, one can make remarkably accurate predictions about the most likely type of defect, and therefore tailor the workup appropriately. (Figure 22A-2 provides a summary of the location of the various deficiencies on the developmental paths of the various cell lineages.) Before any tests are ordered, any infection must be treated. Existing infection may make screening tests abnormal and complicate the search for the underlying immune defect. The first step is to order and evaluate the appropriate screening tests.

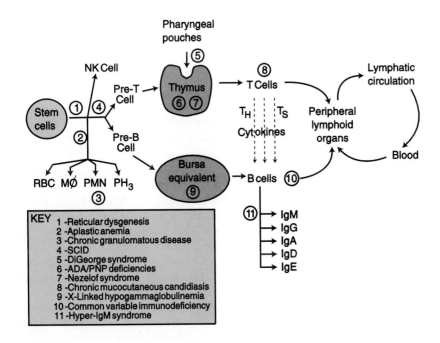

Figure 22A-2   The location of different immunodeficiencies on different cell-lineage developmental paths.

Screening Tests

The basic screening tests are as follows:

Complete blood count. CBC should include differential and platelet count. *The clinician should personally examine the smear!*

Skin tests, using positive controls (antigens derived from microbes to which exposure would be expected). Anergy cannot be properly diagnosed on the basis of one or two skin tests. The clinician should use at least five antigens, selected on the basis of what the patient can reasonably be expected to recognize. For example, it is not useful to use coccidioidomycosis antigens in a patient from central New York who has never been to the southwest desert, nor is it acceptable to use histoplasmin on a patient who has never left Arizona.

Immunoglobulin levels—total IgG, IgA, and IgM. The clinician must be sure to take into account that normal levels of these immunoglobulins are age-related.

IgG functional—antibody titers to polio, rubella, and tetanus. *Note:* If the patient has not been immunized, a negative titer may be clinically meaningless.

IgM functional—isohemagglutinin titers (anti-A and anti-B blood group antibodies). *Note:* If the patient is AB-positive, the titers should be negative.

Complement—CH_{50}, C3, C4 levels

If the screening tests are abnormal *or* the history and physical examination are unusually suspicious, the clinician can proceed to specific tests. The workup may be invasive, but there may be no alternatives; remember that the longer you wait, the sicker the patient is likely to become and the less able to tolerate the necessary procedures. See Table 22A-6.

TABLE 22A-6   Specific Tests for Evaluation of Possible Immunodeficiency Syndromes

Suspected Defect	Test
B cell	B-cell enumeration
	IgD, IgE levels
	IgG subclasses
	Ig response to immunizations
	Ig survival
	Lymphoid biopsies
T cell	T-cell enumeration
	T-cell subsets
	T-cell response in vitro to mitogens, antigens, autologous cells, allogeneic cells
	HIV titers
	Lymphocyte enzyme assays
	Lymphokine production assays
	Thymic hormone assays
	Lymphoid biopsies
NK cell	NK-cell-activity assay
Phagocytic cell	Morphology
	Assays for mobility, chemotaxis, phagocytosis, bactericidal activity
	Leukocyte enzyme assays
	Nitroblue tetrazolium (NBT) reduction assay
	Chemiluminescence assay
	Tuftsin assay
	Adherence molecule assays
Complement	Individual component assays
	Inhibitor assays
	Opsonization assays
	Granulocyte and red blood cell receptor assays

SELF-TEST QUESTIONS*

Match the following diseases with the correct description of the onset of manifestations.

1. Combined variable immunodeficiency
2. Isolated IgA deficiency
3. X-linked hypogammaglobulinemia

a. Often asymptomatic
b. Usually asymptomatic until age 6 months.
c. Onset of symptoms usually in adulthood

Match the following defects with the type of infection a person with that defect is at high risk for.

4. T-cell defect
5. B-cell defect
6. Terminal complement defect
7. Polymorphonuclear cell defect

a. Neisseriae
b. *Staphylococcus aureus, Candida*
c. Varicella-zoster, mycobacteria
d. *Streptococcus pneumoniae, Giardia*

8. Which of the following is *not* a feature of DiGeorge syndrome?
   a. Aortic arch abnormalities
   b. Hypertelorism
   c. Hypothyroidism
   d. Hypocalcemia

9. Common features of common variable immunodeficiency include all of the following *except:*
   a. Nodular lymphoid hyperplasia of the gut
   b. Autoimmune diseases, e.g., SLE, immune thrombocytopenia
   c. Increased risk of malignancy
   d. Rare survival past the fourth decade

10. Patients with all of the following syndromes *but one* may have adverse immunologic reactions upon receipt of blood products. Which is the syndrome in which this is not a major concern:
    a. Isolated IgA deficiency
    b. Common variable immunodeficiency
    c. DiGeorge syndrome
    d. Severe combined immunodeficiency syndrome (SCID)

ADDITIONAL READINGS

Hong R. Histological assessment of immunodeficiency. *Clin Immunol Allergy.* 1981;1:509–541.

Hong R. Evaluation of immunity. *Immunol Invest.* 1987;16:453–499.

Kantoff PW, Freeman SM, Anderson WF. Prospects for gene therapy for immunodeficiency syndromes. *Ann Rev Immunol.* 1988;6:581–594.

McGeady SJ. Transient hypogammaglobulinemia of infancy: Need to reconsider name and definition. *J Pediatr.* 1987;110:47550.

Ochs HD, Wedgwood RJ. IgG subclass deficiencies. *Ann Rev Med.* 1987;38:325–340.

Rosen FS, Cooper MD, Wedgwood RJP. The primary immunodeficiencies. *N Engl J Med.* 1984;311:235–242, 300–310.

Stiehm RE, ed. *Immunologic Disorders in Infants and Children.* 3rd ed. Philadelphia: Saunders; 1989.

Yocum MW, Kelso JM. Common variable immunodeficiency: The disorder and treatment. *Mayo Clin Proc.* 1991;66:83–96.

22

Immunodeficiency Syndromes

B. AIDS

INTRODUCTION

The acquired immunodeficiency syndrome (AIDS) was first recognized in 1981, when young, previously healthy patients presented with *Pneumocystis carinii* pneumonia and Kaposi's sarcoma, both very rare diseases in young, immunocompetent individuals. In 1984, Robert Gallo and Luc Montagnier discovered that AIDS was caused by infection with the human immunodeficiency virus (HIV, at first called HTLV-III/HLV). Two strains of this virus, HIV-1 and HIV-2, have been described. HIV-2 infection is mostly restricted to Africa.

EPIDEMIOLOGY

In 1993 AIDS was the leading cause of death in American males 25 to 44 years of age and the fourth leading killer of women in the same age group. Nearly 340,000 Americans had developed AIDS and over 200,000 had died of AIDS by October 1993. The number of cases of the disease is increasing at 3 to 5 percent a year, a rate that has been steady since 1990. Many more people are infected with the virus but have not developed AIDS. For example, in a pilot study performed in December 1989, about 4 percent of residents of Dallas County, Texas, from 18 to 54 years old, were HIV-seropositive. HIV is transmitted by blood, by sexual contact, and in utero from mother to child. About 50 percent of patients with AIDS are men who have sex with men (a definition *not* synonymous with being a homosexual), and about 25 percent are intravenous drug abusers. Other high-risk groups include recipients of contaminated blood products, particularly hemophiliacs, and sexual contacts of people at high risk for developing AIDS (about 37 percent of all new AIDS cases in 1993), such as prostitutes and the sexual partners of intravenous drug abusers. About 5 percent of patients with AIDS deny any known risk factors. For the past 9 years all blood products have been screened for the presence of anti-HIV antibodies before use in transfusions. Serum antibodies to HIV are detected by the commercially available enzyme-linked immunosorbent assay (ELISA) and the more sensitive and specific immunoblot assay.

MOLECULAR BIOLOGY

Microbiology

HIV is a member of the cytopathic and non-transforming lentivirus family of retrovirus. Other lentiviruses include simian immunodeficiency virus (SIV), feline immunodeficiency virus (FIV), visna or maedi virus, and caprine arthritis-encephalitis virus. Another retroviral family is Oncovirinae, which contains the human T-cell leukemia virus (HTLV-I), feline leukemia virus (FeLV), and the avian leukosis sarcoma group of viruses. HIV has a dense cylindrical core which contains two copies of the approximately 10-kb long viral ribonucleic acid (RNA) genome (Fig. 22B-1). The viral genome contains the three characteristic retroviral genes *gag*, *pol*, and *env* (Table 22B-1). The *gag* gene is responsible for structural capsid protein production. The *pol* gene directs the production of reverse transcriptase, integrase, and protease. The *env* gene directs the production of envelope glycoproteins. The *tat* and *rev* gene products regulate viral replication and protein synthesis.

Infection

HIV uses the CD4 surface molecule as its receptor. A 120-kd viral envelope glycoprotein called gp120 first binds to the CD4 molecule on the surface of a host cell. The primary binding site is at the carboxy terminus gp120 which binds to residues 37–53 at the amino-terminus of the CD4 molecule within a sequence which resembles the immunoglobulin variable (V) domains. Soluble forms of recombinant CD4 competitively inhibit

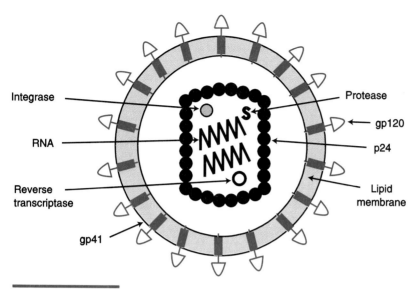

Figure 22B-1   Schematic representation of the human immunodeficienc virus showing the major structural and functional components.

TABLE 22B-1   Major Components of HIV

Genome	Consists of double-stranded RNA
env gene	Directs production of envelope glycoproteins
gag gene	Responsible for structural capsid protein production
pol gene	Directs production of reverse transcriptase, integrase, and protease
tat gene	Directs production of the regulatory protein *tat*
tat protein	Promotes retroviral transcription and translation
rev gene	Directs production of regulatory protein *rev*
rev protein	Promotes export of viral mRNA from nucleus for translation
RRE (*rev*-responsive element)	A *cis*-acting sequence needed for *rev* activity
CRS (*cis*-acting repression sequence)	Required for *rev* activity
LTR (long-terminal repeat)	A highly compressed promoter which contains the signals for retroviral transcription
Reverse transcriptase	Heterodimer with 61- and 52-kd units which is used to transcribe retroviral RNA into DNA
Integrase	Endonuclease required to integrate the viral DNA into the host's chromosomal DNA
Protease	Viral enzyme which cleaves *gag-pol* and *gag* polyproteins
nef protein	Negatively regulates viral transcription
gp160	Large envelope glycoprotein cleaved into gp120 and gp41
gp120	Envelope glycoprotein which binds to the CD4 receptor on host cells
gp41	Envelope glycoprotein which is believed to be important in fusion of virion with host cell membrane
vif	Affects posttranslational modification of retroviral proteins, promotes viral infectivity
vpu	Promotes export of viral particles, important in spread of infection
vpr	Protein which accelerates viral replication
p24	Major capsid protein produced by the *gag* gene

this binding and prevent infection in vitro. Other, minor, low-affinity HIV receptors have been postulated to exist in neuronal or other tissues to explain the ability of HIV to infrequently infect glial cells, in a process which is not inhibited by the presence of recombinant soluble CD4.

After binding, the viral envelope fuses with the cell membrane and the virus is internalized into the host cell. A hydrophobic amino-terminal domain on the envelope protein gp41, which is partly homologous to the fusion molecules of paramyxoviruses, is believed to be important in membrane fusion. The virus is then uncoated. The retroviral genome, encoded in RNA, is transcribed into deoxyribonucleic acid (DNA) using the viral enzyme reverse transcriptase. The reverse transcriptase is a heterodimer with 61- and 52-kd subunits. The subunits are cleaved from a large polyprotein produced by the HIV *pol* gene. This reverse transcriptase is relatively inaccurate. Since transcription errors are not subject to proofreading, errors produced during viral DNA synthesis become immortalized. Transcription errors may explain the significant genetic variation of HIV strains isolated from different patients or from a single patient at different times. The viral DNA is integrated into the host cell's chromosomal DNA in a process dependent on integrase, a viral endonuclease. Although the mechanism of chromosomal integration is not known, it has been shown in vivo that the retroviral murine leukemia virus uses the linear and not circular form of DNA for integration.

Activation

After proviral integration, the infection may become latent until the infected cell is activated. HIV replication is closely linked to the growth state of the host cell. Noncycling infected CD4 cells express little virus. Host cellular transcription factors including NF-KB and SP-1 are important for viral activation. Mitogens such as phytohemagglutinin (PHA) and concanavalin A (conA) can stimulate the host T cell and induce viral repli-

cation in vitro. It has been speculated that antigenic stimulation in vivo by herpes simplex virus, Epstein-Barr virus (EBV), or cytomegalovirus (CMV) infection can induce HIV expression by the same mechanism. For example, HIV-infected cells actively express virus when coinfected in vitro with plasmids containing genes from herpes simplex virus. The physiologic immune response to HIV infection could also produce signals which induce viral expression. For example, recombinant granulocyte-macrophage colony-stimulating-factor (GM-CSF) induces viral expression in vitro.

Replication

When activation occurs, the integrated viral DNA uses the host's cellular apparatus to synthesize retroviral messenger RNA, to process and transport the RNA to the cytoplasm for translation, and to synthesize retroviral proteins. The HIV long-terminal repeat (LTR) is a promotor, which contains the signals for initiation of retroviral transcription (Table 22B-1). HIV RNA transcription is regulated both by cellular transcription factors and by the HIV *tat* protein. It has been hypothesized that *tat* acts either by increasing initiation of HIV transcription or by promoting the elongation of HIV RNA transcripts. The net effect of *tat* action is to markedly increase HIV RNA production.

The HIV *rev* gene plays a role in the regulation of processing of HIV RNA. It is thought that *rev* promotes export of viral RNA from the nucleus for translation. The *rev* activity requires a *cis*-acting sequence, the *rev*-response element (RRE). Other potential HIV regulatory proteins include *vpr* and *nef*. The *vpr* protein accelerates viral replication by an unknown mechanism. The function of the 27-kd *nef* protein is unclear. While several studies suggested that *nef* acts as a negative factor in HIV infection, possibly reducing transcription of HIV RNA through an inhibitory effect on the LTR, other studies have failed to demonstrate this negative function. In fact in SIV-induced simian AIDS, *nef* is required for high levels of SIV replication in vivo and for disease induction.

The structural components of the virion are self-assembled on the host's cytoplasmic membrane. Host enzymes help attach a fatty acid (myristic acid) to the amino-terminal end of viral structural proteins. These proteins are thereby rendered more hydrophobic and more likely to associate with cytoplasmic membrane. During viral assembly, the *gag-pol* polyproteins are cleaved by the viral protease and become associated with the viral RNA. This protease is part of the *gag-pol* polyprotein. The mature virion contains p24, the major capsid *gag* protein, around the viral RNA and other *gag* proteins (Fig. 22B-1).

The *vif* and *vpu* proteins encode two additional HIV accessory genes that play a role in efficient viral replication. The *vif* protein is believed to play a role in posttranslational modification of viral proteins. In the absence of *vif*, virus particles released from the host cell are poorly infectious.

The *vpu* protein promotes export of viral particles from an infected host cell. This protein is therefore important in viral dissemination in an infected person and in viral transmission to uninfected persons.

The envelope protein gp160 is glycosylated in the endoplasmic reticulum and Golgi complex. About half of the molecular weight of gp160 is composed of these attached carbohydrates. Glycosylation is required for envelope-mediated syncytium formation, a process described below. The gp160 is cleaved by host proteases in the Golgi apparatus into gp120 and gp41. This proteolytic cleavage is necessary for viral infectivity. The mature virion buds from the infected cell's surface. The viral envelope consists of a lipid bilayer containing the viral envelope proteins gp160, gp120, and gp41, and the host's plasma membrane proteins retained after viral budding.

Cytotoxicity

The host cell is usually killed during viral replication. The viral envelope protein gp41 is believed to be cytopathic. An unusual feature of HIV infection is that large amounts of unintegrated viral DNA accumulate in infected cells. Proposed cytopathic mechanisms include intracellular accumulation of unintegrated viral DNA, viral takeover of the cellular apparatus for protein synthesis, and increased cell membrane permeability caused by viral envelope fusion with the host cell membrane. The host immune system may generate cytotoxic cells specific for retroviral proteins present on the surface of infected cells. Also, HIV-infected cells can fuse with uninfected host cells to form multinucleated giant (syncytial) cells which have a very short life span.

HIV-2

The amino acid sequences for the *gag* and *pol* genes are about 58 percent identical for HIV-1 and HIV-2. HIV-1 and HIV-2 contain a few different proteins. The clinically available enzyme-linked immunosorbent assays (ELISAs) for HIV-1 will cross-react with from 59 to 91 percent of HIV-2 antibody-positive sera. HIV-2 appears to be transmitted in the same manner as HIV-1. Although clinical experience with HIV-2 is limited, HIV-2, like HIV-1, is known to produce decreased CD4-cell counts, lymphadenopathy, immunosuppression, and AIDS. Some researchers have suggested that HIV-2 may have a longer incubation period than HIV-1 infection and that HIV-2 infected patients may have a somewhat longer survival.

IMMUNOPATHOLOGY

CD4 Lymphocytes

CD4 (helper) lymphocytes are the most commonly infected cell type because these cells express the highest levels of the CD4 receptor. Still, only a small percentage of CD4 cells in the peripheral blood of infected individuals express virus, as detected by polymerase chain reaction (PCR). In previous studies, in situ hybridization detected HIV in 1 in 100,000 cells. With PCR, a much more sensitive technique, we now know that 1 in 50,000 cells are infected in early infection, and 1 in 100 during full-blown AIDS; there is a 5- to 10-fold higher infectivity rate in lymph nodes.

TABLE 22B-2   Immunologic Derangements Produced by HIV

CD4 CELLS

Quantitative defects
  Cytotoxic and latent HIV infection produces progressive decline in number.
  Decreased in vitro ability to generate CD4-cell colonies.
  Can be bound by retroviral glycoproteins without infection.
Functional defects
  Defective proliferation in response to soluble protein antigens.
  Abnormally small increase of immunoglobulin production in PWM-stimulated
    B lymphocytes.
  Infected T4 cells do not express CD4 molecules on their cytoplasmic membrane.
  Decreased production of IFN-γ and IL-2.

CD8 CELLS

Generally little effect on number.
Impaired cytotoxicity against intracellular viral infections.
Cytotoxic function improved by IL-2.
Relatively normal cytotoxic responses against alloantigens.

MONOCYTES AND MACROPHAGES

Occasionally infected by HIV.
Latently infected monocytes may be the major retroviral reservoir in host.
Infected circulating monocytes may permit retroviral dissemination.
Main infected cell in central nervous system.
Defective chemotaxis.
Defective IL-2 secretion.
Defective antigen presentation to cells.
Defective killing of microorganisms including *T gondii*.

NK CELLS

Decreased cytotoxicity due to absent inductive signals.
Cytotoxicity can be normalized in vitro by inductive signals.

CD4 cells are rapidly killed after viral activation, but nonstimulated CD4 cells may survive for long periods of time while harboring the latent virus. Despite the small percentage of infected CD4 cells, infection produces a gradual, progressive, and relentless decline in the population of CD4 lymphocytes. One hypothesized mechanism is that AIDS patients may have a decreased capacity to generate CD4-cell colonies due to destruction of CD4 precursor or stem cells. Alternatively, AIDS patients can develop autoantibodies directed against an 18-kd protein located on the surface of activated CD4 cells. This antibody is cytotoxic in vitro. Another possible mechanism is lysis by cytotoxic lymphocytes or antibody-dependent cellular cytotoxicity (ADCC) of uninfected CD4 cells which have bound free viral envelope proteins.

Although it is thought that the main immunologic deficiency is due to depletion of CD4 cells, these lymphocytes also exhibit decreased activity. CD4 cells exhibit a defective proliferative response to soluble protein antigens such as tetanus toxoid or to stimulation by macrophages in vitro. CD4 cells from AIDS patients induce an abnormally small increase in vitro of immunoglobulin production in B lymphocytes stimulated by pokeweed mitogen (PWM). In vitro addition of syngeneic monocytes from healthy seronegative identical twins to CD4 cell cultures from AIDS patients does not reconsti-

TABLE 22B-2 *Continued*

B LYMPHOCYTES

Transformed B cells may be infected by HIV (not known whether nontransformed cells
  can be infected by HIV).
Polyclonally activated.
Lymphadenopathy and follicular (B-cell) hyperplasia in lymph nodes.
Elevated serum levels of IgG, IgA, and IgD in adults.
Elevated serum levels of IgG, IgA, IgD, and IgM in children.
Circulating immune complexes.
Poor specific response to novel antigens.
Attenuated responses to primary and secondary immunizations.
Enhanced B-lymphocyte transformation by EBV.
Increased frequency of B-cell lymphomas.

CLINICAL MANIFESTATIONS

Immune-mediated thrombocytopenia.
Cutaneous anergy.
Opportunistic infections normally controlled by cell-mediated immunity.
Frequent development of Kaposi's sarcoma.
Increased risk of B-cell lymphoma.
Possibly increased risk of other malignancies.

OTHER

Infection of dendritic cells in lymph nodes.
Elevated serum level of IFN-γ.
Elevated serum level of α_1-thymosin.
Elevated serum level of β_2-microglobulin.
Elevated serum level of lysozyme.

tute this response. These functional defects frequently occur in HIV-infected patients before significant declines in the CD4 cell population occur. CD4 expression on the cell surface in infected cells is down-regulated. This is probably due to binding of CD4 molecules to viral envelope proteins in the cytoplasm.

Interleukin 2 (IL-2), which is important for CD8-lymphocyte activation, is reduced in the circulation because of decreased production by CD4 lymphocytes. With progressive CD4-lymphocyte decline, cellular immunity, which is the main defense against infection by fungi, parasites, mycobacteria and certain viruses, is compromised.

Recent work drawing on a murine model of AIDS suggests that the type of T-helper-cell response that occurs in HIV-infected pa-

tients might determine the course of infection. TH2 response may predispose to the development of retrovirus-induced immunodeficiency (care to venture a thought as to why?).

The immunologic changes induced by HIV are listed in Table 22B-2.

CD8 Lymphocytes

HIV infection generally has little effect on the number of CD8$^+$ T cells. Some HIV-seropositive patients, even mildly immunocompromised patients, have elevated levels of CD8 cells. This may be due to activation by HIV or by opportunistic pathogens. In healthy subjects the ratio of CD4$^+$ to CD8$^+$ cells is about 2 : 1. Patients with AIDS have an inverted ratio. Patients with advanced

AIDS often develop depletion of all lymphocytes, including the $CD8^+$ population, because of bone marrow or thymic suppression. CD8 cells from AIDS patients exhibit impaired cytotoxicity against cells infected with herpesvirus or cytomegalovirus (CMV). This observed defect may be secondary to CD4-cell dysfunction. In fact, this CD8-cell function can be restored in vitro by adding IL-2. CD8-cell cytotoxic responses against alloantigens are not dependent upon CD4 cells and are relatively well preserved in AIDS patients.

Monocytes

Some monocytes and macrophages have a low concentration of CD4 receptors on their cell surface. In vivo infection of monocytes and macrophages by HIV has been demonstrated. Langerhans cells, monocyte-derived cells present in the skin, also express CD4 on their surfaces and can be infected in vivo and in vitro by HIV. Monocytes and macrophages may be the major reservoir of HIV in the host. Monocytes and macrophages are relatively refractory to the cytopathic effects of HIV, possibly because of a low density of CD4 receptors. Also, these phagocytic cells can engulf the virus. HIV may be able to reside in phagosomes without integrating into the cellular DNA (without forming a provirus). HIV can be transported in infected circulating monocytes to internal viscera, such as the lung or brain. The monocyte or macrophage may then secrete live virus after induction. Macrophages and monocyte-derived microglia appear to be the central nervous system cells most commonly infected by HIV. The neuropsychiatric manifestations of chronic advanced HIV infection may be due to neurotoxic monokines or enzymes released by infected monocytes, or to neuronal inflammation mediated by chemotactic factors released by infected monocytes.

Monocytes in AIDS patients exhibit defective chemotaxis, IL-1 secretion, and antigen presentation to T cells. For example, monocytes in vitro exhibit abnormal chemotaxis to N-formylmethionylleucyl-phenylalanine (FMLP), or lymphocyte-derived chemotactic factor (LDCF). Monocytes in AIDS patients also exhibit defective killing of microorganisms such as *Giardia lamblia*, *Toxoplasma gondii* and *Chlamydia psittaci*. These defects are not primarily due to HIV infection of monocytes because circulating monocytes are infrequently infected by HIV. They are probably due to deficient inductive signals normally produced by CD4 lymphocytes. Indeed, interferon gamma (IFN-γ) can partly restore defective monocyte functions. The level of IFN-γ which is important in activating macrophages, B lymphocytes, and natural killer (NK) cells, is reduced in the circulation in AIDS patients because of decreased production by CD4 cells. In some AIDS patients, however, monocytes spontaneously secrete increased amounts of IL-1 despite deficient inductive signals. Fever and cachexia in AIDS patients may be related to increased secretion of IL-1 and tumor necrosis factor (cachectin).

NK Cells

NK cells kill virally infected cells, tumor cells, and allogenic cells in an HLA-unrestricted manner. It is not known whether HIV can infect NK cells. The number of circulating NK cells is not significantly reduced in HIV-infected individuals, and these cells bind normally to their target cells. However, NK cells exhibit decreased cytotoxicity; the cytotoxicity can be normalized in vitro by inductive signals, such as IL-2, concanavalin A, or phorbol ester and calcium ionophore. Thus once activated by alternative signals, NK cells are able to kill their target cells. These findings are consistent with defective NK-cell activity secondary to absent inductive signals normally produced by CD4 lymphocytes.

B Lymphocytes

Transformed B cells may have a low concentration of CD4 receptors on their surface and may be infected by HIV. Infection of nontransformed B cells has not been demonstrated. B lymphocytes in HIV-infected individuals often exhibit polyclonal activation. An increased percentage of circulating B cells from AIDS patients spontaneously secrete immunoglobulin. Lymph nodes from AIDS patients exhibit marked follicular (B-cell) hyperplasia and an increased concentration of B immunoblasts and plasma cells. HIV and components of HIV can polyclonally activate B lymphocytes in vitro. Also, AIDS patients are frequently infected with EBV and CMV; these infections induce polyclonal B-lymphocyte activation and may contribute to this phenomenon. Polyclonal B-cell activation results in circulating immune complexes, autoantibodies, diffuse lymphadenopathy and elevated serum levels of IgG, IgA, and IgD. Children with AIDS frequently develop IgM hypergammaglobulinemia.

Despite this polyclonal activation, B lymphocytes respond poorly to novel antigens and mitogens. For example, the in vitro antibody response to keyhole limpet hemocyanin (KLH) or PWM is deficient. This is an intrinsic B-cell dysfunction in addition to B-lymphocyte malfunction due to CD4-lymphocyte dysfunction. This defect may be related to an inability of polyclonally stimulated B cells to mount a specific response to new antigens. Consequently, patients develop attenuated responses to primary and secondary immunizations with protein and polysaccharide antigens. For example, HIV-infected patients develop markedly diminished antibody titers and attenuated immunity after hepatitis B vaccination. The serologic diagnosis of acute pyogenic infections may be unreliable in AIDS patients because of a decreased humoral response.

B-lymphocyte transformation by EBV is enhanced in AIDS patients. This may be due to impaired T-cell and NK-cell activity and not due to intrinsic B-cell dysfunction. This phenomenon may be related to the increased frequency of B-cell lymphomas in AIDS patients.

Other Immunologic Abnormalities

Healthy subjects develop a local cutaneous reaction around a site where recall antigens (antigens to which patients have been previously exposed) are injected. Patients with advanced HIV infection develop no cutaneous reaction, a phenomenon called *cutaneous anergy*. Thus skin testing, as is often used to diagnose tuberculosis, may be falsely negative.

Dendritic cells in the lymph nodes or in the circulation can be infected in vivo by HIV. Dendritic cells may permit early systemic spread of HIV infection.

HIV-infected patients develop elevated serum levels of IFN-α. This interferon is commonly elevated in systemic lupus erythematosus (SLE), other autoimmune diseases, viral infections, and neoplasms. The serum level of IFN-α has been proposed as a convenient indicator of the severity of immunosuppression in HIV-infected patients. The serum level of β_2 microglobulin, the nonpolymorphic β chain of HLA class I antigens, is increased in AIDS and in numerous autoimmune, neoplastic, and inflammatory diseases, reflecting increased cell turnover. The serum level of lysozyme, an enzyme present in granulocytes and macrophages, is elevated in patients with HIV infection. This may be due to concurrent infections.

Some patients with HIV infection develop an immune-mediated thrombocytopenia (a depressed platelet count). They may present with petechiae and easy bruisability. Hypothesized mechanisms of this phenomenon include precipitation of immune complexes on platelets with subsequent clearance by fixed macrophages, or antibodies directed to a 25-kd platelet antigen.

Immunologic Responses to HIV

The host mounts both humoral and cellular immune responses to HIV infection. B lymphocytes produce antibodies to the major structural and functional viral proteins, particularly to protein p24 and glycoprotein gp41. Some of the antibodies are able to neutralize the virus in vitro, but are not able to eradicate the infection. Clinically, patients have active, progressive disease despite high titers of these antibodies. Because the initial site of infection frequently is at mucosal surfaces, secretory immunoglobulin A may be an important first defense.

The cellular immune response mounted by CD8 cells, macrophages, and NK cells is believed to be the major antiviral defense. For example, cell-mediated cytotoxic responses but not neutralizing antibodies to the Friend leukemia virus will protect an infected laboratory animal against the development of leukemia. Healthy HIV-seropositive patients tend to have greater ADCC than patients with AIDS. Cytotoxic T cells against the virus and against HIV proteins, particularly envelope and *gag* proteins, have been demonstrated in the lungs and circulation of infected patients.

Currently a number of phase I trials of candidate AIDS vaccines, using the envelope glycoproteins gp160, gp120, or the p17 component of the core protein, are under way to determine safety and immunogenicity. A vaccine containing recombinant envelope protein in vaccinia virus has induced significant T-cell proliferation and significant neutralizing antibodies in preliminary clinical trials.

STAGES OF HIV INFECTION

Primary HIV infection usually presents as a transient illness resembling mononucleosis that lasts 3 to 14 days with fever, sweats, fatigue, sore throat, arthralgia, myalgia, lymphadenopathy, and a truncal maculopapular rash. Patients may develop headache or an encephalitis. The infection then becomes latent. Infection can be detected by the presence of antibodies against the virus using an ELISA or a Western blot, a more sensitive test.

AIDS is an advanced stage of HIV infection in which the patient's immunity is severely compromised (Table 22B-3). The Centers for Disease Control (CDC) criteria for AIDS are documented HIV infection and a prior or current opportunistic infection or other specific disease associated with HIV infection, including Kaposi's sarcoma, lymphoma, wasting syndrome, and AIDS dementia (Table 22B-4). Microorganisms of low virulence typically do not produce disease in immunocompetent patients but may produce chronic, severe, and progressive infections in immunocompromised patients; these are called *opportunistic infections*. These organisms may infect unusual viscera or disseminate throughout the body in im-

TABLE 22B-3 Classification System for Human Immunodeficiency Virus Infection

Group I (acute infection)	Syndrome resembling mononucleosis, with HIV seroconversion
Group II (asymptomatic infection)	HIV infection demonstrated by a serum antibody test or viral cultures
Group III (lymphadenopathy)	At two or more extrainguinal sites for more than 3 months
Group IV	
Subgroup A (constitutional disease)	Fever or diarrhea for >1 month, or involuntary weight loss >10 percent
Subgroup B (neurologic disease)	Dementia, myelopathy, or peripheral neuropathy
Subgroup C1	Infectious diseases indicative of defective cellular immunity (Table 22B-4)
Subgroup C2	Other infectious diseases: multidermatomal herpes zoster, recurrent *Salmonella* bacteremia, nocardiosis, tuberculosis, oral candidiasis, oral hairy leukoplakia
Subgroup D	Neoplasms: Kaposi's sarcoma, non-Hodgkin's lymphoma, primary CNS lymphoma
Subgroup E	Other conditions in HIV infection

Source: Modified from Centers for Disease Control, United States Department of Health and Human Services, Atlanta, Georgia. Classification system for human T-lymphotropic virus type III/lymphadenopathy-associated virus infections. *Ann Intern Med.* 1986; 105:234–237.

TABLE 22B-4   Secondary Infections Indicative of Defective Cellular Immunity

Type of Agent	Disease
Protozoan	*P carinii*
	Toxoplasmosis
	Crypotosporidiosis
	Chronic isosporiasis
Fungus	Candidiasis: esophagus, bronchi, lung
	Cryptococcosis
	Aspergillosis: CNS or disseminated
	Histoplasmosis
Virus	CMV
	Herpes simplex: mucocutaneous or disseminated
	Progressive multifocal leukoencephalopathy (presumed due to papovavirus infection)
Bacteria	Atypical *Mycobacterium*, especially *M avium-intracellulare*
Nematode	Chronic extraintestinal strongyloidiasis

Source: Modified from Centers for Disease Control, United States Department of Health and Human Services, Atlanta, Georgia. Classification system for human T-lymphotropic virus type III/lymphadenopathy-associated virus infections. *Ann Intern Med* 1986; 105:234–237.

munocompromised patients. HIV-seropositive patients become particularly susceptible to opportunistic infection when the CD4 T-lymphocyte count is less than 200/mm³. The diseases associated with AIDS are described below.

CLINICAL PROBLEMS IN HIV-INFECTED PATIENTS

With progressive loss of CD4-cell function and attendant dysfunction of other immune mechanisms, the immune deficiency of HIV infection develops. As discussed in Chap. 22A, T-cell deficiency predisposes to certain types of bacterial, fungal, viral, and parasitic infections, as well as malignancy. The rest of this chapter is devoted to a review of these clinical problems.

Opportunistic Infections

Bacteria

Mycobacterium avium-intracellulare   Although *Mycobacterium avium-intracellulare* (MAI) is ubiquitous, immunocompetent patients rarely develop a localized pulmo-

nary infection. Patients with MAI infection typically are elderly and have chronic obstructive pulmonary disease. In contrast, up to one-half of patients with AIDS develop widely disseminated infection. Infection most commonly occurs in homosexual men. The patients are typically severely immunocompromised, and have multiple prior opportunistic infections and leukopenia. Symptoms include fever, malaise, anorexia, cough, and weight loss. Diarrhea commonly occurs with gastrointestinal infection. Hepatosplenomegaly, a highly elevated serum alkaline phosphatase, and a normal serum total bilirubin level occur with hepatic infection.

Infection is most commonly diagnosed from bone marrow, liver, or blood specimens. MAI may also be recovered by biopsy from the alimentary tract or from stool. Samples should be sent for culture and histologic stains for acid-fast bacteria. Histologic staining is a rapid and straightforward way of demonstrating mycobacterial infection, but does not permit species identification. Histologic findings include abundant acid-fast bacilli with a poorly organized granulomatous response, possibly due to the associated immunodeficiency. Species isolation requires several weeks. While awaiting speciation, antibiotic therapy should include antituberculosis therapy. The prognosis is dismal due to the ineffectiveness of therapy and the advanced stage of compromise of the immune system associated with MAI infection.

Mycobacterium tuberculosis AIDS patients, particularly intravenous drug abusers, have a significant risk of developing tuberculosis, usually from reactivation of a latent infection. AIDS patients who develop tuberculosis tend to be black or Hispanic, although this is likely a reflection of socioeconomic, rather than genetic, background. The infection tends to be unusually aggressive. Patients without AIDS typically develop pulmonary tuberculosis. In contrast, about half of AIDS patients develop extrapulmonary tuberculosis, frequently involving peripheral lymph nodes, bone marrow, or blood. Chest roentgenogram frequently reveals no lesions or hilar and mediastinal lymphadenopathy. Symptoms and signs include fever, night sweats, weight loss, cough, sputum production, pleuritic chest pain, dyspnea, localized rales, lymphadenopathy, and hepatosplenomegaly. Due to the defective delayed-type hypersensitivity reaction in patients with AIDS, cutaneous anergy with a negative tuberculin skin test typically occurs. An unusual feature in patients with AIDS is the development of visceral abscesses due to exuberant mycobacterial growth with severely compromised immunity.

The diagnosis is usually made by histologic stains for acid-fast bacilli or by culture of sputum, urine, blood, lymph node, bone marrow, or liver. Patients with AIDS may develop surprisingly well-formed caseating granulomas because tuberculosis tends to occur before severely compromised immunity develops (Fig. 22B-2a and b). Patients typically respond well to antituberculosis therapy, but the prognosis is poor due to AIDS. AIDS patients frequently develop adverse reactions to these medications. HIV-seropositive individuals with a positive tuberculin skin test, even without evidence of active tuberculosis, should receive prophylactic isoniazid therapy for at least 6 months.

Unusual Mycobacteria   Atypical mycobacteria, excluding MAI, are rare causes of pneumonia, lymphadenitis, cutaneous infections, osteomyelitis, and endocarditis. Infections are generally associated with a predisposing local condition such as emphysematous lungs or prosthetic heart valves. Disseminated disease occurs in patients with genetic immunologic disorders, hematologic malignancies, and chronic renal failure.

Patients with AIDS have developed infection due to *Mycobacterium xenopi, M kansasii,* and *M cheloni.* Symptoms include fever, weight loss, cough, diarrhea, and night sweats. The chest roentgenogram is usually abnormal. The most common abnormality is a bilateral interstitial infiltrate. The diagnosis is most commonly made by histologic stains or culture of sputum or specimens obtained by bronchoscopy.

Other Bacteria   Patients with HIV infection are at high risk of developing infections due to *Salmonella typhimurium* or other *Salmonella* species. These infections, which may occur before the diagnosis of AIDS, are controlled in healthy individuals by cell-mediated immunity. Symptoms include diarrhea, headache, abdominal pain, bloating, nausea, and fever. Cultures of blood or stool are diagnostic.

AIDS patients frequently develop extraintestinal salmonellosis with bacteremia and frequently relapse despite appropriate antibiotic therapy. Chronic carriers in patients without HIV infection typically have residual biliary infection with cholelithiasis. In a previous era, Typhoid Mary was a famous carrier, known to have caused at least 10 outbreaks of typhoid fever while working in different households as a cook. However, recurrent infection in AIDS patients does not appear to be due to residual biliary infection. HIV-infected patients must receive antibiotic therapy for salmonellosis.

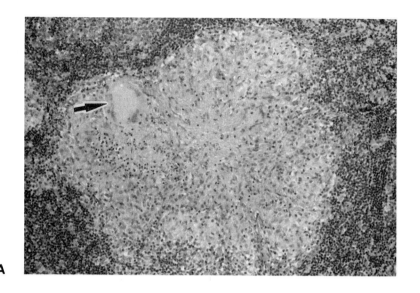

A

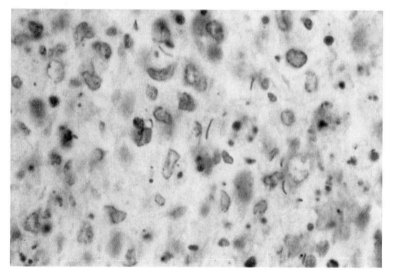

B

Figure 22B-2   (*a*) Photomicrograph taken from a resected peripancreatic lymph node in a patient with AIDS reveals a well-organized granuloma containing mild central necrosis. A characteristic Langhans giant cell (arrow) contains numerous nuclei disposed in a ring surrounding an eosinophilic cytocenter. Note the well-defined border between the granuloma and the inflammatory infiltrate present at the periphery of the photomicrograph. Although this granuloma is well formed, the granulomas in patients with AIDS may sometimes be poorly organized. Stained with hematoxylin and eosin, ×90.; (*b*) Ziehl-Neelsen stain from the same area as in (*a*) reveals numerous acid-fast slender bacilli, one of which is in clear focus in the center of this photomicrograph, ×350. (From Cappell MS, Javeed M. Pancreatic abscess due to Mycobacteria associated with the acquired immunodeficiency syndrome. *J Clin Gastroenterol.* 1990;12:423–429, with permission.)

HIV-seropositive individuals are also at increased risk of developing bacterial pneumonias due to pneumococcus or *Haemophilus influenzae*. Patients with sickle cell disease or asplenia are also at increased risk of developing infection from these encapsulated bacteria. The clinical presentation may be typical except that patients frequently develop bacteremia and do not subsequently develop protective specific antibodies. Infections with *Shigella, Campylobacter,* and *Treponema pallidum* are prevalent in homosexual men.

Fungi

Cryptococcus neoformans *Cryptococcus neoformans* is the second most common opportunistic neurologic infection in patients with AIDS. Symptoms and signs include chronic low-grade fever, headache, an altered sensorium, and meningismus. Pulmonary infection may produce fever, cough, dyspnea, and pleuritic chest pain with a diffuse interstitial or localized infiltrate on chest roentgenogram. Patients with AIDS develop severe infection with a heavy infectious burden as demonstrated by a strongly positive India ink examination or high titers of cryptococcal antigen present in cerebrospinal fluid. The inflammatory response is attenuated with a low-grade mononuclear pleocytosis and a scant cellular infiltrate in infected viscera. Hematogenous dissemination may occur with infection of lymph nodes, pericardium, mediastinum, skin, bone marrow, joints, and liver.

The diagnosis may be made by an India ink preparation, latex agglutination test to detect cryptococcal polysaccharide antigen, cultures, mucicarmine stain, or the Grocott-Gomori methenamine-silver stain. Pathologic examination reveals a budding yeast with a prominent capsule. Poorly formed granulomas may occur. *Cryptococcus* may be detected in the cerebrospinal fluid, pulmonary tissue, skin, blood, urine, or other body fluids.

Therapy includes amphotericin B and flucytosine. Patients with AIDS frequently re-lapse after initially successful therapy; long-term therapy may help prevent relapse. Patients with AIDS on average survive only 5 months after diagnosis despite antibiotic therapy.

Candida *Candida albicans* normally colonizes the alimentary tract in low numbers without producing disease. Neutrophils and macrophages are important in preventing infection. Patients with neutropenia from chemotherapy or lymphoreticular malignancies may develop severe disseminated disease. Patients who are diabetic or who are receiving antibiotics or immunosuppressive therapy may develop thrush or oral candidiasis. HIV-seropositive patients frequently develop thrush. The oropharynx is erythematous, with a white, curdlike exudate. Females may develop vaginal candidiasis.

Patients with AIDS frequently develop *Candida* esophagitis. Patients have pain on swallowing, called *odynophagia*, or difficulty swallowing food, called *dysphagia.* Patients usually also have thrush. Barium studies may demonstrate mucosal ulcers. Esophagogastroduodenoscopy reveals cheesy white plaques and mucosal ulceration. Microscopic examination of a biopsy with a silver stain or of tissue scrapings after washing the specimen with potassium hydroxide (KOH) reveals the typical budding yeast and pseudohyphae. Culture of gastrointestinal tissue is not as specific because *Candida* is a constituent of normal oral flora. Therapy includes nystatin, clotrimazole, or ketoconazole.

Patients with AIDS infrequently develop lung, brain, liver, and gallbladder infection. Cultures of blood or urine may be positive with disseminated infection. Deep-seated infections require therapy with amphotericin B.

Histoplasma capsulatum Histoplasmosis is endemic in the midwestern United States river valleys and in Puerto Rico. Infection most frequently occurs in areas near bird roosts such as urban parks, chicken coops, abandoned buildings, caves, and chimneys. Immunocompetent patients typically develop no symptoms or a transient, self-limited, acute pulmonary disease. Symptoms include fever, chills, headache, myalgia, a nonproductive cough, and pleuritic chest pain.

Disseminated histoplasmosis, defined as extrapulmonary spread of infection, is rare in healthy patients but frequently occurs in patients with lymphoma, leukemia, or AIDS. Lymphadenopathy, hepatosplenomegaly, cutaneous lesions, and oropharyngeal ulcers frequently occur. About half of patients with disseminated histoplasmosis have an abnormal chest roentgenogram. Patients with AIDS may develop a meningoencephalitis.

Bone marrow infection may produce pancytopenia. Hepatic infection typically produces mildly elevated alkaline phosphatase and aspartate and alanine aminotransferase serum levels. Patients occasionally present in shock with multiorgan failure and disseminated intravascular coagulation. Bone marrow biopsy with histologic examination and culture is the most sensitive diagnostic procedure. The diagnosis may also be made by biopsy of liver, lymph node, or lung. Blood cultures or smears may be diagnostic. The oval budding yeast, typically within the cytoplasm of histiocytes, is well demonstrated using the Grocott-Gomori methenamine-silver stain. Patients with AIDS develop a minimal granulomatous response and frequently have falsely negative serologic tests. Isolation of the organism may require culture for up to 6 weeks. Patients typically respond dramatically to therapy with amphotericin B but relapse frequently. Prophylaxis with ketoconazole may help prevent relapse.

Sporothrix schenkii   *Sporothrix schenkii* is a dimorphic fungus which is of low virulence in immunocompetent humans. Infection most commonly occurs in midwestern river valleys in the United States. Immunocompetent patients may develop lymphatic sporotrichosis with erythematous, ulcerated cutaneous nodules distributed along peripheral lymphatic vessels, a fixed cutaneous lesion at a site of trauma, a tenosynovitis, or rarely arthritis. Patients with hematologic malignancies or who are receiving immunosuppressive therapy may develop disseminated disease. Several patients with AIDS have developed systemic sporotrichosis. The diagnosis may be suspected by finding lymphangitic cutaneous disease. Pathologic examination reveals granulomas with a central asteroid body containing eosinophilic material. The diagnosis is made by culture or by the presence of a high serum antibody titer. Disseminated infection is treated with amphotericin B.

Coccidioides immitis   Coccidioidomycosis is caused by the dimorphic fungus *Coccidioides immitis*, which is endemic in the southwestern United States, where it is often called San Joaquin Valley fever. It usually produces a subclinical illness. Symptoms with clinical illness include a dry cough, pleuritic chest pain, fever, and night sweats. Immunocompetent patients rarely develop chronic pulmonary nodules or cavities. Patients who are receiving corticosteroids, have cancer, or have AIDS can develop disseminated disease, involving lungs, lymph nodes, liver, spleen, and kidneys. Dissemination in patients with AIDS is believed to be caused by reactivation of a latent infection. Symptoms include malaise, fever, weight loss, cough, and fatigue. Patients with AIDS frequently have a diffuse nodular pattern on chest roentgenogram and negative serologic and coccidioidin skin tests.

The diagnosis is usually made by histologic examination, using the periodic acid–Schiff (PAS) stain, of sputum or of specimens obtained at bronchoscopy. Bone marrow, blood, urine, and lymph node cultures are frequently positive. Infection produces a granulomatous response. AIDS patients require long-term therapy with amphotericin B and may require long-term suppressive therapy with ketoconazole. The prognosis is poor.

Viruses

Cytomegalovirus (CMV) CMV usually produces subclinical disease in healthy adults. Healthy adults occasionally develop a clinical syndrome resembling infectious mononucleosis. Fever, hepatomegaly, and mildly elevated serum alkaline phosphatase and aminotransferase levels may occur. CMV infection may remain latent after primary infection and recur as the immune system becomes progressively compromised.

About 95 percent of homosexual men have serologic evidence of prior CMV infection. With HIV infection, CMV may produce retinitis, proctitis and colitis, esophagitis, pneumonitis, and hepatitis. Symptoms and signs of retinitis include blurred vision, decreased visual acuity, and visual-field deficits. Fundoscopy reveals fluffy, white retinal exudates with hemorrhages. CMV produces necrosis of the entire thickness of the retina. If untreated, this infection leads to blindness in AIDS patients.

Colitis may produce diarrhea, abdominal pain, weight loss, and *hematochezia*, or red blood in the stool. Esophagitis or gastritis produces dysphagia, odynophagia, or epigastric pain. Endoscopy reveals mucosal erythema, edema, friability, erosions, and ulceration. Pneumonitis may produce fever, dyspnea, and a nonproductive cough. Chest roentgenogram typically reveals an interstitial infiltrate. Most patients have another pulmonary infection, particularly due to *P carinii*. The diagnosis is most commonly made by bronchoscopy. With hepatitis the serum alkaline phosphatase and aminotransferase levels may be moderately elevated. CMV produces focal hepatic necrosis.

CMV infection has been associated with irregular narrowing and dilation of the biliary tree, resembling the cholangiographic pattern found in idiopathic sclerosing cholangitis. Typical clinical findings include right upper quadrant pain, fever, and an elevated serum alkaline phosphatase level. Endoscopic sphincterotomy may provide short-term symptomatic relief. CMV may produce acalculous cholecystitis, or gallbladder in-

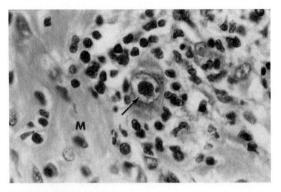

Figure 22B-3   High magnification reveals a large degenerating cell containing intranuclear and cytoplasmic basophilic inclusions which are characteristic for CMV (arrow). Tissue is from the terminal ileum which has been severely damaged by CMV infection. Smooth muscle cells (labeled M), lymphocytes, plasma cells, macrophages, and a few polymorphonuclear cells are present. Stained with hematoxylin and eosin, ×685. (From Wajsman R, Cappell MS, Biempica L, Cho KC. Terminal ileitis associated with cytomegalovirus and the acquired immunodeficiency syndrome. *Am J Gastroenterol.* 1989;84:790–793, with permission.)

flammation not due to gallstones. Patients present with typical findings of cholecystitis, including fever, right upper quadrant pain and tenderness, and a positive Murphy's sign. (Murphy's sign consists of interruption of a patient's deep inspiration due to pain when the physician's fingers are pressed beneath the right costal arch and hepatic margin.)

The diagnosis of localized CMV infection generally requires demonstrating the typical intranuclear inclusions or culturing the virus from tissue biopsied from the specific organ (Fig. 22B-3). Microscopic examination of biopsied tissue reveals large intranuclear inclusions surrounded by a clear halo producing an "owl's eye" appearance and small cytoplasmic inclusions in infected cells. Immunocompromised patients tend to have more frequent intracellular inclusions and less inflammation than immunocompetent patients. In situ DNA hybridization and immunofluorescence with specific antibodies can rapidly detect infection. CMV may be cultured from urine, blood, or tissue from infected sites, especially the rectum. Ganciclovir stabilizes the clinical course of infected patients but may produce neutropenia. Foscarnet holds promise as an alternative therapy without this toxicity.

Herpes simplex   Herpes simplex virus (HSV) infection typically produces cutaneous or mucosal vesicles which ulcerate. HSV type 1 produces an acute gingivostomatitis and pharyngitis. HSV type 2 produces an acute genital infection. Healthy patients have a brief self-limited disease but may develop less severe recurrences, due to latent nerve root infection.

Greater than 95 percent of homosexual men with AIDS have serologic evidence of HSV infection. With progressive deterioration of the immune system, virus reactivation and internal infection may occur. Chronic orolabial or genital ulcerative lesions may develop and penetrate into deep cutaneous layers and produce local tissue destruction and pain. Severe anorectal pain, perianal ulceration, constipation, and tenesmus may develop with proctitis. Sigmoidoscopy reveals mucosal friability and ulcerations. Esophagitis may produce retrosternal pain, odynophagia, and dysphagia. Encephalitis, which rarely occurs, may produce headache, fever, lethargy, personality changes, and confusion. Hepatitis is associated with fever, very high elevation of serum aminotransferase [aspartate aminotransferase (AST) and alanine aminotransferase (ALT)] levels, and leukopenia.

A Tzanck preparation obtained from mucocutaneous lesions may demonstrate typical multinucleate giant cells. Histochemical analysis with specific HSV antibodies is diagnostic. Serologic tests document prior infection. The virus may be cultured from blood, urine, mucocutaneous lesions, or infected viscera. Acyclovir is the recommended therapy.

Varicella-Zoster   The varicella-zoster virus in immunocompetent children produces chickenpox, an acute, ubiquitous, and benign illness characterized by a vesicular rash. Most adults have previously had primary varicella infection. The virus, latent in sensory ganglia, may reactivate years later to produce shingles, a vesicular eruption within one or more dermatomes. Immunocompromised patients are particularly susceptible to reactivating herpes zoster. Patients develop the typical erythematous rash of shingles which covers a few dermatomes. Maculopapules and then fluid-filled vesicles develop within the rash. Usually the lesions heal by crusting and reepithelialization. Occasionally a more widespread cutaneous infection develops, sometimes with dissemination to lungs, liver, or central nervous system, or throughout the skin. Varicella pneumonia may produce severe hypoxemia with a diffusely nodular infiltrate on chest roentgenogram. AIDS patients with disseminated infection require treatment with intravenous acyclovir.

Protozoa

Pneumocystis carinii   *Pneumocystis carinii* pneumonia is the most common life-threatening opportunistic infection associated with AIDS. Indeed, a large increase in requests for pentamidine, to treat this infection, played an important role in the initial description of AIDS. This pneumonia usually occurs only in immunocompromised patients. Symptoms and signs include fever, fatigue, a nonproductive cough, dyspnea, tachypnea, and rales. Extrapulmonic infection is rare. Chest roentgenogram typically reveals a diffuse interstitial infiltrate. Pleural effusions or intrathoracic lymphadenopathy are uncommon. Gallium scans generally reveal uptake throughout the lung parenchyma. Examination of sputum, produced after inhaling a mist of hypertonic saline, identifies *P carinii* in most cases. Fiberoptic bronchoscopy with bronchoalveolar lavage and transbronchial biopsy are highly sensitive diagnostic procedures. Open-lung biopsy is occasionally required for diagnosis. Histologic identification using Giemsa or silver stains are diagnostic. Histologically, an amorphous, foamy material composed of parasites and cellular debris fills the alveolar spaces. Culture or serologic tests are not clinically available. Prophylaxis with inhaled aerosolized pentamidine may facilitate extrapulmonic spread.

Therapy includes trimethoprim-sulfamethoxazole or pentamidine. Patients with mild immunodeficiency and preserved pulmonary function often respond well to antibiotic therapy but frequently relapse. An aerosolized form of pentamidine has been used successfully as prophylaxis against *P carinii* pneumonia in AIDS patients.

Cryptosporidium   *Cryptosporidium* species are coccidian protozoa that are taxonomically related to *Toxoplasma gondii.* Coccidia, members of the class Sporozoa, have alternating sexual and asexual reproductive cycles within the gastrointestinal tract of a single host. After ingestion, cryptosporidia attach firmly to intestinal epithelial cells and destroy the microvilli. Immunocompetent patients develop an acute self-limited diarrhea. Patients with AIDS develop a chronic, voluminous watery diarrhea associated with abdominal pain, weight loss, and dehydration.

Patients with AIDS also develop gallbladder and biliary tree infection associated with cholestasis, cholangitis, and acalculous cholecystitis. Endoscopic retrograde cholangiopancreatography (ERCP) may demonstrate beading or focal strictures and dilation of the biliary tree. This cholangiographic pattern is similar to that found in idiopathic sclerosing cholangitis. Patients typically develop greatly increased serum alkaline phosphatase levels. A coincident CMV infection may contribute to the clinical findings. Biopsy reveals organisms along the luminal mucosal surface. Although the light-microscopic appearance is sufficiently characteristic to establish the diagnosis, electron microscopy is helpful for confirmation. Oocysts may be identified after concentration of stool specimens. Serologic tests have been used on a research basis.

Antibiotic therapy for cryptosporidiosis is currently experimental.

Isospora belli   *Isospora belli*, like *Cryptosporidium*, is a coccidian protozoan. After ingestion, the parasite invades enterocytes in the proximal small bowel. Immunocompetent patients develop a brief, self-limited diarrheal disease. AIDS patients develop a protracted, usually intermittent illness with profuse watery stools, weight loss, nausea, and crampy abdominal pain. The diagnosis may be made by finding oocysts in the stool. Concentration techniques include sugar or zinc sulfate flotation. Oocysts are acid-fast. They are larger and more ellipsoidal than cryptosporidial oocysts. Isosporiasis responds well to treatment with trimethoprim-sulfamethoxazole. However, patients with AIDS frequently relapse. Long-term prophylaxis with trimethoprim-sulfamethoxazole is recommended to prevent relapse.

Microsporidia   Protozoa of the order Microsporidia commonly produce disease in small laboratory mammals, especially rabbits. Infected rabbits commonly develop encephalitis and occasionally hepatitis. Several patients have developed infection with *Encephalitozoon (Nosema) cuniculi*, a species of this protozoan order. Infections have been localized to the cornea or to the muscle, or have been disseminated.

Homosexual men have a high incidence of exposure to these protozoa. Numerous patients with AIDS have developed this infection. Many patients with chronic diarrhea had *Enterocytozoon bienusi* infecting small bowel enterocytes, although asymptomatic carriage of the organism has been described recently and may be quite common. One patient had hepatic *E cuniculi* infection.

Histologic examination reveals extracellular parasites or parasites within histiocytes. The oval 1.5- to 2.5-μm-wide spores stain poorly with hematoxylin and eosin but well with Goodpasture's or Giemsa's stains. They are argyrophilic. At one pole is the polar cap, a PAS-positive granule. Electron microscopy demonstrates a polar filament which *Toxoplasma* species lack. Serologic tests detect prior exposure.

Toxoplasma gondii This protozoan, usually spread to humans from the feces of cats who spend time out-of-doors, produces a subclinical or a self-limited febrile illness with lymphadenopathy in immunocompetent adults. *Toxoplasma gondii* is the most common cause of focal intracerebral lesions in patients with AIDS. Clinical findings include fever, headache, an altered sensorium, and focal neurologic deficits. Computerized tomography typically reveals multiple, bilateral, round isodense or hypodense lesions with either ring or nodular enhancement. Lesions most commonly occur at the corticomedullary junction or in the basal ganglia. Magnetic resonance imaging (MRI) is a more sensitive radiologic test than computerized tomography.

The presence of serum immunoglobulin G (IgG) antibodies, determined using the Sabin-Feldman dye or other assays, documents prior infection but cannot distinguish active from latent infection. AIDS patients in the United States rarely develop IgM antibodies with active infection because the infection almost always arises from reactivation of a latent chronic infection. Patients with encephalitis may produce intrathecal antibodies.

The need for early brain biopsy in patients with typical lesions and a positive serology is controversial. However, a failure of clinical and radiographic improvement within 10 days of initiating appropriate therapy should prompt further diagnostic studies. Needle biopsies of the brain are subject to sampling error. Also, an atypical mononuclear cell infiltrate in small biopsy specimens may be erroneously diagnosed as lymphoma. The diagnosis may be made by microscopic examination of Wright-Giemsa-stained slides of a brain aspirate or biopsy or of a cerebrospinal fluid concentrate after centrifugation. Isolation of the organism requires culture for 1 to 6 weeks. The recommended therapy is pyrimethamine and sulfadiazine. These medications may produce a rash or leukopenia. Clindamycin may be substituted for sulfadiazine in patients who have a severe reaction to sulfonamides. Lifelong suppressive therapy after primary therapy is recommended to prevent relapse.

Malignancies

Kaposi's Sarcoma

Kaposi's sarcoma (KS) is the most common malignancy associated with AIDS. It occurs primarily in homosexual men. Unlike the classic nonepidemic form of KS in older males which typically presents as an indolent malignancy with only cutaneous lesions, KS associated with AIDS presents as a more aggressive malignancy with visceral and cutaneous lesions. Cutaneous lesions are palpable, painless violaceous nodules typically about 1 cm in diameter.

Lymph nodes are frequently involved. About half of AIDS patients develop enteric lesions, which appear as hemorrhagic, violaceous macules or nodules at endoscopy. Lesions may occur in lung, liver, pancreas, adrenal gland, spleen, testis, larynx, and brain. The pathologic diagnosis is usually made by a small punch biopsy of a cutaneous lesion. Histologic examination reveals a proliferation of abnormal vascular structures lined by large endothelial cells and surrounded by spindle-shaped cells.

Treatments include radiotherapy or administration of vinblastine, vincristine, etoposide, or other chemotherapeutic agents. Chemotherapy may produce leukopenia and increase the risk of opportunistic infection. Therapy with INF-α has produced significant tumor reduction in up to one-half of cases. AIDS patients with KS usually die from associated opportunistic infections. A poorer prognosis is associated with more severe immunologic impairment, prior opportunistic infections, widespread disease, pulmonary involvement, and systemic symptoms such as fever, weight loss, and night sweats.

Lymphoma

Patients with AIDS are, like other immunosuppressed patients, at high risk of developing non-Hodgkin's lymphoma. These lymphomas most commonly occur in homosexual men. Persistent generalized lymphadenopathy with diffuse follicular abnormalities often precedes the development of lymphoma. AIDS patients typically develop extranodal involvement, with involvement of unusual sites such as the central nervous system or rectum. The lymphomas typically are of B-cell origin and are frequently high grade according to the Working Formulation of the Non-Hodgkin's Lymphoma classification.

Patients typically have lymphadenopathy, hepatomegaly, and B (systemic) symptoms. B symptoms associated with lymphoma include fever, involuntary weight loss, and night sweats and are correlated with a poor prognosis. Neurologic involvement may produce confusion, lethargy, memory loss, seizures, and focal deficits. With neurologic involvement, computerized tomography typically demonstrates single or multiple hypodense and contrast-enhancing lesions. Patients with AIDS typically respond less well to chemotherapy than do immunocompetent patients.

Several patients with AIDS have developed Hodgkin's disease. It is not known whether patients with AIDS are at increased risk of developing Hodgkin's lymphoma. However, patients with HIV infection develop an unusually aggressive form of Hodgkin's disease. These patients usually present with stage III disease, defined as involvement of lymph nodes on both sides of the diaphragm, or stage IV disease, defined as involvement of an extralymphatic organ. The bone marrow and liver are the most commonly involved extranodal sites. The outcome of chemotherapy in these patients has been disappointing. The median survival is less than 1 year after diagnosis.

Other Malignancies

Anal carcinomas are more common in homosexual men, including those with AIDS. This increased frequency may be related to receptive anal intercourse and chronic human papillomavirus or herpes simplex virus type 2 infection. Other cancers reported in HIV-seropositive patients include esophageal squamous cell cancer, renal cell carcinoma, astrocytoma, lung adenocarcinoma, breast adenocarcinoma, colonic adenocarcinoma, squamous cell cancer of the head and neck, cutaneous squamous cell cancer, gastric adenocarcinoma, adenosquamous carcinoma of the lung, small cell cancer of the rectum, metastatic basal cell cancer, and malignant melanoma.

HIV infection has not been shown to increase the risk of developing any of these cancers other than anal cancer. However, these cancers present atypically in association with AIDS; they tend to develop in young patients, develop at unusual locations, have a highly malignant histology, grow rapidly, and disseminate widely.

Organ-Specific Diseases

AIDS Dementia

Patients with AIDS frequently develop HIV encephalopathy. This dementia may be the sole manifestation of AIDS. Early clinical findings include forgetfulness, confusion, loss of concentration, social withdrawal, and motor abnormalities. Intellectual function usually declines severely within 6 months of diagnosis. Computerized tomography demonstrates cerebral atrophy, dilated ventricles, and diffuse hypodensity of the white matter. Pathologic findings include marked cerebral atrophy, with diffuse white matter pallor, gliosis, and perivascular inflammation. HIV can penetrate through the blood-brain barrier and infect monocyte-derived microglial cells. AIDS dementia is thought to be directly due to HIV infection.

Progressive Multifocal Leukoencephalopathy

Progressive multifocal leukoencephalopathy (PML) is caused by a papovavirus. Clinical findings include focal deficits, ataxia, and cognitive impairment. Computerized tomography reveals hypodense, nonenhancing white matter lesions. Microscopic examination reveals demyelination, enlarged oligodendrocytes containing intranuclear inclusions, and bizarre astrocytes.

Viral Hepatitis
About 90 percent of patients with AIDS have serologic evidence of hepatitis B infection, and about 10 to 20 percent are chronic carriers. Patients with AIDS and prior hepatitis B infection have normal or mildly elevated serum aminotransferase levels. Histologic examination typically reveals minimal hepatic inflammation and necrosis in chronic carriers. This attenuated immune response may be due to AIDS. Patients with AIDS who develop acute hepatitis B may have increased viremia and are at increased risk of becoming chronic carriers of hepatitis B virus. Patients with HIV infection develop a suboptimal antibody response to plasma-derived hepatitis B virus vaccines.

Delta hepatitis is a hepatotropic RNA virus dependent upon hepatitis B for replication and survival. Intravenous drug abusers with hepatitis B surface antigenemia have a high prevalence of antibodies to delta virus, regardless of whether they have HIV infection. However, patients with HIV infection develop mildly higher serum AST levels with delta hepatitis infection. A case has been reported of suspected reactivation of delta hepatitis after developing HIV infection. Several patients with HIV infection have developed hepatitis C.

Antiretroviral Therapy

Zidovudine (azidothymidine, AZT) is a slightly modified chemical analogue of the normal chemical substrate for thymidine synthesis. This molecule competes with the normal retroviral substrate for thymidine synthesis during retroviral DNA synthesis. This thymidine analogue can also be erroneously incorporated into retroviral DNA during synthesis and thereby arrest the further growth of viral DNA because this analogue prevents normal DNA-phosphodiester linkage.

Zidovudine in patients with advanced HIV infection improves immunologic function, decreases the frequency of opportunistic infections, and lengthens the median survival time. Zidovudine improves cognitive function in patients with AIDS-related dementia. Several studies suggest that zidovudine may also benefit asymptomatic HIV-seropositive patients. Zidovudine is effective against a wide cross section of HIV genotypic variants. However, HIV strains resistant to zidovudine may develop in patients receiving this medication for more than 6 months. The side effects of zidovudine include bone marrow suppression, nausea, headaches, and rarely myopathy or seizures.

Other nucleoside analogues such as ddI and ddC are undergoing investigation as antiretroviral compounds. Soluble CD4, synthesized using recombinant technology, binds to HIV and inhibits HIV infectivity in vitro. Dextran sulfate also has some antiretroviral activity.

SUMMARY

The human immunodeficiency virus binds to the CD4 receptor on the surface of host cells. Infection produces a gradual, relentless decline in the population of CD4 cells and severely compromised cellular immunity. Due to the importance of CD4 cells in the immune response, many immunologic phenomena are defective or decreased including the delayed-type hypersensitivity reaction, serum levels of IL-2 and INF-γ, NK-cell function, and monocyte chemotaxis and secretion of IL-1. B cells develop a perpetual polyclonal activation but respond poorly to novel antigens.

Primary HIV infection may produce a transient illness resembling mononucleosis. AIDS is an advanced stage of HIV infection in which the patient's immune system is severely compromised. The classic CDC criteria for AIDS were documented HIV infection and a prior or current opportunistic infection or other specific disease associated with HIV infection including Kaposi's sarcoma, lymphoma, wasting syndrome, and AIDS dementia. The new CDC criteria for AIDS are documented HIV infection and a CD4 cell count less than 200/mm³. Opportunistic infections are due to microorganisms which do not produce disease in immunocompetent patients but can produce chronic, severe, and progressive infections in immunocompromised patients. *Pneumocystis carinii*, the most common life-threatening opportunistic pathogen, produces a pneumonia. Infection with *M avium-intracellulare* commonly occurs in the advanced stages of HIV infection and is frequently widely disseminated. Patients with AIDS may develop cytomegaloviral retinitis, colitis, esophagitis, pneumonitis, and hepatitis. Although patients with HIV infection develop oral candidiasis, only patients with AIDS develop *Candida* esophagitis. Kaposi's sarcoma presents as an aggressive vascular malignancy with widespread cutaneous and visceral lesions. Patients with AIDS are also at high risk of developing severe, chronic, or disseminated infection with *M tuberculosis*, atypical mycobacteria, *H capsulatum*, *S schenkii*, *C immitis*, *C neoformans*, herpes simplex, varicella-zoster, *Cryptosporidium*, *I belli*, *T gondii*, and microsporidia. The multifarious clinical manifestations of HIV infection have provided a dramatic demonstration of the mechanisms and importance of the immune system.

SELF-TEST QUESTIONS*

For each of the following incomplete statements or questions, choose the letter of the appropriate combination of correct completions or responses:

    A. Only a, b, and c are correct.
    B. Only b and c are correct.
    C. Only b and d are correct.
    D. Only d is correct.
    E. All are correct.

1. HIV:
   a. Binds to the CD4 receptor on the surface of host cells
   b. Most commonly infects the CD8 (T suppressor) cell
   c. Produces an abnormal ratio of CD8 (T suppressor) to CD4 (T helper) cells
   d. Binds to gp120 (120-kd glycoprotein) on the surface of host cells

2. The following are true of HIV:
   a. HIV must infect cells of a host to survive.
   b. Infection leads to a polyclonal activation of B lymphocytes.
   c. Infection leads to a decreased production of antibodies to novel antigens.
   d. Patients with latent HIV infection typically exhibit hypergammaglobulinemia.

3. Primary HIV infection
   a. May produce a mononucleosis-like syndrome
   b. Never leads to a latent infection
   c. May produce lymphadenopathy
   d. Does not produce headaches or an encephalitis

4. The following are true about risk groups for acquiring AIDS:
   a. Homosexuals are at high risk for AIDS.
   b. Hemophiliacs who have classical hemophilia (hemophilia A) are at high risk for AIDS, but patients who have Christmas disease (hemophilia B) are not, because only the former require blood product transfusions.
   c. Intravenous drug abusers are at high risk for AIDS.
   d. The largest group who develop AIDS have no known risk factors.

5. Immunologic phenomena in patients with AIDS include:
   a. Preserved or increased delayed-type hypersensitivity (DTH)
   b. Decreased production of IL-2 and IFN-γ

c. Defective monocyte secretion of IL-2 and antigen presentation with preserved chemotaxis

d. Infection of circulating monocytes with HIV

6. Infection with *Mycobacterium avium-intracellulare* (MAI):
   1. Can be reliably differentiated from infection by *Mycobacterium tuberculosis* only by isolation of the organism by culture of bodily fluids or tissue
   b. Typically occurs in patients whose immune system is severely compromised
   c. Usually produces poorly organized granulomas in patients with AIDS
   d. Usually responds well initially to antituberculosis therapy

7. *M tuberculosis* in AIDS patients:
   a. Rarely produces extrapulmonary tuberculosis
   b. Typically is associated with a negative PPD test
   c. Almost always produces a significant pulmonary abnormality on chest roentgenogram
   d. More frequently produces well-formed granulomas than does MAI in patients with AIDS

8. Patients with HIV infection are at increased risk of developing bacterial infection due to:
   a. *Salmonella typhimurium*
   b. *Haemophilus influenzae*
   c. *Streptococcus pneumoniae*
   d. *Salmonella typhimurium* but not other salmonella species

9. The following are true:
   a. *Cryptococcus neoformans* is the most common cause of opportunistic neurologic infection in patients with AIDS.
   b. *C neoformans* has a prominent capsule which can be detected by an India ink preparation.
   c. *Toxoplasma gondii* is the second most common cause of opportunis-

tic neurologic infection in patients with AIDS.
   d. The Sabin-Feldman dye test usually cannot distinguish active from prior toxoplasmosis in patients with AIDS.

10. The following are true:
    a. *Herpes simplex* virus infection may be diagnosed using immunohistochemistry.
    b. Cytomegalovirus (CMV) infection may be diagnosed using immunohistochemistry.
    c. About 95 percent of homosexual men have serologic evidence of prior *herpes simplex* or CMV infection.
    d. CMV and cryptosporidium produce a secondary sclerosing cholangitis due to the development of autoimmune phenomena.

11. The following infections indicate a severe immunologic impairment and are qualifying for AIDS in patients who have known HIV infection:
    a. Salmonella bacteremia
    b. Oral candidiasis
    c. Strongyloides infection lasting longer than 2 weeks
    d. Cryptosporidiosis lasting longer than 1 month

12. Infections which almost always produce a poorly formed granulomatous response in HIV-infected patients include:
    a. *Histoplasma capsulatum*
    b. *M tuberculosis*
    c. *M-avium-intracellulare*
    d. *Candida albicans*

13. The following pathogens can remain latent after primary infection in immunocompetent hosts and can produce severe secondary infection in patients with AIDS:
    a. *Coccidioides immitis*
    b. *T gondii*
    c. *Herpes simplex virus*
    d. *M tuberculosis*

14. The following typically remain latent after primary infection in immunocompetent hosts and can reactivate with the development of AIDS:
    a. CMV
    b. Salmonella
    c. Varicella-zoster
    d. *Pneumocystis carinii*

15. The following are true of Kaposi's sarcoma in AIDS patients:
    a. AIDS patients with Kaposi's sarcoma usually present with extensive cutaneous lesions but rarely with visceral lesions.
    b. Kaposi's syndrome occurs primarily in homosexual men with AIDS.
    c. Once an AIDS patient develops Kaposi's syndrome, death follows rapidly, except when the lesions involve only the lungs.
    d. Kaposi's syndrome usually involves frequent gastrointestinal lesions.

16. The following are true of lymphomas and AIDS:
    a. Most lymphomas of AIDS are of B-cell, not T-cell, origin.
    b. Patients with AIDS who develop Hodgkin's lymphoma have stage III or IV disease.
    c. The risk of developing non-Hodgkin's lymphoma is greatly increased in AIDS.
    d. The risk of developing Hodgkin's lymphoma is greatly increased in AIDS.

ADDITIONAL READINGS

Broder S, Mitsuya H, Yarchoan R, Pavlakin GN. Antiretroviral therapy in AIDS. *Ann Intern Med.* 1990;113:604–618. Fine discussion of therapy for AIDS.

Cann AJ, Karn J. Molecular biology of HIV: New insights into the virus life-cycle. *AIDS.* 1989;3(suppl 1):S19–S34. Detailed review of the microbiology of the human immunodeficiency virus.

Cappell MS, Schwartz MS, Biempica L. Clinical utility of liver biopsy in patients with serum antibodies to the human immunodeficiency virus. *Am J Med.* 1990;88:123–130. Hepatic manifestations of AIDS.

Fauci AS. The human immunodeficiency virus: Infectivity and mechanisms of pathogenesis. *Science.* 1988;239:617–622. Very fine discussion of immunologic derangements in AIDS.

Friedman S, ed. Gastrointestinal manifestations of AIDS. *Gastroenterol Clin North Am.* 1988; 17(3):451–653. Entire issue devoted to gastroenterologic manifestations of AIDS.

Gallo RC, Montagnier L. AIDS in 1988. *Sci Am.* 1988;259:41–48. Good overall review of the biology of HIV.

Hawkins CC, Gold JWM, Whimbey E, Kiehn TE, Brannon P, Cammarata R, Brown AE, Armstrong D. *Mycobacterium avium* complex infections in patients with the acquired immunodeficiency syndrome. *Ann Intern Med.* 1986;105:184–188. The authors' experience with infection by this important opportunistic pathogen.

Imagawa DT, Lee MH, Wolinsky SM, et al. Human immunodeficiency virus type 1 infections in homosexual men who remain seronegative for prolonged periods. *N Engl J Med.* 1989;320:1458–1462. Examines sensitivity of serologic tests at detecting HIV infection.

Jacobson MA, Mills J. Serious cytomegaloviral disease in the acquired immunodeficiency syndrome (AIDS): Clinical findings, diagnosis and treatment. *Ann Intern Med.* 1988;108:585–594. Review of disease produced by this important opportunistic pathogen in AIDS.

Ma P, Armstrong D, eds. *AIDS and Infections of Homosexual Men.* 2nd ed. Stoneham, Ma.: Butterworth Publishers; 1989. Comprehensive textbook of AIDS.

Sande ML, Volberding PA. Medical management of AIDS. *Infect Dis Clin North Am.* 1988;2(2):285–555. Good review of entire spectrum of medical manifestations of AIDS.

23

Psychoneuro-immunology

INTRODUCTION

The conventional wisdom imparted by most immunology texts is that an immune response following the administration of an antigen is the direct consequence of, and solely determined by, the activities of leukocytes within an autonomous immune system. Although immune responses can occur and be analyzed in vitro (i.e., they can be regulated autonomously), in fact, the immune system functions in an intact organism where it interacts with other physiologic systems. The past decade has witnessed a veritable explosion of information at the organismic, cellular, and molecular levels revealing that immune responses are subject to regulation by the central nervous system (CNS) through neurohormones of the hypothalamo-pituitary target organ axes, central and peripheral neurotransmitters, and secondary mediators under their influence (Fig. 23-1). The realization that the CNS has immunomodulatory potential has been derived from many different lines of evidence. For example, primary and secondary lymphoid organs are innervated by postganglionic noradrenergic nerve fibers of the sympathetic nervous system and by neuropeptide-containing fibers, and lymphoid cells express cell-surface β_2 adrenoceptors as well as receptors for many peptide neurotransmitters. Discrete lesions in specific central autonomic sites have been associated with alterations in immunologically relevant parameters. Learning, as exemplified by classical Pavlovian conditioning, can effect enhanced or depressed immune responses. And, finally, "stress" has immunomodulatory effects in both animal and human subjects under experimental and naturalistic conditions.

In this chapter, we will first review some of the evidence indicating that behavioral factors are capable of affecting immune function in man and experimental animals. We will then describe some of the neural and endocrine circuits that link the brain

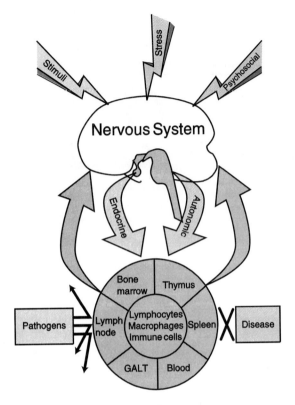

Figure 23-1   Cartoon overview of behavior, nervous system, endocrine system, and immune system interactions. The cartoon points out that stimuli received by the brain are processed and translated into the release of endocrine and autonomic nervous system neurochemicals (via the pituitary and hypothalamus). These neurochemicals, in turn, act directly or indirectly on the lymphoreticular organs and cells of the immune system, which, of course, are also modulated by antigens. The bidirectionality of nervous system–immune system interactions is indicated by the arrows (representing, for example, cytokines) going from the antigenically stimulated immune system to the brain.

and the immune system. We will also present some of the evidence revealing the bidirectionality of CNS–immune system interactions.

BEHAVIORAL REGULATION OF IMMUNITY

Classical (Pavlovian) Conditioning and Immunomodulation

Classical or Pavlovian conditioning is perhaps the first behavioral approach that has been used experimentally to reveal a relationship between the CNS and the immune system. Originally, Pavlov repeatedly exposed dogs to a pairing of food, a stimulus that unconditionally elicits the physiological response of salivation, with a neutral stimulus such as the sound of a bell. Eventually, the neutral stimulus became a conditioned stimulus, since it elicited salivation in the absence of food, the unconditioned stimulus. Since Pavlov conducted his experiments in the 1920s, a wide range of behavioral, physiologic, and pharmacologic processes have been conditioned in a wide diversity of species. The first conditioning studies that involved nonspecific arms of the defense system were conducted by Soviet investigators in 1926, as extensions of Pavlov's work on the conditioning of physiologic responses. In these early studies, Metal'nikov and Chorine conditioned an increase in polymorphonuclear leukocytes (PMNs) in the peritoneal exudate of guinea pigs by repeatedly pairing the intraperitoneal injection of foreign material with scratching or heating of the animals' skin. After multiple pairings, and after waiting until the number of PMNs returned to baseline levels, they reexposed the animals to only the conditioned stimulus, and observed an increase in the number of PMNs. Several variations on this experimental theme, plus experiments in which increased levels of specific antibody were attributed to conditioning, were published in the Russian literature in the 1930s and the 1950s.

The first rigorously controlled and immunologically relevant conditioning experiments in the west were published in 1975 by Ader and Cohen. In those experiments,

rats were injected once with cyclophosphamide (CY), a potent immunosuppressive drug that unconditionally depresses immunity. Just prior to CY administration, the experimental rats consumed a novel, distinctively flavored drinking solution of saccharin, the conditioned stimulus. Subsequently, the conditioned rats were reexposed to the conditioned stimulus at the same time they were injected with an antigen, sheep red blood cells (SRBCs). The anti-SRBC antibody titers of the experimental rats, determined 6 to 8 days later, were significantly depressed relative to antibody titers in the appropriate control animals (i.e., nonconditioned animals, or conditioned animals that were not reexposed to the conditioned stimulus).

Experiments reproducing conditioned immunopharmacologic effects have now been performed worldwide using different species of animals, several immunosuppressive drugs as unconditioned stimuli, and different conditioned stimuli. These studies have revealed conditioned alterations of a variety of immune responses that include antibody responses to both thymus-independent and thymus-dependent antigens; mitogen- and alloantigen-induced lymphocyte proliferation; graft-versus-host (GVH) reactions; skin graft rejection; numbers of white cells; severity of arthritic inflammation; growth of a plasmacytoma; delayed-type hypersensitivity (DTH) responses; and activity of natural killer (NK) cells.

In most of the conditioning studies performed to date, the degree of conditioned suppression (or enhancement) has been small, albeit statistically significant and reproducible. However, the biologic impact of such "small" conditioned immunopharmacologic effects can be great. This was shown clearly in a study using the inbred (NZB × NZW)F$_1$ hybrid mouse (NZB/W), which spontaneously develops an autoimmune disease resembling systemic lupus erythematosus (SLE). A regimen of chronic (weekly) CY administration was found to unconditionally delay the onset of lupus and prolong the life of the NZB/W animals. A similar delay in disease onset and a striking decrease in mortality were observed when conditioned NZB/W mice were exposed to the conditioned stimulus instead of receiving active drug therapy on some weeks (what would be referred to, in behavioral terms, as a partial schedule of pharmacologic reinforcement). In other words, conditioned mice showed a significant delay in the onset of lupus that was associated with a cumulative dosage of CY that was, by itself, too small to alter the course of the autoimmune disease in nonconditioned animals. In another series of experiments, some of the conditioned NZB/W animals were exposed to the conditioned stimulus after the course of therapy with active drug was stopped. Conditioned mice repeatedly reexposed to the gustatory conditioned stimulus survived significantly longer than control conditioned animals that received no additional CY during the same period of time.

Experiments with the conditioned lupus-prone mice raise the intriguing possibility that conditioned immunopharmacologic effects in humans may be beneficial in situations in which it would be desirable to reduce the amount of actual drug administered to a transplant recipient or to a patient with an autoimmune disease such as rheumatoid arthritis or SLE.

Despite its potential clinical usefulness, the immunopharmacologic model of conditioned immunosuppression may provide little insight into the basic impact and physiology of conditioning on immune responses in healthy individuals. A more revealing model would be one in which an immune response can be conditioned by pairing a conditioned stimulus with a naturally occurring immunologic response modifier (e.g., a cytokine) or with a substance that itself unconditionally elicits an immune response, namely an antigen. Although only a few conditioning studies of this type have been published, the single report of a conditioned change in the numbers of cytotoxic T lymphocytes in the absence of the direct administration of antigen (see Clinical Aside 23-1) highlights the physiologic importance of

conditioning alterations of immunity during the normal life of an organism.

Clinical Aside 23-1
Conditioned Changes in Immunity: Antigen As an Unconditioned Stimulus for Generation of Cytotoxic T cells

Gorczynski, Macrae, and Kennedy consecutively grafted CBA mice with allogeneic skin from C57BL/6J mice. During the 40-day interval between first-, second-, and third-set grafting, the number of CTL precursors specific for the alloantigens of the sensitizing donor increased and then returned to baseline levels. The transplantation procedure itself provided for a constellation of conditioned stimuli (e.g., anesthesia, shaving the flank, surgical preparation of a graft bed onto which the skin allograft was placed, and bandaging). On the fourth (test) trial, animals in all groups were exposed to just the conditioned stimuli (i.e., they were sham-grafted). Only conditioned mice displayed an increase in CTL precursors in response to the stimulus conditions associated with the grafting procedure in the absence of an actual graft.

In each of several replications of this experimental protocol, approximately half the conditioned mice showed the aforementioned conditioned change in CTL precursors. These "responder" mice were then divided into subgroups that either experienced two additional learning trials (i.e., two separate trials in which conditioned and unconditioned stimuli were paired) or two extinction trials (unreinforced exposures to the conditioned stimulus). All responder animals that received additional conditioning trials displayed an increase in CTL precursors following reexposure to the conditional stimulus, whereas none of the responders given extinction trials showed the conditioned response. *See* Gorczynski RM, Macrae S, Kennedy M. Conditioned immune response associated with allogeneic skin grafts in mice. *J Immunol.* 1982;129:704.

We do not yet fully understand the constellation of mechanisms involved in conditioned alterations of immunity (see Clinical Aside 23-2). It is clear, however, that such learning involves sensory input to the higher forebrain processing centers and subsequent outflow from the CNS (either directly and/or indirectly) to the immune system.

Clinical Aside 23-2
Mechanisms Mediating Conditioned
Immunomodulation

Any analysis of mechanisms underlying conditioned immune changes must address (1) the nature of the neurochemical consequences of various conditioned stimuli in the nervous systems, (2) which (and how) relevant internal physiologic consequences of an antigenic or pharmacologic unconditioned stimulus become associated internally with the neurologic sequelae of a conditioned stimulus, and (3) how presentation of the conditioned stimulus evokes the immunomodulatory responses that many investigators have observed. Given the complexity of these research areas, it should come as no surprise to learn that we are rather ignorant of the mechanisms underlying conditioned immunomodulation. Thus far, we do know that the presentation of saccharin to animals that have been conditioned by the pairing of saccharin with cyclophosphamide creates an "immunomodulatory milieu." This was first suggested by experiments in which conditioned rats were still immunosuppressed when they were immunized with sheep erythrocytes a few weeks after being exposed to the conditioned stimulus. More recent and more direct evidence that conditioning alters the internal milieu (and may primarily affect T cells) comes from the use of classic lymphocyte-transfer and cell-mixing protocols. In conditioning studies in which the unconditioned stimulus is the injection of an immunosuppressive drug, it is unlikely that reexposure to the conditioned stimulus elicits the direct effects of the drug on the lymphocyte (i.e., alkylation of DNA in the case of cyclophosphamide). Rather, it would appear that the actual unconditioned stimuli being perceived by the CNS as deviations from homeostasis are some immunologic consequence(s) of this direct drug effect on the lymphocyte, such as a change in lymphocyte number and/or traffic. See Gorczynski RM. Analysis of lymphocytes in, and host environment of, mice showing conditioned immunosuppression to cyclophosphamide. *Brain Behav Immun.* 1987;1:21.

Conditioning is perhaps the best example of "feed-forward" regulation of physiologic processes, a situation in which a response recurs in anticipation of a need. For example, competitive runners who display increased cardiovascular output prior to actually running a race exhibit a conditioned response. Patients undergoing cancer chemotherapy who display nausea as a drug side effect often display a conditioned or anticipatory nausea when they enter the hospital prior to actually undergoing a chemotherapy session. Given our knowledge that immune responses also can be conditioned, it does not seem unreasonable to suggest that during the influenza season, environmental stimuli (e.g., people sniffling and bemoaning the flu, television advertisements for flu medications) can trigger or facilitate the development of a protective anamnestic anti-influenza immune response.

Stress and Immune Function

For years, psychologists (and now immunologists) have argued over the proper definition of "stress." For purposes of this chapter, we will adopt the definition of the physician-scientist Hans Selye, who thought of stress as a deviation from homeostasis, the normal resting condition. It is well known that the administration of a stressor (anything that causes a deviation from homeostasis) results in complex neurophysiologic and neurochemical changes as the host tries to adapt. As described below, these CNS changes regulate many physiologic processes including those involved in the generation of an immune response.

Animal Studies

Immunomodulatory "stress" protocols in experimental animals have involved different periods of exposure to either psychosocial stressors (e.g., maternal separation, differential housing, handling) or physical stimuli (e.g., restraint, electric shock, rotation, noise). Immunologic outcomes measured in such studies include the development of primary and secondary antibody- and cell-mediated immune responses to experimental antigens, microbial pathogens, and tumor cells in vivo; the numbers of B cells and numbers of T cells in various subsets in different lymphoid compartments; the magnitude of mitogen- and/or antigen-induced lymphocyte proliferation in vitro (see Clinical Aside 23-3); the production of and response of cytokines; NK-cell cytotoxicity; and macrophage activation. Despite the phylogenetic constancy of the fact that the stress response can affect the immune system, which in many studies translates into a reduction in the response parameter being measured, it is misleading to speak categorically about the nature and "direction" of these stress effects. Indeed, numerous published studies in this area indicate that stressors can be associated with an enhancement as well as a depression of an immune response and that different stressors can have different qualitative, and perhaps even quantitative, effects on a single immune parameter. Moreover, the magnitude and direction of behaviorally driven changes in immune function appear to be related to factors such as:

1. The duration of exposure to the stressor
2. The intensity of the stressor
3. The timing of stress administration relative to the timing of antigenic exposure
4. The length of time between the immunologic assay and exposure to the stressor
5. The age and immune status of the animal
6. The concentration of antigen used to elicit an antibody response
7. The lymphoid compartment examined
8. The coping behavior of the organism

Experimental evidence regarding the relationship of several of these factors to behaviorally driven changes in immune function is presented in Clinical Aside 23-4.

Clinical Aside 23-3
Stress and in Vitro Mitogen Responses of Lymphocytes

One of the most commonly chosen outcome measurements of the effects of stress on the immune system is the proliferative response of lymphocytes cultured either with standard T-cell mitogens such as phytohemagglutinin and concanavalin A (conA) or with B-cell mitogens such as lipopolysaccharide. Although many authors write as if stress-associated alterations in mitogen-driven lymphoproliferation are synonymous with altered immune *function*, it should be understood that mitogen-stimulated lymphocyte division, in contrast with antigen-specific poliferation, does not reflect specific immune function per se. Thus, in principal, one could observe a 25 percent change in tritiated thymidine incorporation in polyclonally stimulated splenocytes or peripheral blood lymphocytes from a stressed animal that is quite capable of responding to a thymus-dependent antigen by producing specific antibody with the same kinetics and the same titer as an unstressed control. On the other hand, stress-altered mitogenesis may well provide some indication of significant physiologic changes in either the numbers of leukocytes in a particular lymphoid compartment, a limited availability of different leukocyte-derived cytokines needed for polyclonal proliferation, and/or an altered physiologic state of the responding lymphocytes itself (e.g., altered expression of relevant cytokine and/or antigen receptors).

Clinical Aside 23-4
Experiments on Factors Affecting the Magnitude and Direction of Behaviorally Driven Changes in Immunity

1. The ability to visualize an effect of stress on specific immunity may depend on the concentration of antigen used to elicit an immune response: Moynihan and colleagues have demonstrated an antigen concentration–dependent suppressive effect on the secondary antibody response following primary immunization of mice with a very small amount of keyhole limpet hemocyanin (KLH). Mice were injected with 1 μg (or less) of this thymus-dependent protein antigen. This concentration of antigen did not elicit a primary antibody response detectable by an enzyme-linked immunoassay, but it did prime animals so that a subsequent injection of the same amount of antigen evoked a detectable secondary antibody response. Animals were subjected to foot-shock stress. A suppressive effect on the development of the secondary response to 1 μg KLH (injected about

3 weeks after priming) was demonstrated when shock was delivered 24 h after low-dose antigen priming. This foot-shock effect on the secondary response was also dependent on the amount of antigen used to evoke the secondary response. That is, a depressed secondary anti-KLH antibody response was demonstrable when the primed and stressed mice were challenged with 1 µg KLH but not with 5 µg KLH. These observations suggest that some immunomodulatory effects of a stressor may be subtle and could be masked when an investigator selects a concentration of antigen to inject based on what elicits an optimal response in the laboratory rather than on the physiologic concentrations of antigens that might be encountered in the real world. *See* Moynihan JA, Ader R, Grota LJ, Schachtman TR, Cohen N. The effects of footshock stress on the development of immunological memory following low dose antigen priming in mice. *Brain Behav Immun.* 1990;4:1.

2. Different stressors can affect the same parameters of immunity quite differently: Solomon examined the influence of three different stressors on the primary and secondary antibody responses to polymeric flagellin in rats. At the concentrations of antigen used, no differences in either primary or secondary antibody titers were noted when animals were subjected to chronic foot-shock stress. In contrast, rats subjected to a change in housing from two per cage to five to six per cage for 1 week prior to immunization did display a significantly depressed primary and secondary antiflagellin response. Finally, rats that were sleep-deprived for 2 days before and 2 days after primary and secondary immunization with flagellin had a depressed primary but an unaffected secondary antiflagellin antibody response. Solomon GF. Stress and antibody response in rats. *Int Arch Allergy.* 1969;35:97.

3. There appear to be critical periods relative to immunization when the physiologic responses to a stressor can culminate in a demonstrable effect on antibody formation: Esterling and Rabin subjected mice to rotation stress beginning either on the day of or the day after immunization with sheep red blood cells (SRBCs). There was no effect of stress when it was administered beginning at the time of immunization; however, the number of splenic antibody-

forming cells and the titers of serum antibody titers were significantly depressed in mice for whom rotational stress began 24 h after immunization.

Zalcman and colleagues have also provided evidence of a critical period when foot shock of mice affects humoral immunity. Mice were subjected to shock sessions at either 0, 24, 48, 72, or 96 h after immunization with SRBCs. The anti-SRBC plaque-forming cell response (i.e., the number of individual antibody-forming cells) was assayed 96 h after immunization. Only when the foot-shock session was initiated 72 h after immunization was a significant reduction of serum antibody titers and the number of plaque-forming cells noted. *See* Esterling B, Rabin BS. Stress-induced alteration of T-lymphocyte subsets and humoral immunity in mice. *Behav Neurosci.* 1987;101:115. Zalcman S, Minkiewicz-Janda A, Richter M, Anisman H. Critical periods associated with stressor effect on antibody titers and on the plaque-forming cell response to sheep red blood cells. *Brain Behav Immun.* 1988;2:254.

4. The same stressor may differentially affect antibody responses to different antigens, and the efficacy of the timing of a given stressor on an in vivo immune response may depend on whether one is evaluating cellular or humoral immunity: Okimura and Nigo reported that restraint stress depressed the plaque-forming-cell response of mice to SRBCs, but did not affect their antibody response to ficoll, a type 2 thymus-independent antigen. Thus, whether a given restraint protocol affects humoral immunity may depend on the nature of the antigen being used to evoke antibody production.

An immunodepressive effect of restraint on the anti-SRBC antibody response was noted when the animals were restrained before, but not after, immunization. However, when the same stressor was administered either for the first 2 days before or for the 2 days immediately following priming with SRBCs, a delayed-type hypersensitivity response to a subsequent challenge with SRBCs was depressed. *See* Okimura T, Nigo Y. Stress and immune responses. I. Suppression of T cell functions in restraint-stressed mice. *Jpn J Pharmacol.* 1986;40:505.

5. Short- and long-term stress can evoke different effects on immune responses: Monjan and Collector demonstrated that stress can be

associated with enhanced as well as depressed in vitro mitogenesis. In these early studies, mice were subjected to auditory stimulation for 5 s every minute during a 1- to 3-h period for various periods of time before being killed. Spleen cells were cultured with conA or LPS. Short-term exposure to noise produced a striking suppression of mitogen responses. After approximately 3 weeks of auditory stress, mitogen responses returned to control levels. Between 3 and 6 weeks of stress, however, there was actually an enhanced response to both the T-cell and B-cell mitogens. Thus, there appeared to be an interaction between the number of exposures to the auditory stressor and the direction of the modulated mitogen response. *See* Monjan AA, Collector MI. Stress-induced modulation of the immune response. *Science.* 1977;196:307.

The observation that physical and psychosocial stressors can modify both disease progression and the immune response has led to the idea that stress plays an important role in the pathogenesis of immunologically relevant diseases (e.g., cancer, viral and bacterial infections, autoimmunity, and allergy). However, animal studies have yet to demonstrate a cause-and-effect relationship among a stressor, altered immune reactivity, and subsequent disease progression that can be taken as hard fact. That is, sufficient experimental evidence has not yet been accumulated demonstrating that stress-associated alterations of some facet of immunocompetence are directly responsible for particular pathophysiologic effects.

Stressors elicit a multiplicity of distinctive neuroendocrine consequences, and, as described below, immune responses are affected by the neuroendocrine milieu in which leukocytes normally function. However, it is not clear which (and how) stress-associated neuroendocrine changes may be related to which stress-associated immunomodulatory events. Five illustrative examples can be cited.

1. Although the hypothalamo-pituitary-adrenal axis is activated during many stressful situations, and there are numerous reports of stress-induced adrenocortically mediated immunosuppression, stress-induced alterations of immunologic reactivity also have been noted in adrenalectomized animals.

2. Although hypophysectomy obviates the effects of stress on some immune functions, stress-induced suppression of other functions can be potentiated by this procedure.

3. The hypothalamo-pituitary-adrenal axis plays a role in stress-induced analgesia. This has led investigators to set up experiments which demonstrate that endogenous opioids can play a role in stress-associated immunomodulation in a variety of species. However, not all stress effects on immunity can be blocked by opioid antagonists such as naloxone or naltrexone and/or mimicked by exogenous opioids such as endorphins and morphine.

4. Although levels of catecholamines from the adrenal medulla and postganglionic sympathetic neurons and other neurotransmitters are known to be altered in response to stressors (and many studies have revealed a functional role for catecholamine in immune function), few studies have attempted to correlate stress-induced changes in plasma catecholamines or in catecholamine activity in lymphoid organs with altered immune function.

5. Finally, there is conflicting evidence that neurotransmitters such as γ-aminobutyric acid (GABA) may play a role in stress effects on immune function.

Clinical Studies

The earliest data suggesting a clinically relevant link between behavior and immunity are observations of a relationship between psychosocial factors, including stress, and susceptibility to disease processes that involve the immune system. For example, there are abundant clinical data documenting an association between psychosocial factors associated with the loss of a family member or loved one and an increased morbidity and mortality associated with infectious diseases or cancer. Such conjugal bereavement can be associated with a reduction in the mitogen-induced proliferative responses of peripheral blood lymphocytes and a reduction in the activity of NK cells.

More recent clinical studies involving a different stressful situation should be of particular interest to students who use this text. Medical students at Ohio State University have been evaluated immunologically before, during, and after basic sciences examination periods. Glaser and Kiecolt-Glaser reported that the following were all reduced in samples they collected from students during the examination period relative to samples obtained during a relatively unstressful interim period: mitogen reactivity, NK-cell activity, percentages of total T cells and CD4$^+$ helper and CD8$^+$ cytotoxic/suppressor T cells in the peripheral blood, and production of interferon gamma (IFN-γ) by stimulated lymphocytes. Examination stress in the same medical student population was also associated with an increased titer of antibody to specific protein components of Epstein-Barr virus (EBV), an immunologic event apparently resulting from an increase in free virus (or its constituent antigens) attributed to a stress-associated decrease in the cellular immune response that normally holds the virus in check. Although there was an increase in the students' self-reported symptoms of infectious illness during examinations, a cause-and-effect relationship between the observed immune changes and actual disease has not been firmly documented, nor is it likely that such mechanistic associations can be ascertained in noninvasive studies with humans.

Stress-associated alterations in the immune system have been noted in many other recent clinical studies. In a study of marital quality and divorce, Kiecolt-Glaser and colleagues found that women who had been separated 1 year or less had poorer mitogen responses of their peripheral blood lymphocytes, decreased cell-mediated responses to EBV (i.e., an increased anti-EBV antibody titer), and a significantly lower number of peripheral blood CD4$^+$ helper T cells than a matched control group. No differences between the two groups in the percentage of cytotoxic/suppressor CD8$^+$ T cells or in the helper-suppressor ratio were apparent. Higher antibody titers to both EBV and herpes simplex virus 1 (HSV) were also seen in separated or divorced men compared with a demographically matched group of married men. Some of the same immunologic changes have also been seen in individuals who provide primary care for a family member with Alzheimer's disease. Six years after the Three Mile Island power plant incident, individuals who had lived in the vicinity of the nuclear reactor had more neutrophils; a depressed number of B cells, NK cells, and CD4$^+$ T cells; and an increased antibody titer to HSV and cytomegalovirus compared with matched controls.

Other recent studies have reported immediate immunologic effects following exposure to severe stressor. For example, the number of NK cells and CD8$^+$ cells were increased in the peripheral blood of individuals sampled within a few hours after an earthquake in Los Angeles when compared with samples drawn 6 and 12 months later. This may be attributable to physiologic changes in compartmentation and lymphocyte trafficking brought about by hormones and neurotransmitters activated by the stressor, as may many of the changes in peripheral blood measures following stress. The stress of performing simulated battle tasks for 3 days resulted in an increase of interferon production following viral stimulation of leukocytes in vitro. A rapid increase in the number and activity of NK cells was also seen in young subjects performing mental arithmetic under examiner pressure. It is intriguing to note that in these few examples, long-term stress resulted in a depression of the immune parameter being investigated, whereas immediate stress resulted in its enhancement.

One cannot assume that every immediate or long-term stressful situation is associated with a significant and reproducible set of comparable immune changes in every individual or in an experimental cohort. As mentioned previously, in both retrospective and prospective studies of bereaved individuals, some investigators have observed a decrease in mitogen reactivity and/or NK-cell cytotoxicity. However, other studies have reported no changes in these particular parameters. In fact, what does appear to be consistent in all studies of bereaved subjects is a lack of change in DTH, levels of serum IgM, IgG, and IgA, and absolute numbers or percentages of B cells and T cells (both CD4$^+$ and CD8$^+$ T cells). Similarly, an association between affective disorders such as major depression and diminished mitogenic responses of peripheral blood lymphocytes or other immunologically relevant changes has been described in some reports, but has not been consistently demonstrated. In general, studies on such clinical populations are complicated by numerous variables including the nature of the depression, the inpatient versus outpatient status of the subject, the severity of the disease, the patient's age, recent and past medical history, and the nutritional status of the subject. The design of such studies must also take into consideration the status of the control subjects (age, sex, job, exercise level, hospitalization status, etc.) against which the immunologic values of the experimental cohort will be compared (see Clinical Aside 23-5). In addition, the nature of social relationships and resources during the period of stress may influence the immunologic outcome. These features are a necessary complication of all human studies, particularly those involving psychosocial variables. In the medical student–examination stress paradigm mentioned above, the effects of the stressor on NK-cell activity was greatest in those medical students who exhibited the highest level of loneliness. Similarly, the extent to which separation or divorce in women was associated with immune changes appeared to be related to the nature of the ongoing social relationship to the former husband.

Clinical Aside 23-5
Depression and Immune Function

Schleifer and colleagues assessed several immune parameters in 91 drug-free hospitalized and ambulatory patients with major depressive disorder who were representative of a range of ages, severity of illness, and sex. There were no significant mean differences between the patients and age- and sex-matched controls in number of peripheral blood lymphocytes, T and B cells, T-cell subsets, mitogen responses, and NK-cell activity. However, when multiple regression analyses were conducted to investigate the contribution of age, sex, severity, and hospitalization status to the immune measures, a subgroup of depressed patients—the oldest and the most severely depressed—emerged whose immunologic values did deviate significantly from control values. *See* Schleifer SJ, Keller SE, Bond RN, Cohen J, Stein M. Major depressive disorder and immunity: Role of age, sex, severity and hospitalization. *Arch Gen Psychiatry*. 1989;46:81.

The many studies documenting immunologic changes during immediate and long-term stress have led to the reasonable idea that some forms of behavioral intervention might attenuate or facilitate reversal of stress-associated changes in immune function (and, perhaps, in subsequent morbidity and mortality). By and large, intervention studies using guided imagery, relaxation, biofeedback, laughter, and other putative coping strategies that have become increasingly popularized in self-help books have not been rigorously (i.e., scientifically) designed and such results are mainly anecdotal. In the absence of both a control population and a clear explanation of selection criteria for the experimental subject, any study claiming therapeutic success for such interventions must be viewed with appropriate caution, if not skepticism. At the same time, however, the possibility that such therapies may influence the immune system or disease process should not be discarded out of hand, and indeed is being seriously explored by some scientists. A few intriguing, albeit preliminary, studies are noteworthy.

1. Relaxation intervention in the Ohio State University medical student population undergoing examination stress was associated with an increased number of peripheral blood CD4$^+$ cells.
2. Relaxation intervention in geriatric residents in independent living facilities was

associated with an increase in NK-cell cytotoxicity and a decrease in anti-HSV antibody titers.

3. In a 12-month longitudinal study, cancer patients who practiced relaxation and imagery showed increases in mitogen and mixed lymphocyte responsiveness, NK-cell cytotoxicity, and production of IL-2.

4. A retrospective review of the 10-year history of patients with metastatic breast cancer who received group psychotherapy (as an adjunct to a standard regimen of chemotherapy and radiation therapy) for the first year after clinical diagnosis revealed a strikingly increased survival of this group when compared with age-matched control patients with the same diagnosis (37 months versus 19 months). However, as pointed out by David Spiegel, the senior author of the study, these survival differences do not *necessarily* reflect a direct or even an indirect involvement of the immune system. Other factors, such as better compliance with chemotherapeutic regimens or any of a host of other variables, may have contributed to the differences in survival between the experimental and control groups.

5. Fawzy and colleagues have recently found that a 6-week period of psychosocial intervention aimed at increasing coping skills in patients with malignant melanoma was associated with an increase in interferon-augmented NK-cell activity and numbers of NK cells relative to a control population measured at a 6-month follow-up point. Changes were most notable in those patients who reported increased levels of anger and decreased levels of anxiety and depression during the 6-month period.

It is important to emphasize that although stressors can influence the behavior of human peripheral blood leukocytes in vitro, and stress is associated with increased morbidity and mortality resulting from such problems as infectious disease, there is a paucity of data establishing a causal relationship between such stress-altered leukocyte function and increased morbidity in humans or in experimental animals. However, some correlative data are consistent with such a cause-and-effect relationship. For example, Kemeny and colleagues studied individuals with chronic recurrent HSV infection and found that depressed mood was associated with a high number of genital herpes recurrences. Depressed mood was also associated with a decrease in the level of CD8$^+$ T cells, an immunologic event which, for some individuals, precedes an outbreak of herpes.

In addition to numerous specific unanswered questions about stress, immune changes, and disease, there are several very general, yet fundamental, issues that have never been addressed. Two of these are worth mentioning. First, in humans, we do not know whether a significant stress-associated in vitro change in some function of lymphocytes in the peripheral blood is reflective of the altered behavior of lymphocytes in another lymphoid compartment (e.g., spleen, nodes). Compartmentation of stress effects has been reported for experimental animals where corticosteroid-, norepinephrine-, and opioid-related changes in different specific measures of immune reactivity were seen following exposure of rats to a single stressor. Second, the immunologic consequences of a given stressor in a patient with an autoimmune disease, or in a patient who is already immunocompromised because of an age-related decline in immunocompetence, immunosuppressive drug or radiation therapy (e.g., a bone marrow transplant recipient), or a viral infection (e.g., HIV) may be of greater clinical significance than the same stressor applied to an immunologically normal individual.

CNS–IMMUNE SYSTEM INTERACTIONS

The fact that stress and conditioning can alter various immune reactivities means that the CNS must be capable of playing some role in regulating immunity. Two additional sets of observations pointing directly to CNS–immune system interactions are those that describe the immunologic effects of discrete electrolytic lesions in the brain and those that describe innervation of lymphoid tissues and its consequences. Results from each of these approaches will be summarized separately.

Lesions

Lesions of the preoptic/anterior hypothalamic region of the hypothalamus result in a transient depression of several immunologic parameters. Among these are the numbers of nucleated splenocytes and thymocytes, proliferative responses of T cells to mitogens, NK-cell cytotoxicity, and antibody production. Hypophysectomy of animals with lesions of the anterior hypothalamus reverses these immunologic effects, suggesting that they are mediated by hypothalamopituitary neuroendocrine changes. Lesions of the medial or posterior hypothalamus are associated with reduced numbers of T and B cells and a decrease in the CD4/CD8 ratio. Lesions in these areas have also been associated with an enhanced rejection of allografts. In contrast to the suppressive effects of hypothalamic lesions, lesions in some limbic forebrain structures lead to enhanced immune responses. For example, lesions of the dorsal hippocampus or amygdaloid complex result in a transient increase in numbers of splenocytes and thymocytes and an increase in mitogen-induced T-cell proliferation that is reversible by hypophysectomy. Lesions of the lateral septal system and its connections to the hippocampus have been associated with chronic alterations in T-cell responses. Lesions of the caudal reticular formation in the medulla and caudal pons result in inhibition of DTH responses, whereas lesions in rostral medial reticular formation and raphe nuclei lead to an enhanced DTH. Lesions of the reticular formation are also followed by thymic involution. Recently, Renoux, Biziere, and coworkers published data indicating a laterality associated with an immunomodulatory role of the cerebral cortex. Specifically, large lesions in the left cerebral

hemisphere of mice resulted in decreased T-cell numbers, impaired T-cell responses to mitogens and alloantigens, a depressed T cell–dependent IgG antibody response to SRBCs, and depressed NK-cell cytotoxicity. No effects were noted on B cells and macrophages. In contrast, lesions of the right cerebral hemisphere were associated with enhanced T cell–mediated immune reactivities. The cerebral cortex is involved in conscious interpretation of the outside world and in responses to psychosocial factors and stressors. Thus, the influence of the cerebral cortex on immune responses may provide an important link between these phenomena and the outflow of neuroendocrine transmitters and neurotransmitters to the immune system.

Innervation of Lymphoid Tissues

It has long been known that the autonomic nervous system, particularly the postganglionic sympathetic noradrenergic nerves, provide innervation to the vascular and capsular/trabecular smooth muscle in lymphoid organs (see Chap. 1). Only recently, however, have the immunocytochemical and fluorescence histochemical studies of David and Suzanne Felten and their colleagues and from other laboratories clearly demonstrated the presence of noradrenergic sympathetic nerve fibers and peptidergic nerve fibers in the parenchyma of primary (thymus, bone marrow) and secondary (spleen, lymph nodes, gut-associated lymphoid tissues [GALT]) lymphoid organs of rodents (Figs. 23-2 and 23-3). These nerve fibers are in direct contact with lymphocytes and macrophages, forming close neuroeffector junctions. In addition, neurotransmitters released from these nerves appear to diffuse and act at considerable distances from the terminal release site (paracrinelike effects) extending the physiologic range of CNS-immune system contacts. The pattern of innervation of primary and secondary lymphoid tissues can be summarized as follows. In the bone marrow, plexuses of noradrenergic fibers travel in with

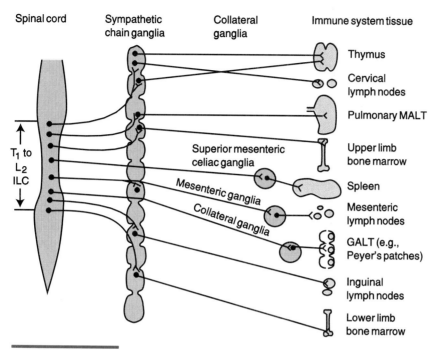

Figure 23-2 Sympathetic noradrenergic innervation of the immune system. These sympathetic nervous system two-neuron connections from the CNS to target lymphoid organs have been mapped in detail for the thymus, some lymph nodes, spleen, and GALT of the rat. The other organs have been shown to receive extensive noradrenergic innervation, but the precise preganglionic levels and ganglionic sources have not been determined yet. The presence of both noradrenergic and peptidergic nerve fibers in lymphoid organs shown in this diagram has been established by immunohistochemistry or fluorescence histochemistry, often in conjunction with neurochemical analysis of norepinephrine or the neuropeptides. Nerve terminals and varicosities using norepinephrine or neuropeptides are found adjacent to lymphocytes, macrophages, reticular cells, and other cell types in secondary lymphoid organs, and adjacent to thymocytes or bone marrow stem cells in primary lymphoid organs. These connections are better established than those for peptidergic innervation, shown in Fig. 23-3.

the vasculature and then distribute into the parenchyma. In the thymus, postganglionic sympathetic nerve fibers from neurons in the superior cervical ganglion and the upper sympathetic chain distribute with the capsular/septal system and arborize directly into the cortex where they end among thymocytes and along the vasculature of the corticomedullary junction. Nerve fibers containing neuropeptide Y (NPY) show a similar pattern of localization to that of norepinephrine and tyrosine hydroxylase (TH), the rate-

limiting enzyme in the synthesis of catecholamines, suggesting they are colocalized. Substance P (SP), calcitonin gene–related protein (CGRP), and vasoactive intestinal peptide–like (VIP-like) immunoreactive nerve profiles have been identified in the thymic capsular/septal system, closely associated with mast cells; SP and CGRP appear to be colocalized. Oxytocin and vasopressin appear in a nonneural thymic compartment.

In secondary lymphoid organs, noradrenergic fibers (and TH-positive fibers) arising

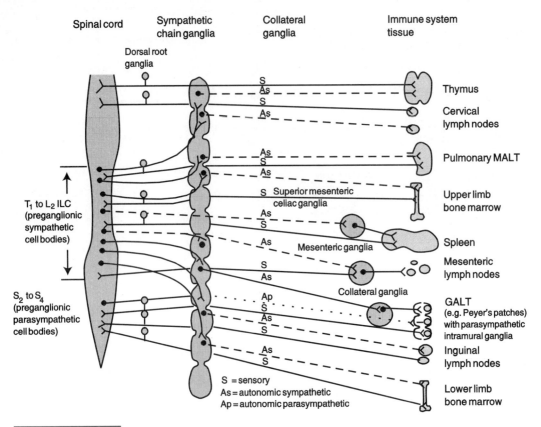

Figure 23-3   Possible peptidergic and cholinergic innervation of the immune system. Although peptidergic nerve fibers have been found in lymphoid tissues (SP and CGRP are usually colocalized; NPY is usually colocalized with norepinephrine; VIP, Met-E, CCK, and other peptides are less well described), careful tracing studies with peptide labeling are needed to determine whether they derive from primary sensory neurons, autonomic neurons, or other sources (e.g., gut enteric neurons). Dorsal root ganglia are primary sensory cell bodies. Sympathetic chain ganglia and collateral ganglia are sympathetic ganglia.

primarily from ganglion cells in the sympathetic chain or from collateral ganglia distribute mainly in the white pulp of the spleen, the medullary cords, and the paracortical and cortical zones of lymph nodes, and in the lamina propria and thymus-dependent areas of GALT. Electron microscopic studies have revealed TH-positive noradrenergic nerve terminals forming direct synaptic contacts with T lymphocytes and macrophages in the thymus-dependent periarteriolar lymphatic sheath (PALS) area and along the marginal sinus of the spleen, the organ in which these contacts have been most intensively studied.

NPY-containing nerve fibers in the rodent spleen appear to be colocalized with noradrenergic fibers. Nerve fibers containing SP and CGRP are also present in the spleen where they distribute around the central arterioles and large venous sinuses, travel in the trabeculae, and extend into both the red pulp and the PALS. Additional putative neurotransmitters found in the murine spleen include somatostatin, cholecystokinin (CCK), neurotensin, methionine-enkephalin (Met-E), and VIP.

The observations described in the preceding text are illustrated in Figs. 23-4 to 23-10.

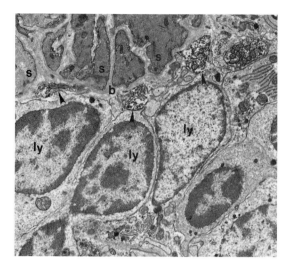

Figure 23-4 Electron micrograph showing tyrosine-hydroxylase positive (TH⁺) sympathetic nerve terminals (arrowheads) in the adventitial zone between the smooth muscle cell(s) along a central artery of the white pulp of a rat spleen, and T lymphocytes (ly) in the periarteriolar lymphatic sheath (PALS). The nerve terminals are separated from the smooth muscle cells by at least a basement membrane (b), but demonstrate close apposition (tips of the arrowheads) with membranes of the lymphocyte.

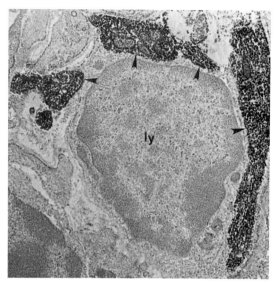

Figure 23-5 Electron micrograph showing numerous TH⁺ noradrenergic sympathetic nerve terminals (arrowheads) adjacent to a single lymphocyte (ly) in the periarteriolar lymphatic sheath of the white pulp of a mouse spleen. Long zones of direct apposition between nerves and lymphocytes are present.

Neurotransmitters, Neuropeptides, and Immunity

As just discussed, noradrenergic sympathetic nerve fibers innervate primary and secondary lymphoid tissues, ending in compartments where T lymphocytes and antigen-presenting cells are present. Sympathetic denervation surgically (by ganglionectomy) or chemically (with the neurotoxin 6-hydroxydopamine) depletes splenic norepinephrine by 90 percent or more, indicating that the neurotransmitter is derived almost entirely from the neural compartment of the spleen. Electrical stimulation studies and turnover studies reveal that the noradrenergic transmitter, norepinephrine, is released into the extracellular fluid of the spleen where it is available to act as a neurotransmitter in a paracrine fashion.

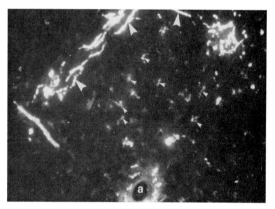

Figure 23-6 Fluorescence histochemical micrograph of fluorescent noradrenergic nerve fibers in the white pulp of a rat spleen. Fibers surround the central arteriole (a) (although some of these terminals also abut adjacent lymphocytes), extend along the outer periarteriolar lymphatic sheath near the marginal zone (large arrowheads), and distribute in scattered profiles among cells in the periarteriolar lymphatic sheath (small arrowheads).

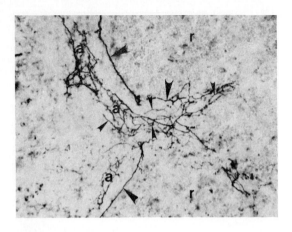

Figure 23-7 TH⁺ nerve fibers in the white pulp of a rat spleen. These fibers course adjacent to a central artery (a) in longitudinal profile, along the marginal sinus at the outer edge of the periarteriolar lymphatic sheath (large arrowhead), and among lymphocytes in the parenchyma of the white pulp (small arrowheads). TH⁺ nerve fibers are not present in the adjacent red pulp (r).

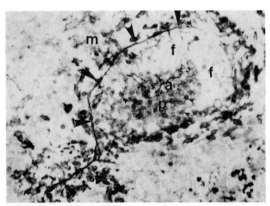

Figure 23-8 TH⁺ fibers in the white pulp of a rat spleen, in the same sites as in Fig. 23-7. In this section, a second immunocytochemical staining of T lymphocytes (using the OX-19 monoclonal antibody) demonstrated TH⁺ fibers among T lymphocytes near the central arteriolar system (a), and although stain for ED3⁺ macrophages along the marginal sinus demonstrates TH⁺ fibers at the outer periarteriolar lymphatic sheath (p), TH⁺ fibers are also present in the parenchyma of the white pulp. A few fibers (arrowheads) course along a follicle (f) populated by B lymphocytes (unstained). [Triple-label immunohistochemistry for TH⁺ nerves (nickel-enhanced to show the nerves as dark black), OX-19 for lymphocytes, and ED3 for macrophages; rat spleen.]

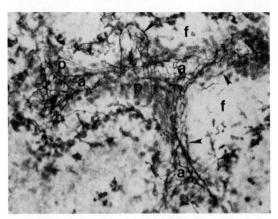

Figure 23-9 TH⁺ fibers (large arrowheads) course along the marginal sinus of the white pulp of a rat spleen. The macrophages along the marginal sinus are doubly counterstained with antibody for ED3 (macrophages). T lymphocytes are counterstained with antibody for OX-19, and show up as small circular cells (small arrowheads) in the center of the white pulp. Key: a = central artery, p = PALS, f = follicle, m = marginal zone. [Triple-label immunohistochemistry for TH⁺ nerves (nickel-enhanced), ED3⁺ macrophages (large dark cells), and OX-19⁺ T lymphocytes (small cells in the PALS); rat spleen.]

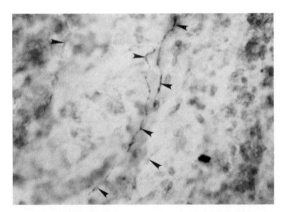

Figure 23-10 SP⁺ nerve fibers (arrowheads) coursing through the cortex of the thymus in a rat. The thymocytes are counterstained with OX-19 monoclonal antibody. SP⁺ nerves course adjacent to thymocytes in the cortex, regardless of whether they run through small extensions of the septa or run directly through the parenchyma. There are no barriers to diffusion of neurotransmitter between nerves and thymocytes. [Double-label immunohistochemistry for SP⁺ nerves and thymocytes (OX-19); rat thymus.]

Norepinephrine may also be available in higher concentrations from direct interactions resembling synapses with specific lymphocytes in the PALS. Beta adrenoceptors, particularly those of the β_2 subclass, are present on B and T lymphocytes, on monocytes and macrophages, and on granulocytes. Sympathectomy in adult rodents results in upregulation of β adrenoceptors on splenocytes; such upregulation on β adrenoceptors following denervation also is seen on cells of nonimmunologic relevance in the periphery. Beta adrenoceptors on lymphocytes are linked through a cyclic-AMP (cAMP) second messenger system, providing strong evidence of an immunomodulatory role for norepinephrine, possibly through cAMP generation and subsequent phosphorylation events. Although a comprehensive review of all examples of this role is beyond the scope of this chapter, a few basic findings are worth highlighting. Norepinephrine interacts with β adrenoceptors on thymic lymphocytes to inhibit thymocyte mitogenesis and enhance expression of cell surface differentiation antigens. Physiologic concentrations of norepinephrine enhance the primary in vitro IgM anti-SRBC antibody response; β blockers, but not α blockers, prevent this enhancement. Chemical sympathectomy of adult rodents results in diminished primary antibody responses in the spleen following systemic challenge and in popliteal lymph nodes following footpad challenge. The cytotoxic T-lymphocyte (CTL) response to allogeneic cells can be enhanced by mixed agonists and β agonists, and suppressed by chemical sympathectomy. Norepinephrine has also been reported to inhibit synthesis of complement components through an α-adrenoceptor mechanism and to inhibit activation of macrophages in a tumor cell lysis model. Chemical sympathectomy in adult rodents also has been associated with a suppressed DTH response, with an enhanced in vivo proliferation of lymphocytes in some but not all lymph nodes, with enhanced NK-cell activity in vivo and in vitro, and with increased severity of experimental autoimmune encephalomyelitis and adjuvant-induced arthritis in sus-

ceptible strains of rats. Finally, the egress of activated lymphocytes from secondary lymphoid organs appears, at least in part, to be under noradrenergic control. Before one can categorically attribute any altered immunologic activity associated with a particular behavioral state to an effect of norepinephrine, one first must know:

1. Whether norepinephrine is involved in the particular immune response being measured
2. The state of noradrenergic activity in the organism (high norepinephrine release in stress, low release in a poststress interval)
3. Numbers and kinetics of β adrenoceptors on lymphocytes
4. The magnitude of the antigenic challenge
5. Levels of immunomodulatory cytokines and hormones
6. Diurnal influences

Although the criteria for identifying an immune system–associated neurotransmitter have been formally satisfied only for norepinephrine, lymphocytes bear receptors for other neurotransmitters, and other neurotransmitters appear to play an immunomodulatory role. For example, T and B lymphocytes and macrophages possess receptors for SP, somatostatin, and VIP. SP enhances vascular permeability and increases local vasodilation. Both of these effects enhance the ability of lymphocytes to migrate to areas of inflammation. SP is a T-cell mitogen and can enhance T-cell proliferative responses to lectins. SP can enhance concanavalin A (conA)-induced IgA production by lymphocytes from mesenteric lymph nodes, spleen, and Peyer's patches. In addition, SP enhances phagocytosis by macrophages and chemotaxis by polymorphonuclear leukocytes. Systemic SP fiber denervation by capsaicin (neurotoxin) can result in diminished inflammation associated with herpes zoster infection (shingles) or rheumatoid arthritis in humans or rats. Selective denervation of SP fibers from lymph nodes can delay the onset of adjuvant-induced arthritis in rats as well as diminish the severity of inflammation. Somatostatin, acting through receptors on lymphocytes, inhibits many of the actions of SP. Somatostatin inhibits release of SP from the peripheral terminals of primary afferent neurons. It also has a direct receptor-mediated effect on lymphocytes and monocytes. Somatostatin exerts an inhibitory effect on phytohemagglutinin (PHA)-induced human T-cell mitogenesis, suppresses endotoxin-mediated leukocytosis, and suppresses release of colony stimulating factor activity by splenic lymphocytes. In general, VIP also inhibits a variety of immune functions (e.g., depresses T-cell but not B-cell proliferative responses to mitogens). The down-regulation of VIP receptors on T lymphocytes following incubation of these cells with VIP alters the interaction of T cells with the specialized high endothelium on the postcapillary venules where lymphocytes enter mesenteric lymph nodes and Peyer's patches, thereby diminishing T-cell ingress to these sites. Thus, lymphocyte traffic into GALT depends on the integrity of the high-affinity VIP receptor system on T cells. A VIP-nerve plexus is present in GALT just adjacent to the high endothelium.

CNS Recognition of Immune Reactions

Convincing evidence that the CNS monitors changes in immunity comes from studies in which neuronal firing rates in certain brain regions have been shown to change during the course of an immune response. During the peak of an antibody response, for example, increased firing rates in the paraventricular and ventromedial nuclei of the hypothalamus, and the preoptic/anterior hypothalamic area, have been described by several investigators. Neurochemical measurements of monoamines provide further support for the idea that the CNS monitors the immune status of an organism. Norepinephrine levels in the hypothalamus (a key regulator of neuroendocrine outflow and autonomic activity) were shown to be diminished during the peak of an antibody response, probably the result of increased norepinephrine turnover. Supernatants from mitogen-stimulated lymphocytes can effect a decrease in hypothalamic norepinephrine levels within 2 h after administration. Analyses of microdissections of specific regions of the brain of immunized animals during the peak of an antibody response have revealed decreased norepinephrine in the paraventricular nucleus of the hypothalamus but not the supraoptic nucleus, the anterior hypothalamus, or the medial hypothalamus. It is likely that IL-1 mediates such norepinephrine changes; Dunn has demonstrated that IL-1 can enhance norepinephrine in the paraventricular nucleus. Decreased levels of norepinephrine and serotonin were seen in the dorsal hippocampus and an increase in serotonin in the nucleus solitarius during the rising phase of immune response. No changes in monoamine metabolism were seen in other discrete locations, and no changes were noted during the decline of the antibody response. These immunologically communicated changes in central monoamine metabolism are consistent with the notion (discussed elsewhere) that cytokines generated during an immune response are in direct or indirect communication with specific hypothalamic, limbic forebrain, and brainstem autonomic sites.

There is also an accumulating body of data pointing to behavioral consequences of an immune state. For example, pituitary-deficient dwarf mice have a deficit in maze-learning performance relative to normal controls. Viral infections of mice and immune complex disease in rats have been associated with altered "emotionality" and/or learning abilities. Finally, recent data are consistent with the notion that immunologic abnormalities of the autoimmune strain of MRL/lpr-lpr mice can modify the animals' behavior which, in turn, operates to "correct" the immunologic abnormality.

ENDOCRINE INFLUENCES ON IMMUNITY

No immunologist questions the fact that, in vitro, productive interactions among subsets of T and B lymphocytes and accessory cells can result in the production of antibody and effector T cells. However, students of immunology must not ignore the fact that the neuroendocrine milieu in which these cells normally live can influence these interactions. The cell surface and/or cytoplasmic receptors for a diversity of hormones and the neuropeptides they express provide the opportunity for leukocytes to receive and transduce potentially modulatory and interactive signals from outside what has been traditionally viewed as "the immune system." In this section we will summarize data indicating that (1) hormones of the anterior pituitary and the adrenal gland are immunomodulatory, (2) lymphocytes and accessory cells receive neuroendocrine cues, and (3) products of the leukocyte components of the immune system can communicate with and modulate endocrine and nervous system responses. We shall even more briefly mention the immunomodulatory roles of hormones produced by the posterior pituitary, the thyroid gland, the pineal, the gonads, and the thymus.

The Anterior Pituitary Gland

Studies in the 1960s first pointed out that a strain of pituitary-deficient dwarf mice were immunologically abnormal. These animals displayed thymic involution, hypoplasia of bone marrow and secondary lymphoid tissues, and depressed cell-mediated and humoral immunity. An interrelationship between the pituitary and the immune system was substantiated by hypophysectomy and reconstitution protocols. The critical questions then became which of the many hormones produced by or stored in the pituitary, and which of the hypothalamic releasing hormones, could modulate immunity.

The hormones produced by the anterior lobe of the pituitary are grouped into three major classes according to their amino acid sequence identity. One group of hormones includes growth hormone (GH) and prolactin. Adrenocorticotropin (ACTH), α-melanotropin, and β-lipotropin constitute a second

group of peptides, which are derived from the precursor protein proopiomelanocortin. β-Lipotropin is the prohormone for a class of opioid peptides, the endorphins. The third group includes thyroid stimulating hormone (TSH) and the gonadotropin releasing hormones, luteinizing hormone (LH) and follicle stimulating hormone (FSH).

Growth Hormone

In several species, GH deficiencies consequent to hypophysectomy (hypox) have been associated with abnormal cellularity of the bone marrow and thymus, and depressed T-cell function, NK-cell activity, and antibody responses. These deficiencies can be corrected to some extent by the administration of GH. The injection of hypox rats with GH also causes marked increases in superanion production by resident zymosan-stimulated peritoneal macrophages. GH also has immunologic effects when it is administered to normal as well as to hypox animals and when it is added to cultures of leukocytes harvested from intact animals. Kelley and colleagues grafted aged rats with a pituitary cell line that produces both GH and prolactin, and observed a change in the architecture of the aged thymus and a reversal of age-associated changes in immunocompetence (e.g., decreased cell mitogen-induced proliferative responses and IL-2 synthesis). GH can increase the in vitro proliferation of transformed and normal lymphocytes and the activity of alloantigenic specific cytotoxic T cells from intact animals. Macrophages from the peripheral blood and lungs can be activated in vitro by GH to produce superoxide anions that nonspecifically kill ingested bacteria. This effect can be inhibited with a specific antibody to GH. As might be inferred from all these observations, high-affinity receptors for GH are expressed on thymocytes, resting and activated peripheral lymphocytes, and monocytes.

The impact of GH on immunity is influenced by the CNS, other hormones, products of pathogens, and the immune system itself. For example, secretion of GH is increased by viruses, bacterial endotoxin, and IL-1.

Thymosin fraction V, a group of low molecular weight peptides extracted from bovine thymuses, causes pituitary cells to increase their secretion of GH (and prolactin). This suggests a feedback loop between the thymus and pituitary (see below). The restoration of immunity in hypox rats can be antagonized by ACTH. Finally, at least some immunomodulatory effects of hypothalamic lesions may be mediated through the pituitary gland.

Prolactin

Although prolactin is best known for its role in mammalian reproduction and lactation, it also influences immunologic processes. Inhibition of pituitary prolactin secretion in rats with the dopamine receptor agonist bromocriptine (see Clinical Aside 23-6) results in suppressed antibody and DTH responses. Hypoprolactinemia has been associated with (1) a failure of the immune system to effectively deal with a challenge of *Listeria monocytogenes*, (2) a depressed lectin-induced mitogenesis of T and B cells that is independent of IL-2 production or IL-2 receptor expression, (3) a suppressed T cell–dependent activation of macrophages, and (4) a suppressed microbially induced T-cell production of IFN-γ. These effects can be reversed by administration of exogenous prolactin. In vivo administration of antibodies to prolactin can inhibit lymphocyte proliferation, and administration of exogenous prolactin or dopamine antagonists (to stimulate endogenous prolactin release) results in increased mitogenic responsiveness of lymphocytes and DTH responses and can reverse immunosuppression effected by cyclosporine.

Clinical Aside 23-6
Prolactin, The Dopaminergic System
and Immunity

Release of prolactin from lactotrophs is under the negative control of dopamine from tuberoinfundibular dopaminergic neurones. That is, the binding of dopamine to dopamine-2 receptors on lactotroph cells inhibits prolactin release. Dopamine-2–receptor agonists (e.g., bromocriptine or pergolide) mimic dopamine in that they also suppress prolactin release, whereas inhibition of the dopaminergic system, or the use of dopamine-2 antagonists (e.g., with haloperidol), stimulates prolactin secretion.

The complexity underlying prolactin–immune system interactions is just beginning to be appreciated. The interactions include the dopaminergic system (see Clinical Aside 23-6) and cells of the immune system itself. Some stimulated lymphocytes can produce immunoreactive prolactin directly, but IL-1 can stimulate the pituitary to inhibit prolactin release in vitro and in vivo. In addition, prolactin interacts with other products of the endocrine system. Circulating prolactin negatively regulates its own release by stimulating dopaminergic neurons. Thyrotropin releasing factor, some opioid peptide, VIP, and steroid hormones regulate (estrogens elevate, corticosteroids depress) prolactin levels. It is noteworthy that elevating exogenous or endogenous prolactin levels in mice whose cortisone has also been elevated can reverse some (e.g., mitogen responsiveness), but not all (e.g., lymphoid tissue atrophy), of the immunosuppressive effects of this corticosteroid. Immediate physical or behavioral stressors induce a rapid rise in prolactin levels, and prolactin, like ACTH and the catecholamines, is a "stress hormone." Unlike ACTH, however, the stress-associated prolactin increase is followed by decreased prolactin secretion and then refractoriness to further stimulation with repetition of the stressor.

Corticotropin (ACTH), Endorphins, and Enkephalins

ACTH and the endogenous opioid peptides α-, β-, and γ-endorphin are generated by enzymatic processing of the proopiomelanocortin precursor molecule (see Clinical Aside 23-7). ACTH, which can be released by corticotropin-releasing hormone (CRH) produced by neurons in the paraventricular nucleus of the hypothalamus, increases the output of corticosteroids from the adrenal cortex. This increase in plasma cortisol causes a decrease of the hypothalamic releasing factor CRH, which, in turn, decreases ACTH secretion from the pituitary and allows circulating cortisol levels to return to normal. This circuit is known as the *hypothalamo-pituitary-adrenal (HPA) axis* (Fig. 23-11).

Clinical Aside 23-7
ACTH, Enkephalins, and Endorphins

ACTH and the endogenous opioid peptides α-, β-, and γ-endorphin are generated by enzymatic processing of the proopiomelanocortin (POMC) precursor molecule. β-Endorphin is composed of 31 amino acids; α- and γ-endorphin are composed of the first 16 and 17 amino acids, respectively, that make up β-endorphin.

The enkephalins (methionine-enkephalin, or Met-E, and leucine-enkephalin, or Leu-E) are pentapeptides that originate from the 236 amino acid precursor molecule proenkephalin A. This prohormone, like POMC, is stored in the chromaffin cells and is released into the bloodstream during activity of the pituitary gland. Proenkaphelin A (as well as POMC) is also found in the adrenals. These prohormones release various intermediate peptide fragments (peptides E and F) as well as the final end products, Met-E, Leu-E, and β-endorphin. The main action of the enkephalins is on nerve cells that have opioid receptors (i.e., naloxone specifically antagonizes the opioid activities of enkephalins). *See* Lundblad JR, Roberts JL. Regulation of proopiomelanocortin gene expression in pituitary. *Endocrine Rev.* 1988;9:135.

The HPA axis is involved with the immune system in two ways. As will be described below, adrenal corticosteroids are potent immunomodulatory steroids. In addition, activation of the HPA is influenced by cytokines such as IL-1, IFN-γ, tumor necrosis factor, IL-2, and platelet-activating factor. The best-studied cytokine in this regard is IL-1. Direct administration of IL-1, either peripherally or intracerebroventrically, results in enhanced release of CRH from the hypothalamus into the hypophyseal portal circulation where it can trigger the release of ACTH from the anterior pituitary and the subsequent release of corticosteroids. It is unclear whether peripherally produced IL-1 can cross the blood-brain barrier directly via the relatively permeable circumventricular organs such as the organum vasculosum of the lamina terminalis and/or whether peripherally produced IL-1 acts centrally to cause the release of another signal molecule such as prostaglandin. Within the brain itself, microglial cells (and possibly astrocytes) as well as specific groups of neurons in the hypothalamus have been reported to produce IL-1. These cells of the CNS are in an appropriate anatomic position to modulate hypothalamic CRH secretion. Although binding sites for IL-1 (and some other cytokines) have been detected in the CNS, the cell types bearing such a binding site (e.g., specific subsets of neurons, glia, and other supporting cells) have not been fully elucidated, nor have the specific criteria for binding sites being receptors been fulfilled.

IL-2 can stimulate production of ACTH from pituitary cells. IL-2 administered to humans in clinical cancer immunotherapy trials has been associated with a rise in plasma ACTH and cortisol. It also has been associated with fever, hypotension, and neuropsychiatric symptoms, suggesting a central effect.

In vivo, ACTH can suppress both humoral (e.g., antibody responses, Arthus-type reactions, and anaphylactic hypersensitivity) and cell-mediated (allograft rejection) immunity. At least some of these and other in vivo immunomodulatory sequelae of the exogenous administration of ACTH can be attributed to the corticosteroid products of the target adrenal gland (discussed below) rather than to a direct effect of the pituitary-derived ACTH on cells of the immune system. However, in cell culture systems where endogenous corticosteroids are not present, ACTH itself can suppress antibody production, interfere with macrophage tumoricidal activity, modulate B-cell function, and suppress IFN-γ production.

Endorphins are produced by all lobes of the pituitary gland, the adrenal medulla, macrophages, antigen- or mitogen-activated lymphocytes, and T cells incubated with anti-CD3 antibody (CD3 is part of the T-cell antigen receptor complex). Endorphins (and

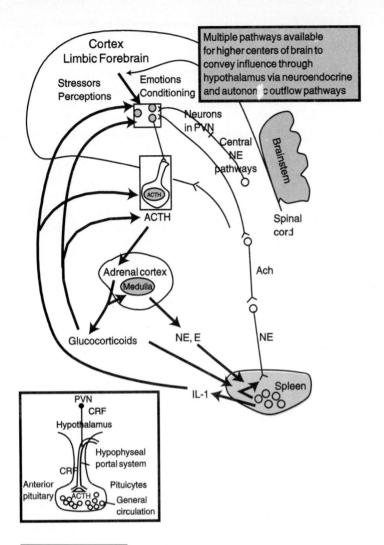

Figure 23-11 Integrated circuitry of the brain, the pituitary-adrenal axis, the sympathetic nervous system, and the immune system, using the spleen as an example. The CNS processes information from a wide range of sensory and molecular sources. The perception of those inputs depends on the animal's present state and past experience for interpretation and reactivity. Outflow from the CNS travels via the hypothalamo-pituitary axis and autonomic outflow. In the case of adrenal corticosteroid regulation, CNS pathways converge on the paraventricular nucleus (PVN), which contains the corticotropin-releasing factor (CRF) cell bodies. These cells send axons to the hypophyseal portal blood vessels in the median eminence, and release CRF into those vessels, resulting in a very high concentration of CRF reaching the pituicytes. The pituicytes that secrete adrenal corticotropic hormone (ACTH) react to CRF by releasing ACTH into the general circulation. Circulating ACTH acts on target gland cells in the adrenal cortex, resulting in glucocorticoid secretion first into the adrenal portal system (stimulating induction of phenylethanolamine N-methyltransferase, resulting in increased epinephrine synthesis and release) and then into the general circulation. Glucocorticoids can suppress the proliferation and activity of unstimulated or nascent lymphocytes, while permitting activated cells to react

enkephalins) can modify antigen-specific or mitogen-dependent in vitro proliferation of lymphocytes, NK-cell activity, antibody responses, IFN-γ production, and chemotaxis of phagocytes. The net effect of an endorphin on a given immune parameter may be depression or enhancement. For example, ACTH and α-endorphin inhibit, whereas β-endorphin either enhances or has no effect on the primary anti-SRBC antibody response. The direction of endorphin-associated immunomodulation may depend on which amino acid sequence binds to the rel-

evant opioid or nonopioid receptor and/or on the stage of activation or differentiation of the particular lymphocyte that binds the endorphin in question. In addition, some of the literature is contradictory.

Several mechanisms have been proposed to explain the immunomodulatory activity of endorphins. Endorphins and ACTH may alter the immunologically relevant receptors on the lymphocytes to which they bind. Indeed, Heijnen, Ballieux, and colleagues have demonstrated that β-endorphin and ACTH modulate the CD2 (SRBC receptor) and CD3

---

vigorously, thereby enhancing signal-to-noise immune reactivity. Glucocorticoids also have a wide range of other functions, many of them suppressive, on cells in the immune system (see text). It now appears that IL-1, acting directly or secreted at the peak of an immune response, can act either directly on the hypothalamic CRF neurons or indirectly through secondary mediators via one of the circumventricular organs (such as the organum vasculosum of the lamina terminalis), to activate them and enhance the activity of the CRF-ACTH-glucocorticoid axis. The PVN of the hypothalamus, as well as other descending pathways from the limbic forebrain, hypothalamus, and brainstem, can also activate or alter the activity of the autonomic nervous system. In the case of the spleen, these descending pathways act on preganglionic autonomic neurons in the intermediolateral cell column of the spinal cord in the T6 to T12 regions. These neurons act on cells in the superior mesenteric celiac ganglion (a prevertebral, or collateral sympathetic ganglion), which in turn sends its axons into the white pulp of the spleen, where those axons end adjacent to lymphocytes (particularly T cells) and macrophages (see text for full description of distribution). The action of norepinephrine (NE), the principal postganglionic sympathetic neurotransmitter, is very complex and depends upon the specific timing of its release and the status of the adrenoceptors of the target cells. It is clear that norepinephrine can influence individual cellular functions of lymphocytes and macrophages (proliferation, differentiation, production and secretion of products, and trafficking), collective actions of immunocytes (primary and secondary antibody responses, CTL activity, NK-cell activity, DTH responses), and subsequent fate of the challenged host (response to tumors, viruses, autoimmune disease). Norepinephrine and epinephrine (E) from the adrenal medulla are taken into sympathetic NE terminals by a high-affinity uptake carrier, and augment and reinforce the sympathetic response. Colocalized neurotransmitters also may be released during sympathetic activation (e.g., NPY). Both short and long neurochemical and direct fiber links (via afferents) may provide feedback at all levels of the neural axis. Thus, endocrine hormones, neurotransmitters or their secondary mediators, and cytokines or their secondary mediators may act on neurons to orchestrate the adaptive responses generated by the CNS. Clearly, there are direct and indirect links and feedback communication at all steps in this system.

epitopes on human peripheral blood T cells. Another mechanism may relate to the recent observations of Heijnen and colleagues that incubation of PHA-stimulated T cells with γ-endorphin results in a total disappearance of IL-2 receptors on T cells. Finally, γ-endorphin has been reported to bind preferentially to certain HLA class I antigens, suggesting an immunogenetic component of the effects of endorphins on immune responses.

Enkephalins (see Clinical Aside 23-7) bind to specific opioid receptors in brain tissue and may also bind to receptors on lymphocytes. Enkephalins are reported to be immunomodulatory with respect to (1) antibody formation in vitro and in vivo, (2) the numbers of peripheral blood leukocytes, (3) the number of T-cell SRBC rosettes, (4) thymic weight, (5) resistance to viral and tumor challenges, (6) leukocyte migration, (7) antibody-dependent cell-mediated cytoxicity, and (8) production of IL-2 and expression of the IL-2 receptor. The dose and nature of the enkephalin, the dose and route of antigen administered, and the timing of enkephalin administration relative to antigen all play a role in determining the direction and extent of the immunomodulation seen.

Behavioral states such as stress can be associated with increased levels of endorphins and enkephalins. In a paradigm that involved either intermittent (naloxone-sensitive or opioid-mediated) or continuous (naloxone-insensitive) foot-shock stress, enhancement of tumor growth occurred only when opioid-mediated intermittent stress (which also depressed NK-cell cytotoxicity) was applied. These observations reinforce the point made previously that all stressors need not involve the same mediators.

The Adrenal Gland

Corticosteroids

Following early demonstrations that corticosteroids caused lymphoid involution and exerted clinically important anti-inflammatory and immunosuppressive effects, studies of the mode and site of action of these steroids grew exponentially as did our understanding of the complexity of the immune system. Some of the dose- and regimen-related effects of exogenous corticosteroids in different species include (1) growth retardation and wasting, (2) lymphopenia, (3) increased catabolism of immunoglobulins and an associated decreased concentration in serum, (4) depression of antibody formation, (5) inhibition of adjuvant effects of *Corynebacterium parvum* on IgM antibody formation, (6) prolongation of tolerance, (7) inhibition of skin and renal allograft rejection, (8) retarded DTH reactions, (9) inhibition of contact sensitivity, (10) inhibition of the generation of cytotoxic effector cells, (11) reduction of mixed leukocyte reactions, (12) reduced generation of helper T cells, (13) alteration in lymphocyte recirculation pathways, and (14) depressed NK-cell reactivity.

The in vivo and in vitro effects of corticosteroids on monocytes and macrophages are as profound and immunologically relevant as the effects of corticosteroids on lymphocytes. These include a suppression of (1) numbers of circulating monocytes, (2) class II major histocompatibility complex (MHC) antigen expression, (3) phagocytosis and intracellular killing of certain microorganisms, (4) cytokine production and secretion, (5) cytotoxicity by interferon-treated macrophages, (6) numbers of epidermal Langerhans cells, (7) biosynthesis of some complement components, (8) expression of Fc receptors, (9) chemotaxis, (10) antigen presentation, and (11) production of inflammatory mediators such as plasminogen activator, elastase, and collagenase.

Corticosteroid effects are mediated via soluble cytosolic and nuclear corticosteroid receptors. Both activated lymphocytes and immature lymphoid cell express greater numbers of corticosteroid receptors than do either resting lymphoid cells or more mature lymphocytes. The corticosteroid-receptor interaction results in a complex that inhibits transcription and activation of specific genes such as those that encode for IL-1. Given that corticosteroids can impair IL-1 production, its broad effects on the immunologic consequences of activity of this cytokine should not be surprising.

Many of the aforementioned immunosuppressive activities of corticosteroids were ascertained from studies that involved pharmacologic rather than physiologic concentrations of hormone. However, there are at least two lines of evidence pointing out that these adrenal steroids actually do play an important immunoregulatory (physiologic) role in vivo. The first comes from recent experiments of Besedovsky and colleagues who reported a transient elevation of serum corticosterone in mice and rats during the peak of the antibody response and following the parenteral administration of soluble products of conA-activated T cells. They suggested that the antigen-induced increase in corticosteroids regulates overproduction of antibody and, as such, may explain the phenomenon of "antigenic competition" (the depressed primary antibody response to an antigen administered within a few days after the primary immunization of that animal with an unrelated antigen). Adrenalectomy partially abolished antigen competition and was also associated with enhanced B-cell activity. These observations led to the proposition that the immune system itself can regulate the HPA axis by means of cytokines released from activated monocytes. As discussed above, this idea has received significant support in that IL-1 stimulates secretion of hypothalamic CRH and increases the concentration of ACTH in plasma. Thus the HPA axis may be an integral part of immunologic circuitry involved in immune responses.

The second indication that corticosteroids and the HPA axis play an important physiologic role comes from the recent studies of Sternberg and others who have investigated the role of the HPA axis in the manifestation of experimentally induced autoimmune inflammatory diseases. In response to a single intraperitoneal injection of streptococcal cell wall peptidoglycan polysaccharide, LEW/N strain rats develop a biphasic arthritis characterized by an initial acute thymus-independent and a subsequent chronic thymus-dependent phase. LEW/N rats are also susceptible to a variety of autoimmune inflammatory diseases including orchitis, uveitis, thyroiditis, collagen- and adjuvant-induced arthritis, and experimental allergic encephalomyelitis. By contrast, Fisher 344 strain rats are remarkably resistant to the development of arthritis induced by streptococcal cell wall peptidoglycan polysaccharide, as well as to the other autoimmune inflammatory diseases just listed. These observations led to the hypothesis that susceptible LEW/N rats, but not resistant Fisher rats, have a defect in their immune system–HPA axis response to inflammatory and other stress mediators. The logic underlying this hypothesis is that if increased systemic corticosteroids constitute the final effector stage in the immune system–HPA axis and if physiologic levels of corticosteroids play a critical role in preventing inflammation, then a defect in the HPA axis could result in an increase in an inflammatory response. This hypothesis was supported by several facts. First, the plasma ACTH and glucocorticoid responses to injections of either streptococcal cell wall peptidoglycan polysaccharide or IL-1 are reduced dramatically in LEW/N female rats relative to Fisher 344 rats. Second, treatment of LEW/N female rats with physiologic levels of a synthetic corticosteroid (dexamethasone) significantly suppresses the severity of the inflammatory response. Third, interruption of the HPA axis of Fisher 344 female animals with a corticosteroid receptor antagonist results in a striking systemic inflammatory response to streptococcal cell wall peptidoglycan polysaccharide in this normally inflammatory disease–resistant strain. Subsequent studies have shown that the defect in the ACTH in the LEW/N females appears to be the secondary result of a defect in regulation of CRH secretion and biosynthesis in the paraventricular nucleus of the hypothalamus.

An avian model of human Hashimoto's autoimmune thyroiditis is also associated with an abnormal glucocorticoid response to inflammation. The obese strain of chickens develops autoimmune thyroiditis and displays T-cell hyperreactivity to antigens and mitogens. When chickens of this strain are immunized, they do not show the increase in corticosteroids seen in other strains. Similarly, they do not display the corticosteroid response following an injection of cytokines that was described above. However, when they are treated with physiologic concentrations of hydrocortisone, their T-cell hyperreactivity and the lymphoid infiltration of their thyroids are ameliorated.

It has long been known that stress activates the HPA axis, thereby elevating corticosteroids. It is also apparent that the effects of stress are associated with some alterations of immune function. In addition, at least some forms of stress are associated with an altered susceptibility to infection and neoplastic disease. Despite the fact that the corticosteroid-induced down-regulatory modulations of the immune system are extensive, it would be simplistic to attribute all immunologic consequences of altered behavioral states solely to increased adrenocortical steroids. At low concentrations, corticosteroids exert stimulatory effects on certain immunologic responses; higher concentrations routinely appear inhibitory. Also, the effects of opioid peptides and catecholamines that are produced in the adrenal medulla are subject to hypothalamic and pituitary influences and are themselves immunomodulatory. Finally, as noted earlier in this chapter, stress-induced immunosuppression has been observed in adrenalectomized animals, and some aspects occur in hypophysectomized rats. Therefore, it appears that both the hypothalamo-pituitary systems and direct nervelike connections are involved in translation of behavioral states into alterations of immunologic functions.

The adrenal medulla is the site of synthesis of the catecholamines, serotonin, and opioid peptides. Hormones as well as nerve stimulation are involved in the normal regulation of catecholamine synthesis by the adrenal medulla. Nerve stimulation releases acetylcholine from the preganglionic nerve endings, which stimulates catecholamine release from adrenal medulla cells. Corticosteroids control production of medullary TH,

the rate-limiting enzyme of catecholamine synthesis, as well as phenylethanolamine N-methyltransferase, the enzyme that converts norepinephrine to epinephrine. The increased rate of synthesis of catecholamines during stress is integrated with, but not entirely dependent upon, production of ACTH, corticosteroids, and perhaps other trophic hormones produced by the pituitary. Epinephrine, in turn, stimulates the release of ACTH from the pituitary gland and has a synergistic effect with CRH. At the same time, catecholamines inhibit the release of other pituitary hormones such as prolactin, GH, LH, and FSH. Therefore, there is a mutual regulatory interaction between catecholamines and the pituitary. The immunologically relevant effects resulting from norepinephrine produced and released locally in the nerves innervating lymphoid organs or from circulating norepinephrine and epinephrine acting transiently from the circulation or taken up by the catecholamine-specific high-affinity carriers on sympathetic nerve terminals and subsequently released are described elsewhere in this chapter.

The Posterior Pituitary Gland

The two neuroendocrine or neurohypophyseal hormones, arginine vasopressin (AVP) and oxytocin, and their carrier neurophysins, are synthesized by neurons in supraoptic and paraventricular nuclei of the hypothalamus and transported to nerve endings in the posterior pituitary gland (neurohypophysis). Very little information about possible immunomodulatory roles of these neuroendocrine hormones is available. Antagonist studies suggest that there is an AVP-type receptor on lymphocytes. Although AVP is neither mitogenic nor costimulatory for thymocytes, it, as well as oxytocin, can replace IL-2 requirements for T-cell-mitogen induction of IFN-γ in mouse spleen cell cultures. That is, it can provide helper signals. The structural basis for these helper signals appears to reside in the six N-terminal amino acids of AVP.

The Gonads

Immunologic dogma holds that females are generally less prone to infection, produce higher antibody titers, reject skin allografts across so-called weak histocompatibility barriers more rapidly, respond better to mitogens and particulate antigens, and have a higher frequency of certain autoimmune diseases than do males of the same outbred species or inbred strain. Ablation studies and replacement protocols in which animals receive either estrogens or androgens have revealed that gonadal steroids may contribute to this sexual dimorphism in immunologic reactivity. The nature of the effects reported in the literature are variable and, to some extent, depend on species, strain, concentration and nature of antigen, and the hormonal and estrous cycle status of the animal. Overall, however, suppressive effects are dominant. Thymectomy and gonadectomy studies have revealed that many of these effects may be attributable to an interrelationship between the development and function of the gonads and the thymus (see below). For example, female nude mice, which are athymic as part of the nude phenotype, have atrophic ovaries. Neonatal thymectomy also leads to ovarian dysgenesis which can be restored by grafting either the thymus, thymocytes, or splenocytes. Prepubertal orchidectomy of mice delays thymic involution and is associated with enlarged nodes and spleens. Marked effects of prepubertal orchidectomy on the thymuses of strains of mice prone to autoimmune disease also have been noted. Oophorectomy has been reported to enhance in vivo alloimmune reactivity of females. In such studies, females with transplanted testes showed a significantly lower incidence of rejection than oophorectomized animals without testicular grafts. The nature of this thymus-gonad interaction may be related to the fact that specific sex hormone cytoplasmic receptors are found in thymic epithelial cells. Both ovarian and testicular hormones exert a modulating effect on the thymic epithelium via these receptors. Estrogen-receptor concentrations are significantly higher in female mice than in male mice. Castration elevates thymic estrogen receptors in males to levels that are nearly equivalent to those in females. It is proposed that effects of gonadal steroids on the thymic epithelium secondarily influence the behavior of thymocytes and that this, in turn, regulates the immune response. In addition to this indirect effect on developing T cells, sex hormones may directly or indirectly affect B cells and macrophages. In addition, sex hormones may exert hemopoietic influences by regulating the differentiation pathways of pluripotent stem cells in the bone marrow.

The Thyroid Gland

The surgical removal of the thyroid from perinatal rats, or feeding young chicks thiouracil, a goitrogen which interferes with thyroid function, has been reported to cause a reduced number of lymphocytes, decreased antibody responses in vivo, and diminished proliferative T-cell responses in vitro. When adult rats were thyroidectomized, antibody production and cell proliferative responses were still reduced, but the loss of cells in the lymphoid tissue did not alter the histologic appearance of these organs and no wasting occurred. As previously mentioned, a strain of pituitary-deficient dwarf mice are immunologically compromised. Their immune function can be restored to nearly normal or above normal levels after administration of thyroxine (T_4) or T_4 plus growth hormone. It has also been suggested that the relative deficiency of thyroid hormones that accompanies aging may contribute to the age-related decline in immune function.

When normal animals are given T_4, or when normal lymphocytes are cultured in T_4-containing medium, the number of lymphocytes (particularly T cells) is increased, as are antibody responses. Triiodothyronine (T_3) is thought to be antagonistic to T_4 in vitro (but not in vivo), since it causes decreased proliferative responses to B- and T-cell mitogens.

The Thymus

For reasons that are unclear, most immunologists have not paid much attention to the endocrine function of the thymus, a function that was known long before this organ became recognized as a central lymphoid tissue involved in positive and negative selection of maturing T cells. It is clear, however, that various thymic peptides can modulate lymphocytes directly and/or mediate changes on the immune system via hormonal and neural pathways. For example, thymosin fraction 5 (TF5), a partially purified extract from bovine thymuses, and two of its sequenced constituent peptides, thymosin α_1 and thymosin β_4, can (1) induce lymphopoiesis, (2) stimulate maturation of T cells, (3) restore full T-cell reactivity in adult thymectomized mice, and (4) enhance in vitro mitogen responses, alloreactivity, antibody production, and IL-2 production. These thymic peptides also can alter the activity of neuroendocrine circuits. TF5 increases secretion of ACTH, β-endorphin, corticosteroids, GH, and prolactin; and TF5 also can block binding of corticosteroids to their receptors in lymphocytes. TF5 and thymosin β_4 can stimulate secretion of LHRF from the hypothalamus. Intracerebroventricular injection of thymosin β_4, but not thymosin α_1, into the lateral ventricles of the mouse causes significant increases in circulating corticosterone. These and other data argue for a thymus-pituitary-adrenal axis modulated by thymosin α_1 and a thymus-pituitary-gonadal axis modulated by thymosin β_4.

The Pineal Gland

Circulating levels of melatonin, a major hormonal secretory product of the pineal gland, reflect a diurnal rhythmicity (highest in the dark cycle) that is controlled by a circadian clock in the suprachiasmatic nucleus of the hypothalamus. This nucleus influences the pineal gland via descending pathways that regulate sympathetic outflow from the T1 preganglionic neurons to the superior cervical ganglion and then to the pineal gland. Pinealectomy or pharmacologic disruption of melatonin biosynthesis depresses antibody synthesis. Moreover, administration of exogenous melatonin to normal mice has been reported to increase the primary and secondary antibody responses to SRBCs (but not to a thymus-independent antigen), providing it is given during the animals' dark cycle when melatonin synthesis is maximal. Although melatonin administration does not appear to influence the development of a primary CTL response in vaccinia virus–infected animals, injections of melatonin during viral priming is associated with a significantly enhanced secondary CTL response. According to recent studies of Maestroni and colleagues, the opioid antagonist naltrexone antagonizes the immunoaugmentary effects of exogenously administered melatonin. Additional data from this laboratory are consistent with the possibility that melatonin actually stimulates activated T cells to release opioid agonists (see below), which in turn, enhance the immune response of normal mice.

HORMONES PRODUCED BY LYMPHOCYTES

One of the more intriguing observations in psychoneuroimmunology is that some leukocytes can produce a variety of bonafide neuroendocrine peptides. Blalock, Smith, and colleagues were the first to convincingly demonstrate that murine lymphocytes treated with lipopolysaccharide (LPS) or Newcastle disease virus can produce ACTH and endorphins. A small number of T cells, B cells, and NK cells produce ACTH in response to Newcastle disease virus; only B cells cultured with LPS produce ACTH. These same proopiomelanocortin-derived peptides also are produced constitutively by a subpopulation of mouse macrophages. Interestingly, lymphocytes, like cells of the anterior pituitary, produce ACTH and β-endorphin in response to CRH. Whether leukocyte-derived ACTH is capable of eliciting corticosteroid responses in hypox mice injected with virus and whether this response can be inhibited by a synthetic corticosteroid are points of controversy in the literature. It is likely that ACTH and other anterior pituitary peptides produced by lymphocytes or other leukocytes, when released, exert their main effects within the local lymphoid microenvironment.

The neuroendocrine peptide repertoire of leukocytes is not restricted to proopiomelanocortin-derived peptides. ConA-stimulated leukocytes produce Met-E, immunoreactive GH, and immunoreactive prolactin. Some human T lymphocytes and cell lines stimulated with staphylococcal enterotoxin A or thyrotropin-releasing hormone (TRH) can produce TSH, and chorionic gonadotropin has been detected in supernatants of mixed lymphocyte reactions.

These observations have led Blalock to propose that leukocyte-derived peptide hormones serve as endogenous regulators of the immune system as well as conveyors of information from the immune to the neuroendocrine system. His proposal that the immune system plays a sensory role in which leukocytes recognize stimuli such as viral and bacterial products, and secrete signal molecules that report this to the central and peripheral nervous system, is indeed provocative. It remains to be determined, however, whether leukocyte-derived hormones reach threshold levels in the serum consistent with communication with distant organs or whether they act locally as paracrine or autocrine regulators. In addition, direct stimulation of primary sensory nerve fibers may be elicited by cytokines or other secretory products such as histamine from mast cells.

CONCLUSION

The traditional view of the immune system held that the immune system is autonomous, i.e., self-regulatory, and therefore independent of the rest of the body. The contents of this chapter should make it abundantly clear that this view is no longer tenable. In general terms, experimental and clinical data and conditioning phenomena and stress effects demonstrate that behavior can influence immunity. Neural and endocrine signals can be received and acted upon by the immune system. Conversely, neural, endocrine, and behavioral responses are set into motion by signals from the immune system. No longer can we think of the lymphoid tissues as mere collections of leukocytes. Rather, we now know that the lymphoid microenvironment contains immunomodulatory products of nerve fibers and paracrine, endocrine, and autocrine secretions. The paracrine environment includes cytokines as well as other secretions of accessory or supporting cells such as serotonin, histamine, prostaglandins, and probably lymphocyte-derived neuropeptides. The endocrine environment includes hormones derived from the pituitary (ACTH, endorphins, GH, prolactin, LH, FSH, TSH), its target organs (corticosteroids, gonadal steroids, thyroid hormones, and others) and from the immune system proper (thymic peptides, lymphocyte-produced hormones). While most immunologists focus their attention on cell-cell interactions, these newly emerging data compel one to consider the immunomodulatory influences of blood-borne signals that do not depend on cell-cell interactions. Neurotransmitters are salient signal molecules with respect to cells of the immune system. Norepinephrine and several other neuropeptide neurotransmitters are present in physiologically effective concentrations as paracrine secretions and are available to interact with nearby cells. The direct contact of nerve terminals with lymphocytes and macrophages constitutes a new form of synapselike communication that may provide more direct signals in addition to paracrine communication, and may be superimposed upon the neuroendocrine milieu. Further, cells of the immune system may secrete substances, including hormones, that modulate their own function (autocrine regulation), neurotransmitter secretion from adjacent nerve terminals, or receptor expression on target lymphoid cells.

The immune system, endocrine system, and nervous system are communicating and interacting systems. Hormones may alter the expression of neurotransmitter receptors.

Neurotransmitters may alter the activity of hormones and cytokines interacting with lymphocytes or macrophages. Cytokines may stimulate nerve terminals to release neurotransmitters, in addition to their "primary" effects on cells of the immune system. Clearly, there are both long and short feedback loops between the nervous and immune systems. Short loops may be represented by a direct exchange, such as nerve terminal release of a neurotransmitter, such as norepinephrine, that modulates cytokine (e.g., IL-1) production, which in turn interacts with the nerve terminal to alter neurotransmitter metabolism and releases. Long loops may be illustrated by the CRH-ACTH-glucocorticoid axis, which alters lymphoid cell secretion of cytokine, which in turn feeds back to the CNS (limbic-hypothalamic) communication channel. IL-1 may be the most salient cytokine in this loop, based on its central effects on CRH neurones and on monoamine metabolism related to the HPA axis. Understanding all the circuits and channels of communication among the brain, behavior, and the immune system will continue to provide challenges in the twenty-first century; clinical application of what we already know about these interactions may well offer therapeutic benefits early in the last decade of this century.

SELF-TEST QUESTIONS

1. Design a study (clinical or basic) to determine whether a psychosocial stressor with its attendant neuroendocrine consequences might play a role in the development and/or progression of an autoimmune disease.

2. A recently published retrospective review of the 10-year history of patients with metastatic breast cancer revealed that those individuals who received group psychotherapy (as an adjunct to a conventional regimen of chemotherapy and radiation therapy) for the first year after clinical diagnosis demonstrated a strikingly increased survival time compared with age-matched control patients with the same diagnosis who received the same conventional therapy. How would you determine whether this observation was, at least in part, a reflection of immunologic differences between the two populations?

3. Outline evidence supporting the proposition that IL-1 can serve as a mediator of nervous system–immune system interactions.

4. Discuss how a growth hormone dysfunction might contribute to an altered susceptibility to a bacterial and/or viral pathogen.

5. Provide a definition of immunity that incorporates the fact that the generation of an immune response involves neural and endocrine contributions.

ADDITIONAL READINGS

Ader R, Felten DL, Cohen N, eds. *Psychoneuroimmunology.* 2nd ed. San Diego: Academic Press; 1991.

Blalock JE, ed. *Neuroimmunoendocrinology.* 2nd ed. Basel: Karger; 1992.

24

Aging, Nutrition, and the Immune System

A. Aging and the Immune System:
The Effects of the External Environment on the Internal Immunologic Milieu

INTRODUCTION

Individuals have differing capabilities to mount an immune response, and these differences are accentuated as they get older. As an individual ages, the immune response decreases, particularly the level of T-cell activity. A major challenge to research into the relation of aging and immunity is to determine whether a high level of response is correlated with increased survival. If this is the case, methods for modulating these declining immune responses using biologic response modifiers or pharmaceuticals may be indicated for the elderly.

Although many of the physiologic changes that occur with age have been known for centuries, the full nature and causes of these age-associated changes have been investigated only recently and have not yet been clearly defined. One of the most difficult aspects of studying aging is to differentiate between changes due to "normal" aging and those which are due to an underlying disease state. Many investigators feel, however, that even in the absence of disease, specific age-associated changes would occur. There is probably a unifying cause of these changes, regardless of the organ system affected. It has been proposed that the changes seen with aging are due to a lifetime of accumulating mutations that are debilitating but not lethal. Pronounced changes in the immune system associated with age may reflect the ability of immune cells to respond quickly and effectively to foreign antigens via cellular proliferation. This high rate of DNA synthesis may allow environmental stresses to be manifested more easily in the immune system than in other tissues. The inability to accurately and efficiently repair such mutations may result in the changes associated with age. It is unclear if mutation rates increase with increasing age. However, since DNA repair mechanisms appear to decline with age, it is logical to postulate that increasing numbers of DNA changes do occur.

An inability to effectively neutralize free radicals in the body may also contribute to the age-associated decline of the organism. The activities of the enzymes glutathione reductase, catalase, and superoxide dismutase have all been shown to decrease with age. However, the factors that cause the changes in these enzymes have not been delineated. Another mechanism of age-associated changes may be that as decalcification occurs with aging the toxic metabolites that have been stored in the bone during an individual's lifetime are released and the liver cannot adequately remove them.

The previous chapters in this book have presented the complexity of interactions between cells and their products during an immune response. In this chapter numerous observations regarding changes in the immune system with increasing age will be outlined. It is important to recognize that loss, or decline, of one of the immune components can affect all other areas of the immune response, resulting in a decreased ability to respond to foreign stimuli (resulting, e.g., in increased cancer and severity of infections) and/or an increased frequency of responses to self-antigens and thus an increase in autoimmune reactions.

CLINICAL OBSERVATIONS

Epidemiologic studies reveal that elderly individuals have an increased incidence of many diseases, including some infectious diseases, e.g., urinary tract infections, respiratory infections, and wound infections. Although deficits in particular components of the immune system may be involved, changes in the primary immune barriers of the body may be equally responsible for the increased susceptibility of the elderly to infections. Mucosal surfaces, skin, ciliated cells, tears, gastrointestinal pH, and mechanical activities (e.g., flushing and breathing) all provide important barriers to infection. With increasing age, secretion of mucus slows in the oral mucosa and in the nasopharynx; rate of clearance and total amount of mucus cleared from the lungs by cilia are reduced; sebaceous secretion slows; skin tends to dry; increases in gastric pH occur. All of these can lead to increased colonization by inefficient removal of bacteria and viruses, even in fully immunocompetent individuals.

In addition to increases in infectious diseases, elderly individuals demonstrate an increase in immune disorders. *Monoclonal gammopathies* are a group of related disorders of overproduction of a homogeneous immunoglobulin by a single clone of plasma cells. Table 24A-1 shows the spectrum of monoclonal gammopathies. All of these disorders are most prevalent in the elderly. For example, idiopathic monoclonal gammopathy is the overproduction of a single clone

---

TABLE 24A-1   The Monoclonal Gammopathies

Lymphoproliferative disorders associated with
  gammopathies
  Plasmacytomas
  Multiple myeloma
  Waldenström's hyperglobulinemia
  Chronic lymphocytic leukemia
  Lymphoma
Nonlymphoid disease associated with gammopathies
  Cancer
  Autoimmune disease
  Liver disease
  Collagen vascular disease
  Persistent infection
Idiopathic monoclonal gammopathy
Monoclonal gammopathies with undetermined
  clinical relevance

---

of immunoglobulin without associated disease. It occurs in about 1 percent of the population below age 50 and in 10 percent of persons over age 75, and progressively increases afterward. Although not by itself a clinical problem, a significant number of people with this finding may subsequently develop a lymphoproliferative cell disease, such as lymphoma or multiple myeloma, or may develop amyloidosis (see Clinical Aside 16-2).

The incidence of multiple myeloma also shows a marked increase with age. In this highly malignant form of monoclonal gammopathy, malignant proliferation of plasma cells results in pathology in many different organ systems due to the tumor products and the host response to them. Bone lesions are caused by osteoclasts responding to an osteoclast activating factor produced by the tumor cells. This factor, classically referred to as OAF, is now known to be interleukin 1 (IL-1). IL-1 causes bone fragility and hypercalcemia in these patients, and renal failure can occur due to hypercalcemia or to hyperuricemia. The increased protein load due to monoclonal light-chain secretion (Bence-Jones protein) may lead to the formation of intratubular casts of these proteins complexed with smaller amounts of other serum proteins such as albumin or fibrin and large amounts of Tamm Horsfall protein (derived from the tubule cells). Multinucleate giant cells surround these casts, causing further blockage. There is often a decrease in serum levels of the nonmyeloma immunoglobulin due to decreases in normal antibody secretion. There are also decreased production and increased destruction of normal antibodies, since breakdown and production rates are dependent upon serum concentration. Electrophoresis of the patient's serum shows a sharp spike in the γ region of serum proteins (see Appendix C); this spike is referred to as an *M protein*. A decrease in the amounts of each of the other immunoglobulin classes will also be seen.

Autoimmune reactions, with or without

associated disease, also occur more frequently in elderly individuals. Antinuclear antibody (ANA) and anti-DNA antibody, common in diseases like systemic lupus erythematosus (SLE), are examples of autoantibodies more often found in the elderly than in younger individuals. The mechanisms of control of antibody synthesis are incompletely understood, so the exact nature of age-related changes in these controls is still unclear. Mechanisms such as faulty suppressor T-cell function, change in the anti-idiotype network, and altered production of T-cell factors that control self-reactive cells have been suggested.

The frequency of the presence of rheumatoid factor in serum also increases with age; 10 to 20 percent of people over age 65 have circulating rheumatoid factor. Rheumatoid factor is an autoantibody to the Fc region of IgG. Although not a test diagnostic of rheumatoid arthritis, rheumatoid factor is often found in rheumatoid arthritis, where a high level of serum rheumatoid factor usually means more severe and progressive disease. These autoantibodies, produced in

the synovial membrane, can bind complement and may contribute to the cartilage destruction and bone erosion seen in rheumatoid arthritis. Although the exact mechanisms behind monoclonal gammopathies and autoantibody production are not clear, it seems that normal regulation of immunoglobulin synthesis by the appropriate immune cell networks is no longer in operation.

Cancer is the only disease that has a strict correlation with increasing age. Over 50 percent of all malignancies occur in persons over the age of 65. Since the exact causes of cancer have not been defined, it is not possible to delineate the age-associated changes that contribute to the increased incidence of cancer in the elderly. It may be that a fairly long period of time after exposure to the inducing agent is needed for the development of cancer. Therefore, the immunologic changes that occur with age may have no impact on development of cancer. It is more likely, however, that inefficient DNA repair, increase in free radicals, and decrease in immune response associated

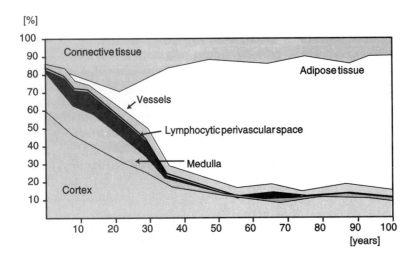

Figure 24A-1   Age-related changes of relative volumes (%) of thymic tissue compartments.

with aging do contribute to tumor induction and promotion.

IMMUNE SYSTEM-RELATED ORGAN AND TISSUE CHANGES WITH AGING

The Thymus

The organ that appears to undergo the most pronounced changes as it ages is the thymus. As described in Chap. 7, T-cell progenitors leave the bone marrow and circulate to the thymus, where they mature under the influence of the thymic hormones, e.g., thymosin. The age-related change that occurs in the thymus is referred to as *thymic involution*. In humans, involution is accompanied by the replacement of lymphoid tissue with adipose tissue. Due to this replacement, the actual size of the thymus does not change significantly, but the proportion of lymphocytes greatly decreases (Fig. 24A-1). Thymic involution starts at puberty and continues throughout life. By age 45 or 50, only 10 percent of the original lymphoid mass is left. Although hormone-secreting cells remain, thymic hormone production decreases with age, falling drastically at age 25 and continuing to decline steadily thereafter. While the ability of the thymus to produce hormones and thus allow maturation of T cells is decreased, there appears to be no deficiency in the ability of the bone marrow to produce T-cell precursors. The ability of these T-cell precursors to home to the thymus is also unaltered, as demonstrated by the presence of numerous immature T cells in the aged thymus. In addition, several investigators have detected an increase in immature T cells in peripheral blood of elderly subjects. Thus, even in the aged, the thymus may be an immunologically active organ, albeit at levels far lower than in the first three decades of life.

The Lymph Nodes, Peyer's Patches, and the Spleen

The secondary lymphoid organs, such as the spleen, lymph nodes, and Peyer's patches, are the sites where mature lymphocytes respond to foreign antigens. All of the secondary lymphoid organs contain a wide array of immune cells. Often B cells and T cells are separated geographically within the organ, with antigen-presenting cells (APCs) such as macrophages interspersed throughout the organs. Age-related changes in these compartments would be expected to have obvious immunologic consequences.

It is important to discuss the concept of compartmentalization before proceeding. Immune cell responses are often studied by isolating, or *compartmentalizing*, the relevant cells [B cells, T cells, natural killer (NK) cells, etc.] from a specific tissue. Each of these tissue "compartments" studied has a different proportion of immune cells, as well as a different microenvironment, and so the observed changes of one of the compartments may not always reflect similar changes in another. For example, studies of human lymphocytes have been generally limited to peripheral blood lymphocytes (PBLs), yet the PBL compartment may not be an accurate indicator of the changes occurring with increasing age in the secondary lymphoid organs, where most interaction with antigen occurs. Most of the studies describing organ-specific changes have been obtained from animal studies. Unfortunately, these studies generally have not been performed in parallel with investigation of changes in PBLs.

Although no major morphologic changes have been observed in any of the secondary lymphoid organs with age, changes in immune function have been observed. The general consensus is that in tissue with a preponderance of B cells, age-associated changes are not as pronounced as in those tissues dominated by T cells. Mucosal-associated lymphoid tissue (MALT) accounts for about one-third of all lymphoid tissue, and includes the Peyer's patches, tonsillar lymph tissue, and adenoids. Immune response in these tissues is effected primarily by B cells, mediating humoral defense. Some studies have indicated that aged individuals have fewer immunoglobulin molecules on the B-cell surface, but this may not be functionally significant. When B cells from elderly donors are mixed with T cells from young donors, T-dependent antibody synthesis is normal. However, T cells from elderly donors mixed with young B cells from young donors do not support normal levels of T-dependent antibody synthesis. Although small increases in the number of IgA-secreting B cells have been observed in these tissues in animal models, overall T-independent antibody response in these tissues is not significantly altered with increasing age. See Chap. 11.

In contrast to MALT, lymph nodes do show changes with aging. Composed of approximately 75 percent T cells, lymph node cells demonstrate a decreased ability to proliferate in response to the T-cell mitogens phytohemagglutinin (PHA) and concanavalin A (conA) in aging mice. In addition, specific antibody responses to various antigens are significantly decreased in the lymph nodes of aged mice as determined by plaque-forming cell assays. This decrease in the number of antibody-producing cells in vitro is reflected in a decreased systemic level of specific antibody. Humoral changes evidenced in these tissues are often due to changes in the T cells that are required for initiation of antibody responses. It appears that this decrease is due to diminished helper T-cell function rather than to an increase in suppressor T-cell activity. However, experiments to directly address this issue have not been performed.

Some morphologic changes with age have been described for the spleen, but these changes have not been consistent. Reported increases in splenic size with age may be secondary to underlying diseases. Functional decreases in T-cell response from splenic lymphocytes to mitogens with increasing age have been shown in mice and rats. T-independent B-cell function in the spleen is, however, unaltered with age. Some investigators have noted a decrease in the number of B cells expressing surface IgG, but, again, there appears to be no functional significance to this finding.

CELL-SPECIFIC EFFECTS OF AGING

T Cells

The relatively recent advent of experimental techniques to identify specific T-cell subsets, coupled with the ability to perform functional assays on immune cells, has allowed accumulation of significant information regarding the effects of age on immunologic parameters. Chapter 7 described current T-cell surface markers and functions ascribed to different subsets of T cells. This section will describe age-related changes of T-cell populations and of lymphokines that modulate T-cell functions.

A fundamental question is whether or not changes occur with increasing age in the percentage or absolute numbers of T cells or T-cell CD4$^+$ or CD8$^+$ subsets. Although inconsistencies among the results of the various studies exist, the following general statement can be made: There are no large changes in the percentage or absolute number of any of the T-cell populations with increasing age. Studies indicate that there is an increase in the number of memory T cells (CD4$^+$, CD45RA$^-$) in the peripheral blood of both mice and humans.

Although there are no major changes in the number or percentage of various populations of T cells, there is a consistent decrease observed with increasing age in the functional ability of these T cells. As described in Chap. 7, once T cells interact with an appropriate stimulus, the responding T

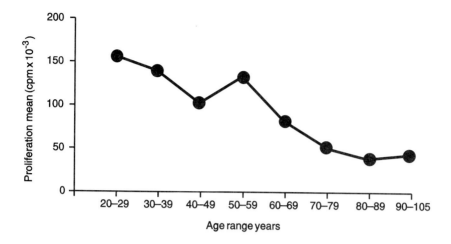

Figure 24A-2   Age-related decline in T-cell responsiveness to the mitogen phytohemagglutinin. Proliferation assessed by uptake of radiolabeled DNA precursors and expressed as counts per minute (cpm).

cells will proliferate. Using the T-cell-specific mitogens PHA and conA to induce T-cell proliferation, it has been demonstrated that the proliferation of lymphocytes from the spleen, lymph nodes, and peripheral blood of mice and rats, and from the peripheral blood of humans, decreases with increasing age (Fig. 24A-2). Similar decreases in lymphoproliferation are observed using anti-CD3 antibody as the stimulus. This decreased ability of lymphocytes from elderly subjects to proliferate is not due to differences in the amount of stimulus or the period of incubation needed for optimal proliferation, since lymphocytes from both young and elderly subjects demonstrate the same requirements for maximal proliferation.

Suppressor T cells have been implicated in both the decline of antibody production and the increase in autoantibodies. Pokeweed mitogen (PWM) causes polyclonal B-cell activation and the production of immunoglobulin. Significantly fewer PBLs of aged humans were stimulated to produce immunoglobulin in response to PWM than observed in the PBLs of young controls. The decreased response of the elderly was attributed to suppressor T cells, since depletion of CD8+ cells from the culture significantly enhanced the number of immunoglobulin-producing cells. In other studies, similar increases in immunoglobulin-producing cells after PWM stimulation have been obtained by depletion of monocytes. Therefore, several cell types may inhibit B-cell function in the elderly.

Whereas T suppressor cells decrease antibody response of B cells with increasing age, it has been postulated that a *decline* in the number T suppressor cells or in the function of these cells is responsible for the increased autoantibody levels observed with increasing age. Although a decrease in the number of suppressor T cells has not been a consistent finding among the numerous studies of T-cell populations, it is possible that there is a specific decline in the number of suppressor T cells specifically reactive with self-antigens. In addition to a decline in suppressor T cells, a decline in autoreactive anti-idiotypic antibodies has been suggested as a mechanism for the development of autoantibodies with age. Neither of these hypotheses, however, has been definitively supported experimentally.

A major point to consider is that although

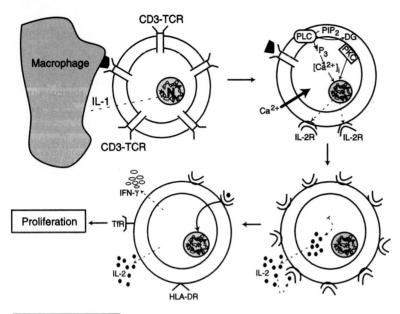

Figure 24A-3   Lymphocyte activation. The macrophage (or other antigen-presenting cell) processes and then presents the antigen to the T cell. After the antigen interacts with the TCR (T cell antigen receptor), the CD3-TCR complex initiates cellular changes, including liberation of diacylglycerol (DG) and inositol trisphosphate (IP$_3$) from phosphatidyl inositol bisphosphate (PIP$_3$) by the action of phospholipase C (PLC), increase in intracellular calcium, and activation in the nucleus (N) of the genes encoding interleukin 2 (IL-2), interleukin 2 receptor (IL-2R), the transferrin receptor (TfR), and HLA-DR.

most of the data regarding changes in immune function with age represent the mean response of a group of individuals, great heterogeneity exists in the responses of elderly individuals. Although 50 to 60 percent of any elderly population demonstrate about half the proliferative response of young controls, as many as 40 percent of elderly *individuals* can have proliferative responses comparable to responses of young subjects. The remaining elderly subjects (generally 10 to 20 percent) demonstrate responses at <20 percent of the mean response of young controls. A recent study further demonstrates the importance of determining the response of an individual. Although

the investigators found that the mean percentage of T cells of an elderly *population* of men did not significantly decrease with increasing age, the percentage of T cells of an *individual* did significantly decrease relative to earlier assessments of the individual's cells within 3 years before death. This decrease in T cells was observed in all causes of death.

Since decreased lymphoproliferation is a characteristic of lymphocytes from many elderly subjects, the mechanism of this decline has been investigated. In order to define the changes observed in lymphocytes of elderly subjects in the proper context, a review of the material presented in Chaps. 6 and 7 on the events that occur during lymphocyte activation may be helpful (Fig. 24A-3). The foreign substance (i.e., antigen or mitogen) must interact with a specific receptor on the surface of the T cell. In a classic interaction, an antigen-presenting cell (APC) would process the antigen and present it in the context of major histocompatibility complex (MHC) class II molecules to the T cell. The interaction of T cells with the APC leads to T-cell activation. Lymphokines such as IL-1 are involved in the process, which results in the expression of IL-2 or IL-4 receptors on T cells and further production of these lymphokines. The activation signal in T cells involves activation of phospholipase C, increase in intracellular Ca^{2+} concentration, translocation and activation of protein kinase C (PKC), and gene activation of coding regions for IL-2, IL-2R, and transferrin receptor. Alterations in any of these steps can result in decreased proliferation. Below is a discussion of age-related changes in the events that occur during lymphocyte activation.

1. Interaction with antigen or mitogen. Studies of the number and the affinity of receptors for T-cell mitogens in the elderly have revealed no changes in either. Similar studies are currently being performed for anti-CD3 antibodies and specific antigens. Related findings show that the number of T cells entering the first round of cell division is not different in the elderly, but there is a significant decline with age in the number of cells that progress through repeated divisions.
2. Changes in APCs. To date, no differences in the ability of APCs (e.g., macrophages) either to present antigen or to produce IL-1 have been observed. Differences in the level of MHC class II antigen expression on APC, however, have not been examined.
3. IL-2 and IL-2R. Production of IL-2 is significantly decreased in elderly humans and mice. Addition of exogenous IL-2 to cul-

tures of lymphocytes has restored the lymphocyte proliferative responses of old mice to the level of young, untreated control lymphocytes in some, but not all, studies. In humans, such treatment can increase the lymphocyte proliferative responses of the elderly, but not to the levels of young controls. Further, only about a third of the elderly humans demonstrating decreased lymphoproliferation will respond to the addition of exogenous IL-2. This may reflect an inability to bind IL-2. Examination of IL-2R in both humans and mice has demonstrated that there is a decrease in the number of both low- and high-affinity IL-2R. This reduction was more pronounced in the number of high-affinity receptors. Since the percent of IL-2R-positive lymphocytes after culture with mitogen has been directly correlated to the level of lymphoproliferation in both young and elderly subjects, the decreased ability of lymphocytes to produce IL-2R upon appropriate stimulation may be an important reason for the decrease in lymphoproliferative ability observed with increasing age.
4. Intracellular activities. Studies in mice have demonstrated a decrease in accumulation of cytosolic Ca^{2+} upon activation of T lymphocytes. These studies, however, have not been confirmed in humans.

In an effort to determine if the decrease in Ca^{2+} accumulation and subsequent decrease in proliferation is due to deficient transmembrane signaling via specific receptors, studies have utilized phorbol esters and calcium ionophores, agents that bypass the normal physiologic stimulation of membrane receptors. Phorbol esters directly stimulate PKC, while calcium ionophores open plasma membrane calcium channels and thereby increase intracellular calcium levels. The combination of these events leads to activation of nuclear events that occur during a normal immune response. These methods of T-cell stimulation have been shown to partially restore proliferation in aged T cells. The restoration of IL-2 secretion and IL-2R expression was of greater magnitude. Since only a small fraction of proliferative function is restored, a block at the membrane transduction of growth signals cannot be the only factor in the decrease in lympho proliferation with age.

More work must be done to delineate the biochemical mechanism of cell cycle activation before the effects of age-related changes can be determined. Studies of whether certain aged T-cell subsets show differential effects in activation at the subcellular level must be done before any therapies designed to augment T-cell function can be evaluated.

B Cells

The parameters studied most frequently for possible changes with age in B cells are cell number and immunoglobulin synthesis. Although it is possible to consider B cells independently, many B-cell functions are regulated by T cells. Therefore, in reports of changes in B cells with increasing age, the role of T cells must be carefully considered.

The absolute numbers of B cells found in the PBLs of elderly humans, as well as in the spleen of elderly mice and rats, are not significantly different from the numbers observed in young controls. This is also true for B-cell-rich tissues, such as Peyer's patches. However, this does not mean that B-cell functions are not affected by increasing age. It has been recognized clinically for many years that there is a decreased ability of elderly subjects to produce antibody in response to vaccination. The frequency of seroconversion following influenza vaccination is generally decreased in the elderly. In addition, the magnitude and duration of antihemagglutinin antibodies is lower in elderly individuals compared to young adults. Con-

comitant with this decreased antibody response to foreign antigens, there is an increase in autoantibodies.

The development of T-independent antibody responses has also been investigated. Carbohydrates, which are important antigens on the surfaces of some encapsulated bacteria, are T-independent antigens. Using the phosphorylcholine determinant of pneumococcal teichoic acid as a model polysaccharide antigen, a consistent, progressive decline in antibody levels was observed until age 70, when leveling off occurred. This pattern of response was confirmed using other T-independent polysaccharides. It has been suggested that leveling off of antibody decline may be a reflection of natural selection against the low-antibody responders, leaving the high responders as subjects. These studies appear to suggest that B cells alone demonstrate decreased response with age. However, several investigators have demonstrated that although T cells are not required for initiation of T-independent antibody responses, T cells can amplify or suppress these responses. Therefore, it remains to be determined whether the described decrease in T-independent antibody response with increasing age is a B-cell defect alone.

Nonspecific Immunity

It is tempting to speculate that nature can compensate for the shortcomings in one compartment of immune function in an individual by having another flourish, much in the same way a blind person acquires a more acute sense of hearing. Just as it is not clear whether the blind person actually hears better or is just more aware of that sense, so too it is difficult to say that nonspecific immunity can compensate for a declining specific immunity. In at least one situation, however, compensation for altered specific immunity appears to occur by an increase in nonspecific immunity. The athymic nude mouse, which congenitally lacks a thymus and thus lacks mature T cells, has a much higher level of NK-cell activity than does its euthymic relatives with mature T-cell function. Presumably, this is to compensate for lack of mature T cells. Many people approach the study of the nonspecific immune responses in elderly subjects with the hypothesis that these activities may be greater than those in the young as a way to compensate for decline in other immune defenses.

Macrophages

The macrophage and monocyte population of cells controls many different aspects of both specific and nonspecific immunity. Macrophages and monocytes are important in regulation of both B- and T-cell responses by the production of many soluble factors. They also direct the immune response by direct contact, such as when presenting antigen to T and B cells. They are important immunosurveillance cells and are a primary defense against tumors and bacteria.

As stated above, neither IL-1 production nor the ability to present antigen by macrophages is significantly altered with increasing age. Related to the efficiency of antigen presentation is the actual uptake of foreign materials by macrophages. Alterations in this ability will affect antigen clearance, removal of immune complexes, and antigen presentation. Studies of monocytes of humans and mice have shown no significant differences with aging in either Fc-receptor-dependent or nonspecific phagocytosis.

Infection and case fatality rate due to *Streptococcus pneumoniae* are estimated to be three- to fivefold greater in the elderly than in the young adult population. Given these facts, studies examined whether bactericidal activity of alveolar macrophages is decreased in old mice. These studies indicated that bactericidal activity is not decreased with aging; in fact, in some instances

older animals actually demonstrate increased ability to kill internalized bacteria. The ability of macrophages to kill internalized pathogens has been linked to the generation of the "respiratory burst" by these cells. No age-related changes in the ability to generate respiratory burst have been reported. In summary, the function of macrophages of elderly subjects is at least comparable, and possibly better, than that observed in young controls.

NK Cells

NK cells are another cell type involved in nonspecific immunity. They are important in tumor surveillance and in defense against bacteria, viruses, and parasites. NK cells comprise a large part of the *null cell* population, which is defined as those mononuclear blood cells that are non-B, non-T, non-monocyte. Since null cells are readily available from peripheral blood, many human studies have been performed. Most of the studies have indicated that NK-cell activity of the elderly either increases or is not significantly different from NK-cell activity in young controls. In some of these studies, aged individuals demonstrated both an increased number of NK cells and increased cytolytic activity per NK cell. Like mature T cells, NK-cell subsets have been defined by differences in cell surface markers and cell function. The most important NK-cell surface markers are CD56 and CD16. Different combinations of these two markers identify subsets that are functionally distinct. CD56$^-$CD16$^+$ cells are the most active subset and do not seem to change with age. CD56$^+$CD16$^+$ and CD56$^+$CD16$^-$ cells show lower NK-cell activity in young individuals than CD56$^-$CD16$^+$ cells, but selectively and progressively increase in number with advancing age. Table 24A-2 provides an overview of changes in the immune system with age.

Different strains of animals demonstrate varying levels of innate NK-cell activity. In some strains, increased activity of the

TABLE 24A-2   Overview of Immune Responses with Age

Activity	Human	Mouse	Rat
T-cell proliferation	↓	↓	↓
B-cell proliferation			
T-cell-dependent	↓	↓	↓
T-cell-independent	NC	NC	NC
IFN-γ production	↓	↑	↑
IL-2 production	↓	↓	NC
Macrophage	NC	↑	NA
NK cell	↑	↓	NA

NC = no significant change; NA = not well studied.

NK cells has been correlated with increased survival. This has not been studied in humans to date. It would be interesting to see if the immunologic fitness of a person could be gauged in part by NK-cell activity. Perhaps those who can compensate for age-related declines in specific immunity by increases in nonspecific immunity will live longer.

There is little, if anything, known about changes in polymorphonuclear cell function with aging.

SELF-TEST QUESTIONS*

1. Which of the following clinical findings is not observed with increasing frequency with increasing age?
   a. Idiopathic monoclonal gammopathy
   b. Autoantibodies
   c. Rheumatoid factor
   d. Mucous secretions
2. A white male, age 88, is immunized with influenza vaccine. He is exposed to influenza about 6 weeks later, develops influenza, becomes secondarily infected with *Streptococcus pneumoniae*, and dies. The most likely explanation for this scenario is:
   a. He did not respond to the influenza vaccine.
   b. Although antibody was in the serum, no anti-influenza antibodies were in the respiratory tract.
   c. The *S. pnuemoniae* bacteria were resistant to the host defenses.
   d. Nonspecific host defenses were nonfunctional.
3. Which of the following defects in host defenses *could not* be responsible for the above scenario:
   a. Decreased bacteriocidal activity of macrophages
   b. Decreased helper T-cell activity
   c. Increased suppressor T-cell activity
   d. Decreased NK-cell activity
4. Considering the normal activation scheme of T cells, all of the following have been shown to be decreased in elderly subjects *except*:
   a. Intracellular Ca^{2+}
   b. IL-1 production
   c. IL-2 receptor expression
   d. IL-2 production

ADDITIONAL READINGS

Cohen HJ. Monoclonal gammopathies and aging. *Hosp Prac.* March 1988:87–94.

Ershler WB. Why tumors grow more slowly in old people. *J Natl Cancer Inst.* 1986;4:837–839.

Krishnaraj R, Blandford G. Age associated alterations in human natural killer cells. *Cell Immunol.* 1988;114:137–148.

Makinodan T, Kay MMB, eds. *Handbook of Immunology in Aging,* Boca Raton, Fla.: CRC Press; 1981.

*Answers will be found in Appendix E.

Meydani SN, Blumberg JB. Nutrition and immune function in the elderly. In: Munro, Danford, eds. *Nutrition, Aging and the Elderly*. New York: Plenum; 1989.

Murasko DM, Nelson BJ, Silver R, Matour D, Kaye D. Immunologic response in an elderly population with a mean age of 85. *Am J Med.* 1986;81:612–618.

Rabinowich H, Goses Y, Reshef T, Klajman A. IL-2 production and activity in aged humans. *Mech Ageing Dev.* 1985;32:213–226.

Steinmann GG, Klaus B, Muller-Hermelink. Involution of the aging human thymic epithelium is independent of puberty. *Scand J Immunol.* 1985;22:563–575.

24

Aging, Nutrition, and the Immune System

B. Nutrition and Immunity

INTRODUCTION

Malnutrition is a worldwide problem, not only in third world or developing countries, but also in the United States, especially in those surviving on fixed or limited incomes, e.g., the elderly. Starvation in America is a greater problem in times of general economic downturn. A great deal is known about the relationships among malnutrition, impaired immunity, and susceptibility to infection in people living in developing countries. Animal studies suggest that undernutrition, as opposed to malnutrition, may actually have a *beneficial* effect on immunity—preserving or even increasing resistance to infection, malignancy, and autoimmune diseases. These observations raise questions about what level of nutrition is optimal for normal immune function and good health.

It is generally thought that undereating and excessive thinness are associated with an increased risk of illness, particularly infections. This is probably because infectious diseases are very prevalent in malnourished populations in developing countries, and underweight persons with chronic debilitating illnesses are at risk for infections. Our societal concerns about undereating are demonstrated by adults often warning children of the dangers of not eating properly.

Before we continue, a few important points must be made. First, malnutrition rarely occurs in a clinical vacuum. Many of the studies of the effect of malnourishment were done in the third world, where coincident chronic infection, especially parasitic, may occur. As seen elsewhere in this volume, chronic inflammation can have immunomodulatory effects, and parasites seem specially adept at altering host defenses. In addition other factors must be considered, such as crowding, unsanitary conditions, and extreme psychological stress (Chap. 23). Second, the timing of malnourishment is crucial in understanding the ultimate effects; prenatal and early childhood seem to be times when the immune system is particularly vulnerable. Postnatal dietary deficiencies may cause alteration of lymphoid organ development, intestinal localization of lymphocytes, or decreased mucosal immune responses. Thus, malnutrition that occurs while the immune system is developing might in part explain the high incidence of mucosal surface infections seen in malnourished children. Finally, the *type* of malnutrition is important. An individual may have a diet deficient in protein, calories, minerals, fatty acids, or vitamins, or any combination of these. Each type of deficiency may have a different associated immune problem.

MALNUTRITION AND IMMUNITY

Studies in Humans

It is known that people in developing countries, particularly children, have increased frequency and severity of infections (notably diarrhea and respiratory infections). It was once thought that this susceptibility was due solely to the protein deficiency of their diet. It is now clear that multiple nutritional deficiencies—protein, calories, fat, vitamins, and minerals—often coexist; each class of nutrients plays a major role in normal immune function. The facts that these malnourished populations are chronically exposed to or infected with a variety of infectious agents, and that infection, especially parasitic infection, is itself immunosuppressive have already been noted.

Malnourishment is associated with depressed cell-mediated immunity (CMI) and humoral immunity (HI) and with different phagocytic defects (Table 24B-1). The defects in CMI are especially prevalent and serious,

TABLE 24B-1 Immune Abnormalities Described in Humans with Protein and Calorie Malnutrition

Component	Tests	Immunologic Abnormality
Cell-mediated immunity	Lymphocyte count	Often ↓
	T-cell count	↓
	Interferon level and production	↓
	Proliferative responses to mitogens	↓
	Delayed hypersensitivity skin tests	↓
	Graft rejection	↓
	Helper T-cell count	↓
Humoral immunity	B-cell count	↓ or nl
	Serum immunoglobulins	Variable, often ↑
	Antibody affinity	↓
	Secretory IgA	↓
	B-cell homing	↓
Phagocytes	Neutrophil mobility and chemotaxis	↓
	Phagocytosis	↓
	Bactericidal activity	↓
	IL-1 production	↓
	Bone marrow reserve	↓
Complement	C_3	↓

but any of the abnormalities can predispose to infection. The majority are found in all starved persons, regardless of the reason for the starvation, and revert to normal with refeeding and a return to normal weight.

Several studies shed light on how semistarvation can alter immune function. In their classic work, *The Biology of Human Starvation*, Keys et al. reviewed many of the studies of victims of starvation—in particular, prisoners of war, victims of famine, and volunteers in human experiments. It is difficult to generalize about these studies because the circumstances of each differ markedly. However, leukopenia with relative lymphocytosis and atrophy of the thyroid and lymphoid tissue were among the more frequently noted abnormalities. Anecdotal reports about children living in the Warsaw ghetto noted that those who were the most malnourished had fewer and less severe infections (especially measles). This would suggest that there may be *heightened* resistance to infection in subgroups of malnourished persons; this seeming paradox will be expanded upon later.

At the University of Minnesota, Keys et al. studied volunteers who had an average weight loss of 25 percent of their initial body weight during a 24-week period of semistarvation. Leukopenia (with a normal white blood cell differential) was noted at the time of weight nadir, while total serum protein, albumin, and transferrin levels remained normal. There was no difference in the number or severity of colds during weight loss or the 12-week recovery period, as compared with normal controls. The study subjects lived in a relatively disease-free, comfortable environment, with medical and other support personnel readily available. Keys speculated that these salubrious circumstances allow the body to tolerate a greater degree of wasting than could be borne under natural, nonvoluntary conditions of starvation. In a study of prolonged fasting in 27 obese men, a rapid decrease in the peripheral blood neutrophil count was noted. After 1 month of fasting, the neutrophil count stabilized at about one-third to one-half of the prestarvation levels and did not return to normal until the subjects were fed more than 1000 calories per day. Eight of the subjects developed infections (type not specified) during the fast, but were able to mount a reactive leukocytosis and granulocytosis. It was suggested that the observed neutropenia might be secondary to an increase in the pool of marginated neutrophils rather than to a defect in production. In another study of fasting for 10 days, a progressive decrease in polymorphonuclear cell killing activity and decreased mitogen-induced peripheral blood lymphocyte proliferation were seen by the end of the fast. (See Clinical Aside 24B-1).

Clinical Aside 24B-1
Can Undernutrition Be Advantageous?

Drawing upon animal data, historical accounts of decreased frequency and severity of infections in the more malnourished of starvation victims, and their own observations in developing countries, Murray and Murray speculate that undernutrition may have a salutary biologic effect. They propose that undernutrition, within limits, is associated with decreased susceptibility to intracellular pathogens, a contention which has been supported by others. This is an attractive premise, from a teleologic perspective. Human beings have been hunter-gatherers and growers for millennia. In all that time we have always been subject to the whims of nature, with famine and drought following times of plenty. Yet human beings have survived. Given humanity's long history of undernutrition, it seems unlikely that malnourishment has led to immunodeficiency, which would predispose to infection, morbidity, and mortality. Rather, it seems reasonable that this "usual" level of nutrition should correlate with optimal immune responsivity, ensuring survival of the species during times of famine.

In addition, the Murrays suggest that low-weight persons have increased resistance to tumorigenesis. They propose that undernutrition leads to a generally growth-suppressing host environment; interferon and hypometabolism (including decreased T_3 and impaired somatomedin activity) simultaneously conserve energy and thwart cellular proliferation. Thus, leanness may actually exert a favorable effect on immune defense mechanisms.

Studies in Animals

Animal studies have examined the effect of nutrient-deficient diets on immune function and the subsequent development of infection, malignancy, or autoimmunity. These studies vary in animal species, design, diet, and the mitogens, antigens, or infectious agents used as stimuli. Thus, the results have been variable. The diet-related immunologic changes found are summarized in Table 24B-2. Isolated protein deficiency has been associated with increases, decreases, or no change in CMI and HI. In general, however, CMI is increased while HI is decreased in animals maintained on protein-deficient diets.

Animal diets deficient in protein and total calories may cause an increase in resistance to infection in the early stages of starvation. Later, the effect on immunosurveillance may be deleterious or helpful, depending on the assay used. Of note, protein-calorie deprivation increases the life-span of short-lived mouse strains, delays or ameliorates the activity of autoimmune disease in the lupus-prone MRL/lpr-lpr mouse, blunts the age-related decrease in immune function commonly seen in aged mice, and is associated with fewer spontaneous tumors.

Diets deficient in total fat are associated with increased murine cellular immune function and decreased lupus activity. Essential fatty acid deficiency interferes with inflammatory responses and with lupus and arthritis activity in the mouse models of these diseases; it is also associated with decreased allograft rejection, decreased antibody responses, and increased mixed lymphocyte and graft-versus-host reactions. The effects of linoleic acid deficiency include a decreased inflammatory reaction but increased allograft rejection and increased resistance to methylcholanthrene-induced tumors. Linoleic acid supplementation decreases allograft rejection, decreases cytotoxicity, and protects the animal against autoimmune damage in the experimental autoimmune encephalomyelitis model. (See Clinical Aside 24B-2)

TABLE 24B-2 Immune Abnormalities Described in Animal Models of Specific Dietary Deficiencies

Deficiency	Immunologic Abnormality	
Protein and calories	↑ Life-span of short-lived mice ↓ Autoimmunity in lupus-prone mice; blunts age-related changes in CMI ↓ Spontaneous tumors	↑ Resistance to *Babesia, Plasmodium* ↓ Resistance to *Listeria* ↓ Natural cytotoxicity ↑ NK-cell activity
Protein	↑ Graft rejection ↑ T-cell-mitogen responses ↓ Spontaneous tumors ↑ Resistance to viral infections ↑ CMI or resistance to *Listeria* ↓ Delayed-type hypersensitivity ↓ NK-cell activity	↓ Antigen-presenting cell function ↓/Nl Helper T cells for IgG production ↓ IgA response Nl Antibody response to *Brucella* ↓ Antibody response to sheep RBCs ↑ In vitro antibody response ↑ Phagocytosis of *Listeria*
Essential fatty acids	↑ T-cell-mitogen responses ↓ T-cell-mitogen responses ↓ Graft rejection ↑ Graft rejection ↑ Mixed lymphocyte reaction ↓ Cytotoxicity	↓ Experimentally induced arthritis ↓ Lupus activity in NZB/W mice ↓ Plaque-forming cells ↓ Antibody response ↓ Macrophage motility
Linoleic acid	↑ Graft rejection ↓ Inflammatory reactions	↓ Resistance to induced tumors

Clinical Aside 24B-2
Dietary Therapy of Rheumatoid Arthritis

From animal models we know that modification of fat in the diet may alter inflammation. We know that a low-fat diet can diminish the risk of atherosclerosis, but can a change in dietary fat alter human inflammatory disease? The most studied example is rheumatoid arthritis, a chronic inflammatory joint disease usually affecting the small joints of the hands and feet, the wrists, the ankles, and other joints. The serologic marker for this disease is rheumatoid factor (described in Clinical Aside 31-2). As noted above, one can modify the lupus experienced by MRL/lpr-lpr mice by modifying the fat intake. Likewise, by giving NZB/W mice (also a lupus-prone strain) a diet rich in coconut oil (deficient in essential fatty acids) or by giving them prostaglandin E₁, one can extend their life relative to mice fed a safflower oil–rich diet (which is replete with essential fatty acids). Mice fed a diet supplemented with menhaden oil (derived from an Atlantic cold water fish) also lived longer. Menhaden oil contains eicosapentaenoic acid (EPA; see Fig. 24B-1), a fatty acid which can be metabolized by the same enzymes which produce prostaglandins and leukotrienes from arachidonic acid; the compounds derived from EPA, however, are not proinflammatory, which is the likely explanation for the effect seen in mice. The same diet has a suppressive effect on collagen-induced arthritis, as well. Eskimos eat a diet rich in fish oil and they have mild platelet dysfunction and prolonged bleeding time, on the basis of impaired thromboxane synthesis (they also have a very low incidence of atherosclerosis—care to speculate on a biochemical connection?). Menhaden oil and other sources of EPA have been used in patients with rheumatoid arthritis. Modest but encouraging diminution of activity of disease has

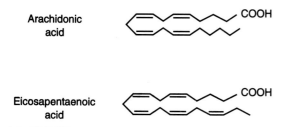

Figure 24B-1 Chemical structure of arachidonic acid and eicosapentaenoic acid.

been found in some studies. Reduction in the production of leukotriene LTB_4 and abnormalities of platelet activation were found in these patients.

Another possible dietary manipulation is the use of γ-linolenic acid, found in the oil of the evening primrose, as a supplement. Although the precise biochemistry is somewhat unclear, use of this oil has been associated with reduction in the severity of experimental autoimmune encephalomyelitis and arthritis in rats and rheumatoid arthritis in humans.

In general, deficiencies of minerals have been associated with decreased immune function (Table 24B-3). Iron deficiency was immunosuppressive in some studies. However, other studies suggest that iron deficiency may increase resistance to infection and that giving iron supplements to iron-deficient animals can cause worsening of infection. (Recall that transferrin is a negative

acute phase response protein [see Chap. 16, on the acute phase response]; denying iron to a microorganism can decrease the growth of the pathogen.) One folk remedy calls for the use of copper bracelets to decrease the severity of, or prevent, rheumatoid arthritis. No studies have demonstrated the effectiveness of oral or topical mineral preparations on this or other diseases.

It is clear that vitamins are necessary for the development of normal immune responses (Table 24B-4). Vitamin B_6 is involved in normal HI and CMI. In both young and aged animals, deficiency of vitamin B_6 is associated with lymphopenia and decreased antibody production. Supplementation with this vitamin has been reported to increase lymphocyte mitogen responses in animals and humans. Vitamin A deficiency has been associated with diminished NK-cell activity and interferon production.

TABLE 24B-3   Mineral Deficiences Induces Human and Animal Immune Abnormalities

Deficiency	Human	Animal
Iron	Lymphopenia ↓ Mitogen responses ↓ DTH ↓ Antibody response ↓ Phagocytosis, bacterial killing ↓ Chemotaxis	↓↑ Mitogen responses ↓ Killer-T cell activity ↓ NK-cell activity ↓ Antibody responses ↓ Bacterial killing
Zinc	Lymphopenia Lymphoid atrophy ↓ Mitogen responses ↓ DTH ↓ NK-cell number ↓ PMN chemotaxis	Thymic and lymphoid atrophy Lymphophenia ↓ Mitogen responses ↓ DTH ↓ NK-cell activity ↓ ADCC activity ↓ Killer-T cell activity ↓ Antibody production, especially to T cell–dependent antigens
Copper	No evidence of effect	Lymphoid atrophy ↓ Antibody responses
Magnesium	No evidence of effect	Eosinohilia and leukocytosis ↓ Graft rejection ↓ Antibody responses
Selenium	No evidence of effect	↓ Mitogen responses ↓ CTL activity ↓ Antibody responses, especially to T cell–dependent antigens ↓ PMN bactericidal activity
Excess	No evidence of effect	↑ Mitogen responses ↑ Mixed lymphocyte reaction ↑ CTL function ↑ Lymphotoxin (TNF-β) production

TABLE 24B-4   Vitamin Deficiencies Induce Human and Animal Immune Abnormalities

	Human-Disease Model	Animal Model
Vitamin A	Loss in the functional integrity of mucosal surfaces ↓ Lysozyme production locally	Lymphoid atrophy Lymphopenia ↓ Mitogen responses ↓ Antibody responses
Vitamin D	↓ PMN motility and phagocytosis	
Vitamin E Deficiency	No evidence of effect	↓ Mitogen responses ↓ DTH ↓ Antibody responses
Excess	No evidence of effect	↑ Mitogen responses ↑ Antibody production
Vitamin C Deficiency	↓ DTH ↓ Mitogen responses ↓ PMN chemotaxis	↓ Mitogen responses ↓ DTH ↓ Graft rejection ↓ Antibody production ↓ PMN chemotaxis, migration, and phagocytosis
Excess	↑ Mitogen responses ↑ Interferon production	
Vitamin B_1 (thiamine)	No evidence of effect	Lymphopenia ↓ DTH ↓ Antibody production
Vitamin B_2 (riboflavin)	No evidence of effect	Lymphoid atrophy Lymphopenia ↑ Growth of spontaneous tumors ↓ Antibody responses
Niacin	No evidence of effect	No evidence of effect
Pantothenic acid	No evidence of effect	Lymphoid atrophy Lymphopenia ↓ Antibody production
Biotin	↓ DTH ↓ Mitogen responses ↓ Antibody production, especially IgA	↓ Antibody production
Vitamin B_6 (pyridoxine)	Lymphoid atrophy ↓ DTH ↓ Graft rejection ↓ Mixed lymphocyte reaction ↓ Antibody responses (especially if combined with panthothenic acid deficiency)	Lymphoid atrophy Lymphopenia ↓ Mitogen responses ↓ Mixed lymphocyte reaction ↓ DTH ↓ Skin transplant rejection ↓ Antibody production
Vitamin B_{12}* (cobalamine)	Lymphopenia ↓ Mitogen responses ↓ DTH ↓ Phagocytosis and bactericidal activity	Lymphoid atrophy Lymphopenia ↓ Mitogen responses ↓ DTH ↓ Antibody production ↓ Phagocytosis

*Folate deficiency produces the same findings as seen in vitamin B_{12} deficiency.

Little is known about the effects of vitamin D deficiency on immune reactivity, but vitamin D has a profound impact on the function of B and T cells and macrophages. The addition of vitamin D to cell cultures decreases the production of IL-2, GM-CSF, and INF-γ, decreases antibody production (likely due to suppression of T-helper T-cell function), and increases (in some studies) production of IL-1, tumor necrosis factor, and prostaglandin E_2, while increasing the ability of macrophages to fuse and mediate cytotoxicity. Recall that vitamin D_3 is 25-hydroxylated in the liver and then 1-hydroxylated in the kidney; an anephric individual will have low levels of 1,25-dihydroxyvitamin D_3, the active form of the vitamin. It is of note that in certain diseases, like sarcoidosis, activated macrophages can 1-hydroxylate vitamin D_3, with resulting hypercalcemia, even in patients with no functioning renal tissue. It has been proposed that vitamin D has an active immunologic function, with T- and B-cell regulatory effects (Fig. 24B-2). The therapeutic use of vitamin D_3 analogues may provide physiologic immunosuppressive effects with minimal toxicity.

A great deal of attention has been paid to the role of vitamin C in the normal immune response. Well-designed studies have not been able to show any effect of high doses (some would call them "industrial doses") of vitamin C on the subsequent development of the common cold, although there is evidence that vitamin C may decrease the duration of cold symptoms. Supraphysiologic doses of vitamin C have been reported to increase mitogen responses, especially in the elderly, but the clinical significance of this is unclear. Individual case studies suggest that vitamin C supplementation of patients with the Chédiak-Higashi immunodeficiency syndrome (see Chap. 17) increases their faulty polymorphonuclear cell function into the normal range. Vitamin C has antioxidant activity, and some studies have speculated that vitamin C and vitamin E, another antioxidant, might alter the production of prostaglandins and oxygen radicals by means of their antioxidant activity; this also is pure speculation.

Another antioxidant with a possible immunomodulatory effect is the tripeptide glutathione. Increases in mitogen responses and delayed-type hypersensitivity occur after supplemental glutathione is given to mice and humans, most notably in the elderly. Although intracellular glutathione is normal in the cells of the elderly, there is evidence to suggest that the intramitochondrial pool of glutathione is diminished in the elderly and is replenished by giving exogenous glutathione.

The perfect dietary therapy for an inflammatory disease would consist of a naturally occurring compound, easy to administer, with no toxicity. There is some evidence that such a compound is *capsaicin*, derived from chili peppers. Capsaicin depletes type C unmyelinated nerve fibers of a neurotransmitter known as substance P. When substance P is injected into a joint or subcutaneously, inflammation occurs locally. The distribution of joints affected in collagen-induced arthritis in rats parallels the density of nerve fibers

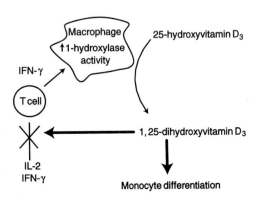

Figure 24B-2   Model for paracrine role of vitamin D in immunoregulation. Macrophage activation by IFN-γ is accompanied by induction of 1-hydroxylase activity and generation of calcitriol from 25-hydroxyvitamin D_3. Local calcitriol production inhibits interferon and IL-2-driven T-cell proliferation. Furthermore, calcitriol increases monokine production and promotes monocytic differentiation of myeloid stem cells.

containing substance P in these joints. When potentially susceptible rats are pretreated with capsaicin, they develop less severe collagen-induced arthritis. Human studies of rheumatoid arthritis have begun; capsaicin is commercially available as a topical treatment for cutaneous herpes zoster (shingles), which can be intensely painful. (No, there is no evidence that people in countries with cuisines rich in chili peppers have a lower incidence of rheumatoid arthritis, but it was a good thought!)

SELF-TEST QUESTIONS

1. How can chronic inflammatory conditions, like parasitic infestations, be immunomodulatory?
2. What factors determine the serum level of albumin? Therefore, what is the significance of a low serum albumin?
3. Anorexia nervosa is a severe psychiatric disorder, in which the patients, usually young women, do not eat; they are especially fat- and carbohydrate-depleted, but are not protein deficient. They are not immunocompromised. How can this unique set of nutritional conditions explain the intact immune systems of anorexic patients?
4. Human beings have been hunter-gatherers and subsistence farmers through much of history, often not optimally nourished. However *Homo sapiens* prevailed, suggesting that the immune response in undernourished individuals did not suffer markedly. How can suboptimal nutrition, or undernutrition, make for a more optimal immune response?

ADDITIONAL READINGS

Beisel WR. Synergism and antagonism of parasitic diseases and malnutrition. *Rev Infect Dis.* 1982; 4: 746–750.

Beisel WR, Edelman R, Nauss K, et al. Single nutrient effects on immunologic functions. *JAMA.* 1981; 245: 53–58.

Corman LC. Effects of specific nutrients on the immune response. *Med Clin North Am.* 1985; 69: 759–791.

Erickson KL, Adams DA, McNeil CJ. Dietary lipid modulation of immune responsiveness. *Lipids.* 1983;18:468–474.

Garre MA, Boles JM, Youinou PY. Current concepts in immune derangement due to undernutrition. *J Parenteral Enteral Nutr.* 1987;11:309–313.

Gershwin ME, Beach RS, Hurley LS. *Nutrition and Immunity.* New York: Academic; 1985.

Keys A, Brozek J, Henschel A, et al. *The Biology of Human Starvation.* Minneapolis: University of Minnesota Press; 1950.

Kubo C, Day NK, Good RA. Influence of early or late dietary restriction on lifespan and immunological parameters in MRL/Mp-lpr/lpr mice. *Proc Natl Acad Sci USA.* 1984;81:5831–5835.

Murray J, Murray A. Starvation suppression and refeeding activation of infection. An ecological necessity? *Lancet.* 1977;1:123–125.

Murray J, Murray A. Toward a nutritional concept of host resistance to malignancy and intracellular infection. *Perspect Biol Med.* 1981;24:290–310.

Wakeling A. Review: neurobiological aspects of feeding disorders. *J Psychiatr Res.* 1985;19:191–202.

25

The Immunology of Neoplasia

INTRODUCTION

Cancer is a disease that results from the unregulated and ultimately harmful growth of a certain cell type or types within an organism. Malignancy is characterized by fast growth, invasiveness into local tissue, progression into more abnormal forms, and dissemination (metastasis) into distant organs. Cancer is very heterogeneous both at the level of the organism, since almost every organ or tissue of the body can be affected, and at the population level, where cells within the malignant population vary greatly both in cell surface phenotype, metastatic potential, and susceptibility to immunologic effector mechanisms. Therefore, each individual type of cancer can represent a unique problem for the organism as a whole and for the immune system in particular.

The advancement of theories regarding the importance of protective mechanisms for controlling the growth of malignantly transformed cells in multicellular organisms has laid much of the foundation for modern immunologic thinking. As early as 1909, Paul Ehrlich theorized that cancer cells arise frequently, but contain "markers" or changes on their cellular membranes that can be recognized as foreign and destroyed by the immune system. This theory led to the formulation of the "immune surveillance" hypothesis by Thomas in 1958, and later by Burnet in 1970, which suggested that the immune system, which constantly "patrols" the organism for evidence of malignant transformation, has developed mechanisms which can specifically recognize and destroy neoplastic cells. This hypothesis led to a significant amount of work in the field of tumor immunology, and a large number of effector mechanisms have been identified which can, under the appropriate conditions, kill malignantly transformed cells.

Studies of the immune response to malignancies in experimental animals and also in humans have identified a number of immunologic components which can eliminate or slow the growth of neoplastic cells. These effector mechanisms include antibody and complement, antibody-dependent cell-mediated cytotoxicity, natural killer cells, cytotoxic T cells, macrophages, polymorphonuclear cells, and lymphokine-activated killer (LAK) cells. Despite the fact that all of these effector mechanisms have been shown to specifically eliminate malignant cells, it is not clear whether any of these mechanisms plays a significant antineoplastic role in vivo. In addition, malignant cells are quite adept at surviving in spite of the presence of these effectors. A large number of escape mechanisms used by malignant cells to resist immunologic attack have been identified. These escape mechanisms include resistance to killing, antigenic modulation, "hiding," production of blocking factors, induction of immune suppression, and selection of immunologically resistant variants (clonal selection).

Despite the questionable relevance of immunologic mediators in controlling and eliminating malignant cells in vivo, there is renewed hope that immunotherapeutic approaches can be used to treat malignant disorders. This hope stems from the fact that treatment of patients bearing tumors with a number of different immunologic mediators, including LAK cells, monoclonal antitumor antibodies, and pharmacologic agents which enhance macrophage activity, has led to significant and even total remission of malignant diseases in some cases. Therefore, the war on cancer continues, and there is a renewed sense of hope that immunology will play a significant role in the ultimate victory.

TUMOR DEVELOPMENT

The development of neoplasia most likely occurs because of the transformation of a single cell from normal to cancerous. A malignant cell must undergo a number of changes, both genotypically and phenotypically, in order to become malignant and to be able to adapt itself to the host environment. The fact that the incidence of cancer increases exponentially with increasing age suggests that these changes must occur over time in order to make cells neoplastic. The period between individual exposure to a neoplastic transforming agent and the emergence of a malignant disease is called the *latency period,* and it may last many years. A number of factors, including genetic factors, environmental factors, and the type of cell being transformed, determine how long the latency period will be. Environmental factors which can cause malignant changes and/or changes in immune function are reviewed in Chap. 32, "Immunotoxicology."

The exact mechanisms by which cells become malignantly transformed is still a mystery. A number of agents have been described which can induce the transformation of a normal mammalian cell into a malignant cell. These agents, called *carcinogens,* can be roughly divided into several categories, including chemical carcinogens (e.g., methylcholanthrene, benzopyrene), ionizing radiation (e.g., ultraviolet irradiation, γ-irradiation), and oncogenic viruses, including oncodna (oncogenic DNA) and oncorna (oncogenic RNA) viruses. In addition, it is believed that cells can change into malignant cells without the action of a transforming agent: an abnormal genetic alteration occurring within a given cell during normal functioning can result in the loss of growth control mechanisms at the genetic or cellular level. These cells give rise to what are classified as *spontaneous tumors,* since they appear to have no known external causative agent responsible for inducing the malignant transformation. It is, of course, impossible to determine exactly whether a tumor is the result of a spontaneous malignancy or has been induced by an unidentified carcinogen, and tumors are normally categorized as spontaneous when no known high risk factor identified with an agent-induced malignant transformation can be identified.

TUMOR ANTIGENS

In order for the immune system to recognize and eliminate neoplastic cells, these cells must express antigens which can be targets of immune attack. These antigens, called *tumor-associated antigens,* are not present on cells from normal tissue. In experimental animal systems, the presence of tumor-associated antigens on most tumors can be demonstrated by experiments much like those shown in Fig. 25-1. The injection of irradiated cells, or cells which have been phenotypically altered to increase immunogenicity, can often protect an individual from the reinfusion of live tumor cells. In addition, when an established tumor is surgically removed, then reinfused into the same individual, these animals are almost always resistant to the outgrowth of that malignancy. The immunity developed by immunization or surgical resection is specific, in that the growth of an unrelated tumor is not inhibited. The antigens responsible for this immunity are called *tumor-specific transplantation antigens (TSTA),* and the existence of TSTA on human tumors is a matter of some debate.

Tumor cells whose antigens have been characterized display a wide variety of different types of antigens. Tumors from different individuals which arose by transformation due to the same oncogenic virus normally express identical tumor-associated antigens. These antigens arise from the genetic material supplied by the virus, and represent either viral antigens or antigens aberrantly expressed by host cells as a result of virus infection. These antigens confer a cross-reactive protection in that immunization with one tumor cell line will protect against a challenge with a different tumor cell line transformed by the same (but not a different) virus. The expression of these cross-reactive antigens allows for the development of therapeutic protocols and vaccinations which will protect against the progressive growth of all tumors transformed by that same virus.

The expression of tumor-associated

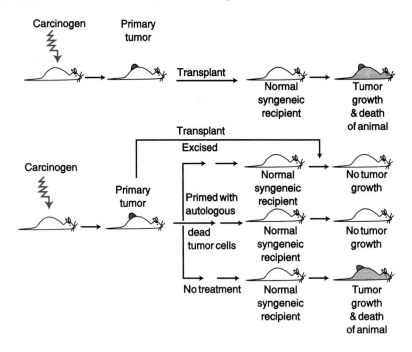

Figure 25-1   Demonstration of tumor-associated antigens that can be targets of immune attack. Live tumor cells biopsied from animals which have developed a spontaneous or carcinogen-induced tumor can normally be transplanted into a normal, syngeneic recipient, resulting in the development of a tumor by the recipient animal. However, transplantation of irradiated tumor cells, or total excision of the primary tumor lesion, leads to an immunologic priming of the recipient animal to that tumor. Therefore, upon subsequent transplantation of live tumor cells into primed animals, these tumor cells are immunologically rejected, and no tumor appears.

antigens on the surface of carcinogen-induced tumor cells is quite different. Tumor cells which arise in genetically identical experimental animals either spontaneously or by the application of chemical or radiation carcinogens normally have antigens that are individually specific for that tumor. It has even been found that application of the same carcinogen to two distinct parts of the same individual results in the development of malignancies which express unique antigens. The origin and biochemical nature of these antigens are for the most part unknown, and consequently the existence of these antigens is quite mysterious and controversial. Therefore, while viruses appear to induce cross-reactive antigens which have for the most part been identified and characterized, carcino-

gen-induced or spontaneously arising tumors normally express unique tumor-associated antigens of unknown etiology.

Tumor cells which express tumor-associated antigens may also express normal antigens in higher or lower amounts than the normal tissue from which they arose, and may express antigens that have been previously expressed during development but are no longer expressed by normal tissue. Antigens in this group are called *oncofetal* antigens because they are expressed by both oncogenetically transformed cells and cells of the developing fetus. Included in this important class of antigens are α-fetoprotein, found on malignancies of the liver, and carcinoembryonic antigens, found on tumors of the stomach and intestine.

GENERATION OF IMMUNITY TO MALIGNANT CELLS

The immunologic response to malignant cells includes a large number of immune effector mechanisms which can be demonstrated to have a cytolytic or inhibitory effect on the growth of tumor cells both in vivo and in vitro. This includes both the innate and the specific immune response, as well as both the humoral and cell-mediated response. The immunologic effector mechanisms which inhibit the outgrowth of malignancies are discussed in the following section.

Humoral Immunity

The generation of antibody responses to malignant cells has been shown to have both a positive and negative effect on the outgrowth of malignant cells. Cytotoxic antibodies which kill tumor cells in the presence of complement can be demonstrated in the sera of patients wth malignant diseases. Upon binding to the surface of a tumor cell, these antibodies can activate the classical pathway of complement, resulting in the death of the tumor cell by osmotic integrity (see Chap. 13). In addition, some antitumor antibodies can cooperate with certain lymphoid cells to kill tumor cells by *antibody-dependent cell-mediated cytotoxicity (ADCC)*. These antibodies can specifically bind to the surface of the tumor cell with its antigen-specific receptor, and a subclass of lymphoid cells, historically called "killer cells," can bind to the Fc portion of these antibodies and kill the tumor cell. In this case, the lymphoid cell takes the place of complement and serves as the lytic agent in tumor cell killing. These killer cells are not T cells, B cells, or macrophages, but belong to a class of lymphocytes termed *null cells* because they do not express cell surface markers of any of these subsets. Under certain circumstances, antibodies can also bind to macrophages and "arm" them. Such "armed" macrophages can bind to and kill tumors (see below).

Not all antibodies to tumors are beneficial, however, Only certain subclasses of antibodies can fix complement or participate in ADCC (see Chap. 3), and consequently not all antibodies are effective at killing tumor cells. Antibodies have been described which bind to tumor cells or tumor cell antigens but which do not mediate killing of tumor cells in the presence of complement. Rather, these antibodies appear to interfere with other, more effective immune responses to tumors, including both humoral and cell-mediated effector mechanisms. These antibodies are called *blocking factors,* and appear to be an important escape mechanism for tumors.

Cell-Mediated Immunity

T Cells

T cells can provide a strong protection against rapidly growing malignancies. *Cytotoxic T lymphocytes (CTLs)* bear receptors which recognize antigens on the surface of tumor cells and specifically kill the cells bearing those antigens. CTLs are primarily CD8$^+$, which means they recognize tumor antigens in the context of class I MHC molecules, although some CD4$^+$ CTLs have been described against class II–bearing tumor cells. Inflammatory T cells are stimulated by soluble tumor antigen and secrete lymphokines which can be directly cytotoxic to the tumor cells or which can generate a local delayed-type hypersensitivity response which results in the recruitment of nonspecific cytotoxic cells such as neutrophils and monocytes.

Macrophages

Macrophages generally inhibit tumor cell growth via two mechanisms. The first is by cytolytic effects, which result in the death of the tumor; the second is by cytostasis, which results in the inhibition of tumor cell growth without cell death. This cytostatic effect on tumor cells has only been described for macrophages, and may represent an important in vivo defense mechanism for controlling tumor cells.

Macrophages can be sensitized to tumor

cells in two ways. The first is through antibody-dependent "arming," which was described above. The second is by activation. Macrophages are activated, or made "angry," by exposure to lymphokines, pharmacologic agents, or natural activators such as bacteria, endotoxin, glycogen, thioglycolate, and even tumor cells themselves. These activated macrophages bind to and kill tumor cells but do not appear to have any cytolytic effect on normal tissue. This specificity for tumor cells is quite remarkable, although the recognition mechanism of macrophages for malignant cells is at present unknown.

Natural Killer Cells

Natural killer (NK) cells are a population of lymphoid cells which demonstrate significant cytolytic activity against a large number of different malignant cells regardless of their origin, tissue type, or transforming agent. NK cells are present in lymphoid tissue of naive individuals, do not proliferate after immunization with any tumor cell type, are not genetically restricted in their cytotoxic activity, and do not appear to have specificity for one particular surface antigen on susceptible target cells. In addition, they have been found in the lymphoid tissues of virtually every species examined. As such, these cells appear to belong to the natural, or innate, immune system.

The ontogeny of NK cells is still a matter of considerable debate. They do not express cell surface markers that would characterize them as T cells (since they lack CD3, CD5, and CD4/CD8), B cells (since they lack surface IgM and C3 receptors), or macrophages (since they lack class II molecules, Fc receptors, and CD11), but rather they express unique cell surface molecules, including CD13 and CD56. However, morphologically they appear to be small resting lymphocytes, and adaptive transfer experiments have suggested that NK cells, like other lymphocytes, are derived from precursors found in bone marrow. They show a strict age-related activity, with NK activity appearing shortly after birth, peaking at young adulthood, and gradually declining with age.

NK cells show a wide range of target specificities. Unlike the cytolytic activity of CTLs, the cytolytic activity of NK cells is not restricted to cells of the same MHC haplotype; NK cells can kill syngeneic, allogeneic (same species, different genotype), or even xenogeneic (different species) tumor cells. Experimental results have shown that NK cells bind to susceptible target cells but not to resistant target cells, and this binding is required for NK-cell killing, although the target structure on susceptible target cells has not been identified. In addition, it is believed that the mechanism of NK-cell cytolysis is identical or very similar to that seen with CTLs (see Chap. 8).

Although NK-cell activity does not appear to increase in individuals exposed to NK cell–sensitive tumor cells, NK cells appear to be under regulatory control by the immune system. Several lymphokines have been identified, including interferon alpha (IFN-α), IFN-β, interleukin 2 (IL-2), and IL-4, which can substantially increase the lytic activity of NK cells. Until just recently, it has been very difficult to establish cloned lines of cells with NK-cell activity, and therefore work in characterizing NK cells has been slow. The NK-cell lines which have been established appear to grow very slowly and often lose their lytic activity after prolonged culture.

The role of NK cells in protecting individuals from the outgrowth of malignantly transformed cells is also a matter of some debate. Although malignantly transformed cells in animals with intact NK-cell activity can still grow, a number of experiments have suggested that NK cells can be important in protecting against the outgrowth of cancerous lesions. Athymic T cell–deficient mice (which exhibit NK-cell but not CTL activity) given treatments of anti-IFN antibodies show decreased NK-cell activity and increased susceptibility to metastatic spread of tumors. Conversely, in animals deficient in NK-cell activity, tumors showed significantly more invasiveness and metastasis than control animals exhibiting normal NK-cell activity.

Lymphokine-Activated Killer (LAK) Cells

LAK cells are another population of lymphoid cells capable of killing malignantly transformed cells. These cells appear to be phenotypically different from T cells, B cells, and NK cells. Like CTLs and NK cells, LAK cells can bind to and lyse malignantly transformed cells. Unlike NK cells, these cells normally show no reactivity against malignant cells unless activated to become cytolytic by incubation with large amounts of lymphokines. The lymphokine which appears to activate LAK cells is IL-2, and IL-4 can synergize with IL-2 to further augment their activity. However, like NK cells, LAK cells show a wide range of specificity for a number of malignantly transformed cells and normal cells do not appear to be targets of their cytolytic activity.

The origin of LAK cells is not known. They appear to be bone marrow–derived lymphocytes, and can be found in the spleen, peripheral blood, and lymph nodes of most species tested. It has recently been found that a better source of LAK cells is *tumor-infiltrating lymphocytes (TILs)*, which are isolated directly from the patient's tumor mass. Both LAK cells and TILs are activated by in vitro incubation with IL-2 and appear to require constant stimulation with IL-2 to maintain their activity.

ESCAPE MECHANISMS OF TUMORS

Genetic Instability and Repopulation

Despite all of the immunologic mechanisms so far identified which have a deleterious effect on the growth of malignant cells, cancerous lesions do appear within individuals and, without therapeutic manipulation by the clinician, will eventually kill the host. This is because neoplastic cells behave as a population, and as such are quite adept at circumventing or overcoming immunologic responses designed to eliminate them. Two properties of malignant cells favor their survival as a population within an unfriendly environment: genetic instability and repopulation.

Genetic Instability

Tumor cells constantly generate progeny which are phenotypic variants of the original transformed cell. These variants can differ slightly from the original parent cell in growth pattern, cell surface antigen expression, and sensitivity to immunologic effector mechanisms. Those variants with the greatest selective advantage to survive will gradually overtake those more susceptible to immune attack, and the variants exhibiting the fastest growth, greatest invasive potential, and weakest immunogenicity will dominate. The theory of *clonal selection* suggests that this mechanism ensures that only tumor cells capable of escaping immunologic destruction, generally by losing their most immunogenic antigens and becoming more like the normal tissue from which they were derived, will survive in a hostile environment of immunologic responsiveness. It is these cells which will appear clinically as a neoplastic lesion and go on to ultimately destroy the host. The principle of clonal selection, illustrated in Fig. 25-2, operates not only in natural immunologic resistance, but also in the resistance developed by progressive malignancies to drug, radiation, and immunotherapeutic interventions.

Repopulation

The second property which favors the survival of populations of malignant cells is known as *repopulation*. While the destruction of a large proportion of bacteria or parasites by the immune system can generally eliminate a potentially lethal infection, a single tumor cell which escapes immunologic destruction has the potential to develop into a malignant lesion. Therefore, it is not sufficient to kill 99 percent or even 99.99 percent of the malignant cells within an individual by natural or therapeutic mechanisms. Rather, the immune system must be capable of eliminating *all* of these cells, since failure to do so may result in the eventual

526 PART III: CLINICAL CONSEQUENCES

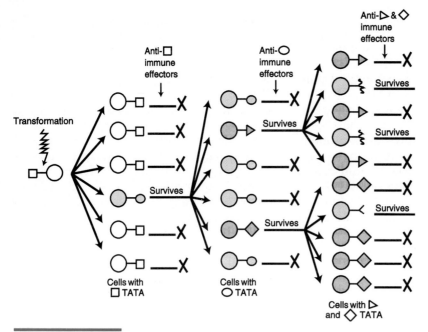

Figure 25-2 Clonal selection theory. Cells undergoing a transformation event begin rapid division and variant generation. The immune system, sensing danger, launches an attack against this neoplastic growth with a potent antitumor effector mechanism. While most of the cells are destroyed by the immune effector mechanisms reactive with the predominant tumor associated transplantation antigen (TATA), one variant is resistant to this effector mechanism and survives. This clone, now resistant to immune effector 1, continues to rapidly divide and generate variants. The immune system launches a second attack with a different effector mechanism, once again leading to the death of a large proportion of tumor cells. However, once again, a clone survives, and this clone is now resistant to both immune effector 1 *and* immune effector 2. This clone continues to rapidly divide and generate variants until it is exposed to immune effector 3. This time, although the majority of cells are killed, several clones survive, and these clones are now resistant to immune effectors 1, 2, and 3. This process of expansion, variant generation, and selection continues until one or several clones survive which are resistant to all immune effector mechanisms. It is these clones that appear as the malignant lesion that is clinically diagnosed.

death of the host. This same principle forms the rationale for combination therapy in the treatment of malignancies, since few therapies by themselves are capable of eliminating the entire population of malignant cells.

Resistance to Killing Mechanisms

Malignant cells often develop mechanisms which aid their survival in the event of im-

mune attack. For example, many tumor cells can modulate their surface antigens, leading to the disappearance of these antigens from the cell surface, or "shed" their antigens, making it difficult for immune cells or factors to reach and destroy tumor cells. Tumor cells can also release factors which serve to "block" effective immunity. These so-called blocking factors are now believed to be either noncytotoxic antibodies, which "cover up" determinants, preventing more effective immune mechanisms from recognizing and destroying the tumor cell, or shed antigen that forms complexes with antibody, preventing membrane fixation of complement. Tumor cells have also been found to secrete anti-inflammatory substances, such as IL-1, IL-2, etc., which inhibit cytokine activity or inhibit the recruitment and activation of macrophages. Some malignant cells have even been shown to be more resistant than the parent cell to antibody plus complement and/or cell-mediated killing, thereby allowing these cells to escape normally effective immunologic destruction.

Antigenic Modulation

Due to their higher level of genetic instability, malignant cells appear to have the capability of modulating their surface antigens to less immunogenic forms. This may involve genetic mechanisms such as point mutations, gene recombination, or gene conversion, or simply changes in the processing and glycosylation of antigens. Although these changes in antigenic structure are random, clonal selection dictates that those changes which result in less immunogenic antigen forms will be favored.

Hiding

It has been observed that the injection of a very small amount of tumor cells into an experimental animal results in the development of a malignant lesion, while the injection of much larger doses of tumor cells results in tumor rejection. It is thought that perhaps the small amount of antigen introduced may be too small to invoke an immune response and that the tumor has time to establish itself and generate variants before the immune system finally begins its attack. However, several experiments have suggested that low doses of tumor cells may actually induce low zone tolerance, leading to an active suppression of the immune response to that malignancy, resulting in tu-

mor escape, also called "hiding," or "sneaking through."

Immune Suppression

Often an individual is capable of mounting an effective immune response to tumors, but is prevented by the activation of immune suppressor cells. These cells actively eliminate or inhibit the ability of immune effector mechanisms, both humoral and cell-mediated, from destroying tumor cells. The major mediator of immune suppression is the suppressor T cell, and the activities of suppressor T cells in preventing immune responses to tumors and ultimately tumor rejection has been demonstrated in both experimental animals and humans. Suppressor T cells have been found to play a role in allowing "sneak through" escape as well as in the shutdown of the immune system that occurs in tumor load (see below). Suppressor T-cell activity is even thought to play a major role in *concomitant immunity*, a phenomenon in which tumor cells in the primary lesion are resistant to immune attack, but these same tumor cells transplanted to secondary sites are immunologically destroyed.

Immunodeficiency

It is well known that individuals under immunosuppressive treatments for autoimmune diseases and/or tissue transplants have a higher incidence of malignancies. In addition, some individuals are genetically incapable of responding to tumor antigens. This inability to respond is analogous to the immune-response (Ir) gene effects seen in the immune response to many protein antigens. Like the Ir gene effects, the inability to respond to tumor antigens has been genetically linked to the MHC.

Tumor Load

When a tumor becomes too large, it has the capability of nonspecifically suppressing the entire immune system. This phenomenon, referred to as *tumor load,* results in the total shutdown of immunologic mechanisms, leading to the host's inability to respond to bacterial, viral, or even mitogenic stimuli. Generally, this phenomenon is strictly related to the physical size of the tumor, and excision of the tumor results in full recovery of the immune response within a few days.

Immunostimulation

While in most cases an active immune response against a tumor is good for the patient, there are cases in which an active immune response is actually harmful. If tumor cells are able to parasitically use the growth and differentiation factors produced by the immune system, namely the lymphokines, as growth factors themselves, then the more active the immune response against the tumor, i.e., the more lymphokines produced by the immune system, the faster the tumor actually grows. This phenomenon, called *immunostimulation of tumor cells,* is especially prevalent in tumors of the lymphoreticular system, such as myelomas, lymphomas, and leukemias.

IMMUNE THERAPY

While many immunologic mechanisms have been identified that can play a role in the destruction of cancerous cells both in vitro and in vivo, it is still not clear what precise role these cells or molecules could play in actually protecting the individual from malignancies. Nonetheless, one could potentially utilize these mechanisms as therapeutic agents in the treatment of malignant diseases. The great potential of immunotherapeutic agents, in contrast to therapies involving irradiation, surgical resection, and/or cytotoxic drugs, is the specificity of such reagents for only those cells or subsets of cells that need to be manipulated to increase tumor immunity.

The main concern of an oncologist is to identify malignant diseases early enough in the progression of the disease for treatment

to be effective. This is also true of immune therapy; one must begin immune therapy before tumor load has rendered the immune system incapable of responding to specific stimulation. Several different types of treatments which have proved to be successful in human or animal model systems are currently being used or are under development.

Nonspecific Immunopotentiators

Early efforts to treat malignancy by means of immunostimulation involved the use of *immunopotentiators,* or *adjuvants.* These potentiators were used in polyclonal stimulation of the immune system, and were designed to generate inflammatory responses at the site of injection. The most often-used potentiators were bacillus Calmette-Guérin (BCG) and *Corynebacterium parvum,* and they were often mixed with killed or inactivated tumor cells. When the potentiator was injected into the tumor-bearing individual, an inflammatory response resulted which often led to rejection of tumor cells at distant sites. However, the potential for harmful immunologic responses, and the relatively low success rate, have made these treatments much less desirable than others currently being used.

Monoclonal Antibodies and Immunotoxins

The advent of monoclonal antibody technology led to an intense effort to generate monoclonal antibodies to tumor antigens to be used in the treatment of malignancy. Often, if a patient's serum contains antibodies to the autologous tumor, lymph nodes or peripheral blood lymphocytes of such a patient are used to generate monoclonal antibodies to the antigens expressed on the tumor cells. These antibodies can then be passively infused into patients, with the hope that they will bind to the tumor cell surface, killing the cell. For such treatment to be effective, two problems must be solved. First, the monoclonal antibodies must be truly tumor-specific, and not work against antigens that are also expressed by normal tissue. Second, the antibodies must be capable of killing the tumor with a high degree of efficiency once they reach their target.

The problem of how to identify tumor-specific antibodies remains to be solved, but attempts have been made to increase the killing potential of antibodies by attaching a lethal agent to the antibody that will only kill the appropriate target cell. These agents may be toxins, such as ricin, choleratoxin, and bungerotoxin, or cytotoxic drugs such as daunomycin. These "immunotoxins" are only lytic upon entry into cells, and only enter the cell when the antibody engages the appropriate antigen on the surface of the target cell. They have thus proved to be highly specific for tumor cells, and quite effective, under some conditions, in eliminating tumor cells.

Cytotoxic Lymphocyte Lines and Clones

Even more effective than immunotoxins at killing tumor cells are the cytotoxic lymphocytes. Therefore, treatments are being developed where cloned cytotoxic T cells specific for tumor cells are infused into patients. This treatment has the disadvantage that these cells often do not home properly to the malignant lesion, and are therefore not effective in treating metastatic spread of disease.

Removal of Immune Suppressor Cells

Since it has been shown that immune suppressor cells can effectively eliminate tumor-specific immunity, therapeutic treatments have centered around the removal of suppressor cells rather than the generation of effector mechanisms as a treatment for cancer. Such treatments involve the use of drugs (such as cyclophosphamide) or monoclonal antibodies to remove suppressor cells in vivo, thereby allowing the natural immunity to proceed unabated. These treatments have shown great promise and, in

combination with other immune therapies, represent a potentially important avenue for future therapeutic interventions.

LAK and TIL Therapy

Use of LAK cells or TILs as therapeutic agents involves the use of autologous peripheral blood lymphocytes (for LAK cells) or lymphocytes from tumor biopsies (for TILs) stimulated for varying periods of time in vitro with IL-2. These cells are then passively reinfused into the tumor-bearing patient, along with repeated doses of IL-2 over an extended period of time. This treatment has proved very successful for certain types of tumors, but also carries with it several drawbacks. The first is the tissue toxicity of the large doses of IL-2 that are infused into the patient to maintain LAK-cell or TIL activity. The infusion of large doses of IL-2 has been shown to cause headaches, fever, and general malaise, in addition to other more serious complications in some patients. In addition, this regimen is costly and difficult to perform, and only certain tumors appear to respond routinely to treatment. Therefore, it is questionable whether this technique will be widely used in the future.

SELF-TEST QUESTIONS

1. Consider the theory of immunosurveillance. Do you think the immune system plays a major role in the natural elimination of malignancy? What evidence supports your conclusion? What evidence refutes it?
2. What are the major immunologic effector mechanisms which may play a role in protection against malignant diseases?
3. Consider at least 10 different mechanisms tumor cells use to escape immune destruction. How does each play a role in tumor resistance to immune attack?
4. Combination therapies are often more successful than single therapies in treating malignancy. In light of the clonal selection theory, why might this be the case?

5. What are some of the more successful therapies being used today to stimulate immunity against malignancy?
6. What are some of the major problems connected with the use of cytokines and cytokine-induced cells to treat human malignancy?

ADDITIONAL READINGS

Heberman RB. Multiple functions of natural killer cells, including immunoregulation as well as resistance to tumor growth. *Concepts Immunopathol.* 1985;1:96.

Mule JJ, Shu S, Rosenberg S. The anti-tumor efficacy of lymphokine-activated killer cells and recombinant interleukin-2 *in vivo. J Immunol.* 1985;135:646.

Naor D. Suppressor cells: Permitters and promoters of malignancy? *Adv Cancer Res.* 1979;29:45.

North RJ. The murine anti-tumor response and its therapeutic manipulation. *Adv Immunol.* 1984;35:89.

Oldham RK. Natural killer cells: Artifact to reality, an odyssey in biology. *Cancer Metastasis Rev.* 1983;2:323.

Rosenberg SA et al. Cancer immunotherapy using interleukin-2 and interleukin-2-activated lymphocytes. *Ann Rev Immunol.* 1986;4:681.

Rosenberg SA. Immunotherapy of cancer using interleukin-2: Current status and future prospects. *Immunol Today.* 1988;9:58.

Tanaka K et al. The role of the major histocompatibility complex class I antigens in tumor growth and metastasis. *Ann Rev Immunol.* 1998;6:359.

Vitetta E et al. Immunotoxins. *Ann Rev Immunol.* 1985;3:197.

26

Transplantation Immunology

INTRODUCTION

Clinical organ transplantation requires a delicate balance: induction of tolerance to foreign antigens present on the graft with maintenance of the host's ability to respond to other nonself-antigens, such as pathogenic microorganisms. In order to understand the immunologic principles governing this balancing act, we must first understand the principles of basic immunology—the biology and inheritance of the major histocompatibility complex (MHC) antigens, the mechanisms and regulation of cell-mediated and humoral immunity, the regulatory molecules of the immune system, and the inflammatory response. Throughout this chapter repeated reference will be made to these principles.

Experimental transplantation has a centuries-old history, dating to the mythical exploits of Hua T's and Pien Ch'iso in China during the second century B.C., but modern clinical transplantation began in 1954 with a kidney transplant between identical twins. Development of 6-mercaptopurine in 1959 by Schwartz and Dameshek (and subsequent development of azathioprine by Elion and Hitchings) dramatically increased the success of organ transplantation between nonidentical donors. Cyclosporin A (cyclosporine), introduced by Borel in 1976, further increased graft survival. These drugs are described in more detail in Chap. 33A, "Immunopharmacology." Today, successful transplantation of the cornea, bone marrow, kidney, heart, and liver occurs at many medical centers around the world. Increasing success with lung, heart-lung, pancreas, and small bowel allografts is gradually being achieved.

The induction of tolerance to a foreign organ by an intact immune system is the goal of modern clinical transplantation. Class I and class II antigens seem to be the most important in graft survival, and histocompatibility testing for these, as well as ABO antigens, is performed. Acute rejection by cell-mediated immune reactions is common, but hyperacute rejection due to antibody present before transplantation is rarely seen if adequate histocompatibility testing is done.

Since only grafts from identical twins are not rejected without immunosuppression, nonspecific immunosuppression is used extensively in transplantation medicine. Multiagent protocols are common, with corticosteroids, azathioprine, cyclosporine, antilymphocyte globulin, and/or monoclonal antibodies employed in combinations. Antigen-specific immunosuppression would engender the fewest deleterious effects, but this technique is still in the experimental stages.

As the number of transplants increases, so does the requirement for organ donors. The need for solid organs has increased at a greater rate than the available pool of brain-dead donors. In part, this is because certain criteria must be met for organ donation. First, there must be clinical brain death (defined by absence of any detectable neurologic function on physical examination) without concomitant death of organ systems. In addition, there must be absence of transmissible infection (and risk factors for these infections) and malignancy; absence of autoimmune and metabolic diseases; and age and size requirements specific for each organ. Shortage of organs has also been due to lack of public awareness, and to the moral and ethical questions surrounding declaration of brain death. Legislation requiring notification of next-of-kin that organ donation is possible has been enacted in some states, and has increased organ donation in California by an estimated 25 to 33 percent. Living donors are used routinely for bone marrow transplants, and, at many centers, relatives may donate a kidney to a family member. Recently, segmental liver transplants from living donors have been performed. Obviously, the use of living-related donors is not an option for heart, whole liver, or whole pancreas transplants.

Ischemic damage to potential donor organs is an ever-present possibility. Warm ischemia time for organs from living donors is minimized by coordinating organ harvest with surgical preparation of the recipient. However, since organs from brain-dead donors are often harvested at one institution and shipped to recipients at distant centers, techniques for organ preservation become essential. Current techniques for organ preservation are based on the observation that hypothermia suppresses metabolism. Therefore, the majority of organs are preserved on ice. The recently developed UW solution (University of Wisconsin, or Belzer's, solution) approaches preservation from another perspective. With organ storage in cold UW solution, tissue injury is decreased by including components such as ATP to increase cell membrane stabilization. Preservation techniques also offer the opportunity for immunomodulation leading to a decrease in the number of passenger leukocytes (particularly interstitial dendritic cells) or for treatment with pharmocologic agents aimed at preservation of cell composition.

THE LANGUAGE OF TRANSPLANTATION IMMUNOLOGY

Discussion of transplantation immunology requires the definition of some commonly used terms. An *autograft* refers to a transplant from one region to another in the same individual. This may also be referred to as *autologous* transplantation. A transplant from one genetically identical individual to another (i.e., monozygotic twins) is termed an *isograft*. (*Isogeneic* and *syngeneic* are synonyms.) Allografts (*homografts* or *allogeneic* transplants) are performed between genetically nonidentical individuals of the same species; *xenografts* or *heterografts* (*xenogeneic* grafts) are transplants from one species to another.

THE GENETICS OF TRANSPLANTATION

The Laws of Transplantation

The basic law of transplantation may be stated succinctly: Permanent acceptance of a graft without immunosuppression is possible only when all major and minor antigens present in the graft are also present in the recipient. This situation occurs in monozygotic siblings and inbred animals. If antigens in the donor and the recipient are not identical, rejection of the transplanted organ will occur. When immunocompetent organs, such as bone marrow or small bowel, are transplanted, not only can the graft be rejected by the host, but the host can be rejected by immunocompetent cells in the graft (*graft-versus-host disease [GVHD]*). Tolerance of nonidentical grafts requires manipulation of the immune system with specific and/or nonspecific immunosuppression.

The Effects of MHC Antigens

Although it is possible to define many histocompatibility loci, the major histocompatibility loci are the most significant for organ transplantation (Table 26-1). Class II antigens (HLA-DR, HLA-DP, and HLA-DQ) are probably the primary antigens eliciting host immune response and subsequent rejection of the graft. Class I antigens (HLA-A and HLA-B, but apparently not HLA-C) also play a role in graft rejection.

Occasionally, an HLA-identical kidney will be rejected. This suggests that non-MHC minor antigens can also induce host immune response. These antigens have been extensively studied in rodents, with at least 40 defined in mice, but have not been as well defined in humans. Experimental data in humans correlate the presence of polymorphic non-MHC antigens on vascular endothelial cells and monocytes with rejection of HLA-identical grafts. Minor antigens are very important in bone marrow transplantation, and

TABLE 26-1 Types of Immunosuppresssion

Antigen-Nonspecific	Antigen-Specific
Cytotoxic drugs	Neonatal tolerization
Corticosteroids	Enhancing antibodies
Azathioprine	Anti-idiotypic antibodies
Antilymphocyte globulin	Blood transfusions
Cyclosporine	
Monoclonal antibodies	
Total lymphoid irradiation	
Thoracic duct drainage	

may also be responsible for GVHD in HLA-matched transplants.

Graft-versus-Host Disease

GVH reactions are a problem associated with the transplantation of immunologically competent tissue (such as bone marrow) into an immunodeficient or immunosuppressed host. If the immunocompetent cells within the graft recognize the host as foreign tissue, the graft cells will in effect reject the host by the same mechanisms seen in host rejection of the graft. Both $CD4^+$ and $CD8^+$ cells can mediate GVH reactions. For poorly understood reasons, the primary manifestations of GVHD are sloughing of the intestinal mucosa and infiltration of skin epithelium. Mononuclear cell infiltrates are also seen in the hepatic bile ducts and in the bronchial mucosa. GVHD occurs to some degree in virtually all bone marrow transplant recipients, even in siblings with HLA-identical matches (See Clinical Aside 26-1). In this case, the antigens responsible are probably minor rather than major histocompatibility antigens.

Clinical Aside 26-1
Kidney Transplant in Glomerulonephritis

Bob Smith is a 24-year-old white male who was first noted on route urinalysis to have proteinuria. His physician noted that he also had hypertension, hypercholesterolemia, hypoalbuminemia, a creatinine clearance of 30 mL/min, and a serum creatinine of 1.9 mg/dL (normal 0.7 to 1.2 mg/dL).

Suspecting membranous glomerulonephritis, on the basis of the clinical scenario, the physician performed a renal biopsy. Light microscopy demonstrated subepithelial proteinaceous deposits on hematoxylin-eosin staining.

Because of the immunoglobulin deposition, hypertension, and deteriorating renal function, Mr. Smith was referred to a nephrologist who treated his autoimmune illness with cyclophosphamide and prednisone. Initially the therapy was effective in decreasing his hypertension and proteinuria. Unfortunately, despite initial success, Mr. Smith continued to slowly lose renal function.

At age 27, Mr. Smith developed unremitting hypertension, nausea, and chronic renal failure. His BUN was 150 mg/dL and his creatinine was greater than 12 mg/dL. Mr. Smith's nephrologist also noted that he was losing weight, and had severe pruritus associated with his uremia. Hemodialysis was begun. An arteriovenous fistula was created by connecting the cephalic vein of the left forearm to the radial artery. This provided access to a high-flow conduit for hemodialysis.

Although Mr. Smith's uremia was adequately controlled by hemodialysis, he and his nephrologist decided that kidney transplantation would be preferred for long-term treatment. In preparation for transplantation, Mr. Smith's blood was sent to the laboratory to determine his blood type and his HLA type. Mr. Smith was also screened for antibodies to white blood cell antigens. Finally, before addition to the waiting list for a cadaveric kidney, Mr. Smith underwent blood transfusion from five random donors to induce formation of anti-idiotypic antibodies for its immunosuppressive effect.

When a suitable donor became available, Mr. Smith entered the hospital. A final cross-match screening of his serum for antibody against the antigens of the cadaveric kidney was completed, to avoid a hyperacute rejection. Mr. Smith had no preformed antibody to the donated kidney, and the process of renal transplantation began. He was given immunosuppressive doses of cyclosporine, azathioprine, and corticosteroids, as well as his first dose of polyvalent antilymphocyte globulin.

The operation went well, and Mr. Smith's uremia was corrected immediately. His induction immunosuppression was completed by tapering doses of cyclosporine, azathioprine, and prednisone, and cessation of antilymphocyte globulin. One month after leaving the hospital, Mr.

Smith's creatinine began to rise again and the renal allograft became tender. A biopsy of the kidney showed intense infiltration of lymphocytes between the tubular cells. Increased immunosuppression was begun, including reinstitution of monovalent antilymphocyte globulin therapy. The graft became less tender, and his creatinine once again dropped into the normal range. Thereafter, Mr. Smith's renal function remained stable, and he was tapered to minimal doses of cyclosporine, azathioprine, and prednisone.

Histocompatibility Testing

Histocompatibility testing involves identification (or *tissue typing*) of the class I and class II antigens of both the donor and the recipient of the organ. Recipients of cadaver kidneys have traditionally been selected by matches with donor antigens. Recent advances in tissue typing have demonstrated as much as a 15 percent increase in kidney transplant survival when epitope matching (see below, under "Transplantation Today— State of the Art") rather than conventional HLA-A, HLA-B, and HLA-DR matching was performed. (Tissue matching does not seem to be as critical in heart and liver transplantation, but is imperative in bone marrow transplantation.) Since current immunosuppression techniques provide excellent graft survival without HLA-identical matches, some centers no longer attempt strict tissue matching.

Conversely, because anti-class I or anti-class II antibodies present in the recipient can cause hyperacute rejection of the transplant, these antibodies must be detected before transplantation by *cross-matching*. The laboratory tests used for tissue typing and in cross-matching depend either on cytotoxicity or cell proliferation.

Tissue typing is generally performed by a lymphocytotoxic test (Fig. 26-1) for HLA-A, HLA-B, HLA-C, and HLA-DR antigens. Antisera of defined class I or class II specificity are used in combination with cells of donor or recipient origin (usually peripheral blood or splenic lymphocytes). Cross-matching is done by a similar technique, but with cells of defined specificity and test serum.

Proliferative tests give a predictive in vitro correlate of the response to the prospective allograft, but are not widely used clinically. Mixed lymphocyte culture (MLC), with donor cells as targets and recipient cells as responders, has been used in some centers to predict the success of living-related-donor kidney transplants. However, the long incubation time (5 to 6 days) required for the MLC limits its usefulness. Because class II antigen–primed typing cells may be prepared and stored in liquid nitrogen, the primed lymphocyte test (PLT) can identify disparate HLA-DR and HLA-DP antigens in 12 to 24 h, but development of lymphocytotoxic tests for class II antigens has made the PLT obsolete. Cell-mediated lympholysis assays, which may be an in vitro correlate of allograft rejection, remain the province of research.

In addition to tissue typing and cross-matching, ABO typing is routinely performed on both donor and recipient. While individuals of blood types A, B, or AB can receive organs from type O individuals, presence of anti-A or anti-B antibodies causes hyperacute rejection of the graft.

HOST AND GRAFT IMMUNE RESPONSE

Types of Rejection

Even with immunosuppression, many, if not all, organ transplants are rejected. Rejection may be classified as hyperacute, accelerated, acute, or chronic. Many rejection episodes may be reversed by increased immunosuppression.

Hyperacute rejection occurs within minutes of vascular anastomosis and is due to preformed host cytotoxic antibodies to donor HLA or ABO antigens. Preformed anti-HLA antibodies are the result of exposure to the relevant antigens through blood or blood product transfusion, previous organ transplant, or pregnancy. These antibodies

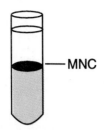

1. Mononuclear cells (MNC) are separated by density centrifugation.

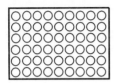

2. MNC are added to a panel of antibodies.

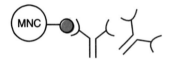

3a. Antibody binds to antigen on MNC.

3b. The appropriate antigen is not present on MNC. Antibody does not bind.

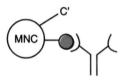

4a. Complement is fixed.

4b. Complement is not fixed.

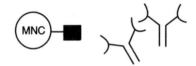

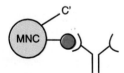

5a. MNC are killed; eosin is admitted.

5b. MNC remain viable; eosin is excluded.

Figure 26-1 Lymphocytotoxicity assay. Using a panel of different antibodies specific for different class I and II MHC markers, one can determine the tissue type of the lymphocyte. If the antibody binds to the MHC antigen on the cell, 3a, 4a, and 5a occur. If the antibody does not recognize and bind to the MHC antigen, 3b, 4b and 5b occur.

interact with the vascular endothelium of the organ. Complement is activated, followed by heavy platelet deposition and thrombosis. Infiltrating cells are predominantly neutrophils, with relatively few lymphocytes. The final result is acute ischemic necrosis. Cell-mediated immunity plays no part in hyperacute rejection. Since the initiation of histocompatibility testing (crossmatching) prior to transplantation, hyperacute rejections are no longer common.

Accelerated rejection occurs within 2 to 5 days after transplantation. Both humoral and cell-mediated responses due to previous sensitization with donor antigens are implicated. Rarely, accelerated rejection is caused by antibodies to minor antigens present on donor kidney cells or to antiendothelial cell antibodies.

Most HLA-mismatched grafts require treatment for *acute rejection* 7 to 21 days after transplantation. A complex series of cell-mediated mechanisms is initiated in the lymphoid tissues, blood vessels, lymphatics, and interstitium of the graft. Mononuclear cell infiltrates cause arteritis and perivascular cuffing, and, along with occasional granulocytes, heavily infiltrate the interstitium. The most severe vascular lesions are generally located in the arterial intima. Class I and class II antigen expression is up-regulated, and initiates extensive endothelial damage. Some antibody-complement-mediated vascular damage probably also occurs, but cell-mediated immunity is the primary cause of acute rejection.

Chronic rejection (occurring more than 1 year after transplantation) reflects a disturbance of host-graft tolerance not treatable by increased immunosuppression. In contrast to acute rejection, chronic rejection is an indolent process resulting in fibrosis and scarring with limited inflammatory response. The most striking abnormalities are in the arteries and arterioles, where, in addition to progressive ischemia, there is also a cumulative loss of structural and functional integrity due to earlier acute rejection episodes. Humoral response is predominant in chronic rejection, although cell-mediated mechanisms such as antibody-dependent cellular cytotoxicity may also play a part.

The extent and rate of each type of rejection vary, since tissues are rejected by different mechanisms and at different rates. For example, bone marrow and skin grafts are extremely susceptible to rapid rejection, heart and kidney tissue are intermediate in immunogenicity, and liver grafts are relatively insensitive. It is interesting that hyperacute rejection is not common in liver allografts, even with blood-group mismatch or preformed antibodies to donor HLA antigens. (The liver, however, can undergo vigorous cellular rejection with involvement of bile duct epithelium. This cellular rejection may

be distinguished from primary biliary cirrhosis by the absence of ductular proliferation, the absence of granulomas, and the accumulation of copper-binding protein in the periportal hepatocytes.) Some factors influencing susceptibility to rejection include presence and extent of lymphatic drainage, access of host circulation to the graft, the amount of vascular endothelium present, the extent of contact between recipient alloreactive cells and donor alloantigen-presenting cells, and the degree of expression of class I and class II antigens.

The Mediation of Rejection by Specific and Nonspecific Responses

The mechanisms by which grafts are rejected are complex (Fig. 26-2), but primarily involve classical primary or secondary immune responses. Generally, acute and chronic rejection are a response to the first exposure to the disparate antigens, while hyperacute rejection illustrates the acquisition of memory and the rapid secondary response.

Rejection follows a conventional pattern of recognition, cellular proliferation, and tissue destruction. All allografts exhibit mononuclear cell infiltration within hours of transplantation, even in the presence of immunosuppression. Immunologically specific responses leading to rejection are initiated when foreign antigens on the graft are recognized by infiltrating host T cells. Class I antigens act as targets for CD8$^+$ cells, while CD4$^+$ cells recognize class II antigens. Both humoral and cell-mediated rejections are dependent on this small population of T cells. T-cell activation and proliferation are a result of the interaction in the host of the donor-specific T cells with graft antigens.

Do these infiltrating T cells actually cause rejection? One model suggests that after antigen-specific T cells enter the graft, clonal proliferation of CD4$^+$ cells occurs and lymphokines are released. However, full-blown rejection is generated by a cascade requiring more than these antigen-specific cells. Macrophages are activated, either by direct

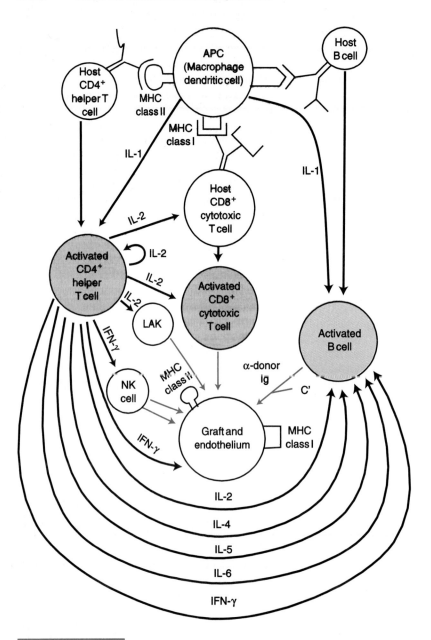

Figure 26-2   Mechanisms of graft rejection. Many different mechanisms may be active, including natural killer (NK), lymphokine-activated (LAK) and cytotoxic T cells, as well as killing mediated by anti-donor immunoglobulin plus complement (C'). Modification of the endothelium by the direct effect of lymphokines contributes, as well.

contact with the antigen-activated T cells or with T-cell lymphokines. Activated T cells secrete more IL-2 (which acts both as a growth factor and as a stimulus for production of other lymphokines by the antigen-activated T cells) and express receptors for IL-2. IL-2 also induces proliferation of activated class I–specific CD8$^+$ T cells, generates lymphokine-activated killer cells, and acts as a growth and differentiation factor on B cells. The IFN-γ released by activated helper T cells stimulates NK-cell activity and up-regulates class II antigen expression on donor tissues such as the vascular endothelium, while IL-4 and IL-5 act on B cells.

There is controversy about which cells actually cause the tissue damage seen in rejection. Grossly, patchy cellular infiltrates are seen throughout vessel walls. Mononuclear cells are seen in the interstitium, and endothelial swelling and vacuolation occur. In general, cells expressing class I or class II antigens seem to be most vulnerable. For example, the endothelium of the capillaries, arteries, and veins, and the glomeruli of the kidney, may be extensively damaged by rejection, while the parietal cells of Bowman's capsule are relatively unaffected. CD8$^+$ cytotoxic T cells have long been considered to be the effector cells in graft destruction, and can, in animal models, cause rejection on their own. However, experimental data show that rejection and tissue destruction can proceed without CD8$^+$ cells. In fact, the physical manifestations of rejection (endothelial damage, necrotizing arteritis, mononuclear cell infiltration, and intimal proliferation and fibrosis) are due primarily to cytokines released by infiltrating cells rather than to antigen-specific immune injury. Macrophages in particular produce cytokines which increase vascular permeability and contribute to local tissue necrosis. Neutrophils are also present in allografts undergoing rejection and may cause some tissue damage, but are probably bystanders rather than active participants in rejection.

As we have seen, rejection encompasses both cellular and humoral components. The humoral response to an allograft depends on the extent of antigenic disparity, the immunogenicity of the antigens, the target organ, and the ability of the host to produce antibody. The main target of humoral immunity is the organ vasculature, and injury can be extensive. Complement- and antibody-dependent cytotoxicity are the primary mechanisms of humoral tissue injury. The susceptibility of grafts to antibody depends on whether antigen-antibody complexes are internalized and whether there is a repair mechanism present in the graft. Some antibodies may actually *enhance* rather than decrease allograft survival, leading to speculation that donor antigen-specific antibody might be useful for clinical immunosuppression.

Immunologic Monitoring of Host and Graft Response

Since rejection is common but very often treatable in allograft transplants, accurate and early diagnosis of rejection is essential (see Clinical Aside 26-2). Monitoring may be of biochemical criteria (i.e., creatinine levels in kidney transplant patients, liver enzymes for liver transplants), histologic criteria (needle core biopsies or fine needle aspirations), or immunologic parameters.

Clinical Aside 26-2
Bone Marrow Transplant in Leukemia

Mary Jane Dunn is a 5-year-old white female who presented to her pediatrician with fever, fatigue, and numerous ecchymoses on her extremities. Blood work demonstrated a white blood count of 11,000 with 75 percent juvenile blast forms, a platelet count of 42,000, and a hematocrit of 18 percent. Suspecting acute myelogenous leukemia (AML), Mary Jane's pediatrician obtained histochemical and immunologic confirmation.

After confirmation of the diagnosis of AML, Mary Jane underwent antineoplastic chemotherapy. She went into complete remission from her leukemia, with no blast forms identified in either her peripheral blood or marrow. Because the relapse rate in AML despite successful therapy is extremely high, Mary Jane proceeded on to bone marrow transplantation. Initially her siblings were screened, and one of her brothers was found to be HLA-identical as well as ABO-compatible.

Before transplantation, Mary Jane was given very-high-dose cyclophosphamide and whole-body radiation to obliterate any remaining malignant cells, and to obliterate her own marrow so that she could accept the transplant. After transplantation, with bone marrow donated by Mary Jane's brother, Mary Jane's peripheral complete blood counts demonstrated initial restoration of her hemopoietic system. One month later, Mary Jane was noted to have bloody bowel movements, ulceration in her mouth, and open wounds involving the skin of the extremities and trunk. Mary Jane also developed jaundice and began having hemoptysis.

It became apparent that Mary Jane was developing acute graft-versus-host disease (GVHD), with the donated blood cells infiltrating the epithelium of a number of systems in her body. She was treated aggressively with cyclosporine and methotrexate, and the acute GVHD resolved. From that point on, Mary Jane's hemopoietic system remained stable without rejection or further GVHD.

Immunologic monitoring of the peripheral blood is relatively noninvasive (as opposed to tissue biopsy). Mixed lymphocyte culture, response to mitogenic stimuli, cytotoxic and suppressor assays, phenotypic analysis of mononuclear cells, and cytokine levels have all been used clinically with limited success. These parameters are not totally specific for rejection, and are affected by outside influences, such as infection or immunosuppression. Measuring serum levels of soluble IL-2 receptors seems to be the most promising method of immunologic monitoring presently available, with moderately elevated levels correlating with rejection.

IMMUNOMODULATION— THE ESTABLISHMENT OF TOLERANCE?

Nonspecific Immunosuppression

Immunosuppression generally begins at the time of transplantation and continues

throughout the life of the graft. Nonspecific immunosuppression (Table 26-1) down-regulates host response to the graft and occasionally induces tolerance of donor antigens. Multiagent protocols including corticosteroids, azathioprine, antilymphocyte globulin (or anti-CD3 monoclonal antibody), and cyclosporine are common.

Unfortunately, nonspecific immunosuppression also disrupts the host response to pathogens. Chemoprophylaxis directed against common opportunistic pathogens (e.g., trimethoprim-sulfamethoxazole to prevent *Pneumocystis* infection, high doses of nystatin to prevent infection with *Candida*, and immunoglobulin to prevent cytomegalovirus [CMV] infection or reactivation) may be employed. Obviously, the lowest effective doses of immunosuppressive agents are used. Many of the agents used in transplantation maintenance therapy are also used in the treatment of immune and autoimmune diseases (see Chap. 33A).

Corticosteroids (e.g., prednisolone or methylprednisolone) impair cellular rejection mechanisms, but are rarely used as the sole source of immunosuppression because of significant side effects (Table 26-2). Corticosteroids also suppress macrophage production of IL-1 by blocking activation of the IL-1 gene, and therefore indirectly inhibit IL-2 production and release, with resulting inhibition of cytotoxic T-cell proliferation and differentiation. Corticosteroids may also lyse T cells and inhibit immune cell migration. While corticosteroids are used in low doses for maintenance of immunosuppression, high-dose pulses reduce the fever and inflammation occurring in rejection and are very effective in reversing rejection episodes.

For the past 20 years, corticosteroids have been used in conjunction with *azathioprine*, a 6-mercaptopurine analogue which inhibits synthesis of both DNA and RNA by preventing the synthesis of adenylic and guanylic acids from inosinic acid. Azathioprine affects rapidly dividing cells in the lymphoid organs, bone marrow, skin, and gastrointestinal tract. At therapeutic doses (limited by side effects), immunosuppression is partial,

TABLE 26-2 Side Effects of Nonspecific Immunosuppression

Corticosteroids	*Azathioprine*
Lymphocytopenia	Bone marrow depression
Cataract formation	Megaloblastic anemia
Cushing's syndrome	Gastrointestinal disturbances
Hypertension	Hepatotoxicity
Osteoporosis	
Growth suppression	*Antilymphocyte globulin*
Delayed wound	Thrombocytopenia
healing	Granulocytopenia
	Leukopenia
OKT3	Antigen-antibody-induced
"Flulike" symptoms	glomerulonephritis
Pulmonary edema	Complement-mediated
Hypotension	hypersensitivity
	Serum sickness
Cyclosporine	
Nephrotoxicity	*Total lymphoid irradiation*
Hepatotoxicity	Leukopenia
Lymphoma	Fever
Hirsutism	CMV infection or
Tremor	reactivation
Hypertension	Lymphoma
Nausea, vomiting	Gastrointestinal disturbances
Gum hyperplasia	

Note: All nonspecific immunosuppression carries a risk of increased infection from pathogenic and opportunistic organisms.

and cell-mediated immunity is suppressed more than humoral immunity. Azathioprine is not particularly useful in reversal of acute allograft rejection.

Corticosteroids and azathioprine both affect multiple organ systems while inducing immunosuppression. The search for more specific immunosuppressants has led to the prophylactic use of antilymphocyte globulin (ALG) in conjunction with other agents and for treatment of rejection episodes. ALG is the IgG fraction of a heterologous antiserum prepared by injecting horses, rabbits, or goats with purified human peripheral blood lymphocytes, thymocytes, or splenocytes. ALG acts as an opsonin and facilitates clearance of lymphocytes through the mononuclear phagocyte system. Some complement-mediated lysis of lymphocytes may also occur. Continued ALG therapy may lead to the generation of nonspecific suppressor T cells. ALG is more specific in its targets than corticosteroids and azathioprine, but there are still significant side effects.

Monoclonal antibodies operate through mechanisms similar to those of ALG, but with much greater target specificity. OKT3, produced by murine hybridomas, is specific for the delta protein of the T cell–antigen recognition complex. Treatment with OKT3 effectively blocks T-cell effector functions primarily by opsonization followed by clearance of the antigen receptor–CD3 molecular complex. Once again, side effects are significant. OKT3 is primarily used for treatment of corticosteroid-resistant rejections. Some clinicians are assessing prophylactic use of OKT3 in high-risk patients, but patient production of antimurine antibodies is not uncommon, and has important therapeutic implications such as loss of effectiveness of the drug for further use. Therapeutic use of monoclonal antibodies to the IL-2 receptor, the T-cell-antigen receptor, certain cell surface activation markers (e.g., CD5) and CD4 is currently under investigation.

Major increases in graft survival occurred following the introduction of *cyclosporine*, a very hydrophobic 11-amino acid polypeptide (with the novel amino acid C9-onine) produced by *Tolyprocardium inflatum.* By selectively inhibiting production and/or release of IL-2 from activated T cells (and possibly by blocking production of other lymphokines such as IL-4 and IL-5), cyclosporine suppresses both humoral and cell-mediated immunity. Cyclosporine is highly immunosuppressive when used prophylactically, but has not been useful in treating established rejection, partly because activation of the IL-2 receptor gene is not blocked. Increased incidence of nephrotoxicity and other side effects from the original high-dose therapy has led to employment of low-dose cyclosporine in conjunction with other immunosuppressants.

Nonspecific immunosuppression has also been approached, at least experimentally, by *total lymphoid irradiation (TLI)* and *thoracic duct drainage.* Both of these techniques cause systemic depletion of T lymphocytes. TLI is based on the highly radiosensitive nature of most T lymphocytes, and results in decreased T-cell function and number and in tolerance to the graft. Improved graft function has been achieved in some high-risk patients, but transplantation must occur within a few weeks of TLI, and patients still require immunosuppression. Use of TLI to help establish donor-specific tolerance has potential, but the treatment is very expensive and side effects are severe.

Thoracic duct drainage may be accomplished by inserting a catheter into the thoracic duct. Removal of mononuclear cells from the lymph decreases the number of circulating lymphocytes. Clinical trials using thoracic duct drainage in conjunction with corticosteroids, azathioprine, and/or ALG have been successful in increasing allograft survival, but technical problems make this a difficult and very expensive procedure.

Establishing Antigen-Specific Tolerance

Establishing donor-specific immunosuppression would eliminate many of the difficulties associated with nonspecific immunosuppression. In some animal models transferable specific tolerance (dependent on T suppressor cells) can be induced in neonates. Unfortunately, establishment of specific tolerance in adult animals has proven elusive.

Establishment of tolerance requires two distinct phases: (1) induction by immunization with antigen or antibody and (2) maintenance. Antigen-specific antiserum has been used to induce tolerance in animals. In clinical practice, tolerance induction has been attempted by the use of blood transfusions (random or donor) or, less commonly, anti-idiotypic antibodies.

In 1960 Brent and Medawar proposed three possible mechanisms for immunologic enhancement by specific antiserum:

1. Antibody coats the graft antigens, thereby preventing recognition by the host.
2. Antibody blocks the immune effector mechanisms.
3. Antibody present at the time of transplantation blocks the host's response to

the graft antigens, leading to specific B-cell tolerance.

In addition, the antibody may suppress cell-mediated immunity by opsonizing helper or cytotoxic T cells reacting with specific class I or class II antigens. Immunologic enhancement has been successful in animal studies, particularly in rats with low class II antigen expression on vascular endothelium. Unfortunately, benefit in humans (who have high class II expression) may be limited by the titer of antibody tolerated without antigen-antibody complex damage to the endothelium.

Blood transfusion from random donors significantly improves kidney allograft survival. Five to ten transfusions are required for maximum effect. Potential recipients of grafts from live donors derive benefit from three spaced transfusions of donor blood. However, with both random and donor-specific transfusions, there is substantial potential for the development of cytotoxic anti-HLA antibodies. For example, about 30 percent of potential live-donor graft recipients become sensitized to donor antigens during the transfusion protocol. The factors responsible for maximum graft survival as opposed to those leading to sensitization are not understood.

Why do blood transfusions increase graft survival? Both specific and nonspecific mechanisms may operate:

1. The red cell breakdown products themselves may be nonspecifically immunosuppressive.
2. The white blood cells present in the transfusions may elicit a primary antibody response while the HLA-bearing graft maintains this protective antibody response—a mechanism very similar to that proposed by Brent and Medawar for immunologic enhancement. The observation that the presence of antibody-blocked Fc receptors on B cells correlates with good allograft survival supports this hypothesis.
3. Suppressor cells (or suppressor factors) may be generated. These cells inhibit helper T

cells and B cells, prevent IL-2 action of responsive cells, prevent recruitment of naive cells, and prevent differentiation of immature cytotoxic T cells.

4. Blood transfusions may help identify recipients who make cytotoxic antibody in large amounts, so-called high responders. These cytotoxic antibodies would be detected by the routine cross-matching carried out before the transplant, and would preclude transplantation of particular class I and class II antigens.

5. Anti-idiotypic antibody may be induced. Blood transfusions in humans do generate both anti-HLA antibodies and anti-idiotypic HLA antibodies. Anti-idiotypic antibodies may be responsible for the successful transplantation of individuals with historically positive crossmatches where anti-HLA antibodies detected at some time before transplantation are undetectable by the time of transplantation. Anti-idiotypic antibodies affecting both humoral and cellular immunity have the potential to be a very effective means of specific immunosuppression, although occurrence of anti-anti-idiotypic antibody could override the benefits of anti-idiotypic antibody.

Antigen-specific immunosuppression is the *sine qua non* of successful transplantation.

TRANSPLANTATION TODAY—STATE OF THE ART

Over 50,000 organ transplants were performed in the United States in 1989 (Table 26-3). Graft survival has been increasing over the past decade, and the advent of new generations of immunosuppressive agents such as FK506, antibodies to cytokines and cytokine receptors, and multiagent therapy should allow continued improvement.

HLA matching, once the *sine qua non* of organ transplantation, does not seem to be as essential in patients treated with cyclo-

TABLE 26-3 Organ Transplants and Estimated Survival Rates in the United States in 1989.

Organ	No. of Transplants	1-Year Survival, %
Kidney	8,886	90–95
Heart	1,673	82
Liver	2,160	77
Pancreas	412	44
Heart-lung	70	68–70
Lung	89	35
Cornea	36,900	90–95
Bone marrow	1,659	14–70

Source: United Network for Organ Sharing.

sporine. An analysis by UCLA of kidney graft survival showed a difference of only 11 percent between HLA-identical matches and zero matches in patients treated with cyclosporine. Matching is not common in heart, heart-lung, liver, pancreas, or cornea transplants (although a 10 percent increase in corneal graft survival has been observed with HLA-matched grafts). Current thinking suggests that cross-matching to determine reactivity with defined epitopes on HLA molecules, called *epitope matching*, rather than antigen matching may be more meaningful. In standard cross-matching, incompatibilities are detected by serologic or cellular reactivity with the entire class I or class II MHC molecule. Within every protein molecule there are multiple epitopes, and MHC molecules are no exception. Epitope matching allows one to measure reactivity with the set of epitopes unique to that MHC molecule, rather than with the entire molecule. This allows for more sensitive detection of mismatches at the HLA locus. In addition, a proposed match which is acceptable by standard techniques but unacceptable by epitope mapping may predict trouble with engraftment. Patients whose grafts had no epitope mismatches had a 15 percent increase in graft survival when compared to patients transplanted with tissue with more than 25 epitope mismatches. An even newer approach is to use the polymerase chain reaction (PCR) as a means of determining an even better match. (How would you use PCR to assure such a match?)

Although graft survival of kidney, heart, liver, and cornea transplants is excellent, improvement in heart-lung, pancreas, and small bowel allografts is desirable. Heart-lung transplants have been complicated by breakdown or stenosis of the bronchial anastomoses. In addition, obliterative bronchiolitis and occlusive vascular disease account for 50 percent of the deaths.

Combined pancreas-kidney transplants have been more successful than pancreas transplantation alone. Pancreas transplantation with bladder drainage of exocrine secretions has improved survival by allowing early diagnosis of rejection based on urinary amylase activity. Pancreatic islet cell transplantation would be ideal and would decrease the morbidity seen with pancreas transplantation, but the survival of the highly immunogenic islets has been poor and human islets for transplantation have been difficult to obtain.

Transplantation of the small bowel has been pursued sporadically over the past 30 years, but the 1-year graft survival is still less than 10 percent. Rejection of this highly immunogenic organ has been the rule, and adequate bowel function without total parenteral nutrition has been the exception.

Bone marrow allograft survival depends on the underlying disorder. Survival has improved to 50 to 70 percent in patients with aplastic anemia but is as low as 14 percent in patients with chronic myelogenous leukemia with blast crisis. Complete HLA matching is no longer required in all cases, and the survival of nonidentical marrow is comparable to that of HLA-identical marrow. However, the incidence of acute GVHD is much greater in patients transplanted with nonidentical marrow.

Acute GVHD remains the greatest problem in bone marrow transplantation, and carries a 50 percent mortality rate. Twenty to fifty percent of patients receiving HLA-identical bone marrow from a sibling develop significant acute GVHD. An equal number of patients may develop chronic GVHD, either independently or as a sequelae of acute GVHD. The incidence of GVHD may be decreased by treatment of the recipient with cyclosporine and methotrexate, or by depletion of T lymphocytes from the donor bone marrow before transplantation. However, increased graft failure has been observed with the use of T cell–depleted marrow, suggesting that T cells are necessary to destroy host cells causing rejection. Moderate GVHD actually has a beneficial effect on disease-free survival in leukemic patients—a "graft-versus-leukemia" effect.

SELF-TEST QUESTIONS

1. Sibling A (age 42) donated a kidney to sibling B (age 28). The HLA laboratory results indicated that the two siblings were matched at the HLA-A, HLA-B, HLA-D, and HLA-D/DR loci. Sibling B received triple immunosuppressive drug therapy, but rejected the graft after 2 months. Why?

2. A kidney from an AB-positive, Rh-negative, HLA-A2,12: HLA-B1,27; HLA-DR3,4 donor was transplanted into an O-positive, RH-positive, HLA-A2,5; HLA-B1,21; HLA-DR3,5 recipient. The graft underwent hyperacute rejection 15 min after establishment of blood flow. What was the most likely cause of this rejection?

3. Endothelial damage and necrotizing arteritis are seen during acute rejection. What is the direct cause of this tissue damage?

4. After a kidney allograft, a patient received quadruple immunosuppressive therapy with azathioprine, corticosteroids, OKT3, and cyclosporine. Three weeks after transplantation, the patient's serum creatinine increased to 3.5 mg/dL (normal range is 0.6 to 1.2 mg/dL). A biopsy of the transplanted kidney showed lymphocytic infiltration with vascular lesions in the arterial intima. What was the *most likely* cause of the increase in serum creatinine?
   a. Chronic rejection of the graft
   b. Acute rejection of the graft
   c. Accelerated rejection of the graft

d. Cyclosporine nephrotoxicity
e. Antimurine antibody formation
5. Following bone marrow transplantation between two strains of inbred rats, GVHD is most likely in which combination?
a. Lewis donor → Lewis recipient
b. Brown Norway donor → Lewis recipient
c. Lewis–brown Norway F_1 donor → Lewis recipient
d. Lewis–brown Norway F_1 donor → brown Norway recipient
e. Brown Norway donor → Lewis–brown Norway F_1 recipient

ADDITIONAL READINGS

Bevan MJ. High determinant density may explain phenomenon of alloreactivity. *Immunol Today.* 1984;5:128–130.

Calne RY, ed. *Transplantation Immunology: Clinical and Experimental.* New York: Oxford University Press; 1984.

Kahan B, ed. *Cyclosporin A: Biological Activity and Clinical Applications.* New York: Grune & Stratton; 1984.

Klein J. *Natural History of the Major Histocompatibility Complex.* New York: Wiley; 1987.

Lechler RI, Lombardi G, Batchelor JR, Reinsmoen N, Bach FH. The molecular basis of alloreactivity. *Immunol Today.* 1990; 11:83–88.

Parkman R. Graft-versus-host disease: An alternative hypothesis. *Immunol Today.* 1989; 10:362–364.

Roopenian DC. What are minor histocompatibility loci? A new look at an old question. *Immunol Today.* 1992; 13:7–10.

Schreiber SL, Crabtree GR. The mechanism of action of cyclosporin A and FK 506. *Immunol Today.* 1992; 13:136–142.

Williams GM, Burdick JF, and Solez K, eds. *Kidney Transplant Rejection: Diagnosis and Treatment.* New York: Marcel Dekker; 1986.

27

Pregnancy and the Fetal-Maternal Relationship

INTRODUCTION

Pregnancy becomes established through a complex process, a critical period of which is the implantation stage. Optimally coordinated interaction between the conceptus and the maternal decidua allows the blastocyst to attach so that the trophoblast can invade the endometrium to develop nutrient vessels for the conceptus. In humans this process is inefficient and results in significant embryo and fetal wastage. It is believed that 75 percent of all human conceptions fail to become established pregnancies that produce viable offspring. Preimplantation loss is common and affects 50 to 60 percent of embryos. After implantation, approximately 30 percent of pregnancies undergo spontaneous abortion; about two-thirds of these losses occur before the pregnancy has been clinically recognized. Thus there are approximately two occult pregnancy failures for each clinically observed spontaneous abortion. It has been suggested that these two types of pregnancy loss represent distinct pathophysiologic states, since occult losses arise before fetal chorionic circulation has been established, whereas clinical spontaneous abortions usually occur after a vascular supply to the fetus has been initiated.

Spontaneous abortion is the most common complication of pregnancy, occurring at a frequency of 10 to 15 percent. In most instances it is an isolated, nonrecurring event, but in some women it occurs repeatedly. When a woman has had three or more consecutive abortions, she is categorized as suffering from "habitual abortion." Several causes of recurrent abortion have been suggested, including chromosomal anomalies in one or both parents, uterine anatomic defects, genital tract infections, the presence of antiphospholipid antibodies such as anticardiolipin antibody, and hormonal deficiency resulting from inadequate corpus luteum function. Women are described as having "unexplained" habitual abortion when an obvious cause cannot be established. In these women one cause is believed to be an impairment in maternal immunologic recognition resulting in failure to produce a protective response toward the fetus.

For your assistance in reading this chapter, the following embryologic terms are defined here.

GLOSSARY

Blastocyst: The fertilized ovum undergoes cell division (producing smaller cells, known as *blastomeres*) to yield a cell mass with the appearance of a mulberry, called the *morula*. The more centrally placed cells (the *inner cell mass*) are surrounded by a layer of superficial cells (the *trophoblast*, occasionally called the *outer cell mass*). With accumulation of interstitial fluid within the morula, the spaces between the cells on one side of the inner cell mass become larger and then merge to form an inner cavity, known as the *blastocele*. This stage of development of the morula is called the *blastocyst*.

Chorion: The outermost of the extraembryonic membranes, which contributes to the formation of the placenta.

Decidua: A process of alteration of the pregnant endometrium in which stromal cells increase in size and number and blood vessels and glands undergo modification. These changes in the uterine mucosal connective tissue are elicited by the implanting blastocyst and are dependent on progesterone. Part of the tissue from which the placenta is derived is decidual in origin.

Embryo: Describes the early stage of prenatal development, during which time organogenesis occurs; in humans this extends from week 4 to week 8 of gestation.

Endometrium: A layer of tissue lining the cavity inside the uterus, which contains glandular structures and blood vessels, among other structures.

Fetus: Describes the developing soon-to-be baby at a stage where the body structures are recognizable; in humans this stage extends from approximately week 9 to the end of gestation.

Placenta: The organ that provides nutrition for the fetus, formed from the membranes of the fetus, which attaches to the uterine endometrium/decidua.

Trophoblast: At the site of implantation, the portion of the blastocyst which comes in contact with the endometrium begins to proliferate. This area of thickening of the blastocyst is called the *invading trophoblast*. The inner layer of cells differentiates into an inner *cytotrophoblast*, immediately adjacent to the inner cell mass. On the uterine side of the cytotrophoblast that invades the endometrium and contacts maternal blood directly is a thick outer layer in which the cells merge to form a syncytium, with loss of the separating cell membranes; this layer is the *syncytiotrophoblast*. Thus, the trophoblast is tissue derived from the outer cell of the blastocyst, which attaches the fertilized ovum to the uterine wall, forms the placenta, and separates extraembryonic membranes from decidua.

IMMUNOLOGIC CONSIDERATIONS IN FETAL-MATERNAL INTERACTION

Mammalian fertilization involves the fusion of sperm and oocyte surface membranes, following which sperm surface antigens continue to move freely over the zygote membrane. The conceptus also inherits and expresses on the surface of its cells the father's histocompatibility antigens, which are usually foreign to the mother. Other fetal cell surface markers represent organ-specific and embryonal (oncofetal) antigens. The pregnant female may recognize and mount immune responses against some of these antigens. In some instances, an antigen-specific

response may result in immunity that "rejects" the embryo. However, recent studies indicate that spontaneous abortion may also be initiated by effector cells such as natural killer (NK) cells, lymphokine-activated killer (LAK) cells, and macrophages from the mother's innate (or natural) immune system that recognize primitive embryonic and tumor cells. Thus, the hypothesis that abortion may represent rejection of the fetus as a foreign body by the mother is plausible.

Several observations support a role for the specific immune response. For example, some women who abort lack serum factors which block the reactivity of their lymphocytes to placental and/or paternal leukocyte antigens. Immunization of these women with paternal lymphocytes that stimulate production of blocking antibodies is associated with a reduction in the rate of subsequent abortion. Studies of pregnancy failure after in vitro fertilization demonstrate infiltration of embryos by maternal mononuclear cells. Similarly, lymphocytic infiltration of villi and decidua is also observed in a significant proportion of tissue samples obtained from first trimester spontaneous abortions. These findings are not unlike those identified in graft rejection by both specific and natural effector mechanisms.

Survival of the conceptus at each stage of its development depends upon avoidance of harm from maternal graft rejection cells. This may come about by lack of generation of harmful types of immunity, by lack of accumulation of the effectors of immunity at the implantation site, or by lack of fetal susceptibility to damage by maternal effector mechanisms. Alternatively, a protective environment may be generated by active suppression of maternal immune and innate effector cell activation by maternal cells, by the conceptus itself, or as a consequence of an interaction between them. The latter model is particularly appealing, since both specific and innate systems are paralyzed.

Most of the available information on immunologic issues relating to maternal-fetal interaction has been obtained from murine and other animal studies, because human tissue is seldom accessible for investigation during early peri- and postimplantation phases of pregnancy. Human studies, nevertheless, have usually paralleled the findings from murine studies. The developmental kinetics of pregnant laboratory mice mated with genetically nonidentical mice of the same species are such that the first four postimplantation days correspond to the first 16 to 18 days of human postimplantation embryo growth (4 to 5 weeks gestational age, where the onset of the last menstrual period is defined as the onset of pregnancy and a 4-week menstrual cycle is assumed). Therefore, pregnancy failure during the 4-day postimplantation phase of murine pregnancy corresponds roughly to the time period during which occult pregnancy failure occurs in humans, whereas failure of mouse pregnancy on or after day 9.5 (5 days postimplantation) corresponds to the timing of most human first-trimester abortions.

THE FETUS-TROPHOBLAST UNIT AS TWO SEPARATE GRAFTS

The developing blastocyst at implantation (Fig. 27-1) consists of an inner cell mass that will become the fetus and an outer trophoblast layer that will become the placenta at the fetal-maternal interface. The fetal tissue and the trophoblast may be viewed as two separate grafts of the conceptus, and maternal immune reactions can be directed against either.

Immune Response to Fetal Tissue

Fetal tissue is immunogenic and susceptible to immunologic recognition and rejection by the mother even while she is pregnant, provided that contact occurs between cells of the fetus and the maternal lymphomyeloid system. This phenomenon was clearly demonstrated in experiments in which fetuses transplanted to the thigh of a pregnant ro-

dent were rejected but those remaining in her uterus were unharmed.

Models of interspecies pregnancy, such as goat-sheep matings and transfer of donkey embryos into horses, are associated with pregnancy failure in which there is mononuclear cell infiltration of the fetus. In addition, there is an accelerated failure in repeated interspecies pregnancies, which is indicative of immunologic memory. Similarly, transfer of *Mus caroli* blastocysts into the uterus of *Mus musculus* recipients has been associated with postimplantation maternal cytotoxic-T-lineage infiltration of the *M caroli* fetus, which is resorbed within its trophoblast shell. This phenomenon is similar to the frequently occurring situation in which an anembryonic sac is found in patients with spontaneous abortion. However, despite these observations, entry of maternal lymphocytes into the fetus is relatively uncommon due to a barrier at the maternal-fetal interface where maternal cells are effectively blocked. Therefore, the conceptus behaves in a manner different from conventional allografts, and this may be due to the properties of its trophoblast.

Immune Response to the Trophoblast

At the time of blastocyst implantation, the invading conceptus is analogous to a locally invasive tumour. The trophoblast cells contiguous to and invading the endometrium coalesce to become an amorphous, multinucleated mass called the *syncytium*, which is made up of syncytiotrophoblast cells derived from an inner layer of cytotrophoblast cells. The trophoblast is, therefore, made up of two clearly distinguishable layers of cells: the syncytiotrophoblast cells, which are contiguous with maternal decidua, and the cytotrophoblast cells, which form an inner layer covering the fetal vessels as they traverse into the placental villi. As invasion by the trophoblast proceeds, maternal blood vessels are trapped to form lacunae, which become filled with maternal blood. Consequently, mater-

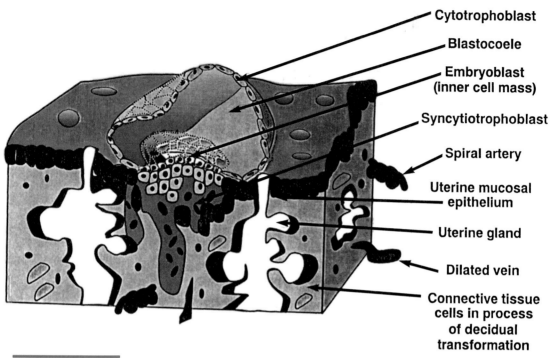

Cytotrophoblast

Blastocoele

Embryoblast
(inner cell mass)

Syncytiotrophoblast

Spiral artery

Uterine mucosal
epithelium

Uterine gland

Dilated vein

Connective tissue
cells in process
of decidual
transformation

Figure 27-1 Diagrammatic relief presentation of the blastocyst implanting in the uterine mucosa.

nal blood directly bathes the syncytiotrophoblast layer, but fetal blood is separated from trophoblast cells by the endothelium of the fetal vessel in the intravillous space. As the placenta grows, the cytotrophoblast outside the villi (extravillous or invasive cytotrophoblast) anchors the placenta to and directly contacts maternal decidua.

The fetal trophoblast is a unique tissue, the development of which is dependent upon the presence of paternal genetic material. Extensive immunologic studies on the trophoblast have confirmed that the syncytiotrophoblast fails to express class I major histocompatibility complex (MHC) antigens. However, trophoblast-specific TA-1 and TA-2 antigens have been detected on trophoblast cells. In contrast, early invasive cytotrophoblast tissue express a modified form of class I MHC antigen. These cells also in-

vade the maternal spiral arterioles of the placental bed as an essential step in early placentation, thus coming into direct contact with maternal blood. Therefore, even though the syncytiotrophoblast does not express MHC antigens, the cytotrophoblast, which comes into contact with maternal decidua and maternal blood, does in a modified form. Interestingly, class II MHC antigens are absent from both types of trophoblast at all stages of gestation.

Trophoblast tissue is not susceptible to lysis by cytotoxic T lymphocytes and appears to be resistant to rejection by antigen-specific immune effector mechanisms. Similarly, gestational trophoblast neoplasms, in which the trophoblast genes are entirely paternal, are not rejected by the female even when high levels of paternal human leukocyte antigens (HLA) are expressed.

Nevertheless, murine placental function can be compromised by antibody to paternal MHC antigens in the presence of highly active xenogeneic (rabbit) complement. Isolated trophoblast cells can be lysed by antibody and rabbit complement. Also, it is becoming increasingly apparent that trophoblast tissue may be sensitive to certain types of nonspecific effector cells that are part of the innate defense system that selectively acts as a surveillance system against primitive cells such as tumor cells and embryonic cells. Included among the effector cells with the potential to kill trophoblasts are macrophages and LAK cells. These cells employ primitive recognition mechanisms and do not require exposure to antigen to be cytotoxic, but they have no memory that would enable a more vigorous response on second exposure. In the case of macrophages, killing may be mediated by peroxide and enzymes, and by release of tumor necrosis factor α (TNF-α), which also has the ability to cause thrombosis of the vascular supply. In addition, the cytotoxic capacity of the innate effector cells can be boosted by lymphokines. This is especially relevant as trophoblast cells have been reported to produce interleukin 2 (IL-2).

Experimental evidence from immunodeficient mice (*nu/nu* and *SCID/SCID* genotypes) strongly supports the belief that nonspecific immune mechanisms are involved in trophoblast failure. The mice were found to possess killer cells capable of in vitro lysis of trophoblast-type target cells. The effector cells do not appear to be conventional NK cells, since the trophoblast is resistant to lysis by such cells, but they may be LAK cells, which can cause lysis of the trophoblast. Further support for the latter hypothesis comes from observations in the CBA/J × DBA/2 murine model of spontaneous abortion in which the abortion rate was reduced by injecting antibody to asialo-GM1, which is a marker on NK cells and other precursors of cells capable of becoming killer cells (LAK cells) after activation by cytokines. In contrast, treatment with anti-T-cell antibodies

(e.g., anti-L3T4 or anti-Lyt-2) or with antibodies to the IL-2 receptor did not prevent abortion. These observations emphasize the role of innate maternal immune mechanisms rather than antigen-specific mechanisms in fetal rejection of the fetal-placental unit.

Cytokines such as TNF-α may also play a role in trophoblast destruction. Trophoblast cells express receptors for TNF-α, and this factor has been shown to cause lysis of a murine placental cell line with trophoblast features. TNF-α levels are elevated in the decidua of aborting murine (CBA/J × DBA/2) matings compared with nonaborting matings, and injection of recombinant human TNF-α doubles the resorption rate. Abortion can also be increased by injecting lipopolysaccharide, which induces TNF-α production. Since TNF-α causes vascular thrombosis, trophoblast failure may result from thrombosis of the villus blood supply causing fetal death. In addition, macrophages and polymorphonuclear leukocytes are attracted to areas where TNF-α is being produced and can release lytic enzymes and toxic peroxide radicals to which all cells are susceptible. Finally TNF-α (in concert with IL-2) may activate LAK cells. Thus, locally produced TNF-α may be involved in fetal loss through its effect on trophoblast function.

It is now apparent that fetal "rejection" appears to be mediated both by antigen-specific mechanisms of graft rejection and by non-antigen-specific mechanisms directed against the trophoblast and possibly its vascular supply. Therefore, for pregnancy to be successful, *both* the antigen-specific and innate systems must be inhibited. How does the fetus avoid these harmful effects? One possible explanation is that active *suppression* of host rejection mechanisms at the fetal-maternal interface is crucial for fetal survival, and the necessity of such suppression is greatest at the time of and shortly after implantation, when the fetal-maternal interaction is most intimate. Other theories have implicated the role of prostaglandins and growth factors at the implantation site.

DEFENSE MECHANISMS PROTECTING THE FETAL-PLACENTAL UNIT

Decidualization of the endometrium is important in preparing a suitable milieu for implantation and nutrition of the conceptus. There is good evidence that the decidua might also have an important role in impairing certain aspects of graft rejection. Allografts placed on hormonally primed endometrium or in the endometrium of pregnant animals implant and survive for a much longer period of time than allografts placed at nonuterine sites. However, in presensitized animals, skin grafts on the endometrium are promptly rejected. In contrast, grafts placed at the chorion-decidua junction of pregnant mice mated with genetically nonidentical mice of the same species were protected to a significant extent even in immune hosts. These findings suggest that decidualization may protect allografts in nonimmune hosts by preventing the stimulation of maternal immunity. Second, a potent mechanism appears to exist at the chorion-decidua junction that prevents the passage of maternal graft-destroying cytotoxic effector cells into the fetus per se.

During normal pregnancy, cells with immunosuppressive activity accumulate at the implantation site scattered among decidual cells in the compact layer of the decidua. It is generally agreed that some of the cells in the decidua originate in the bone marrow, but the proportion of these cells is still debated. Two functionally distinct types of suppressor cell have been isolated from the uterine lining. One suppressor cell type, which is hormone-dependent, has been recovered from the endometrium; the second type, which is trophoblast-dependent, is found in the decidua during early pregnancy. A similar bimodal pattern of suppressor cell activity is observed in the lymph nodes draining the pregnant murine uterus, but it is delayed by 24 to 48 h relative to the uterine suppression.

Endometrial Suppressor Cells

Prior to implantation, a novel population of hormone-induced suppressor cells appears in the uterus of both humans and mice. This cell is large in size and may bear the T-cell marker Lyt-2. It does not appear to be a classic suppressor T cell, since it is restricted to the endometrium, its activity is induced by hormones rather than by antigen, it lacks antigen specificity, and it does not release any soluble suppressor factors. This suppressor cell is not a macrophage, as it does not bear the characteristic Mac-1 marker. Also, its suppressive activity cannot be eliminated by the addition of indomethacin or by treatment with complement and a monoclonal antibody directed against macrophage surface determinants.

The suppressor cell appears to block maternal sensitization, thereby inhibiting the generation of cytotoxic cellular immune responses against non-MHC antigens which are expressed by cells of the early conceptus. These antigens may play an important role at the maternal-fetal interface. Immunization of rodents against these antigens results in a lower frequency of successful pregnancy and reduced litter size. Also, mucosal immunization of C3H mice against syngeneic sperm (which may share antigens with early embryos) may lead to a reduced litter size because of spontaneous resorption associated with maternal lymphocyte infiltration.

Inhibition of innate effector cell function by these suppressor cells may also be possible, as seen in the CBA/J × DBA/2 murine model. Activation of nonspecific effector cells by injection of poly I:poly C produces rapid postimplantation failure. The failure rate can be dramatically increased by administration of anti-Lyt-2 antibody to pregnant mice 2 to 3 days after implantation.

The activity of the large suppressor cell is short-lived, subsides as pregnancy continues, and is replaced by a trophoblast-dependent suppressor cell. The endometrial suppressor cell, therefore, plays a transient role in the cascade of regulatory events that ensure fetal survival.

Decidual (Trophoblast-Dependent) Suppressor Cells

Early in the postimplantation phase in the mouse, a small suppressor cell with cytoplasmic granules appears in the decidua and replaces the large endometrial suppressor cell. This new cell lacks conventional T-cell and macrophage markers but possesses Fc receptors for IgG. The mechanism of activation of the small suppressor cell appears to be dependent on signals from the trophoblast. Such activation seems to be restricted to the implantation site in the uterus, since no small-cell activation is observed when the pregnancy is located at a site remote from the uterus. The localization and trophoblast dependence suggest that the small suppressor cell might be associated with those events at the chorion-decidua junction that lead to inhibition of graft rejection and survival of the fetus.

The non-T suppressor cell releases soluble factors that have potent inhibitory action on a variety of specific and nonspecific effector mechanisms. These factors inhibit the development of cytotoxic T lymphocytes (CTLs), NK-cell activation, and generation of LAK cells by interfering with the action of IL-2. They also inhibit the response of natural cytotoxic cells to activation by IL-3, inhibit the cytotoxic respiratory burst of monocytes and macrophages, and block the cytotoxic action of TNF-α on certain target cells. In vivo, sponges treated with suppressor cells or their soluble products and implanted into the peritoneal cavity of C3H mice were not infiltrated by CTLs, whereas sponges treated with unconditioned medium showed significant CTL activity. The soluble immunosuppressive molecule is highly sticky and associated with a variety of carrier proteins. It can be neutralized by antibody to transforming growth factor β (TGF-β), which is known to have inhibitory action against cytokine activation of a variety of effector cells. Therefore, TGF-β or a closely related molecule has the potential to block both antigen-specific and innate effector mechanisms capable of attacking the fetus-trophoblast unit.

Suppression of effector cells by prostaglandin E$_2$ (PGE$_2$) has been proposed as a mechanism in decidua. However, it is important to note that the method of disaggregation of decidua affects the type of suppressor molecules detected. PGE$_2$-mediated suppression is seen primarily when decidua is disaggregated with enzymes. Such techniques tend to destroy the TGF-β-producing activity of decidua but liberate macrophage-like cells that produce PGE$_2$-type suppressor molecules. Further, PGE$_2$ production is suppressed in human endometrium after ovulation and in early pregnancy decidua by progesterone. In fact, kinetic experiments on human endometrium and early decidua suggest that the endogenous rate of PGE$_2$ synthesis is well below a level required for suppressive effects. These observations and the fact that prostaglandin synthetase inhibitors (such as acetylsalicyclic acid and other nonsteroidal anti-inflammatory drugs) do not cause abortion in humans suggest that the in vitro generation of PGE$_2$-mediated suppression may be an artifact. Finally, the suppressive activity of the factor produced by the small suppressor cell could not be removed with activated charcoal or neutralized by antibody to prostaglandin or progesterone, indicating that it is not related to these two factors.

TROPHOBLAST-DEPENDENT SUPPRESSOR CELLS AND FETAL SURVIVAL

Evidence that suppressor cells play a role in fetal survival is provided by animal and human models of spontaneous abortion. In pregnancies established by the transfer of *M caroli* blastocysts into *M musculus* uteri and in pregnancies established in CBA/J females mated by DBA/2 males, there is deficient suppressor cell activity at the implantation site. Even in mating combinations with low abortion rates, there is a distribution curve of suppressive activity among implantation sites such that spontaneous resorption is seen at sites where suppressor cell activity is low. In contrast, mouse embryos dying from the action of lethal genetic mutations are not associated with deficient suppressor cell activity in the decidua prior to fetal death. Additional information suggesting that the absence of suppressor cell factors (which block IL-2) may be causative in spontaneous abortion comes from the findings that IL-2 is a key lymphokine in allograft rejection; injection of IL-2 into primigravid mice mated with genetically nonidentical mice of the same species causes pregnancy failure. Also, injection of an antibody against pregnancy-associated null-type suppressor cells (i.e., cells typical of the trophoblast-dependent suppressor cell) produces spontaneous abortion. Finally, in the murine model of recurrent abortion, immunization of the female mouse with paternal antigens is associated with a boosting of local suppressor cell activity which results in successful pregnancy.

Clinical studies of the decidua in early pregnancy found that suppressor cell activity was absent in some women with missed abortion. There was also a deficiency of mononuclear cells with cytoplasmic granules in the placental beds prior to spontaneous abortion. In addition, significantly less immunosuppressive activity was observed in the supernatants obtained from placental bed biopsies in the abortion group when compared with a normal pregnancy group. Collectively, these observations suggest that a deficiency of local suppressor cell activity is probably the precipitating cause of maternal rejection of the fetus, reflecting trophoblast failure, and not a nonspecific result of fetal death.

During normal pregnancy there is evidence for activation of NK cells, natural cytotoxic (NC) cells, and macrophage-type cells, which may be the immune system's way of ensuring that the least fit of the implants (i.e., those whose trophoblasts have subnor-

mal ability to activate suppressor cells) are eliminated. Indeed, spleen cells of mice were shown to contain low levels of cells capable of killing a trophoblast target in vitro. Thus the balance between trophoblast-dependent suppressor activity and the level of intensity of maternal effector activity during the post-implantation period seems to determine whether the newly implanted conceptus will be successful or not. However, this balance can be tipped toward a favorable outcome with immunization of abortion-prone females using allogeneic cells bearing paternal antigens. In this situation, a specific immune response against antigens on the trophoblast exerts a helpful rather than harmful effect.

IMMUNOTHERAPY FOR RECURRENT SPONTANEOUS ABORTIONS

Attempts have been made to reduce spontaneous abortion in animals and humans using immunization against paternal antigens to stimulate appropriate maternal responses. Immunization of CBA/J female mice before mating against the $H-2^d$ MHC antigens of the DBA/2 male can prevent abortion and increase litter size. DBA/2 itself is not immunogenic, and immunization with BALB/c (also $H-2^d$) is required to induce protection. In the CBA/J × DBA/2 model, protection against abortion is mediated by soluble antigen-specific factors that increase local suppressor activity at the implantation site. A similar benefit has been noted in B10 females immunized with spleen cells before mating with B10.A males; here, the B10.A male is effective. In horses carrying extraspecies transfer of donkey conceptuses, immunization against donkey lymphocytes is effective. In some women with unexplained recurrent abortion and with no antipaternal cytotoxic antibodies, immunization with paternal or third-party donor lymphocytes reduces the probability of subsequent spontaneous abortion.

The rationale for immunization as a treatment for recurrent abortion is to prevent rejection of the conceptus by stimulating the production of serum factors which lead to blockage of the reactivity of maternal lymphocytes against trophoblasts and/or paternal leukocyte antigens. The exact mechanisms whereby immunization confers its apparently beneficial effects are not clearly understood, and blocking effects in vitro do not necessarily reflect the mechanism of action in vivo. Indeed, this blocking activity may be only a correlate and is not always associated with clinical effect. This may be due to the beneficial biologic effect resulting from another antibody that is directed against trophoblast antigens. It has been shown that one effect of successful immunization is the boosting of local trophoblast-dependent suppressor cell activity by serum factors. This could be due to a local effect of antibody in the uterus, enhancing trophoblast function. A second mechanism could be improved trophoblast growth as a result of increased suppression of TNF-α-activated cells which show elevated activity in the decidua of abortion-prone mice.

Preliminary reports of lymphocyte immunization in humans were of case series which lacked suitable controls. Subsequently, a randomized controlled trial demonstrated a significantly higher success rate with paternal lymphocyte immunization (77 percent) compared with a control group (37 percent). Similar high success rates have since been reported by many others, and presently there are several ongoing controlled trials testing the efficacy of this treatment. The "cure" rate without treatment appears to be quite low, ranging between 25 and 37 percent, with an average rate of 31 percent. This rate is much lower than that expected from epidemiologic studies of habitual abortion and indicates that the subset of women with unexplained habitual abortion (in whom a maternal allogeneic recognition defect is assumed) is particularly prone to recurrent losses without treatment. Immunotherapy appears to be efficacious in this group, resulting in a 2.5-fold increase in successful pregnancy (Table 27-1).

Source of Lymphocytes for Immunization

In most centers, paternal lymphocytes are used to immunize the women prone to recurrent spontaneous abortions, in an attempt to develop the appropriate protective antipaternal immune responses. However, in some centers, lymphocytes are pooled from the blood of several healthy donors with success rates that are similar to the rates obtained with paternal lymphocyte immunization (Table 27-1). The rationale for such treatment is based on the theoretical importance to the allogeneic recognition process of antigens which are carried on both trophoblasts and lymphocytes (the *trophoblast-lymphocyte cross-reactive [TLX]* antigen). Some trophoblast antigens must be shared by lymphocytes, as many in vitro blocking assays used in pregnancy research depend for their targets upon lymphokine release or measurement of responses to allogeneic cells in mixed lymphocyte culture reactions. Earlier experimental studies indicated the presence of TLX antigens, and it has now been shown that rabbit antisera to human syncytiotrophoblastic microvilli are cytotoxic to peripheral blood lymphocytes (PBLs). In addition, common bands have been identified upon electrophoresis of solubilized preparation of PBLs and trophoblast membranes. These antigens have been shown to be polymorphic. Also, antisera are cytotoxic for PBLs

TABLE 27-1 Summary Data on Pregnancy Outcomes Following Immunotherapy

Treatment	Successful Pregnancy	
	%	RANGE
Paternal lymphocyte immunization	77	63–85
Donor lymphocyte immunization	80	72–83
Placebo or no treatment	31	25–37

from some people but not from others, and these reactions cannot be correlated with the HLA types of the donors. Since syncytiotrophoblasts are devoid of MHC antigens, these findings suggest that trophoblast cells have their own histocompatibility complex and that these antigens are manifest on PBLs as TLX antigens. It has been suggested that if the mother and the father share the same TLX, the conceptus will not be antigeneic and will not stimulate a protective immune response in the mother. Exposure to lymphocytes from several donors would increase the probability of stimulating a protective "blocking" anti-TLX response that may be missing in the woman prone to spontaneous abortions.

There are some problems with the TLX theory as initially formulated, since an immune reaction against a shared TLX antigen would represent autoimmunity; i.e., the mother, in making an antibody to the TLX antigens of the father and fetus, would also make antibodies against her own lymphocytes which express the same antigens. If sharing does occur, it seems more likely that the cells of the father and fetus may not have all of the important antigenic determinants present in the mother's antigen complex. They are still viewed as foreign to the mother, but not sufficiently so to elicit an intrauterine immune response; i.e., the paternal TLX antigen is insufficiently immunogenic. Immune responses to TLX antigen may also depend on "helper antigens," and if there is an immune response defect, this can be overcome by addition of helper effect. Unless the husband is TLX-homozygous and shares an antigen in common with his partner (in which case a 100 percent failure rate would be expected), there would still be a 50 percent or greater chance of success based on simple Mendelian genetics, even after numerous spontaneous abortions. Given the low spontaneous cure rate in this group of women (Table 27-1), the hypothesis of shared TLX antigens seems unlikely.

The issue regarding the best source of lymphocytes for immunization has still not been resolved, especially since 70 to 75 percent of women experiencing failure after paternal lymphocyte immunization may achieve success through immunization with third-party donor lymphocytes. Also, it has been observed that women who have experienced abortion only with one partner may have successful pregnancies with another. The use of third-party lymphocyte immunization is complicated by the risks of viral transmission. In addition, the possibility that there will be more efficient maternal sensitization to erythrocytes or platelet antigens (which often contaminate the lymphocyte preparation) makes the use of donor lymphocytes less appealing.

Dose of Cells for Immunization

The dose of cells used for immunization affects the success rate in a dose-dependent fashion. The optimal dose necessary to achieve a successful outcome has not yet been established, but appears to be at least 100 million cells since the success rate drops significantly with lower doses.

In most centers, repeated doses are given at fixed intervals (which vary from center to center) before conception is attempted. The frequency of injections is usually determined by serum testing for the presence of circulating cytotoxic antibodies directed against paternal or donor lymphocytes. Although this test may not be the best predictor of success, it has been shown that women who develop antibodies to the immunizing cells are better protected. In centers where donor lymphocytes are used, reimmunization is usually carried out as soon as a pregnancy is confirmed, and treatment is continued at regular intervals until the end of the second trimester.

Interval between Immunization and Conception

The time between immunization and conception appears to influence prognosis. The sooner conception occurs after immunization, the more favorable the outcome. In two studies, pregnancy losses after treatment occurred only when the immunization-to-conception interval was greater than 47 days and 80 days, respectively, indicating that pregnancy immediately after immunization optimizes the results.

Possible Risks from Immunotherapy

The immediate short-term effects of maternal immunization are local pruritus and sometimes erythema and swelling around the injection sites. Occasionally, skin pigmentation is observed due to contamination of the lymphocyte preparation by erythrocytes. Sensitization to red cell antigens is a theoretical risk. Rh-negative women are given prophylactic anti-Rh immunoglobulin injections at the time of immunization. To date, no adverse sequelae from rhesus antigen sensitization have been reported.

Some authors have raised concerns over the possibility that immunotherapy results in intrauterine growth retardation (IUGR) of the fetus. However, IUGR may be an inherent feature in couples with recurrent spontaneous abortion, and the occurrence of IUGR may be related to the use of a relatively low dose of cells. With higher cell doses, the frequency of IUGR has not exceeded the normal expectation. The majority of studies support the idea that immunotherapy leads to the delivery of normal, healthy offspring. The physical-development parameters for the first year of life have all been within the normal range, and no adverse effects on immunologic development have been identified in these infants.

THE IMMUNOTROPHIC HYPOTHESIS

The discussion so far in this chapter has focused on antigens produced by the fetus-trophoblast unit and their recognition by maternal effector cells. The basic assumption, which has been supported in part by experimental and clinical evidence, is that if protective responses are not generated, the fetus-trophoblast unit will be destroyed by the mother's graft rejection system through specific and innate effector mechanisms. Recently, however, an *immunotrophic hypothesis* has been proposed as an alternative explanation of the maternal-fetal interaction which results in fetal survival. The basis for this hypothesis is the observation that increased fetal survival following immunotherapy in the CBA/J × DBA/2 system was accompanied by an increase in placental and fetal weight. The hypothesis states that maternal immune recognition of the fetus and the trophoblast by T cells leads to placental and fetal growth and viability via local release of lymphokines such as IL-3 and granulocyte-macrophage colony-stimulating factor (GM-CSF). If the immune response is deficient, subnormal levels of growth factors will be secreted, resulting in increased susceptibility to spontaneous abortion.

Several experimental observations lend some support to the idea of immunotrophism. For example, GM-CSF and IL-3 promote growth of trophoblastlike cells in vitro. The injection of anti-T-cell antibodies such as anti-CD4 and anti-CD8 leads to reduced placental growth and function and increased fetal resorption. The administration of low doses of semipurified and recombinant GM-CSF to abortion-prone mice in midgestation produces protective effects on the pregnancy, resulting in an abortion rate reduced to levels comparable with those following active immunization.

Recent studies have exposed a number of potential problems with the immunotrophic hypothesis. First, using surface markers, few T cells are identifiable in the decidua, and these cells are unable to perform typical T-cell functions such as proliferating in response to mitogens like concanavalin A, perhaps because of the effects of local suppression. Secondly, *SCID* mice, which lack both mature T cells and B cells, may have successful pregnancies and produce adequate levels of placental cell growth stimulating activity. Furthermore, the spontaneous resorptions in this strain of mice are associated with a deficiency of suppressor activity in their decidua and the presence of antitrophoblast killer cells in their spleens.

From the evidence presented, it can be concluded that recognition of trophoblast antigens by maternal T cells does not seem to be necessary for cytokine-dependent placental growth and fetal survival. However, cytokines which are present in decidua do appear to have an important role at the fetal-maternal interface. Further study is needed to elucidate the interactions among these molecules, suppressor cells, and suppressor factors to try to explain the mechanisms that determine success or failure of the conceptus and how these mechanisms can be modulated by immunotherapy.

TRANSPLACENTAL IMMUNITY

The maternal-fetal immunologic relationship extends beyond the question of fetal graft rejection by the mother. In order for the newborn to survive in the germ-filled environment when it is born, the mother provides the fetus with a wide repertoire of antibody developed by her immune system against antigens to which she has become immune. These immunoglobulins are actively transported from the maternal to the fetal circulation, a process that is mediated by receptors on the surface of the trophoblast. The antibody levels gradually decline after birth and are replaced by the newborn's own antibody production. (See also Chap. 28, "The Immune Response of Normal Children.") If the mother has antibodies that can be detrimental to the fetus, autoimmune or isoimmune diseases can become manifest. Usually the disease in the newborn is transient and resolves as the maternal antibody is catabolized. However, in some situations severe symptoms can occur in utero or immediately after birth, giving rise to life-threatening conditions for the fetus (e.g., Rh disease, autoimmune thrombocytopenic purpura, systemic lupus erythematosus [SLE], myasthenia gravis, Graves' disease). Thus, even though the mother's immune system does not reject the fetus and its trophoblast, maternal immunity (or autoimmunity) can affect the baby either systemically (as in Rh isoimmunization) or in an organ-specific manner (as seen in neonatal lupus, which is associated with congenital complete heart block).

The human Rh blood group system is extremely complex and several major antigens have been identified. The Rh_0 (D) antigen is present in fetal red blood cell membranes. Rh-negative women develop anti-Rh_0 (D) antibodies only when exposed to Rh_0 (D)-positive cells, a situation which can occur during pregnancy when an Rh-negative mother is carrying an Rh-positive fetus. The maternal immune system responds to Rh-positive cells by producing IgM antibodies and later IgG anti-Rh_0 (D) antibodies. The reaction of anti-Rh_0 (D) antibodies with Rh_0 (D) antigens results in destruction of Rh-positive cells. In the fetus, severe anemia and hyperbilirubinemia result, leading to a condition known as *erythroblastosis fetalis*. In the neonate, the primary clinical problem is hyperbilirubinemia. Immunization to the Rh_0 (D) antigen can be prevented by the administration of Rh-immune globulin, either before or within 72 h of exposure to Rh_0 (D)-positive cells.

SLE is a chronic, multisystem inflammatory disease in which autoantibodies to autologous DNA are produced. These antinuclear antibodies can be found in the blood of infants born to women with SLE. The two most common manifestations of neonatal SLE are dermatologic and cardiac in nature. In recent years, antibodies to tissue ribonucleoproteins have been found; such antibodies cross the placenta and show a clear and marked association with congenital complete heart block in the infant. If the baby survives the neonatal period, the prognosis is good.

Occasionally, patients with SLE or with no evidence of lupus will produce autoantibodies which bind to phospholipids. Some of these antibodies are of no clinical significance, representing nothing more than a serologic abnormality. In others, the antiphospholipid antibodies may induce tissue damage of a unique sort, called the *antiphospholipid syndrome* or the *anticardiolipin antibody syndrome*. (See Clinical Aside 27-1).

Clinical Aside 27-1
Anticardiolipin Antibodies

One of the major infectious scourges of the early part of this century was syphilis, also known as lues. In the same year that the cause of syphilis, *Treponema pallidum*, was discovered Osler described systemic lupus erythematosus (SLE). Shortly thereafter a serologic test for syphilis was developed by Wassermann which used extracts of luetic organs to demonstrate binding of serum antibodies. Two facts quickly became clear. First, normal organs could be used rather than organs from patients with syphilis (one of the current tests for syphilis, the VDRL, uses and extract of beef heart, known as cardiolipin). Second, nonluetic SLE patients could test positive in Wasserman's test. This biologic false-positive (BFP) also occurred in about 1 percent of the normal population. Over the next 30 to 40 years it became clear that between 5 and 44 percent of patients with SLE had BFPs; occasionally the BFP was noted years before the clinical features of SLE. In the 1950s SLE patients with BFPs were also noted to have a prolonged whole-blood bleeding time that was not correctable with normal plasma. These represented the first reports of a "lupus anticoagulant," an antibody which interfered with the coagulation cascade. Paradoxically, patients with this "anticoagulant" activity did not have clinical problems with bleeding; rather they experienced a tendency to thrombosis.

In the last decade, it has become apparent that BFP and anticoagulant activities are serologic markers for a clinical syndrome. With more sophisticated testing, we now know that this syndrome is associated with antibodies against a variety of phospholipids, most notably cardiolipin, and so the syndrome is known as the *anticardiolipin antibody syndrome*. The clinical syndrome consists of:

Thrombosis, both venous (recurrent deep vein thromboses) and arterial (cerebrovascular, peripheral, coronary, and retinal).

Abortion (spontaneous intrauterine death, with placental thrombosis and infarction). Increased risk of premature labor and babies small for gestational age.

Thrombocytopenia.

Endocardial lesions (lesions of Libman-Sacks endocarditis. (A nonbacterial marantic endocarditis, seen in SLE, may be linked to antiphospholipid antibodies.)

Coombs' positive hemolytic anemia.

Livedo reticularis.

Migraine, chorea, epilepsy.

A likely explanation for fetal loss and obstetric problems is placental damage, perhaps due to vasculopathy induced by the autoantibodies and platelet fixation. A similar mechanism may underlie the cardiac endothelial damage noted above.

Thus, a new subset of autoimmune disease has been established in the last decade. Physicians realized that the BFPs really represented a serologic reactivity which might be pathogenic and could thereby explain previous clinical observations, e.g., Libman-Sacks endocarditis and spontaneous intrauterine death.

SELF-TEST QUESTIONS

For the following incomplete statements choose the letter of the combination of responses that correctly complete the statement.

A. a, b, and c are correct.
B. a, c, and d are correct.
C. b, c, and d are correct.
D. all are correct.

1. Trophoblast
   a. Is made up of two clearly distinguishable layers of cells in which the syncytiotrophoblast fails to express class I MHC antigens
   b. Cells are susceptible to lysis by antigen-specific immune effector mechanisms
   c. Failure may occur by TNF-α through its action on the villus blood supply
   d. Cells are susceptible to lysis by LAK cells

2. During normal pregnancy, the decidua exerts a protective effect on the fetus-trophoblast unit because:
   a. Lymphoid cells with immunosuppressive activity accumulate at the implantation site
   b. The trophoblast is necessary to activate decidual suppressor cells which produce TGF-β or a closely related molecule which has the potential to block both antigen-specific and innate effector mechanisms capable of attacking the fetus-trophoblast unit
   c. Grafts placed at the chorion-decidua junction of pregnant mice mated with genetically nonidentical mice of the same species are protected even in immune hosts
   d. Suppression of maternal effector cells occurs by PGE_2

3. Paternal lymphocyte immunization treatment:
   a. Appears to produce a better chance of success if the interval between immunization and conception is long
   b. Is associated with an increase in decidual suppressor cell activity
   c. Appears to be an effective therapy for women with unexplained recurrent abortion

   d. Seems to have a dose-dependent effect on pregnancy outcome

4. Unexplained spontaneous abortion appears to be:
   a. Mediated by antigen-specific mechanisms of graft rejection
   b. Mediated by non-antigen-specific mechanisms directed against trophoblast and possibly its vascular supply
   c. Caused by fetal chromosomal anomalies which result in poor trophoblast function
   d. A frequent clinical problem

ADDITIONAL READINGS

Chaouat G, ed. *The Immunology of the Fetus*. 2nd ed. Boca Raton, Fla.: CRC Press; 1993.

Clark DA. Controversies in reproductive immunology. *Crit Rev Immunol*. 1991; 11:215–247.

Gleicher N, ed. *Principles and Practice of Medical Therapy in Pregnancy*. Norwalk, Conn.: Appleton & Lange; 1992.

Gleicher N, ed. *Reproductive Immunology*. Immunology and Allergy Clinics of North America, vol. 10, no. 1. Philadelphia: Saunders; 1990.

28

The Immune Response of Normal Children

INTRODUCTION

The development of the normal immune response begins early in fetal life and proceeds through childhood. The immune response depends on complex interactions between cellular and humoral components of the immune system, with each component maturing at its own rate in the fetus, newborn, and child.

The ontogeny of T and B lymphocytes is reviewed elsewhere in this text (Chaps. 6 and 7). In this chapter we focus on the developing organism as a whole, tracing the *function* of the individual elements of the immune system from early fetal life through adulthood. The "immunodeficiencies" of the normal newborn and premature infants will be reviewed. Differences between the immune responses of normal children and adults will be highlighted.

GENERAL CONSIDERATIONS

The immune system of the developing child does not act in isolation from other organ systems. The skin and mucous membranes serve as important barriers to infection and may be more permeable in the neonatal period. Similarly, relative immaturity of cardiovascular and pulmonary systems may also contribute to the fragile health of the newborn. The status of the mother with regard to immunocompetence and infection (especially systemic infection or infection of the birth canal) needs to be considered in assessing immunocompetence of the neonate. The effects of infection on the developing host should be considered. Rubella infection is relatively benign in the child but can have devastating systemic effects in the fetus. Conversely, herpesvirus infection can be overwhelming in the neonate but usually is more benign in the child and adolescent.

HUMORAL IMMUNE RESPONSES

The capacity to produce antibodies is present early in fetal life. Cells bearing surface immunoglobulin are present in fetal spleen, blood, and lymph nodes at relative isotype frequencies similar to those in normal adults. IgM synthesis has been demonstrated in the fetus by 10 weeks of gestation; IgG synthesis occurs later, and IgA synthesis occurs at 30 weeks. This implies that cells are present very early in fetal life which are committed to IgG or IgA production but which have not matured to acquire the ability to synthesize large amounts of immunoglobulin. At birth, serum from normal neonates contains one-tenth the amount of normal adult IgM and very little IgA. IgG levels in the newborn are near those found in adults; however, this represents maternal immunoglobulin which has crossed the placenta (Table 28-1). The bulk of maternal immunoglobulin is transferred in the last trimester and attains full-term newborn levels by 33 weeks of gestation. IgM levels increase to adult levels by 2 years of age. IgG levels drop in the developing infant to about a third of normal adult levels over the first 4 to 6 months of life. This represents catabolism of maternal IgG. IgG levels then gradually increase in children to become indistinguishable from adult levels by 7 years of age. IgA levels, which are usually not detectable in the newborn, increase gradually to 25 percent of adult levels by 1 year, 50 percent of adult levels by age 3 to 4, and adult levels by age 7 (see Table 28-1).

Specific secretory IgA and IgM antibodies appear in saliva during the first few days of life. Specific secretory IgA antibodies reach adult levels by 12 months of age. There is relative lack of secretory IgA in the saliva and other secretions of infants in the first month of life. Milk secretory IgA antibodies may neutralize or prevent the mucosal attachment of pathogenic bacteria in the breast-fed infant.

TABLE 28-1   Levels of Immunoglobulins in Sera of Normal Subjects, by Age

Age	IgG mg/dL	IgG Percent of Adult Level	IgM mg/dL	IgM Percent of Adult Level	IgA mg/dL	IgA Percent of Adult Level	Total Immunglobulin mg/dL	Total Immunglobulin Percent of Adult Level
Newborn	1031 ± 200*	89 ± 17	11 ± 5	11 ± 5	2 ± 3	1 ± 2	1044 ± 201	67 ± 13
1 to 3 months	430 ± 119	37 ± 10	30 ± 11	30 ± 11	21 ± 13	11 ± 7	481 ± 127	31 ± 9
4 to 6 months	427 ± 186	37 ± 16	43 ± 17	43 ± 17	28 ± 18	14 ± 9	498 ± 204	32 ± 13
7 to 12 months	661 ± 219	58 ± 19	54 ± 23	55 ± 23	37 ± 18	19 ± 9	752 ± 242	48 ± 15
13 to 24 months	762 ± 209	66 ± 18	58 ± 23	59 ± 23	50 ± 24	25 ± 12	870 ± 258	56 ± 16
25 to 36 months	892 ± 183	77 ± 16	61 ± 19	62 ± 19	71 ± 37	36 ± 19	1024 ± 205	65 ± 14
3 to 5 years	929 ± 228	80 ± 20	56 ± 18	57 ± 18	93 ± 27	47 ± 14	1078 ± 245	69 ± 17
6 to 8 years	923 ± 256	80 ± 22	65 ± 25	66 ± 25	124 ± 45	62 ± 23	1112 ± 293	71 ± 20
9 to 11 years	1124 ± 235	97 ± 20	79 ± 33	80 ± 33	131 ± 60	66 ± 30	1134 ± 254	85 ± 17
12 to 16 years	946 ± 124	82 ± 11	59 ± 20	60 ± 20	148 ± 63	74 ± 32	1153 ± 169	74 ± 12
Adults	1158 ± 305	100 ± 26	99 ± 27	100 ± 27	200 ± 61	100 ± 31	1457 ± 353	100 ± 24

*One standard deviation.
Source: Stiehm ER, Fudenberg HH. Serum levels of immune globulins in health and disease. *Pediatrics* 1966; 37:715. Used with permission.
Values shown were derived from measurements made in 296 normal children and 30 adults. Levels were determined by the radial diffusion plate method using specific rabbit antisera to human immunoglobulins.

IgE-bearing cells have been observed in fetal lung and liver tissue by the 11th week of gestation; however cord serum contains little IgE. The finding of IgE antibodies to penicillin in the absence of these antibodies in the mother suggests that intrauterine sensitization is possible. Serum IgE concentrations increase to reach adult levels at 6 years of age.

Antigenic stimulation in the form of intrauterine infection can accelerate the maturation of antibody production such that IgM levels in the newborn increase to greater than 20 mg/dL and may even approach adult values. Therefore, measurement of neonatal IgM or cord IgM levels is useful in clinical practice to determine the presence of intrauterine infection. Similarly, specific IgM antibodies to potential infectious agents are commonly assayed (i.e., *toxoplasmosis, syphilis* (other), *rubella, cytomegalovirus, herpes simplex virus* infections—the so called TORCH titers) to aid in the diagnosis of congenital infections. (See Clinical Aside 28-1.)

The neonatal humoral immune response differs from that in adults in that it is primarily an IgM response, which is persistent; IgG and IgA responses are relatively deficient. The mechanism of this defect is not known with certainty. Precursor cells, i.e., those bearing surface IgG and IgA, are present in the neonate. IgG and IgA antibody responses are more T-cell dependent than are IgM responses (the T cell is involved in isotype switching), and there is evidence of impaired helper T-cell function in the neonate (see below). Impaired IgG and IgA responses have also been confirmed in vitro. Newborn B cells stimulated by pokeweed mitogen (PWM) or nocardiae do not make IgG or IgA responses at normal adult levels. Maturation of IgG and IgA responses occurs by age 5.

Clinical Aside 28-1
Congenital Anomalies and Intrauterine Infections

In the infant with encephalitis, microcephaly, cerebral calcifications, cataracts, chorioretinitis, patent ductus arteriosus, hepatosplenomegaly, thrombocytopenia, jaundice, or prematurity, congenital infection with toxoplasmosis, syphilis, rubella, cytomegalovirus, or herpes simplex virus (TORCH syndrome) needs to be considered. As the bulk of neonatal IgG is maternally derived, total IgM or antigen-specific IgM, of neonatal origin (i.e., cord blood), should be tested to aid in making this diagnosis.

IgG subclass levels and responses to antigens have been recently studied. IgG2 and IgG4 responses are relatively deficient in the neonate. Antibodies to carbohydrate antigens are primarily IgG2 in the normal host; deficiency of this subtype of IgG may partially explain the poor antibody responses to polysaccharide vaccines (e.g., pneumococcus, *Haemophilus influenzae*), as well as frequent infections with these and other encapsulated organisms in neonates and young children. Thus, with *H influenzae* type B immunization the polysaccharide antigen is coupled to a protein antigen—hapten (diphtheria)—in order to induce a greater humoral immune response in infants and toddlers.

The young child is relatively naive with regard to antigenic exposure, and is exposed to neoantigens throughout life. Primary immune responses in young children are virtually all IgM, and reach their peak concentrations at 2 weeks. (See Clinical Aside 28-1.) Isotype switch to IgG and amplification in the concentration of antibody occur after secondary exposure. During the secondary immune response antibodies may be more efficient in neutralization because of higher affinity.

In summary, neonates have poor humoral immune responses with regard to amplification and isotype switching, deficient responses to polysaccharide antigens, and low levels of circulating immunoglobulins. Children are exposed to neoantigens throughout early life, and the lack of a mature humoral immune response may contribute to the high incidence and mortality rates of neonatal sepsis. (See Clinical Aside 28-2.)

Clinical Aside 28-2
Neonatal Sepsis

Serious life-threatening sepsis occurs in approximately 0.1 to 1.0 percent of all neonates, and mortality can approach 75 percent. The incidence of neonatal sepsis is related to relative immunodeficiency of the infant as compared to adults, to maternal factors such as uterine infections, and to iatrogenic factors such as invasive procedures, indwelling catheters, and nosocomial pathogens. The outcome of infection in the newborn is related to timeliness of diagnosis, timeliness of administration of antibiotics, prematurity, and immunocompetence of the host. Clinical manifestations of sepsis include hyper- or hypothermia, jaundice, respiratory distress, hepatomegaly, abdominal distension, anorexia, vomiting, and lethargy.

CELLULAR IMMUNE RESPONSES

T Cells

There are fewer T cells in cord blood than in normal adult blood, although results depend on the method used to enumerate T cells. Using T cell–specific monoclonal antibodies, decreased percentages of T lymphocytes are found in cord blood, as compared to adults. Newborn venous blood contains decreased percentages of T cells as determined by E-rosetting; however, due to neonatal lymphocytosis the absolute number of T cells is normal. Surface marker analysis reveals immature populations of T cells present in cord blood. The helper-suppressor ratio is decreased in cord blood (1.71 compared with 1.98 in adult blood).

Because determination of T-cell function is more difficult than quantifying and determining function of immunoglobin, less is known about the maturation of T-cell function in the developing fetus, neonate, and child. T cells have been identified in human fetuses as early as 11 weeks of gestation in the liver, and then subsequently in the bone marrow, thymus, and spleen. T cell antigen–specific responses have been demonstrated at 12 weeks of gestation, graft-versus-host (GVH) reactivity at 13 weeks, and response to mitogens at 12 weeks. Mixed leukocyte culture (MLC) reactions have been detected by the 12th week of gestation. The MLC is used to assess the ability of T cells to respond to allogeneic MHC antigens. Proliferative responses of cord blood T cells to phytohemagglutinin (PHA) (mitogen), streptokinase-streptodornase (SK-SD), and *Candida* (antigens) have also been studied. Unstimulated and mitogen-stimulated proliferation were greater than in adults, SK-SD responses were lower, and *Candida* responses were similar. Values approached adult levels by 20 months of age. Concanavalin A (conA) responses were delayed in the infant, as compared to PHA responses.

Lymphokine production by cord blood mononuclear cells is impaired in some experimental systems. Production of mitogen-induced macrophage inhibitory factor, IFN-γ, macrophage activating factor, and IL-2 is lower than in adults.

Impaired T-cell cytotoxicity in the newborn has also been demonstrated. Antigen-specific T cell–mediated cytotoxicity of B cells infected with Epstein-Barr virus was shown to be decreased as compared with adult T cells; similarly, cell-mediated lympholysis of allogeneic cells was impaired. Natural killer cell (NK-cell) activity is diminished as compared with adults, but can be augmented in vitro by treating mononuclear cells with interferon. Antibody-dependent cell-mediated cytotoxicity (ADCC) is almost undetectable at birth and approaches adult values at 6 years of age.

Many studies have demonstrated an excess in suppressor T-cell function in the cord blood of neonates. Human newborn's T cells suppress adult lymphocytes in several in vitro assays, including the differentiation of adult B cells to plasma cells after exposure to PWM.

Neonatal T cells function poorly as helpers, especially in providing help for isotype switching to IgA and IgG production (see above). T cells from human newborns inhibit division of their mothers' lymphocytes, by releasing soluble suppressive factors. This increase in suppressor tone of the cellular immune system in neonates may reflect a role in the development of self-tolerance and/or the maintenance of the fetal allograft in the mother.

Thus increased suppressor tone; impaired proliferation, cytotoxicity, and lymphokine production; and relative T lymphocytopenia are evident in the newborn. It is not surprising that delayed-type hypersensitivity (DTH) skin test responses are also impaired. Therefore, DTH testing is of limited usefulness in assessing immunocompetence in the young infant even when the infant has been exposed to the antigen in question.

Macrophages

Monocytes are first seen in fetal spleen and lymph nodes at about 4 to 5 months gestational age, about 2 months after the first granulocytes are seen. Studies in rabbits and monkeys show that alveolar macrophages are few in number at birth; postnatally they increase rapidly in healthy animals but not in those with hyaline membrane disease. Studies in the neonatal mouse and rat show impaired antigen processing in macrophages. In the human there is evidence of decreased expression of class II antigens on neonatal macrophages. Some studies suggest that there may be a relative deficiency of neonatal monocyte chemotaxis. Neonatal macrophage killing function varies with the type of assay and organisms used as target. Normal killing of *Toxoplasma gondii* but decreased killing of group B streptococci and *Staphylococcus aureus* have been described. Production of IL-1 by human neonatal macrophages appears to be the same as in adults. Production of tumor necrosis factor has not been studied.

Impaired T-cell lymphokine production (see above) may be in part responsible for some decreased macrophage function. In vitro, neonatal macrophage functions can be improved by IFN-γ and other macrophage stimulants.

In summary, neonates exhibit impaired antigen processing and chemotaxis. Results obtained in cytotoxicity assays vary, depending upon the experimental system.

Polymorphonuclear (PMN) Cells

Granulocytopoiesis is demonstrable during the second month of gestation, and the neutrophil is therefore an early cell in ontogeny. The bone marrow neutrophil storage pool in the premature and full-term infant is substantially less than that of adults, so it can be exhausted faster during bacterial infections. In examining PMN function in the neonate and young child, one must be aware of certain serum factors which play a major role in their function. It is difficult to differentiate true cellular deficiencies from deficiencies in serum components (see below) in certain assay systems. In low concentrations of adult serum, neonatal PMNs are less effective phagocytes than adult PMNs; however in studies using 10 percent or more of adult serum, neonatal PMN phagocytosis was normal. PMNs from premature infants phagocytose normally but are deficient in bactericidal activity when compared to those of full-term babies; full-term PMNs are slightly deficient when compared to those of adults. This defect appears to be due to poor oxygen radical generation.

A more profound defect exists in neonatal PMN chemotaxis. It is the most clearly established defect in phagocytic defenses and contributes to the failure of the neonate to produce and deliver adequate numbers of phagocytes to the site of a serious infection. This defect appears to be due to decreased deformability of neonatal PMNs, and is demonstrated by impaired conA-induced capping. This may be secondary to developmental membrane differences affecting C5a receptors and/or the functional activity of the cytoskeleton. Decreased expression of CR3 (C3bi receptor), which may contribute to impaired chemotaxis and adhesion of neonatal PMNs, has also been demonstrated. Neutrophil chemotaxis finally reaches adult levels at 16 years of age.

In summary, neonatal PMNs show decreased chemotaxis, deformability, adhesion, and killing when compared to those of normal adults.

SERUM FACTORS

Complement

Most complement components are synthesized in early fetal life before the onset of immunoglobulin synthesis. Plasma concentrations of complement components gradually increase throughout gestation. Plasma concentrations of the components of both the classical and alternative pathways are decreased in neonates when compared to those in adults. This relative deficiency is more pronounced in premature infants. Complement-mediated opsonization and generation of chemotactic factors from neonatal serum are decreased. Serum of neonates contains increased amounts of a factor which inhibits complement-dependent chemotactic activity.

Fibronectin

Fibronectins are glycoproteins present in the extracellular matrix, in plasma, and on the surface of fibroblasts. There are two forms of this molecule: a soluble form which exists in blood and other body fluids, and an insoluble form which exists in extracellular spaces of connective tissue and as a component of basement membranes. Fibronectin is produced by fibroblasts, endothelial cells, macrophages, and epithelial cells, and functions as an opsonin, stimulating reticuloendothelial clearance of particles. Fibronectin may decrease bacterial adherence to the mucosa and thus prevent its invasion, presumably by occupying important sites on the microorganism which are necessary for binding to cells. Cord blood monocytes synthesize less fibronectin than monocytes derived from adult blood. Term and premature newborns have lower fibronectin levels than normal adults. Children less than a year of age have lower plasma fibronectin levels than older children.

IMMUNODEFICIENCY IN THE PREMATURE INFANT— NEONATAL SEPSIS

In considering the status of the immune system in the premature infant, one must take into account the maturational state of the immune system, as presented above. An infant born before 33 weeks of age will be deficient in maternal immunoglobulin and will have markedly impaired PMN and macrophage functions with regard to adherence, chemotaxis, and killing. Other factors contributing to a high incidence of sepsis in the premature infant, as well as a poorer prognosis, are immaturity of the developing respiratory and gastrointestinal systems, which offer poor barriers to infection, and iatrogenic causes of infection (e.g., indwelling catheters, endotracheal tubes, humidified incubators, hospitalization). (See Clinical Aside 28-2.) Uterine infection per se can be a cause of prematurity, further illustrating the need to seek a cause of infection in the premature infant and treat it aggressively.

Since the most profound immunologic defects are in function of the PMNs and the humoral immune system, interest in reconstitution of these functions is keen (reviewed in Cairo, 1989). Recently, neutrophil transfusions in the septic neonate have been attempted, and preliminary data suggest a role for this therapy in reducing mortality in the septic infant, especially when neutrophil pools in the host are depleted. Potential problems associated with use of this therapy, however, include GVH disease due to contaminating T cells, fluid overload, and exposure to transfusion-related infections, and thus neutrophil transfusion is still considered experimental. Other options being explored include administration of lymphokines with growth-promoting function for hematopoietic progenitor cells.

Similarly, prophylactic treatment of the small premature infant with intravenous immunoglobulin has been tested, and preliminary data suggest a role in decreasing mortality from sepsis. (See also Chap. 34 on the clinical use of intravenous γ-globulin.) However, the interference of this therapy with the therapeutic benefit of penicillin in the newborn rat infected with group B streptococcus has tempered enthusiasm, and this therapy is also considered experimental.

IMMUNIZATION IN CHILDREN

The goal of immunization in children is twofold: one is to prevent disease in individuals; the other is to eradicate disease globally. The eradication of smallpox illustrates the ultimate goal of immunization: to make further immunization against the agent unnecessary. Immunization can be accomplished by stimulating the individual to develop an immunologic response to the infectious agent (active immunization), or by providing to the individual specific antibody already formed in another host (passive immunization). Vaccination programs have been extremely effective in decreasing the incidence of diphtheria, measles, mumps, pertussis, poliomyelitis, rubella, and tetanus in the United States. Immunizations for measles, mumps, and rubella (MMR) are often given together, as are immunizations for diphtheria, pertussis, and tetanus (DPT).

Active immunization may result in protective antibodies which are antitoxic, antiinvasive, or neutralizing for the infectious agent. Vaccines can contain intact, attenuated organisms, killed organisms, or only a part of the microorganism or its biologic product (e.g., toxin). For some infections, the presence of serum antibodies does not guarantee protection. Some responses to vaccines are protective for life; protection in others, especially when killed rather than attenuated organisms are used, requires repeated exposure to the antigen(s) (boosters).

Scheduling of immunizations (Table 28-2) is dependent upon the maturation of the immune response in the host, as well as the incidence, morbidity, and mortality of the infection in the developing host. For example, although the DPT and polio vaccines

TABLE 28-2   Recommended Schedule for Active Immunization in Children

Age	Immunization
Birth	Hepatitis B
1 month	Hepatitis B
2 months	DTP, OPV, HbOC or PRP-OMP
4 months	DTP, OPV, HbOC or PRP-OMP
6 months	DTP, OPV, HbOC or PRP-OMP
12 months	PRP-OMP
15 months	MMR,* HbOC
18 months	DTP, OPV
4–6 years	DTP, OPV, MMR
14–16 years	Td

*At 12 months of age, if endemic.
Abbreviations: DTP—diphtheria and tetanus toxoids with pertussis vaccine; OPV—oral poliovirus vaccine containing attenuated poliovirus types 1, 2, and 3; HbOC or PRP-OMP—*Haemophilus influenzae* type B vaccines; MMR—live measles, mumps, and rubella viruses in a combined vaccine; Td—adult tetanus toxoid (full dose) and diphtheria toxoid (reduced dose) for adult use.

are more immunogenic when administered in late infancy, the risks of the infections targeted by these vaccines are greatest in young infants, and vaccination of the young infant (2 months of age) is recommended.

IMMUNOLOGY OF BREAST MILK

Another potential source of immunocompetence in the human neonate is breast feeding. Some studies have suggested that breast feeding has protective effects against gastroenteritis, respiratory infections, otitis media, and atopy. Studies have been flawed, and inconsistent results have been reported. Thus the protective effects of breast feeding in the neonate and developing child must be considered controversial.

Colostrum and early breast milk contain extremely high levels of secretory IgA, with the capacity to deliver up to 100 mg/kg per day to the infant. After maternal enteric antigen exposure, specific secretory IgA antibodies appear in milk. Because of this so-called enteromammaric link, the infant receives antibodies to common bacterial antigens likely to be encountered, and this may prevent colonization as well as infection from potentially pathogenic bacteria. Secretory IgA antibodies are not absorbed into the blood, except during the first days of life, and remain on mucous membranes and function there. Human milk also contains IgG and IgM antibodies, but at concentrations much lower than IgA. There is some evidence that secretory IgA binding to antigens diminishes foreign protein absorption from the gastrointestinal tract and thus prevents allergic sensitization.

Colostrum contains up to 3×10^6 leukocytes per milliliter, which decreases to 10^5 cells per milliliter by 3 months after birth. Approximately 20 percent are neutrophils, 60 percent monocytes, and 10 percent lymphocytes. The lymphocyte population is made up mostly of T cells, with relatively more $CD8^+$ cells than in maternal peripheral blood. Milk-derived T cells have been shown to function in antigen-induced proliferation and in the production of lymphokines. IL-1 has also been demonstrated in human milk. The protective role of maternal T cells in the young infant is not known. Human milk also contains lactoferrin (iron-binding protein) and a B_{12}-binding protein, which can deprive bacteria of these factors which are necessary for growth. This is another potential mechanism whereby breast feeding may be protective against infection.

Thus humoral and possibly cellular immunity are delivered to the neonate who is breast-fed. Additionally, the breast-fed neonate may not be exposed to foreign antigens either because of secretory IgA binding of proteins or because of decreased exposure to cow's milk or soy proteins in commercial formulas. Other aspects of the mammary gland immune system and the transfer of immunoglobulin to breast milk are discussed in Chap. 3, on antibodies, and Chap. 11, on mucosa-associated lymphoid tissues.

SUMMARY

Infants may be predisposed to bacterial infections because of a relative deficiency of specific antibody and because of impaired ability to deliver competent phagocytes to the site of infection. Viral infections may occur because of impaired production of INF-γ or deficiencies of NK-cell or antigen-specific cell-mediated cytotoxicity. Immunocompetence in early neonatal life is largely maternally derived through transplacental passage of immunoglobulins, and potentially through breast feeding. The age at which most immune functions reach maturity is unknown; however the risk of severe, overwhelming infection appears to decrease by 3 months of age. The maturational state of the immune system in the developing child must be considered in the planning of vaccinations as well as in the interpretation of immunologic diagnostic testing such as DTH testing.

SELF-TEST QUESTIONS

1. Characterize the serum concentrations of the three major immunoglobulin isotypes in the normal newborn as compared to the normal adult.
2. The normal 8-month-old infant will be deficient in which IgG subtype? What are the functional or clinical implications of this deficiency?

3. What is the most profound defect in neutrophil function in the normal newborn?
4. Why is DTH testing to assess immunocompetence or antigenic exposure in the neonate of limited usefulness?
5. Breast milk is a potential source of immunocompetence in the human neonate because it contains what potential immunologically active components? By what mechanisms can it delay the appearance of atopy in the child?

ADDITIONAL READINGS

Allansmith M, McClellan H, Butterworth M, Maloney JR. The development of immunoglobulin levels in man. *J Pediatr.* 1968;72:276–290.

Cairo MS. Neonatal neutrophil host defense. *Am J Dis Child.* 1989;143:40–46.

Gotoff SP. Neonatal immunity. *J Pediatr.* 1974;85:149–154.

Stiehm ER, Fudenberg HH. Serum levels of immune globulins in health and disease. *Pediatrics.* 1966;37:715.

Wilson CB. Immunologic basis for increased susceptibility of the neonate to infection. *J Pediatr.* 1986;108:1–12.

INTRODUCTION

The word *atopy* comes from the Greek "atopos," meaning "out of the way, uncommon." Atopy describes conditions in which exposure to commonly encountered substances causes an individual to produce a clinical IgE-mediated hypersensitivity response. This exposure may occur through ingestion or inhalation or by a topical or parenteral route. For an allergic response to occur, sensitization or prior exposure is required. The development of the atopic state, although not the ability to respond to a specific allergen, appears to be influenced by heredity, but the pattern of inheritance is not yet known.

Scientists have been studying the phenomenon of immediate hypersensitivity throughout the twentieth century. In 1901, Portier and Richet found that dogs injected with the toxin of the sea anemone developed mild symptoms of toxicity. However, when the dogs were injected a second time, they developed a severe reaction, with vomiting, dyspnea, and death. Scientists felt that this phenomenon was the "opposite" of immunity and called it *anaphylaxis,* from the Greek *ana* meaning "backward" and *phylaxis* meaning "to guard." Another important experiment, described in the introduction to this book, was done by Carl Prausnitz and Heinz Küstner in 1922. Küstner was known to be allergic to fish. He injected his serum intradermally into Prausnitz's arm, and 24 later injected fish extract into the same site. Prausnitz experienced an immediate local reaction with a wheal and erythema in the pretreated area. Thus, allergic reactivity could be transferred from an atopic person to a nonallergic individual. The Prausnitz-Küstner, or passive transfer test, became important in the diagnosis of allergies in the early days of the field. It is rarely used today due to the risk of viruses being transferred via the serum. It was not until 1967 that the Ishizakas identified IgE as the immunoglobulin in the transferred serum responsible for the development of wheal-and-flare reactions.

CLASSIFICATION OF HYPERSENSITIVITY REACTIONS

Various reactions can occur under the broad classification of hypersensitivity. Gell and Coombs devised a system to divide these reactions into four general types based upon the immune mechanisms involved (Fig. 29-1).

Type I—Anaphylactic or immediate-type hypersensitivity. These reactions involve IgE formed in response to a specific antigen. IgE binds to mast cells and basophils via the Fc receptors on the cells. When antigen is again introduced and reacts with the cell-bound IgE, immediate release of mediators occurs. These mediators are then capable of affecting various organ systems. This type of reaction is important in many conditions, including anaphylaxis, extrinsic asthma, and allergic rhinitis.

Type II—Antibody-dependent cytotoxic reactions. These reactions involve antibody, usually of the IgG or IgM isotype. The antibody combines with an antigen which is either part of the cell or is already bound to the membrane of the target cell. This antigen-antibody reaction makes the cell susceptible to lysis through effector mechanisms involving complement or effector cells bearing Fc receptors. This type of reaction plays a role in transfusion reactions, autoimmune hemolytic anemia, and some drug allergies.

Type III—Immune complex hypersensitivity. These reactions involve the formation of circulating antigen-antibody complexes.

When exposure to antigen occurs, antibody is produced and reacts with the antigen to form immune complexes. The immune complexes then deposit in tissues or on blood vessel endothelial surfaces and cause damage through the activation of complement and the attraction of polymorphonuclear leukocytes to the site. Examples of this type of reaction include immune complex glomer- ulonephritis, serum sickness, and Arthus-type reactions.

Type IV—Delayed or cellular hypersensitivity. These reactions involve T lymphocytes. Antigen is presented to the antigen receptors of T lymphocytes, stimulating them to release lymphokines. The lymphokines activate monocytes and macrophages, which

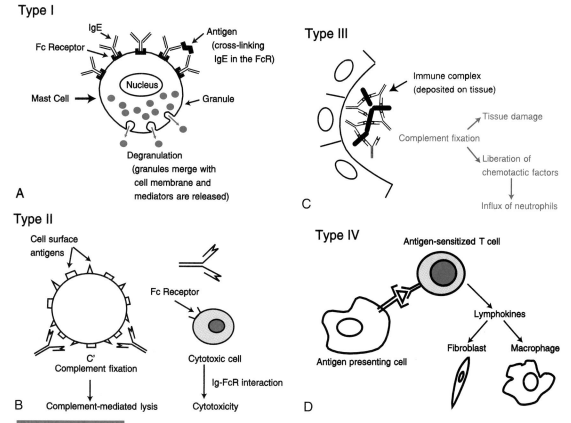

Figure 29-1 The four different types of hypersensitivity reactions, according to Gell and Coombs. *(A) Type I*—Immediate hypersensitivity reaction due to antigen interaction with cell-bound IgE. The antigen-antibody interaction causes degranulation of the cell, with liberation of inflammatory mediators. *(B) Type II*—Free antibody binds to an antigen. If the antigen is part of a cell, the antibody–antigen interaction can lead to complement-mediated cell lysis or to engagement of a cell capable of mediating antibody-dependent cellular cytotoxicity. *(C) Type III*—Antigen-antibody interaction causes the production of immune complexes, which can deposit on tissues or in blood vessels and cause inflammation and tissue damage, at least in part mediated by the complement cascade. *(D) Type IV*—Delayed type hypersensitivity (DTH), whereby an antigen-sensitized T cell is activated to produce cytokines and cause cell-mediated immune changes.

subsequently cause tissue damage. Since lymphokines must be produced and must then act upon other cells, these reactions occur 24 to 72 h following an encounter with the antigen. This type of reaction is responsible for the cutaneous response in tuberculin skin testing, as well as graft-versus-host (GVH) disease and contact dermatitis.

It is important to remember that these varied manifestations of hypersensitivity do not exist as totally separate entities. Several types of reactions may occur in the same clinical condition, each contributing to local tissue damage.

The rest of this chapter focuses mainly on the mechanisms and consequences of the type I hypersensitivity reaction.

IMMUNOLOGY OF THE TYPE I HYPERSENSITIVITY REACTION

IgE Antibody

Structure
IgE antibodies mediate type I hypersensitivity reactions. The basic structure of IgE is formed from two ε heavy chains and two light chains, either κ or λ (Fig. 29-2). This immunoglobulin has a molecular mass of 190 kd and a carbohydrate content of 12 percent. Each ε heavy chain has a molecular mass of 72.5 kd and is composed of five domains. IgE has the lowest concentration in serum of any of the human immunoglobulin classes. The half-life of IgE is 2 to 3 days in the circulation and 8 to 12 days in the skin. IgE does not cross the placenta.

Measurement of the total serum IgE level is not a valuable screening test for allergic disease. Although the majority of atopic individuals will have a higher serum IgE than normal individuals, this is not uniformly seen. Even among nonatopic individuals, the levels of serum IgE vary widely.

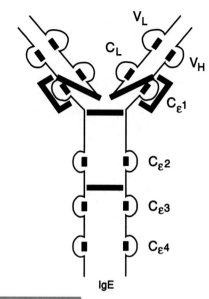

Figure 29-2 Schematic diagram of an IgE molecule. Of note, IgE's ε heavy chain has four constant domains (in common with the μ heavy chain) rather than three constant domains, as in the other immunoglobulin heavy chains. The "extra" domain lies between what corresponds to C_H1 and C_H2 of γ chains.

Production
The regulation of IgE production has been demonstrated by Vercelli and Geha (1991) to require two signals and involve both T and B lymphocytes. How these signals interact to affect IgE synthesis is currently the focus of intense study.

In order for IgE to be synthesized, a B lymphocyte must be induced to "switch" to IgE production. Interleukin 4 (IL-4), produced by T lymphocytes, is necessary for this isotype switching to IgE to occur. IL-4 acts at the gene segment encoding the constant region of the immunoglobulin heavy chain to initiate transcription through the ε locus. However, for IgE synthesis to occur, a second signal is also required. This signal can be delivered by helper T cells through direct contact between their T-cell receptor complexes and MHC class II antigens on B lymphocytes. It is not, however, essential that the second signal involve direct T- and B-lymphocyte contact. Epstein-Barr virus (EBV), for example, has been demonstrated to interact with IL-4 to induce IgE production in a T cell–independent manner.

Once IgE production is induced, it can be regulated by cytokines other than IL-4. For instance, IL-5 and IL-6 enhance the effect of IL-4 on B lymphocytes, while IFN-γ inhibits the IL-4 effect (Fig. 29-3).

Target Cells for IgE

Mast cells and basophils are the primary cells involved in the course of immediate hypersensitivity reactions. Mast cells are chiefly

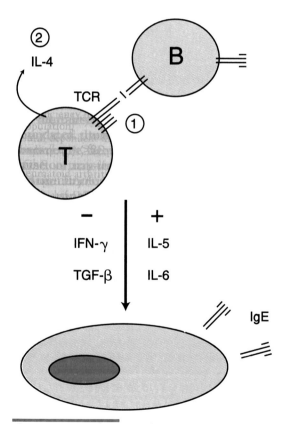

Figure 29-3 Schematic diagram of cytokine influences on the production of IgE. After interaction with a T cell, B cells' development into IgE-secreting plasma cells is enhanced by IL-5 and IL-6 and suppressed by IFNγ and TGFβ. IL-4 is a T cell cytokine involved in promotion of secretion of IgE or IgG.

found in connective tissues of the skin, the respiratory and gastrointestinal tracts, the nervous system, lymphoid tissues, blood vessels, and bone marrow. There are two distinct subpopulations of human mast cells, which differ in the type of enzymes contained (see Chap. 19a). The fact that these mast cells contain different enzymes may signify that they play different roles in immunologic reactions. Basophils make up a very small percentage of the polymorphonuclear leukocytes found in the circulation and bone marrow. They enter tissues and accumulate at the sites of certain immunologic or inflammatory reactions, where they make up a very small proportion of the total leukocytes present.

Both mast cells and basophils have high-affinity surface receptors for IgE, in contrast with the low-affinity IgE receptors found on such cells as monocytes, eosinophils, and platelets. The IgE receptor is a complex composed of four polypeptide chains—α, β, and two identical disulfide-linked γ chains (α β γ_2). The α chain has two nonidentical domains and appears to protrude from the cell surface; it is this protruding part of the molecule that binds to IgE. Bound noncovalently to the α chain is the β chain, which is also composed of two nonidentical domains. Both the β chain and the two γ chains are intramembranous, with minimal exposure to the exterior of the cell. Recent work has revealed that the site on IgE that binds to the Fc receptor lies at the $C_\varepsilon 2$-$C_\varepsilon 3$ junction of the ε heavy chain.

Mediator Release

It is generally believed that the cell membrane of mast cells and basophils is in a fluid state and that the cell surface receptors with bound immunoglobulin are movable. The triggering of these cells relies upon this physical characteristic. IgE can bind with high affinity to Fc receptors on mast cells and basophils, and exposure to antigen can "bridge" the cell-bound IgE molecules, causing them to move closer together. It appears to be the interaction between these apposed IgE receptors, rather than between the IgE molecules themselves, that triggers the subsequent mediator release from the cells.

Once two IgE receptors are cross-linked, a series of biochemical events involving multiple pathways begins. These pathways involve substances such as inositol lipids and diacylglycerol and the mobilization of calcium in the cell. The end result of these events is the fusion of mast cell and basophil granules with the cell plasma membrane, thus allowing the discharge of their contents.

Mediators

The granules of mast cells and basophils contain mediators; some of these are preformed and others are newly generated upon cell activation. The mediators which have been isolated from human mast cells are listed and discussed in Chap. 19A. Clinically, what we see as an immediate hypersensitivity reaction is due to the combined actions of mediators such as histamine, prostaglandins, leukotrienes, and platelet-activating factor (PAF). (See also Chapter 15, describing lipid mediators of inflammation.) It is likely that with further study, other mediators will be identified that will provide us with more opportunities to manipulate the system. Are you able to think of currently available therapeutic agents which affect these mediators and might prevent or modify allergic symptoms?

DIAGNOSIS OF THE TYPE I HYPERSENSITIVITY REACTION

Some of the more common disorders for which allergists are consulted are anaphylaxis, asthma, rhinitis, conjunctivitis, sinusitis, headaches, atopic dermatitis, and urticaria. It is the physician's task to ascertain whether allergies are contributing to the patient's symptoms. A good history, including a complete medical evaluation but focusing on characterization of the "allergic" symptoms, is essential to making this determination. It is important to determine when

the symptoms occur (what time of day and what time of year), their frequency, and other associated features which the patient may not think of as being related, such as decreased hearing or sense of smell. The history should afford a comprehensive view of the patient's environment, allowing identification of possible offending allergens. The confirmation of a person's sensitivity to a specific agent requires diagnostic testing.

In addition to the evidence of allergic disease obtained from the history, characteristic features can be seen on the physical examination. These include allergic "shiners" (dark discolorations beneath the eyes), allergic nasal crease (a transverse line at the junction of the nasal bridge and lower nose), Dennie's line (a wrinkle beneath the lower eyelid), and allergic facies (an open-mouthed, gaping expression). Examination of the nose reveals swollen, moist turbinates with a watery discharge.

Skin testing—prick, intradermal, or scratch—is the principal method used for diagnosing allergy.

Prick testing involves placing drops of allergen extracts (aqueous solutions of the allergen) on the skin of the patient's back or volar surface of the forearm. The skin is pricked through the drops with a small needle. This should abrade the skin, but not draw blood. A drop of histamine and a drop of saline serve as the positive and negative controls, respectively. After 15 min, the wheal and erythema are measured at each allergen site. Table 29-1 is a representative classification system for prick-test reactions.

TABLE 29-1 Grading System for Prick Testing

Grade	Reaction
0+	No difference from negative control
1+	Erythema < 21 mm
2+	Erythema ≥ 21 mm without wheal
3+	Wheal with surrounding erythema
4+	Wheal with pseudopods and surrounding erythema

TABLE 29-2 Grading System for Intradermal Testing

Grade	Erythema, mm	Wheal, mm
0	<5	<5
+/−	5–10	5–10
1+	11–20	5–10
2+	21–30	5–10
3+	31–40	10–15 (or pseudopods)
4+	>40	>15 (or with many pseudopods)

The advantage of prick testing is that it is easy to perform and allows multiple tests to be placed simultaneously. It is also safe because minimal allergen is absorbed and there is only a small chance of a systemic reaction occurring. The disadvantage of this method is its relative insensitivity. Therefore, a negative prick test (< 2+ reaction) should be followed by intradermal testing. Scratch testing is similar to prick testing except that the skin is scratched rather than pricked beneath the extracts.

Intradermal testing involves injecting 0.02 mL of extract into the skin to produce a small bleb; histamine and saline again serve as controls. The wheal and erythema are measured at each site after 15 min. Table 29-2 shows an example of criteria used for interpretation of intradermal testing.

Intradermal testing is more sensitive than prick testing but also has a greater risk of inducing a systemic reaction.

False-negative and false-positive results can occur with any form of skin testing. These result from recent use of medications, such as antihistamines, which suppress skin reactivity; use of poorly prepared extracts; or dermatographism, in which some normal persons develop wheals upon scratching of their skin. Skin test results must therefore be correlated with the clinical history.

In some instances, skin testing is not possible. These include patients with severe skin disease and those who are extremely anxious. In these cases, an in vitro procedure for measuring antigen-specific serum IgE is available. This radioallergosorbent test (RAST) is a radioimmunoassay in which the antigen of interest is bound to a paper disk to which the serum to be tested is added. If IgE antibodies specific for the antigen are present in the serum, they will bind. After washing away any unbound nonspecific IgE, radiolabeled anti-IgE antibodies are added, forming a complex of paper-bound allergen–IgE with the labeled anti-IgE. The amount of bound radioactivity measured is proportional to the specific IgE in the tested serum. Although RAST is a safe and convenient test, it is more expensive and less sensitive than skin testing, which remains the procedure of choice in most situations.

CLINICAL MANIFESTATIONS OF ALLERGY

Anaphylaxis

Anaphylaxis is a severe generalized allergic reaction. Similar clinical syndromes which are not immunologically mediated are termed *anaphylactoid*. The true incidence of anaphylaxis is difficult to estimate, as it may not be clear that a patient's clinical symptoms, especially in the case of sudden death, were due to an anaphylactic reaction to an antigen. However, in 1978 the incidence of fatal anaphylaxis in Ontario, Canada, was estimated to be 0.4 cases per million population per year. Anaphylaxis does not seem to occur more frequently in atopic individuals.

Many agents have been implicated in the etiology of anaphylaxis, with penicillin and Hymenoptera stings being among the most common. Other causes include other antibiotics, foods, and drugs. Exercise-induced anaphylaxis is called a "physical allergy" and is triggered by vigorous exercise. Cases have been described in which anaphylaxis occurs when exercise is preceded by food ingestion. Anaphylaxis that occurs in the absence of an identifiable cause is called idiopathic anaphylaxis. Although antigens administered through parenteral, oral, inhalant, or topical routes may precipitate anaphylaxis, the parenteral route is the most likely to cause such a reaction.

Anaphylaxis is a systemic reaction which affects chiefly the skin and the cardiovascular, respiratory, and gastrointestinal systems. The clinical course is variable. Early symptoms are nonspecific and include anxiety, weakness, sneezing, coughing, and generalized pruritus. Skin manifestations range from diffuse erythema to urticaria and angioedema. Respiratory symptoms of hoarseness, dyspnea, and wheezing may progress to severe lower airway obstruction and laryngeal edema. Associated gastrointestinal complaints include nausea, vomiting, abdominal cramping, and diarrhea. Finally, cardiac arrhythmias and hypotension may occur. (Refer to the section of Chap. 19A on mast cell mediators and try to determine which of these mediators might be responsible for these manifestations.) In one series of 400 fatal anaphylactic reactions from Hymenoptera stings, 69 percent of deaths were attributed to respiratory complications and 24 percent were due to cardiovascular causes.

The diagnosis of anaphylaxis is a clinical one. Identification of the precipitating agent involves use of skin testing or RAST to determine the presence of IgE to the suspected allergen. For agents that induce anaphylactoid reactions, a provocative challenge test is the only way to identify the causative factor. This is a dangerous procedure and is rarely performed.

Treatment of anaphylactic reactions consists of both short- and long-term management. For short-term management, epinephrine, a sympathomimetic amine, is the drug of choice. It is administered in a dose of 0.1 to 0.3 mL of a 1:1000 solution intramuscularly and may be given repeatedly. Epinephrine acts as a potent vasopressor to increase blood pressure and as a cardiac stimulant. If anaphylaxis occurs after a Hymenoptera sting or immunotherapy with an allergen extract and an injection site is visible, a tourniquet should be placed proximal to it. Other therapy which may be necessary includes intramuscular or intravenous diphenhydramine, administration of fluids and/or pressors, in-

travenous aminophylline and corticosteroids, intubation, and cardiopulmonary resuscitation. Due to the possibility of symptom recurrence, the patient should be observed at least 12 h after an anaphylactic reaction.

The most important step in preventing repeated reactions is to avoid the offending agent. The patient must be aware of all products which contain the antigen as well as any potentially cross-reacting substances. For example, a patient who has a severe reaction after aspirin ingestion must carefully read medication labels, as a large number of over-the-counter products contain aspirin. If use of an anaphylaxis-provoking drug is unavoidable, desensitization can be undertaken. This involves the serial administration of gradually increasing doses of the drug. Why this procedure works is not entirely clear. Another successful treatment, useful for sensitivity to hymenopterans, is venom immunotherapy which produces protective IgG "blocking" antibody, i.e., IgG which may interact with the allergen, preventing it from binding to the cell bound-IgE. Finally, in many cases, patients who have experienced anaphylaxis should carry injectable preloaded epinephrine.

Asthma

Asthma is a chronic respiratory disorder characterized by recurrent airway obstruction. The obstruction is manifested clinically as dyspnea, wheezing, and/or cough and is at least partially reversible. Asthmatic airways demonstrate hyperresponsiveness to a variety of nonspecific stimuli.

When an asthmatic person is exposed to a provoking stimulus such as an allergen, an IgE-mediated asthmatic response occurs within 15 min. This early response is a classic allergic reaction, with mast cell mediator release leading to bronchoconstriction, mucus secretion, and mucosal edema. Bronchodilators, such as β_2-adrenergic agonists, can reverse the early response. In at least 50 percent of asthmatics, the early response is followed 4 to 6 h later by a late-phase response. The late-phase asthmatic response is also dependent on IgE and the release of mediators, probably from basophils rather than mast cells. The unique feature of the late-phase response is that the mediators attract inflammatory cells, primarily eosinophils and neutrophils, to the airways. It is believed that the late-phase response is accountable for the nonspecific airway hyperreactivity that continues long after exposure to the triggering stimulus has ended. This has important implications for treatment. The late-phase asthmatic response is not fully reversed by bronchodilators. Cromolyn sodium and corticosteroids are anti-inflammatory and therefore affect the late-phase response and reduce airway hyperresponsiveness.

Acute episodes of asthma can be triggered by a variety of stimuli. These include exercise, cold air, viral infections, air pollutants, emotional factors, and allergens. Exposure to allergen appears to be an important factor in the development of both the asthmatic condition and acute asthmatic episodes. Therefore, in addition to bronchodilators and anti-inflammatory therapy, avoidance of or treatment for allergic stimuli can be of great benefit to the asthmatic person. The percentage of asthmatics with an allergic component to their disease is probably underestimated. In fact, the classification of asthma into distinct groups called allergic (or extrinsic) and nonallergic (or intrinsic) is being questioned. Some researchers believe that there is a close link between atopy (occasionally manifested as only an elevated IgE level, without clinical evidence of atopic disease) and airway hyperresponsiveness. This association has been demonstrated in children with no history of atopy and no symptoms of airway disease.

Allergic Rhinitis

Rhinitis is inflammation of the mucous membranes of the nose. It can be either infectious or noninfectious, with the latter being further divided into allergic and nonallergic types.

Allergic rhinitis is a very common disorder, with onset of symptoms most frequently in childhood or adolescence and an estimated prevalence in the United States of between 3 and 19 percent. Symptoms of allergic rhinitis are intranasal pruritus, sneezing, nasal congestion, and rhinorrhea with clear watery discharge. Symptoms may be seasonal or perennial depending on the causative environmental factors. Seasonal allergic rhinitis is due to exposure to pollen from wind-pollinated plants such as ragweed, trees, and grasses. Perennial allergic rhinitis is due to inhalation of allergens such as house dust mites, animal dander, and mold spores. Sensitization by recurrent exposure to an allergen, for example, during two to three pollinating seasons, is required before allergic rhinitis develops. Once symptoms begin, they tend to persist for many years, although spontaneous remissions do occur.

While the diagnosis of allergic rhinitis is usually not difficult, in the case of the perennial type it may be impossible to determine from the history and physical examination whether allergy is present. In questionable cases, laboratory studies can be useful. Nasal secretions can be stained with Hansel's stain and examined microscopically. A predominance of eosinophils suggests an allergic cause, while the presence of many neutrophils is characteristic of infectious rhinitis. When present, peripheral blood eosinophilia and elevated total serum IgE can be helpful in diagnosing allergic rhinitis. The best way to determine a patient's sensitivity and the specific causative allergens is skin tests or RAST.

It is important to adequately treat allergic rhinitis not only for symptom relief, but also to prevent complications. Although data are inconclusive, it appears that nasal polyps, sinusitis, and otitis media with effusion may occur secondary to untreated allergic rhinitis. Nasal polyps develop from recurrent inflammation and edema of the nasal mucosa leading to hyperplasia which then causes obstruction of the nasal passage. Sinusitis occurs when chronic edema of the nasal mucosa causes obstruction of the nasal ostia, through which the sinuses drain. Increased mucus production and decreased ciliary action accompany the obstruction, thereby establishing a favorable environment for secondary bacterial infection. In the case of otitis media with effusion, edema of the nasal mucosa may lead to obstruction of the nasopharyngeal orifices of the eustachian tube. This results in an effusion in the middle ear with subsequent infection. When allergy is involved in the etiology of these disorders, both the acute process and the underlying allergic condition must be treated.

TREATMENT OF ALLERGIC DISORDERS

The approach to the treatment of patients with allergic diseases must encompass three areas: minimizing exposure to symptom-producing allergens, pharmacologic management, and, in selected patients, the use of immunotherapy.

Clearly, the best way to "treat" allergic symptoms is to avoid provoking them in the first place. A patient with allergic rhinitis which occurs only following exposure to cats will be symptom-free if cat allergens are avoided completely. However, it is often impossible to eliminate entirely many clinically significant allergens due to their widespread distribution. In these cases, decreasing the patient's exposure through environmental manipulations will aid in controlling symptoms. For instance, house dust mites, *Dermatophagoides farinae* and *Dermatophagoides pteronyssinus*, are found year-round in homes. They grow especially well in warm temperatures with 70 percent relative humidity and heavily infest mattresses, carpets, and upholstered furniture. Reducing exposure to dust mite allergens includes removal of carpets, enclosing mattresses in plastic covers, washing bedding frequently in hot water, and eliminating upholstered furniture. Mold spores are also difficult to avoid. Limiting exposure around the home requires using an air-conditioner or dehumidifier to decrease humidity, avoiding freshly cut grass or raked leaves, and keeping

refrigerator drip trays and garbage containers clean and dry. Pollen exposure can be reduced indoors by using an air-conditioner and keeping windows closed.

Pharmacologic agents are frequently required in conjunction with these environmental interventions. Antihistamines, cromolyn sodium, and glucocorticoid preparations form the basis for symptomatic therapy of allergic diseases.

The classic H_1-receptor antagonists are most useful in treating allergic symptoms. (Refer back to the discussion of histamine in Chap. 19 and review the actions of histamine on H_1 receptors.) They are available in many varieties, often in combination with decongestants (see Table 29-3) and are used to treat anaphylactic reactions, allergic rhinitis, urticaria, pruritus, and allergic conjunctivitis. All the classes of H_1 blockers are well absorbed after oral administration, but differ in their duration of action, intensity of side effects, and amount of symptomatic relief in individual patients. The main side effects involve the central nervous system and anticholinergic actions. These include sedation, dryness of the mouth, urinary retention, gastrointestinal upset, and dizziness. Newer antihistamines lack anticholinergic effects and do not penetrate the blood-brain barrier to produce sedation. The response to a particular antihistamine is very variable, with a patient often responding better to one class of H_1 blockers than to another.

Cromolyn sodium is not well absorbed through the gastrointestinal tract and is therefore used mainly as an aerosol or locally applied solution. It is effective for the prophylactic treatment of asthma, allergic rhinitis, and allergic ocular disorders and is becoming a first-line therapy for these conditions. The precise mechanism of action of cromolyn has not been completely elucidated but is thought to involve inhibition of the release of mast cell mediators by stabilization of the cell membrane. Side effects are minimal and include throat or nasal irritation, headache, dizziness, nausea, and rash.

Corticosteroids in oral, parenteral, and topical forms have proved to be efficacious

TABLE 29-3   Representative Antihistamines

Class	Generic Name	Trade Name
Ethylenediamines	Antazoline	Vasocon-A
	Tripelennamine	PBZ
Ethanolamines	Clemastine	Tavist
	Diphenhydramine	Benadryl
Alkylamines	Brompheniramine	Dimetane
	Chlorpheniramine	Chlor-Trimeton
	Triprolidine	Actidil, Actifed
Piperazines	Hydroxyzine	Atarax
Phenothiazines	Methdilazine	Tacaryl
	Trimeprazine	Temaril
Piperidines	Azatadine	Optimine, Trinalin
	Cyproheptadine	Periactin
Miscellaneous agents (nonsedating)	Astemizole	Hismanal
	Terfenadine	Seldane

in the treatment of a variety of allergic disorders. Among their numerous effects, corticosteroids selectively inhibit the late-phase response to antigen challenge in the nose and lung, reduce the number of mast cells in the nasal mucosa, and inhibit chemotaxis of leukocytes into the nose and lung. In the past, the use of corticosteroids was hampered by concerns about their serious side effects, including osteoporosis, hypertension, cataract development, and hyperglycemia. Newer topical preparations for use in rhinitis and asthma are associated with fewer adverse effects, while offering many of the same therapeutic advantages.

In those patients whose asthma, rhinitis, or conjunctivitis can be attributed to or exacerbated by exposure to aeroallergens, immunotherapy may be of benefit. Immunotherapy involves the administration of increasing doses of allergenic extracts over a period of time. Patients selected for this therapy should have both a clinical history and positive skin test or RAST showing response to the specific aeroallergens with which they are to be treated. Avoidance methods and pharmacologic therapy should have been previously attempted without adequate improvement. The goal of immunotherapy is to allow the patient to be exposed to allergens in the environment without developing allergic symptoms. Treatment is begun with low doses of aqueous extracts injected subcutaneously every 7 days and is increased in amount until an adequate maintenance dose of injected allergen is reached. Maintenance doses are usually administered monthly and are continued year-round for a minimum of 3 to 5 years. Clinical improvement is both allergen-specific and immunotherapy dose-dependent, with high cumulative doses of allergen having the greater effectiveness. The mechanisms for clinical improvement with immunotherapy are not entirely clear. However, several immunologic changes have been consistently demonstrated during this therapy, including an increase in the serum level of IgG "blocking" antibodies to a plateau level, an initial rise followed by a gradual decrease in antigen-specific IgE antibodies, a suppression of the usual seasonal rise in antigen-specific IgE, and an increase in allergen-specific IgG and IgA in nasal secretions. In addition, in some patients basophil reactivity to allergen as measured by histamine release is reduced, in vitro lymphocyte proliferation in response to antigen is diminished, and antigen-specific suppressor T cells develop. For patients with allergic rhinitis, immunotherapy will lead to clinical improvement in 80 to 85 percent of those treated. Its benefit in the treatment of asthma may vary depending on the allergens involved.

Future trends in the therapy of allergic

diseases will likely proceed in several directions. Work is being done with modified extracts for use in immunotherapy. These would provoke fewer systemic reactions while continuing to stimulate IgG "blocking" antibody production. Other potential therapies involve the utilization of immunomodulators such as cytokines derived from T lymphocytes and/or macrophages, or drugs which act by preventing the actions of allergic mediators. Although these therapies are not currently available, they provide exciting possibilities for furthering both the understanding and treatment of allergic diseases in the future.

SELF-TEST QUESTIONS

1. Immunologic changes seen with immunotherapy include all of the following *except:*
    a. An initial rise in allergen-specific IgE with a return to pretreatment level
    b. A rise in allergen-specific IgG "blocking" antibodies
    c. Normal seasonal peak in allergen-specific IgE
    d. Development of allergen-specific suppressor T cells
2. Mast cell mediator release can be triggered by all the following *except:*
    a. Two IgE molecules plus anti-IgE antibody
    b. Multivalent antigen plus two IgE molecules
    c. Two IgE molecules plus two monovalent haptens
    d. One anti-IgE receptor antibody

For the following problem choose the correct letter of the combination of answers that correctly completes the statement:
A   a, b, and c are correct
B   a and c are correct
C   b and d are correct
D   d is correct
3. The regulation of specific-IgE production involves:
    a. T helper cells
    b. IgE-bearing B cells
    c. Repeated exposure to antigen
    d. High-affinity Fc receptors for IgE

Match each of the following effects of histamine with the letter of the agent(s) listed below that will antagonize that effect.
4. Cutaneous flush
5. Increased skin temperature
6. Increased gastric acid secretion
7. Increased heart rate
    a. Diphenhydramine
    b. Cimetidine
    c. Both diphenhydramine and cimetidine
    d. Neither diphenhydramine nor cimetidine.

ADDITIONAL READINGS

de Shazo RD, Smith DL, eds. *Primer on Allergic and Immunologic Diseases.* 3rd ed. *JAMA;* 1992:268.

Sears MR et al. Relation between airway responsiveness and serum IgE in children with asthma and in apparently normal children. *N Engl J Med.* 1991;325:1067–1071.

Vercelli D, Geha RS. Regulation of IgE synthesis in humans: A tale of two signals. *J Allergy Clin Immunol.* 1991;88:285–295.

30

Immunohematology

Immune Mechanisms, Both Natural and Physician-Induced, Which Influence the Formed Elements of the Blood

INTRODUCTION AND GENERAL CONCEPTS

The human hematopoietic system produces cells (erythrocytes, platelets, neutrophils) that have a unique capacity to interact with components of the human immune system. For example, the neutrophil and platelet possess Fc receptors for antibody and all three cell types circulate widely throughout the body both in vascular and immune system compartments (e.g., lymph nodes, spleen). They are therefore "ready" to encounter and engage a functioning immune system.

Circulating autoantibodies of different isotypes may bind to either granulocytes, platelets, or erythrocytes, and are believed to be the primary component in the genesis of immune system–mediated hematologic disease. After binding, the antibody-cell complex is then highly likely to be recognized by cells of the monocyte-macrophage system (see below and Fig. 30-1), with subsequent ingestion and destruction. In addition, natural killer (NK) cells have membrane Fc receptors and are also capable of recognizing this antibody-cell complex. However, it is not as clear that NK cells mediate the destruction of the target cells in autoimmune hematologic diseases.

Clinically significant anticellular serum antibodies may be subdivided into two general groups: *idiopathic* (usually autoantibodies) and *antigen-induced* (usually alloantibodies). The latter group is seen in individuals given mismatched blood components, postpartum females, and individuals who have been exposed to certain drugs. In both groups, antibody is capable of reacting with specific membrane antigens on the granulocyte, platelet, or erythrocyte. The presence or amount of detectable levels of auto- or alloantibodies does not strictly predict clinical disease. High levels of autoantibody may be associated with no alteration in blood cells; conversely, there may be minimal numbers of antibody molecules binding to the target cell, yet significant clinical changes occur.

Clearly, there are additional factors that assist in mediating the impact of antibody-induced hematologic diseases. These may include, affinity of antibody for antigen, distribution and quantity of membrane antigens, and ability of antibody to fix complement (see Table 30-1). The isotype and subclass of antibody will also alter the potential fate of antibody-coated cells (Table 30-2). Further discussion of isotypes and subclasses of antibodies and their characteristics can be found in Chap. 3, "Antibodies."

In general, IgM-isotype auto- or alloantibodies are more effective at fixing complement than other Ig isotypes. Thus, pathologic conditions where IgM antibodies are primarily involved may result in more damage to blood cells through complement fixation and activation. Alternatively, if the

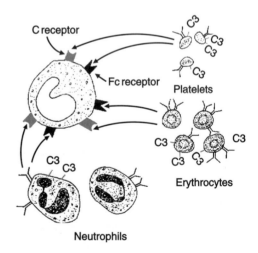

Figure 30-1 Blood cells coated with antibody or complement (C_3) will be recognized and then bound to cells of the monocyte-macrophage system. This recognition occurs through binding to either Fc receptors (for antibody) or complement receptors (C receptors). After binding, the blood cells will either be released, partially ingested, or completely destroyed.

TABLE 30-1 Some Factors That Modulate Immune System–Mediated Blood Cell Destruction

> Number of antigen sites on membrane
> Mobility of antigens within membrane
> Class of immunoglobulin
> Subclass of IgG
> Quantity of antibody-sensitizing blood
> Equilibrium constant of antibody
> Ability of antibody to activate complement
> Thermal range of antibody (especially for
>   erythrocytes)
> Activity of recipient's reticuloendothelial system
>   (macrophages)

pathologic antibody is IgG, the specific IgG subclass (IgG1, IgG2, IgG3, IgG4) is critical in determining the impact of the antibody. IgG1 and IgG3 subclasses are more efficient at fixing complement, and there are Fc receptors on monocyte membranes for these subclasses. Finally, the presence of both Ig and complement components on blood cells is usually indicative of an active destructive process. The combined presence of IgG and complement may enhance the recognition and destruction of immunoglobulin-coated blood cells by effector cells (e.g., monocytes and macrophages or lymphocytes). Thus, evaluation of disease processes that involve antibody and/or complement molecules should include detailed analysis of these effector molecules. This will aid both the diagnostic and prognostic information.

The detection of both immunoglobulin and complement on erythrocytes is routinely evaluated by the direct antiglobulin or Coombs' test (see Fig. 30-2).

In the following sections we examine some disease states and immune system mechanisms which alter granulocytes, erythrocytes, and platelets. The parameters of the hematopoietic cell that render it susceptible to immune system manipulation, the immune mechanisms of different clinical diseases, and possible therapeutic maneuvers will be emphasized here.

IMMUNE SYSTEM–MEDIATED GRANULOCYTOPENIA

Cell Target—Granulocytes

Granulocytes circulate in peripheral blood in both a marginating (along vessel wall) and circulating pool. Both pools are available to immune effector molecules. Polymorphonuclear leukocytes (granulocytes) are capable of interacting with circulating antibody or immune complexes. One autoimmune mechanism involves the generation of autoantibodies to granulocyte membrane antigens. Fetal granulocytes may induce maternal (anti-HLA) antibodies (isoimmune neutropenia), and leukoagglutinins may be seen following transfusion of blood products.

TABLE 30-2 Fc-Dependent Characteristics of Immunoglobulins*

Class	Binding Complement		Placental Transport	Binding to Monocytes
	CLASSICAL	ALTERNATIVE		
IgG1	+ +	+	+ + +	+ +
IgG2	+	0	+	0
IgG3	+ + +	+	+ +	+ + +
IgG4	0	0	+	0
IgA	0	+ +	0	0
IgM	+ + +	+	0	±
IgD	0	0	0	0
IgE	0	ND†	0	0

*Strength of Ig characteristics assessed from no activity (0) to strongest detected activity (+ + + +).
†ND = not determined.

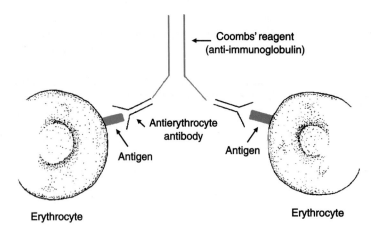

Figure 30-2 Direct antiglobulin test. This scheme depicts the mechanics of the serologic test. Antigen (open column) present on the erythrocyte membrane is reactive for IgG antibody. To detect the presence of antierythrocyte antibody on erythrocyte membranes, a developer called Coombs' reagent (anti-immunoglobulin) is added. The bivalency of the anti-immunoglobulin results in binding of two separate cells by the reagent. This results in agglutination or clumping, which is detected either macroscopically or microscopically. To detect other immune components (e.g., complement, Ig isotypes), specific types of Coombs' reagent are added (e.g., anticomplement, anti-IgG, anti-IgG3).

At present, two neutrophil-specific antigens are known to be potentially involved in autoimmune neutropenia, NA2 and ND1. However, it is still unclear what role specific antigens play in various pathologic states.

Granulocytes express two receptors that are crucial for interaction with immune complexes; Fc receptor for IgG molecules and receptors for the C3b and C5a components of complement. These two membrane receptors greatly facilitate recognition and binding of circulating antibody or immune complexes (e.g., antibody-antigen or complement-containing complexes) to the granulocyte. Thus there may be dramatic changes in neutrophil levels if a significant antineutrophil immune process intervenes by virtue of the cell's availability to interact with immune effector molecules and the rapid turnover (half-life of 12 h in blood) of the cell. In addition, Fc or complement receptor occupancy may subsequently result in altered basal neutrophil function (e.g., increased metabolic activity or phagocytosis).

Mechanism and Classification of Immune Granulocytopenia

Antibody and/or complement-coated granulocytes are removed from circulation through increased interaction with the monocyte-macrophage system (Fig. 30-1). The type of antibody involved relates very closely to the classification of diseases associated with granulocytopenia (see below).

Alloantibodies, autoantibodies, and drug-induced antibodies are formed in reasonably distinct clinical situations. Careful clinical and laboratory studies help to characterize these separate disorders.

Alloantibodies

Posttransfusion Immune Granulocytopenia

Repeated transfusions may result in production of HLA-reactive alloantibodies or alloantibodies that react to granulocyte-specific antigens of the donor(s). A febrile reaction to transfusion in patients who have had multiple transfusions is usually due to granulocyte-specific antibodies and is called a *leukoagglutinin reaction* (see Clinical Aside 30-1). Thus, blood bank studies would demonstrate that the patient's serum causes clumping of the patient's neutrophils. The presence of granulocyte antibodies may result in shortened granulocyte survival.

Clinical Aside 30-1
Leukoagglutinin Reaction—Transfusion-Induced Fever

A 55-year-old white male had emergency appendectomy following acute appendicitis. During the surgery a major blood vessel was nicked; and the patient suffered approximately 1000 mL of excess blood loss. Immediately following surgery, the surgeon recommended transfusion of 2 units of blood. As the patient was being given the second unit, his temperature began to rise. The temperature continued to rise for approximately 4 h after the transfusion and persisted for a further 12 h. In addition, the patient had a mild drop in blood pressure, suffered nausea, and had one vomiting episode. Because of the apparent transfusion reaction, the blood bank was consulted.

The blood bank determined that this was a nonhemolytic febrile reaction. They explained to the surgeon that febrile reactions without hemolysis are frequently due to sensitization to white cell or platelet antigens. In fact, nonhemolytic febrile reactions account for as many as one-third of all recognized transfusion reactions. The diagnosis rests on laboratory demonstration of HLA or non-HLA antibodies to white cell antigens. These are usually called *leukoagglutinins*, or *lymphocytotoxins*. Most reactions of this type are associated with sensitivity to granulocytes. However, sensitivity to other cells, such as lymphocytes or platelets, may also be the culprit. The blood bank consultant explained that no treatment would be necessary. Only supportive therapy would be required, since this is a self-limiting reaction. In addition, the blood bank recommended that in the future leukocyte-poor blood be obtained, i.e., blood that had been stored for over 1 week and that had been subjected to microaggregate filtration.

Postpregnancy Immune Granulocytopenia

This disease occurs in newborn infants due to the transplacental passage of maternal IgG antibodies to the neutrophil-specific antigens inherited from the neonate's father. The disease occurs in approximately 1 in 2000 neonates, and the neutropenia may last for 2 to 4 months. It is usually not detected unless there is an obvious infection in the newborn. Since the granulocytopenia may resolve in a few weeks, supportive antibiotic therapy is usually sufficient.

Autoantibodies

Idiopathic Autoimmune Neutropenia Patients diagnosed with autoimmune neutropenia are usually selectively neutropenic and have positive tests for neutrophil antibodies. The syndrome of chronic autoimmune neutropenia is more prevalent in young children (6 to 24 months) than in adults. The granulocyte-specific antibodies are usually IgG or IgM. The clinical course of autoimmune neutropenia is typically benign, of relatively short duration, and usually does not require therapy. Idiopathic autoimmune neutropenia may be seen in infants and young children, and it is important to differentiate this disorder from granulocytopenia caused by maternally derived alloantibodies.

Granulocytopenia with Other Disorders In adults there are a number of autoimmune diseases with associated granulocytopenia. The more common ones are rheumatoid arthritis (RA), systemic lupus erythematosus (SLE), Evan's syndrome, and Felty's syndrome. Rheumatoid arthritis and SLE are both systemic diseases with detectable circulating autoantibodies, rheumatoid factor in RA and antinuclear antibodies in SLE. Occasionally antigranulocyte antibodies are found which may be implicated in granulocytopenia. Evan's syndrome is the combination of autoimmune hemolysis and thrombocytopenia, while Felty's syndrome is defined as long-standing rheumatoid arthritis with splenomegaly and granulocytopenia. The splenomegaly is believed to be involved in the etiology of neutropenia. This is not typically a serious clinical complication, but in certain situations very low persistent granulocytopenia may result in repeated infections. Treatment to alleviate the persistent granulocytopenia is steroids, splenectomy, or both. The etiologic agent in these clinical disorders is believed to be circulating autoantibodies or perhaps immune complexes. Finally, in some patients, an autoantibody directed against bone marrow myeloid progenitors may be present. Most recently, involvement of T cell–mediated component of the immune system directed against myeloid precursors has been implicated in the generation of clinically important granulocytopenia.

Drug-Induced Granulocytopenia

There are frequent reports of drug-related immune granulocytopenia. However, until recently, there were no reliable in vitro methods to directly establish the presence of drug-dependent antibody. There are laboratory tests that rely upon membrane immunofluorescence to detect granulocyte-specific drug-induced immune complexes. Several mechanisms have been described in drug-related granulocyte destruction.

Immune Complex A drug like quinine can induce drug-specific IgG1 or IgM antibodies (usually complement fixing), and the immune complexes formed (drug-Ig) can then associate with granulocyte membranes or circulate in the patient's sera. These drug-immune complex-coated cells are presumably cleared at an increased rate by the reticuloendothelial system. This mechanism has been most clearly detected and analyzed in drug-induced thrombocytopenia (see below).

Drug Absorption High serum concentrations of a drug like penicillin may result in nonspecific absorption of the drug to cell membranes. Antipenicilillin antibodies then bind to the penicillin on the membrane, with subsequent removal of the cell from the circulation. Again, both platelet and granulocyte cell membranes may be coated with the drug, with resultant granulocytopenia and thrombocytopenia. The mechanism of cell clearance for drug-coated cells is not well defined.

Autoantibodies There are several drugs which may result in membrane-directed autoantibodies, including aprindine, levamisole, and gold. In such cases, the drug is not required in the assay system to detect autoantibody. The mechanism by which drugs induce autoantibody production is not known but may include ablation of a T subset function. This in turn may result in stimulation of autoantibody secretion by B cells. (See Clinical Aside 30-2.)

Clinical Aside 30-2
Drug-Induced Granulocytopenia

In clinical assessment of drug-related granulocytopenia it is important to remember the following:

1. Discontinuation of drugs usually results in tapering and/or complete disappearance of cytopenia.
2. Drug-induced antibodies may not only perturb circulating mature peripheral cells but also marrow progenitor cells.
3. In order to prove that the drug(s) is involved in granulocytopenia, you should perform granulocyte immunofluorescence tests (or other relevant in vitro tests) and collect sera both at the acute stage and when the patient is convalescing (with and without drug) to determine if drugs played an essential role in cell destruction.

IMMUNE SYSTEM–MEDIATED HEMOLYSIS

Cell Target—Erythrocytes

Immune hemolysis (literally, lysis of red blood cells) is best characterized as a premature shortening of the normal erythrocyte life span

(100 to 120 days). It is possible to tag circulating erythrocytes with a radiolabel (chromium 51) and subsequently measure erythrocyte survival. Anemia may not be present if the bone marrow is proliferating (erythroid hyperplasia) to compensate for hemolysis, although an increased number of reticulocytes (young red blood cells) will be seen in the peripheral blood smear. Immune complex–mediated injury is usually due to antibody binding to specific erythrocyte antigens. The production of these antibodies may occur spontaneously (idiopathic), may be associated with certain diseases, or may arise in conjunction with drug ingestion.

Mechanism and Classification of Immune Hemolysis

The critical factor in induction of hemolysis is the binding of an antibody to the surface of the erythrocyte. Once antibody reactive with human erythrocytes is bound, the potential for erythrocyte interaction with the monocyte-macrophage system is enhanced. If the erythrocyte-bound antibodies also fix and activate complement, the circulating erythrocyte has an even greater chance of binding to and being ingested by splenic or hepatic macrophages through interaction with receptors for the Fc region of immunoglobulin and/or complement receptors. In most clinical circumstances it is the latter cell-cell interaction (extravascular) that results in hemolysis. There are occasional (fortunately rare) clinical diseases where a marked intravascular erythrocyte injury predominates (e.g., major transfusion mismatch, paroxysmal cold hemoglobinuria). The very high rate of intravascular hemolysis in these diseases is associated with increased patient symptoms usually related to low hemoglobin (e.g., shortness of breath and fatigue). There are several immune system parameters that modulate erythrocyte removal (see Table 30-1). In general immune hemolysis may be subdivided into autoimmune, drug-induced, or alloantibody-induced (see Table 30-3).

TABLE 30-3 Classification of Immune Hemolysis

AUTOIMMUNE
Warm antibody
Idiopathic
Secondary (associated with chronic lymphocytic leukemia, lymphoma, SLE)
Cold antibody (agglutinin)
Idiopathic
Secondary (associated with *Mycoplasma pneumoniae,* infectious mononucleosis, lymphoma)
Paroxysmal cold hemoglobinuria
Idiopathic
Secondary (associated with viral infections, syphilis)

DRUG-INDUCED
Hapten (e.g., penicillin)
Innocent bystander (e.g., quinidine)
Autoimmunelike (e.g., α-methyldopa)

ALLOANTIBODY-INDUCED
Hemolytic transfusion reactions
Hemolytic disease of newborn
ABO disease
Rh disease

Autoimmune Hemolysis

The main immune aberration in autoimmune hemolysis is the generation of autoantibodies specific for autologous red cell antigens. These antibodies are subdivided into *warm-reactive* and *cold-reactive* types, the names referring to the temperature of optimum binding of the antibodies to erythrocytes in vitro. Warm-reactive antibodies, which occur twice as frequently as cold-reactive antibodies, are usually IgG and bind more efficiently to their antigen at or near 37°C. These antibodies may have specificity for antigens of the Rh system. Cold-reactive antibodies are typically IgM and have optimum binding to antigen at or around 4°C. These IgM molecules may preferentially react with adult rather than fetal erythrocytes. The erythrocytes bound by IgG autoantibodies are usually recognized and removed by splenic macrophages, while erythrocyte-IgM autoantibody complexes are handled by hepatic macrophages. It is important to remember that *if* these IgG or IgM autoantibodies fix and/or activate complement, the severity of hemolysis is worse.

An important distinction between the two types of antibody is that warm-reactive antibodies frequently result in spherocytes (loss of erythrocyte membrane, due to partial ingestion by macrophages, yields an erythrocyte with nearly normal volume but less surface area, explaining the transition from the normal biconcave disk to a sphere) on peripheral smear, whereas cold-reactive antibodies often generate rouleaux ("coin stacks") of erythrocytes on smear. The rouleaux are seen because the IgM antibody binds at lower temperatures, and the large size and multivalency of IgM permit bridging between erythrocytes. It is important to note that the pathologic (i.e., clinical disease causing) cold IgM agglutinins frequently have a broad thermal amplitude for reactivity with erythrocytes. That is, they bind to erythrocytes over a wide range of temperatures (4°C to 20°C, or even higher). Thus they may have the capacity to agglutinate erythrocytes in the circulation and cause obstruction in small veins and arteries (see Raynaud's phenomenon, below).

There are additional features (laboratory and clinical) that help to distinguish the two types of immune hemolysis. Hemolysis associated with IgG is often detected by falling hemoglobin and a positive antiglobulin (Coombs') test (see Fig. 30-2). Rarely, this test may be negative. In addition, the specific components (immunoglobulin or complement) detected on erythrocytes by the direct antiglobulin test are helpful in confirming specific pathologic processes (see Table 30-4). In half the patients, an underlying clinical disease is present or emerges, such as lymphoma, chronic lymphocytic leukemia, and vasculitis. The hemolysis is best treated by prednisone, splenectomy, or both. Most patients (70 percent) respond to prednisone alone. The remaining 30 percent require splenectomy, and after splenectomy, half of those patients may require addition of prednisone to help induce a remission in hemolysis. The use of intravenous γ-globulin for hemolytic anemia and immune thrombocytopenia is described in Chap. 34. Finally, even in remission, the patient may still have a positive antiglobulin test.

IgM cold-reactive hemolysis (cold agglutinin syndrome) is not associated with a positive antiglobulin, but large aggregates of erythrocytes are seen at room temperature. The major factor in determining hemolysis

---

TABLE 30-4 Direct Antiglobulin Test Results in Various Immune Hemolysis Types

Hemolysis Type	Direct Antiglobulin Test Results
AUTOIMMUNE	
Warm antibody autoimmune hemolytic anemia (most common type)	IgG and/or complement (C3)
Cold-agglutinin syndrome	Complement (C3) alone
Paroxysmal cold hemoglobinuria	Complement (C3) alone
DRUG-INDUCED	
α-Methyldopa (Aldomet)	IgG alone
Penicillin	Usually IgG alone, but complement (C3) may also be detected
Other drugs (e.g., quinidine, phenacetin—usually reactive due to immune complex formation)	Usually complement (C3) alone, but IgG may also be detected)

is the upper limit of the temperature at which the IgM on the red blood cells can interact with complement. The higher this temperature limit, known as *thermal amplitude,* the greater the chance that the IgM can activate complement in vivo and result in clinically significant hemolysis. Diseases associated with IgM cold-reactive immune hemolysis include lymphomas, infectious mononucleosis, and viral illnesses for which the common underlying mechanism is the production of IgM cold agglutinins (see Table 30-5). These cold agglutinins, because of impaired circulation secondary to aggregated erythrocytes, may result in Raynaud's phenomenon. Raynaud's phenomenon is a disorder in which circulation to the distal portion of the fingertips, nose, and ears is severely reduced due to local vasospasm. This may result in ischemic changes to these areas with pain, discoloration, edema, ulceration, and even loss of tissue, but more often is isolated to what is called the *tricolor response.* (The word *tricolor* refers to the fact that initially the skin turns blue, due to local cyanosis, then white, due to decreased blood flow. With the resolution of the vasospasm, hyperemia develops and the area turns red, often with throbbing.) Treatment is usually preventive (avoid cold, dress warmly, etc.), because prednisone and splenectomy are seldom helpful. Plasmapheresis is an alternative therapeutic maneuver for this form of hemolysis. This is a process where several units of blood are removed from the patient, the plasma removed and discarded, and only the erythrocytes returned to the patient. Since most of the IgM is found intravascularly, this is a reasonable but temporary means of treating cold agglutinin disease.

Drug-Induced Immune Hemolysis

There are three recognized mechanisms for drug-induced hemolysis (see Fig. 30-3). Antibodies are the ultimate cause of hemolysis, but the mechanisms described for each of the following three drugs are very different: true autoantibodies, antidrug antibodies, and an innocent-bystander mechanism.

α-Methyldopa   This is the drug most commonly associated with autoimmune hemolysis. It is believed that α-methyldopa induces formation of true autoantibodies reactive with the patient's erythrocytes. A strikingly high percent of patients (15 percent) have a positive antiglobulin test following long-term ingestion of this antihypertensive drug, but most do not develop hemolysis and only a few patients (<10 percent) actually have clinical hemolysis. Usually only IgG is detected on erythrocyte membrane. Following cessation of the drug, the hemolysis usually disappears, although the antiglobulin test may remain positive.

Penicillin   Patients who receive large doses ($>20 \times 10^6$ units per day) of intravenous penicillin for a long time may also develop immune hemolysis and a positive antiglobulin test. Penicillin binds to the erythrocyte membrane and acts as a hapten. Subsequently drug-specific antibody is produced and attaches to the drug-erythrocyte complex.

TABLE 30-5   Cold Agglutinin in Clinical Disease

IgM Antibody		
CLONALITY	BLOOD GROUP SPECIFICITY*	*Clinical Disease*
Polyclonal (κ and λ)	Anti-i	*Mycoplasma pneumoniae* infection
Polyclonal (κ and λ)	Anti-i	Infectious mononucleosis
Monoclonal (κ and λ)	Anti-i	Lymphoma
Monoclonal (κ)	Anti-i or anti-P	Idiopathic cold-agglutinin disease

*i and P are two different blood group antigen families found on human erythrocytes.

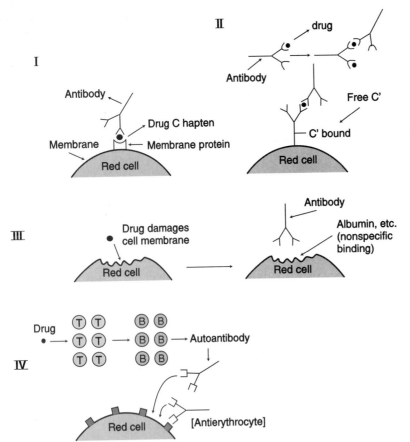

Figure 30-3 Mechanisms of immune hemolysis caused by drugs. (I) The drug acts as a hapten, binding to the membrane with subsequent hapten-antihapten (antibody) binding. (II) Drug-antidrug immune complexes form in the circulation and then attach to the erythrocyte with subsequent complement (C') fixation (innocent bystander). (III) Drug damages the erythrocyte membrane, and there is subsequent nonspecific binding by different plasma proteins (e.g., albumin, immunoglobulin). (IV) The drug stimulates T cells, which in some fashion promote B cells to produce autoantibodies that are erythrocyte-specific.

An antipenicillin antibody–penicillin complex is thus formed on the surface of the erythrocyte. These immune complex–laden erythrocytes are recognized by the splenic macrophages, where they may be phagocytosed and destroyed.

Quinidine and Stibophen   In this type, the drug (e.g., Stibophen) binds to a carrier protein (albumin) which acts as a hapten. Drug-specific complement-fixing antibodies are produced. These antibodies react with the drug in plasma and may result in activation of the complement pathway in the circulation. Certain complement activation molecules (e.g., C3b molecules) in the plasma may surround and bind to the erythrocyte (an innocent bystander). If C3b binds, there may be subsequent activation of the alternative complement pathway. Occasionally the activation of complement will proceed to the terminal components (i.e., C7, C8, C9; see Chap. 13) and intravascular hemolysis will result. Hemolysis may be explosive, and the antiglobulin test (Fig. 30-2) is positive only with anticomplement serum, since there is no membrane-bound IgG or IgM.

Alloantibody-Induced Immune Hemolysis
This type of hemolysis may result if compatibility testing by the blood bank is faulty. The recipient's red blood cells (RBCs) are tested for ABO and Rh antigens, and the serum is tested for unexpected antibodies to erythrocytes (other than naturally occurring anti-A or anti-B). Blood is infused into a recipient only if it is ABO- and Rh-compatible and no unexpected circulating antibodies that may

react with donor erythrocytes are detected, i.e., the recipient's serum does not cause in vitro hemolysis of the donor RBCs. However, despite the best efforts of modern blood banks, there are still two major types of posttransfusion immune hemolysis.

Acute Posttransfusion Immune Hemolysis
Routine blood bank procedures preclude a major erythrocyte antigen mismatch (i.e., ABO antigens). Such cross-matching is necessary because the ABO antigens are highly immunogenic and the recipient's serum may contain naturally occurring anti-A or anti-B. It is usually a clerical or administrative error rather than a technical error that results in transfusion of ABO-incompatible blood. If the transfused unit is ABO-incompatible, a major antigen-antibody reaction (e.g., A antigen on the RBCs with anti-A antibodies) results and there is significant, life-threatening hemolysis with activation of both complement and coagulation systems.

Delayed Posttransfusion Immune Hemolysis   This usually results because incompatible erythrocytes (not ABO-incompatible) are transfused. The recipient develops a low-level but gradual immune response, so that after a few days to several (1 to 3) weeks there is enough antierythrocyte antibody to result in clinically detectable hemolysis. Usually delayed transfusion reactions are seen in patients who have been previously transfused or who were pregnant. The hemolysis in delayed transfusion reactions is usually of mild to moderate severity.

Neonatal Isoimmune Hemolysis
The ability of fetal erythrocytes to cross the placenta and expose their paternal antigens to the maternal immune system may lead to maternal sensitization. Maternal IgG antibodies directed against fetal antigens may then in turn cross the placenta into the fetal circulation and destroy the fetal erythrocytes. The most important fetal erythrocyte antigen involved in such a process is the Rh D antigen. This is because the Rh antigens are

capable of generating potent, destructive antibodies. When there is maternal-paternal Rh incompatibility (Rh-negative mother and Rh-positive father), there is great potential to generate severe intrauterine hemolysis and hemolysis induced by fetal wastage. The Rh incompatibility does not cause hemolysis in the first pregnancy, but hemolysis can occur in the subsequent Rh-incompatible pregnancy and worsens with succeeding pregnancies. Treatment for this potentially serious disorder is prevention, by administering anti-Rh IgG to all Rh-negative women after they have given birth to an Rh-positive newborn. It is probable (but not certain) that the anti-Rh IgG binds to fetal erythrocytes (Rh-positive) in the maternal circulation and removes them before the maternal immune system can mount a response.

To a much lesser extent, fetal-maternal ABO incompatibility may result in hemolysis of the fetal erythrocytes. This is usually not clinically as serious for two main reasons: (1) antibodies are of the IgM class and thus do not penetrate the placenta, and (2) the basic molecular components (carbohydrates) of A and B antigens are found in maternal bodily secretions. These fluid phase antigens partially bind and neutralize the anti-AB antibodies.

Paroxysmal Cold Hemoglobinuria
This disorder was first described in tertiary syphilis patients, who, when placed in cold environments, developed a fulminant clinical syndrome of chills, fever, headache, and pain, along with hemoglobinuria. The hemolysis is caused by a cold-reactive IgG immunoglobulin (also called Donath-Landsteiner antibody) with specificity for the P antigen on erythrocytes. It is unclear why the specificity for P antigen occurs in this disease. This antibody is an efficient activator of the classical complement pathway in vivo. This generates considerable intravascular hemolysis and associated clinical symptoms. More recently the clinical syndrome due to the Donath-Landsteiner antibody has been noted in patients with viral infections.

IMMUNE SYSTEM–MEDIATED DESTRUCTION OF PLATELETS

Cell Target—Platelets

Platelets cells circulate in blood at a concentration of 250,000 ± 50,000 per μL in normals individuals, with two-thirds of all platelets in systemic circulation and one-third in the spleen. The latter exchange freely with the circulatory pool. Platelets have a half-life of 9 to 10 days and a turnover of 35,000 per day. Thus, as with neutrophils, any significant immune system–mediated process directed against platelets will quickly result in thrombocytopenia. The membrane antigens that are involved in immune system–mediated destruction include the platelet antigen PLA-1 and the HLA antigens. PLA-1 is a platelet antigen found on the majority of human platelets (see below).

Mechanism and Classification of Platelet Destruction

Immune system–mediated removal of human platelets is primarily a result of anti-platelet antibodies which increase platelet clearance by the monocyte-macrophage system. These antibodies may be subgrouped into three general types: alloantibodies, true autoantibodies, and antidrug antibodies.

Alloantibodies

These are usually directed against the PLA-1 antigen or histocompatibility (HLA) antigens of the platelet.

PLA-1 Antigen About 2 percent of the population have platelets which lack PLA-1. Persons who lack PLA-1 and receive transfusions of PLA-1-bearing platelets are at risk for posttransfusion purpura (PTP). After transfusion, patients develop anti-PLA-1 antibodies, which bind to PLA-1 antigens released from transfused platelets. The antigen-antibody complex may then bind to the patient's PLA-1-negative platelets (innocent

bystander), with increased removal of the PLA-1-negative platelets. This disease is usually short-lived and does not require treatment.

Pregnant mothers with PLA-1-negative platelets may be sensitized by fetal PLA-1-positive platelets. The resulting IgG anti-PLA-1 antibodies traverse the placenta and cause neonatal isoimmune thrombocytopenia.

HLA Antigen Patients who require frequent massive platelet transfusions (e.g., patients with aplastic anemia, leukemic patients on cytotoxic therapy), usually receive platelets from HLA-unmatched donors. Since platelets have membrane HLA antigens, the recipients often develop anti-HLA antibodies. The presence of such antibodies is directly correlated with the lack of effect of subsequent platelet transfusions in these patients (i.e., no increase in platelet count, no hemostatic benefit). To avoid such isoimmunization, a careful HLA antigen match with potential platelet donors is needed, which helps prevent the production of anti-HLA antibodies by the recipient.

True Autoantibodies

IgG autoantibodies reactive with platelets may result in shortened platelet survival and thrombocytopenia. The reduction may be severe and life-threatening and can arise spontaneously with or without associated diseases. These include SLE, chronic lymphocytic leukemia, lymphoma, and, rarely, solid tumors. The platelet antibody is directed against undefined platelet antigen(s). In severe cases, the few available platelets have membrane coated with IgG, C3, or both. IgG antiplatelet antibodies may traverse the placenta; therefore, newborns of mothers with circulating IgG anti-platelet antibodies may suffer from thrombocytopenia.

Autoimmune thrombocytopenic purpura may be either acute or chronic. In children it is usually a postviral, acute form, and the patients generally do very well (80 percent recover with no therapy). In contrast, adults usually have the chronic form. It is rare to define the cause and adults often have a prolonged course with continued production of platelet autoantibodies. Therapy for this latter disorder is initially corticosteroids and/or splenectomy (see Chap. 18, on monocytes, for a description of the mechanisms underlying this therapy). (See Clinical Aside 30-3.) In refractory cases, additional immunosuppression is tried with alternate drugs like cyclophosphamide or vincristine.

Clinical Aside 30-3
Idiopathic Thrombocytopenic Purpura (ITP) in Adults

A 28-year-old woman presented to her physician with complaints of small scattered bruises on her lower limbs and arms as well as scattered petechiae. She complained of a bruising tendency and menorrhagia (i.e., excessive menstrual bleeding) and recurrent nosebleeds for several months before coming to the doctor. Otherwise, she felt quite well. Her past medical history was otherwise unremarkable. She was not taking drugs, and no serious medical disorders had previously been diagnosed.

On physical exam, there were no abnormalities other than a palpable spleen tip in the left upper quadrant on deep inspiration. Laboratory examination revealed a platelet count of 35,000/mL; her hemoglobin, white blood cell count, and differential were normal. However, peripheral smear demonstrated frequent bizarre giant platelets. No other laboratory abnormalities were detected.

Her physician considered the diagnosis of ITP. Because of the frequent association of platelet-associated immunoglobulins in this disorder, the physician ordered tests for both serum- and platelet-associated antiplatelet antibodies. These tests both came back positive. (Note that platelet-associated immunoglobulin levels are elevated in more than 90 percent of patients.) Her physician elected to follow this patient with no intervention for several weeks because 10 percent of adults with ITP recover spontaneously. In addition, since her platelet count was greater than 30,000, he did not feel that she required platelet transfusions. Follow-up 7 days later revealed that her platelet count had dropped to 20,000. The physician elected to start prednisone at 1 mg/kg of body weight. (Prednisone is often used in order to prevent removal of antibody-coated platelets by the monocyte-macrophage system.) The patient's platelet count increased to 100,000/mL after 2 weeks of prednisone therapy. However, prolonged follow-up demonstrated that it was impossible to reduce the prednisone level without a significant reduction in platelet count and further petechiae and ecchymoses. It was therefore decided to subject the patient to splenectomy. The spleen is the major site of platelet destruction as well as an important site of antibody production. Intravenous immunoglobulin appears to be effective in temporarily elevating platelet count in patients with ITP, and this patient was given intravenous immunoglobulin immediately prior to surgery. Splenectomy was performed, and the patient's post-surgery platelet counts were significantly elevated.

From 70 to 90 percent of patients improve after splenectomy, and platelet levels are restored permanently to normal in approximately 70 percent. For the minority of patients who do not respond to splenectomy, it may be necessary to place them back on maintenance prednisone.

Not infrequently idiopathic thrombocytopenic purpura (ITP) is the first manifestation of a multisystem autoimmune disease like SLE. Platelet transfusions are not indicated because the transfused platelets are rapidly removed in ITP, unless it is a life-threatening case. Especially in children, intravenous γ-globulin may be curative; see Chap. 34.

Antidrug Autoantibodies

Several drugs are implicated in thrombocytopenia. The primary mechanism is production of drug-antidrug immune complexes which may bind to innocent platelets. The immune complex–coated platelet is then cleared rapidly by the monocyte-macrophage system. The list of drugs reported to result in clinically significant thrombocytopenia includes gold salts, quinine, sulfonamide analogues, quinidine, and heparin. Usually, once a patient is sensitized to a medication, repeat administration of the drug results in platelet drops within 24 h. Heparin and gold are potential exceptions, where thrombocytopenia may be seen weeks (heparin) to months (gold salts) following drug ingestion or infusion. Discontinuing the offending drug is the treatment of choice; further therapy is rarely needed.

SELF-TEST QUESTIONS

1. Which of the following group of IgG subclasses would potentially give more severe hemolysis?
   a. IgG1 and IgG2
   b. IgG1 and IgG3
   c. IgG2 and IgG4
   d. IgG2 and IgG3
2. Which of the following mechanisms best explains α-methyldopa ingestion in a positive direct antiglobulin test?
   a. α-Methyldopa acts as a hapten.
   b. α-Methyldopa induces immune complexes.
   c. α-Methyldopa binds to the red cell membrane.
   d. α-Methyldopa induces excessive B-cell production of autoantibodies.
3. Which of the following serologic parameters is consistent with a pathologic (clinically aggressive) cold agglutinin?
   a. Broad thermal amplitude
   b. High-titer cold agglutinin
   c. Presence of complement on the membrane
   d. All of the above
4. As a consulting hematologist, you are told the patient has a positive direct antiglobulin test with a markedly shortened red cell survival as measured by chromium 51 survival. The patient's hemoglobin is 0.07 (7.0 g/dL), and you know that a previous hemoglobin done 6 months ago was normal. Which of the following therapeutic approaches would you recommend?
   a. Observation
   b. Begin prednisone on a daily basis and observe the patient carefully for change in hemoglobin
   c. Use transfusions only
   d. Proceed to splenectomy immediately
5. You are informed as a consulting hematologist that a pregnant female who is now in her seventh month of pregnancy has a diagnosis of ITP. You are about to explain the possibilities of this disease on the newborn's platelet population. Which of the following represents the best explanation?
   a. You tell the mother there is nothing to worry about since the process is confined to her immune system.
   b. You explain to the mother that certain antibodies can pass through the placental barrier and potentially affect the child's platelets.
   c. Even though the antibody can passage the placental barrier, the antibody cannot bind to the fetal platelets.
   d. If the newborn fetus has significant thrombocytopenia, it will be necessary to remove the newborn child's spleen in order to stop the process.

ADDITIONAL READINGS

Dacie JV. Autoimmune hemolytic anemia. *Arch Int Med.* 1975;135:1293.

DiFino SM, Lachant NA, Kirshner JJ, Gottlieb AJ. Adult idiopathic thrombocytopenic purpura. Clinical findings and response to therapy. *Am J Med.* 1980;69:430.

Hegde UM, Suiable A, Ball S, Roter BLT. The relative incidence of idiopathic and secondary autoimmune thrombocytopenia: A clinical and serological evaluation in 508 patients. *Clin Lab Haematol.* 1985;7:7.

Lalezari P, Khorshidi M, Petrosova M. Autoimmune neutropenia of infancy. *J Pediatrics.* 1986;109:764.

Leddy JP, Swisher SN. Acquired immune hemolytic disorders (including drug-induced immune hemolytic anemia). In Samter L, ed. *Immunologic Diseases.* Boston: Little, Brown; 1978.

VanderVeen JPW, Hack CE, Engelfriet CP, et al. Chronic idiopathic and secondary neutropenia, clinical and serological investigations. *Br J Haematol.* 1986;63:161.

31

Autoimmune Disorders: Systemic and Organ-Specific

INTRODUCTION

"Horror autotoxicus": The immune system does not attack self; it is in horror of autoaggression. Ehrlich's concept of the nineteenth century molded the thinking of immunologists for decades. As has been described elsewhere, the reciprocal concepts of tolerance and autoimmunity were at first thought to hinge on the total avoidance of autoreactivity in normal individuals. This was articulated in Burnet's "forbidden clone theory"—autoreactive clones are normally *eliminated* in fetal development. The escape of such clones from fetal elimination represents a rare, potentially pathogenetic event.

All of the above is predicated upon the concept that autoimmunity is synonymous with *autoaggression.* Recent studies have demonstrated that many immunologic and developmental processes include *autorecognition.* This, then, is probably a better definition: autoimmunity is a process whereby the immune system recognizes "self." From this perspective, autoimmunity can be viewed as a part of normal physiologic mechanisms, not necessarily related to autoaggression. A moment's thought will allow you to recall many examples of immunologic molecules recognizing other molecules on pathogens, immune effector or control cells, or in the circulation.

There are many examples of pathology possibly due to autoimmunity and such mechanisms have been proved pathogenic in some diseases. This breaking of tolerance probably represents the activation of previously quiescent clones—an escape from the multiple control systems, both global and organ-specific, that are usually quite successful. There is some evidence to support the contention that an "autoimmune carrier state" may exist as long as these control systems hold sway. However, one must be cautious in interpreting autoimmunity. Often, tissue damage releases antigens which then serve as the target of newly produced immunoglobulin or T cells; this then represents

nonpathogenetic autoimmunity—in essence, "ex post facto" autoimmunity.

This chapter will describe some of the mechanisms behind autoimmunity—how the natural, often complex control systems occasionally do break down to allow self-destruction—and will describe some human diseases where these mechanisms may be active. There are two types of autoimmunity, organ-specific and systemic, and examples of both will be discussed. Certain animal models are of value in understanding human disease, and some of these will be described. HLA and hormonal associations of autoimmunity will be discussed. Some of the means currently being used and others proposed for use in restoring immune homeostasis will be explored.

As preparation for the following discussion, please review the following examples of physiologic or salutary autoimmunity:

Idiotype network (Chaps. 3 and 9)

Recognition of self (MHC) in immune response and histogenesis (Chap. 4 and Appendix B)

Antigen-specific suppressor cells and factors (Chap. 9)

Ligand-receptor interactions (Chaps. 7, 12, and 20)

MECHANISMS BEHIND AUTOIMMUNITY

Pathogenic autoimmunity represents a loss of control over the immune system. Many mechanisms can be postulated to explain this, some of which have been demonstrated, some simply theorized. In any event, discussing them allows a review of the immunologic mechanisms already discussed, helps to explain the nature of these syndromes, and may suggest therapeutic modalities which might be explored in the treatment of disease. Table 31-1 lists some examples of autoimmune diseases due to organ-specific autoantibod-

TABLE 31-1   Clinical Syndromes Due to Autoantibodies

Abnormality	Effect of Autoantibody	Clinical Disorder
	ENDOCRINOLOGIC SYNDROMES	
Thyroxine		
Excess	Stimulates TSH receptor	Grave's disease
Deficiency	Blocks TSH receptor	Hypothyroidism
Cortisol		
Excess	Stimulates ACTH receptor	Cushing's syndrome
Deficiency	Blocks ACTH receptor	Addison's disease
Insulin		
Excess	Stimulates β cells, blocks insulin receptor	Hypoglycemia
Deficiency	Blocks β cells, stimulates insulin receptor	Hyperglycemia
Gastric acid		
Excess	?Stimulates H_2 receptor	Duodenal ulcer
Deficiency	Blocks gastrin receptor	Achlorhydria
Calcium		
Excess	Stimulates PTH receptor	Secondary hyperparathyroidism
Vitamin B_{12} deficiency	Binds intrinsic factor, alters parietal cell function	Pernicious anemia
	NONENDOCRINOLOGIC SYNDROMES	
Neuromuscular	Acetylcholine receptor destruction or down-regulation	Myasthenia gravis
Renal and pulmonary	Anti-basement membrane antibody	Goodpasture's syndrome
Uveal tract	Antibodies formed post-ocular trauma	Sympathetic ophthalmia
Cardiac	Antibodies formed post-cardiac surgery	Postpericardiotomy syndrome
Cutaneous	Antibodies to keratinocyte surface protein	Pemphigus vulgaris
	Antibodies to normal epidermal basement membrane 230-kd protein of hemidesmosomes	Bullous pemphigoid

ies. What follows is a discussion of some mechanisms thought to underly these organ-specific autoaggressive syndromes.

Newly MHC-Positive Cells

Most nonimmune cells in the body do not express MHC class II molecules on their surface. But what would happen if, say, a thyroid cell were to suddenly express class II? Resident or passing CD4$^+$ T cells could possibly recognize thyroid-specific surface antigens on these cells (especially antigens which are not expressed elsewhere in the body, e.g., the thyrotropin receptor) (Fig. 31-1). With the addition of interleukin 1 (IL-1), *antigen presentation* could take place, and suddenly a local immune reaction could occur. Were this to be the case, organ-specific autoimmune damage might occur. In fact, IFN-γ can in-

duce the production of class II antigens in a number of cells, including thyroid. Class II positivity has been demonstrated on the surface of thyroid cells in patients with autoimmune thyroiditis. Autoantibody production is thought to result and may cause disease. But two quite distinct types of clinical problems may occur. If the autoantibody produced can fix complement or link with a cell capable of antibody-dependent cell-mediated cytotoxicity (ADCC), tissue damage may occur. If the antibody blocks or interferes with a vital surface component of the cell, the cell may not appear damaged but it may not function normally. If surface molecules are cross-linked by these antibodies, that molecule may be down-regulated or internalized. In any of these cases, to go back to our example, hypothyroidism might develop. But a second possibility exists: the antibody may not block

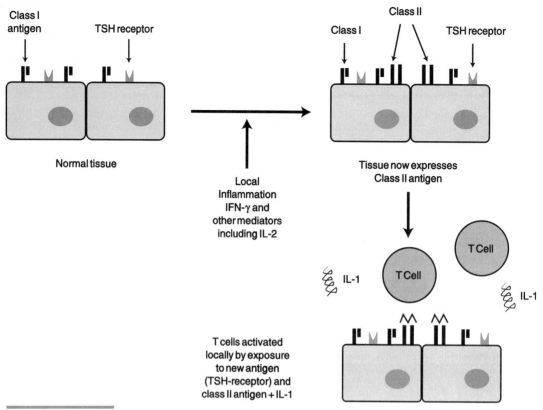

Figure 31-1   Newly expressed MHC on cell not previously MHC-positive can now present antigen.

a surface component or receptor; rather it may act as an *agonist*, mimicking the effect mediated by the ligand of that receptor. If an antibody can act as an agonist while attaching to the thyrotropin receptor, hyperthyroidism may occur. This actually does occur; an antibody to the thyrotropin receptor which acts as an agonist was originally called LATS (for long-acting thyroid stimulator), and is found in Graves' disease, a form of autoimmune hyperthyroidism. Other examples of autoantibodies causing increased or decreased function of their target cells are listed in Table 31-1.

Anti-Idiotype Antibody—Internal Image

Another way to explain autoantibodies with antigen specificities for individual cell sur-

face antigens is by invoking the id network. Recall that antibodies made to an antigen will then elicit anti-idiotype autoantibodies, anti-anti-idiotype antibodies, etc. Let us visualize an antibody made to a virus particle. This particular virus uses a cell surface component as its means of entry into the cell; there are many examples of this (see Chap. 21). Antibodies to the part of the virus which plugs into the "receptor" could very well resemble the receptor itself. An anti-idiotype antibody directed against the antigen-binding pocket of the antibody could plug into the receptor in just the way that the original ligand did. The language used to describe this phenomenon is that the anti-idiotype antibody produces an "internal image" (Fig. 31-2); the net result is that the anti-idiotype antibody interacts with the receptor with one of two possible effects. The resulting anti-

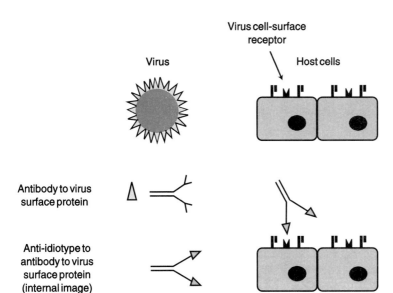

Figure 31-2   Anti-idiotype antibody—internal image.

receptor antibody might block the receptor or it might have agonist activity. Were a virus to bind to the insulin receptor, the resulting anti-idiotype internal image might cause hyperglycemia (by blocking insulin or down-regulating the receptor), or it might cause hypoglycemia (by acting as an insulin agonist). Other examples of agonist and antagonist antibodies have been described (Table 31-1).

Anti-Idiotype Antibody— Intersecting Chains

If an anti-idiotype antibody serves as a part of an immunoregulatory mechanism, it is possible that such an antibody could up- or down-regulate responses, depending on the relative amounts of antigen, idiotype, and anti-idiotype. Recognition of the idiotype on the surface of B cells causes cross-linkage and possible stimulation with expansion of the clone, differentiation, and secretion of immunoglobulin. Recall that the network is complex and not entirely specific. A "chain" of idiotype–anti-idiotype antibodies leading from one antigen could include antibodies involved in other idiotype–anti-idiotype "chains." (See Fig. 31-3.) This "cross-talk" between chains could conceivably result in

the activation of autoimmune clones. A possible example of this is found in the work of Dwyer, Vakil, and Kearney on the immunopathogenesis of myasthenia gravis (see Chap. 35D for a description of this neuromuscular syndrome). Monoclonal antibodies were made to different antigens, including the acetylcholine receptor and α-1,3-dextran, a constituent of various bacteria, including *Serratia* and *Enterobacter*. Anti-idiotypes were made to the antiacetylcholine receptor and anti-dextran antibodies, and anti-anti-idiotypes were made, as well. Some of the antibodies cross-reacted between the networks emanating from the two original antigens, suggesting cross-talk between the two chains. Further, a monoclonal antibody was made from the B cells of a patient with myasthenia. This human monoclonal antibody bound to a murine monoclonal antibody directed against the acetylcholine receptor. However, the human antibody also bound to dextran and, furthermore, it agglutinated dextran-containing bacteria! With these findings, the researchers looked at normal and myasthenic sera: 10 of 60 patients had antibodies to dextran, but none of the 40 normal sera had such reactivity. Is this an example of parallel sets? Does this suggest that an infection can set off myasthenia by perturbing a hitherto quiescent autoreactive clone?

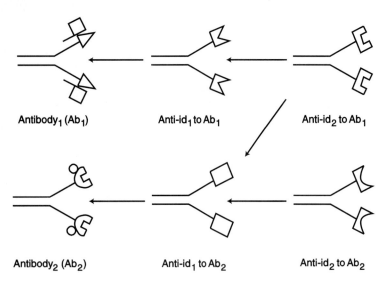

Antibody$_1$ (Ab$_1$)   Anti-id$_1$ to Ab$_1$ Anti-id$_2$ to Ab$_1$

Antibody$_2$ (Ab$_2$)   Anti-id$_1$ to Ab$_2$ Anti-id$_2$ to Ab$_2$

But Anti-id$_2$ to Ab$_1$ can bind to Anti-id$_1$ to Ab$_2$

Figure 31-3   Idiotype–anti-idiotype intersecting chains.

Molecular Mimicry

We know that the immune response is not absolutely precise. Different antigens which resemble each other can be bound by the same antibody. Thus if one makes an immune response to an antigen, reactivity to a related antigen may occur. This has major advantages; if you have antibodies and B cells against one *Streptococcus pneumoniae* and get infected with another *S pneumoniae*, there may be enough cross-reactivity so that your antibodies will help fight off the new infection. Now, what if a microbial structure resembles a component of human tissue? The immune response to that microbe might recognize the host. Such *molecular mimicry* may result in autoreactivity (Fig. 31-4). This precise mechanism may be active in a number of diseases (Table 31-2).

Rheumatologists have developed a number of animal models of rheumatoid arthritis. One of these is adjuvant-induced arthritis, produced by injecting susceptible strains of rats or mice with complete Freund's adjuvant, an oil base containing antigens from *Mycobacterium bovis*. T cells from animals with adjuvant arthritis transfer the disease to naive animals; further, T-cell clones to

mycobacterial antigens from affected animals can also transfer the disease. These clones also react with proteoglycan from the cartilage found in the joints of animals. Does this mean that the T cells are reacting with cross-reactive rodent antigen and that this causes the arthritis? This has not been established, but it is interesting to note that patients with rheumatoid arthritis have T cells which are reactive with mycobacterial antigens, most notably heat-shock proteins. Perhaps the immune response to a pathogen's heat-shock proteins could result in a cross-reacting response to human heat-shock proteins. Could this be an example of molecular mimicry, one with potentially widespread clinical consequences?

Modified Self-Antigens

Adult animals and humans are tolerant to self-antigens in normal circumstances. But what if an environmental agent or drug is introduced which alters a self-antigen? The result might be a new antigenic determinant eliciting an immune response to the altered self, which in turn leads to the destruction of self. Altered self-antigens expressed on a

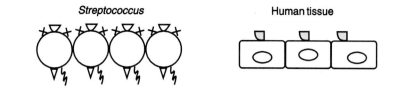

Antibody is made to each of the *Streptococcus* surface components.

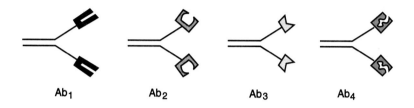

Ab₁ Ab₂ Ab₃ Ab₄

Ab₃ can bind to a surface component on human tissue which resembles but is not identical to a *Streptococcus* component.

Figure 31-4 Molecular mimicry.

cell surface or released locally may, then, explain autoimmunity, although this has never been demonstrated.

Release of Sequestered Antigens

Early in development certain organs (e.g., the brain and, in general, organs derived from the ectoderm and endoderm) are isolated from the rest of the circulation; the constituent proteins are said to be *sequestered*, in that the immune system does not see them, i.e., these proteins are found in immunologically isolated, or privileged, sites. If an infection or trauma causes damage to such an organ, the release of a previously sequestered antigen may elicit an autoimmune reaction. The release of such sequestered antigens is not, strictly speaking, a loss of tolerance, but the

autoreactivity is no less real. The release of these antigens causes ex post facto autoimmunity. In most circumstances the autoimmunity is not the cause of tissue damage. However, such a mechanism is the likely cause of the postcardiotomy syndrome. (See Clinical Aside 31-1.)

Clinical Aside 31-1
Dressler's Syndrome and the
Postcardiotomy Syndrome

Patients who have open heart surgery or, occasionally, patients who have had a myocardial infarction may make an immune response to newly liberated heart-derived antigens. These autoantibodies can bind to the pericardium and may cause local inflammation; the postcardiotomy syndrome (after surgery or penetrating trauma) and

TABLE 31-2   Molecular Mimicry in Clinical Medicine

Disease	Organism	Human Component
Rheumatic fever	*Streptococcus*-M proteins	Cardiac myosin
		Subthalamic nuclei
Chagas disease	*Trypanosoma cruzi*	Nonmyosin cardiac proteins
Lyme neuropathy	*Borrelia burgdorferi*	Axonal protein

Dressler's syndrome (after myocardial infarction) are the result; patients with these syndromes present with fever, pericarditis, pleuritis, pneumonic infiltrates, and occasional arthritis. A number of studies have documented antibodies against a variety of heart-derived antigens in these patients. Other studies have found circulating immune complexes, which may be implicated in the pathogenesis. On the basis of your knowledge of the timing of the primary antibody response, when would you expect to find these antibodies and therefore the onset of these syndromes? (The above are to be differentiated from a syndrome much like serum sickness which can develop during or immediately after cardiac bypass surgery but which does not represent autoimmunity. Complement component 3 (C3) is activated in the bypass machine, and the clinical problems are a manifestation of infusing the patient with active component C3a.)

Loss of Suppressor Cell Function

Recall that immunologic control is accomplished by the balance of positive and negative, or helper and suppressor, influences; this constitutes the Yin and Yang of the immune encephalomyelitis. If one assumes that suppressor activity might control dormant autoreactive clones, the loss of such suppressor activity (or the loss of sensitivity to such effects) might unleash autoimmunity. Animal models of autoimmune disease are of value in looking at the role of suppression. The model noted above, adjuvant-induced arthritis, is a T cell–mediated disease. Other animal models of the same sort include experimental autoimmune encephalomyelitis (EAE) and experimental autoimmune thyroiditis (EAT). In EAE inoculation of susceptible mice with myelin basic protein causes a neurologic syndrome which mimics human multiple sclerosis. In EAT thyroglobulin inoculation in the appropriate strain causes thyroiditis. In EAT, one can isolate T cells from the affected mouse which can transfer the disease. The C57BL/6 mouse strain is relatively resistant to EAT (it is a nonsusceptible strain). One can isolate T cells from inoculated but asymptomatic C57BL/6 mice which are capable of transferring EAT (Fig.

31-5). What does this mean? If there are potentially virulent T cells in the C57BL/6 mice, why don't the mice get thyroiditis? It seems likely that something in that strain prevents these T cells from causing damage—something is suppressing their potential for autoimmunity. It would not be unreasonable to postulate an autoimmune "carrier state," where the potential for autoreactivity is present but is kept under control. There is evidence of organ-specific control in humans (T cells in the eye which suppress autoreactivity to uveal antigens), and systemic mechanisms are probably active, as well. If an environmental or infectious influence modifies this, autoimmunity may result; perhaps aging causes a gradual decrease in some of these mechanisms. There is, in fact, evidence to suggest that autoreactive T-cell clones are present, but under control, in normal humans.

Thymus and Bursa Equivalent Abnormality

The theory that autoreactive clones are not allowed into the adult immune repertoire led to the thought that autoimmunity was the result of faulty filtering of T and B cells by the sites where these two lymphocyte populations are educated, the thymus and the bursa equivalent. We now know that the forbidden clone theory as described previously is not entirely correct and that autoreactive clones can be found, but the possibility that abnormalities of these organs may predispose to autoimmunity is still being investigated.

Other Mechanisms

Before we proceed, can you think of other possible mechanisms which might unleash autoreactivity? We have already invoked the new expression of class II antigens, the idiotype–anti-idiotype control network, molecular mimicry, and loss of suppressor cell function, among others.

Other plausible explanations might include an isolated abnormality of high endo-

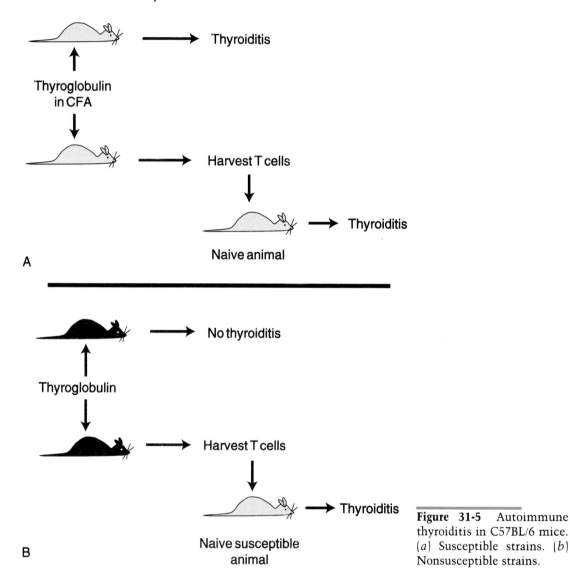

Figure 31-5 Autoimmune thyroiditis in C57BL/6 mice. (*a*) Susceptible strains. (*b*) Nonsusceptible strains.

thelial venules, which might cause local accumulation of activated T cells and their proinflammatory lymphokines (see Chap. 12 on homing mechanisms of lymphocytes), polyclonal activation of B and/or T cells with nonspecific activation of autoreactive clones, systemic abnormalities in the production of lymphokines or their inhibitors, or some abnormality of the repertoire of T cell–antigen receptor or immunoglobulin genes. No evidence exists in support of any of these mech-

anisms, but the latter has been the focus of much study of antinuclear antibodies and rheumatoid factors. (See Clinical Aside 31-2 and Fig. 31-6.)

Clinical Aside 31-2
Rheumatoid Factor

Many years ago, the serum of a patient with rheumatoid joint disease was found to agglutinate. Analysis showed that the serum contained an

Rheumatoid Factor

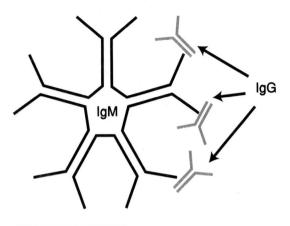

Figure 31-6   Rheumatoid factor.

antibody which bound to the patient's own antibodies, specifically IgG. This factor, named *rheumatoid factor* (*RF*), is an IgM which binds to IgG and is frequently found in rheumatoid arthritis (RA), but can also be found in a number of other diseases typified by chronic immunologic activity, including malaria, infectious mononucleosis, subacute bacterial endocarditis, and sarcoidosis, among others. Thus, the presence of RF is not diagnostic of RA. The key here is chronic immunologic reactivity. There needs to be a way to remove immune complexes and debris in physiologic conditions. An IgM which can bind to IgG seems tailormade for this purpose: IgG and attached antigen are bound by RF and removed from circulation. Antinuclear antibodies (ANA) may serve a similar purpose. Of interest is that ANA and RF sequences often represent genomic sequences, unmodified by the usual changes seen in immunoglobulin gene rearrangements. Perhaps these antibodies were so important that they needed to be produced rapidly and without delay. But what if the ANA or RF sequences were modified, or isotype switching from IgM to IgG occurred, or the IgG subclass were changed, e.g., to an IgG which better fixes complement? The unmodified genomic sequence–related RF or ANA might not have been capable of causing tissue damage, but this new antibody might.

Other factors seem to be involved in the development of autoimmunity, as well. It is quite clear that hormonal influences play a role; systemic lupus erythematosus (SLE) and other autoimmune diseases are more common in women, and certain mouse models of SLE can be modified by alteration of the hormonal milieu of the mouse. In the (NZB × NZW) F₁ (standing for a cross between New Zealand black and New Zealand white mice) mouse model of SLE, oophorectomy decreases disease severity and delays its onset—this effect can be reversed by treating the mouse with estrogens and accentuated by giving the mouse androgens.

There is also an apparent genetic influence. Certain HLA types are more frequently represented in the patients with autoimmune disease than in the general population (Table 31-3), and there is an increased prevalence of autoantibodies in the first-degree relatives of patients with SLE. (Might this represent a predisposition to the development of autoimmunity in these individuals, requiring a trigger or second exogenous stimulus in order to become a clinical problem?) The exact nature of this linkage is not yet clear. See Chap. 4 for a discussion of the MHC and its role in immune responsiveness.

TABLE 31-3   MHC Antigens and Linkage with Diseases

Disease	HLA Linkage	Relative Risk
Idiopathic hemochromatosis	A3	8
	B14	5
Behçet's syndrome	B 5	6
Ankylosing spondylitis	B27	100
Reiter's syndrome	B27	40
Acute anterior uveitis	B27	10
Psoriasis	B17	6
	B13	4
	Cw6	7
	B27	1
Psoriatic arthritis	Bw38	9
	Bw39	3
	B27	1
Psoriatic spondylitis	B27	12
Inflammatory bowel disease (IBD)	None	
IBD with arthritis	None	

TABLE 31-3   Continued

Disease	HLA Linkage	Relative Risk
IBD with spondylitis	B27	12
Subacute thyroiditis	B35	14
Congenital adrenal hyperplasia	B47	15
Goodpasture's syndrome	DR2	16
Multiple sclerosis	DR2	5
	DR3	4
SLE	DR2	1–3
	DR3	3–6
	DQw1	3
	C4A*QO	3
	C4A*QO (homozygous)	17
	C4A*QO and DR2	25
Idiopathic membranous nephropathy	DR3	12
Myasthenia gravis	DR3	2.5
Dermatitis herpetiformis	DR3	15
Celiac disease	DR3	11
Sjögren's syndrome	DR3	10
Addison's disease	DR3	6
Graves' disease	DR3	4
IgA deficiency (normal population)	DR3	13
Insulin-dependent diabetes mellitus	DR3	5
	DR4	5
	DR3 and DR4	20
Rheumatoid arthritis	DR4	8
	DRw53	4–6
	DQw3	4–6
Pemphigus vulgaris	DR4	14
Hydralazine-induced lupus	DR4	6
Idiopathic IgA nephropathy	DR4	4
Hashimoto's thyroiditis	DR5	3
Pernicious anemia	DR5	5
Pauci-articular juvenile rheumatoid arthritis	DR5	5

CLINICAL EXAMPLES OF AUTOIMMUNITY: ORGAN-SPECIFIC AND GENERAL

As described above, single-organ autoimmune damage can be produced in a number of animal models. By inoculating the appropriate animal with central nervous system myelin, one can produce experimental allergic encephalomyelitis, a model for the human disease multiple sclerosis (see Clinical Aside 31-3); by using peripheral nerve myelin, lesions of experimental allergic neuritis can be produced, a model for the human disease Guillain-Barré syndrome. Thyroglobulin in adjuvant can induce thyroid destruction, as noted above. Finally, two models of human rheumatoid arthritis are of interest. Adjuvant-induced arthritis has been described previously. If one gives collagen in adjuvant to an animal which is not susceptible to adjuvant-induced arthritis, one can produce collagen-induced arthritis. In each case, T cells and/or immunoglobulin specific for the inoculated protein can be found in the animal; in some cases transfer of the disease can be accomplished by transfusing antibody or cells to naive animals.

Clinical Aside 31-3
Experimental Autoimmune Encephalomyelitis

Experimental autoimmune encephalomyelitis (EAE) is an animal model for T cell–mediated demyelinating disease of the central nervous system (CNS).* EAE resembles in many ways the human disease multiple sclerosis (MS) and therefore serves as an animal model for it. The disease is readily induced in many experimental animals by immunization with spinal cord homogenate or purified myelin proteins like myelin basic protein (MBP) or myelin proteolipid protein (PLP) emulsified in complete Freund's adjuvant (CFA). In mice, induction of EAE with antigen/CFA also requires the injection of pertussigen (or killed pertussis organisms) as a second adjuvant. The exact function of pertussis here is still speculative. EAE is characterized by perivascular leukocytic infiltration into the CNS and a subsequent inflammatory reaction thought by many to represent a typical T cell–mediated delayed-type hypersensitivity (DTH) reaction to myelin antigens. Others believe that demyelination is due to direct tissue damage induced by MHC class II–restricted cytotoxic T lymphocytes. The inflammatory reaction (or direct T cell–mediated damage) results in areas of demyelination often described as "plaques," which in severe cases cause paralysis. EAE is usually an

*Zamvil SS, Steinman L. The T lymphocyte in experimental allergic encephalomyelitis. *Ann Rev Immunol.* 1990;8:579.

acute, self-limiting disease but it can also take the form of a chronic, relapsing disease like MS when induced in young animals or in animals with a suppressed immune system. Chronic, relapsing EAE can also be induced in normal adult animals by the adoptive transfer of antigen-specific T-cell lines or clones.

It is widely accepted that EAE has a cellular pathogenesis and that the disease is mediated by MHC class II–restricted CD4$^+$ T cells ("helper" phenotype) specific for antigenic determinants on MBP or PLP. T cells that induce EAE and the antigenic determinants to which they are specific are called *encephalitogenic T cells* and *encephalitogenic determinants*, respectively. The encephalitogenic determinant can be different for different species and even for different MHC haplotypes within a species. For example, in H-2^s (SJL and A.SW) mice at least two encephalitogenic determinants have been defined at the C terminus of MBP between residues 89–169 and one between residues 17–27 at the N terminus. For H-2^u (PL/J and B10.PL) mice at least three encephalitogenic determinants have been identified at residues 1–9, 9–16, and 35–47 of the N terminus. The role of class II–restricted CD4$^+$ T cells in EAE induction has also been demonstrated by the ability to strongly inhibit the induction and progression of EAE in vivo by the administration of monoclonal antibodies specific for CD4 (35–38), class II antigens, or T-cell receptor (TCR) molecules used by the encephalitogenic T cell.

Interestingly, in most cases, encephalitogenic T-cell clones in a particular mouse or rat strain use a very restricted pool of TCR genes and an even more restricted pool of Vβ gene families. This prompted the proposal of the "V-region disease hypothesis," which suggests that the contribution of the TCR to the encephalitogenicity of T cells is not due only to its antigenic specificity, but has somehow also to do with the TCR family utilized in the MBP-specific T-cell clones. In other words, even the recognition of an encephalitogenic determinant by a T-cell clone does not necessarily make it encephalitogenic. It would also have to belong to a particular TCR family in order to induce the disease. The fact that having a self-recognizing T-cell population in a particular individual does not necessarily mean that it will develop an autoimmune disease is further demonstrated by experiments in which a foreign transgene is driven by an inducible promotor such

that it can be expressed at any time after birth. The expression of such a gene in a particular organ in mature mice will induce a potent immune response against it, which will cause an autoimmunelike disease; however, this response is transient and the responding cells are either deleted or anergized (see Chap. 7 for more details on T-cell clonal anergy).

Perhaps the biggest enigma in demyelinating autoimmune diseases like EAE or MS—and in fact in most other autoimmune diseases—is what induces the onset of the disease. If MS is indeed similar to EAE and is induced by MBP- or PLP-specific T cells, it is hard to understand how antigen ever becomes available to the immune system in an immunogenic state. Some believe that a viral infection could cause cell damage that could result in antigen leakage or that a response to a pathogen like a virus might cross-react with some myelin antigens. Why the disease is chronic and why it usually follows a course of remission-relapse cycles is unclear.

Autoimmune disease may affect a single organ (an autoimmune response to that organ), may affect a few organs (immune reactivity to components shared by different organs), or may be systemic.

Autoimmune damage to individual organs is relatively common in clinical medicine. The thyroid gland (Hashimoto's thyroiditis, primary myxedema, or thyrotoxicosis) and the adrenal gland (Addison's disease) may be damaged by autoaggressive immune behavior, as can the neuromuscular junction (myasthenia gravis). Likewise, the circulating formed elements of the blood may be destroyed by autoantibodies. Autoimmune hemolytic anemia, thrombocytopenia, and leukopenias are discussed in Chap. 30. Premature ovarian failure (early menopause) and primary testicular failure can be due to autoimmune damage, just as rare cases of infertility can be ascribed to antisperm antibodies found in the female's genital secretions (see Chap. 27). Transplacental passage of autoantibodies can occur, occasionally causing neonatal thyrotoxicosis, thrombocytopenia, or myasthenia gravis in the infants of mothers with these conditions. Autoimmune damage to the stomach can cause chronic atrophic gastritis, which may be a premalignant condition (care to speculate on that association?). Another function of the stomach is to produce a protein known as intrinsic factor (IF), which binds vitamin B_{12} to allow its absorption in the terminal ileum. Some patients make an antibody to IF; these patients cannot absorb vitamin B_{12} and will ultimately develop a syndrome known as pernicious anemia (see Clinical Aside 31-4).

Clinical Aside 31-4
Pernicious Anemia

Vitamin B_{12} is absorbed from the gut by means of a protein known as intrinsic factor (IF), which is produced by the gastric parietal cells. In the gut lumen the vitamin is bound by IF, and the complex is absorbed in the terminal ileum (small intestine) (Fig. 31-A1). If the terminal ileum is defective or surgically removed (as can happen in Crohn's disease), if there is *no* dietary vitamin B_{12} (as in strict vegetarians), or if there is some interference with the production of binding with IF, vitamin B_{12} deficiency can occur. (Vitamin B_{12} is stored in the liver, where a normal individual has about three years' supply; thus deficiency syndromes do not appear for a long time, even after an individual has ceased absorbing vitamin B_{12}. Now for an aside within an aside: If the liver contains so much vitamin B_{12}, what do you think might happen to serum vitamin B_{12} levels in the presence of hepatitis? What is the significance of a normal serum vitamin B_{12} level in a patient with active hepatitis?)

Studies of patients with pernicious anemia have found serum antibodies to IF in about 60 percent of afflicted individuals, and in 90 percent of patients there are serum antibodies to gastric parietal cells. There are two types of antibodies to IF—one blocks the binding of the vitamin to the factor and the other blocks intestinal uptake of the IF-vitamin complex. Patients with pernicious anemia often have antibodies to other organs, including the thyroid and adrenal glands.

Why is it called "pernicious" anemia? The consequences of vitamin B_{12} absence include a megaloblastic (large red blood cells) anemia, weight loss, anorexia, and weakness; this nonspecific combination of problems often causes these pa-

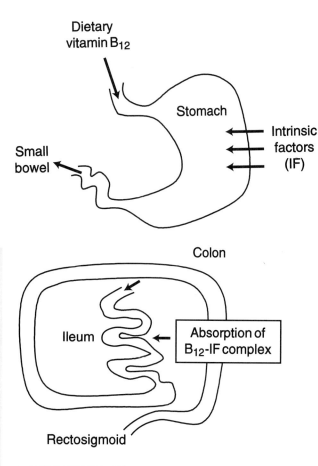

Figure 31-A1   Absorption of dietary vitamin B_{12}.

tients to be misdiagnosed as having a malignancy. It is the insidious development of neurologic disease caused by this deficiency, known as "subacute combined degeneration" of the dorsal and lateral columns, which is the most severe problem. Symmetric peripheral neuropathy occurs, with progressive ataxia, spastic paraplegia, and loss of sphincter tone. CNS defects may develop, including memory loss and even dementia. A potential problem in diagnosis is that folate therapy can repair the anemia, while the neurologic disease progresses. (Never give folate to a patient with megaloblastic anemia without considering possible coexisting vitamin B_{12} deficiency.)

Another example of single organ–specific autoimmunity is insulin-dependent diabetes mellitus, explained in great detail in Chap.

35B. However, occasional diabetic patients may have other endocrinologic abnormalities, including hypothyroidism, hypoadrenalism (Addison's disease), and pernicious anemia, among others. Two "polyglandular failure syndromes" have been described. The first starts in childhood, with siblings often affected, but no genetic linkage has thus far been identified. The other starts in early adulthood through middle age and affects multiple generations. The latter syndrome is thought to represent an autosomal dominant, HLA-B8/DR3 linked phenomenon. In both, multiple endocrine organs are damaged by autoreactivity; the molecular explanation for why these organs are affected in the same individual has not been determined. Reflecting back on the contents of this chapter, can you suggest some plausible mechanisms for the polyglandular failure syndromes?

Many patients with thyroiditis have antibodies to their own stomachs with no overt dysfunction of the stomach; patients with pernicious anemia often have antithyroid antibodies but no thyroid inflammation. Examples of autoimmunity damaging more than one organ include Schmidt's syndrome (autoimmune thyroiditis and adrenal insufficiency), Evans' syndrome (autoimmune thrombocytopenia and hemolytic anemia, and Goodpastures syndrome (see Clinical Aside 31-5).

Clinical Aside 31-5
Goodpasture's Syndrome

Antibodies to the glomerular basement membrane can cause local damage and leakage of protein into the urine. There are certain antigens in the glomerular basement membrane which cross-react with or are identical to antigens in the basement membrane of pulmonary capillaries. It is this cross-reactivity which pathogenetically links the pulmonary hemorrhage and glomerulonephritis seen in Goodpasture's syndrome. Usually seen in young men often after a viral syndrome, Goodpasture's syndrome represents an example of in situ antibody binding, with subsequent tissue disruption. The antibody eluted from renal tissue from these patients binds to lung and vice versa. If one takes this antibody and infuses it into a monkey, the monkey will experience an identical pulmonary-renal syndrome.

Systemic autoimmunity can be a very severe clinical problem, affecting many organ systems sequentially or simultaneously, with occasionally disastrous consequences. It is difficult to invoke as an explanation a specific immune response to a single specific antigen found on or in a number of disparate organs. One possible mechanism might be that a clone or clones of immune cells now recognize "self" as being foreign, presumably by means of interaction with "self" MHC markers. The rogue clone(s) act as if they were not of "self"; this is analogous with graft-versus-host reactions mounted by transplanted T cells, either resident in transplanted organs or found in donor bone marrow (see Chap. 26). This phenomenon has been suggested as the cause of progressive systemic sclerosis, an autoimmune disease manifested by the development of sclerosis of the skin (scleroderma) and internal organs. The theory is that tissue modification occurs, presumably due to the local production of cytokines and growth factors.

Systemic disease may occur if the individual produces large quantities of *immune complexes,* defined as aggregations of antibody bound to its relevant antigen. Immune complexes are part of normal immune function (this would be a good time to review the function and means of activation of the complement system described in Chap. 13). After antibody binds to its target, the complexes are taken up by the reticuloendothelial system, binding to Fc receptors on the surface of phagocytic cells, especially in the liver, spleen, and bone marrow. Viruses are bound, inactivated, and cleared this way. Thus, immune complexes are part of normal immune function. They may have immunoregulatory function as well, down-regulating B cells by cross-linking surface-bound immunoglobulin and occupied Fc receptors.

Some special examples of immune complex production should be described. If you have circulating antibodies to a certain antigen and this antigen is injected subcutaneously, you will make local immune complexes at the injection site. Complement fixation causes release of chemotactic factors, with inflow of polymorphonuclear and other inflammatory cells, as well as the activation of the kinin and coagulation cascades. Local release of inflammatory mediators, including serotonin (from platelets), eicosanoids, platelet-activating factor, and oxygen radicals, causes local tissue destruction. Clinically, there are edema, erythema, and local necrosis, usually reaching a maximum in 4 to 6 h. This is called the *Arthus' reaction.* A related phenomenon is the Prausnitz-Küstner reaction, as described in Chaps. 1 and 29. The serum of an individual who has a known allergy, e.g., to seafood, is injected subcutaneously into a nonallergic person. If the recipient should eat seafood, he or she will develop a local allergic reaction, with a wheal and flare, and may experience a systemic anaphylactic reaction. Here, IgE to the seafood is transferred and binds to local mast cells; the potential to reproduce this response persists for up to 90 days, since the active principle here is the persistence of mast cells with the relevant bound IgE.)

The Arthus' reaction may be of clinical relevance. If someone has antibodies to antigens found in his or her tissue, an Arthus'-type reaction may occur. The antigen may be an intrinsic part of that tissue or may be a newly associated endogenous or exogenous compound. Local, or in situ, immune complex formation can then cause fixation of complement, etc. If an antigen is an intrinsic part of a tissue and fixes antibody and complement locally, the inflammation is termed a Gell and Coombs type II reaction (in situ immune complex); some examples of this include transfusion reactions (see Chap. 30), myasthenia gravis (see Chap. 35D), and Goodpasture's syndrome. Alternatively, if a new antigen is inhaled and stays in the alveoli, one might develop in situ immune complexes and inflammation. This, plus coexisting T-cell reactivity (Gell and Coombs type IV hypersensitivity), may be at the root of extrinsic allergic alveolitis. (Examples are farmer's lung—antigen derived from mold-

ing hay; bagassosis—moldy pressed sugar cane; pigeon breeder's disease—pigeon droppings; and humidifier lung—fungi growing within air ducts.) If the antigen is bound by antibody in the circulation, with ultimate deposition and tissue destruction, the inflammation is termed a Gell and Coombs type III reaction (see Chap. 29). The former may be at the root of damage to a single tissue (e.g., myasthenia) or to multiple tissues all of which share a common antigen (polyspecific disease, e.g., Goodpasture's syndrome), whereas the latter may be the cause of multisystem disease with no recurring or common antigenic theme to the organs affected (polydiffuse disease).

Immune complexes can be formed in the circulation, as noted above, after antibody binds to endogenous antigens (e.g., malignant cell-derived antigens) or exogenous antigens (e.g., infectious antigens). The phenomenon of circulating immune complexes causing diffuse tissue damage was first described by von Pirquet and Schick as a toxicity of the use of horse antiserum to combat tetanus. The syndrome included arthritis, glomerulonephritis, and inflammation of blood vessels (causing vasculitis), all due to deposition of immune complexes at these sites. Unknown to von Pirquet and Schick at that time was the fact that the antibody response to a new antigen passes through three phases: antigen excess, antigen equivalence, and antibody excess (Fig. 31-7). In the early phase, there is very little antibody formed; the antigen is part of soluble immune complexes of the right size to evade clearance and become deposited in blood vessel walls. In antigen equivalence or antibody excess the complexes are cleared as described above. Only under certain circumstances will immune complex–mediated damage occur.

The antigen at the root of immune complex–mediated vasculitis (inflammation of blood vessels) is usually unknown. Some patients with hepatitis B virus infection will experience vasculitis in the prejaundice phase, i.e., in the early phase of their infection, while still in antigen excess. Other infections known for the shedding of antigens and occasional

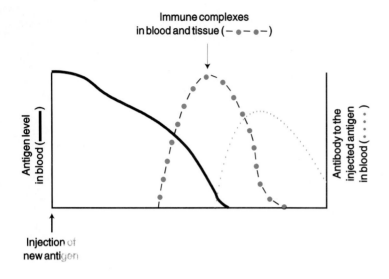

Figure 31-7   Antibody response to a new antigen.

vasculitis include subacute bacterial endocarditis, leprosy, and certain parasitic infections, including malaria and schistosomiasis mansoni. (I suppose that a philosophical question emerges at this point. A vasculitis occurring because of immune complex deposition with the complexes formed around an exogenous antigen is not an antigen-specific autoreactive phenomenon. Complexes fix complement, thereby causing inflammation, and tissue damage results. Strictly speaking, this is not autoimmunity; it is self-destruction due to inflammation. We consider this mechanism here [see Clinical Aside 31-6] because we use a broader definition of autoimmunity.)

Clinical Aside 31-6
Cryoglobulinemia

Immune complexes may settle in tissues or blood vessels and cause tissue damage. Some immune complexes will precipitate if the complex-containing serum is placed at 4°C; the material at the bottom of the cooled tube is called a *cryoprecipitate*, and it contains immunoglobulin, fibronectin, other serum proteins, including complement, and (presumably) the antigens which are the targets of the antibodies.

Cryoglobulins are found in many infectious diseases (bacterial sepsis, leprosy, hepatitis B virus, cytomegalovirus, poststreptococcal glomerulonephritis, syphilis, Lyme disease, malaria, toxoplasmosis, coccidioidomycosis), autoimmune diseases (SLE, rheumatoid arthritis, Sjögren's syndrome, scleroderma, sarcoidosis), and lymphoproliferative diseases (Waldenström's macroglobulinemia, lymphoma). Cryoglobulins have been divided into three types:

Type I, about 25 percent of cases: Monoclonal immunoglobulin, usually IgM; usually in large quantity, often associated with a lymphoproliferative syndrome

Type II, about 25 percent of cases: Monoclonal immunoglobulin, usually IgM; mixed with other polyclonal immunoglobulins, IgM often has rheumatoid factor activity

Type III, about 50 percent of cases: IgM-IgG mixture; polyclonal, often in very small quantity

Types II and III are termed "mixed" cryoglobulins. About 30 percent of patients with cryoglobulinemia have an idiopathic process, i.e., a primary process, known as "essential" cryoglobulinemia.

Essential mixed cryoglobulinemia primarily affects women in the fifth to sixth decade, as in the following case.

A 57-year-old female presents with a 15-year

history of Raynaud's phenomenon, chronic anemia, and intermittent joint pain and fever. She was diagnosed as having rheumatoid arthritis 4 years ago. Two years ago she developed skin rash ("little red dots on my legs"), dry mouth and eyes, fatigue, weakness, and muscle soreness. On examination, her arterial blood pressure is normal; she has a fever of 103.2°F. She has blotchy, purpuric maculopapular lesions on the neck, brown discoloration over the pretibial area, petechiae on the legs, and well-marginated erythematous lesions on the feet, with three 2- by 4-cm ulcers. The parotid glands are slightly enlarged. Muscle wasting is noted diffusely, and there is inflammation of the ankles, fingers, and wrists. There is a mild left foot drop (peroneal nerve damage, with inability to dorsiflex the foot). The WBC is normal; the hematocrit is 20 percent; urinalysis reveals 10 to 15 WBC, 40 to 50 RBC per high-powered field, and a urine reaction for protein of 3+. Blood chemistries are normal (sodium, potassium, chloride, carbon dioxide); the BUN and creatinine are likewise normal. ESR is 70 mm/h. Rheumatoid factor is weakly positive at 1:40. All blood and urine cultures are negative. There was 5.2 g of protein in a 24-h urine collection; the calculated creatinine clearance was 77 mL/h. Cryoglobulins were found, the "cryocrit" being 3 percent. (Blood is clotted at 37°C and the resulting serum is cooled to 4°C for 2 to 3 days. The cooled serum is spun, with the cryoprecipitate in the pellet; the cryocrit, like the hematocrit, is the percentage of the original serum volume taken up by the precipitate.) Analysis of the material revealed monoclonal IgM with rheumatoid factor activity and polyclonal IgG, i.e., a type II mixed cryoglobulinemia. A skin biopsy revealed vasculitis, with destruction of capillaries and small venules. A lip biopsy of a minor salivary gland showed many foci of lymphocytes, with one germinal center; the architecture of the gland was distorted. (The complaints of dry eyes and mouth, called *sicca syndrome*, plus this biopsy appearance, are diagnostic of Sjögren's syndrome.) Kidney biopsy revealed diffuse glomerulonephritis, with granular deposition of IgG, IgM, and complement. She was treated with high-dose prednisone and the later addition of cyclophosphamide and has had no further skin lesions. Her foot drop has improved somewhat, and her proteinuria has diminished. Her arthritis has improved. To summarize: This patient has rheumatoid arthritis and Sjögren's syndrome, a common association, with cryoglobulinemia causing a vasculitis affecting the skin, muscles, nerves, and glomeruli; significant proteinuria; and mild renal insufficiency. What are the molecular and cellular mechanisms of the vasculitis?

Why do certain people get immune complex–mediated vasculitis and most do not? Host susceptibility certainly depends on the efficiency of the reticuloendothelial system; on the antigen dose, valence, and persistence; on the avidity and affinity of the antibody being made; and on the isotype, subclass (e.g., IgG1 and IgG3 fix complement well, IgG2 and IgG4 less so), and charge of the antibody (complexes containing positively charged antibodies are more likely to cause glomerulonephritis). Genetic factors which determine whether an individual is a "high responder" or "low responder" also influence the chances of developing disease. Solubilization of the complexes is crucial in avoiding disease. (What keeps complexes in solution, rather than allowing them to precipitate in tissues and blood vessels?) Vascular permeability is another major influence; the local presence of vasoactive amines, derived from mast cells, basophils, and platelets, may influence deposition. Finally, the hemodynamics of individual organ system vascular beds play a major role; areas of high blood pressure gradients (as where renal, choroid, and ciliary body filtration take place) or areas of turbulence (as where vascular bifurcations occur) predispose to complex deposition. The methods used to measure immune complexes in serum are described in Appendix C.

SLE is a multisystem, nonorgan-specific autoimmune disease. It primarily affects women in their child-bearing years, causing arthritis, kidney disease, skin lesions, CNS damage (e.g., stroke, dementia, seizures), pleurisy and pericarditis, and various cytopenias. This female predominance strongly suggests a hormonal influence. This is certainly the case in the (NZB × NZW) F_1 mouse model of SLE, described earlier. In addition, human females with SLE may experience an exacerbation of disease in the postpartum period. All of this indirect evidence suggests a hormonal influence on disease activity. A genetic predisposition to SLE has been defined. There is an excess of HLA-DR2 and HLA-DR3 in patients with SLE, and having the null C4A allele also increases the risk of developing SLE. (Among the many functions of complement is *solubilization of immune complexes*—see a possible association?) The precise initiating event in SLE is not known in most patients; antecedent therapy with drugs (including procainamide, hydralazine, penicillamine, and chlorpromazine) causes some people to make antinuclear antibodies and in some of these a lupuslike syndrome will develop. What is known about SLE is that autoantibodies are formed against nuclear and cytoplasmic antigens, including DNA, ribonucleoprotein particles, and histone, as well as against certain cells, including T cells and neurons; antithyroid or antiadrenal antibodies are relatively uncommon. Precisely how these autoantibodies might cause the disease is not clear, although it seems likely that immune complex deposition is involved. The best example of this is lupus glomerulonephritis, where complexes of DNA and anti-DNA antibodies have been eluted from affected kidneys. It is possible that free DNA (which bears a negative charge, due to its phosphate residues) has an affinity for the positively charged glomerular basement membrane, thus increasing the trapping of these complexes. Alternatively, recent studies suggest that free circulating DNA is, in fact, tightly bound to histone and it is the histone which has a strong affinity for the basement membrane. Using indirect immunofluorescence testing, immune complexes can be identified in different areas of the glomeruli associated with unique syndromes.

Immune complexes may also cause arthritis, pericarditis, and pleuritis in lupus. (SLE was first described by Kaposi, who called it *polyserositis*, meaning inflammation of the serosal lining of many organs. Polyserositis was a descriptive name for the syndrome, as is lupus: the erythema over the malar eminences was thought to look like the facial markings of a wolf—*lupus* is Latin for "wolf.") Vasculitis may cause damage to the kidneys, brain, and skin, as well. Direct toxic effects of autoantibodies are probably more important in CNS lupus than in vasculitis.

Another interesting autoantibody is the "lupus anticoagulant," one of the most glaring misnomers in medicine (see Clinical Aside 31-7).

Clinical Aside 31-7
The "Lupus Anticoagulant": The Antiphospholipid Syndrome

It has been known for some time that certain patients with SLE have a positive test for syphilis, but they do not have syphilis; when further testing is done, their positive VDRL or RPR is not corroborated by the fluorescent treponemal antibody-absorption test (FTA-ABS). This false-positive test is due to serum antibodies to cardiolipin, a phospholipid derived from beef heart, which is a reagent used in the test. Many of these patients also have a prolongation of the PTT coagulation test, also due to antibodies to phospholipids. The clinical associations of this serologic reactivity are fascinating. These patients do not have excessive bleeding, as one might suspect from the prolonged PTT; rather, they experience thrombosis and thrombophlebitis! This may present as pulmonary embolization (blood clots breaking off, or embolizing, to the lung), stroke, or, in pregnant women, placental damage and recurrent loss of pregnancy. Thrombocytopenia is also frequent. Some of these patients may have a clinical syndrome much like multiple sclerosis. Finally, many of these patients will have thrombi on their heart valves, which ultimately can cause dysfunction of the valve. These deposits were described by Libman and Sacks earlier this century, and the endocardial lesions of this nonbacterial endocarditis bear their name, *Libman-Sacks endocarditis*. Some of these patients do not have SLE by the standard criteria. Thus the "lupus anticoagulant" is not an anticoagulant and it can occur in patients who do not have lupus—not a very helpful descriptive name, is it?

NOW THAT WE KNOW A DISEASE IS AUTOIMMUNE, WHAT CAN WE DO ABOUT IT?

If the clinical problem due to autoimmune disease is the absence of a hormone, e.g., hypothyroidism, one can replace that hormone. This works well for Hashimoto's thyroiditis, but it is well known that even adequate control of diabetes mellitus with insulin therapy does not totally prevent the late complications of this disease (see Chap. 35B).

In Chap. 33A a variety of therapeutic modalities in autoimmune disease are described. They are, for the most part, nonspecific. If one can identify the offending agent at the root of pathogenic immune complexes, one can eliminate it; stopping intravenous penicillin in someone with serum sickness due to the penicillin is one example of this. However, because we usually do not know the offending agent(s), we often have to try nonspecific therapeutic modalities. In order to remove circulating immune complexes, plasmapheresis (removal of plasma with replacement by albumin) has been tried, usually with disappointing results. Total nodal irradiation has been tried (as was thoracic duct drainage many years ago), or monoclonal antibodies to T cells, in order to deplete T cells. All these modalities are nonspecific and will remove the good antibodies or T cells along with the bad. Just as with steroids and cytotoxic agents, immunosuppression is global, with attendant problems.

The obvious answer is to develop specific therapeutic agents, with narrowly defined targets. An example of this might be the definition of the specific HLA-DR molecule which is expressed on the surface of autoimmune damaged cells. (Recall that interferon may elicit the production of class II markers on cells previously devoid of these molecules; the subsequent chain of events is described above.) If one could target this specific DR molecule with monoclonal antibodies, one might abrogate the autoimmune damage. This has, in fact, been done in the mouse (allergic autoimmune encephalomyelitis and experimental autoimmune myasthenia gravis) and in the BB/W rat (insulin-dependent diabetes mellitus). The key word here is "specific," however; monoclonal antibodies to an inappropriate class II target made diabetes worse.

Other strategies for controlling autoimmune disease due to T-cell reactivity have been suggested. One might try to induce anergy by oral administration of the critical self-antigen, as has been done in studies of patients with rheumatoid arthritis and multiple sclerosis. Alternatively, one might try to induce anergy by eliminating or blocking the costimulatory signal from the antigen-presenting cell or by interfering with the T cell–antigen-presenting cell interaction, perhaps by inhibiting the TCR-MHC complex (anti-MHC, CD4, or TCR antibodies) or by blocking accessory molecule interactions (antibodies to LFA-1, LFA-2, ICAM, or CD2). The influence of lymphokines could be modified; blocking antibodies to IL-1 or IL-2 receptors, soluble IL-1 or IL-2 receptors, or IL-1 inhibitory proteins like the IL-1 receptor antagonist (IL-1RA) could be given. If one were to bind a cellular toxin to IL-2 or to another molecule capable of interacting with immune cells, one might delete that population. Lymphokine production could be blocked, by cyclosporine or FK 506, or other inhibitory lymphokines could be given, e.g., TGF-β. All of these are feasible, but please pause a moment to consider the potential drawbacks.

Since the autoimmune specificity is defined by the T-cell-antigen receptor, it might be possible to engineer an antibody or peptide which would interact with the receptor. A peptide which binds to and blocks the receptor might work. Alternatively, one might produce a peptide which mimics the combined MHC molecule–antigenic peptide complex; such molecules, which require a great deal of information about the autoimmune process in question, have induced anergy in certain animal models.

Finally, recall the idiotype–anti-idiotype network. If one could produce or purify the proper anti-idiotype, one could down-regulate the offending clone of antibody. This may be the reason that intravenous γ-globulin is effective in the therapy of certain autoimmune diseases (see Chap. 34).

Our appreciation of autoimmunity as a part of normal physiology has provided insights into normal immune function. We now understand that a large number of diseases have autoimmunity as part of the pathogenesis. We are still a long way from full appreciation of these mechanisms and have little if any insight into the initiation of autoimmunity in most cases. Nonetheless, as our understanding of the molecular biology of the cell expands and our ability to identify viral and other pathogens increases, the answers to autoimmune disease will come.

Let's end on a note to ponder: There is an increased incidence of malignancy, especially lymphoproliferative disease, in autoimmune diseases, e.g., rheumatoid arthritis, Sjögren's syndrome, and Hashimoto's thyroiditis. Why should this be? Give this some thought before you proceed with your reading.

It is possible that both autoimmune and malignant diseases are due to proliferation of the same clone(s) of immune cells and that the autoimmunity is merely a premalignant manifestation. This seems unlikely: there is a very long lag time between the onset of autoimmunity and the malignancy. Is it possible that there is an innate, or acquired, susceptibility to both? Or that both are due to the same external influences? Finally, could it be that the chronic antigenic stimulation in autoimmunity causes a "malignant degeneration" of lymphocytes? In favor of this is the fact that the malignancy is often found at the site of the primary tissue damage, e.g., lymphoma of the thyroid in thyroiditis, or of the parotid glands in Sjögren's syndrome. Another possibility is that some of the therapeutic interventions used may somehow predispose to malignancy. This could be the case in SLE or rheumatoid arthritis, where

cytotoxic agents are often used (see Chap. 33A). But what of cases where these agents are not used, or diseases like thyroid disease or diabetes, where it seems unlikely that hormonal replacement would cause malignancy? There may be multiple explanations for the association of malignancy and autoimmunity, but at this time the full story is not known. It is striking and thought-provoking, however, that immunodeficiency syndromes and diseases of "excess immunity" (autoimmunity) both predispose to malignancy.

SELF-TEST QUESTIONS

1. Give three examples of physiologic "autoimmunity." Give three examples of mechanisms of pathologic autoimmunity.
2. Describe the anti-idiotype "internal image" and how this can be involved in the evolution of an autoimmune reaction.
3. If potentially autoimmune T cells are found in the peripheral blood of normal animals, there must be some mechanisms whereby these cells are "controlled." What might these mechanisms be?
4. In 25 words or less (or more, if you insist), describe the concept of "molecular mimicry."
5. What would be the systemic ramifications of production of immune complexes which can fix complement? Where might these complexes deposit? What would determine if they deposit, stay in solution, or are cleared? How would they be cleared?
6. How might you explain the pathogenesis and hormonal and MHC linkages of SLE on the basis of a viral (perhaps retroviral) etiology?

ADDITIONAL READINGS

Kumar V, Kono DH, Urban JL, Hood L. T-cell receptor repertoire and autoimmune diseases. *Annu Rev Immunol.* 1989;7:657–682.

Cohen IR. Autoimmunity to chaperonins in the pathogenesis of arthritis and diabetes. *Annu Rev Immunol.* 1991;9:567–589.

Cohen IR. Autoimmunity: Physiologic and pernicious. *Adv Intern Med.* 1984;30:147–165.

Hansen BL. Why do some individuals produce autoreactive antibodies against receptors and/or their ligands? A possible answer to the question. *Scand J Immunol.* 1986;24:363–370.

32

Immunotoxicology

How the Environment Can Affect the Normal Immune System

INTRODUCTION

The immune system is an intricate combination of mechanisms which, when in balance, maintain health. It may be helpful to review those chapters on immune mechanisms prior to studying this chapter.

Briefly, in the short term, the body handles acute insults by its repair and recuperative mechanisms. If repeated acute episodes occur, they can lead to severe tissue damage (e.g., fibrosis of the lung) or to a chronic debilitative state (e.g., somatic mutation leading to cancer). The repair process itself can cause tissue damage (e.g., development of chronic bronchitis) or formation of scar tissue resulting in organ dysfunction such as liver cirrhosis. Broadly speaking, major deleterious effects on the immune system lead to cancer, allergic and autoimmune diseases, or increased susceptibility to infection. Approximately 85 percent of all cancers are due to environmental factors. Theoretically, one molecule can cause the damage that results in a tumor. Therefore there are no threshold values (a level below which no effect is anticipated) for carcinogens, even though in actuality threshold values may exist. Cancer is a multistage process that can be promoted by chemicals which do not appear to react directly with DNA. A non-cancer end point does have a threshold value.

In addressing the role of the environment on the immune system, it is important to consider the route of exposure.

The skin is the first defense against foreign substances. In the dermis, immunologic components, including macrophages, mast cells, and lymphocytes, make up what some investigators call "skin-associated lymphoid tissue." In the epidermis are Langerhans cells, major members of the skin's immune system. The potential for transcutaneous absorption differs in different parts of the body, with the highest levels on the abdomen, scrotum, and neck and the lowest on the palms of the hands and soles of the feet. The skin is the site of most occupational and household exposures and is the major site for primary irritation and localized allergic reactions.

The respiratory system provides a very large surface area to the environment, approximately 80 m². It has an active, local immune system, with alveolar macrophages providing a major line of defense in the lower respiratory tract. The bronchus-associated lymphoid tissue (BALT) provides localized antigen-specific protection.

The oral route of exposure can lead to formation of tolerance, as can the intravenous route. Gut-associated lymphoid tissue (GALT) provides local immunity for the gastrointestinal tract. The blood, of course, has the major cell types for immune responses in the white blood cells.

The route of exposure does not always determine the target organ, a point that will be brought out later.

RADIATION

Radiation is measured in Système Internationale units. The joule (J) is the unit of energy; the gray (Gy) is the unit of absorbed dose, replacing the rad which equals 10^{-2} J/kg; the sievert (Sv) is the the unit of ionizing radiation absorbed dose equivalent; and the becquerel (Bq) is the unit of activity, replacing the curie (Ci) which equals 3.7×10^{10} Bq. The sievert (Sv) (equivalent to 100 rems, for roentgen equivalent mammal) is, for X or γ radiation, equal to the gray. To put these units in perspective, a chest x-ray results in exposure to about 0.03 to 0.1 mGy.

Natural sources of radiation include the following:

1. Cosmic rays: 85 percent protons, 14 percent α particles, and about 1 percent nuclei. Less than 0.05 percent of the primary cosmic protons penetrate to sea level. Cosmic rays originate from galactic sources. Only a small fraction are normally solar in origin. However, solar flares

occur with cyclic sun spot activity, at which time an increase in cosmic rays from the sun occurs.

2. Cosmogenic nuclides: reaction products from the interactions of high-energy cosmic ray primary particles with atmospheric nuclei.

3. Primordial radionuclides: Radioactive elements found in the earth's crust with half-lives comparable to the age of the universe (greater than 10^{10} years).

Together these three sources result in both external and internal radiation exposure, and vary substantially throughout the world. Doses range from 1.2 mGy/year (120 mrad/year) in Washington, D.C., to 70 mGy/year (7000 mrad/year) in Ramsar, Iran, to 175 mGy/year (17,500 mrad/year) in Guarapari, Brazil. The average outdoor absorbed dose rate in air from terrestrial sources is 5 × 10^{-8} Gy/h (5 × 10^{-6} rad/h) with decay from uranium 238 accounting for more than half the effective dose equivalent. Indoor exposure to radon gas (which decays to other radioactive elements), prevalent especially in well-sealed houses, is an important cause of lung cancer. Radon is more fully discussed below.

Consumer products that contain various radionuclides include radioluminous timepieces, electronic and electrical devices (e.g., television sets), antistatic devices, and smoke detectors; dose equivalent rates range from 0.01 to 0.03 mSv/year (1 to 3 mrem/year) for luminous wristwatches to 80 mSv/year (8000 mrem/year) for tobacco products (lead 210 and polonium 210 in tobacco smoke).

Over 1000 nuclear explosions have occurred worldwide, with more than half occurring underground. Well-contained underground explosions deliver an extremely low dose commitment. The annual per capita absorbed dose from fallout radionuclides is approximately 0.045 mSv (4.5 mrem).

Occupational exposure to radioactivity occurs in the management of nuclear fuel, medicine, research, industry, aviation, and nonuranium mining; phosphate fertilizers contain the radionuclide uranium 238 decay series. About 1.3 million persons are potentially exposed on an occupational basis, with half of these receiving a measurable dose. The mean equivalent for all workers is 1.1 mSv/year (110 mrem/year), and the total annual collective dose equivalent in the United States is about 1500 mSv (150,000 mrem).

Survivors of the atomic bombs dropped at Hiroshima and Nagasaki represent an important group because they are the largest number of significantly exposed persons of any of the epidemiologic studies. No life shortening in survivors has been documented from any cause except cancer, with the risk of breast cancer extending to women less than 10 years of age at the time of the explosion.

Following exposure to large doses of whole-body irradiation, different syndromes may develop depending on the level of radiation. For a whole-body dose of more than 50 Gy (5000 rad) a central nervous system syndrome results, and survival time is usually less than 48 h. Disorientation, apathy, ataxia, prostration, tremors, and convulsions occur. Death is caused by vascular damage, meningitis, myelitis, and encephalitis. Fluid is retained in the meninges, brain, and choroid plexus, causing marked edema.

For those exposed to a whole-body dose of 7 to 50 Gy (700 to 5000 rad), a gastrointestinal syndrome results with lethargy, diarrhea, dehydration, and sepsis, and degenerative abnormalities in the small bowel epithelium occur. Bile enters the intestinal lumen. Abnormalities in secretion of fluid into the bowel and reabsorption may cause a large loss of fluid and electrolytes. Infection occurs as early as 24 h after exposure because there is direct killing of mature lymphocytes with a decrease of cells in bone marrow, peripheral blood, and Peyer's patches.

A hematopoietic syndrome results in those exposed to 2 to 7 Gy (200 to 700 rad). There is a prodromal, asymptomatic period of 1 to 3 weeks during which bone marrow, lymphatic organs, and immune responses are markedly affected. Lymphocytes decrease in number rapidly, with a somewhat more delayed reduction of polymorphonuclear cells, platelets, and red blood cells. Major consequences of exposure are increased rates of infection and of neoplasms. Small lymphocytes are very radiosensitive, with 0.02 to 0.04 Gy (2 to 4 rad) causing significant changes in motility and morphology. Antigen-activated lymphocytes are more resistant to ionizing radiation. Plasma cells are very resistant and can continue to secrete antibody at doses in excess of 100 Gy (10,000 rad). B lymphocytes are more sensitive to radiation than T cells. The amount of radiation that causes damage to B lymphocytes is 1 Gy (100 rad); for T lymphocytes, it is 20 Gy (2000 rad). Therefore, de novo antibody production is more sensitive to radiation toxicity than delayed-type hypersensitivity or graft-versus-host disease. The order of decreasing sensitivity of antibody production to irradiation is IgA, IgM, and IgG. Exposure in utero causes at least a temporary decrease in the child's antibody-producing competence.

There is an increased rate of leukemia in those with occupational exposure to radiation, especially radiologists and x-ray technologists. The risk of cancer can be passed to offspring through damage of the germ cells. A population-based case-control study conducted on 338 patients under 15 years of age who had primary tumors of the central nervous system revealed a positive association between central nervous system tumor risk and paternal exposure to ionizing radiation. Thus, the true toll of the Chernobyl accident has not yet been realized.

ENVIRONMENTAL POLLUTANTS

The effect of environmental pollutants on human health is of increasing concern.

Atmospheric Gases

It is well documented that nitrogen dioxide (NO_2) and sulfur dioxide (SO_2) increase the susceptibility of humans to respiratory diseases. Photochemical oxidants and sulfates at places of residence cause measurable impairment of lung function, as does living in a home where gas stoves provide heat (and liberate NO_2). There is some controversy over the effect of NO_2 on asthmatics. With long-term exposure to NO_2 asthmatics have been reported to become more susceptible to attack from bronchoconstrictive agents. However, for short-term exposure, no effect on pulmonary function of humans with asthma or bronchitis has been documented.

Mechanisms involved in increased infection caused by NO_2 are not easy to sort out because so many concomitant effects are involved, including direct lung damage, decreased production of prostaglandins, and immune modulation. The prostaglandins regulate many physiologic parameters, including bronchial tonus, and affect immune responses. The primary antibody response is suppressed by NO_2, but the secondary response is slightly stimulated. Cell-mediated immunity is suppressed after long-term exposure to NO_2 but enhanced after shorter exposure. Inhalation of NO_2 plays a role in facilitation of blood-borne cancer cell spread, while ozone (O_3) inhalation does not. In a mouse model, antibody to influenza virus increased after chronic exposure to NO_2. The increase could have been the result of increased viral growth due to a suppression of interferon production. Mice have been used as animal models to study many aspects of the effect of NO_2 on the response to various infectious agents such as *Klebsiella pneumoniae* and influenza virus.

Sulfur dioxide is often found in atmospheres containing NO_2. Some studies of SO_2 alone have been performed to study its effect. In a hematologic and immunologic study of humans exposed to SO_2, percentages of monocytes decreased and lymphocytes increased, but no changes were seen in numbers of blood erythrocytes or immunologic parameters, including lymphocyte transformation in response to B- and T-cell mitogens and numbers of lymphocytes with receptors for sheep red blood cells or the Fc portion of IgG.

Photochemical oxidants are chemical products of reactions between hydrocarbons and oxides of nitrogen that are initiated by sunlight (smog). Ozone is one of the most prevalent of this group of chemicals found in the natural atmosphere. When oxidants exceed 0.25 ppm, the number of asthma attacks is significantly increased.

The combined effects of ozone and NO_2 have been studied in humans. There was a decrease in vital capacity, inspiratory capacity, and several flow-related measures of lung function during exposure. The response to exposure to the combined pollutants O_3 and NO_2 was similar to that observed in O_3 exposures alone. No synergism was observed.

In a separate study, humans were exposed to 0.15 ppm each of O_3, SO_2, and NO_2 alone and in combination, with intermittent light exercise. Among the various indices of pulmonary function, specific airway conductance (the most sensitive index) was significantly decreased, with a slightly greater decrease for the mixture than for O_3 alone.

Exposure of mice to ozone after challenge with *Mycobacterium tuberculosis* resulted in significant enhancement in the number of bacteria in the lungs. In the same study, exposure to ozone after challenge with *M tuberculosis* resulted in suppression of cutaneous delayed hypersensitivity without affecting serum antibody titers to the microorganisms in guinea pigs. In a rabbit model, following unilateral lung exposure, low levels of ozone (0.5 to 3 ppm) decreased viability of alveolar macrophages, depressed various intracellular hydrolytic enzymes (lysozyme β-glucuronidase, acid phosphatase), and increased the absolute number and percent of polymorphonuclear leukocytes within pulmonary lavage fluid.

Indoor Air

Buildings produce their own pollutants. Common pollutants of indoor air include radon gas, tobacco smoke, asbestos, fungi and bacteria, carbon monoxide and nitrogen oxides, formaldehyde, benzene, and styrene. Sources of these pollutants range from pipe insulation and carpets to cigarette smoke.

Perhaps the most serious of the indoor pollutants is radon gas. Produced by the decay of uranium 238, radon accumulates in tiny air pockets in soil. It is pulled into houses by pressure differences created by the rising of warm indoor air. Radon decays to other radioactive elements, e.g., polonium, that bind to dust and are inhaled into the lungs, where they can cause cancer. Researchers have extrapolated from rates of lung cancer in uranium miners who are exposed to known amounts of radon and its products and calculated that 2000 to 20,000 cases of lung cancer each year may be caused solely by indoor radon pollution.

Passive smoking, i.e., breathing the smoke generated by others, is responsible for 30 percent more lower respiratory illnesses in children of smokers than those living in nonsmoking families. Although half of the nonsmokers in a study believed they had not been exposed to smoke, 85 percent had measurable levels of tobacco substances in their urine. An experimental and theoretical investigation was made into the range and nature of exposure of nonsmokers to respirable suspended particles from cigarette smoke. It was found that nonsmokers are exposed to significant air pollution burdens from indoor smoking. Rates of respiratory illness in children were studied in six cities. It was found that maternal smoking was associated with a 20 to 35 percent increase in rates of eight respiratory illnesses in children, and paternal smoking with a lesser but substantial increase.

In smokers themselves there is more in vitro extracellular release of hydrogen peroxide by alveolar macrophages. In those smokers with recent lower respiratory tract infection, even more significant increases in H_2O_2 release occurred. These findings are consistent with the hypothesis that H_2O_2 of alveolar macrophage origin contributes to the development of emphysema in smokers. In a separate study, alveolar macrophages from smokers were found to release significantly more elastase, which would also contribute to the development of emphysema. Cigarette smoking was found to be associated with a twofold increase in total number of pulmonary dendritic and/or Langerhans cells. Most Langerhans cells found in the parenchyma of smokers' lungs were observed in close association with areas of type II pneumocyte hyperplasia.

Occupational Exposure

The workplace may present concentrated exposure to compounds that, under ordinary usage, are at non-toxic levels. Most exposures are via the dermal and respiratory routes, with distant target organs sometimes affected. Of increasing importance in occupational lung diseases are low molecular weight compounds used in the manufacture of epoxy resins, plasticizers, adhesives, etc. Formaldehyde, used as a disinfectant or in the production of resin products for the wood, shoe, and clothing industries, causes dermatitis, urticaria, bronchitis, and reactive airway disease. Colophony (pine resin), used in soft soldering fluxes, and p-phenylenediamine, used in the fur, paint, and rubber industries, have also been implicated in the generation of industrial asthma. Of particular concern are the phthalates used in the manufacture of epoxy resins, plasticizers, and adhesives. Tetrachlorophthalic anhydride has been shown to cause asthma as a result of occupational exposure.

Trimellitic Anhydride (TMA)

TMA, perhaps the most completely studied of these low molecular weight compounds in humans, has been shown to cause at least four occupational respiratory syndromes:

1. Asthma: requires a latent period of exposure before onset of symptoms, which occur almost immediately after second exposure.
2. Late respiratory systemic syndrome: characterized by cough, mucus production, occasional wheezing, and dyspnea, as well as by systemic malaise, chills, arthralgias, and myalgias. Symptoms [TMA flu, accompanied by high levels of serum antibody to trimellitic (TM)–human serum albumin] appear 4 to 12 h after the second exposure.
3. Pulmonary disease-anemia syndrome: manifested by hemoptysis, dyspnea, pulmonary infiltrates, restrictive lung disease, and hemolytic anemia; requires a latent period of exposure (correlated with antibody to TM protein and TM erythrocytes).
4. Irritant syndrome: occurs at the first high-dose exposure to TMA powder or fumes and is manifested by upper airway irritation and cough with little or no antibody to TM protein.

The relationship between antibody and TMA-induced disease is complex. All individuals with serious lung disease caused by the hapten TMA had antibody to it, but not all individuals with antibody developed disease. In fact, of 61 workers observed for over 4 years, 41 percent developed serum antibody, but only 20 percent developed an immunologic syndrome, i.e., late respiratory systemic syndrome, asthma-rhinitis, or both. Therefore, if workers were removed from the workplace based on levels of antibody to the hapten, twice as many workers would be removed than would be necessary. A study isolating reagenic antibody has not clarified the situation. When IgE was examined separately, it was apparent that even a low serum level of biologically active IgE could be associated with significant clinical symptoms and skin-test reactivity, especially when total serum antibody to TMA was low. Presence of IgE and skin-test results did not always correlate with lung disease, however, as shown by examples of workers who had erythema on prick testing as well as significant amounts of total and IgE antibody to TMA, but manifested only mild rhinitis. Interestingly, in the absence of antibody, workers did not develop disease but only an irritant response.

Isocyanates

Isocyanates, used in the production of polyurethane foams, adhesives, paints, and plastics, are known to cause lung disease. Many studies have cited cases of sensitization resulting from exposure to isocyanates. Inhalation of aerosols or skin contact as a result of accidental spills causes sensitization. It should be noted that sensitization is not limited to the route of exposure; for example, pulmonary hypersensitivity and systemic sensitization can result from topical exposure. It is interesting that inhalation exposure required one-thousandth the amount of toluene diisocyanate, compared with dermal exposure, to produce an equivalent antibody response. In a separate study, allergic contact dermatitis was induced by intratracheal administration of hapten.

Although methylisocyanate has not been shown to be a sensitizer, the toxic and subtoxic effects of the compound predispose recipients to other diseases. An accident provides an example. In late 1984, leakage of methylisocyanate in Bhopal, India, caused devastating effects. At least 5000 people died, and many of the survivors suffered blindness and lung damage. Even many years after the exposure, the lungs of moderately affected people still show profound abnormalities in a variety of pulmonary function tests. There is great concern that the survivors will be more susceptible to lung diseases, including tuberculosis and filariae.

Pesticides

Of the different classes of compounds among the pesticides, organophosphates and organocarbamates present major problems to the immune system. The organocarbamates share with organophosphates the property of inhibition of cholinesterase. Therefore, some of the symptoms caused by exposure to these compounds can be explained by excess cholinergic activity. These include excessive salivation and lacrimation, sweating, urinary urgency, abdominal cramps, nausea, and bronchospasm. These compounds also affect other esterases involved in chemotaxis, phagocytosis, complement activation, and release of histamine.

An example of the carbamate family of pesticides is aldicarb. Aldicarb is acutely toxic; its mechanism of action consists of reversible inhibition of acetylcholinesterase activity. There is no evidence that aldicarb has any long-term adverse health effects. However, a report in 1985 suggested that aldicarb may cause a suppression of the humoral immune response in an inverse dose-response fashion. Following that report, a human epidemiologic study showed evidence of immunomodulation in women drinking water from wells contaminated with low concentrations of aldicarb. Exposed individuals showed an increased peripheral blood lymphocyte response to *Candida albicans* in vitro, increased numbers of T8 cells (suppressor lymphocytes), and a decreased ratio of T4 to T8 cells (helper-suppressor ratio). In contrast, two studies conducted in mice showed that aldicarb at a wide range of concentrations in drinking water was not immunomodulatory as measured by body and relative organ (spleen, thymus) weights, blood counts, differential leukocyte counts, antibody formation, lymphocyte response to mitogens or allogeneic lymphocytes, natural killer cell function, cytotoxic T-lymphocyte function, and percent and absolute numbers of splenic B cells, T cells, helper T cells, and suppressor T cells.

Organic phosphates are most often used as insecticides. They are also used as gasoline additives, hydraulic fluids, defoliants, fire retardants, plastic components, growth regulators, and industrial intermediates. Skin is the most common route of exposure followed by the respiratory tract; oral exposure is rare. Symptoms include the "cholinergic" symptoms described above, as well as headache, vertigo, blurred vision, muscular weakness and ataxia, diarrhea, vomiting, coma, and pulmonary edema. Death can result from two causes: (1) paralysis of the respiratory muscles and paralysis in that portion of the brain responsible for respiration and (2) cardiovascular failure. Workers exposed to sublethal levels of phosphoorganic pesticides have an increase in infectious disease (tonsillitis, bronchitis, pyelonephritis, and adnexitis). A decrease of cholinesterase activity was observed both in serum and in the red blood cells of workers, dependent on the degree of exposure. A marked impairment in vitro of neutrophil chemotaxis was observed in all groups of workers. Function of other cell types was not measured. Upper respiratory infection frequency was greater and the timing of recurrence of infection was dependent on time of exposure to the pesticides. In contrast, infections outside the respiratory tract were normal in frequency.

Polychlorinated Organic Compounds

Polychlorinated biphenyls (PCBs) are extremely stable compounds and are poorly metabolized. Exposure results in immune modulation, but whether this takes the form of suppression or stimulation depends on the conditions of exposure and the species exposed. Mice exposed to hexachlorobenzene (HCB) had reduced serum immunoglobulins and increased sensitivity (reduced host resistance) to endotoxin and *Plasmodium berghei*. In contrast, rats had marked increases of lymphoid organ weights and increased immunoglobulin levels.

Perinatal exposure to polychlorinated organic compounds, many of which cross the placenta, is more devastating to the immune response of an individual than is adult exposure. However, thymic atrophy results in either age group, and there is suppression of both cell-mediated and humoral immunity. The mechanism of action of 2,3,7,8-tetrachlorodibenzo-*p*-dioxin (TCDD) has been studied. TCDD binds to specific cytosolic receptor sites, triggering pleiotropic biochemical responses, some of which result in altered patterns of cell growth and differentiation and/or tumor promotion. The immune system is a particularly sensitive target. Although TCDD is profoundly immunosuppressive in rodents, there is no clear evidence that it is immunosuppressive in humans.

Polybrominated biphenyls (PBBs) have been shown to be immunomodulatory in humans. Again, an accident has provided humans for study. In 1973, a commercial preparation of PBB was used instead of magnesium oxide in preparation of feed for lactating cows and was also used in chicken feed. Thymic atrophy occurred in animals, and PBBs were shown to be tumorigenic. Not only were the animals badly affected, with death within 6 months of ingestion, but humans who ate the contaminated meat or milk and egg products were also affected. PBBs are stored in the thymus, liver, brain, and adipose tissues, where they persist for long periods. Peripheral blood lymphocytes from humans who were exposed to the PBBs had suppressed responses to T- and B-cell mitogens and to allogenic antigens in vitro. In addition, there was a marked increase in the number of lymphocytes without detectable surface markers and elevated levels of IgG, IgM, and IgA. Suppression of T-cell and B-cell function persisted for at least 8 years.

Trichloroethylene, used to degrease metals, was found to cause mutations in chromosomes of metal workers. Although no significant differences were found in sperm counts and sperm morphology between workers and nonexposed controls, lymphocytes from exposed workers showed a significant increase in frequency of breaks, gaps, translocations, inversions, and hyperdiploid cells.

Metals and Minerals

Heavy metals of environmental concern include cadmium, lead, mercury, manganese, and arsenic. Cadmium, lead, and mercury have no known essential role in metabolic pathways, and at certain concentrations they are toxic. Manganese is an essential element at very low concentrations and is toxic at higher levels. Arsenic is also an essential element for some animal species at low concentrations, but toxic at higher levels. Each heavy metal can exist in a variety of forms, each form differing in its toxic action. Heavy metal cations can eliminate the effectiveness of other mineral cofactors by substituting for cations essential in normal metabolism.

Inorganic heavy metals form coordinated

complexes, via ionic bonds, with various chelating agents, peptides, proteins, and other compounds. The toxic effects of heavy metals vary depending on the strength of the bonds formed with the target site. Heavy metals have high affinity to negatively charged groups of proteins and may cause changes in protein conformation leading to inhibition of various enzymes.

Organic heavy metals form organometallic compounds by binding covalently to carbon molecules, e.g., tetramethyl lead and methyl mercury. In comparison to inorganic heavy metals, they are bulkier and considerably less soluble in aqueous solutions. Neither competes with or binds to Ca^{2+}-binding sites.

There are different modes of release of metals to the environment. Wear and corrosion release alloys or amalgams. Flaking and volatilization are involved with metals in paints, pigments, and batteries (when burned). Metals are lost in manufacturing processes, e.g., copper and mercury in the manufacture of chlorine; copper, zinc, and chromium mordants used in dyeing; mercury in felt manufacturing; chromium in tanning; lead in desulfurization of gasoline; zinc in rayon spinning; and mercury fulminate and lead azide in the manufacture of detonators and explosives. Use of certain consumer products releases metals. For example, when gasoline containing lead is burned, the lead is largely dispersed into the atmosphere. Copper, chromium, and arsenic are used as wood preservatives and are dispersed when the wood is burned. Heavy metals in pesticides are largely immobilized by the soil, with the exception of arsenic and mercury, which are volatile. Metals in pharmaceuticals, including cosmetics and dental filling material and germicides, are mostly dissipated to the environment via waste water. Mercury dental fillings are likely to be buried with cadavers. The effects of individual metals are described below.

Gold

Little is known about adverse effects from industrial exposure to gold. However, many studies have established gold as a therapeutic agent, particularly in producing clinical remission in rheumatoid arthritis. Gold is cumulative and must be given in gradual increases for maximum efficacy and avoidance of reactions. Toxic effects include stomatitis and pruritus with or without rash. Albumin and red cells may be found in the urine, and blood changes, usually thrombocytopenia, but occasionally leukopenia or eosinophilia, may occur. Gold compounds have been shown to inhibit antigen- and mitogen-induced lymphocyte proliferation and are considered immunosuppressive.

Asbestos

Patients exposed to asbestos display alterations in cell-mediated and humoral immunity. Inhalation of asbestos fibers is associated with a marked increase in the risk of developing pulmonary malignancy, with a concomitant suppression of natural killer cell function. One study has suggested that mineral dust (asbestos and silica) modulates the production of inflammatory and fibrogenic cytokines.

Mercury

Mercury causes toxicity to the central nervous system and lysis of red blood cells. Inhaled mercury vapor easily diffuses across the alveolar membrane. Mercury vapor is oxidized to divalent mercury by red blood cells and is deposited in many tissues, with the highest concentration occurring in the kidneys. A portion of the oxide is transported to the brain, where biotransformation from the oxide to bivalent mercury may occur. Mercury levels in hair correlate with levels in the blood, and can serve as an indicator of mercury absorption by humans.

The effects of mercury on humans are revealed by accidents. In one such accident, workers were exposed to methyl mercury in the manufacture of seed fungicides. Symptoms began 3 to 4 months after onset of exposure and continued after exposure had ceased. Most frequent initial symptoms were paresthesia of the extremities, ataxia of gait, dysarthria, and impaired peripheral vision. In

Iraq, methyl mercury–treated wheat, intended for planting, was fed to animals. When no adverse effects were noted, the wheat was used in baking bread for human consumption. Over 6000 individuals died of methyl mercury poisoning, not as a direct result of the poisoning, but from intercurrent infections. In Minamata and Niigata, Japan, industrial pollution of water led to mercury poisoning of fish, which then led to poisoning of humans who ate the fish.

Twenty-three fetal cases were reported from the accident in Minamata. The mothers were asymptomatic during pregnancy except that five experienced paresthesia. The children born of these pregnancies had severe psychomotor retardation. None could crawl, stand, or say recognizable words until 3 years of age. All were ataxic, and most had increased deep tendon reflexes and tone, involuntary movements, and incontinence.

Cadmium

Major sources of cadmium in the environment include release during smelting of lead, zinc, or copper; burning of cadmium-containing materials such as scrap metal, plastics, cigarettes, coal, gasoline, motor oil, and tires; water that has leached cadmium from galvanized or plastic pipes; and treatment of crops with cadmium-containing fertilizers and pesticides.

Epidemiologic evidence has revealed direct associations between cadmium levels and mortality from myeloma, lymphoma, and cancers at several other sites, including the mouth and pharynx, esophagus, large intestine, larynx, lung, breast, and bladder. A separate investigation found direct associations with leukemia and cancers of the intestine, breast, uterus, prostate, and skin, but an inverse association with liver cancer. In mice, cadmium chloride was found to be immunomodulatory: Following exposure to cadmium chloride, there was a dose-related increased susceptibility to herpes simplex type 2 virus, T- and B-lymphocyte proliferation in response to mitogens was reduced, and macrophage phagocytosis was increased.

Lead

Lead sources in the environment include the burning of coal, the combustion of "leaded" gasoline, and air-borne effluents of smelting. Lead compounds are used in printing, plastics, putty, plaster, paint, solder, ceramic glazes, and batteries. Lead can be inhaled or ingested (e.g., liquids from cans sealed with lead solder, moonshine whiskey [moonshine is often distilled in old automobile radiators, which contain lead solder], foods stored in improperly glazed earthenware, paint). Overall, lead is immunosuppressive, causing decreased ability to fight infectious microorganisms, decreased synthesis of antibodies, and decreased cell-mediated immunity. Lead also causes increased tumor growth, with alterations of the reticuloendothelial system. Although known to be immunosuppressive, lead was shown to increase responses of lymphocytes to thymic-dependent mitogens and to stimulate macrophage activity.

Other Metals

There is epidemiologic evidence that selenium has a protective effect against cancer. A potential mechanism of action is suggested by data indicating that selenium in vitro and in vivo decreases the activity of hydroxylating enzymes that activate procarcinogens and may increase a detoxifying enzyme, glucuronyl transferase, thus acting during the early stages of tumor initiation.

Zinc is essential for life, functioning in nucleic acid polymerases and playing a dominant role in nucleic acid metabolism, cell replication, tissue repair, and growth. However, a direct correlation was found between estimated zinc intake and age-adjusted mortality from leukemia and cancers of the intestine, breast, prostate, and skin. Inverse correlations between zinc and selenium concentrations in blood suggest that zinc increases cancer risk by its antagonism of selenium. However, experimental evidence is contradictory, showing that zinc can either enhance or retard the growth of tumors. In a study with mice it was found that a high dietary intake of zinc made the animals more resistant to infection with *Candida albicans* and increased their capacity to elicit delayed-type hypersensitivity (DTH) responses. In contrast, low zinc intake resulted in increased susceptibility to infection and less capacity to elicit DTH reactions.

Arsenic is unique among the metals in that it has been associated with cancer in humans but not in laboratory animals. Cancers of the skin, lung, and liver occurred in German and French vineyard workers who suffered from chronic arseniasis. In addition, there was a direct relationship between the arsenic content of well water and the prevalence of skin cancer in the population drinking the water.

Cobalt caused lung fibrosis in tool grinders as well as increased susceptibility to virus infection.

Zinc, selenium, and other metals are necessary for the proper function of a number of organ systems. Their roles in the normal function of the immune system is discussed in Chap. 24B.

CONCLUSIONS

The immune system is an important target for environmental toxins. Animal studies suggest that environmental agents can alter the immune system both by depressing and increasing function, resulting in immunosuppression or increased hypersensitivity and autoimmunity. Several animal models are considered good predictors of human immunotoxicity, with the mouse being the most commonly used. In dealing with models, it should be remembered that following exposure to a compound, in vitro tests show modulation much more readily than in vivo tests such as host resistance to microorganisms. It is difficult to extrapolate from animals to humans because the metabolism, biodistribution, excretion, etc., are different.

In addition, many of the immunomodulatory effects of compounds are species-specific; e.g., TCDD is very immunotoxic to rodents, but there is little evidence that it has much effect on humans. In contrast, humans can be very sensitive to compounds to which animals are not susceptible; e.g., thalidomide is tolerated by laboratory animals, but can cause profound congenital anomalies in humans. Those farm animals in Iraq that were fed wheat treated with methyl mercury appeared unaffected, but when the grain was ground into flour and used for bread for human consumption, the humans suffered methyl mercury poisoning and many died. Testing in animals gives important information about the immunotoxicity of xenobiotics, but extrapolating the data to humans is risky. Our best data on humans come from careful epidemiologic studies in the workplace and from accidents. An increased awareness of the importance of monitoring the environment for toxic effects on animals as well as humans is mandatory.

ADDITIONAL READINGS

Ayree RU, McMichael FC, Rod SR. Measuring toxic chemicals in the environment: A materials balance approach. In Lave LB, Upton AC, eds. *Toxic Chemicals, Health, and the Environment.* Baltimore: Johns Hopkins University Press; 1987:38–70.

Bekesi JG, Roboz J, Fischbein A, et al. Immunological, biochemical, and clinical consequences of exposure to polybrominated biphenyls. In Dean J, et al. *Immunotoxicology and Immunopharmacology.* New York: Raven Press; 1985:393–406.

Hermanowicz A, Kossman S. Neutrophil function and infectious disease in workers occupationally exposed to phosphoorganic pesticides: role of mononuclear-derived chemotactic factor for neutrophils. *Clin Immunol Immunopath.* 1984;33:13.

Karol MH. Immunological response of the respiratory system to industrial chemicals. In Leong BJK, ed. *Inhalation Toxicology and Technology,* Ann Arbor, Mich.: Ann Arbor Science; 1981:233–246.

Mettler RA, Jr, Moseley RD, Jr, eds. *Medical Effects of Ionizing Radiation.* New York: Grune & Stratton; 1985.

Repace JL, Lowry AH. Indoor air pollution, tobacco smoke, and public health. *Science.* 1980;208:464.

Zeiss CR, Wolkonsky P, Chacon R, et al. Syndrome in workers exposed to trimellitic anhydride. A longitudinal clinical and immunologic study. *Ann Intern Med.* 1983;98:8.

SELF-TEST QUESTIONS

1. Exposure to radiation results in different syndromes depending on the amount of exposure. A hematopoietic syndrome (exhibited by a decrease in peripheral blood lymphocytes, polymorphonuclear cells, platelets, and red blood cells) occurs after exposure to:
   a. 50 Gy
   b. 7G–50 Gy
   c. 2–7 Gy
   d. 0.1–2 Gy
   e. All of above
   f. None of above

2. Of the pollutants of indoor air, the most serious is (are):
   a. Cigarette smoke
   b. Asbestos
   c. Fungi and bacteria
   d. Carbon monoxide
   e. Nitrogen oxide
   f. Benzene
   g. Styrene
   h. Radon

3. In the workplace, occupational lung diseases result from inhalation of haptens found in paints and resins. The best way to identify patients at risk is to study the following:
   a. Presence of antibody to the hapten in the serum
   b. Presence of cell-mediated immunity to the hapten
   c. Presence of flulike symptoms
   d. Shortness of breath
   e. Asthma
   f. All of above
   g. None of above

4. The organophosphate pesticides cause immune modulation by the following mechanisms:
   a. Alter lymphocyte response to specific antigens.
   b. Cause increased production of prostaglandins.
   c. Inhibit antibody formation.
   d. Inhibit esterases involved in chemotaxis, phagocytosis, complement activation, and release of histamine.
   e. All of above
   f. None of above

5. Methyl mercury is toxic to humans but not to farm animals. Characteristics of toxicity include:
   a. Paresthesia of extremities
   b. Ataxia of gait
   c. Dysarthria
   d. Impaired vision
   e. Effect on fetus without symptoms in mother.
   f. All of above
   g. None of above

33

Immunomodulatory Therapy

A. Immunopharmacology

INTRODUCTION

The era of human immunopharmacology was ushered in in the late 1940s with the clinical use of cortisone (compound E) in the management of rheumatoid arthritis (RA) by Hench and colleagues. The discovery that corticosteroids could make an immediate (albeit short-lived) major change in the signs and symptoms of RA (and other immune system–mediated diseases) was so revolutionary that it warranted the awarding of the Nobel Prize in Physiology and Medicine in 1950. It soon became apparent, however, that prolonged use of corticosteroids could lead to severe problems. This markedly dampened the enthusiasm for use of the corticosteroids.

Because prolonged use of corticosteroids was associated with significant toxicity, attention was diverted to other compounds which could control immunologically mediated disease while reducing the need for corticosteroids. In 1951 Diaz-Jimenez reported the beneficial effects of nitrogen mustard (an agent borrowed from cancer chemotherapy) on RA. Over the next 20 or so years a variety of cancer chemotherapy agents (cytotoxic agents) were employed experimentally in the management of RA and other immunologically mediated diseases. The ones which proved most effective and durable were azathioprine (replacing 6-mercaptopurine, its metabolite), chlorambucil, cyclophosphamide, and methotrexate (Fig. 33A-1). Unfor-

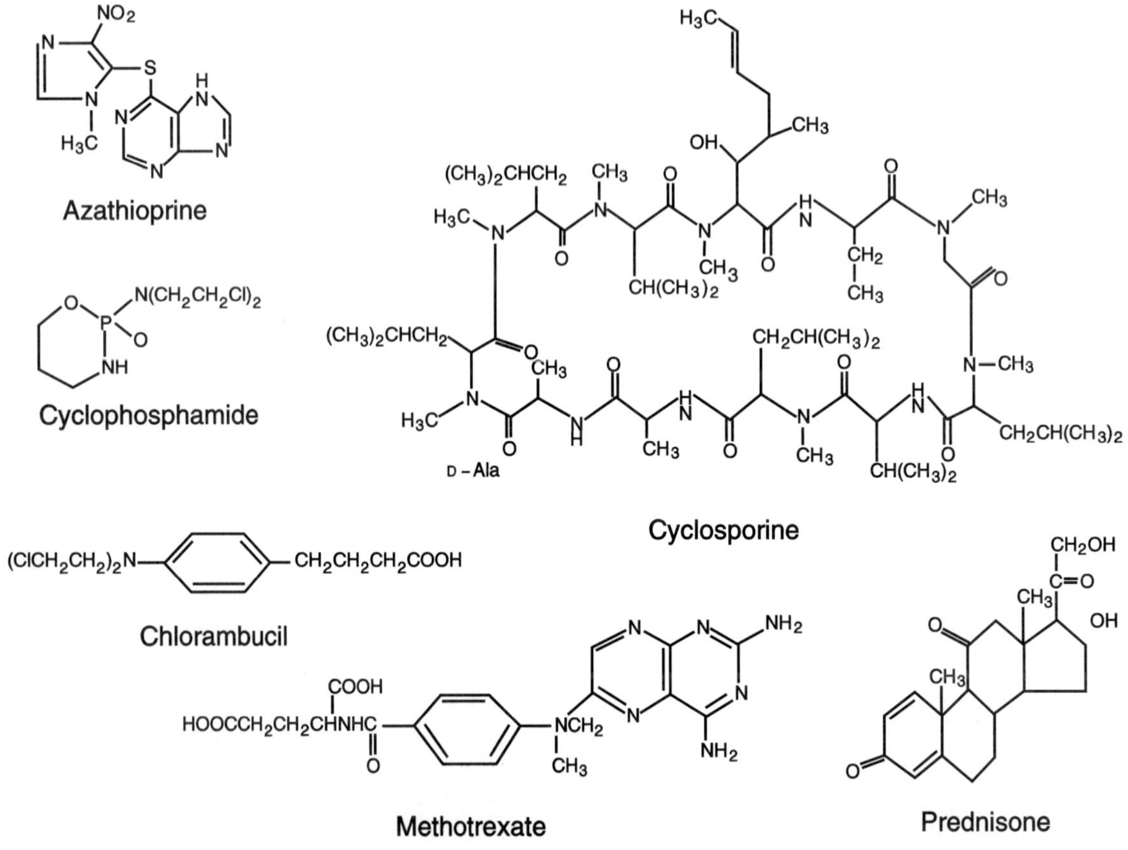

Figure 33A-1. Chemical structure of azathioprine, chlorambucil, cyclophosphamide, cyclosporine, methotrexate, and prednisone.

tunately the "honeymoon" with the cytotoxic drugs came to an end in the 1970s with the realization that they too were often associated with serious toxicity. In some instances the toxicities were more formidable than those of corticosteroids.

It was not until the introduction of cyclosporine (cyclosporin A) in 1978 for the prevention of renal transplant rejection that a useful, truly specific immunosuppressive agent became available for treatment of immunologically mediated disease (Fig. 33A-1). Corticosteroids and the cytotoxics were nonspecifically immunosuppressive: immunosuppression is only one of the many actions of these agents and there is little specificity about which immune responses are altered. This "shotgun" approach is in large part responsible for the most serious side effects. Unlike the cytotoxic drugs, which affect all dividing cells in the body, and corticosteroids, which also affect many cell types, cyclosporine specifically down-regulates the helper T subset of T cells and also interferes with the process of T-cell differentiation in the thymus.

To be balanced, therefore, any discussion of immunopharmacology must address not only the potential benefits but also the potential adverse effects of any given drug. The benefits must outweigh the risks in order to justify the use of these agents. The present chapter will address the following issues:

1. *Pharmacology:* how the body absorbs, metabolizes, and disposes of the drug and its metabolites, along with a discussion of the factors which alter the absorption, metabolism, and disposition of the compound (Table 33A-1).
2. *Mechanism of action:* how the drug is thought to work; more than one mechanism may be operative.
3. *Adverse effects:* the potential toxicity of the drug and its metabolites.
4. *Illustrative case using the compounds:* a longitudinal look at a patient with systemic lupus erythematosus illustrates the rationale and judgments needed in managing a difficult immune-mediated disease over a 15-year period of time.

AZATHIOPRINE (AZA)

Pharmacology

About 60 percent of AZA (Fig. 33A-1) is absorbed when the drug is administered orally. Following absorption, it is rapidly metabolized to 6-mercaptopurine (6-MP) which, like AZA, is not cytotoxic. 6-MP is then metabolized by xanthine oxidase to other metabolites, two of which are cytotoxically active: 6-thioinosinic acid and 6-thioquanylic acid (both 6-MP ribonucleotides). AZA is metabolized within 10 h (primarily by erythrocytes and the liver) to inactive metabolites which are excreted in the urine. Minute amounts of metabolites appear in cerebrospinal fluid (CSF), breast milk, and feces. Active metabolites may cross the placenta.

Since AZA is metabolized by xanthine oxidase, concomitant administration of allopurinol, an inhibitor of xanthine oxidase (often used to treat gout), delays AZA inactivation and may increase AZA toxicity; in these cases, the AZA dose should be reduced to one-fourth the usual dose. The presence of liver disease increases the likelihood of AZA toxicity. Since metabolites of AZA accumulate in the presence of renal failure, a dose reduction of 25 to 50 percent is needed initially.

Mechanism of Action

AZA is an inactive prodrug which is rapidly metabolized to another inactive prodrug (6-MP) before it is metabolized to cytotoxically active 6-MP ribonucleotides. These metabolites competitively inhibit purine biosynthesis both by feedback inhibition of the first step in de novo purine biosynthesis and by blocking the interconversion of the ribonucleotide inosinic acid to adenylic acid or guanylic acids. These metabolites are incorporated into DNA and as a result they block cell replication.

AZA is a cell cycle–nonspecific drug which primarily affects proliferating but not resting lymphocytes. It therefore inhibits all immune reactions that require cell proliferation prior to exertion of function.

TABLE 33A-1 Pharmacokinetic Characteristics of Cytotoxics, Corticosteroids (Prednisone), and Cyclosporine

	AZA	Chlorambucil	Cyclophosphamide	MTX	Cyclosporine	Prednisone (corticosteroid)
Absorption after oral dosing	60%	70%	100%	39%	20–50%	80%
Active agent						
Parent drug	Inactive	Inactive	Inactive	Active	Active	Inactive
Metabolite	6-thioinosinic acid	Phenylacetic acid mustard	Phosphoramide mustard	7-hydroxy-methotrexate	Probable (?)	Prednisolone
Sites						
Activation	RBCs, liver	Unknown	Liver	Parent active	Parent active	Liver
Inactivation	Liver	Unknown	Liver	GI tract	Liver	Liver
Excretion	Largely urine: <10% AZA, 20–35% metabolite	Largely urine: 1% chlorambucil, 20–70% metabolite	Largely urine: <25% cyclophosphamide, 35% metabolite	Largely urine: 70% MTX, 5–29% metabolite	Largely biliary; In urine: <1% cyclosporine, 6% metabolite	Largely liver; small metabolite in urine
Dosage adjustment						
Liver dysfunction	↓ dosage	?	↓ dosage	Contraindicated	↓ dosage	↓ dosage (with hypoalbuminemia)
Renal failure	↓ dosage	?	↓ dosage	Contraindicated	No change	No change
Drug interactions	Allopurinol increases toxicity	?	Allopurinol increases toxicity; enzyme inducers decrease efficacy*	NSAIDS, sulfa, salicylates, PAH, probenecid increase toxicity	Enzyme inducers decrease efficacy Enzyme inhibitors increase toxicity†	Enzyme inducers decrease efficacy

*Hepatic enzyme inducers, e.g., phenobarbital, rifampin, phenytoin.
†Hepatic enzyme inhibitors, e.g., ketoconazole.

Comparable degrees of T and B lymphocyte depletion are noted with this drug. If the drug is given immediately after antigen exposure, primary and secondary antibody responses can be suppressed. AZA can block de novo cutaneous delayed hypersensitivity but it affects secondary delayed hypersensitivity to a much lesser extent. AZA has little effect on established graft rejections or secondary responses. No effect on production and/or release of most lymphokines is observed. In vitro proliferative responses of lymphocytes to mitogens are not impaired.

AZA inhibits proliferation of promyelocytes in bone marrow, thus decreasing the number of circulating monocytes available to become macrophages in peripheral blood. Also, AZA decreases the number of mono-cytes and granulocytes available for migration into an area of inflammation. A major immunosuppressive effect of AZA may in fact be its inhibition of mononuclear cells and inflammatory responses.

CHLORAMBUCIL

Pharmacology

Seventy percent of orally administered chlorambucil (Fig. 33A-1) is absorbed, and absorption is rapid. It is rapidly and almost completely metabolized in unknown sites to its major metabolite, phenylacetic acid mustard, which is cytotoxically active, and several other poorly characterized inactive metabolites. Within 24 h 20 to 70 percent of the chlorambucil dose is eliminated in the urine, largely as poorly characterized metabolites. Less than 1 percent of chlorambucil and phenylacetic acid mustard appear in the urine. Neither fecal excretion nor the effect of renal or liver disease on the metabolism or efficacy of chlorambucil has been studied.

Mechanism of Action

This is not a well-studied area. Since chlorambucil is an alkylating agent, the mechanisms of action are considered to be similar to that of cyclophosphamide.

CYCLOPHOSPHAMIDE

Pharmacology

Orally administered cyclophosphamide (Fig. 33A-1) is almost completely absorbed. The pharmacokinetics of orally and intravenously administered cyclophosphamide are therefore similar. Cyclophosphamide is almost completely metabolized by the hepatic mixed-function oxidases in the liver to active (phosphoramide mustard) and inactive metabolites. Thirty-five percent of cyclophosphamide appears as inactive metabolites and up to 25 percent appears as cyclophosphamide itself in the urine, with small amounts appearing in feces, expired air, CSF, sweat, saliva, and synovial fluid. Cytotoxic material appears in breast milk and may induce leukopenia in breast-fed babies. Hemorrhagic cystitis is caused by the urinary metabolite acrolein, a side effect which can usually be abrogated by concurrent administration of Mesnex, a sulfhydryl compound which chemically binds and detoxifies these urotoxic metabolites.

Because some retention of cyclophosphamide and metabolites occurs in renal failure, initial doses of cyclophosphamide should be reduced by 25 to 50 percent. Hepatic enzyme induction (i.e., by phenobarbital) shortens the half-life of cyclophosphamide, but clinically

relevant cytotoxicity or toxicity is not altered. For reasons which are not understood, concomitant administration of allopurinol increases the chances of leukopenia.

Mechanism of Action

Although cyclophosphamide itself is not cytotoxically active, it is metabolized in the liver into active metabolites which cross-link DNA so that it cannot replicate. The drug is cell cycle–nonspecific in its action: cyclophosphamide is directly cytotoxic to dividing lymphocytes as well as to resting lymphocytes. Cyclophosphamide induces lymphocytopenia: B cells are apparently more affected than T cells; the effects on various T-cell subpopulations have not been well studied in humans. In the mouse, low doses (20 µg/kg) were shown to affect mainly suppressor T cells. Administration of such a low dose before antigen priming will augment antibody responses, and if injected after the drug, may interfere with the generation of suppression of a tolerogen.

Cyclophosphamide readily suppresses the primary immune response (cellular and humoral), especially if administered immediately after antigen challenge, but it also can inhibit an established immune response (both humoral and cellular). Cyclophosphamide effectively suppresses many cell-mediated immune responses such as delayed hypersensitivity skin tests, graft-versus-host reactivity of lymphoid cells, cell-mediated cytotoxicity, mitogen- and antigen-induced blastogenesis, and production of soluble mediators. Cyclophosphamide also has anti-inflammatory properties.

METHOTREXATE (MTX)

Pharmacology

The percent of orally administered MTX (Fig. 33A-1) which is absorbed decreases as the oral dose increases, with a range of 39 to 90 percent, in part because active absorptive transport becomes saturated and in part because MTX may be metabolized by the intestinal bacteria (10 to 35 percent of orally administered MTX may be so metabolized). Intracellular polyglutamation and enterohepatic recirculation may prolong retention and delay elimination of MTX and metabolites. Circumstances which prolong retention and delay elimination (e.g., ascites, azotemia, concomitant use of certain drugs) may markedly increase toxicity. The parent drug and the 7-hydroxy-MTX metabolite are cytotoxically active. The major route of excretion of MTX and its metabolites is through the kidney, with minute amounts of MTX appearing in breast milk, CSF, and saliva.

Concomitant administration of salicylates, other nonsteroidal anti-inflammatory drugs, probenecid, sulfonamides, and para-aminohippurate (PAH) may increase MTX toxicity by delaying MTX excretion and/or by displacing MTX from plasma proteins. By supplying folic acid in its active, reduced form, thereby bypassing the MTX-induced blockage of DNA synthesis, citrovorum factor (Leucovorin) can reduce the toxicity of MTX, particularly if administered within 24 h.

Mechanism of Action

MTX inhibits dihydrofolate reductase (DHFR), an enzyme necessary for the reduction of dihydrofolic acid (FH_2) to tetrahydrofolic acid (FH_4). FH_4 is converted to coenzymes required for 1-carbon transfer reactions involved in the synthesis of thymidine and thus DNA. The inhibition of DHFR by MTX therefore results in inhibition of the synthesis of DNA, RNA, and proteins, thereby decreasing cellular proliferation. MTX acts primarily in the S phase of the cell cycle (cell division), being active only in the period of maximal cell proliferation and DNA synthesis.

MTX can prevent, prolong, or delay a primary or secondary antibody response, but the suppression of the secondary response occurs to a lesser degree than that of the primary response. MTX may also prevent induction of a primary delayed hypersensitivity reaction, but it is a weak inhibitor of the secondary response. MTX has anti-inflammatory properties, which may in fact be responsible for much of its immunosuppressive action. It is a weak inhibitor of graft rejection.

CYCLOSPORINE

Pharmacology

Only 20 to 50 percent of orally administered cyclosporine (Fig. 33A-1) is absorbed—and erratically at that. Cyclosporine disappears slowly from the serum. Cyclosporine is very lipophilic, being associated with plasma lipoproteins (80 percent), other plasma proteins, and erythrocytes. It is widely distributed throughout the body and persists in body tissues for a considerable time after therapy is discontinued. Cyclosporine is metabolized by the hepatic mixed-function oxidases into at least 15 metabolites. Cyclosporine and metabolites are excreted largely via the biliary system, with only 6 percent of administered cyclosporine appearing in the urine.

Compounds which induce hepatic enzyme metabolism (i.e., rifampin, phenobarbital, and phenytoin) may lower cyclosporine concentrations, whereas drugs which inhibit hepatic metabolism (i.e., ketoconazole) may raise cyclosporine levels. Liver dysfunction may increase cyclosporine toxicity. Cyclosporine may induce nephrotoxicity, resulting in declining renal function, a situation which may necessitate reducing the dose or discontinuing cyclosporine to prevent further renal damage. Cyclosporine toxicity is not increased in the presence of renal failure. Very low cyclosporine concentrations appear in CSF and breast milk. Cyclosporine crosses the placenta.

Mechanism of Action

Cyclosporine passively crosses the cellular membrane into the cell, binding to a protein called cyclophilin. This cyclophilin-cyclosporine complex initiates inhibition of DNA transcription. That inhibition then prevents accumulation of mRNA for several cytokines. In this way cyclosporine abrogates several pathways for T-cell proliferation induced by antigen or mitogen. The specific sites of cyclosporine action include:

1. Inhibition of T-cell interactions with macrophages, which decreases their synthesis of IL-1
2. Prevention of the ability of IL-2-producing T lymphocytes to express IL-2 receptors
3. Suppression of synthesis and release of IL-2 by helper T cells
4. Rendering T cells unresponsive to IL-2

Cyclosporine inhibition of T lymphocytes occurs in the G_0 or G_1 phase (resting phases), during antigen-induced proliferation. It thus interferes with the differentiation of cytotoxic T-cell precursors into mature cytotoxic T cells. Cyclosporine does not inhibit cytotoxic activity of mature, proliferating cytotoxic T cells already generated. In essence, cyclosporine blocks the amplification of cellular immune responses and the generation of T-cell effectors (helper and cytotoxic) as well as other functions dependent on IL-2: i.e., cyclosporine inhibits production of antibody to T cell–dependent antigens by B cells, inhibits production of IFN-γ, and inhibits natural killer (NK) cells. Since T cells already primed are resistant to cyclosporine, cyclosporine must be present within the first 24 h of antigen stimulation for optimal suppression, since this is a critical period in the induction of the immune response (i.e., against an allograft).

The growth of bone marrow–derived myeloid, erythroid, or B-lymphocyte cell lines is not inhibited, and B-lymphocyte responses to T cell–independent antigens are not affected. Cyclosporine does not impair macrophage responses to lymphokines, but it is a strong inhibitor of delayed hypersensitivity.

PREDNISONE (PROTOTYPE CORTICOSTEROID)

Pharmacology

About 80 percent of prednisone (Fig. 33A-1) is absorbed when administered in 5- to 10-mg oral doses. Lesser percentages may be absorbed with higher oral doses. Prednisone is rapidly absorbed and rapidly transformed to its active metabolite, prednisolone. About 70 percent of circulating prednisolone is bound to transcortin (corticosteroid-binding globulin) and to a lesser extent to albumin. In the presence of hypoalbuminemia, however, the frequency of steroid side effects increases (i.e., serum albumin concentrations less than a 2.5 g/dL are associated with a doubling in the frequency of steroid side effects) presumably because more unbound corticosteroid is available. Prednisolone is inactivated (reduced and conjugated) in the liver by the hepatic mixed-function oxidase system and the metabolites are excreted in the urine. Induction of this enzyme system (as by phenobarbital) may reduce prednisolone's efficacy because prednisolone is more rapidly inactivated. Although liver dysfunction may delay conversion of prednisone to prednisolone, it does not appear to affect prednisone's efficacy or toxicity.

Mechanism of Action

Corticosteroids passively enter a target cell and bind to a hormone-specific cytoplasmic protein receptor which is then activated by dephosphorylation. The "activated" form is transferred to the nucleus where it binds to the nuclear chromatin. The bound activated complex then induces alterations of specific mRNAs. These hormone-regulated mRNAs then carry out the response to the corticosteroids by altering the rates of synthesis of protein.

In humans, corticosteroids act at multiple sites. The observed clinical actions undoubtedly reflect the net effect on different effector limbs of the immune network. The actions of corticosteroids can be grouped into the following three areas: (1) effects on leukocyte traffic; (2) effects on the preprogrammed functional capabilities of leukocyte effector cells; and (3) effects on soluble mediators of inflammation.

Leukocyte Traffic

Although cytolytic for lymphocytes in some species, corticosteroids are usually not cytolytic in humans. One major action of corticosteroids is induction of shifts in the traffic of leukocytes: the absolute and relative numbers of circulating eosinophils, basophils, monocytes, and lymphocytes are decreased and the absolute and relative numbers of granulocytes are increased at 4 to 8 h after administration of corticosteroids. All the cellular elements return to normal levels within 48 h. Among the lymphocyte populations affected by corticosteroids, T lymphocytes (CD4$^+$ helper lymphocytes in particular) leave the circulation and are sequestered in the bone marrow and lymph nodes, while B lymphocytes and most CD8$^+$ (suppressor) lymphocytes remain in the circulation.

Neutrophilic leukocytosis results from increased circulatory half-life of the neutrophils, increased release of neutrophils from bone marrow, and diminished emigration from circulation of neutrophils into inflammatory sites.

Function

Corticosteroids primarily alter the functions of monocytes, macrophages, and T lymphocytes; they have minimal effects on B lymphocytes. The effects of corticosteroids on the functions of monocytes and macrophages include inhibition of Ia expression, production of IL-2, antigen presentation, response of macrophages to migration inhibition factor, phagocytosis, digestion of antigen, and ability of monocytes to differentiate into macrophages. Corticosteroids also inhibit delayed hypersensitivity skin tests and decrease binding of immune complexes by Fc receptors on phagocytic cells.

Corticosteroids inhibit T-cell proliferation in the following ways: (1) by inhibiting IL-2 production, thereby decreasing the ability of T lymphocytes to proliferate and respond to antigens and mitogens; (2) by inhibiting the entry of T lymphocytes into the G_1 phase and the progression of activated cells from the G_1 to the S phase of the cell cycle; and (3) by rendering the IL-2-producing T-lymphocyte population unresponsive to IL-1.

Administration of corticosteroids decreases serum IgG, IgA, and IgM levels (maximally at 2 to 4 weeks). Corticosteroids can inhibit new antibody production, but they are poor inhibitors of secondary antibody responses.

Mediators

Corticosteroids do not block the interaction of antibodies with sensitized lymphocytes or the release of histamine or kinins that is initiated by this process. They do, however, block multiple tissue responses to these stimuli. For example, corticosteroids inhibit production and release of prostaglandins and leukotrienes (by inhibiting the enzyme phospholipase A), increase the number of β-agonist receptors on cell membranes, stabilize lysosomal membranes, and promote maintenance of capillary integrity and vascular tone.

ADVERSE EFFECTS OF IMMUNOSUPPRESSIVE AND IMMUNOMODULATORY DRUGS

On a theoretical basis it would seem reasonable to treat diseases manifesting significant autoimmune features with immunosuppressive or immunomodulatory drugs. There is now little doubt that many autoimmune diseases (including RA and SLE, as well as graft rejection) can be down-regulated by immunosuppressive drugs. Even though these drugs are clearly effective, the fact that they are terribly toxic markedly restricts their use (i.e., to patients with severe or fatal disease who have failed to respond to other, less toxic medications).

When using the immunosuppressive drugs available today, it is important to remember the history of their use in the past. Their clinical use was often dictated not so much by a clear understanding of their molecular mechanisms of action, but rather on whether their use in a few patients "worked." It was a purely empiric approach. The first well-known use of corticosteroids was in treating RA in the 1940s. The discovery and use of corticosteroids in clinical trials was a significant advance in medicine, ushering in the era of immunosuppressive therapy. It soon became evident, however, that corticosteroids are a double-edged sword: on the one hand, lives and vital organ functions can be saved by corticosteroids; on the other hand, their use is attended by significant morbidity and mortality, particularly when used for long periods of time and/or in moderately high doses (e.g., >20 mg prednisone per day). Because corticosteroids affect many metabolic and immunologic functions, their use is similar to using a shotgun to kill a flea: they are not specific in their immunosuppressive action. Of the adverse side effects of corticosteroids (see Table 33A-2), the problems with cataracts, hypertension, premature arteriosclerosis, myopathy, avascular necrosis, osteoporosis, and increased susceptibility to infection are the ones with gravest consequences.

The cytotoxic drugs (AZA, chlorambucil, cyclophosphamide, and MTX) were initially developed for treatment of cancer, mainly leukemia. During the period of early use, it was discovered (largely by serendipity rather than by plan) that they might be useful in the management of immune system–mediated disease. Their use also was empiric. The cytotoxic drugs were called "cytotoxic" because their key action relates to inhibition of cell division, which prevents new cell formation while allowing senescence and eventual death of the remaining cells. The tissues

TABLE 33A-2   Corticosteroid Toxicity

System	Effect
CNS	Psychiatric
	Benign intracranial hypertension
Ophthalmologic	Cataracts
	Glaucoma
Cardiovascular	Hypertension
	Premature arteriosclerosis
Gastrointestinal	Ulcerogenicity
	Intestinal perforation
	Pancreatitis
Musculoskeletal	Myopathy
	Avascular necrosis
	Osteoporosis
Metabolic-endocrine	Glucose intolerance
	Iatrogenic Cushing's syndrome
	Sodium retention
	Potassium wasting
	Growth failure (children)
	Obesity
Integumentary	Thinning
	Capillary fragility
	Acne
Immune	Increased susceptibility to infection

most susceptible to the cytotoxic effects of the drugs are those undergoing the most rapid cellular turnover, namely bone marrow cells, fetal cells, dermal epithelium, buccal and intestinal mucosa, mucosal cells of the urinary bladder, and hair follicles.

It is obvious, therefore, that the cytotoxicity of these drugs extends to tissues not involved in autoimmunity. This "shotgun" action accounts for many of the side effects listed in Table 33A-3. Among the most ominous adverse effects of the cytotoxic immunosuppression drugs are increased susceptibility to infection, hepatic toxicity with or without cirrhosis (especially with MTX and to a lesser extent AZA), infertility (with chlorambucil and cyclophosphamide), hemorrhagic cystitis and bladder cancer (with cyclophosphamide), teratogenicity (especially with MTX and to a lesser extent with chlorambucil and cyclophosphamide), and neoplasia (in treatment of conditions other than transplant, neoplasia occurs up to 2 to 10 times more frequently than normal with

TABLE 33A-3   Frequency of Toxicity of Cytotoxic Drugs

Toxicity	AZA	Cyclophosphamide	Chlorambucil	MTX
Toxicity common to all cytotoxic agents				
Dose-related marrow suppression	+ to + +	+ to + + +	+ + to + + +	+ to + +
Susceptibility to infection	+	+	+ +	+ to + +
GI intolerance	+ +	+ +	+	+ +
Rash	+	+ +	+ +	+
Toxicity not shared by all drugs				
Hepatic damage	+	0	0	+ to + + (m)
Oral ulcers	0	0	0	+ +
Hair loss	0	+ + +	+ to + +	+ to + +
Azoospermia or anovulation	0	+ + +	+ +	±
Cystitis (hemorrhagic, fibrotic)	0	+ + (m)	0	0
Teratogenesis	0	+ (m)	+ (m)	+ + + (m)
Neoplasia	+ (m)	+ (m)	+ (m)	0

Key: 0 = considered not to occur. + = toxicity present, but in <5%. + + = toxicity in 5–30%. + + + = toxicity in >30%. (m) = toxicity of major concern.

chlorambucil and cyclophosphamide and up to 3 times more frequently with AZA).

In contrast to the corticosteroids and the cytotoxic drugs (which are nonspecifically immunosuppressive in their modes of action) cyclosporine is truly an immunosuppressive drug: its major mode of action is to down-regulate the synthesis, release, and response to two lymphokines—IL-1 and IL-2. Nevertheless, it is in its own right a toxic medication, with the most significant tox-

icities being nephrotoxicity, neurotoxicity, and hepatotoxicity (Table 33A-4).

Because the toxicity of corticosteroids, cytotoxic drugs, and cyclosporine is so great, the indications for their use must be very compelling. It was the risks of cytotoxic therapy that prompted Schwartz to outline in 1971 the general guidelines for using cytotoxic therapy, most of which are still applicable today (Table 33A-5). Although his recommendations applied specifically to cy-

TABLE 33A-4   Cyclosporine Toxicity

System	Effect
Kidney	Azotemia (interstitial fibrosis)
	Hypertension
	Hyperkalemia
Neurologic	Tremor
	Convulsions
	Headache
	Paresthesias
GI System	Hepatotoxicity
	Anorexia
	Nausea, vomiting, diarrhea
	Gum hyperplasia
Integument	Hypertrichosis
	Acne
Neoplasia	Lymphoma
Miscellaneous	Flushing
	Cramps
	Breast fibroadenomas
	Increased susceptibility to infection

TABLE 33A-5   Guidelines for Use of Cytotoxic Therapy in Rheumatic Diseases

1. The disease being treated should be life-threatening or seriously crippling.
2. The lesions should be at least partially reversible.
3. The disease should be unresponsive to, or the patient intolerant of, conventional (less toxic) therapy.
4. Active infection should be absent when immunosuppressive therapy is instituted.
5. Objective parameters should be measured before and during therapy. If no response is evident, immunosuppressive therapy should be discontinued.
6. The patient should be fully informed of the potential risk of starting therapy as well as the potential consequences if immunosuppressive therapy is not employed.
7. Meticulous follow-up for signs of acute or chronic toxicity and infection is mandatory.

totoxic drugs, they apply in almost equal measure to corticosteroids and cyclosporine as well. The most important points to remember are as follows:

1. The level of treatment should equal the level of greatest morbidity and mortality of the disease in its untreated state.
2. The benefits should be greater than the risk.
3. Patients must be informed of the risks of immunosuppressive therapy and participate fully in the decision to institute therapy.

Clinical Aside 33A-1
Immunopharmacological Therapy of Systemic Lupus Erythematosus

May 1975

Mary Smith, a 24-year-old secretary, presents with a 3-month history of poorly described musculoskeletal aches and pains with stiffness in the joints in the morning, erythematous rashes on the face and extremities, and afternoon fevers. Six weeks ago she noted the onset of loss of hair and the first in a series of sores in her mouth. Laboratory tests reveal the following abnormal values: a low white blood cell count (WBC) of 2700, mild anemia (hemoglobin of 10.5 g/dL), positive antinuclear antibody, elevated levels of antibody to double-stranded DNA, and decreased levels of complement components. Normal pertinent laboratory values include urinalysis, renal function tests (creatinine of 0.8 mg/dL), chest x-ray, and electrocardiogram.

Ms. Smith meets American College of Rheumatology criteria for the diagnosis of systemic lupus erythematosus (SLE), a multisystem disorder commonly acknowledged to be the product of a deranged hyperactive immune system. When managing a multisystem autoimmune disorder such as SLE, it is important to remember that the level of treatment should be adjusted to the greatest level of morbidity and mortality expected from the disease in its untreated state: the benefit should clearly outweigh the risk. Although serologically her SLE is active, the level of clinical activity at this point is relatively minor. There is a reasonable expectation that her disease may not worsen and that the risks of starting corticosteroids or

other immunosuppressive drugs outweigh the potential benefits. A course of treatment with less risk is warranted: mild hydrocortisone cream for rashes; hydroxychloroquine (a noncytotoxic agent which may modify or lessen disease activity) for arthralgias, rashes, and alopecia; and anti-inflammatories for musculoskeletal pain. Her disease is nevertheless active and she will require close follow-up.

October 1978

Following her initial visit 3 1/2 years ago, Mary has done well using local skin creams and ibuprofen. She chose not to begin hydroxychloroquine because she feared the risk of damage to her eyes. In the interval, Mary has gotten married and is interested in having children. About 3 weeks ago, however, she reported the onset of mild fevers, increased joint pains, easy bruisability, and bleeding of the gums with tooth brushing. Two days ago she began coughing; she has chest pain on the left side which becomes worse when she coughs or takes a deep breath. Examination shows petechiae and purpura scattered over the body, a pleural friction rub, and evidence of pleural effusion. Chest x-ray confirms a pleural effusion on the left. Laboratory testing reveals a low WBC count of 2500, a platelet count of 10,000, and elevated levels of serum antibody to double-stranded DNA. Urinalysis and creatinine are normal.

Mary's SLE is again active; this time she has serositis with pleural effusion and severe thrombocytopenia, with evidence of a bleeding diathesis, that is potentially life-threatening (i.e., intracranial hemorrhage may occur). Clearly the risks are great enough to warrant the use of corticosteroids (but not cytotoxic agents at this time). Corticosteroids usually produce rapid results by raising the platelet count at the same time that anti-inflammatory effects normalize body temperature and correct serositis and pleural effusions. Corticosteroids can also be indicated for other complications as well, e.g., glomerulonephritis, cerebritis, myositis, pericarditis, and hemolytic anemia—all of which may lead to serious morbidity or early mortality.

For some of these complications, use of corticosteroids will result in normalization within several months or less, at which time the dosage can be reduced or the drug stopped altogether. Others are not so easily managed, and normalization would require large doses of corticosteroids for long periods, risking complications from the corticosteroids themselves. For such patients, the use of cytotoxic therapy is considered. In Mary's case, a short course of corticosteroids was anticipated.

September 1980

Mary responded well to prednisone 20 mg tid with normalization of platelet count and control of serositis, fever, and arthralgias. Within several months her prednisone was tapered to 20 mg qd and within 6 months to 10 mg qd. Attempts to lower corticosteroids further were met with recurrence of fevers, arthralgias, oral ulcers, and fleeting chest pains. The patient developed moon facies early in the course of corticosteroids along with increased blood pressure and glucose intolerance; these adverse effects disappeared when her prednisone was tapered to 10 mg qd. In the interval Mary had become pregnant, but had miscarried at 3 months. Within the last 2 weeks she has noted the onset of ankle swelling, increased rash, nocturia, fevers, body aching, and lymphadenopathy. Laboratory values now show leukopenia, anemia, hypoalbuminemia, RBCs and RBC casts in the urine, proteinuria (4+), and serum creatinine of 1.8 mg/dL. Glomerulonephritis secondary to SLE was suspected. A kidney biopsy confirmed that she had diffuse proliferative glomerulonephritis, a lesion which significantly increases the risk of renal failure and death.

Again Mary's SLE has flared. This time she has developed serious renal disease, a complication which usually worsens if not treated, resulting in death or renal failure and dialysis in a high percentage of patients. High-dose corticosteroids alone can improve the prognosis, but the high doses are required for long periods of time. Even with high doses of corticosteroids, a significant percentage of patients go on to death or renal failure. In the 1970s and 1980s several controlled studies of prednisone (with and without cytotoxic agents) were conducted. The results of long-term follow-up of patients studied at the National Institutes of Health (studies which account for about half the total number of patients in the United States who have been part of studies) are shown in Fig. 33A-A1. The studies show a trend toward benefit with prednisone coupled with AZA or cyclophosphamide over prednisone alone. The only regimen which was clearly superior to prednisone alone was the combination of oral prednisone with pulse cyclophosphamide (given as intravenous pulses once every 3 months). Unfortunately the advantages of the cytotoxic regimens were not really evident until years after they were instituted, at which time it became clear that the incidence of late renal failure was reduced by earlier treatment with cytotoxic drugs (particulary intravenously administered cyclophosphamide). At this time in the course of Mary's disease, intravenous cyclophosphamide plus prednisone is likely to have more benefit than risk, despite the fact that the risks of cyclophosphamide for a childless

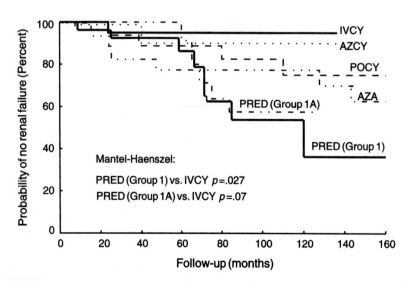

Figure 33A-A1 Probability of maintaining life-supporting renal function in 107 patients with active SLE-related nephritis, according to treatment group. (PRED denotes prednisone; AZA azathioprine; POCY oral cyclophosphamide; AZCY combined oral azathioprine and cyclophosphamide; and IVCY intravenous cyclophosphamide).

27-year-old female are considerable (probable sterility, possible hemorrhagic cystitis, increased susceptibility to neoplasia, increased risk of infection, acute hair loss, etc).

October 1987

Mary had refused to take cyclophosphamide in 1980 because of the potential side effects. She had, however, agreed to take AZA as well as oral prednisone. She was also given 1.0-g methyl prednisolone pulses IV periodically from 1980 to 1982 in an attempt to control her SLE nephritis. Initially she seemed to do reasonably well, but over the past 2 years her serum creatinine has climbed from 2.0 mg/dL to 5.6 mg/dL. Other features of her SLE have been relatively quiescent recently, and she is now no longer taking either prednisone or AZA. Her chronic azotemia is being managed by diet alone. She is hypertensive, but her blood pressure is controlled by medication. She has had three miscarriages and has no children of her bearing; however, she and her husband adopted a newborn 3 years ago.

Unfortunately, Mary's kidney disease was not controlled by our presently available immunosuppressive therapies. She is facing the prospect of dialysis in the near future and is being educated with that eventuality in mind. Her SLE is quiescent otherwise, an event that often accompanies azotemia in SLE. Further down the line, a renal transplant may be an option for her, an option she will probably be eager for since she is now a young mother. With a transplant she will again be faced with the prospect of taking immunosuppressive medication: namely prednisone, cyclosporine, and AZA. The management of renal transplantation is covered in Chap. 26.

SELF-TEST QUESTIONS

1. All of the following immunopharmacologic drugs are known to be associated with an increased risk of neoplasia except:
   a. Azathioprine
   b. Chlorambucil
   c. Cyclophosphamide
   d. Cyclosporine
   e. Prednisone

2. In contrast to the other immunopharmacologic drugs which interfere with many and multiple immunologic functions, this drug's main site of action is to interfere in the release of IL-2, a lymphokine essential in amplifying T-cell proliferation:
   a. Azathioprine
   b. Chlorambucil
   c. Cyclophosphamide
   d. Cyclosporine
   e. Methotrexate

3. Match the drug in the left column with the characteristic in the right:

   Column A

   a. Azathioprine
   b. Cyclophosphamide
   c. Cyclosporin
   d. Methotrexate
   e. Prednisone

   Column B

   ____ 1. Its introduction in the 1940s sparked the age of immunosuppressive therapies

   ____ 2. As the most specific immunopharmacologic drug discussed, it has as one of its major actions inhibition of IL-2 synthesis and release

   ____ 3. Concomitant administration of allopurinol increases its toxicity by inhibiting its metabolism by xanthine oxidase

   ____ 4. Is cytotoxic by virtue of its inhibition of the enzyme dihydrofolate reductase

   ____ 5. Its metabolites are cytotoxic by virtue of their ability to alkylate DNA

   ____ 6. Induces changes in leukocyte traffic (CD4$^+$ helper lymphocytes leave peripheral blood while CD8$^+$ suppressor lymphocytes remain in the circulation)

4. Which of the following is/are important guideline(s) when using cytotoxic drugs?
   a. The level of greatest morbidity and mortality of disease dictates the level of treatment
   b. Meticulous follow-up of patients for signs of toxicity and infection is essential
   c. Patients must be fully informed of the possible risks of therapy as well as of the consequences if cytotoxic therapy is withheld
   d. Patients should be intolerant of, or unresponsive to, less toxic therapy
   e. Organ dysfunction caused by disease should be at least partially reversible
   f. All of the above

5. The following is/are true statement(s) about cyclosporine treatment:
   a. Because cyclosprine is metabolized by xanthine oxidase, toxicity increases with allopurinol therapy
   b. Inhibits cytotoxic activity of mature, proliferating cytotoxic T cells
   c. Suppresses synthesis of IL-2 by helper-T lymphocytes
   d. Alters lymphocyte traffic by causing CD4$^+$ lymphocytes to leave the circulation while CD8$^+$ lymphocytes remain in the peripheral blood
   e. All of the above

6. The following is/are true statement(s) about corticosteroid actions:
   a. Inhibit Ia expression, production of IL-1, antigen presentation, and phagocytosis and digestion of antigen by monocytes
   b. Inhibit T-cell proliferation by inhibiting IL-2 production
   c. Render IL-2-producing T-lymphocyte population unresponsive to IL-1
   d. Decrease serum immunologlobulins
   e. Inhibit production and release of prostaglandins and leukotrienes
   f. All of the above

ADDITIONAL READINGS

Arnold M, Schreiber L, Brooks P. Immunosuppressive drugs and corticosteroids in the treatment of rheumatoid arthritis. *Drugs* 1988;36:350–363.

Britton S, Palacios R. Cyclosporin A—Usefulness, risks, and mechanism of action. *Immunol Rev.* 1982;65:5–22.

Clements PJ, Davis J. Cytotoxic drugs: Their clinical application to the rheumatic diseases. *Semin Arthritis Rheum.* 1986;15:231–254.

Katz P: Immunosuppressant therapy. *Adv Intern Med.* 1984;29:167–192.

Kovarsky J. Clinical pharmacology and toxicology of cyclophosphamide: Emphasis on use in rheumatic diseases. *Semin Arthritis Rheum.* 1983;36:359–372.

Tsukos GC. Immunomodulatory treatment in patients with rheumatic diseases: Mechanisms of actions. *Semin Arthritis Rheum.* 1987;17:24–38.

33

Immunomodulatory Therapy

B. Transfer Factors

INTRODUCTION

Transfer factors are families of small peptides that have the property of transferring the ability to express antigen-specific cell-mediated immunity from immunized donors to nonimmune recipients. To put this phenomenon in the proper context, one must briefly describe some of the observations that antedated the discovery of transfer factors (see Chap. 1). In the early 1900s it was shown that an intense inflammatory response developed when filtrates from cultures of mycobacteria were injected into the skin of animals with tuberculosis. If the injection site contained living mycobacteria, they were usually killed by the inflammatory response. Many attempts were made to transfer this form of immunologic inflammation to unimmunized recipients with the serum from immune donors, but the experiments always failed, and the nature of this form of immunity was not understood.

In 1942, Karl Landsteiner and Merrill Chase of the Rockefeller Institute for Medical Research reported that delayed-type hypersensitivity (DTH) to tuberculin and contact allergy to picryl chloride could be transferred from sensitized guinea pigs to unsensitized recipients with cells from peritoneal exudates. Thus, the "cell-mediated" basis of these reactions was established. Subsequent experiments established certain ground rules for transfer of cell-mediated immune responses. For example, it was found that to achieve successful transfers it was essential to use living, intact cells from hypersensitive donors. Moreover, for the recipient to remain sensitized to the test antigen for a long period of time, it was necessary to use syngeneic donor-recipient pairs.

Experiments that led to the discovery of transfer factors were begun in 1949 when H. Sherwood Lawrence of New York University Medical School reported that it was possible to transfer DTH from sensitized human donors to unsensitized human recipients with leukocytes from the peripheral blood. In contrast to the firmly established observations in guinea pigs, in human recipients the hypersensitive state persisted for many months even though the cell donors and recipients were unrelated. Subsequently, Lawrence and coworkers discovered two additional features of transfer of cell-mediated immunity in humans that were in contrast to the findings in guinea pigs. Transfer of DTH to recipients could be accomplished even when the donor cells were killed or disrupted by freezing and thawing. Especially surprising was the finding that a dialyzable material from the lysed leukocytes would transfer reactivity. These observations in humans were not readily accepted by the immunologists of the time, and even today the phenomenon of transfer factors is viewed with skepticism by some.

Fortunately, transfer factors have been the subject of careful scientific studies during the past decade, and many of their properties have been defined. Moreover, several carefully conducted clinical trials have shown that specific transfer factors have application in medicine as methods for correcting immunologic defects in patients with certain immunodeficiency diseases and for inducing prophylactic immunity against certain viral infections.

PROPERTIES OF TRANSFER FACTORS

Transfer Factors Are Derived from Antigen-Specific T Cells Transfer factors are products of specific antigen-primed T lymphocytes of immune donors. They are preformed in the cells of immune donors and are released by disrupting the cells. They may be separated from cell membranes and macromolecules such as histocompatibility molecules, polynucleotides, and large proteins by dialysis; the transfer factor molecules have low molecular weights and will pass through dialysis membranes. A rigorous procedure for final purification of transfer factors has been developed, but most of the clinical trials have been done with crude transfer factor–containing dialysates.

Transfer Factors Modify Cell-Mediated Immunity Only The immunologic effects of transfer factors are limited to cell-mediated immune responses. Transfer factors do not enhance antibody responses. Most of the clinical studies on the effects of transfer factors on immune responses have been conducted in immunodeficient patients with chronic or recurrent infectious diseases. Prior to treatment the patients were unable to express DTH to the infecting organism, and when their lymphocytes were exposed to antigens from the organism in vitro, they did not respond by proliferation, secretion of lymphokines, or expression of cytotoxic activity. After treatment with a specific transfer factor the recipients respond to the antigen by expressing DTH. Moreover, when their T lymphocytes are stimulated with the antigen in vitro, they respond by secreting lymphokines and expressing cell-mediated cytotoxicity. In most studies, recipients of transfer factors did not develop T lymphocytes that respond to antigens by proliferating. Thus, the pool of antigen-responsive cells does not expand (Fig. 33B-1). This may explain why sustained clinical benefits from transfer factor therapy require repeated administrations of the materials.

In vitro studies have shown that transfer factor–containing leukocyte dialysates may induce antigen responsiveness in T lymphocytes from unsensitized subjects. After incubation in the dialysates, the cells respond to stimulation with antigen by secreting a lymphokine known as *leukocyte migration inhibition factor (LMIF)*. However, the cells do not proliferate in response to the antigenic stimulation.

Transfer Factors Are Active against the Sensitizing Antigen Only The immunologic properties of transfer factors are antigen-specific. To obtain a specific transfer factor from T lymphocytes, the donor must have been sensitized to that antigen by immunization or natural exposure, and the sensitization must have produced cell-mediated immunity (in contrast to antibody synthesis) in the donor. Only the cell-mediated immune responses of the donors appear in the recipients. Unsensitized donors do not produce transfer factors. For example, a patient with chronic mucocutaneous candidiasis (an immunodeficiency syndrome described in Chap. 22A) who responds nicely to *Candida*-specific transfer factor may have a relapse of the infection when the regular donor is out of town and the patient receives transfer factor from a different, non-*Candida*-sensitized, donor. This is usually not a problem, however, as transfer factors are stable in the freezer for years.

The Antigen Specificity of Transfer Factors May Be Mediated by Antigen Binding Transfer factors bind to antigens in an immunologically specific manner. This property may be the mechanism that determines the antigen specificity of a transfer factor, and it must be closely related to the mechanism of action of transfer factors. In addition, these interactions have provided the basis for answering a key question about transfer factors. Some investigators had proposed that transfer factors were nonspecific adjuvants that functioned by amplifying cell-mediated immune responses. However, by exploiting the affinity of a transfer factor for its antigen, it has been possible to separate transfer factor molecules of a given specificity from mixtures containing several transfer factors. Not only does this finding argue strongly against the "adjuvant activity" hypothesis, but it also suggests that there are many transfer factors, probably one for each

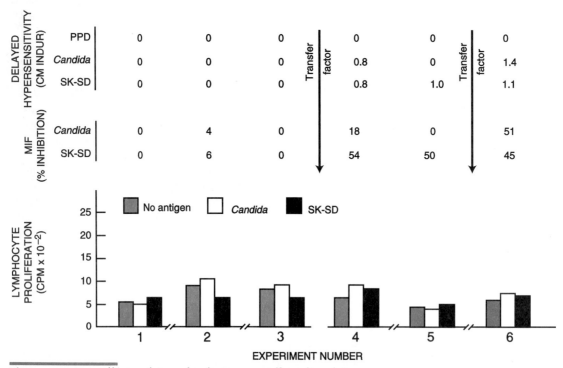

Figure 33B-1.   Effects of transfer factor on cell-mediated immune responses in chronic mucocutaneous candidiasis. The donor had cell-mediated immune responses to *Candida* and to streptokinase-streptodornase (SK-SD), but not to purified protein derivative (PPD). Antigen-specific delayed hypersensitivity and lymphokine production were transferred to the recipient, but the recipient's lymphocytes remained unresponsive to both antigens in the T-lymphocyte proliferation assay. Note that responsiveness to *Candida* was temporary but could be restored by administering more transfer factor.

antigenic determinant (epitope) that evokes a cell-mediated immune response.

Transfer Factors are Distinct from the Other Antigen-Binding Proteins Produced by B Cells and T Cells   Transfer factors are not antibodies or T-lymphocyte receptors. Even though transfer factors bind specifically to intact antigen molecules (like antibodies), they have several properties that make them unlike antibodies. For example, their molecular masses (about 5 kd) are much smaller than the smallest known antibody molecules (IgG molecules have a molecular mass of 160 kd). In addition, careful studies of serum from donors who had transfer factors in their T lymphocytes failed to demonstrate the presence of transfer factors in the serum. This is not the case with antibodies, which are found in the serum.

The direct interaction between transfer factors and intact antigen molecules is strong evidence against the notion that transfer factors are soluble T-lymphocyte receptors, since T-lymphocyte receptors do not bind free antigen (Chap. 7).

Transfer Factors Can Alter Genetically Determined Responses to Antigens   The intensity of immune responses by inbred animals is controlled by genes in the major histocompatibility complex (Chap. 4). Thus, a given strain of mouse or guinea pig may be a "low responder" to one antigen and a "high responder" to another antigen. A similar situation may occur in patients in whom poor responsiveness to antigens from an infectious organism may make them susceptible to chronic or repeated infections with that organism.

To learn about genetic factors that regulate production of transfer factors and the effects of transfer factors on recipients of high- or low-responder phenotypes, a series of experiments was done in inbred mice that were either high or low responders to the test antigens. The studies were done with synthetic antigens to rule out the possibility that the experimental animals had had any natural exposure to them. Briefly, it was found that high-responder donors made large amounts of transfer factor that was specific for the immunizing antigen. Low-responder donors made little or no transfer factor. The most important finding was that when a specific transfer factor from a high-responder donor was given to a low-responder recipient, the recipient responded to the antigen like a high responder. Thus, administration of this transfer factor changed the phenotype of the recipient to that of the high responder. While the mechanism of this effect is not yet known, it is probably important for understanding the effects of transfer factors in genetically-determined immune deficiency diseases.

Transfer Factors Are Polypeptides   Two transfer factors have been purified and have undergone chemical analysis although the primary structures are still unknown. Both are polypeptides with a molecular mass of approximately 5 kd (this corresponds to approximately 40 amino acids). These data are compatible with the reports that show that certain proteases are capable of degrading transfer factors to inactive molecules.

TRANSFER FACTORS IN CLINICAL MEDICINE

There have been several controlled clinical trials in which transfer factors were evaluated in patients with unusual susceptibility to infections with certain viruses or fungi. In a disease known as *chronic mucocutaneous candidiasis,* in which patients have subnormal immune responses to the yeast known as *Candida albicans,* a transfer factor from donors with cell-mediated immunity to this yeast was very effective in correcting the immunologic defect and prolonging remissions that were induced by antifungal drugs. Identical preparations from a donor who did not have cell-mediated immunity to *Candida albicans* were not effective, and beneficial effects only occurred in the recipients who acquired and maintained specific cell-mediated immunity.

The herpes simplex virus can cause chronic and recurrent skin, mucous membrane, and genital infections that have significant morbidity. Three independently conducted clinical trials have shown that a transfer factor from herpes simplex–immune donors will dramatically reduce the frequency and severity of exacerbations of these infections. In some patients complete remissions were observed.

In one study patients were treated alternately with transfer factor from a herpes-immune donor and an identical preparation from a donor who lacked such immunity. When they received the material from the nonimmune donors, relapses occurred. However, when they were retreated with the material from the immune donors, remissions were observed.

Chickenpox can be a serious, even life-threatening, infection in patients with defective cell-mediated immunity. A few years ago, transfer factor from a donor who had recovered from an infection with varicella-zoster virus was evaluated as a means for *prevention* of chickenpox infections in children with acute leukemia. This material was compared with a placebo preparation. Of the children who received the placebo, 15 had significant exposures to chickenpox and 13 of these developed infections. In contrast, in the transfer factor–treated patients, 16 had significant exposures and only 1 developed a clinical infection. These highly significan findings indicate that transfer factors ma provide a means for inducing prophylactic immunity in diseases for which there are no effective vaccines.

Certain patients with acquired immuno-deficiency syndrome (AIDS) become parasi-tized with cryptosporidia and have severe diarrhea and weight loss. Recently a transfer factor from donors with immunity to cryp-tosporidia was evaluated in AIDS patients with intestinal cryptosporidiosis. Six of seven patients had beneficial responses. A placebo preparation was not effective. These findings indicate that transfer factors may be helpful in treatment or even prevention of oppor-tunistic infections, even in patients with AIDS.

HOW DO TRANSFER FACTORS WORK?

The mechanisms by which transfer factors affect the immune system are still unknown. However, from the properties of transfer fac-tors described above, it is possible to make some speculations. First, all models for the mechanisms of action must consider the evi-dence that the effects of transfer factors are antigen-specific. It has also been appreciated that the effects are limited to the effector functions of T lymphocytes such as produc-tion of lymphokines and cell-mediated cy-totoxicity. Therefore, the ultimate target cells for the action of transfer factors must be T lymphocytes.

The finding that transfer factors interact with antigens in an immunologically spe-cific manner must be essential to the mech-anism of action. Since the classical T-lym-phocyte receptors do not interact with native antigens, transfer factors may serve as or in-duce an alternative pathway for antigen rec-ognition by T cells. This mechanism would explain the induction of specific antigen re-sponsiveness in genetically determined low-responder animals. Identification of such a

pathway, if it exists, could be an important discovery in cellular immunology.

SELF-TEST QUESTIONS*

For each of the following, choose the letter of the appropriate combination of correct completions or responses
  A. a, b, and c are correct.
  B. a and b are correct.
  C. b and d are correct.
  D. d is correct.
  E. All are correct.

1. Transfer factors are antigen-specific pro-teins that have the following immuno-logic properties:
   a. Specificity
   b. Induction of delayed-type hypersen-sitivity
   c. Induction of lymphokine production
   d. Induction of antibody production
2. By correcting specific immunologic de-fects, transfer factors have been shown to have efficacy in treatment and/or pro-tection of:
   a. Fungal infections such as chronic mucocutaneous candidiasis
   b. Recurrent infections with herpes simplex
   c. Treatment of cryptosporidiosis
   d. Bacterial meningitis

ADDITIONAL READINGS

Kirkpatrick CH. Delayed hypersensitivity. In Samter M, Talmage DW, Frank MM, Austen KF, Claman HN, eds., *Immunological Diseases.* Bos-ton: Little, Brown; 1988: 261–277.

*Answers will be found in Appendix E.

Kirkpatrick CH. Transfer factor. *J Allergy Clin Immunol* 1988; 81:803–813.

Lawrence HS. Transfer factor in cellular immunity. In *The Harvey Lectures*, Series 68. New York: Academic Press; 1974: 239–350.

Rozzo SJ, Kirkpatrick CH. Purification of transfer factors. *Mol Immunol.* 1992; 29:167–182.

Rozzo SJ, Merryman CF, Kirkpatrick CH. Murine transfer factor, IV: Studies with genetically regulated immune responses. *Cell Immunol* 1988; 115:130–145.

34

The Clinical Use of Intravenous Gamma Globulin

INTRODUCTION

Our contemporary approach to the use of antibodies for passive protection developed rapidly when all aspects of fluid replacement for the severely injured became matters of such urgency in the early days of the Second World War that a special laboratory to study such problems was established in New York. It was here in 1940, under the leadership of Cohn, that the antigen-specific immunoprotective properties of serum ("antibodies"), known since 1938 to reside in the gamma globulin (γ-globulin) fraction of the serum proteins, were further studied. Serum proteins could be separated according to their mobility in an electric field. Globulins could be subdivided by such a technique into clearly distinct, although overlapping, α-, β-, and γ-globulin bands. The New York scientists found that they could extract and concentrate γ-globulins from serum without damaging their antibody properties and prepare the therapeutically useful concentrated (16 g/100 mL) γ-globulin product still widely used today. Concentrated from pooled and convalescent serum, such γ-globulin preparations were shown to be of use for the prophylaxis and treatment of many infections such as measles, poliomyelitis, and hepatitis A.

It was immediately obvious that a γ-globulin preparation which could be administered intravenously would be advantageous, as the viscosity and the necessary limitation on the volume which could be administered intramuscularly compromised the usefulness of the product. Cohn's "fraction II" could not be administered intravenously as all too often such attempts, whether deliberate or inadvertent, led to an anaphylactoid response with the potential for inducing shock. Today, we understand that protein aggregates in the concentrated preparation can spontaneously activate the complement cascade. Two components of the classical pathway for complement, C3 and C5, when activated, affect smooth muscle and blood vessels in the airways in a manner similar to histamine and the other vasoactive compounds that can be released from mast cells and basophils.

Many years of immunochemical research were to be required before a concentrated, biologically active and safe preparation of γ-globulin suitable for intravenous (IV) use was to become available.

IMMUNOGLOBULIN ANATOMY

The γ (*gamma*) in γ-globulin refers to a specific region on an electrophoretic strip wherein one may find certain proteins when serum is subjected to an electric current; this clustering is due to the similar mobility properties of the γ-globulin proteins. There are five distinct immunoglobulins that overlap in this region; they are designated by the letters M, G, A, D, and E, each of which refers to a specific class of immunoglobulin. By far the predominant class in serum is IgG, and the immunoprotective properties of γ-globulin are almost entirely due to the presence of this molecule. For this reason, immunochemists preparing γ-globulin for IV use attempt to supply only purified IgG. However, even in our most sophisticated products, small amounts of other immunoglobulin classes will be found.

The basic anatomy of immunoglobulins is described in detail elsewhere in this book (Chap. 3). It is important to emphasize here, however, that the antigen-binding site for a given antigenic determinant is identical throughout the five immunoglobulin classes. This fact is important when considering the immunomodulatory properties of intravenously administered IgG. Amino acid sequences in the Fc portion determine the class of the molecule and, perhaps more importantly, the abilities that the molecule has to remove and destroy bound antigen and to interact with regulatory loops that control immune responses (Fig. 34-1).

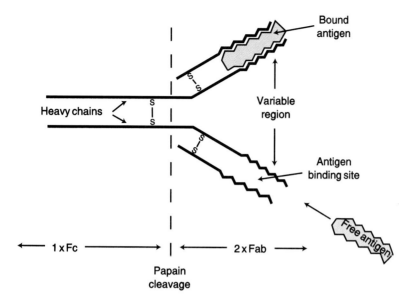

Figure 34-1   The basic anatomy of an immunoglobulin molecule. Two heavy and two light chains of amino acids are linked, shown by disulfide (S—S) bridges. At one end of the molecule, three-dimensional steric configuration (idiotypic determinant) allows one (and only one) antigen to enjoy best-fit status (complicated key into complicated lock). The molecule can be further subdivided by digestion with papain. Two fractions that have antibody activity will be formed (Fab), and one fraction that tends to crystalize (Fc) will be formed. The amino acid sequence of the latter determines the major functional activity of the molecule.

During evolution, four subtle variations on the IgG theme resulted in the production of four subclasses of the molecule. Subtle changes in the amino acid sequence and disulfide-binding arrangements create these differences. The clinical importance of these subclasses has become clearer in recent years, and this new appreciation of their specific roles is of considerable importance in developing ideal replacement and immunomodulatory strategies with γ-globulin. The major distinctions of the four subclasses are presented in Table 34-1.

From the 12th week of gestation, the human fetus is capable of producing immunoglobulin. At birth, the challenge initiated by encounters with antigens activates an obligatory maturational sequence in which babies must make IgM immunoglobulins before they can produce IgG, and indeed, IgG before they can product IgA. It is not until the third month of life that IgG production is adequate. To ensure protection during these vulnerable phases, all classes of maternal IgG cross the placenta from the 8th week of gestation. Transplacental passage accelerates toward the end of pregnancy so that full-term babies are normally born with adult levels of serum IgG, all of maternal origin. Premature babies are born with proportionately reduced amounts of IgG. Secretory IgA, contained in colostrum and breast milk, is necessary to complete the humoral immune protection of a neonate. For further discussion of the capacity of infants and children to make antibodies, refer back to Chap. 28.

TABLE 34-1   Immunoglobulin Subclasses

Subclass	Function	Half-Life, Days × 10⁻³	Molecular Weight per Cell of RES*	Receptors, mg/dL†	Serum
IgG1	Tissue protection, activation of complement	21 ± 5	146	31×10^3	900
IgG2	Response to polysaccharide antigens, activation of complement	20 ± 2	146	100×10^3	300
IgG3	Tissue protection, virus neutralization,‡ activation of complement	7 ± 1	165§	34×10^3	100
IgG4	Tissue protection, binding to mast cells, protection of respiratory tract	21 ± 2.5	146	21×10^3	50

*Cells of the RES have receptors for the Fc protion of IgG subclasses.
†There is considerable physiologic variation in these values.
‡*Virus neutralization* refers to the property of binding viruses before they gain entry to potential host cells; this neutralizes the viruses.
§IgG3 is unique in having 10 or more disulfide bridges binding the heavy and light chains together.

CHEMICAL MODIFICATION OF IgG FOR INTRAVENOUS USE

The challenge to the chemists attempting to produce a concentrated form of IgG for intravenous use was considerable. The first essential was to avoid the formation of spontaneously occurring IgG aggregates in the concentrated material. Such aggregates could spontaneously activate the complement cascade. Some activated complement components, especially C3 and C5, can produce an anaphylactoid-like response because of their affects on smooth muscle. The specific geographic regions of the IgG molecule, referred to as *domains*, are detailed in Chap. 3. For our purposes here, it is important to realize that the three constant domains and the one variable domain must all remain intact if concentrated IV preparations of γ-globulin (IVIG) are to retain all the biologic activity of the natural products. In addition, while concentrating IgG, special care had to be taken to protect the hinge region which gives the molecule flexibility, an essential property for a two-armed (bivalent) molecule that must be able to bind to moving membranes.

The second and third constant domains of the heavy chain of IgG must be intact if immunoglobulin is to bind to receptors for the Fc portion of IgG found on many cells of the reticuloendothelial system (RES). The binding of IgG to phagocytic and cytotoxic cells expressing Fc receptors is an essential step if antigen is to be destroyed and eliminated. Numerous cells in the body carry on their membranes receptors for the Fc portion of an IgG molecule (FcR). While some FcRs bind free IgG, most bind Fc more efficiently if the antibody molecule has bound antigen. When this occurs, a configurational change develops in the Fc fraction which facilitates binding to FcR. Three distinct forms of receptor for the Fc portion of IgG are recognized, and their distribution is compartmentalized. More is known of the structure of these Fc receptors and the cells which bear them than of the functional mechanisms activated when they bind. We do know, however, that the binding of antigen-antibody complexes by such receptors has at least three important functions:

1. The cells of the RES (scavenger cells) can bind complexes and subsequently experience an intracytoplasmic oxidative burst

that is important if phagocytosis is to proceed efficiently.

2. Lymphocytes are driven to make an antigen-specific response when antigen cross-links receptors for antigen on their surface. A lymphocyte can either be activated or deactivated if an immune complex of antigen and IgG is able to link membrane receptors for antigen and the Fc portion of IgG.

3. Some regulatory thymus-derived T cells have receptors for the Fc portion of IgG, and indeed other classes of immunoglobulin, and binding of critical concentrations of antigen-antibody complexes may activate important regulatory mechanisms which can block antigen-specific as well as class-specific reactions. All these mechanisms are likely to be important when large amounts of IgG are infused intravenously to treat an immunopathologic process. The Fc portion of the concentrated material also appears to be essential when complexes consisting of antibody and idiotype and anti-idiotype must interact with regulatory T cells to manipulate the immune system (see below).

At this writing, a number of commercially available preparations of γ-globulin suitable for IV use can be rated as excellent. A partial list appears in Table 34-2. These immunoglobulins meet, and in many cases exceed, the WHO criteria for such products, listed in Table 34-3. Most successful approaches to the production of a concentrated form of IgG

TABLE 34-3 WHO Standards for IVIG

1. At least 90% IgG as monomer
2. Less than 10% split products
3. Less than 5% aggregates
4. Minimal spontaneous anticomplementary activity
5. Free of pyrogens and vasoactive molecules
6. Subclass representation similar to normal serum
7. Fc and C3b mechanisms for opsonization activated
8. No isohemagglutin activity
9. Biologic half-life that exceeds 14 days

suitable for IV use have utilized (1) gentle enzymatic degradation of the immunoglobulin molecule using either pepsin or plasmin; (2) chemical modification of the base molecule using sulf-β-propriolactone; (3) reduction and alkylation; or (4) a concentration under low-pH conditions and treatment with polyethylene glycol (PEG).

The best products currently available have all four subclasses of IgG present and biologically active in near-normal concentrations.

RELEVANT ASPECTS OF IMMUNOREGULATION

There is a similarity between control of the human immune system and control of the human autonomic nervous system. A complex, simultaneous, and vital interplay of stop-and-go signals provides the balance and appropriateness to the degree of inflammation generated at any given time in response to antigen. Discipline is essential, given the de-

TABLE 34-2 IgG Preparations Suitable for IV Administration

Producer	Country of Origin	Process Used
Sandoz	Switzerland	pH₄; pepsin
Cutter	United States	pH₄; sugar
Scottish Blood Transfusion Service	United Kingdom	pH₄; pepsin
Green Cross Glycol (PEG)	Japan	Polyethylene
Armour	United States	PEG
Immuno	Austria	PEG/hydrolase
Alpha Therapeutic	United States	PEG
Baxter Travenol	United States	Chromatography

struction of innocent-bystander tissue which can result if an overenthusiastic immune response occurs. In addition, there is a constant need to ensure that we only attack foreignness. Current thinking about immunopathology is that inadequate immunoregulation is the fundamental cause of clinical immunologic problems, except in cases of primary and secondary immunodeficiency states. Immunoregulation is discussed in detail elsewhere in this book; only the major concepts relevant to our discussion are included here.

Immunologic control involves many separate and interacting mechanisms, but specific regulatory T cells appear to carry the major responsibility for keeping our immunologic house in order. This concept is important for our discussion, for as we will see, IgG appears to be involved in the regulation of both allergic and autoimmune responses. *Allergy* (*allos*, "altered"; *ergos*, "energy") is commonly equated with IgE-mediated immediate hypersensitivity reactions, although this was not the intent of the originator of the term. With the increasing recognition that undisciplined and even chronic release of cytokines may produce disease in a manner analogous to the problems associated with the undisciplined release by IgE-antigen complexes of the histaminelike reagents of basophils and mast cells, the concept of T-cell allergy has become increasingly relevant.

While there is no doubt that direct antigen binding to a receptor for that antigen on the membrane of regulatory T cells (T-cell receptor [TCR]) activates those cells, many other important immunoregulatory loops are known. IgG is involved in immunoregulation via at least two distinct mechanisms.

1. The manipulation by antigen-antibody complexes of FcR for IgG on phagocytic B and T cells
2. The manipulation of the idiotype network by IgG anti-idiotypic antibodies

Imagine you administer a shot of tetanus toxoid. To any one of the thousands of antigenic determinants injected, a specific inducer T and B cell will react with the eventual production of IgG antibody to antigen. While such antibody will bind with antigen, a specific family of inducer T and B cells are present within our antigen recognition repertoire that can recognize the idiotypic portion of the antitetanus antibody just described. In many cases, an anti-idiotypic antibody will carry an idiotypic region of its own that must be identical, in a three-dimensional sense, to the antigen that initiated the reaction in the first place ("internal image" idiotype). Such antibodies can be used as antigen and have indeed been used as vaccines. (See Figs. 34-2 to 35-5.)

We constantly make small amounts of antibodies to sequences of our own tissue proteins. We constantly make anti-idiotypic antibodies to these autoantibodies to prevent any significant immunologic attack on self. In normal serum, we can find trace amounts of both autoantibodies and anti-idiotypic antibodies capable of binding to these autoantibodies. It follows that the concentrated IgG preparations available for IV use will contain a vast library of antibodies capable of reacting with thousands of determinants because of the diversity of the experience of the thousands of donors who contribute to the pool. Among such antibodies will be many molecules with anti-idiotypic specificity. Anti-idiotypic antibodies manipulate the immune system in at least three ways. First, they can have a "neutralizing" effect; e.g., they can "neutralize" autoantibody by forming an idiotype–anti-idiotype dimer. This may prevent autoantibody binding to antigen and facilitate the clearance of the antibody complex when the Fc portions involved bind to FcR on cells of the RES. Secondly, anti-idiotypic antibodies may bind to the B-cell receptor for antigen (an immunoglobulin) and down-regulate the immune response. This may occur when dimers consisting of idiotype and anti-idiotype in the serum bind to the B-cell FcR or when an anti-idiotypic antibody "bridges" the receptors for antigen and the FcR portion of IgG. It has been shown that under certain circumstances, such binding may inhibit antibody synthesis by a

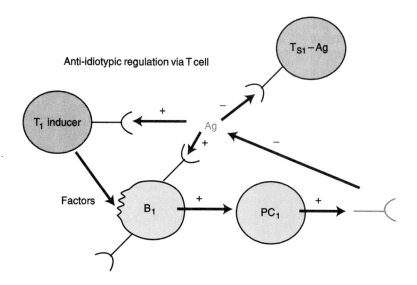

Figure 34-2 The secretion of antibody specific for antigen. Antigen (Ag) binds to specific receptors on the inducer T cell (T_1) which supplies permissive signals to the B cell (B_1) that allows it to divide to form a plasma cell (PC_1) that will secrete antibody. Simultaneously, Ag interacts with a specific suppressor T cell (T_{s1}–Ag) that regulates the response.

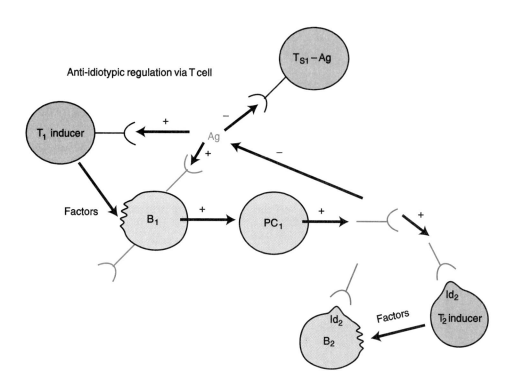

Figure 34-3 Initiation of an anti-idiotypic response. Antibody secreted by PC_1 is recognized by a second inducer T cell (T_2), which carries a membrane-specific receptor for the antibody. It gives permissive signals to a B cell (B_2) capable of recognizing the idiotypic determinant of the first antibody. The idiotypic determinant on T_2 and B_2 recognizing antibody is Id_2.

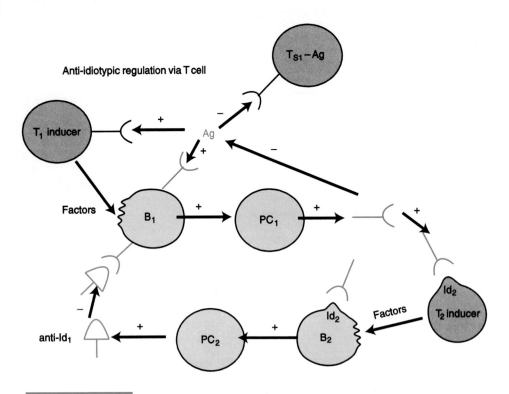

Figure 34-4 Secretion of anti-idiotypic antibody. B_2 divides to form a plasma cell (PC_2) that secretes an anti-idiotypic antibody (reactive with the antibody from PC_1). This second antibody (αID_1) "looks like" antigen and so can bind to the receptor for Ag on B_1. This interaction can augment, but more usually suppresses, the formation of the first antibody.

blockade of the phosphatidyl inositol cascade. Finally, anti-idiotypic antibodies can activate antigen-specific immunoregulatory T cells directly.

MECHANISMS PRODUCING IMMUNOMODULATION BY IVIG

It has been observed that the administration of IVIG alters T-cell, B-cell, monocyte, macrophage, and neutrophil function, but the mechanisms producing these alterations are not at all well defined. Direct analysis of these potential mechanisms in the diseases we have discussed (listed in Table 34-4) lends support

to only two: (1) an interaction of IgG with FcR on the membrane of various cells and (2) the manipulation by anti-idiotypic antibodies of both activated and autoreactive cells and secreted autoantibodies.

Evidence for Immunomodulation by FcR Blockade

Theoretically, cells such as platelets, when coated with autoantibody, would be less likely to be attacked and destroyed by cells of the RES were the receptors for the Fc portion of IgG on reticuloendothelial cells saturated by intravenously administered IgG. FcR blockade can be demonstrated after the administration of IVIG, and the survival time of in-

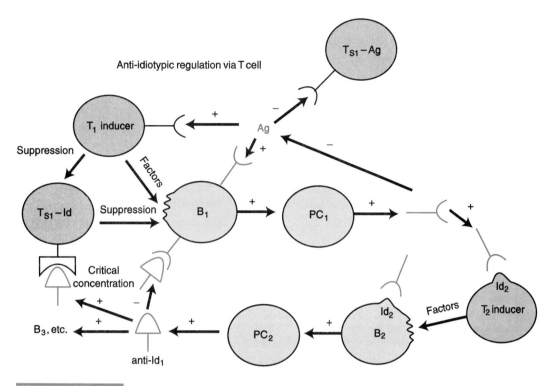

Figure 34-5 Down-regulation by anti-idiotypic antibody. The second antibody (αId_1) will be recognized by a specific B and T cell and so the chain reaction will continue. More importantly, αId_1 binds to a specific receptor for this product on another regulatory T cell (T_{s1}–Id). After interaction this cell can suppress both T_1 and B_1 and block the continuation of the original reaction to Ag.

fused red cells coated with anti-Rh D antibodies is significantly longer if the infusion of these antibody-coated cells follows the administration of IgG. In vitro experiments show that monocyte binding of IgG-

platelet complexes is blocked by IVIG. Thus it is likely that in some clinical situations, blocking of FcRs on cells of the RES produces a clinically beneficial effect. However, such a blockade cannot explain the long-term benefits that follow the administration of IVIG in a number of disease states. The regeneration of certain FcR receptors can be slow, but there is general agreement that while some immediate benefit, such as the rise in the platelet count within hours of the administration of IVIG to patients with autoimmune thrombocytopenic purpura, could represent FcR blockade, other important mechanisms must be operating in the establishment of long-term remissions. In some autoimmune cytopenias, blockade of FcRs is not associated with any clinical

TABLE 34-4 Secondary Immunodeficiencies Requiring IVIG

Malignant states
  Chronic lymphatic leukemia
  Multiple myeloma
  Acute lymphatic leukemia
  Non-Hodgkin's lymphoma
Post-bone marrow transplant
Premature infants
After severe burns or blunt trauma
In combination with antibiotic therapy
Following plasmapheresis

improvement. If the platelets and neutrophils which express FcR bound IVIG via those FcRs, they might be protected from autoantibodies if the bound IgG sterically hindered auto-antibody binding. There are, however, no experimental data to support this possibility.

Evidence for Immunomodulation by Anti-Idiotypic Antibodies

IgG dimers are plentiful in IVIG preparations which may be constituted from a pool contributed to by 10,000 or more donors. Such dimers represent idiotype–anti-idiotype reactions, which demonstrates clearly that anti-idiotypic antibodies are present in these preparations. The likely importance of anti-idiotypic antibodies in IVIG was first considered when it was noted that patients with autoantibodies to factor VIII cleared 95 percent of such antibody from their serum within 36 h of receiving IVIG. Some patients have not reproduced anti-factor VIII antibodies in their serum for 5 years following the administration of IVIG. F(ab')₂ fragments from IVIG could be shown to bind to and neutralize the ability of F(ab')₂ fragments prepared from antibody to factor VIII in the serum of patients. This observation has been extended to a number of other disease-associated autoantibodies. Thus, F(ab')₂ preparations of IVIG have inhibited the binding to their targets of antibodies to thyroglobulin, DNA, intrinsic factor, a target antigen for the autoantibodies present in chronic inflammatory demyelinating polyneuropathy, and the cytoplasmic neutrophil antigen which reacts with autoantibodies present in the serum of many patients with Wegener's granulomatosis. It has been noted that when IVIG F(ab')₂ from a particular batch of IVIG would not bind to the F(ab')₂ of a particular patient's disease-associated autoantibody, clinical improvement did not follow infusion of that IVIG product.

Further evidence for the presence of F(ab')₂ fragments in IVIG, with a high affinity for the F(ab')₂ of autoantibody, has been produced by experiments in which serum containing a known autoantibody was passed over a column of sepharose complexed to F(ab')₂ from IVIG. Acid elution of the F(ab')₂ bound to such a column was associated with a remarkable increase in the concentration of autoantibody.

It is possible that the F(ab')₂ fraction of some antibodies in IVIG could bind to non-idiotypic (allotypic) regions of a particular autoantibody. While such binding would not explain the inhibition of autoantibody binding to a specific target, it could explain the clearance of autoantibody from the serum. However, no antibody to these allotypic regions of IgG have been found in any IVIG product.

Recently, an intriguing study revealed that F(ab')₂ preparations from IVIG products capable of binding to the idiotypic region of a specific autoantibody could in fact bind to the F(ab')₂ region of a number of other autoantibodies, suggesting that there exists some shared privileged sites in the idiotypic region of a number of autoantibodies that can be targeted by immunoregulatory anti-idiotypic antibodies. Thus, an F(ab')₂ molecule in IVIG that can react with the F(ab')₂ region of antibody to thyroglobulin can also react to the F(ab')₂ region of antibody to factor VIII. Shared amino acid sequences in the idiotypic region of a number of autoantibodies would markedly increase the overall efficiency of immunoregulatory anti-idiotypic molecules recognizing such shared sequences.

Anti-idiotypic antibodies capable of binding to the idiotypic region of a specific autoantibody can be found in IVIG and the serum of patients recovering from a disease which featured that autoantibody. They cannot be found in the serum of individual healthy subjects. Healthy individuals do produce anti-idiotypic antibodies capable of binding with autoantibodies in their serum not associated with the production of autoimmune disease. It is likely that this interaction is responsible for the harmlessness of such "naturally" occurring autoantibodies. The idiotypic sequences of disease-associated autoantibodies is different from those of "natural" autoantibodies found in the serum of healthy individuals. Thus it is likely that anti-idiotypes in IVIG capable of interacting with the F(ab')$_2$ region of disease-associated auto-antibodies is provided by donors who have either recovered from a disease associated with a particular autoantibody or who have controlled it at a subclinical level.

INDICATIONS FOR THERAPY WITH IVIG

The advantages of using an IV rather than an intramuscular (IM) γ-globulin preparation are obvious. Indeed, IV preparations are now clearly the choice for the management of severe hypogammaglobulinemic states associated with either primary or secondary immunodeficiencies. We will discuss these and then look at the perhaps more interesting subject of the use of supraphysiologic doses of IgG to produce an immunomodulatory effect. To refresh your memory about immunodeficiency syndromes, review Chaps. 22A and B.

IVIG in the Management of Primary Immunodeficiency States

Of the primary immunodeficiencies, defects in humoral immunity are most common. Early diagnosis and adequate IgG replacement therapy have revolutionized the outlook for individuals troubled by such disorders. Soon after the recognition in 1952 of the existence of antibody deficiency states, replacement therapy with IM γ-globulin began. The difficulty of giving sufficient amounts of IM γ-globulin to maintain adequate levels of IgG, especially in children, was recognized as the major problem with this form of therapy. In the late 1960s attempts to solve this problem involved the infusion of fresh frozen plasma. Certainly, the results in adults were better than those obtained with IM γ-globulin, but volume restrictions limited the use of fresh frozen plasma in very young children. With plasma therapy there was a considerable danger of developing non-A, non-B hepatitis, even when a "buddy system" was used in which a select

population of healthy volunteers repeatedly supplied the plasma for an individual patient. Certainly, the higher IgG levels achieved in adults by this technique, and the better health that resulted, demonstrated the desirability of using a preparation that keeps the IgG level of patients with hypogammaglobulinemia in the physiologic range. The currently available IVIG preparations allow us to safely and effectively supply any desired concentration of serum IgG to patients of any age.

Shortly after infusing IgG intravenously, 100 percent of the γ-globulin can be found in the intravascular space. Over the next 3 days, the infused material equilibrates within the extravascular pool, which is primarily extracellular. At equilibration, as much as 85 percent of the infused material remains within the vascular compartment. The catabolism of the IgG that then circulates is primarily Fc-mediated, since cells of the RES remove IgG after it binds to their Fc receptors. Uptake by such cells is concentration-dependent, and although a half-life for IgG and its subclasses can be calculated, the disappearance curves do not precisely conform to the kinetics of a true equilibrium state. This is probably related to the fact that Fc receptors are regulated up and down by IgG itself and, undoubtedly, to other factors associated with the need to produce an inflammatory response. The half-lives listed in Table 34-2 are accurate for the subclasses as a whole, but it is important to realize that the most important factor modulating half-life will be encounter with antigen. Inherent in the successful use of any sort of passive protection is a realization that additional replacement will be needed should antibody be removed from the circulation by interaction with a specific antigen.

IVIG for the Management of Secondary Immunodeficiencies

Replacement therapy with γ-globulin for secondary immunodeficiency states (listed in Table 34-4) is an important subject, for these secondary deficiencies occur much more frequently than do primary immunodeficiencies. Seventy percent of patients with chronic lymphatic leukemia, a B-cell malignancy, eventually develop significant hypogammaglobulinemia. This secondary immunodeficiency is particularly dangerous when patients are treated with chemotherapeutic and immunosuppressive regimens in an attempt to control the end stages of the leukemic proliferation of B cells. A similar situation occurs in many patients with multiple myeloma. Behind the monoclonal IgG spike, which is most frequently present in such patients, the levels of serum polyclonal IgG may be in the hypogammaglobulinemia range. Again, it is when chemotherapy is used for the treatment of myeloma that there is significant increased hazard of overwhelming infection in such patients. Recent trials strongly suggest that the dangers referred to can be minimized by beginning adequate replacement therapy with IVIG before initiating chemotherapy.

Many preparations of concentrated γ-globulin suitable for IV use have high titers of antibody against the viruses of the herpes family. γ-Globulin, extracted from plasma pooled from a large number of donors, may well have titers of antibody to the varicella-zoster virus that approach those found in zoster immunoglobulin. It seems likely that IVIG will afford significant protection from varicella-zoster infection for patients with acute lymphatic leukemia and non-Hodgkin's lymphoma, who normally experience considerable morbidity and occasionally die from an exacerbation of their infection with this virus. While some controversy still surrounds the ideal way to use IgG to prevent cytomegalovirus infection after bone marrow transplants, a number of studies now suggest that prophylaxis with IVIG may be important, and there seems little doubt that IVIG therapy acts synergistically with the anticytomegalovirus agent ganciclovir.

Premature infants may be born with significant hypogammaglobulinemia because of a failure of sufficient maternal IgG to cross the placenta. In western countries, because of the excellence of nursing care available

and the newer generations of antibiotics, the morbidity associated with infection in premature infants has fallen to such low levels that is has been difficult to establish a clear-cut indication for the use of IVIG in premature infants. Recent studies, however, indicate that for premature infants at highest risk, therapeutic intervention with IgG is indicated. This is particularly true for infants with a group B streptococcal infection. Patients who experience severe burns, and even blunt trauma, may go through a period of weeks when their ability to respond with a normal humoral and cell-mediated response to antigen is compromised. Patients with burns may lose large amounts of serum from their wounds. Ongoing studies will no doubt provide definitive indications for the use of hypogammaglobulinemia following burns or trauma, but already there are studies which indicate that IVIG can be of assistance to such patients.

One of the advantages of IVIG preparations is the availability of a detailed analysis of the antibodies present. Table 34-5 lists antibodies which are usually well represented in pooled products. Manufacturers must be encouraged to continue to supply a detailed analysis with each batch prepared, for it is obvious that with passive protection techniques, the product is only of use to any individual if the antibody he or she requires is actually present. Antibodies to some antigens will vary with the collection sites chosen. For this reason, antibodies to certain *Pseudomonas* serotypes may be regionally restricted. In the near future it appears that computer batching of plasma collected from

TABLE 34-5   Antibodies Usually Well Represented in IVIG

Mycoplasma	Group B streptococci
Staphylococcus aureus	Adenovirus type II
Neisseria organisms	Epstein-Barr virus
Haemophilus influenzae	Cytomegalovirus
Proteus mirabilis	Varicella-zoster virus
Salmonella	

sites where a specific serotypic profile has been generated will supply us with a hyper-immune-type product. IVIG therapy is not recommended for patients with protein-losing enteropathies. It is not possible to keep up with the γ-globulin loss in such patients, and fortunately they do not suffer from the severe infections which one might anticipate, given the profoundly low levels of IgG which are often present. This may result from the fact that they can produce antibodies to specific antigens even though they are rapidly eliminated.

Patients with antibody deficiency syndromes are particularly susceptible to chronic enteroviral infection. A chronic echovirus encephalitis is not at all uncommon and is a most serious complication for such patients. IVIG preparations have been used successfully via an intraventricular route to control enteroviral encephalitis.

Children with AIDS suffer not only from a defect of cellular immunity but also from defects in production of specific antibodies. The hypergammaglobulinemia seen so frequently is virus-driven rather than antigen-driven. Administration of IVIG has been beneficial for children, and indeed, there are a number of studies which suggest that not only do they suffer from fewer bacterial infections, but there is a slowing of the disintegration of the functional integrity of T cells.

The Principles of IgG Replacement Therapy

While the titer of specific antibodies in serum is all-important for any particular encounter with antigen, clinical experience has taught that patients of any age with IgG levels less than 200 mg/dL must be considered candidates for sudden and often overwhelming bacterial sepsis. Levels above 400 mg/dL are usually associated with adequate, but not ideal, humoral immune protection. Thus, the goal of γ-globulin replacement therapy is to ensure that serum levels of IgG never fall below 400 mg/dL. If IgG is to be given as infrequently as possible, to minimize disruption of the patient's normal routine, the postinfusion levels of IgG must be sufficiently high to match the frequency intervals chosen with the half-life of the IgG preparation used. Monthly infusions are used by most clinical immunologists, and infusions are designed to raise the IgG level to a postinfusion high of at least 800 mg/dL. Recent experiments with the administration of IVIG preparations in the home have shown that such an approach may be promising for at least some patients with hypogammaglobulinemia, and the ability to infuse γ-globulin conveniently, even on a weekly basis, minimizes the necessity of having prolonged trough levels at a less than ideal concentration. For most patients, an intravenous dose of 400 mg/kg per month, a larger dose than previously recommended but warranted by recent clinical trials, will be satisfactory.

Individual metabolism of IgG varies, and the half-life of any particular preparation used for a given patient should be calculated initially by measuring γ-globulin levels on a weekly basis.

When using replacement therapy for IgG subclass deficiencies, the above routine is normally satisfactory, although some adjustment is usually required for patients with an isolated IgG3 deficiency before optimum dosage regiments can be determined. The normal half-life of IgG3 is considerably less than that of other immunoglobulin subclasses. IgG2 deficiencies are physiologic in neonates who cannot make adequate amounts of this class of antibody before the end of their first year of life. IgG subclass deficiency is also seen frequently in association with IgA deficiency. A significant number of the more severely immunocompromised patients with IgA deficiency may also suffer from a previously unrecognized deficiency of IgG2, essential for making an adequate humoral immune response to polysaccaride-containing antigens. Care must be taken in administering IVIG preparations to patients with any form of IgA deficiency, since some of these patients make anti-IgA antibodies that can interact with the small amounts of IgA contaminating the IVIG product. In these patients with preformed anti-IgA antibodies, infusion of IVIG can thus eventuate in anaphylactic responses. These anti-IgA antibodies, which are thought to be present as autoantibodies, can be measured in selected laboratories, and such measurements may predict whether it will be safe to use an IVIG preparation on such a patient. IgG2 deficiency has also been found associated with a syndrome of chronic otitis media in children over the age of 3 years in whom this problem persists. The defect is also found in a number of patients with systemic lupus erythematosus (SLE), recurrent pericarditis, and diabetes mellitus.

IgG4 deficiency may occur in situations where IgA is low but IgE is high. Deficiency of IgG4 has also been associated with otitis media, but is more often seen in a syndrome which features sinusitis, recurrent pneumonia, bronchiectasis, or atopic dermatitis. Familial cases have been reported. It is of interest that a number of adult patients suffering from bronchiectasis have been found to have an IgG4 deficiency, and preliminary clinical trials suggest that replacement therapy may well prove of benefit. Such studies suggest that IgG4 may play an important role in protecting the lower respiratory tract from infection. As the molecule appears to be present in only small amounts in the respiratory tract, this association is as yet poorly understood, but it may well be that the very marked decrease in respiratory tract infections seen in patients with hypogammaglobulinemia who are given ideal replacement therapy with high-dose IVIG reflects an increased availability in the airways of IgG4.

CLINICAL EXPERIENCE WITH IVIG AS AN IMMUNOMODULATORY AGENT

Scattered reports during the 1960s noted that some patients with both severe hypogammaglobulinemia and a Coombs-positive hemolytic anemia experienced less hemolysis following replacement therapy with γ-globulin. However, interest in the immunomodulatory properties of IgG only developed with the report of a significant rise in the platelet count of two agammaglobulinemic patients with severe thrombocytopenia who received IVIG. This observation was soon complemented by reports that platelet counts in children with Wiskott-Aldrich syndrome frequently increased after infusion of IVIG. In this rare syndrome, severe humoral and cell-mediated immunodeficiencies are combined with eczema and thrombocytopenia. Platelet-associated antibodies have been causally linked to the development of the thrombocytopenia. A study of the efficacy of IVIG in the treatment of acute autoimmune thrombocytopenia in children requiring therapy followed, and numerous studies have indicated that IVIG is extremely efficient in the management of this condition. It is now the treatment of choice for children with acute autoimmune thrombocytopenic purpura who need treatment.

Studies of chronic autoimmune thrombocytopenic purpura, a condition which more frequently affects adults and is often steroid-resistant, have provided encouraging results, but significantly fewer patients respond to IVIG with a persistant elevation of their platelet count. However, even a transient improvement may allow a splenectomy to be carried out more safely in such individuals. Recently, two distinct glycoproteins have been identified as the targets for autoantibodies in patients with chronic thrombocytopenic purpura. F(ab')$_2$ fragments from IVIG have been shown to be capable of neutralizing these antibodies in situations where the infusion of IVIG is clinically successful, indicating that an anti-idiotypic interaction may be involved.

It has been demonstrated that the thrombocytopenia which results when an individual makes an immune response to infused platelets can be suppressed by high-dose IVIG therapy, as can posttransfusion purpura, neonatal thrombocytopenia, and the acute thrombocytopenic purpura that occasionally occurs during pregnancy. The latter two conditions do not represent autoimmune phenomena but rather a normal immune response to incompatible platelets which have crossed the maternal-fetal barrier. Nevertheless, it is of interest that this normal response is blunted by IVIG. IVIG has also been reported to be of use in gold-induced thrombocytopenia and thrombotic thrombocytopenic purpura.

Initial attempts to treat autoimmune hemolytic anemias with IVIG, particularly of the "warm" (IgG-mediated) type, produced disappointing results. However, there are now a number of studies which have substantiated the clinical usefulness of IVIG in the treatment of autoimmune hemolytic anemias due to hemolytic antibodies of the IgG class. Recently IVIG has been used to successfully treat a patient with Evan's syndrome (refractory autoimmune hemolytic anemia with autoimmune thrombocytopenic purpura) and a similar success was noted with a 75-year-old man with an idiopathic IgG-mediated autoimmune hemolytic anemia who had previously been unsuccessfully treated with immunosuppression and splenectomy. IVIG appears to be most successful in the management of hemolytic anemia when it is associated with severe immunodeficiency syndromes.

Many cases of pure red cell aplasia appear to be due to immune suppression of erythropoiesis by IgG autoantibodies or the presence in bone marrow of abnormally functioning suppressor T cells. A recent case report described the successful treatment of a 4-year-old girl with antibody-mediated pure red cell aplasia. It is of considerable interest that the cytotoxic activity of the patient's IgG for her hematopoietic progenitor cells could be reversed in vitro not only by the intact IVIG product that produced a clinical response but also by $F(ab')_2$ fragments made from this preparation. Antibodies with anti-idiotypic activity may have neutralized her cytotoxic antibodies.

IVIG has had definite but limited success in the management of autoimmune neutropenia. It is of interest that in patients with Felty's syndrome, where the neutropenia appears to be secondary to the production of antineutrophil antibodies, IVIG has consistently failed to be of benefit. This has led to suggestions that the neutropenia of Felty's syndrome must involve different pathologic mechanisms from those operative in isolated autoimmune neutropenia. Further evidence suggesting that cytopenias may be produced by different immunologic mechanisms comes from a case report in which a 15-year-old girl with both neutropenia and thrombocytopenia received IVIG. Initially only her neutrophil count responded and only with subsequent therapy did her platelets also rise. The administration of IVIG to patients with neutrophil dysfunction associated with antineutrophil antibodies has been shown to improve neutrophil chemotaxis, reduce the level of circulating antineutrophil antibodies, and inhibit the ability of the sera of patients with autoimmune neutropenia to suppress the mobility of neutrophils from a normal donor. One case has been reported where a presumed autoimmune pure white cell aplasia was treated with high-dose IVIG. A short-lived but rapid remission was achieved. The immune mechanisms underlying hematologic diseases are described in more detail in Chap. 30.

Acquired inhibitors of antihemophilic factor (factor VIII) may cause a coagulopathy clinically similar to hemophilia. Such inhibitors have been demonstrated to be antibodies and occasionally are active against factor IX as well. The spontaneous appearance of antibodies to factor VIII can be inhibited within 36 h by the administration of IVIG, and in some patients the suppression of the secretion of this autoantibody has lasted for 5 years. Again there is evidence that it is the binding of $F(ab')_2$ fragments from the IVIG preparation to the autoantibody that is responsible for the suppression. Occasionally, replacement therapy with purified factor VIII for the treatment of hemophilia may stimulate an immune response to this factor. Two patients who developed antibodies to infused factor VIII were treated successfully with IVIG, clinical improvement was associated with the disappearance of inhibitory antifactor VIII antibodies, and the remission induced had lasted 7 months at the time of the report (Table 34-6).

IVIG FOR NONHEMATOLOGIC AUTOIMMUNE DISEASES

Myasthenia gravis develops when autoantibodies directed against the receptor for acetylcholine at the myoneural junction block normal transmission of impulses to the muscle fibers. In a number of studies, the administration of IVIG has been associated with improvement in the clinical condition of patients, sometimes but not always associated with diminution in circulating antibodies to

TABLE 34-6   IVIG for Immunohematologic Disorders

THROMBOCYTOPENIA
Hypogammaglobulinemia with thrombocytopenic purpura
Wiskott-Aldrich syndrome
Acute autoimmune thrombocytopenic purpura
Chronic autoimmune thrombocytopenic purpura
Alloimmunization following platelet transfusion
Posttransfusion purpura
Neonatal immune thrombocytopenia
Acute thrombocytopenic purpura of pregnancy
Gold-induced thrombocytopenia
Thrombotic thrombocytopenic purpura

ANEMIA
Autoimmune hemolytic anemia ± immunodeficiency
Hemolytic anemia and thrombocytopenic purpura (Evan's syndrome)
Pure red cell aplasia
Fetal-maternal Rh immunization

NEUTROPENIA
Autoimmune neutropenia
Pure white cell aplasia

HEMOPHILIA (B)

Associated with antibodies to factor VIII
  Spontaneous
  After factor VIII infusion
Associated with antibodies to factor IX

the acetylcholine receptor. In one series, authors noted that concurrent with improvement was an increased number of cells in the circulation expressing the CD16 and CD8 differentiation antigens. Such cells may represent natural killer cells and/or immunoregulatory cells. An increase in T lymphocytes expressing receptors for the Fc portion of IgG was also noted. Such cells usually have an immunoregulatory role. Improvement in the syndrome resembling myasthenia gravis that is occasionally seen with malignancy (Eaton-Lambert syndrome) has also been reported. The immunopathogenesis of myasthenia gravis is described in more detail in Chap. 35D.

IVIG has been reported to shorten the course of the neurologic abnormalities associated with the Guillain-Barré syndrome and chronic inflammatory demyelinating polyneuropathies. The latter neuropathies may be found in association with infections, malignancy, and a number of autoimmune diseases, or their appearance may be idiopathic. The presence of mononuclear infiltrates of affected nerves is usual and suggests immunopathology. In one series, 13 of 17 patients improved markedly after the infusion of IVIG. When IVIG therapy was discontinued, a number of patients deteriorated clinically; however, upon the reintroduction of the IVIG, they again experienced significant improvement.

The demyelination associated with multiple sclerosis is widely thought to be immune-mediated. Therapy for this condition has generally been unsatisfactory and consists of attempts to control the progression of the disease with corticosteroids, ACTH, and immunosuppressive drugs. In one series, 11 of 31 patients with multiple sclerosis given IVIG improved, the condition of 9 others was apparently stabilized, and 11 continued to deteriorate. When compared to the course of the disease in controlled subjects, the degree of improvement noted after IVIG was statistically significant. Subsequent experience has been encouraging but suggests, as is true for most of the trials reported herein, that a double-blind placebo-controlled trial is both warranted and needed.

Experience with IVIG in patients with SLE is still limited, but there are reports that in acute exacerbations of the disease, this therapy may be of assistance. Two infants born to mothers with active SLE, who were both thrombocytopenic and neutropenic, were treated successfully with IVIG soon after birth. Women with SLE who have circulating antibodies to cardiolipin have an increased chance of miscarriage during pregnancy. A recent report suggests that IVIG therapy can markedly reduce this risk. Limited experience in polymyositis and Sjögren's syndrome doesn't allow one to say more than that the steroid-sparing activity noted suggests that further examination of the use of IVIG in such conditions in warranted.

Therapy with IVIG for patients with rheumatoid arthritis has been attempted but no firm conclusions are available at this time. In an early report, the use of IVIG derived from human placentas resulted in significant but transient clinical improvement in 7 of 10 hospitalized patients. In another, larger series, 60 percent of 31 patients with severe rheumatoid arthritis, receiving 1500 mg of placenta-eluted IgG on 7 consecutive days each month, experienced at least a 50 percent improvement in their condition. An increased responsiveness of lymphocytes after such therapy in patients with rheumatoid arthritis was demonstrated, and the authors suggested that the beneficial effects might be mediated by the presence of polyspecific antibodies directed against D-locus antigens of the human leucocyte antigen system (HLA-DR) thought to be linked to the genes regulating reactivity to self.

Bullous pemphigoid develops when autoantibodies attack antigens in the basement membrane of the skin. Severe blistering follows. In one study a rapid but transient improvement in the condition of 8 of 11 patients with bullous pemphigoid followed the administration of IVIG. Only one of these patients had a prolonged remission, but it seems that IVIG can significantly lower the requirement for steroids in this condition.

Thyroid eye disease can develop without autoimmune thyroid disease being obvious, but more usually is a complication of thyrotoxicosis and may become more severe as the thyroid disease is treated. This can be a debilitating and indeed dangerous condition which may result in blindness. Eight patients with thyroid eye disease, a number of whom failed to respond to very high doses of steroids and azathioprine, or even orbital radiation, improved markedly after high-dose IVIG therapy (Table 34-7).

IVIG FOR OTHER DISEASES FEATURING IMMUNOPATHOLOGY

A number of immunopathologic diseases in which the exact mechanisms producing tissue damage are unclear have been found to respond to IVIG. A number of these conditions may well represent immunologically mediated damage to tissues caused by the undisciplined secretion of cytokines from T cells and macrophages. Kawasaki disease and chronic fatigue syndrome are likely to represent examples of such conditions.

Mucocutaneous lymph node syndrome

TABLE 34-7 IVIG for Nonhematologic Autoimmune Diseases

Myasthenia gravis	Recurrent abortions (cardiolipin antibodies)
Eaton-Lambert syndrome	Polymyositis
Guillain-Barré syndrome	Sjögren's syndrome
Demyelinating polyneuropathy	Rheumatoid arthritis
Multiple sclerosis	Bullous pemphigoid
SLE	Thyroid eye disease

(Kawasaki disease) is associated with a fever of unknown cause lasting 5 days or more, inflammation of the conjunctivae, inflammation around the lips and in the oropharynx, a swelling of the cervical lymph nodes, an erythematous edema, and eventually desquamation of the fingers, hands, and feet. Truncal rashes are common. There is a significant incidence of coronary artery abnormalities in patients with this syndrome. A multicenter controlled trial of high-dose IVIG plus aspirin was compared with aspirin alone for the treatment of Kawasaki disease. The IVIG regimen was shown to reduce the frequency of coronary artery abnormalities, results which were subsequently confirmed in another controlled study in the United States. Although circulating immune complexes may be found in the serum of children with Kawasaki disease, the beneficial effects of IVIG are not associated with the disappearance of these complexes from the serum. It seems much more likely that this disease is mediated through an excessive production of cytokines, the secretion or effects of such molecules being modified by IVIG. High-dose IVIG therapy instituted within 10 days of the onset of disease significantly reduces the development of the cardiovascular anomalies that may be fatal.

Chronic fatigue syndrome is a common condition in which a pathologic degree of fatigue following minimal exertion is combined with neuropsychologic disturbances (frequently impaired concentration and short-term memory) and a number of humoral and cellular immune abnormalities. This disorder frequently appears after an illness with features typical of an infection, although organisms are not usually identified. The disorder probably results from the effects on the central nervous system of a number of cytokines. A double-blind placebo-controlled trial has shown that many patients with chronic fatigue syndrome benefit from IVIG, especially those less than 35 years of age who have had the disorder for less than 2 years.

IVIG is of benefit to children with atopic dermatitis or steroid-dependent asthma. In a group of children shown to have both acute and late-phase bronchospasm following airway challenge with antigen, who had required large doses of steroids for the management of their asthma, IVIG was associated with a decreased need for steroids and a marked diminution in late-phase reactivity. Preliminary results in a series of children with juvenile rheumatoid arthritis associated with severe systemic manifestations (Still's disease) indicate that the systemic manifestations, if not the arthritis, can frequently be controlled within 24 h of giving high-dose IVIG. A multicenter trial in the United States is looking at the effect of IVIG in Crohn's disease and ulcerative colitis; very preliminary examination of the data suggests that the effects may be more beneficial in patients with ulcerative colitis. In an interesting study, women who frequently and spontaneously aborted but were otherwise well—and specifically did not have antibodies to cardiolipin in their serum—were able to carry a fetus to term after treatment with IVIG. The beneficial mechanisms are unknown.

A number of studies looking at the benefit of IVIG in patients undergoing bone marrow transplants suggest that not only can IVIG protect the lungs and intestinal tract from cytomegalovirus infection but may suppress the severity of graft-versus-host disease.

It is worth reemphasizing in this section on the immunomodulatory effects of IVIG

TABLE 34-8   IVIG for Other Diseases Featuring Immunopathology

Kawasaki disease	Crohn's disease
Chronic fatigue syndrome	Ulcerative colitis
Childhood steroid-dependent asthma	Recurrent abortions (no cardiolipin antibodies)
Atopic dermatitis	Graft-versus-host disease
Juvenile rheumatoid arthritis	HIV infection in children

that such material seems to *manipulate* the immune system in HIV-positive children so that T cells become more resistant to the cytopathic effects of the virus (Table 34-8).

CONCLUSION

In May 1990 the National Institutes of Health sponsored a Consensus Development Conference on IVIG therapy. The conference noted the excitement generated from numerous clinical reports of a beneficial effect of IVIG on many conditions but highlighted the need for controlled trials in almost all of the conditions mentioned in this chapter. Controlled studies of the immunomodulatory effects of IVIG have only been performed in thrombocytopenic purpura, Kawasaki disease, chronic fatigue syndrome, and relapsing demyelinating polyneuropathy. In many of the conditions we have discussed, the appropriate dosage and treatment schedules for the administration of IVIG have not been elucidated. It is possible that alteration in the amount, frequency, or duration of administration may improve efficacy.

Side effects associated with the administration of IVIG are low, usually occurring in fewer than 5 percent of patients. Most reactions are mild and self-limited. There is no evidence that either the hepatitis B or HIV viruses can be transmitted by IVIG. Adverse reactions can often be prevented by reducing the rate or changing the volume of infusion.

We can expect that current research will soon increase our understanding of the mechanisms of action of IVIG in the numerous conditions in which it appears to be effective. A better understanding of the mechanisms involved will not only supply a rationale for the expansion of such therapy to other disease states, but will no doubt allow us to produce relevant antibodies using monoclonal or molecular engineering techniques, and thus move us away from the expense and the inefficiency of administering millions of unnecessary IgG molecules to be certain that the ones which we want are really present. IVIG is extremely expensive, and

cost-benefit analysis and a careful evaluation of the quality of life should be included in any long-term outcome measures studied during clinical trials.

SELF-TEST QUESTIONS

1. Which of the following statements about the administration and/or use of IVIG is correct?
   a. The administration of high doses may produce remission in autoimmune thrombocytopenic purpura.
   b. It must be administered slowly because concentrated γ-globulin used intravenously has spontaneous anticomplementary activity.
   c. IVIG preparations are safe and effective in the management of patients with selective IgA deficiency.
   d. IVIG preparations have been associated with the development of AIDS.
   e. In calculating the dose of IVIG to be administered, the physician should take into account the fact that the half-life of the immunoglobulin product is 7 to 12 days in vivo.
2. Which of the following statements concerning the management of immune deficiency states with IVIG is correct?
   a. Patients with chronic lymphatic leukemia should have IVIG on a monthly basis from the time of diagnosis.
   b. IVIG should only be administered to patients who are hepatitis B surface antibody positive.
   c. It is important to maintain serum IgG levels between infusions above a trough level of 400 mg/dL.
   d. IVIG does not help patients who contract cytomegalovirus infection after a bone marrow transplant.
   e. IVIG has proved ineffective in minimizing the progression to AIDS of children infected with HIV.

3. Which of the following statements concerning the use of IVIG for the treatment of patients with autoimmune diseases is correct?
   a. The clearance by infused immunoglobulin of circulating viruses plays a major role in minimizing the development of auto-antibodies.
   b. There is evidence to suggest that the binding of infused IgG to receptors to the Fc portion of IgG on cells of the RES may minimize damage to cells coated with autoantibodies.
   c. Anti-idiotypic antibodies are capable of binding to only one autoantibody.
   d. It is likely that the beneficial effects obtained from therapy are mediated through direct effects on B-cell receptors.
   e. Circulating autoantibodies to factor VIII can be reduced by the administration of IVIG but only with the intact product. F(ab')$_2$ fragments do not have any immunomodulatory effect.

ADDITIONAL READINGS

Abdou MI, Wall H, Lindsey HB, Hasley JF, Susuki T. Network theory in autoimmunity: *in vitro* suppression of serum anti-DNA antibody binding to DNA by anti-idiotypic antibody in systemic lupus erythematosus. *J Clin Invest.* 1981; 67:1297–1304.

Dietrich G, Rossi F, Kazatchkine MD. Modulation of autoimmune responses with normal polyspecific IgG for therapeutic use. In: Melchers F, et al, eds. *Progress in Immunology*, VII. New York: Springer-Verlag; 1989:1221–1227.

Fischer SH, Ochs HD, Wedgewood RJ, Skvaril F, Morell A, Hill HR, Schiffman G, Corey L. Survival of antigen-specific antibody following administration of intravenous immunoglobulin in patients with primary immunodeficiency diseases. *Monogr Allergy.* 1988; 23:225–235.

Haque KN, Zaidi MH, Haque SK, Bahakim H, El-Hazmi M, El-Swailam M. Intravenous immunoglobulin for prevention of sepsis in preterm and low birth weight infants. *Pediatr Infect Dis J.* 1986; 5:622–625.

Imbach P, Barandun S, Baumgartner C, Hirt A, Hofer F, Wagner HP. High dose intravenous gammaglobulin therapy of refractory, in particular idiopathic thrombocytopenia in childhood. *Helv Paediatr Acta.* 1981; 36:81–86.

Kearney JF. Idiotypic networks. In: Paul WE, ed. *Fundamental Immunology.* New York: Raven Press; 1989:663–676.

Lloyd AR, Hickie I, Wakefield D, Boughton CR, Dwyer JM. Intravenous immunoglobulin therapy in patients with chronic fatigue syndrome: a double-blind placebo-controlled trial. *Am J Med.* 1990; 89:561–568.

Schwartz S. Intravenous immunoglobulin for autoimmune disorders. *J Clin Immunol.* 1990; 10:81–89.

Sultan Y, Kazatchkine MD, Maisomeune P, Nydegger UE. Anti-idiotypic suppression of autoantibodies to Factor VIII (antihaemophilic factor) by high dose intravenous gammaglobulin. *Lancet.* 1984; ii:765–768.

CHAPTER

35

Immune Mechanisms in Disease

INTRODUCTION

This final section of the text is designed to synthesize all that has come before. We have collected short descriptions of four diseases in order to discuss in more detail the immunopathogenesis of each. The mechanisms behind each of these diseases may not be precisely known as of yet and are certainly not easily dissected into pure form. Immunopathology in the real world of medicine is never found in pure form; the reasons for tissue damage are usually a compounding of the well-known mechanisms you have already learned. As you read, try to think back on the mechanisms described previously; if they are not clear, please go back and review them as they are discussed. The truly important message to get from these short sections is that a host of diseases can be caused by immunologic mechanisms, and that sometimes the immunology of the disease may not be apparent. Increasingly in medicine we are uncovering immunologic mechanisms of disease not previously thought "immune" in nature. It is up to the clinician and the researcher to understand the importance of immunology to that particular disease process, not only to elucidate mechanisms but also to achieve relief and cure.

A. Acute Interstitial Nephritis

DEFINITION AND CLASSIFICATION

Acute interstitial nephritis (AIN) was first described by Councilman in 1898, in association with diphtherial and streptococcal infections. He defined the condition as an acute inflammation of the renal interstitium characterized by a primarily mononuclear cell infiltration and fluid exudates which were sterile by microscopy and culture, accompanied by degeneration of the epithelium. AIN has continued to be observed in association with other infections, as well as in association with some systemic immunologic disorders or in patients using some pharmaceutical products in the absence of underlying infections. In some cases, no infection, systemic disorder, or causative drug can be identified. Therefore, according to the etiology, AIN can be classified into four main groups— infection-related, drug-related, immune disorder–related, and idiopathic (Table 35A-1).

CLINICAL MANIFESTATIONS

The most common initial manifestation of AIN is an acute deterioration of renal function accompanied by laboratory features of proximal or distal tubular dysfunction. Often, patients with drug-induced AIN have symptoms or signs that suggest a hypersensitivity syndrome, such as fever, rash, arthralgias, and lymphadenopathy. Rarely, they have more dramatic anaphylactic manifestations. Urinalysis commonly reveals sterile pyuria and leukocyte casts. Microhematuria can occur, but the presence of red blood cell casts should suggest a different diagnosis, i.e., glomerulonephritis. Eosinophiluria is helpful in the diagnosis of AIN, especially the drug-induced allergic type, but is nonspecific for this diagnosis. Low-grade proteinuria is common, but, unlike glomerulonephritis, it rarely exceeds 1 g per 24-h period. Nephrosis-range proteinuria may be noted in AIN caused by

TABLE 35A-1   Classification of AIN

Infection-related AIN
  Protozoa: toxoplasmosis
  Bacteria: diphtheria, streptococcosis, brucellosis,
    legionellosis, pneumococcus, tuberculosis
  Viruses: cytomegalovirus, Epstein-Barr virus,
    Hantaan virus, echovirus, coxsackievirus,
    adenovirus, mumps, measles, influenza
  Rickettsia: Rocky Mountain spotted fever
  Spirochetes: syphilis, leptospirosis
Drug-related AIN
  Antibiotics
  Sulfhydryl compounds
  Nonsteroidal anti-inflammatory drugs and
    analgesics
  Anticonvulsive agents
  Diuretics
  Other: cimetidine, allopurinol, α-methyldopa,
    interferon
Immune disorder–related AIN
  Systemic lupus erythymatosus
  Sjögren's syndrome
  Mixed cryoglobulinemia
  Primary biliary cirrhosis
  Cutaneous vasculitis
  Wegener's granulomatosis
  Anti-tubular basement membrane disease
  Tubulointerstitial nephritis-uveitis syndrome
  Granulomatous AIN with sarcoidosis
Idiopathic AIN
  No evidence to suggest any of the etiologies noted
    above

nonsteroidal anti-inflammatory drugs or interferon, but rarely with other drugs. Other accompanying laboratory findings may include peripheral blood eosinophilia, thrombocytopenia, autoimmune anemia, and liver function test abnormalities.

COMPOSITION OF THE INFLAMMATORY CELLULAR INFILTRATE

Since the early descriptions of AIN, the immune system has been thought to play a major role in the pathogenesis. The normal renal interstitium contains the two types of cells responsible for the initiation of an immune response to foreign antigens—*antigen-presenting cells (APCs)* and *T lymphocytes.* Studies (usually done in the rat and rabbit) of the cell population in the normal renal

interstitium show that it includes bone marrow–derived macrophages and dendritic cells, which constitutively express class I and class II major histocompatibility complex (MHC) molecules on their cell membrane and can present antigen to T lymphocytes during the early phases of the immune response. Tubular epithelial cells normally express only class I antigens. In AIN, class I expression is enhanced, and there is also new, induced expression of class II antigens on epithelial cells, possibly due to the action of INF-γ. As a result, tubular epithelial cells can act as APCs, and there is an amplification of the local immune response.

The most abundant inflammatory cells in the renal interstitium in AIN are macrophages and T lymphocytes. By using monoclonal antibodies to surface cell markers and biotin-avidin-peroxidase or immunofluorescence techniques, the phenotype of the lymphocyte infiltrate in AIN has been determined. Although there is some controversy, it seems that T cells belonging to the CD4 subset predominate. There are few B cells and slightly more mature plasma cells, the main effectors in the humoral response. Eosinophils are abundant in the cell infiltrate, as detected by conventional staining procedures or by immunofluorescence. Neutrophils are also a component of the cellular infiltrate in AIN of infectious origin, whereas basophils are seen only occasionally.

INITIATION OF THE IMMUNE RESPONSE

The immune response initiated by a foreign antigen or a modified autoantigen is usually self-limited by specific regulatory events; it terminates with the elimination of the antigen. Suppressor and contrasuppressor T lymphocytes may regulate the magnitude of the response. If the response is too vigorous or the antigen cannot be eradicated, the surrounding tissue may be damaged, due to the effect of mediators released during the immune reaction, such as proteolytic enzymes, oxygen free radicals, and factors promoting

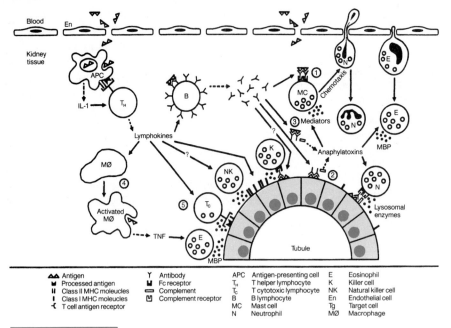

Figure 35A-1   The schematic representation of humoral and cell-mediated immune mechanisms in the pathogenesis of acute interstitial nephritis. 1 = type I hypersensitivity; 2 = type II hypersensitivity; 3 = type III hypersensitivity; 4 and 5 = cell-mediated hypersensitivity. (Reprinted by permission from Ten RM, et al. *Mayo Clin Proc.* 1988; 63:921.)

the growth of connective tissue cells. There are endogenous parenchymal tubulointerstitial antigens that become nephritogenic, possibly because immunologic tolerance to them is lost. Following the priming of CD4 T cells by APCs, which present the processed antigen in association with MHC class II molecules, several immune mechanisms can be triggered, and, therefore, various types of hypersensitivity reaction can occur. Often, multiple immune pathways are simultaneously activated (Fig. 35A-1).

HUMORAL IMMUNE MECHANISMS

Evidence to support the participation of humorally mediated or antibody-dependent hypersensitivity reactions in AIN has been found occasionally. All four of the Gell and Coombs hypersensitivity mechanisms may be in-

volved in the immunopathogenesis of AIN. Type I hypersensitivity or anaphylactic reactions require the production of antigen-specific IgE antibodies by B cells, sensitization of mast cells, and rechallenge with the same polyvalent antigen. Antigen binding leads to the cross-linking of mast cell Fcε receptors and mast cell degranulation. Mediators released from mast cell granules not only stimulate the immune response by attracting and activating other cells (e.g., eosinophil chemotactic factor [ECF]) but also can produce tissue damage by themselves (e.g., various neutral proteinases). (Recall Chap. 19B, on eosinophils, and Chap. 29, on allergy.) Many patients with AIN, especially drug-related AIN, display signs of type I hypersensitivity, including high IgE serum levels, eosinophilia, eosinophiluria, rash, and fever.

In type II hypersensitivity reactions, antibodies directed against tissue antigens (e.g., anti-tubular basement membrane antibodies) result in complement activation and generation of chemotactic factors. Neutrophils and eosinophils are attracted to the area and activated by IgG immune complexes, complement (mainly the C5a component), and several factors released by other leukocytes, such as leukotrienes. The phagocytes cannot ingest their large targets and instead release granule proteins that cause tissue damage. There are animal models of anti-tubular basement membrane interstitial nephritis induced by the injection of tubular basement membrane preparations and mediated by antibody to these antigens. A 48 to 58-kd glycoprotein has been identified in collagenase-solubilized human tubular basement membrane which is selectively recognized by antibodies in the serum of patients with anti-tubular basement membrane nephritis.

Type III hypersensitivity reactions are mediated by the deposition of immune complexes and complement activation in the renal interstitium. This occurs more frequently when large amounts of immune complex material are produced. The accumulation of immune complexes in the renal interstitium can be explained by the in situ formation of immune deposits when the antigen is present on or released from the tubular epithelial cells or by the trapping of antigen, antibody, or immune complexes by nonspecific mechanisms such as charge or interstitial Fc receptor interactions. Other secondary events, such as the cross-linking of the antibody portion of the immune complexes by anti-idiotype antibodies, can also play a role. Granular immune deposits may be detected along the tubular basement membrane in all the immune complex disorders listed in Table 35A-1. This reaction can be reproduced in animals by injection of foreign antigens or kidney extracts.

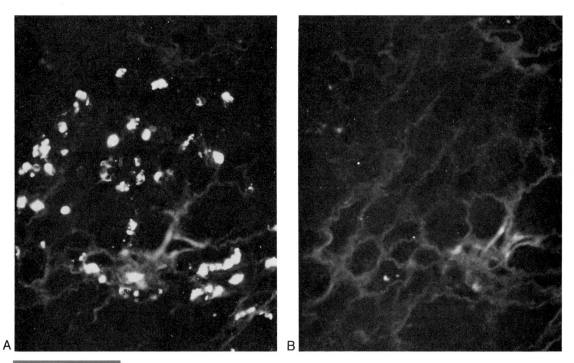

Figure 35A-2 (*a*) Many intact eosinophils and accessible granules in the renal interstitium of a patient with drug-induced AIN stained by rabbit anti-human MBP and fluorescein isothiocyanate goat anti-rabbit IgG (×400). (*b*) Serial section of the same tissue stained by normal rabbit IgG and fluorescein isothiocyanate goat anti-rabbit IgG (×400).

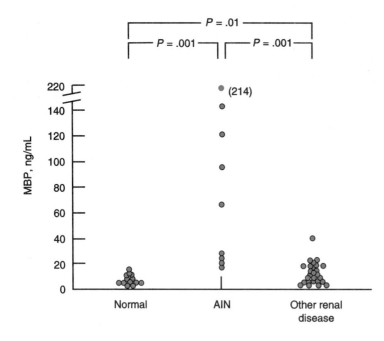

Figure 35A-3 Urinary eosinophil MBP concentration in normal control subjects, patients with AIN, and patients with other renal diseases. (Reprinted by permission from Ten RM, et al. *Mayo Clin Proc.* 1988; 63:921.)

CELL-MEDIATED IMMUNE MECHANISMS

Cell-mediated mechanisms (Gell and Coombs type IV hypersensitivity) seem to be more important than humorally mediated mechanisms in the pathogenesis of AIN. Interaction of primed CD4$^+$ helper T cells with APCs through their antigen receptor results in T-cell activation and release of soluble mediators by the APCs (such as IL-1). Activation of T cells leads to proliferation and release of lymphokines. IL-2, IL-3, and IL-4 amplify the immune response by inducing proliferation and activation of other cells and differentiation of immature precursors. Macrophages are major effectors in cell-mediated immune reactions, not only by phagocytosing their targets but also by generating oxygen free radicals and by releasing factors, such as IL-1 or tumor necrosis factor (TNF), capable of activating other immune cells. Granulomatous reactions with epithelioid and giant cells, which are often observed in interstitial nephritis, result from prolonged antigenic stimulation and macrophage activation. Eosinophils are attracted to the area of inflammation by eosinophil chemotactic factors released by activated T cells. The mechanisms of eosinophil activation and degranulation to release the effector proteins, after they have been attracted to the area of inflammation, are not well known. Platelet-activating factor (PAF), lymphokines such as granulocyte-monocyte colony-stimulating factor (GM-CSF), eosinophil-differentiation factor (EDF), IL-3, IL-5, the recently described HILDA factor, and soluble monokines such as TNF and eosinophil-activating factor (EAF) can promote a respiratory burst and eosinophil degranulation. (*HILDA* stands for human interleukin DA, a 38-kd factor produced by certain T-cell clones which sustains the growth of a murine IL-3-sensitive cell line known as DA. HILDA is a potent activator of eosinophils and can stimulate the growth of bone marrow stem cells.) The eosinophil granule proteins—major basic protein (MBP), eosinophil peroxidase (EPO), and eosinophil cationic protein (ECP)—are very toxic to mammalian cells, and, therefore, lead to tissue damage. Deposition of MBP has been detected by immunofluorescence in the interstitium of patients with AIN (Fig. 35A-2), and high levels of urinary MBP are measured by radioimmunoassay (Fig. 35A-3), presumably due to the leaking of MBP into the tubular lumina. Neutrophils can also be attracted and activated at the site of inflammation by a number of lymphokines or monokines. (Recall Chap. 20, on inflammation, and Chap. 17, on polymorphonuclear cells.) The release of neutrophilic lysosomal enzymes also contributes to the tissue damage. In addition, after activation, eosinophils and neutrophils also release H_2O_2 and oxygen metabolites. These products of the peroxidase-H_2O_2-halide reaction are very cytotoxic. Tubular epithelial cells are sensitive targets for oxidant damage because they have a very active metabolism, as opposed to glomerular cells.

Another form of cell-mediated reaction occurs when $CD8^+$ cytotoxic T lymphocytes are sensitized by the interaction of their receptors with antigen (for example, virus) associated with class I MHC on the target cell. Committed $CD8^+$ T cells are subsequently activated by antigen rechallenge and diverse lymphokines and, therefore, proliferate and release TNF, lymphotoxin, and perforins that are toxic to the tissue.

Natural killer (NK) cells might also play a role by being the main effector cells in antibody-dependent cell-mediated cytotoxicity (ADCC), but their contribution in the pathogenesis of AIN has not been well studied and they are rarely found in the cellular infiltrate of AIN.

ADDITIONAL READINGS

Andres G, Yuzawa Y, Cavalot F. Recent progress in renal immunopathology. *Human Pathol.* 1988; 19:1132.

Gleich GJ, Adolphson CR. The eosinophilic leukocyte: Structure and function. *Adv Immunol.* 1986; 39:177.

Neilson EG. Pathogenesis and therapy of interstitial nephritis. *Kidney Int.* 1989; 35:1257.

Ten RM, Torres VE, Milliner DS, et al. Acute interstitial nephritis: Immunologic and clinical aspects. *Mayo Clin Proc.* 1988; 63:921.

Wilson CB. Study of the immunopathogenesis of tubulointerstitial nephritis using model systems. *Kidney Int.* 1989; 35:938.

35

Immune Mechanisms in Disease

B. Diabetes Mellitus

INTRODUCTION

Diabetes mellitus is a chronic disease characterized by elevated blood glucose levels (hyperglycemia). Over the course of this disease, patients can develop serious medical complications. These include ocular damage (cataracts and diabetic retinopathy), renal damage (diabetic nephropathy), damage to peripheral and autonomic nerves (diabetic neuropathy), and damage to blood vessels (peripheral vascular disease, coronary artery disease, and stroke). Diabetes is a disease with a major public health impact, affecting approximately 14 million people in the United States, and the prevalence is increasing.

There are two major types of diabetes mellitus. *Insulin-dependent diabetes mellitus (IDDM)* usually has its onset in childhood or young adulthood but can present at any age. Over 1 million individuals in the United States have IDDM. There is convincing evidence that in most cases this is an autoimmune disease, with immune mechanisms playing an important role in the specific destruction of insulin-producing β cells in the islets of Langerhans of the pancreas (recall Chap. 31). Since a state of absolute insulin deficiency is produced and insulin is necessary to inhibit ketone production, untreated patients can develop ketoacidosis. Daily insulin injections are required to sustain life. Diabetes which results from the autoimmune destruction of β cells is called type I diabetes mellitus.

Non-insulin-dependent diabetes mellitus (NIDDM) (type II diabetes mellitus) is more common and tends to occur later in life. This is a heterogeneous disorder characterized by insulin resistance and decreased, normal, or elevated serum insulin levels. Many patients with NIDDM are obese and can be treated with caloric restriction alone. Treatment with orally administered sulfonylurea drugs or insulin is sometimes required. Immune mech-

anisms are not recognized to play a role in the pathogenesis of NIDDM.

NATURAL HISTORY OF THE DEVELOPMENT OF TYPE I DIABETES MELLITUS

A genetic predisposition to the development of type I diabetes has been well recognized. This genetic susceptibility is associated with immune response genes within the major histocompatibility complex on chromosome 6. T-cell receptor genes as well as other uncharacterized "diabetogenic" genes may also be important. Since only 30 to 50 percent of identical twins of diabetic patients develop type I diabetes, noninherited factors must be involved as well. The autoimmune process may also be triggered and/or accelerated by viruses, chemical toxins, or other environmental factors. For example, T lymphocyte abnormalities and IDDM develop in approximately 20 percent of the offspring of women infected with rubella during pregnancy.

During the prediabetic stages of type I diabetes mellitus, there are humoral and cellular immune changes, with progressive specific destruction of β cells. These preclinical stages may last for many years. Glucose-stimulated insulin secretion is initially normal but progressively becomes impaired. Only when 80 to 90 percent of the β cells are destroyed does type I diabetes become clinically apparent and hyperglycemia develop.

ASSOCIATION BETWEEN TYPE I DIABETES MELLITUS AND THE MHC

Susceptibility to the development of type I diabetes is strongly associated with genes in the class II locus or D region of the major histocompatibility complex (MHC) on the short arm of chromosome 6. (Recall Chap. 4.) Individuals with haplotypes HLA-DR3 and/or HLA-DR4 are about five times as likely to develop type I diabetes as are individuals in the general population, and up to 90 to 95 percent of caucasian individuals with type I diabetes have these alleles. However, greater than 50 percent of the general population are HLA-DR3- or HLA-DR4-positive. A negative association with type I diabetes has been described for HLA-DR2.

Recent data suggest that the strongest association between the MHC and the development of type I diabetes involves the HLA-DQ region. Amino acid residue 57 of the HLA-DQ β chain appears to be particularly important. The presence of aspartic acid at position 57 is correlated with neutral or decreased likelihood of developing type I diabetes, whereas an alanine, valine, or serine at this position is associated with an increased risk of developing type I diabetes mellitus. Other amino acid residues in the HLA-DQ β chain as well as sequences within the HLA-DQ α chain may also contribute to a predisposition to type I diabetes. Although

the HLA-DQ loci appear to be important, it is likely that multiple genetic abnormalities can influence susceptibility or resistance to type I diabetes mellitus.

The genetics of type I diabetes has been well studied in two animal models, the non-obese diabetic (NOD) mouse and the bio-breeding (BB) rat (see Table 35B-1). In both of these models, the development of diabetes is associated with specific immune response genes within the MHC as well as with genes outside the MHC. For example in the NOD mouse, three different genetic loci are involved. The first is related to the HLA-A β region on mouse chromosome 17, which is analogous to the human HLA-DQ β region on human chromosome 6. The NOD diabetic mouse has a serine substituted for an aspartic acid at position 57 of the HLA-A β chain, again analogous to a substitution associated with increased human susceptibility to type I diabetes. The two other genetic loci involved in the development of diabetes in the NOD mouse are not linked to the MHC. The nature of their gene products is unknown. One of the genes (*IDD-2ˢ*) is near the *Thy-1* locus on chromosome 9 and is recessive. Since it is possible to transfer diabetes

---

TABLE 35B-1   Comparison of Human Type I Diabetes and Two Animal Models of IDDM

	Human Type I Diabetes	NOD Mouse	BB Rat
Hyperglycemia	Yes	Yes	Yes
Ketoacidosis	Yes	Yes	Yes
Female predominance	No	Yes	No
Insulitis	Yes	Yes	Yes
Destruction of β cells	Yes	Yes	Yes
Islet autoantibodies	Yes	Yes	Yes
T-cell lymphopenia	No	No	Yes
Association with MHC genes	Yes	Yes	Yes
Transfer of diabetes by lymphoid cells	?	Yes	Yes
Prevention of diabetes by:			
Bone marrow transplant	?	Yes	Yes
Anti-T-cell antibodies	?	Yes	Yes
Thymectomy	?	Yes	Yes
Silica (toxic to macrophages)	?	Yes	Yes
Immunosuppressive drugs, e.g., cyclosporine	Possible	Yes	Yes

to normal, diabetes-resistant mice by adoptively transferring T cells or by transplanting NOD bone marrow into normal irradiated syngeneic controls, the "diabetogenic" genes need not be present in the β cells of the islets for diabetes to develop.

IMMUNOLOGIC ABNORMALITIES IN TYPE I DIABETES MELLITUS

Some of the earliest evidence suggesting that type I diabetes is an immunologically mediated disease came from histologic observations in which inflammatory cell infiltrates were found surrounding the islets in the pancreases of individuals with this form of diabetes. This was called *insulitis* (literally, inflammation of islands). We now know that these mononuclear cells are mostly CD8$^+$ (cytotoxic/suppressor) T lymphocytes; however, CD4$^+$ (helper/inducer) T cells, B lymphocytes, natural killer (NK) cells, and macrophages are also found. All of these cells are believed to participate in the processes which lead to β-cell destruction. Increased numbers of circulating activated T cells, defects in functional suppressor cells, decreased interleukin 2 (IL-2) production, and hyperexpression of class I MHC antigens on islet cells are some of the abnormalities thought to be important in the development of this disease. The local release of cytokines such as IL-1 and tumor necrosis factor from activated mononuclear cells, and damage by oxygen free radicals, probably also play a role in the destruction of the β cells. The nature of the earliest events in the pathogenesis of IDDM, however, remains unknown.

The importance of the immune system in human type I diabetes is also suggested in studies of identical twins. When a monozygotic diabetic twin received both a kidney and segmental pancreatic transplant from his nondiabetic twin in the absence of immu-

nosuppression, the transplanted kidney functioned well (precluding rejection), but insulitis and diabetes mellitus rapidly redeveloped. The specific autoimmune β-cell destruction recurred despite the fact that the twins had been discordant for diabetes for over 17 years. Conversely, when immunosuppressive drugs were given to a diabetic twin who received a pancreatic transplant from his monozygotic nondiabetic twin, the transplanted islets continued to function well.

The role of cell-mediated immunity in the pathogenesis of type I diabetes has been studied in the NOD mouse and BB rat (see Table 35B-1). In these models, diabetes can be prevented by thymectomy or the administration of antilymphocyte serum, anti-T-cell antibodies or cyclosporine. In the NOD mouse model, the transfer of CD4$^+$ T lymphocytes to T lymphocyte–depleted NOD mice induced insulitis, whereas the administration of anti-CD4$^+$ antibodies prevented diabetes. In another study in NOD mice, both CD4$^+$ and CD8$^+$ T lymphocytes were necessary to transfer diabetes. In addition, macrophages have been found to infiltrate islets early in the development of diabetes in the NOD mouse, and the injection of silica, which is toxic to macrophages, prevents β-cell destruction. Thus, CD4$^+$ T lymphocytes, CD8$^+$ T lymphocytes, and macrophages all appear to contribute to the development of type I diabetes in the NOD mouse.

It had been suggested that the aberrant expression of class II MHC antigens on β cells was important in initiating the anti-islet autoimmune response. However, when class II MHC antigens were expressed in transgenic mice, insulin deficiency developed in the absence of immune system–mediated β-cell destruction. Thus, the expression of these class II antigens is unlikely to be the primary event in the genesis of type I diabetes, but instead may be secondary to the production of lymphokines, such as INF-γ, which are generated during a previously established inflammatory process.

Several autoantibodies to islet cell components and to insulin circulate during the prediabetic stages of type I diabetes. (Recall Chap. 31, on autoimmunity.) The presence of these antibodies, some of which are discussed in more detail in the section below, suggests that antibody-mediated β-cell destruction is also involved in the development of type I diabetes. Some of these antibodies may be formed after the initiation of β-cell damage, thereby being secondary rather than primary in the autoimmune destructive process. The nature of the precise autoantigen or trigger that stimulates the initial immune response against the islet cell remains undefined.

In summary, a model for the pathogenesis of type I diabetes could involve the following events: Susceptible individuals are exposed to a primary triggering event, such as a viral infection or an environmental toxin, which leads to β-cell inflammation. The insertion of viral antigens into the β-cell membrane is one of several mechanisms by which viruses may trigger immune system–mediated destruction. Macrophages infiltrating the islets present β-cell antigens to lymphocytes, resulting in the induction of cytotoxic cells. The specific activated cytotoxic (CD8$^+$) T cells destroy β cells directly as well as through the release of cytokines such as IL-1. Cytotoxic T lymphocytes, NK cells, macrophages, and humoral mediators may all participate in β-cell killing. In addition, there might be an inadequate production of suppressor T cells. The appearance of anti-islet and anti-insulin autoantibodies may be secondary to the autoimmune destruction of the β cells. All of these processes contribute to the death of the β cells and the development of type I diabetes mellitus.

USE OF AUTOANTIBODIES TO PREDICT THE DEVELOPMENT OF TYPE I DIABETES MELLITUS

Several specific autoantibodies are expressed during the development of type I diabetes.

Antibodies to islet cell cytoplasm are present, sometimes for years before the onset of the disease, and levels usually decline after hyperglycemia develops. These polyclonal IgG antibodies, which probably recognize complex gangliosides, can be detected in approximately 65 percent of patients with new-onset type I diabetes and in 2 percent or less of the general population. Anti-insulin antibodies are detected in almost all children less than 5 years of age who develop type I diabetes, but only in one out of eight who are older than 20 years old. These antibodies appear in individuals who have never been exposed to exogenous insulin.

An autoantibody that may be formed in almost all individuals during the early prediabetic stage is directed against a 64-kd β-cell membrane protein, glutamate decarboxylase. The anti-glutamate decarboxylase autoantibody is also detectable in two animal models of type I diabetes, the NOD mouse and the BB rat. The antibody was found at 24 days of life in NOD mice, whereas hyperglycemia did not occur until 150 days. A highly antigenic region of this protein has a similar sequence to a region of the coxsackievirus B4 protein P2-C, supporting the hypothesis that an immune response triggered by a viral protein may contribute to islet cell destruction, i.e., molecular mimicry. An inexpensive assay for anti-glutamate decarboxylase autoantibody is not yet available, but in the future such an assay may allow for identification of individuals early in the development of type I diabetes.

IMMUNOTHERAPY AND TYPE I DIABETES MELLITUS

As reviewed above, there is considerable evidence that type I diabetes is an autoimmune disease in which destruction of the β cells of the pancreas can begin years before the clinical onset of disease. In animal models of IDDM, such as the NOD mice and the BB rat, IDDM can be prevented by immunotherapy using bone marrow transplants, cyclosporine, splenic transfusions, or antithymocyte globulin. (Recall Chap. 33, on Immunotherapy.) Treatment of NOD mice with a monoclonal antibody to the CD4$^+$ determinant on helper/inducer cells stopped the autoimmune destruction of the β cells, preventing the onset of hyperglycemia.

Ideally, in humans, individuals in the prediabetic stages would be accurately identified and specific nontoxic immunotherapy initiated which would halt further islet cell destruction. Although we are close to identifying prediabetic individuals, specific and safe immunotherapy is not yet available. A number of immune intervention trials, however, have been performed, many of which used individuals who had newly diagnosed type I diabetes. At the time of diagnosis, there is still active immunologically mediated destruction of the few remaining insulin-producing β cells. Cyclosporine, a lipophilic cyclic undecapeptide which inhibits T-lymphocyte proliferation, has been one of the agents tested. Some patients with residual β-cell function have responded well to cyclosporine therapy, but the potential toxicities of this drug (such as kidney damage) prevent its use in other than a research setting. Treatment with other immunosuppressive drugs, such as azathioprine (which suppresses T- and B-cell function) and prednisone, may also be helpful in inducing remissions in newly diagnosed individuals with type I diabetes but are also associated with dangerous side effects. When immunosuppressive therapy is discontinued, the natural history of the disease can progress and overt diabetes ensue. Thus, there is a need to develop more specific immunotherapy, such as monoclonal antibodies against the islet-specific activated T cells, which could be safely administered to individuals over prolonged periods of time. Recent studies suggest that if patients can be detected very early in the progressive islet cell destructive process, intensive insulin therapy (islet cell rest therapy, if you will) can retard the insulitis and the development of diabetes.

UNUSUAL DIABETES-RELATED CONDITIONS ASSOCIATED WITH IMMUNE MECHANISMS

Insulin Allergy

Beef, pork, and human insulins are used by all patients with IDDM. Beef insulin differs from human insulin by three amino acids, and pork insulin differs from human insulin by one amino acid. It is therefore not surprising that human insulin is the least antigenic and beef insulin is the most antigenic insulin. In the past, impurities in animal insulin preparations contributed to a significant number of allergic reactions. Since the animal preparations currently used have been highly purified, insulin allergy is now infrequent. Recombinant DNA technology is used to produce much of the human insulin utilized today.

In patients who do develop insulin allergy, localized reactions are most common but generalized insulin allergy can also occur. Humoral and cellular immune responses are responsible for these reactions. In a type I reaction, insulin binds to anti-insulin IgE already present on the FcR on mast cells, resulting in mast cell degranulation. There is a release of mediators of immediate hypersensitivity such as histamine and lymphokines. This process can cause a reaction at the site of injection in which the site is erythematous, swollen, indurated, pruritic, burning, or painful. In the most severe cases, a generalized life-threatening anaphylactic reaction can occur. In these patients, urticaria may quickly spread, and respiratory difficulties (due to laryngeal edema) and circulatory collapse may ensue. Other immune reactions to insulin include type III reactions, resulting in local Arthus-like reactions or serum sickness, and type IV cell-mediated delayed-hypersensitivity reactions. (Recall Chap. 29, on allergy.)

Local reactions most often occur within a few weeks to months after beginning insulin therapy and usually improve with continued insulin usage. Patients with urticaria taking pork or beef insulins should be changed to human insulin. Antihistamine treatment may be required in selected individuals. Severe generalized insulin allergy is a more serious, although fortunately very rare, problem in the management of IDDM. Usually, allergic patients can be desensitized to insulin over 8 to 10 h. During the desensitization process, insulin is commonly administered every 30 min, beginning with very low doses.

Insulin Resistance and Circulating Anti-Insulin Antibodies

Nearly all patients who receive insulin therapy develop anti-insulin antibodies. The lowest titers are found in patients taking human insulins, and higher titers are found in patients injected with beef insulins. These circulating antibodies rarely bind significant amounts of insulin and infrequently cause clinical problems. In some patients, however, circulating anti-insulin IgG antibodies develop which do bind large amounts of insulin and significant insulin resistance develops. These patients require extremely large dose of insulin, and may still remain hyperglycemic.

Type B Syndrome of Extreme Insulin Resistance Associated with Anti-Insulin Receptor Antibodies

This is a rare disorder in which patients are resistant to the action of insulin due to the presence of polyclonal antibodies to the insulin receptor. These antibodies can block the binding of insulin to its cell surface receptor, causing hyperglycemia. In some patients, the antibodies can bind to the insulin receptor and mimic insulin, causing the blood glucose to fall to low levels (hypoglycemia). These patients may have other autoimmune disorders as well.

Autoimmune Polyglandular Syndromes Types I and II

Patients with autoimmune polyglandular syndrome type I can have several autoimmune endocrine disorders, including Addison's disease (loss of the ability of the adrenal glands to produce cortisol), mucocutaneous candidiasis, and hypoparathyroidism (loss of ability of the parathyroid gland to produce parathyroid hormone). In the patients with Addison's disease, lymphocytic infiltration of the adrenal glands and antiadrenal antibodies have been found. Approximately 5 percent of patients develop IDDM. This condition is inherited in an autosomal-recessive fashion, and is not linked to the MHC.

Approximately 50 percent of patients with autoimmune polyglandular syndrome type II have IDDM, and approximately 15 percent of patients with IDDM have this syndrome. An HLA-associated inheritance pattern has been observed. Other autoimmune diseases common in this syndrome include Addison's disease and Graves' disease (an autoimmune thyroid disorder). Some older patients with the type II syndrome develop antibody-mediated hypoparathyroidism. Autoimmune ovarian or testicular failure, pernicious anemia, alopecia, and vitiligo can be present in the type I or type II autoimmune polyglandular syndromes.

CONCLUSION

There is increasing evidence that in type I diabetes, immunologically mediated events are largely responsible for the destruction of the insulin-producing β cells of the islets of Langerhans in the pancreas. Some patients with type I diabetes also have other autoimmune disorders. The HLA-DQ region of the MHC is strongly associated with susceptibility or resistance to the development of type I diabetes. Other genetic loci are probably important as well. Immune abnormalities involving macrophages, T cells, B cells, and cytokine production have been described in patients with type I diabetes, but the precise mechanisms responsible for the initiation and development of the disease remain undefined. Viruses and other environmental factors have been postulated to be triggering agents. In the future, autoantibody assays may be utilized to accurately predict the onset of β-cell destruction, with the goal of intervention with specific immunotherapy to prevent type I diabetes mellitus.

ADDITIONAL READINGS

Clare-Salzler MJ, Tobin AJ, Kaufman DL. Glutamate decarboxylase: An autoantigen in IDDM. *Diabetes Care.* 1992; 15:132.

Eisenbarth GS: Type I diabetes mellitus: A chronic autoimmune disease. *N Engl J Med. 1986; 314:1360.*

Harrison LC, Campbell IL, Allison J, Miller JFAP: MHC molecules and β-cell destruction: Immune and nonimmune mechanisms. *Diabetes.* 1989; 38:815.

Lo D, Burkly LC, Widera G, et al. Diabetes and tolerance in transgenic mice expressing class II MHC molecules in pancreatic beta cells. *Cell.* 1988; 53:159.

Maclaren NK: How, when and why to predict IDDM. *Diabetes.* 1988; 37:1591.

McDaniel ML, Hughes JH, Wolf BA, et al: Descriptive and mechanistic considerations of interleukin-1 and insulin secretion. *Diabetes.* 1988; 37:1311.

Miller BJ, Appel MC, O'Neill JJ, et al: Both the lyt-2$^+$ and L3T4$^+$ T cell subsets are required for the transfer of diabetes in nonobese diabetes mice. *J Immunol.* 1988; 140:52.

Prochazka M, Leiter EH, Serreze D, et al. Three recessive loci required for insulin-dependent diabetes in nonobese diabetic (NOD) mice. *Science.* 1987; 237:286.

Rubinstein P, Rodriguez de Cordoba S: Insulin-dependent diabetes mellitus: Immunogenetic susceptibility, autoimmune components and environmental factors. *Clin Aspects Autoimmun.* 1988; 2:18.

Sarvetnick N, Liggitt D, Pitts SL. Insulin-dependent diabetes mellitus induced in transgenic mice by ectopic expression of class II MHC and interferon-gamma. *Cell.* 1988; 52:773.

Segall M. HLA and genetics of IDDM. *Diabetes.* 1988; 37:1005.

Serreze DV, Leiter EH, Worthen SM, et al. NOD marrow stem cells adoptively transfer diabetes to resistant (NOD NON) F1 mice. *Diabetes.* 1988; 37:352.

Shizuru JA, Taylor-Edwards C, Banks BA, et al. Immunotherapy of the nonobese diabetic mouse: Treatment with an antibody to T-helper lymphocytes. *Science.* 1988; 240:659.

Skyler JS, ed. Symposium on immunology and diabetes: part I. *Diabetes Metabolism Rev.* 1987; 3:723.

Skyler JS, ed. Symposium on immunology and diabetes: part II. *Diabetes Metabolism Rev.* 1987; 3:857.

35

Immune Mechanisms in Disease

C. The Immunopathogenesis of Inflammatory Bowel Disease

INTRODUCTION

The idiopathic inflammatory bowel diseases are ulcerative colitis and Crohn's disease. *Ulcerative colitis* is a predominantly mucosal disease involving the distal or the entire colon. Grossly, friability, ulcerations, and pseudopolyps (islands of residual mucosa surrounded by denuded areas having a polypoid appearance) are seen. Histologically, mucosal inflammation with crypt abscesses, infiltration with plasma cells and neutrophils, mucosal vascular congestion, ulcers, and depletion of goblet cells are the common findings. Clinically, recurrent attacks of bloody diarrhea with associated crampy lower abdominal pain are present.

Crohn's disease, or regional enteritis, is a transmural (involving all layers of the intestine) disease which may potentially affect any segment of the gastrointestinal tract but most often the terminal ileum, the colon, or both, and with characteristic skip areas of normal bowel. Histologically, lymphoid aggregates, typically at crypt bases, submucosal infiltrates with aggregates of lymphocytes and plasma cells, dilated lymphatics, edema, goblet cell preservation, and, in about 60 percent of cases, granulomas are seen. Clinically, the disease may include a large spectrum of manifestations such as abdominal pain, diarrhea, malabsorption, renal calculi, and fistulae formation. The fistulae may involve bowel to bowel, bowel to an adjacent hollow viscus such as urinary bladder or vagina, or bowel to the abdominal or perineal skin.

Pathologically, there is often overlap between the two diseases, making differentiation impossible despite careful gross and microscopic inspection. Extraintestinal manifestations of inflammatory bowel disease include musculoskeletal (seronegative arthritis, sacroiliitis, ankylosing spondylitis), cutaneous (erythema nodosum, pyoderma gangrenosum), biliary (sclerosing cholangitis), ophthalmologic (iritis, episcleritis, uveitis), and vascular (thromboembolic events) disease.

The etiology of inflammatory bowel disease is unknown. Infectious, environmental, genetic, psychological, and dietary factors have been studied. The immune system is clearly involved in the pathogenesis of tissue damage in inflammatory bowel disease. The question remains: Are primary immunologic abnormalities present or are the observed immunologic aberrations a by-product of some other insult to the tissue? In this section, the immunologic abnormalities seen in inflammatory bowel disease are discussed.

HUMORAL IMMUNITY

As early as 1959, Broberger and Perlmann demonstrated that sera from 22 of 30 children with ulcerative colitis gave positive precipitin reactions with extracts of colon from fetuses or newborns. The serum of none of the control patients gave positive precipitin reactions. The factor responsible for the positive precipitin reaction behaved electrophoretically like a γ-globulin.

It was later shown that sera from ulcerative colitis patients, but not from controls or from patients with amebic dysentery, had a high incidence and titer of antibody to colonic tissue extracts. The ability of E Coli 014 antigen to inhibit the colon extract–directed hemagglutination in approximately 30 percent of cases suggested cross-reactivity between the colonic antigen(s) and the E Coli 014 antigen. Healthy first-degree female, but not male, relatives of patients with ulcerative colitis have been shown to have elevated antibody titers to colonic antigen and to E Coli 014 antigen compared with controls.

Using immunoelectrophoresis and immunodiffusion, eluates of resected colons of ulcerative colitis patients were shown to possess significantly higher amounts of tissue-bound IgG when compared to colons of patients with diverticulitis, colon carcinoma, or Crohn's ileocolitis. In the same study, indirect immunofluorescence, using fluorescein isothiocyonate–conjugated antihuman IgG, demonstrated binding of this ulcerative colitis tissue–eluted IgG to antigenic sites on colon epithelium. This colon tissue–bound antibody, the colitis-colon-associated IgG, or CCA-IgG, was found to react to a colon-specific Mr 40-kd antigen present in normal as well as in diseased colon (Fig. 35C-1). Other intestinal tissues, including small intestine, as well as liver did not react with CCA-IgG. IgG antibody eluted from nonulcerative colitis colon tissue did not react with the Mr 40-kd protein. Thus, in patients with ulcerative colitis, autoantibody(s) develops to this organ-specific antigen.

Monoclonal antibodies have been developed against the Mr 40-kd protein. Competitive binding experiments in which CCA-IgG

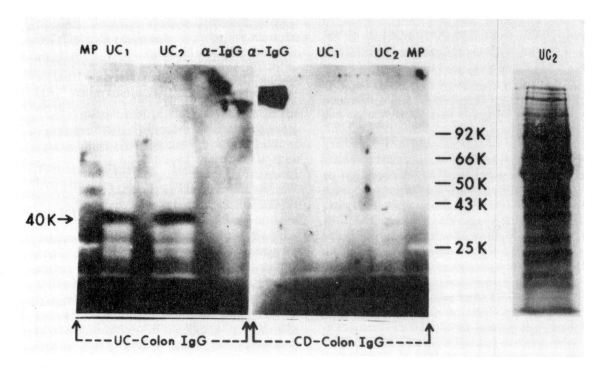

Figure 35C-1 Radiolabeled CCA-IgG (ulcerative colitis [UC]) colon and radiolabeled IgG eluted from Crohn's disease colon tissue (Crohn's disease [CD] colon IgG) are used to probe the colon extracts of two patients with ulcerative colitis (UC₁ and UC₂). Only the CCA-IgG reacts with a colonic protein of molecular mass 40 kd (Mr 40-kd protein) in this autoradiogram of an immunotransblot experiment. Mr 40-kd protein is present in diseased as well as normal colon, but the CCA-IgG is present only in ulcerative colitis. The reactivity of anti-human IgG with both the UC-colon IgG and the CD-colon IgG confirms the maintenance of immunoreactivity following the radiolabeling. The extreme right lane shows the extracted colon tissue proteins stained with Coomassie brilliant blue. MP = marker proteins.

A

B

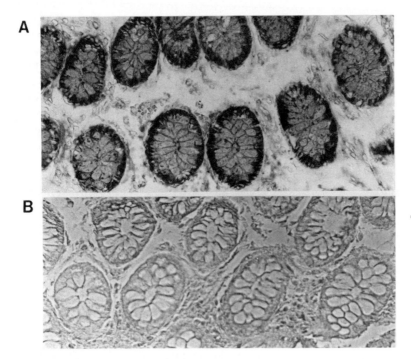

Figure 35C-2   Normal colonic glands (*a*) after and (*b*) before staining with the $7E_{12}H_{12}$ monoclonal antibody using the immunoperoxidase assay. Immunoreactivity is found mainly along the basolateral and apical areas of the epithelial cells.

inhibited the binding of one of the monoclonal antibodies, $7E_{12}H_{12}$ (IgM isotype), suggested the recognition of a common epitope on the Mr 40-kd protein by both CCA-IgG and the $7E_{12}H_{12}$ monoclonal antibody. Using this monoclonal antibody, the Mr 40-kd protein has been localized to epithelial cells both in the crypts and on the luminal surface of the colon. Using the immunoperoxidase assay, the immunoreactivity is predominantly localized to the plasma membrane along the basolateral aspects and the apical areas of the colonic epithelial cells (Fig. 35C-2). The $7E_{12}H_{12}$ monoclonal antibody reacted with all colon specimens tested but not with 13 other epithelial tissues including small intestine, further confirming the organ specificity of the Mr 40-kd protein.

Serum antibodies from patients with active ulcerative colitis and, less frequently, the serum of asymptomatic ulcerative colitis patients, react with the Mr 40-kd protein, whereas the serum of symptomatic patients with Crohn's disease and patients with symptomatic diarrheal syndromes, and normal subjects does not. The patients with symptomatic diarrhea included those with blood and/or mucus in the stool related to various specific pathogens.

These findings suggest an immune abnormality involved in the pathogenesis of ulcerative colitis. If mucosal disruption and exposure of surface antigens to the systemic immune system were all that were necessary for the appearance of CCA-IgG, then any colitis (infectious, Crohn's) would be expected to result in high titers to the Mr 40-kd protein. This has been shown not to be the case. Further questions to be answered are whether there are Mr 40-kd protein–sensitized specific T cells, whether asymptomatic relatives of patients with ulcerative colitis have high titers of these antibodies to the Mr 40-kd protein, whether the presence of these antibodies in asymptomatic patients increases the risk of later developing ulcerative colitis, and whether antigens on the surfaces of the bacteria comprising the normal enteric flora share epitope(s) with the Mr 40-kd protein.

There are qualitative and quantitative differences in the immunoglobulin-producing cells residing in the bowel mucosa. Compared with the colons of control patients, the colons of patients with active ulcerative colitis contain, in areas of persisting glands, approximately 2, 5, and 30 times the normal numbers of IgA-, IgM-, and IgG-producing cells, respectively. The proportions are approximately the same for Crohn's disease patients. However, both in vitro studies using isolated lamina propria lymphocytes and immunohistochemical studies using colon biopsy specimens have shown that the intestinal mononuclear cells of patients with ulcerative colitis contain mainly IgG1-producing plasma cells while in Crohn's disease IgG2-producing plasma cells are more common.

The pathogenesis of Crohn's disease has also been the subject of intense study during the past two decades. Infectious organisms such as viruses, atypical mycobacteria, and cell wall–deficient organisms have been implicated. However, conventional microbial studies have not provided any conclusive results. Recently, *Mycobacterium paratuberculosis* has been implicated as one of the associated pathogen(s) in at least some of the patients with Crohn's disease. This association, however, remains controversial.

Using an unconventional approach, searching for a transmittable agent(s) which may grow better in T cell–deficient animals, athymic nude mice were injected with mesenteric lymph node filtrates from patients with Crohn's disease. It was found that lymphomas and lymph node hyperplasia (with plasma cells predominating) occur in 16 percent of these mice after such injection of Crohn's disease tissue filtrates. Lymphadenopathy occurs in only 4 percent of nude mice injected with control tissue filtrate. On indirect immunofluorescence assay about 50 percent of the serum samples from patients with Crohn's disease reacted with the lymphomas induced by the Crohn's disease tissue filtrate and with hyperplastic lymph nodes. Conversely, only one control serum has reacted with these lymphoid tissues. Spontaneously developing nude mouse lymphomas and lymphomas induced by non-Crohn's disease tissue did not react with the Crohn's disease sera. The indirect immunofluorescence reaction was abolished by the absorption of serum with either lymphomas induced by Crohn's disease filtrate or Crohn's disease tissue, but not by the absorption of serum with control lymphomas or with control intestinal tissue. This specificity suggests the presence of a cross-reactive factor(s) in the Crohn's disease tissue and the filtrate-induced lymphomas.

Using immunoprecipitation experiments it has been shown that intestinal tissue from patients with Crohn's disease contains proteins of molecular masses 200 kd, 160 kd, 120 kd, and 110 kd, which react with the sera of patients with Crohn's disease. Neither control tissue nor the tissue from patients with ulcerative colitis contains these proteins. It has been shown that the 200-kd and 160-kd proteins are glycoproteins and are present both in the colon and in the small bowel tissue of patients with Crohn's disease and not in normal or other diseased intestine. The immunoreactivity has been demonstrated against Crohn's disease sera using immunoblot analysis. The glycoproteins are not immunoglobulins as they do not bind with antibodies against IgG, IgM, or IgA. The source of these glycoproteins, either intrinsic to the bowels or extrinsic, is unknown. Although it was shown in the same study that these tissue glycoproteins from patients with Crohn's disease inhibit the immunofluorescent reaction between Crohn's disease serum and lymphomas induced by the Crohn's disease tissue, while control glycoproteins do not, the relationship between the lymphoma antigens and these newly discovered glycoproteins remains to be determined.

Intestinal permeability to large molecules has been studied in Crohn's disease patients and in their asymptomatic relatives. The intestinal absorption of polyethylene glycol 400 is twice as great in Crohn's disease patients and in their relatives as in controls. The significance of this finding is that the change in permeability is independent of intestinal disease and suggests a genetically transmitted abnormality which may allow absorption of large, potentially immunologically active molecules.

Changes in permeability may be of relevance in the seronegative spondylarthropathies. For example, Reiter's syndrome may occur in association with a postdysentery state. Also, changes in bowel flora have been shown in patients with rheumatoid arthritis, raising the possibility that absorbed intestinal antigens may stimulate a peripherally manifested immune response. It is unclear whether the above findings have a connection with the extraintestinal manifestations of inflammatory bowel disease.

CELLULAR IMMUNITY

In Crohn's disease, there is alteration of normal cellular elements with a relative increase in B lymphocytes and a relative decrease in T lymphocytes in the lamina propria. In the submucosa and the muscularis, there is a relative decrease in B lymphocytes and a relative increase in T lymphocytes. Circulating T lymphocytes are decreased in number and in proportion, whereas circulating B lymphocytes are normal. Conversely, in ulcerative colitis, the number of T lymphocytes in the lamina propria is normal or slightly increased, with an abundance of these cells in the superficial submucosa associated with lymphoid follicles. Plasma cells are the predominant cell type in the inflamed mucosa associated with ulcerative colitis.

Regarding the T-cell populations within the bowel, in both Crohn's disease and in ulcerative colitis CD4$^+$ cells predominate in the lamina propria relative to CD8$^+$ cells and less than half of the CD8$^+$ cells are Leu-1$^+$. This distribution is the same as in normal subjects.

NK cells are absent from the mucosal cell populations of patients with inflammatory bowel disease, as determined by using monoclonal antibodies to the surface markers Leu-7, Leu-11, and Leu-15. However, when lamina propria mononuclear cells are cultured with the lymphokine IL-2, cytotoxicity against the K562 and Daudi cell lines is observed, suggesting the presence of lymphokine-activated killer cell activity.

Cellular cytotoxicity has been demonstrated in inflammatory bowel disease using chicken erythrocytes coated with intestinal epithelial antigens. Peripheral blood lymphocytes from patients with ulcerative colitis and Crohn's disease lyse these coated erythrocytes via antibody-dependent cell-mediated cytotoxicity (ADCC). Lamina propria lymphocytes from patients with inflammatory bowel disease, on the other hand, lyse these coated erythrocytes via a non-MHC-restricted direct T-cell cytotoxic mechanism which is not antibody-dependent.

Using sera from patients with ulcerative colitis, Crohn's disease, and other controls, and peripheral blood lymphocytes from normal individuals, ADCC against a colon cancer cell line has been demonstrated with ulcerative colitis and not with other disorders. This ADCC reaction correlates with disease activity in ulcerative colitis. Taken together, the findings that anti-Mr 40-kd antibodies inhibit this ADCC of the cells, and that CCA-IgG recognizes an epitope(s) on the Mr 40-kd protein expressed on these cells, suggest a role for the CCA-IgG and the Mr 40-kd protein in an autoimmune reaction, perhaps ADCC, contributing to the pathogenesis of ulcerative colitis. It has recently been shown that epithelial cells from patients with ulcerative colitis or with Crohn's disease stimulate CD4$^+$ lymphocytes while epithelial cells from normal controls stimulate antigen-nonspecific suppressor lymphocytes. The fact that tissue from uninvolved areas of bowel in patients with inflammatory bowel disease shares the stimulatory helper effect and that tissue from patients with ischemic bowel disease or diverticulitis shares the stimulatory suppressor effect suggests that this may be a disease-specific and not an inflammation-specific phenomenon.

COMPLEMENT SYSTEM

The metabolism of radioiodine-labeled Clq has been shown to be increased in patients with ulcerative colitis and Crohn's disease. Alternative pathway abnormalities, but not classical pathway abnormalities, have been demonstrated in patients with inflammatory bowel disease. Depression in serum properdin and properdin convertase and decreased consumption of C3–C9 after reaction with cobra venom was noted, and the changes were most significant in patients manifesting extraintestinal disease. The significance of these findings is unclear. Most recently IgG1, along with activated early (C1q, C4c, C3b) and late (terminal complement complex) components of the complement cascade, were localized on the apical face of colonic epithelium in active ulcerative colitis but not in Crohn's colitis. Mr 40-kd antigen was colocalized with IgG1 and C3b apparently targeting an autoimmune attack.

HISTOCOMPATIBILITY ASSOCIATIONS

There have been no consistent histocompatibility associations in ulcerative colitis or Crohn's disease. HLA-B27 is more prevalent among Crohn's disease and ulcerative colitis patients who also manifest ankylosing spondylitis or sacroiliitis. HLA-B27 also correlates with more extensive colonic involvement in both Crohn's disease and ulcerative colitis. HLA-B27 linkage of sacroiliitis and spondylitis not associated with colitis is also found in ankylosing spondylitis and in the axial skeletal disease accompanying some cases of psoriatic arthritis (see Chap. 31, on autoimmunity.)

Among Israeli Jews, there is an increased prevalence of HLA-Bw35 in patients with ulcerative colitis. In this group, HLA-Aw24 is associated with early onset and increased severity of the disease. Among Crohn's disease patients in this group, no HLA associations have been found.

EXTRAINTESTINAL COMPLICATIONS

There has been controversy with regard to the role of circulating immune complexes in the pathogenesis of inflammatory bowel disease and its extraintestinal manifestations. Earlier work supporting an association has been contradicted by later work suggesting no role for immune complexes in the pathogenesis of the disease. Recently, using a monoclonal antibody, a shared and unique epitope(s) related to the Mr 40-kd protein was found in human colon, skin, and biliary tract epithelium. This monoclonal antibody did not react with 15 other types of human epithelial tissue, including tissue from other parts of the gastrointestinal tract.

Because diseases of the skin and biliary tract often complicate ulcerative colitis, it is tempting to speculate that antibodies to shared epitope(s) might play a pathogenic role. However, further studies are needed to understand the pathogenetic mechanism for inflammatory bowel disease and its extraintestinal complications.

CONCLUSIONS

There is extensive literature describing various immunologic phenomena associated with inflammatory bowel disease. Part of the difficulty in finding a reasonable theory is the absence of good animal models for inflammatory bowel disease. It is, therefore, difficult to know which observations are primary and which are secondary to some other insult.

Strober and James have postulated that the mucosal immune system, perhaps as a result of an infection, becomes exposed to mucosal cellular antigens, e.g., Mr 40-kd protein. An ongoing immune response ensues as a result of an abnormality in the antigen-specific immunoregulation, most likely a failure to express adequate antigen-specific suppressor T cell function. This results in formation of autoantibodies and in lymphokine-driven accumulation of secondary inflammatory cells such as lymphocytes, neutrophils, and macrophages.

Despite great advances in the past several years, there is still much to learn about the cellular and humoral immune mechanisms in the inflammatory bowel diseases. These diseases lend themselves to an exciting multidisciplinary approach in which the skills of the immunologist, the rheumatologist, and the gastroenterologist can complement one another in a joint effort to understand the immunopathogenesis of inflammatory bowel disease.

ADDITIONAL READINGS

Bagchi S, Baral B, Das KM: Isolation and characterization of Crohn's disease tissue specific glycoprotein. *Gastroenterol.* 1986;91:326.

Baklein K, Brandzaeg P: Comparative mapping of the local distribution of immunoglobulin-containing cells in ulcerative colitis and Crohn's disease of the colon. *Clin Exp Immunol.* 1975;22:197.

Broberger G, Perlman P: Autoantibodies in human ulcerative colitis. *J Exp Med.* 1959;110:657.

Das KM, Valenzuela I, Williams SE, Soeiro R, Kadish AS, Baum SG: Studies of the etiology of Crohn's disease using athymic nude mice. *Gastroenterol.* 1983;84:364.

Das KM, Vecci M, Sakamaki S: A shared and unique epitope(s) on human colon, skin, and biliary epithelium detected by a monoclonal antibody. *Gastroenterol.* 1990;98:464.

Das KM, Sakamaki S, Vecci M, Diamond B: The production and characterization of monoclonal antibodies to a human colonic antigen associated with ulcerative colitis: Cellular localization of the antigen by using monoclonal antibody. *J Immunol.* 1987;139:77.

Das KM, Dasgupta A, Mandal A, Geng X. Autoimmunity to cytoskeletal protein tropomysin: A clue to the pathogenetic mechanism for ulcerative colitis. *J Immunol.* 1993; 150:1.

Kirsner JB, Shorter RG: *Inflammatory Bowel Disease.* Philadelphia: Lea & Febiger; 1988.

MacDermott RP, Scott MG, Nash GS, Macke K, Bertovich MJ, Nahm MH: Increased spontaneous synthesis and secretion of immunoglobulin G subclass 1 (IgG1) by ulcerative colitis intestinal mononuclear cells. *Gastroenterol.* 1985;88:1483.

Strober W, James S: Immunological basis of inflammatory bowel disease. *J Clin Immunol.* 1986;6:415.

Tekahashi F, Das KM: Isolation and characterization of a colonic autoantigen specifically recognized by colon tissue bound immunoglobulin G from idiopathic ulcerative colitis. *J Clin Invest.* 1985;76:311.

35

Immune Mechanisms in Disease

D. Immunopathogenesis of Experimental Myasthenia Gravis

INTRODUCTION

There has been a revolution in the understanding of myasthenia gravis (MG) in the past decade and a half, resulting from a new understanding of the mechanisms of this disease. MG is the best understood of all autoimmune diseases and is a model for the development of new strategies for the diagnosis and therapy of autoimmunity.

The nicotinic acetylcholine receptor (AChR) is found on a specialized area of skeletal muscle in close proximity to the axon terminus. The nerve releases acetylcholine, which diffuses across the neuromuscular junction to bind to the AChR. The receptor is a large (250-kd) transmembrane protein with five subunits. The pathogenesis of MG is an autoimmune attack of serum autoantibodies on the AChR. The evidence for this pathogenesis is convincing. Significant levels of anti-AChR antibodies occur in about 85 percent of patients with MG and in no normal controls or patients with other neurologic disorders. Experimental disease can be induced in animals by immunization with purified AChR or with the transfer into naive animals of monoclonal anti-AChR antibodies. Immunoglobulins from patients with MG transferred into normal animals induce a myasthenia-like disease. However, there is a lack of understanding of precisely how autoantibodies in this disease effect dysfunction of the AChR. The hallmark of pathology in MG is its absence: i.e., there is no, or at the most very little, muscle inflammation, no vasculitis, and very little, if any, distortion of normal neuromuscular junction architecture. Thus, antibody binding with subsequent complement activation, destruction of the protein in situ, and elicitation of inflammation cascades is *not* a major mechanism. Therefore, other mechanisms such as blocking of neurotransmitter binding and accelerated degradation of AChRs are more likely to be responsible. The evidence for these statements will be summarized below after a review of some important clinical considerations of the disease.

CLINICAL MANIFESTATIONS

The first symptoms of most patients with MG are ocular, and the eyes are almost always involved at some point in the disease. The ocular symptoms are generally ptosis (drooping of the eyelid) or diplopia (double vision), the former due to weakness of the levator palpebrae muscle and the latter due to weakness of one of the extraocular muscles. Since the disease affects the neuromuscular junction and not specific nerves, cranial nerve nuclei, or other parts of the spinal cord, any combination of extraocular muscles can be affected. The extent of involvement of the ocular muscles does not correlate well with generalized symptoms; some patients can have severe ptosis and complete ophthalmoplegia (inability to move their eyes at all) with absence of any other symptoms. Many patients, however, do experience involvement of other muscles. The most commonly involved are other muscles innervated by cranial nerve nuclei, i.e., bulbar musculature such as facial muscles, the tongue, pharynx, respiratory muscles, and neck muscles. Muscles in the extremities are also frequently involved, with some predominance of proximal muscles. The hallmark of myasthenic symptoms is *fatigable weakness*; i.e., the initial muscle effort is often of normal strength, but repetitive use of the muscle leads to rapidly progressive fatigue. Diagnosis is made by the characteristic clinical presentation, and confirmed by ruling out other possible diagnoses, and by appropriate laboratory evaluation such as testing with edrophonium chloride (Tensilon test), repetitive nerve stimulation testing, measurement of anti-AChR antibodies, and imaging of the thymus gland. Abnormalities of the thymus gland are common and include thymitis and thymic tumors, usually nonmalignant thymomas. Although the thymus and thymic pathology are clearly important in MG, their contribution to the course of the disease is unclear.

The natural history of the disease is extremely variable, and the severity of the process early in the course does not always determine the ultimate prognosis. However, usually the most severe manifestations occur early, within the first 3 to 5 years; in the later years, there are fewer and less severe exacerbations. Three-quarters of deaths from MG occur within the first 5 years after disease onset. Many of the deaths are caused by exacerbation of myasthenia by infection, often aspiration pneumonias related to swallowing problems. These infections are sometimes harder to diagnose and treat because of the corticosteroids and other immunosuppressive drugs frequently used in the treatment of MG. Mortality from MG has dropped from 70 percent in the period from 1915 to 1934 to 7 percent in the period from 1966 to 1985 due primarily to a combination of the ability to diagnose less severe cases, to treat infections quickly with antibiotics, and to support patients through crisis by positive-pressure ventilation.

The contribution to decreased mortality of other therapies such as anticholinesterases, thymectomy, corticosteroids, immunosuppressive drugs, and plasmapheresis is less clear, although it is generally felt that these therapies, judiciously used with attention to adverse side effects, can improve the quality of life of patients with MG. The effect of immunosuppressive drugs, corticosteroids, and plasmapheresis on MG is presumably related to their ability to influence antibody production, antibody levels, or effector pathways of immunoglobulin. Preliminary data seem to suggest the efficacy of cyclosporine in MG, although many neurologists are hesitant to use this medication because of its side effects, particularly neph-

rotoxicity. If the preliminary data are confirmed, a role of T cells in the propagation of the autoimmune process in MG would be established since cyclosporine acts predominantly if not solely on T-cell function. This is not surprising, since in the murine model of MG, continued production of anti-AChR antibody requires T-cell help, which can be provided by very low numbers of activated AChR-specific T cells (see the section on experimental models below).

IMMUNOPATHOGENESIS

The precise mechanism by which MG causes weakness is unclear. Many different pieces of evidence point to the AChR as being an important autoantigen in most MG patients. However, there is no proof that it is the only autoantigen or the most important one in *all* myasthenic individuals. In fact arguments exist against the hypothesis that AChR is the sole pathophysiologically important autoantigen in MG. The titer of anti-AChR antibodies as measured by the standard immunoprecipitation assay bears no correlation with severity of clinical involvement in groups of myasthenics. Ten to fifteen percent of patients with MG have no detectable anti-AChR antibodies, and the disease in seronegative patients is clinically indistinguishable from the disease in seropositive patients. Thymic pathology is generally not found in AChR-immunized experimental animals with experimental MG, implying that in the human disease the thymic abnormalities may be primary and not secondary to anti-AChR immunity. Antibodies to other muscle components have been identified in MG, but their pathogenetic significance is unknown. However, there seems little doubt that in a substantial portion of patients with MG, anti-AChR immunity is indeed an important part of the disease process.

Interaction of immunoglobulins with the AChR protein has been detected in a number of ways (see Fig. 35D-1). In most of these systems the immunoglobulins are polyclonal; i.e., anti-AChR antibody activity is a

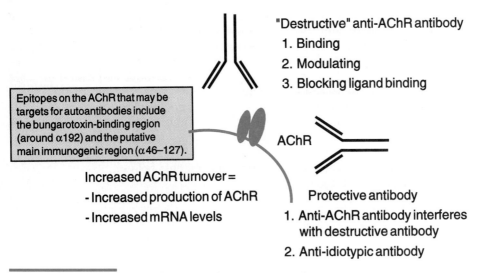

"Destructive" anti-AChR antibody
1. Binding
2. Modulating
3. Blocking ligand binding

Epitopes on the AChR that may be targets for autoantibodies include the bungarotoxin-binding region (around α192) and the putative main immunogenic region (α46–127).

AChR

Increased AChR turnover =
- Increased production of AChR
- Increased mRNA levels

Protective antibody
1. Anti-AChR antibody interferes with destructive antibody
2. Anti-idiotypic antibody

Figure 35D–1   Immunopathogenetic factors in myasthenia gravis.

sum total of a number of different antibody populations, each of a different size. Since in most of these systems there is evidence for some anti-AChR immunoglobulin activity in "normal" sera, *positive* is usually defined as a level of activity above that present in a large number of normal individuals or patients with other neurologic disorders. From these considerations one can thus postulate a number of possibilities for false-negative myasthenic antisera. For instance, a seronegative patient with MG could harbor one or a few clones of anti-AChR immunoglobulins that are very pathogenic (*myasthenogenic*) and a few clones that are nonmyasthenogenic. The presence of a relatively low total number of antibody molecules would mean that this patient's sera might not register above the upper confidence limits of normal controls. Additionally, anti-idiotypic antibodies, which are anti-anti-AChR antibody antibodies, might be present, interfering with the detection of anti-AChR antibodies but not with the interaction of the anti-AChR antibodies in vivo. A large amount of antibody may be present, but may be undetectable in serum because it is bound to the AChR in muscle. Other possibilities exist that might explain our inability to detect anti-AChR antibodies in all patients with MG,

but the wealth of antibody assays available speaks to the continuing search for an understanding of immunopathogenetic mechanisms in MG.

ANTIBODY ACTIVITIES— BINDING

The most commonly used method for detecting antibodies is the indirect immunoprecipitation assay. In this assay AChR is purified from human or rat muscle by detergent extraction of muscle membranes and then labeled with radioiodinated bungarotoxin, which binds to AChR with a very high affinity. Patient serum is then added, followed by an anti-human immunoglobulin precipitating antibody. Radioactive counts in the pellet are determined, a number which correlates with the amount of immunoglobulin in the serum binding to epitopes on the AChR not blocked by the presence of the iodinated bungarotoxin. This assay, the most commonly used for clinical purposes, suffers from two obvious weaknesses: it does not detect antibodies binding at or near the bungarotoxin-binding site and identifies solubilized, and thus somewhat altered, AChR.

These two weaknesses do not interfere to any significant degree with the utility of the assay, which is to confirm the clinical diagnosis of MG. However, these methodologic considerations may contribute to the fact that the amount of anti-AChR antibodies determined in this assay does not correlate with the severity of disease in MG. A number of explanations for this lack of correlation have been invoked, most of which resemble explanations for seronegative myasthenia. One possibility is that the binding immunoprecipitation assay does not measure very pathogenic (myasthenogenic) antibodies present in low concentration.

Since anti-AChR antibodies seem to be involved with disease pathogenesis, but antibodies as measured by the binding immunoassay do not correlate with disease activity, what antibody determination *does* correlate with disease? At least 10 percent of patients with MG are negative by any assay, and these patients are clinically indistinguishable from the seropositive patients, so no single assay or combination of assays is ideal. However, some assays of antibody activity correlate much more closely with disease activity than does the binding assay. Two of these are modulation (accelerated degradation) and blocking assays.

ANTIBODY ACTIVITIES—MODULATION AND BLOCKING

Modulation or accelerated degradation is measured on cultured cells bearing the AChR. Cells are exposed to serum for various amounts of time and then surface AChR is labeled with radioiodinated bungarotoxin. The ability of the serum of a patient with MG to induce accelerated degradation is presumably due to the capacity of anti-AChR immunoglobulin to cross-link receptor, leading to accelerated endocytosis of the receptor. In myasthenic muscle, this increased degradation of AChRs probably leads to a compen-

sated increased production and expression of AChRs; α-subunit mRNA in the leg muscles of myasthenic rats and rabbits is increased four to sevenfold over control animals. However, in vitro this sudden accelerated degradation cannot be compensated for by increased production, and fewer receptors are present on the surface of muscle cells treated with myasthenic serum versus control serum. Antibody titers as determined by modulation assays with cultured rat muscle cells or with cultured human muscle cells correlate better with clinical status than the results of binding assays.

The anti-AChR antibody activity that has consistently correlated best with clinical disease is blocking. In the measurement of blocking, the test serum is incubated with AChR prior to the addition of radiolabeled bungarotoxin; all counts bound to AChR are then measured and compared to a pool of normal sera. The methodology varies among laboratories, with different AChR sources (rat versus human), forms of AChR (solubilized versus unextracted), and times of incubation steps. This assay thus measures those antibody populations binding to a particular epitope (binding at or near the toxin-binding site) and having a high avidity for the AChR (high enough to compete with toxin for binding to the AChR). Anti-AChR antibodies from patients with MG are less likely to block binding to native AChR on the surface of muscle cells than to solubilized AChR, since bungarotoxin binds less avidly to solubilized than in situ AChR. Variations in the percentage of positive results among different laboratories using this assay thus are likely due to methodologic differences. However, despite this variability in the methodology of the blocking assay, a consistent finding in these tests is a relatively low percentage of positive results in patients in remission or with ocular disease and increasing frequency and degree of positive results in patients with worsening clinical status. This conclusion supports the hypothesis that those anti-AChR antibodies that bind at or near the bungarotoxin-binding site and are highly avid for the AChR are the most pathogenic.

ANTI-AChR ANTIBODY ASSAYS—MISCELLANEOUS

A number of other assays, not measuring any particular antibody activity, have been used in an attempt to more accurately measure anti-AChR antibody. For instance, a major weakness of the standard immunoprecipitation assay is its reliance on AChR that is altered in two ways: solubilization and attachment of radioiodinated bungarotoxin. Since antibodies recognize three-dimensional configurations of proteins, solubilization may significantly lower antigenicity, and thus assays using native receptor may be more accurate. A recently published assay makes use of native receptor on the surface of the BC3H1 cell line, a transformed mouse medulloblastoma cell with a high concentration of AChR on its surface. This assay identified anti-AChR antibodies in some myasthenic patients who were antibody-negative by the routine immunoprecipitation assay. A study supporting the importance of native configuration in antigenicity of the AChR was performed by Koethe et al., who documented binding of antibodies from the serum of many myasthenic patients to *Torpedo californica* AChR, but only if the AChR was present on membrane vesicles and not if the AChR was solubilized. Another antibody activity that can be measured on native receptor is complement-mediated lysis. A number of investigators have found that the immunoglobulin of myasthenic patients binds to muscle cells and, in the presence of fresh complement, results in lysis. An antibody activity that is theoretically present but may not correlate with blockade or modulation is one with the ability to induce "stiffening" of the AChR, i.e., an interference with the ability of the AChR to change quickly its three-dimensional configuration in response to ligand, leading to interference with the ability of the receptor to move between sensitized and desensitized states and thus leading to AChR dysfunction. Since AChR is a channel, electrophysiologic measure-

ments can be done to assess the effects of immunoglobulins from patients with MG on receptor properties. These studies are still relatively new, but initial results point to an actual loss of functional AChRs rather than an effect on channel properties such as conductance or open times.

MONOCOLONAL ANTI-AChR ANTIBODIES

The studies summarized above illustrate the inherent difficulty with attempts to deduce pathogenetic mechanisms of autoimmunity when the autoantigen is so complex and the autoantibody response so polyclonal. In order to simplify the system for more precise analysis, a number of investigators have generated monoclonal anti-AChR antibodies and studied their effects in vitro and in vivo. At least two forms of disease have been induced by passive transfer: The first is associated with inflammation at the neuromuscular junction, slowly develops over days, and resembles disease induced by passive transfer of polyclonal antisera. The second is called "hyperacute" disease because it develops within hours after injection and has no inflammatory lesions at the endplate. The latter syndrome has been produced by two different monoclonal antibodies, one mouse and one rat, each directed against the bungarotoxin-binding site on the AChR. The most extensive studies on passive transfer studies of anti-AChR monoclonal antibodies have been performed by Richman et al., using monoclonal antibodies to *Torpedo* AChR transferred into rats. The hope was that the in vitro characteristics of these monoclonal antibodies (i.e., affinity, AChR epitope, subclass, etc.) could be predictive of their in vivo effect. This turned out not to be true. The following conclusions, however, could be made with some confidence. Only monoclonal antibodies identifying extracellular determinants were myasthenogenic. Antibodies to the α chain of the AChR were more pathogenic than antibodies to other subunits. A high antibody affinity for the AChR and ability to fix complement were more common in the pathogenic antibodies.

Although these trends were evident, in vitro activities are, for many monoclonal antibodies, not predictive for pathogenicity. For instance, the monoclonal anti-AChR antibody 5.5, generated by immunization with *Torpedo* AChR, did not cause weakness in mice despite the fact that the antibody bound to the bungarotoxin-binding portion of the AChR, strongly blocked toxin binding to mouse AChR, and caused accelerated degradation of AChR on muscle cells. In addition, the cumulative effect of a number of different subpopulations of anti-AChR antibodies may not be predictably computed from the sum of the effects of each clonal population working alone, since one clone of anti-AChR antibody may affect the AChR in such a way that another, different clone will no longer bind. This was demonstrated in some fascinating monoclonal antibody mixing studies in which monoclonal antibodies directed at the bungarotoxin-binding site on *Torpedo* AChR prevented the binding to AChR of anti-AChR directed to a different epitope. Experiments such as these raise the possibility that some anti-AChR antibodies may actually be protective under certain circumstances. (These "protective" anti-AChR antibodies are obviously distinct from anti-idiotypic antibodies, which may also be protective in human MG.)

Other investigators have been interested in monoclonal antibodies that bind to a special part of the AChR which they call the *main immunogenic region (MIR)*. Antibodies to this area of the α-chain subunit of the AChR, felt to be located between residues 46 and 127, do not directly inhibit AChR function but do induce accelerated degradation. Most of this work has been performed in animal systems, and while some experiments seem to show that the majority of anti-AChR antibodies bind to this area in human disease, the importance of this region in human MG is controversial. The identification of such a region in human MG would be critical

for attempts to develop modalities of immunotherapy more specific than those currently employed.

Areas of the AChR other than the putative MIR have been found to be important in receptor function and MG pathogenesis. A wealth of data have shown that two cysteines at residues 192–193 of the α chain of the *Torpedo* AChR are important in bungarotoxin binding. Antibodies to the bungarotoxin-binding *Torpedo* AChR peptide consisting of residues 173–204 of the α-chain bind to native AChR, and a monoclonal antibody to this peptide blocks bungarotoxin binding to native AChR on the surface of the AChR-bearing mouse cell line BC3H1. Since clinical severity of human myasthenia correlates best with the level of blocking antibody (see above), the bungarotoxin-binding region of the human AChR, which is distinct from the putative MIR, may be a particularly important area in disease pathogenesis.

CONCLUSION

Thus, it is clear that although we know a great deal about MG pathogenesis, there is much that we do not know. On the one hand, the autoantigen is sequenced and fairly well understood and our ability to measure the effects of autoantibody is great. On the other hand, the autoantigen is large with many targets for autoantibodies, the autoantibody response is highly polyclonal, and the effect of autoantibody binding on the cellular metabolism of AChR is poorly understood. In any serum from an individual with MG, the relative roles of antibodies which bind to, accelerate degradation of, or blockade AChR are difficult to measure. It is likely that all of these attributes of anti-AChR antibodies contribute to pathogenicity. The ability of the muscle cells in an individual with MG to increase AChR production in response to increased degradation is also an issue that requires further analysis. The fact that a small percentage of myasthenic individuals have no demonstrable anti-AChR antibodies may signify that antibodies to autoantigens other than AChR or myoactive factors exist in some patients. Myasthenia gravis, experimental myasthenia gravis, and anti-AChR antibodies will continue to be important sources for increasing our understanding of membrane receptors and autoimmunity for many years to come.

ADDITIONAL READINGS

Drachman DB, Adams RN, Josifek LF, Self SG. Functional activities of autoantibodies to acetylcholine receptors and the clinical severity of myasthenia gravis. *N Engl J Med.* 1982;307:769–775.

Gomez C, Richman D. Monoclonal anti-acetylcholine receptor antibodies with differing capacities to induce experimental autoimmune myasthenia gravis. *J Immunol.* 1985;135:234–241.

Grob D, Arsura EL, Brunner NG, Namba T. The course of myasthenia gravis and therapies affecting outcome. *Ann NY Acad Sci.* 1987;505: 472–499.

Linstrom J, Seybold ME, Lennon VA, et al. Antibody to acetylcholine receptor in myasthenia gravis: Prevalence, clinical correlates, and diagnostic value. *Neurology.* 1976;26:1054–1059.

Pachner AR. Experimental models of myasthenia gravis: Lessons in autoimmunity and progress toward better forms of treatment. *Yale J Biol Med.* 1987;60:169.

Summary of Part III: Immune Mechanisms of Disease

Immunology and inflammation represent physiologic activities with a role, often obscure at first glance, in many homeostatic mechanisms. It is the challenge of teaching immunology in this era to provide a forward-looking approach. We must apprise you of what is known about these activities in clinical and research medicine, in order to provide a framework so that you can incorporate "immunologic thinking" into your approach to patients and the study of biologic systems. Part III of *Immunology and Inflammation: Basic Mechanisms and Clinical Consequences* provides some examples to serve both purposes. This text concludes with examples of immunologic mechanisms active in human diseases. We hope that your study of immunology and inflammation will not terminate here but that it will continue in the clinics, wards, and special care units during your medical school and residency training and into practice. We hope that immunology has become a new language, a new mindset, for you and that you will carry it with you into your future. Thus, the success of your immunology course and of this text will not be measured by your current test scores, but by the new approaches you may take in the analysis of physiologic and pathologic processes active in your patients. If we have been able to communicate to you the excitement we, the authors and editors, feel about the topics we have presented, then this textbook has been successful.

Good luck!

A

Glossary and List of Abbreviations

GLOSSARY

A glossary of terms related to infectious diseases is found in Chap. 21, "Immunity to Microorganisms."

ABO: Family of glycoprotein antigens (A, B, AB, or 0 [the absence of A or B]) which constitute the major blood group system in humans. The ABO system was the first to be discovered and is the most important in transfusion practice. Found on red blood cells and other cell types, as well as in a soluble form in body fluids.

Accelerated rejection: See *Rejection.*

Accessory cells: Cells that are not lymphocytes that are required for antigen presentation or IL-1 secretion.

Acquired immunity: Immunity that develops as a result of exposure to a foreign substance or organism or after vaccination.

Acquired immunodeficiency syndrome: AIDS.

Activated macrophage: A macrophage that can kill falcultative intracellular parasites or tumor cells.

Active immunity: Immune protection due to the immune response in the host after exposure to a foreign substance or organism or after vaccination.

Acute inflammation: A process whose hallmarks are edema formation, fibrin deposition, and the presence of neutrophils within the injured tissue.

Acute-phase reaction: Also *acute-phase response.* Change in serum protein levels and homeostasis which results from the elaboration of certain cytokines, including IL-1 and tumor necrosis factor. Serum proteins increased or decreased during the acute-phase reaction are called *acute-phase reactants.*

Acute rejection: See *Rejection.*

Adherent cells: Nonlymphoid cell, usually macrophages, which adhere strongly to glass or plastic surfaces.

Adjuvant: Any of many foreign materials introduced with an antigen to enhance its immunogenicity. These include killed bacteria (*Bordetella pertussis,* mycobacteria) or bacterial products (endotoxin), emulsions (Freund's adjuvant), precipitates (alum), or fine particulate clay (bentonite).

Adoptive immunity: The transfer of the ability to respond to antigen by transplanting immunocompetent cells into a host previously made immunoincompetent, usually by irradiation.

Adoptive transfer: See *Adoptive immunity, Passive immunity.*

Affinity: The strength of binding between an epitope and the antigen-binding site of an antibody molecule (the paratope).

Affinity chromatography: A technique that utilizes the affinity of antibody to antigen to purify specific antigens.

Agglutination: Clumping of particulate antigens, e.g., red blood cells or bacteria, by cross-linking antibody molecules, best accomplished by IgM antibodies. Agglutination may be observed grossly or microscopically and may be used as a test to measure antigen or antibody.

AIDS: Acquired immunodeficiency syndrome. Systemic T-cell immunodeficiency subsequent to infection with the human immunodeficiency virus (HIV).

Allele: The alternative genes which can be present at a specific locus, which then define the characteristics of the individual (the phenotype).

Allergen: Substance capable of inducing a state of specific hypersensitivity as opposed to a beneficial immune response.

Allergy: A hypersensitive state acquired through exposure to a specific allergen.

Alloantibody: Antibody raised in one individual and directed against an antigen (usually cells) of another of the same species. When experimental animals of an inbred strain are immunized with cells of another strain, the antibodies are usually directed against histocompatibility antigens.

Alloantigen: An antigen found only in some members of the species. Such antigens are the result of genetic polymorphism; the histocompatibility antigens are alloantigens.

Allogeneic: Originating from a genetically different individual or inbred cell line of the same species; genetic variation within a species.

Allogeneic effect: The nonspecific enhancement or suppression of an immune response by allogeneic T lymphocytes. It can take the place of helper T cells under some conditions.

Allograft: Transplant from one individual to a genetically nonidentical individual of the same species.

Alloimmunization: Immunization with an alloantigen as, e.g., occurs in hemolytic disease of the newborn.

Allotype: Antigenic determinants on immunoglobulin molecules coded at one genetic locus and inherited as alleles in different members of the same species.

Alternative pathway: A mechanism of complement activation that does not involve the binding of C1, C4, or C2 by antigen-antibody complexes. Contrast with *Classical pathway.*

Anamnestic response: See *Secondary immune response.*

Anaphylaxis: A systemic immediate hypersensitivity reaction caused by the administration of an allergen to a sensitized subject resulting in respiratory distress or vascular collapse; due to antigen-specific IgE present on the surface of mast cells.

Anaphylatoxin: A small fragment of C3 (C3a) or C5 (C5a) capable of degranulating mast cells and liberating vasoactive amines.

Anergy: Absence of a response to skin testing; this lack of delayed-type hypersensitivity may occur because the individual has not been exposed to the antigen injected, or may be the result of loss of reactivity due to, e.g., corticosteroid therapy, protein malnourishment, malignancy, or other severe systemic diseases.

Antibody (Ab): An immunoglobulin molecule capable of combining specifically with a known antigen.

Antibody-dependent cellular cytotoxicity (ADCC): A reaction in which a target cell is bound by the antigen-binding site of an antibody, which in turn is bound to an effector cell by the interaction of the antibody Fc region with the effector cell's FcR and triggers the killing of the target cell. Cells capable of performing ADCC include certain T cells, macrophages and monocytes, eosinophils, and possibly platelets. Also known as antibody-dependent cell-mediated cytotoxicity.

Antigen (Ag): A molecule capable of being the target of an immune response. It may have many determinants.

Antigen-presenting cell (APC): See *Accessory cell.*

Antigen-binding site: That part of the T-cell-antigen receptor or the antibody which binds to antigen. Also known as *paratope.*

Antigenic determinant: See *Epitope.*

Anti-idiotype: An antibody against the idiotype of another antibody.

Antinuclear antibodies (ANA): Antibodies directed against nuclear constituents, usually nucleoproteins; often seen in autoimmune diseases; such as systemic lupus erythematosus.

Apoptosis: Process by which a cell commits "suicide," with chromatin condensation and DNA fragmentation; dependent upon cell protein synthesis. Active in certain developing organs, in thymic selection of pre-T cells, and in cytotoxic T-cell killing of targets. Also known as "programmed cell death."

Arachidonic acid: A fatty acid found in the cell membrane of most mammalian cells. After many types of stimulation arachidonic acid is released and metabolized into prostaglandins and leukotrienes, which are potent biologic mediators.

Arthus' reaction: Local immune (hypersensitivity) reaction mediated by antigen-antibody complexes derived from circulating antibody and antigen injected into the skin. Results in local vascular injury, thrombosis, hemorrhage, and acute inflammation. Contrast with *Passive cutaneous anaphylaxis* (Prausnitz-Küstner) reaction.

Atopy: A genetic tendency to develop sudden hypersensitivity states such as allergic asthma or hay fever.

Autoantibody: Antibody directed at a component of self.

Autocrine: Growth mechanism in which a cell is stimulated by a compound which the cell itself secretes.

Autograft: A transplant from one region to another on the same individual.

Autoimmunity: Immunologic reaction to a component found in one's own body constituents or tissues.

Autologous: Originating from the same individual.

Avidin: A molecule which binds very avidly to many biotin molecules. The avidin-biotin system is used to amplify the readout of ELISA or indirect antibody-binding tests. The first antibody is labeled with avidin; then a second molecule which is conjugated to a radioactive tag or an enzyme is labeled with biotin and added. Many of these molecules will bind to each avidin molecule. Thus, more radioactivity or enzyme will localize at the site bound by the first antibody and increase the signal generated.

Avidity: An imprecise measurement of the strength of binding of antibody and antigen (or receptor and ligand) molecules, usually involving multiple different molecular interactions.

B: Symbol for a component of the alternative pathway; also known as C3 proactivator.

B cell: One of the two major classes of lymphocytes. B cells differentiate in the bursa of Fabricius in birds or the bone marrow of mammals and respond to antigen by differentiating into antibody-producing cells. They express surface immunoglobulins which function as antigen receptors.

Basophil: A polymorphonuclear leukocyte which contains granules that stain deeply when using basic dyes.

Bence Jones protein: A low molecular weight protein found in urine consisting of light chains or light-chain fragments; frequently due to the presence of a malignant overgrowth of one clone of lymphocytes or plasma cells (e.g., multiple myeloma).

Benign monoclonal gammopathy: A monoclonal increase in a single immunoglobulin molecule in the serum, due to an expansion of a single clone of plasma cells. By definition, is not associated with a decrease in other immunoglobulin levels—this benign process is seen in the elderly.

β_2-Microglobulin: A 12-kd polypeptide found in association with histocompatibility antigens on the surface of cells.

Bierbec granules: Rod-shaped granules uniquely found in the cytoplasm of dendritic cells.

Biologic response modifier: A molecule—natural or synthetic—that alters the normal response to a disease, usually through enhancement of the immune system.

Blast transformation: Transition of a small resting lymphocyte to a larger cell with ri-bosome-rich cytoplasm, representing a cell which has been activated and will enter into mitosis. Blast transformation can occur because of exposure of the cell to mitogens or specific antigens.

Blood groups: Alloantigens present at the surface of red blood cells. ABO and Rh are important blood groups in humans.

Bovine serum albumin: A common antigen and carrier in experimental work.

Bradykinin: A potent stimulator of long-standing smooth muscle contraction. Bradykinin, a nine amino acid peptide, is cleaved from a serum alpha globulin, kininogen, by the enzyme kallikrein.

Bursa of Fabricius: A lymphoid organ in the hindgut of birds that influences B-cell development.

Bursa equivalent: In species where a bursa of Fabricius has not been identified, the site of origin of B cells.

C: Abbreviation for the serum complement system. C followed by a number represents a specific component of the complement system, e.g., C3.

C1INH: Symbol for an inhibitor of the activated C1 esterase.

C3bINH: Symbol for an inhibitor of activated C3 (C3b).

C3 receptor: A molecule on the surface of B cells and phagocytes which can specifically bind C3b.

C-reactive protein: One of the acute-phase reactants.

C region: The constant region of light or heavy chains of immunoglobulin.

Cachectin: See *Tumor necrosis factor.*

Capping: The coordinated movement of membrane molecules to one region of the cell surface after binding by a multivalent ligand such as an antibody or an antigen.

Carrier: A large molecule to which haptens are bound, in order to make the hapten immunogenic; the carrier is usually itself an immunogenic protein.

Carrier determinants: Determinants on an antigen which react with helper T cells.

CD4: Phenotypic marker for cells which interact with class II MHC molecules; usually helper cells.

CD8: Phenotypic marker for cells which interact with class I MHC molecules; usually suppressor/cytotoxic cells.

Cellular immunity: Immune phenomena mediated by immune T cells and not by antibody, e.g., delayed hypersensitivity or cytolytic T cell lysis.

Cell-mediated lymphotoxicity: The ability of sensitized T cells (i.e., T cells from an immunized individual) to lyse other cells bearing membrane antigens to which they are sensitized.

Central lymphoid organs: Thymus, bursa of Fabricius (in birds), bone marrow. Important in lymphopoiesis and lymphocyte differentiation; also known as primary lymphoid organs.

Chemokines: Family of proinflammatory cytokines with repair-oriented functions; previously known as *intercrines* and *macrophage inflammatory peptides* (MIPs).

CH$_{50}$: The 50 percent lysis point in a system designed to detect complement by its ability to lyse antibody-coated red blood cells; general measure of the activity of the complement system.

C$_H$ region: The carboxyterminal end or constant region of the heavy chain of immunoglobulins with constant amino acid sequence in different antibodies of the same class and subclass. It comprises three-fourths to four-fifths of the heavy-chain sequence depending upon class.

Chronic inflammation: A process whose hallmarks include the presence of macrophages, histiocytes, lymphocytes, plasma cells, and, occasionally, giant cells and/or eosinophils.

Chronic rejection: See *Rejection.*

C$_L$ region: The carboxyterminal region of the heavy chain of immunoglobulins with constant amino acid sequence for all light chains of a given class. It comprises one-half of the light-chain sequence.

Class: The major molecular types, or isotypes, of immunoglobulin: IgG, IgM, IgA, IgE, IgD. The term is equivalent to *isotype.*

Class I molecules: Tissue antigens, designated as HLA-A, HLA-B, and HLA-C in humans and H-2K and H-2D in mice; include a polymorphic α chain and a monomorphic β$_2$-microglobulin molecule.

Class II molecules: Tissue antigens, designated HLA-D in humans and H-2I in mice; include two polymorphic chains, one α and one β.

Classical pathway: The mechanism of complement activation by antigen-antibody complexes involving the binding of C1, C4, and C2 to activate C3. Contrast with *Alternative pathway.*

Clone: A family of cells which are derived from a single cellular ancestor and which are therefore genetically identical.

Cluster of differentiation (CD): A result of an international conference to simplify the designation of antigens. For example, OKT4 is now CD4.

Cold agglutinin (antibody): Antibody that agglutinates more effectively at temperatures below 37°C.

Colony-stimulating factor (CSF): A substance that specifically stimulates growth of certain types of cells. The expansion of colonies, or clones, of that cell type is the end result of stimulation with CSFs. Many CSFs have been described and are defined by the type of cell population affected, e.g., GM-CSF (granulocyte-monocyte colony-stimulating factor).

Complement (C): A set of serum proteins activated in sequence by antibody-antigen complexes or by bacterial products (alternative pathway) and responsible for many biologic defense mechanisms such as lysis, opsonization, leukocyte chemotaxis, and inflammation.

Complement fixation: Activation of complement by interaction of early complement components with immunoglobulin or surface components of certain pathogens. When complement fixation occurs in vivo, there may be a decrease in the serum levels of complement components.

Complementarity determining region (CDR): The area of the immunoglobulin variable regions which determine the antigen binding of the antibody molecule.

Concanavalin A (conA): A plant substance that binds to mannose and glucose on cell surface glycoproteins and glycolipids and stimulates T cells to proliferate—a lectin.

Contrasuppressor cells: A population of T cells which inhibit suppressor cells.

Coombs' test: Direct or indirect antiglobulin laboratory diagnostic test done as part of the evaluation of hemolytic anemia. The direct Coombs' test can detect the presence of antibody or complement molecules on the surface of red blood cells. The indirect Coombs' test detects antibody in the serum of a patient which is capable of binding to normal red blood cells added in vitro.

Cortex: The peripheral region of a lymph node or the thymus.

Cross-matching: Testing in which a potential blood or organ recipient's serum is incubated with the donor's red blood cells. The end point for this test is agglutination and/or lysis of donor cells, which indicates incompatibility.

Cross-reactivity: Ability of an antibody or cell to react with or bind different antigens because the antigen against which it was made is similar to another antigen. See also *Molecular mimicry.*

Cryoglobulin: A serum globulin which has the property of precipitating upon exposure to the cold (temperature usually used is 4°C). Cryoglobulins may precipitate at more physiologic temperatures and have been implicated in cases of vasculitis.

Cytokine: A substance produced by one cell that causes a change in the function of another cell. A cytokine produced by a lymphocyte is called a *lymphokine* and a cytokine produced by a monocyte is called a *monokine.*

Cytotoxic lymphocytes: Lymphocytes (T cells) that have been sensitized and are able to lyse specific target cells to which they bind.

D: Symbol for a component of the alternative pathway; also pro-C3 proactivator convertase. Also: A region of the immunoglobulin gene.

Degranulation: Process whereby an intracellular granule merges its membrane with the membrane of the cell and disgorges the granular contents into the extracellular space.

Delayed-type hypersensitivity: Antigen-specific inflammatory immune reaction elicited by antigen injected into the skin of immune individuals. It takes 24 to 48 h to develop and subsides over the next 2 to 3 days. It is mediated by T cells and macrophages, not by antibodies.

Dendritic cell: An antigen-presenting cell, probably derived from macrophages or macrophage stem cells, found in the skin (where they are known as Langerhans cells), the lymph node (reticulum cells), afferent lymph (veiled cells), spleen (follicular dendritic cell), and thymus. The cells have abundant spherical dense mitochondria, irregular nuclei, and many long cytoplasmic prolongations. Dendritic cells are estimated to be 10 to 100 times more effective than monocytes as antigen-presenting cells.

Desensitization: A therapeutic intervention which seeks to decrease the patient's reactivity with an allergen. Done when the patient has had an adverse reaction to a drug, but must receive the same compound, e.g., a severe infection requiring treatment with a penicillin in a patient who has previously had an anaphylactic reaction to penicillin.

Determinant: That part of the structure of antigen that binds to an antibody-combining site or an antigen-specific lymphocyte cell surface receptor. See *Epitope.*

Diapedesis: Process by which leukocytes migrate from the blood to the extravascular space by insinuating themselves between endothelial cells.

Direct antiglobulin test: See *Coombs' test.*

Domain: A polypeptide segment of approximately 110 amino acid residues with an internal disulfide bond. The domain is the building block of the molecules which are part of the immunoglobulin superfamily.

DP: Human class II markers (formerly SB).

DQ: Human class II markers (formally DC, MB, and DS).

DR: Human class II markers.

Edema: Escape of fluid from the vascular space into the interstitium, caused by the increased vascular permeability of inflammation. The macroscopic result is tissue swelling.

Electrophoresis: Separation of molecules into discrete bands of different molecular weight, accomplished by use of an electric field to "push" the molecules through a gel with a certain size pore.

ELISA (Enzyme-linked immunosorbant assay): Assay that utilizes an enzyme conjugated to a detector molecule, e.g., a goat anti-human IgG conjugated to an enzyme, such as alkaline phosphatase or horseradish peroxidase, to detect binding to specific antigen in vitro. May be used to quantify either antigen or antibody.

Endocrine: Growth mechanism by which a cell secretes a hormone or growth factor into the circulation to have a general effect on other cells.

Endocytosis: Process of uptake of material by a phagocyte, including the processes known as *phagocytosis* and *pinocytosis.*

Endotoxin: A lipopolysaccharide derived from cell walls of gram-negative bacteria that has multiple biologic effects: it stimulates the immune response nonspecifically, stimulates mouse B lymphocytes, and activates the alternative complement pathway.

Enhancement: A prolongation of allograft or tumor survival by specific antibodies against the foreign tissue.

Eosinophil: A polymorphonuclear leukocyte which contains granules that stain deeply with eosin.

Eosinophil chemotactic factor of anaphylaxis (ECF-A): A molecule released immunologically during immediate hypersensitivity reactions that is able to attract eosinophils.

Epithelioid cell: Cell found in a granulomatous reaction, derived from tissue macrophages.

Epitope: An antigenic determinant, sometimes one that occurs many times on the same antigen.

Epitope matching: A new technique in tissue cross-matching for transplantation, where specific epitopes on HLA molecules, rather than the entire molecule, are detected.

Erythrocyte: Another name for red blood cell (*erythro* is the Greek root for "red").

E-rosettes: A cluster of sheep red blood cells (the E stands for erythrocyte) around a human T cell. It is used to define the human T-cell population, since human T cells can nonspecifically bind to antigens on the surface of sheep red blood cells.

Exon: Portion of the DNA of a gene that is expressed in transcribed RNA.

Exotoxin: Extracellular proteins elaborated by an organism which can then diffuse into surrounding tissues.

Fab fragment: A product of papain digestion of immunoglobulins with one intact light chain and part of one heavy chain. Fab fragments have one combining site for antigen.

F(ab')₂ fragment: A product of pepsin digestion of immunoglobulin with two intact light chains and parts of two heavy chains and two combining sites for antigen but lacking the Fc region.

Fc fragment: A product of papain digestion of immunoglobulin with parts of two heavy chains and no combining sites for antigen. This fragment has sites for activation of complement and for the binding of immunoglobulins to macrophages, lymphocytes, and mast cells and is responsible for many biologic functions of antibodies. C stands for "crystallizable"; only this fragment can be crytallized.

Fc receptor: A molecule on the surface of most lymphocytes and phagocytes able to bind the Fc portion of immunoglobulins.

fMet-Leu-Phe: Formylmethionylleucylphenylalanine. A class of bacteria-derived tripeptides that are highly chemotactic for neutrophils.

Fibrinoid necrosis: A term describing a particular type of tissue destruction, where debris with the appearance of fibrin is present locally. Often used to describe the appearance of the vessel wall, where humorally mediated destruction has caused a vasculitis.

Fluorescent activated cell sorter (FACS): A machine which can measure and sort cells which differentially bind fluorescein-tagged markers.

Follicle: A circumscribed region in lymphoid tissue, usually in the superficial cortex of lymph nodes, containing mostly B cells and dendritic macrophage.

Framework region: The parts of the variable regions of both heavy and light chains which are not involved in antigen binding and are not part of the hypervariable regions.

Freund's complete adjuvant (FCA or CFA): A mixture of mycobacterium and mineral oil that is most commonly used in immunization protocols.

Full-house match: In transplantation medicine, a match in which donor and recipient have an identical match at all HLA loci.

γ-Globulin: A globulin with slow electrophoretic mobility (γ region); includes most of the immunoglobulin molecules. This term is sometimes used to refer to all immunoglobulins of various classes.

Gell and Coombs reactions: The four different types of hypersensitivity reactions:

Type I: Anaphylactic reactions; involves IgE.
Type II: Cytotoxic reactions.
Type III: Immune complex–mediated reactions.
Type IV: Delayed-type hypersensitivity reactions; involves T cells.

Germinal center: A lymphoid follicle with a clear center, representing the site of active immunologic reactivity of B-cell proliferation.

Globulin: Any of a large number of serum proteins distinct from albumin and insoluble at high salt concentrations.

Gm marker: Allotype marker on human IgG heavy chains.

Graft-versus-host (GVH) reaction: The pathologic reactions caused by transplantation of immunocompetent T lymphocytes to an incompetent host. The host is unable to reject the T lymphocytes and becomes the target of attack by them.

Graft-versus-host disease (GVHD): An immunocompetent host is unable to reject transplanted immunocompetent T lymphocytes and becomes the target for these cells. See also *Graft-versus-host reaction.*

Granulocyte: Granular leukocyte; leukocyte with prominent cytoplasmic granules; includes neutrophils, eosinophils, and basophils.

Granuloma: Tissue reaction in chronic inflammation, often elicited by poorly degraded antigens, which results in "walling off" the antigen by macrophages, epithelioid cells, fibroblasts, and multinucleated giant cells.

Gray (gy): SI unit of absorbed dose of ionizing radiation. A routine chest x-ray delivers 0.03 to 0.1 mgy.

H-2: The major histocompatibility complex in the mouse.

H-2K and H-2D: Loci in the major histocompatibility complex in mice coding for class I histocompatibility antigens that are responsible for the rapid rejection of allografts and that serve as targets for T cell cytolysis.

H-2I: Loci in the major histocompatibility complex of mice coding for class II antigens.

Haplotype: A set of genetic determinants coded by closely linked genes on a single chromosome, e.g., MHC haplotype.

Hapten: A chemically defined determinant that, when conjugated to an immunogenic carrier, stimulates the synthesis of antibody specific for itself. It is capable of binding to antibody but cannot by itself stimulate an immune response.

Heavy chain (H chain): The higher molecular weight polypeptide chain in an immunoglobulin molecule; determines the class of the immunoglobulin.

Helper cells: A subpopulation of specific T cells that are necessary to "help" B cells produce antibody to thymus-dependent antigens. They may also provide help in T cell–mediated responses, e.g., killing.

Hematopoiesis: The process of blood cell formation (also *hemopoiesis*).

Hemolysis: Lysis of red blood cell. Reduction in the life span of circulating red blood cells which can be caused by immunologic mechanisms.

Hemolytic anemia: Accelerated destruction of red blood cells due to a variety of abnormalities, including intrinsic defects in the red blood cells, infection, and antibodies to membrane antigens, or passive binding of immune complexes or complement on the surface of the red blood cells. Hemolysis can occur within the vessels (intravascular) or outside the vascular system (extravascular).

Heterograft: A transplant from one species to another. May also be referred to as a *xenograft*.

Heterologous: Originating from a different individual or a different inbred line; sometimes applied to a different carrier molecule.

High endothelial venules (HEVs): Cuboidal endothelium-lined postcapillary venules which are the site where circulating immune cells leave the circulation and enter the surrounding tissue. Often seen at sites of inflammation and in secondary lymphoid organs.

Hinge region: The section of the immunoglobulin molecule that permits bending; found between the Fab and Fc regions of the heavy chains of the antibody molecule.

Histamine: A chemical in the body that causes smooth muscle constriction and dilation of small blood vessels.

Histiocyte: Phagocytic cell derived from macrophages; resident in tissue.

Histocompatibility antigens: Cell surface antigens characteristic of an individual or an inbred line that stimulate the rejection of tissue allografts.

Human immunodeficiency virus (HIV): A class of human T-cell retroviruses which cause AIDS.

HLA (human leukocyte antigen): The major histocompatibility complex in humans.

HLA-A, HLA-B, HLA-C: Three distinct genetic loci in the MHC of humans coding for the major histocompatibility of antigens.

HLA-D: A region of the human major histocompatibility complex coding for antigens expressed primarily on B cells and on activated T cells and macrophages. HLA-D molecules stimulate the specific proliferation of allogeneic T cells in culture.

Hot spots: See *Hypervariable region.*

Humoral immunity: Immune phenomena involving the production of specific antibody.

Hybridoma: A cell line formed by fusion of two cells.

Hyperacute rejection: See *Rejection.*

Hyperemia: Increased local blood flow due to vasodilation.

Hypersensitivity: The state, existing in a previously immunized individual, in which tissue damage results from the immune reaction to a further dose of antigen. If tissue damage is severe, the condition may be referred to as one form of allergy.

Hypervariable region: Defined portions of the variable region of either heavy or light immunoglobulin chains having extreme variability in amino acid sequence in different molecules. The antibody-combining site is made up of the hypervariable regions. There are also hypervariable regions in the T-cell receptor. Hypervariable regions are also known as *hot spots.*

I region: See *H-2I;* murine histocompatibility loci, including I-A, I-B, I-C, I-E, I-J; a region of the MHC where Ir genes are located, encoding Ia antigens.

Ia antigens: Histocompatibility antigens found primarily on murine B cells but also on some macrophages, T cells, and skin. They are encoded by the I region of the major histocompatibility complex.

Idiotype: An antigenic determinant on a specific antibody that is characteristic of that antibody and different from others even of the same isotype and allotype; idiotypes are usually located in or near the combining site; probably determined by the hypervariable regions.

Immediate hypersensitivity: A specific immune reaction that takes place in minutes to hours after the administration of antigen and is mediated by antibodies.

Immune complex: Antigen-antibody complex.

Immunoblot test: Analysis of antigens using electrophoresis to separate the different antigens and then probing the antigens with labeled antibody. Also known as *Western blot analysis.*

Immunogen: A molecule that elicits an immune response.

Immunoglobulin: The various classes of γ-globulin molecules having antibody activity.

Immunoglobulin superfamily: Molecules involved in cell-cell interactions. All members of this multimolecular family are made up of domains.

Incomplete Freund's adjuvant (ICFA): Freund's adjuvant without mycobacteria.

Indirect antiglobulin test: See *Coombs' test.*

Infection: Colonization by organisms in or on a host.

Infectious disease: Pathologic condition, with signs and symptoms associated with frank clinical illness, resulting from infection of a tissue normally free of significant numbers of organisms.

Inflammation: The typical reflexive reaction of the vascularized living tissue to injury. The gross appearance of such tissue reaction is characterized by warmth, pain, redness, swelling, and loss of function. (In the original Latin description: *color, dolor, rubor, tumor, et functio laesa.*)

Innate immunity: Nonspecific defense mechanisms not developed after immunization and not dependent on prior exposure to antigens, e.g., intact skin and mucus membranes, lysozyme in tears, functioning cilia in the respiratory tract.

Intercrines: See *Chemokines.*

Integrins: Families of cell surface accessory molecules involved in cell-cell adhesion.

Interferons (IFN):   A group of cytokines that lead to antiviral activity. The interferons inhibit infection in noninfected cells and modify the functions of those cells. They include IFN-α, IFN-β, and IFN-γ. IFN-α and IFN-β are produced by a variety of cells, including monocytes (leukocyte interferon). IFN-γ is produced by lymphocytes and is also called *immune interferon;* IFN-γ is the major component of macrophage-activating factor.

Interleukin (IL):   One of a group of cytokines. Interleukins 1 through 12 have been described. The term *interleukin* was coined at a time when these cytokines were thought to be active solely in one lymphocyte acting on another. It is now known that interleukins have many actions on nonimmune cells, as well.

Internal image: The region on an anti-idiotypic antibody which binds to the paratope of the idiotype. Thus the anti-idiotype antibody may resemble the original inciting antigen.

Intron: Intervening segment of DNA which is not transcribed into messenger RNA.

Inv marker: Allotype on human κ light chains.

Ir gene: Gene located in the I region of the major histocompatibility complex; Ir genes control the ability to develop specific immune responses to thymus-dependent antigens.

I-A, I-B, I-C, I-E, I-J: Subregions of the I region of the mouse H-2 complex.

Isogeneic: Originating from the same individual or the same inbred strain.

Isograft: A transplant from one genetically identical individual to another, e.g., monozygotic twins or mice from an inbred mouse strain.

Isohemagglutinins: Alloantibodies, usually of the IgM class, that agglutinate red blood cells and are used to type red blood cells.

Isologous: Originating from the same individual or a member of the same inbred strain.

Isotype: The class or subclass of an immunoglobulin common to all members of that species.

J chain: A small polypeptide found in IgM and IgA polymers and responsible for maintaining the polymeric form of the immunoglobulins.

J gene segment: Genetic locus encoding a small segment which joins a variable region gene segment to a constant region gene segment.

K cell: A class of cells, thought to be lymphocytes, able to mediate antibody-dependent cellular cytotoxicity.

Kallikrein: An enzyme, activated by cleavage of prekallikrein by other enzymes of the kinin pathway, which acts on kininogen to liberate kinin, a nine amino acid peptide.

κ chain: One of two possible types of light chains found in immunoglobulin.

Keyhole limpet hemocyanin (KLH):   A polypeptide antigen, derived from an inedible marine snail found off the California coast, used to test the primary immune response.

Killer cells: Cytotoxic lymphocytes.

Kinin: A peptide derived from kininogen by the action of kallikrein; increases vascular permeability.

Kinin system: A collection of serum proteases, mobilization of which is started by activation of coagulation factor XII. Kallikrein formation is the final result of this cascade of proteases, and kallikrein in turn cleaves kininogen to release bradykinin.

Kringle: A Viennese pastry with many intertwined layers of dough; the term is used to describe proteins (usually a peptide with the ends linked by a disulfide bond into a loop) or nucleic acids which fold in a pattern resembling this pastry.

L3T4: A marker found on the surface of murine helper T cells, defined by a monoclonal antibody of this name.

λ chain: One of two possible types of light chains found in immunoglobulin.

Lamina propria: The connective tissue underlying the gastrointestinal epithelium.

Langerhans cells: Dendritic cells in the epithelium of the skin which can act as antigen-presenting cells.

Large granular lymphocyte (LGL): The appearance of a natural killer cell.

Latex fixation test: An agglutination test in which latex beads have an antigen fixed to their surface so that serum can be tested for the presence of antibody capable of cross-linking the beads and causing agglutination.

Lectin: Any of a number of plant products that bind to cells, usually by nature of a combining site for specific sugars.

Leu: Antigen found on human lymphocytes, e.g., Leu-3. The Leu series has been replaced by the CD designation system.

Leukocyte: White blood cell (*leuko* is Greek for "white"); nucleated blood cells which include monocytes, lymphocytes, and the granulocytes (neutrophils, eosinophils, and basophils).

Leukocyte activating factor (LAF): Original name for interleukin 1.

Leukocyte migration inhibition factor (LMIF): A lymphokine produced by antigen-specific T cells in response to antigenic stimulation. Assayed in vitro by measuring inhibition of migration of blood leukocytes from a capillary tube or microdroplets.

Leukopheresis: See *Pheresis.*

Leukotriene: A product of the lipooxygenase pathway of arachidonic acid metabolism that can be a potent chemoattractant or mediator of inflammation.

Ligand: A molecule which binds to another molecule, often designated the receptor.

Light chain (L chain): The lower molecular weight polypeptide chain present in all immunoglobulin molecules.

Linkage: The condition where two genes are present in close proximity to each other on the same chromosome and are inherited together.

Linkage disequilibrium: Certain combinations of alleles (haplotypes) occurring at a higher than expected frequency.

Lipopolysaccharide (LPS): The active component of endotoxin derived from bacterial cell walls; a B-cell mitogen in the mouse. A potent stimulator of macrophages.

Locus: The position on a chromosome where a particular gene is found.

Ly antigen: T cell–specific antigen found in mice.

Lymphocyte: A small mononuclear cell containing a nucleus with densely packed chromatin and a small rim of cytoplasm.

Lymphocyte-activated killer cells (LAK): Multispecific lymphocytes activated in vitro by treatment with IL-2 which have the ability to kill tumor cells.

Lymphocyte function associated (LFA): Pertaining to a series of cell surface molecules which are involved in lymphocyte interactions with other cells.

Lymphokines: Biologically active molecules produced by lymphocytes.

Lymphotoxin: A cytotoxic cytokine produced by T cells. Also known as tumor necrosis factor beta.

Lysosome: A membrane-bound granule containing hydrolytic enzymes found in many cells.

Lysozyme: An enzyme capable of breaking down the cell wall of many bacteria.

Lyt: A system for designating antigens found on murine T cells that distinguishes different functional classes of T cells. Lyt-1 is a helper cell marker; Lyt-2 and Lyt-3 are found on suppressor cells.

M cells: Specialized flattened epithelial cells lining the lumen of the intestine which can take up antigen from the lumen and release the antigen into the subepithelial area of the Peyer's patch.

M component: A large amount of homogenous immunoglobulin detected in urine or serum due to the presence of a malignant overgrowth of one clone of lymphocytes or plasma cells (myeloma).

Macrophage: A general term referring to a ubiquitous nonlymphoid mononuclear phagocytic cell, found in tissues and blood, derived from monocytic stem cells. An important accessory cell in immune responses. Specialized macrophages present in some locations have separate names (e.g., *Kupffer cells* [liver] and *histiocytes* [connective tissue]). Macrophages, which are derived from circulating monocytes, are to be distinguished from the phagocytic granulocytes. In general, macrophages are located in tissues and have relatively little myeloperoxidase compared to monocytes.

Macrophage-activating factor (MAF): Another name for gamma interferon (IFN-γ); a cytokine which increases the phagocytic potential of macrophages.

Macrophage inflammation peptides (MIPs): See *Chemokines*.

Macrophage migration inhibition: See *Migration inhibition factor*.

Major basic protein (MBP): A protein found in the cerebrospinal fluid of some patients with multiple sclerosis. The same abbreviation is also used for myelin basic protein found in peripheral nerve myelin.

Major histocompatibility complex (MHC): A large region of genetic material containing genes encoding the histocompatibility antigens, immune response genes, and lymphocyte surface antigens; responsible for the rapid rejection of allografts (H-2 in mice, HLA in humans).

Margination: Attachment of leukocytes to the endothelium of the blood vessel. Due to the flow characteristics of red and white blood cells, the former occupy a central stream of blood, displacing the leukocytes to the periphery, in contact with the endothelium of the vessel wall. The leukocytes adhere to the endothelial wall and are "removed" from the circulating pool (45 percent of all intravascular leukocytes are circulating and 55 percent are marginated).

Mast cell: A tissue cell, resembling the blood basophil, that has vasoactive amine-containing cytoplasmic granules and membrane receptors for IgE.

Medulla: The central region of the thymus and lymph nodes; in the latter, consists of lymphatic sinuses and medullary cords.

Memory: The ability of the immune system to mount a specific secondary (anamnestic) response to an immunogen that was previously introduced.

Membrane attack complex (MAC): The assembled C5–C9 components of complement that cause cell lysis.

Migration inhibition factor (MIF): A protein produced by lymphocytes upon interaction with antigens that inhibits the motility of macrophages in culture. MIF may be the same as MAF (IFN-γ).

Microvasculature: The vascular network that connects the arterial and the venous circulation; composed of arterioles, capillaries, venules, and arteriovenous anastomoses.

Mitogen: A substance that stimulates lymphocytes to proliferate independently of any specific antigen.

Mitomycin C: A drug used to prevent DNA synthesis in cells; often used in a one-way mixed lymphocyte reaction (MLR).

Mixed lymphocyte reaction (MLR): The proliferative response of allogeneic lymphocytes when cultured together.

Molecular mimicry: Resemblance between two antigens; of immunologic relevance when the antibodies or cells directed against one molecule cross-react with a molecule that the original target resembles or mimics.

Monoclonal: Derived from a single clone.

Monocyte: Circulating phagocytic blood leukocyte with single ovoid or kidney-shaped nucleus and fine granular cytoplasm derived from monocytic stem cells in the bone marrow. It is the precursor of most tissue macrophages.

Monokine: A cytokine produced by a monocyte.

Mononuclear cells: Leukocytes with non-lobulated nuclei, including monocytes, macrophages, and lymphocytes.

Mononuclear phagocyte: Mononuclear cells capable of phagocytosis, including monocytes and macrophages.

Multiple myeloma: A plasma cell tumor producing a characteristic immunoglobulin (*para*-protein); a plasmocytoma.

Natural killer (NK) cells: Cells capable of mediating natural killing, which is killing mediated by large granular lymphocytes without apparent antigenic or major histocompatibility complex specificity.

Nephelometry: A technique used to determine the concentration of a molecule in solution or suspension by measuring the turbidity or lack of light transmission through the solution or suspension.

Neutral protease: A protein-cleaving enzyme with a pH optimum near 7; abundant in phagocytes.

Neutrophil: A granulocyte with a characteristic multilobulated nucleus and a mixture of basophilic and eosinophilic granules. A type of polymorphonuclear leukocyte.

Nonadherent cells: Those cells in suspensions of spleen and other lymphoid tissue that do not adhere to plastic or glass, in contrast to macrophages. Usually lymphocytes.

Northern blot test: A qualitative and quantitative test in which RNA is isolated and separated by electrophoresis. Specific RNA can then be detected by hybridization to a DNA probe.

Nude mouse: Congenitally athymic, nearly hairless, mouse.

Null cell: A class of lymphocyte that does not bear markers for either T cells or B cells. In the older literature this was called "the third population" of cells.

NZB mouse: New Zealand black mouse; an inbred strain that develops autoimmune disease.

NZW mouse: New Zealand white mouse; when bred with NZB mice, the resulting NZB/W [(NZB × NZW)F$_1$] mice develop murine lupus.

OKT: A set of antigens, defined by monoclonal antibodies, found on T-cell populations. This terminology has been replaced by the cluster of differentiation (CD) designation system.

Opportunistic infection: An infection in an immunocompromised host caused by an organism not usually considered pathogenic or virulent.

Opsonization: The enhancement of phagocytosis of a particle or a cell (especially bacteria) by virtue of its being covered by antibody or complement; the phagocytosing cell more efficiently takes the particle up by the interaction of this antibody and/or complement with cell surface receptors on the phagocyte.

Ouchterlony test: A precipitin reaction in a gel in which both antibody and antigen diffuse, bind, and precipitate.

Oxygen metabolites, reactive: Highly reactive compounds of oxygen that are produced by activated neutrophils and mononuclear phagocytes and are highly toxic to host cells and microorganisms.

Paracrine: Growth mechanism by which one cell secretes a factor which then diffuses a short distance to its target cell.

Paratope: See *Antigen-binding site.*

Passive cutaneous anaphylaxis (PCA): Prausnitz-Küstner reaction; the induction of a local, immediate-type immune reaction by injecting antibody into the skin and later injecting antigen intravenously or locally. This reaction is caused by the release of vasoactive amines from mast cells and is manifested by a large increase in vascular permeability.

Passive immunity: Immune protection mediated by cells or antibodies transfused into an immunologically naive host. The host does not produce the protective elements.

Passive transfer: See *Passive immunity.*

Pasteur point: The concentration of oxygen (about 1%) in the earth's atmosphere achieved about 600 million years ago at which organisms were able to shift from fermentation to respiratory metabolism.

Perforin: One name for the cytotoxic molecule of many immune cells that forms a pore in the membrane of the target cell.

Peyer's patches: A collection of lymphoid tissue in the submucosa of the small intestine.

Phagocyte: A leukocyte capable of phagocytosis (ingestion of particles); includes neutrophils, eosinophils, monocytes, and macrophages.

Phagocytosis: Ingestion of particulate matter by a cell.

Phagolysosome: Membrane-lined cytoplasmic vesicle formed by the fusion of a phagosome and a lysosome.

Phagosome: Membrane-bound vesicle enclosing phagocytosed material.

Phenotype: The expressed characteristics of an organism.

Pheresis: A technique in which blood is taken from the vein of a patient; a certain component is removed and the rest is returned by means of another catheter. *Leukopheresis* removes white blood cells, and

plasmapheresis removes plasma (usually to eliminate immune complexes or autoantibodies). *Photopheresis* eliminates activated T cells by giving the patient oral 8-methoxypsoralen, which is taken up by T cells, and then exposing the cells ex vivo to ultraviolet A light.

Phorbol ester: One of a group of potent tumor promoters that can stimulate a variety of cells including those of the immune system by direct activation of protein kinase C (PKC). Examples are PMA (phorbol myristate acetate) and TPA (12-O-tetradecanoylphorbol-13-acetate).

Phospholipase: An enzyme that catalyzes the hydrolysis of phospholipids at various specific bonds. (The phospholipase group consists of phospholipase A_1, A_2, B, C, and D. For example, phospholipase A_2 is responsible for releasing arachidonic acid from plasma membrane lipids.)

Photopheresis: See *Pheresis.*

Phytohemagglutinin (PHA): A compound derived from the red kidney bean which was first described as being able to agglutinate red blood cells (thus its name); later found to be a T-cell mitogen—a lectin.

Pinocytosis: Uptake of soluble macromolecules or colloid by a phagocytic cell.

Plaque-forming cell (PFC): An antibody-secreting cell releasing sufficient antibody against red blood cells to form an area of hemolysis in a layer of agar filled with RBCs with the addition of complement. Antibody reactions are often quantified by counting the number of PFCs. Cells making antibodies to other antigens can be estimated by a modified PFC method in which the protein antigen is bound to indicator red blood cells.

Plasma: The liquid part of unclotted blood remaining after cells have been removed.

Plasmapheresis: See *pheresis.*

Plasma cell: A cell of the B-cell lineage actively secreting large amounts of immunoglobulin. An end cell which no longer divides.

Platelet: Fragments of the bone marrow cell, the megakaryocyte, platelets circulate in the blood and are involved in coagulation and in certain immune mechanisms.

Platelet-activating factor (PAF): A choline-containing phospholipid produced by a variety of cell types that has potent platelet-activating, spasmogenic, vasoactive, and leukotactic properties.

Pokeweed mitogen (PWM): A plant compound which is a lymphocyte mitogen and induces differentiation of B cells with immunoglobulin secretion—a lectin.

Polyclonal: Derived from many clones.

Polyclonal activation: Activation of many clones, as from a mitogen or an antigen which is capable of stimulating many antigen-specific clones.

Polymorphism: Presence in a population of two or more alleles at a given locus at frequencies higher than expected for known mutation rates.

Polymorphonuclear (PMN) cells: Most abundant blood leukocytes in humans; derived from granulocytic bone marrow stem cells. Polymorphonuclear cells have characteristic lobulated nuclei. This type of cell is the hallmark of acute inflammation.

Postcapillary venule: Specialized segment of the microvasculature, immediately distal to the capillary, which is the site of histamine-induced vascular leakage; of major importance for leukocyte emigration into inflamed tissue.

Prausnitz-Küstner (PK) test: A way of detecting antigen-specific IgE in which antigen is injected into skin previously sensitized with IgE antibody.

Primary immune response: The response occurring on first exposure to an immunogen.

Primary lymphoid organs: See *Central lymphoid organs.*

Primed: Previously exposed to an immunogen and capable of making a secondary response to that immunogen; may refer to an animal or to a cell population, or to a macrophage population treated with lymphokine.

Properdin: A component of the alternative pathway.

Prostaglandin (PG): A product of the cyclooxygenase pathway of arachidonic acid metabolism. A potent biologic response modifier. Examples are PGA, PGB, PGC, PGD, PGE.

Protein A: A protein found in the cell wall of *Staphylococcus aureus* which can bind to the Fc region of IgG.

PUVA: Psoralen plus ultraviolet light; a form of therapy for psoriasis.

rad: 100 gy (grays). See *gray.*

Radioallergosorbant test (RAST): Test to detect IgE to specific allergens.

Radioimmunoassay (RIA): A very sensitive assay usually used to detect antigen.

Radioimmunosorbent test (RIST): Test to detect total IgE.

Raji cell assay: A test to measure circulating immune complexes; this lymphoblastoid cell line has Fc receptors which can bind immune complexes.

RBC: Red blood cell.

Reagin: IgE antibody.

Rejection: The destruction of foreign tissue or tumor due to an immune reaction against it. In transplantation medicine, there are different types of rejection:

Hyperacute—within minutes of transplantation; due to preformed cytotoxic antibodies to donor HLA or ABO antigens.

Accelerated—2 to 5 days after transplantation; due to both cellular and humoral reactivity.

Acute—7 to 21 days after transplantation; due to cellular immune reactivity to donor antigens.

Chronic—over 1 year after transplantation; humoral immune recognition plus ADCC; biopsy shows fibrosis of interstitium and vascular degeneration; often not amenable to increased immunosuppressive therapy.

Relative risk: Frequency of disease in individuals with particular HLA antigens compared to the frequency among those who lack that HLA antigen.

rem: 0.01 sievert (Sv). See *sievert*.

Respiratory burst: Sudden increase in oxidative metabolic activity of granulocytes and macrophages following phagocytosis or stimulation by other means.

Restriction enzyme: An enzyme that cuts DNA at a distinct nucleotide sequence.

Restriction fragment polymorphism (RFLP): Different pattern on a Southern blot (between different cells or individuals) resulting from genetic recombination.

Reticuloendothelial system (RES): The collection of fixed phagocytic cells found in the liver, spleen, and lymph nodes.

Rh antigen: Blood group system (cells are either Rh-positive or Rh-negative) determined by the presence or absence of the D antigen. About 15 percent of Caucasians are Rh (D) negative, with other races less often D negative. Rh incompatibility can provide fetal-maternal immunization with intrauterine hemolysis in subsequent pregnancies.

Rheumatoid factor (RF): An anti-immunoglobulin antibody detected against IgG in patients with some rheumatologic diseases. It binds to the Fc region of IgG and is not an anti-idiotypic antibody. Routine laboratory assays usually measure only IgM RF, but RF activity of other classes occurs.

Roentgen: A non-SI unit of radiation γ; a measure of how much ionizing X or γ radiation is in the air.

Sf: Svedberg flotation unit; a sedimentation coefficient.

Secondary immune response: The response occurring on the second and subsequent exposure to an immunogen (memory). An anamnestic response.

Secondary lymphoid follicle: See *Germinal center*.

Secondary lymphoid organs: Peripheral concentrations of lymphocytes; spleen and lymph nodes, for example. Contrast with *Central (primary) lymphoid organs*.

Second-set rejection: Rejection of a graft in an individual previously exposed to the tissue type of the graft. See also *Rejection*.

Secretory component (SC): A polypeptide synthesized by epithelial cells and added to IgA (and some IgM) in secretion of these immunoglobulins; also known as transport piece.

Selectins: A family of leukocyte adhesion molecules.

Serotonin (5-hydroxytryptamine): A catecholamine that is stored in mast cells and platelets and has a role in anaphylaxis.

Serum: The liquid part of blood remaining after cells and fibrin have removed.

Serum sickness: A syndrome resulting from the localization of circulating immune complexes in small vessels and especially the kidney glomeruli.

Sheep red blood cell (SRBC): A common antigen in experimental work.

Shwartzman reaction: A nonimmunologically mediated phenomenon elicited by two dermal injections of endotoxin 24 h apart. There is local inflammation with thrombus formation and systemic disseminated intravascular coagulation.

Sievert (Sv): The SI unit of absorbed dose equivalent, producing the same biologic effect on tissue as 1 gy (gray); replaces the term rem, for roentgen equivalent mammal.

Slow-reacting substance of anaphylaxis (SRS-A): A leukotriene-peptide molecule released immunologically that is responsible for some of the effects of anaphylaxis.

Southern blot test: A test in which DNA is analyzed by first separating the DNA by size electrophoretically and then probing the different size fragments by hybridization with a cloned DNA probe; named after Dr. Southern, who first described the technique.

Specificity: The ability of antibodies or lymphocytes to distinguish between different determinants.

Splenomegaly: The increase in size of the spleen, e.g., the result of a graft-versus-host reaction.

Spondylitis: Inflammation of the spine; often associated with the presence of the HLA-B27 histocompatibility antigen.

Staph protein A: See *Protein A.*

Subclass: Immunoglobulins of the same class but differing in electrophoretic mobility or in an antigenic determinant detectable in the constant heavy-chain region, e.g., IgG1, IgG2, IgG3, IgG4.

Suppressor cells: A subpopulation of T cells (or macrophages) that is able to suppress the immune response. There are specific and nonspecific suppressor cells.

Syngeneic: Pertaining to two individuals of a species that are genetically identical at all relevant transplantation loci, i.e., monozygotic twins or members of intensively inbred strains.

Systemic lupus erythematosus (SLE): An autoimmune disease characterized by the production of autoantibodies to different autoantigens and especially to DNA.

T cell: A class of lymphocytes which differentiate in the thymus, capable of responding to thymus-dependent antigens and MHC gene products. T cells do not produce antibodies; they mediate cellular immune reactions. They express antigen-specific receptors which are related to but different from classic immunoglobulin molecules.

Tac: T-cell receptor on activated cells for IL-2; stands for *T*-cell *ac*tivated.

T-dependent antigen: An immunogen that requires T-cell participation to elicit an antibody response.

T-independent antigen: An immunogen that is able to elicit an antibody response without the participation of T cells.

Theta: An antigen found on T cells in the mouse—the best T-cell marker in the mouse; also called Thy-1.

Thoracic duct lymphocytes (TDL): Circulating lymphocytes obtained from the thoracic duct; predominantly T cells.

Thymectomy: Removal of the thymus.

Thymocyte: Lymphocyte which matured within the thymus.

Thymus-dependent area: A region of peripheral lymphoid tissue such as lymph nodes and spleen containing mostly T cells that atrophies after thymectomy, e.g., the deep cortex of lymph nodes and the periarteriolar sheath of the spleen.

Thymus-independent area: A region within peripheral lymphoid tissue containing mostly B cells, e.g., the follicles of lymph nodes found in the superficial cortex.

TL: A system of mouse T-cell antigens originally found on T-cell leukemia cells and expressed in some mouse strains on normal thymocytes. TL stands for *T*-cell *l*eukemia. A differentiation alloantigen on mouse thymocytes. It is not expressed on mature T cells.

Tolerance: The failure of the immune system, as the result of previous contact with antigen, to respond to the same antigen, although capable of responding to others. Tolerance is best established by neonatal injection of an antigen.

Toxin: Compound produced by pathogens which causes tissue dysfunction or death.

Toxoid: A chemically treated immunogenic exotoxin which can be used for immunization, its toxicity having been removed or altered by the treatment.

Transfer factor: Small molecules extracted from sensitized leukocytes and able to transfer specific delayed hypersensitivity to the recipient. The reactivity is specific for the antigen(s) to which the donor of the leukocytes was sensitized.

Transfusion reaction: Immunologic activation caused by host recognition of transfused cells, e.g., red blood cells. This reaction occurs secondary to alloantibodies that cause hemolysis of the donor erythrocytes. Lesser transfusion reactions may occur with alloantibodies directed against leukocytes (leukoagglutinin reaction).

Transport piece: A polypeptide found associated with secreted IgA but not with serum IgA; synonymous with secretory component.

Tropism: Selectivity by an organism for specific host tissue(s).

Tumor infiltrating lymphocytes (TIL): Lymphocytes cloned from biopsies of tumors, which, when re-infused into the host, can kill the tumor.

Tumor necrosis factor (TNF): Cachectin. A cytokine which was originally named for its ability to lyse tumor cells; two were described: TNF-α from macrophages, and TNF-β from T cells. TNF-α has many more activities than tumor lysis; one striking activity is the induction of cachexia in animals treated with TNF-α (thus the synonym, cachectin).

Tumor-specific transplantation antigen (TSTA): Antigen found on the cell membrane of tumors against which tumor-rejection reactions are directed.

Type I reaction: Anaphylactic reactions; involves IgE.

Type II reaction: Cytotoxic reactions.

Type III reaction: Immune complex–mediated reactions.

Type IV reaction: Delayed-type hypersensitivity reactions; involves T cells.

V region: The variable region of light or heavy chains of immunoglobulin.

Vaccine: An antigen-containing material of an organism which, on introduction into an individual, stimulates active immunity and future protection against infection by that organism.

Valency: The number of antigen-binding sites and therefore the number of antigens which can be bound by an antibody molecule; up to 10 for IgM; 2 for IgG, IgE, and IgD; and variable for IgA. Valency is determined in part by the number of monomers found in the IgA polymer.

Vasculitis: Inflammation and destruction of blood vessels; often described as fibrinoid necrosis or granulomatous.

Vasodilation: Dilation of precapillary arterioles, with subsequent increased blood flow through that vascular bed.

V_H region: The variable amino acid sequence region of the heavy chain.

V_L region: The variable amino acid sequence region of the light chain.

Western blot analysis: Analysis of antigens using electrophoresis to separate the different antigens and then probing the antigens with labeled antibody. Also known as immunoblot test.

Wheal-and-flare reaction: The skin reaction elicited by histamine release. The central raised edema is the wheal; the erythematous surround is the flare. Wheal and flare can be caused by trauma or local cutaneous IgE-mediated reactions.

White blood cell (WBC): Leukocyte.

Xenogeneic: Originating from a different species.

Xenograft: A transplant from one species to another. May also be referred to as a *heterograft*.

LIST OF ABBREVIATIONS

Ab	Antigen
ADCC	Antibody-dependent cellular cytotoxicity (or antibody-dependent cell-mediated cytotoxicity)
Ag	Antigen
AIDS	Acquired immunodeficiency syndrome
AIHA	Autoimmune hemolytic anemia
AIN	Acute interstitial nephritis
Am	Allotypic marker on IgA heavy chains
ANA	Antinuclear antibody
APC	Antigen-presenting cell
B	Symbol for a component of the alternative pathway; also known as C3 proactivator or GBG
BALT	Bronchus-associated lymphoid tissue
Bb	Activated complement component B
BCG	Bacillus Calmette-Guérin
BSA	Bovine serum albumin
BSF	B-cell stimulatory factor
C	Abbreviation for the serum complement system. C followed by a number represents a specific component of the complement system, e.g., C3
CAM	Cellular adhesion molecule
CD	Cluster of differentiation
CDR	Complementarity determining region
CFA	Freund's complete adjuvant
CML	Cell-mediated lymphocytotoxicity
conA	Concanavalin A
CR	Complement receptor
CSF	Colony-stimulating factor
CTL	Cytotoxic T lymphocyte
D	Symbol for a component of the alternative pathway; also pro-C3 proactivator convertase of pro-GBG-ase
DP	Human class II markers (formerly SB)
DQ	Human class II markers (formerly DC, MB, and DS)
DR	Human class II markers
E	Erythrocyte
EA	Erythrocyte coated by specific antibody
EAC	Erythrocyte coated by antibody and complement
EAE	Experimental allergic encephalomyelitis
EAN	Experimental allergic neuritis
EAT	Experimental allergic thyroiditis
EBV	Epstein-Barr virus
ECF-A	Eosinophil chemotactic factor of anaphylaxis
ECP	Eosinophil cationic protein
EGF	Epidermal growth factor
ELAM	Endothelial leukocyte adhesion molecule
ELISA	Enzyme-linked immunosorbent assay
Fab	Antigen-binding component of antibody molecule, product of papain digestion
F'ab	Antigen-binding component of antibody molecule, product of pepsin digestion
FACS	Fluorescent activated cell sorter
FANA	Fluorescent antinuclear antibodies
Fc	Nonantigen-binding component of antibody molecule, product of papain digestion
FCA	Freund's complete adjuvant
FcR	Cell surface receptor for Fc portion of Ig
FITC	Fluorescein isothiocyanate
FMLP	fMet-Leu-Phe
GALT	Gut-associated lymphoid tissues

Gm	Allotypic marker on IgG heavy chains	MBP	Major basic protein *or* myelin basic protein
GVH	Graft versus host	MAC	Membrane attack complex
GVHD	Graft-versus-host disease	MAF	Macrophage-activating factor
Gy	Gray (SI unit of radiation)	MALT	Mucosa-associated lymphoid tissue
HANE	Hereditary angioneurotic edema	MHC	Major histocompatibility complex
HETE	Hydroxyeicosatetraeanoic acid; a metabolite of arachidonic acid	MIF	Migration inhibition factor
		mIg	Membrane-bound Ig
HEV	High endothelial venule	MLC	Mixed lymphocyte culture
HIV	Human immunodeficiency virus	MLR	Mixed lymphocyte reaction
HLA	Human leukocyte antigen; the major histocompatibility complex in humans	NK cell	Natural killer cell
		PAF	Platelet-activating factor
		PCA	Passive cutaneous anaphylaxis
HPETE	Hydroperoxyeicosatetraenoic acid; a metabolite of arachidonic acid	PFC	Plaque-forming cell
		PG	Prostaglandin
		PHA	Phytohemagglutinin
		PK	Prausnitz-Küstner (test)
ICAM	Intercellular adhesion molecule	PKC	Protein kinase C
		PLad	Peripheral lymph node addressin
ICFA	Incomplete Freund's adjuvant	PMA	Phorbol myristate acetate
IFA	Indirect immunofluorescence assay	PMN	Polymorphonuclear neutrophil
IFN	Interferon	PUVA	Psoralen plus ultraviolet A light
Ig	Immunoglobulin		
IL	Interleukin	PWM	Pokeweed mitogen
ITP	Immune (formerly idiopathic) thrombocytopenic purpura	rad	Radiation absorbed dose (supplanted by the SI unit *gray*)
kd	kilodalton; the unit used for measurement of molecular mass	RAST	Radioallergosorbent test
		RBC	Red blood cell
		RIA	Radioimmunoassay
KLH	Keyhole limpet hemocyanin	rem	Radiation emitted dose (supplanted by the SI unit *sievert*)
Km	Allotypic marker on κ light chains		
		RES	Reticuloendothelial system
LAF	Leukocyte-activating factor	RF	Rheumatoid factor
LAK	Lymphocyte-activated killer (cells)	RFLP	Restriction fragment length polymorphism
LFA	Lymphocyte function associated antigen	RIST	Radioimmunosorbent test
LGL	Large granular lymphocyte	Sf	Svedberg flotation unit
LMIF	Leukocyte migration inhibition factor	SBE	Subacute bacterial endocarditis
LT	Lymphotoxin		
LTB$_4$	Leukotriene B$_4$	SC	Secretory component

SCID	Severe combined immunodeficiency	TGF	Transforming growth factor
sIg	Secreted immunoglobulin	TIL	Tumor-infiltrating lymphocytes
sIgA	Secretory IgA	TLI	Total lymphoid irradiation
SLE	Systemic lupus erythematosus	TMA	Trimetallic anhydride
SRBC	Sheep red blood cell	TNF	Tumor necrosis factor
SRS-A	Slow-reacting substance of anaphylaxis	TNI	Total nodal irradiation
		TPA	12-*O*-tetradecanoylphorbol-13-acetate
Sv	Sievert (SI unit of radiation)	TSTA	Tumor-specific transplantation antigen
Tac	T-cell receptor for IL-2	TX	Thromboxane
Tdt	Terminal deoxynucleotidyl transferase		
TCR	T-cell receptor	VLA	Very late activation antigens
TDL	Thoracic duct lymphocyte		
TF	Transfer factor	WBC	White blood cell

B

The Phylogeny of the Immune System: A Review

INTRODUCTION

The human immune system consists of layers of complexity and specificity accreted over time. Certain of these mechanisms suggest that the purposes apparently served are not the original or primary reason for their development. As well, certain functions considered "immune" in nature may actually be mediated by ancient mechanisms of a nonspecific sort.

Figure B-1 is a simplified phylogenetic tree, charting invertebrate evolution from protozoa to coelenterates, chordates, and finally to the immediate ancestor of vertebrates, the tunicate. The other path from the coelenterates leads to the annelids, arthropods, and mollusks, all valuable in the study of immunophylogeny (and, occasionally, in the kitchen), but not on the path to vertebrate development.

The first vertebrates (Fig. B-2), the agna-

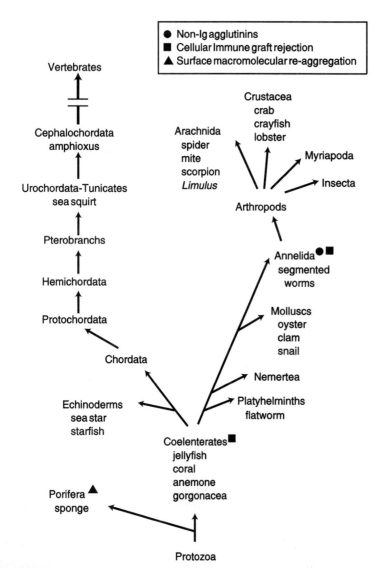

Figure B-1 Phylogenetic tree, tracing development from unicellular organisms to the prevertebrates. Symbols refer to appearance of cellular immune-mediate graft rejection, surface macromolecules mediating cellular cooperation, and nonimmunoglobluin agglutinins.

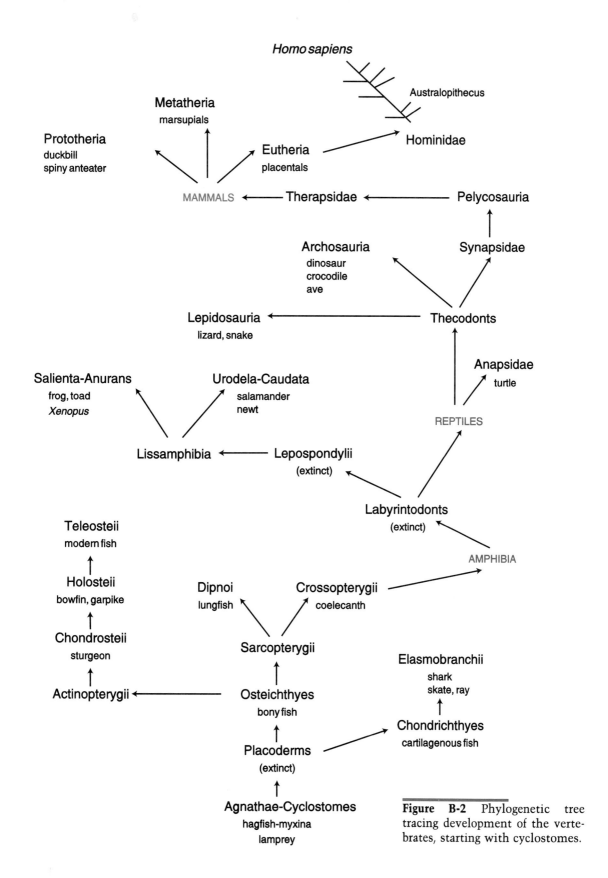

Figure B-2 Phylogenetic tree tracing development of the vertebrates, starting with cyclostomes.

thae, gave rise to the placoderms and thence to the bony and cartilaginous fishes. From a subset of the bony fish, Sarcopterygii, developed amphibians and then reptiles. The reptilian group Archosauria included the now-extinct dinosaurs and gave rise to birds and to the group Therapsida, which ultimately developed into mammals. Within mammalian development, placentation developed and evolved in the Eutheria. The evolutionary path from unicellular organisms to *Homo sapiens* thus stretches 500 million years (Table B-1).

DEFINITIONS

An effective, functional immune system should be able to differentiate between self and nonself, a difference crucial in multicellular organization and histogenesis as well as defense. More precisely, such a system should possess these abilities:

Response: to react and adapt to environmental changes.

Restructuring: to put in place adaptive mechanisms and keep them in the individual's immune repertoire, changes accomplished on both a physiologic and geologic time frame.

Recall: to make use of previous experiences, i.e., memory, to improve the efficiency and rapidity of onset of future responses.

Restraint: to regulate responses once mounted, preventing the system from going out of control.

Three potential pitfalls exist in the study of the phylogeny of the modern immune system: First, modern descendants of more primitive species only give us a hint about the immune response of their ancestors. Second, only a few modern species have been studied intensively. Third, the transitional phases of developmental breakthroughs are

TABLE B-1   Phylogeny of the Species, with Approximate Epoch of Emergence

Epoch	Millions of Years Ago	Species Appearing
Cenozoic Era		
Present		
Pleistocene	1–	
Pliocene	11–1	
Miocene	26–11	Hominoidea
Oligocene	36–26	Anthropoidea
Eocene	55–36	
Paleocene	70–55	
Mesozoic Era		
Cretaceous	130–70	Metatheria, Eutheria
		Prototheria, Aves
Jurassic	165–130	Mammals
		Teleosts
Triassic	200–165	Therapsidae
Permian	230–200	Synapsidae
Paleozoic Era		
Carboniferous	280–230	Reptiles
		Amphibia
Devonian	320–280	Actinopterygii
		Ichthyes
Silurian	350–320	Cyclostomes
Ordovician	420–350	Amphioxus
		Tunicates
Cambrian	500–420	Metazoans, Echinoderms

often missing; this may be the result of the first two factors or, alternatively, Darwinian evolution may not be a smooth, continuous process, but rather a series of fits and starts. (See Stephen Jay Gould's book of essays *Ever Since Darwin*—relevant to this issue, but also terrific reading, in general.) Evolving species exist for only a short time compared to the preceding and following phases, so there is only a slight chance of a representative skeleton surviving. Similarly, it is not reasonable to expect that all immunologic transitional stages survived to this day.

LEVELS OF "IMMUNE" RESPONSE SYSTEMS

It is tempting to anthropomorphize the immune response seen in less advanced species—to read specificity into nonspecific molecular interactions. If the definition of a truly "immune" reaction includes *specificity* and *the acquisition of memory*, then the allograft rejection reactions seen in coelenterates and tunicates cannot be classified as part of an immune surveillance system, since they lack memory. However, they should not be ignored in our studies, either. The function served—maintenance of the individual—suggests that these interactions might be the forerunners of true immunologic events to come. A three-level classification system of immune or "immunelike" reactivity has been developed to take this into account. First, there is *quasi-immunorecognition*; an example of this would be the allogeneic incompatibilities alluded to above. These interactions are not specific, nor do they evoke memory. The mechanisms are obscure, but likely involve macromolecular interaction, with activation of a nonspecific nature occurring at the cell surface, e.g., the nonspecific cytotoxic and agglutinating factors found in the coelomic fluid of worms. Quasi-immunorecognition is not a true immune response, but an unrefined and global response to a "threat." Later in development the *primordial cell-mediated immune response* occurs. Here, differentiated effector cells are

the active principle; specificity and memory are seen in responses to infectious agents, as well as in incompatibility reactions. This level of sophistication is seen in more advanced invertebrates, such as earthworms and starfish. Finally, *integration of the cell-mediated and humoral immune responses* occurs in the vertebrate immune system. Here, cellular cooperation mediates a coordinated response. These three levels have been added, layer on layer, to the recognition repertoire, discernible much as different strata of artifacts in an archaeologic excavation. Earlier examples of "immunoreactivity" have been retained and are still identifiable in the evolution and diversification of the immune system. Remnants of "quasi-immune" systems may be appreciated in humans; these often provide a less exactly tuned, but more prompt, response to infectious assault on the nonimmune host. An example of this is the *alternative* or *properdin* (from the Latin word meaning "to destroy") *pathway* for complement activation, giving the naive host a natural defense against infection and amplifying antibody-dependent (specific) responses in the immune host (See Chap. 13).

QUASI-IMMUNORECOGNITION

Quasi-immunorecognition, the first level of immunologic development, can be found in the earliest of multicellular organisms. Enzyme incompatibilities allow protozoa to reject foreign nuclear transplants. Sponge (Porifera), a marine multiorganism colony, demonstrates tissue-based incompatibilities. Sponges must be able to recognize "same" or "self" in order to build colonies; they use surface-based mechanisms to allow binding to or rejection of another cell. Suspensions of disaggregated sponge cells will reaggregate, usually in a species-specific fashion. Two different sponges, for example, purple and red, can be disaggregated by altering the calcium and magnesium levels in the water bath. When they are mixed together, they will re-form as separate purple and red sponges, not a mixed sponge. This process can be inhibited by adding antisera to cell surface factors, which are complex 800-Sf heat-labile glycoproteins. If such antisera to the surface-bound aggregation glycoproteins of each are added, the reaggregated sponge will now be a uniform mixture of the two cell types. Alternatively, if one attempts a xenograft, there will be "sponge-tissue bridging," followed by cell invasion and host encapsulation of the graft with ultimate necrosis. There is a definable sponge-sponge incompatibility hierarchy, suggesting some degree of molecular specificity. Graft rejection is inhibited if protein or RNA synthesis is blocked. There are examples of apparent accelerated second graft reactions, suggesting that at this level truly immune mechanisms may be emerging. In the absence of memory, however, the response is accomplished by a reaction not truly immune in nature. Nonidentical sponges may live in intimate contact, at peace with each other, perhaps by elaborating suppressor factors or by erecting a physical barrier between each other. In the coelenterates (coral, jellyfish, and anemone) graft incompatibility causes hyperplastic growth by the recipient and necrosis of the graft. This hyperplastic growth potential is also hierarchical, again suggesting interactions which are specific.

Another mechanism of "graft rejection" is found in the coelenterate, Gorgonacea. If two colonies, one large, the other small, are put in the same tank, but not necessarily touching, the smaller will disintegrate. The process starts within hours of first exposure; there is no secondary response. Pretreatment of the larger "killer" colony with inhibitors of protein or mRNA synthesis does not affect the process, but pretreatment of the target colony markedly diminishes the destruction. Treatment of the victim as long as 12 h after exposure can suppress target damage. Such autodestruction, or suicide, may be part of mammalian lymphocyte function, as well. Thus, the phylogenetic roots of apoptosis are long and deep.

CELLULAR IMMUNITY

At the level of the more advanced invertebrates, including echinoderms (starfish) and annelids (earthworms), a cellular immune recognition system appears. Second-set engraftment elicits accelerated rejection, with the allograft surrounded by connective tissue and cell masses as rejection occurs; autotransplantation is unchanged by these manipulations. Mobile cells which accumulate at sites of engraftment and are apparently active in rejection phenomena are found in the coelomic cavities of these organisms. These coelomocytes, also known as hemocytes, undergo blastogenesis after stimulation by a variety of mitogenic lectins and allogeneic cells, properties which suggest that coelomocytes occurring 450 million years ago may be "protolymphocytes." It is more likely that these cells, which are morphologically different from lymphocytes, are undifferentiated stem cells, capable of giving rise to a variety of mobile cells. Thus, circulating through tunicates are a number of types of cells including hemocytes, leukocytes (hyaline or granular), vacuolated cells, pigmented cells, and nephrocytes, the first three of which take part in inflammatory reactions.

With the emergence of the first vertebrates, a true cellular immune response mediated by cells morphologically classifiable as lymphocytes occurs, coincident with the appearance of structures suggestive of thymus, lymph nodes, and spleen. Primitive antibodies are also produced in low titer, although it is not clear if cellular and humoral responses are mediated by different cells. In fish and more advanced vertebrates discrete populations of B and T cells can be identified and there is cellular cooperation in the production of antibodies.

In the coelenterates, small cells, called *amebocytes*, are noted in the body wall. These cells are the first phagocytes, able to differentiate between functioning self and damaged self, between foreign materials and food. They combine nutritive and defensive functions, passing into the lumen of the gut to ingest and, by use of intracellular proteolytic enzymes, digest particles; only later in evolution do nutrition and defense become independent. If they cannot engulf the particle, amebocytes will often spread and "wall it off." Phagocytic cells are also found lining the sinuses of the hepato-pancreas, the ancestral reticuloendothelial system.

Proteolytic enzymes, which were originally digestive in nature, have undergone an evolution of function and specificity starting over 1 billion years ago. Trypsin, chymotrypsin, elastase, and thrombin probably evolved from gene duplication of an ancient protease with subsequent amino acid changes at or near the active site; pancreatic kallikrein is also related to these enzymes. The serine proteases that make up the coagulation cascade are related to pancreatic trypsin; factors IX and X share homologies with prothrombin and trypsin, at both the C terminal (catalytic region) and the N terminal (calcium-binding region). These enzymes and their interrelatedness are described in more detail in Chaps. 13, 14, and 16.

Another offshoot of these proteins is the series of serine esterases which, when activated in a cascade fashion, constitute the complement (C) system. The alternative complement pathway actually developed phylogenetically earlier than did the so-called classical pathway; components are found in invertebrate sera, and a functional alternative pathway is found in amphibians, fish, and the chicken (which lacks a classical pathway of complement activation). Complement-like activity can be demonstrated in elasmobranchs, but not in the more primitive vertebrate, the lamprey.

Six classical pathway components are functional in the shark, suggesting that this means of complement activation is at least 350 million years old. Components C3, C4, and C5 are homologous, probably derived form a single ancestor. The expansion into nine components may represent further fine-tuning of the system. The end result of these molecular evolutionary steps is multiple sets of interrelated but separate enzymes which

are central to the physiologic control and activation of the inflammatory process, allow prohormone activation, and serve digestive functions.

LYMPHOCYTES AND EPITHELIAL CELLS

An effective immune system must be able to differentiate self from nonself. The first place where this became a vital issue was on body surfaces—the gut and the epidermis. These epithelia turn over rapidly; thus the actively proliferating self and the constantly changing environment—the nonself—were presented for immune considerations at one site. These surfaces were logical locations for instructing immunocompetent cells in the differences between self and nonself, places where "response" and "restraint" were brought together. Gut epithelial cells may have been the first antigen-reacting or antigen-presenting cells; later, these cells and their enzymes evolved toward a purely digestive role as the lymphocytes became the immune effector cells. In the primitive agnathan vertebrate, the lamprey, large numbers of lymphocytes are seen diffusely throughout the gut in apposition with epithelial cells; it has been suggested that this epithelium-lymphocyte association may be instructive in nature. Later in evolution compartmentalization of such cell-cell interactions occurs, leading to the development of a discrete thymus, gut-associated lymphoid tissues, and the bursa of Fabricius. Both the thymus and bursa are mesenchymoepithelial organs which originate as offshoots of the gastrointestinal tract; subsequent arrival of extrinsic lymphoid cells completes the organ. Thymus, spleen, and the other lymphopoietic organs (including lymph nodes, the pronephros of myxinae, the jugular body in amphibians, the bursa of Fabricius in birds, and the gut-associated lymphoid tissues in mammals) develop with evolution beyond the agnathans.

EVOLUTION OF CELLULAR RESPONSES

With evolution, cells looking like lymphocytes developed and organs where these cells might learn self from nonself were established. These cells were no longer digestive in nature, but began interacting with nonself in a more active, distinctly immune, way. Activity resembling mixed lymphocyte reaction is found in annelids, and specificity and short-term memory are demonstrable in amebocyte-mediated responses in the snail. Molluskan hemocytes have surface binding sites, with different cells having differing types of receptors. Many species have circulating cells with surface receptors for opsonins or agglutinins; these receptors bind oligosaccharides, often produced by other circulating cells. The cell binding of such lectins then provides for direct hemocyte interaction with the lectin–foreign material complex and increased efficiency of phagocytosis.

The tunicate and the hagfish have circulating cells which respond to phytohemagglutinin, have sheep red blood cell receptors, and are x-ray-sensitive. Frogs have cells morphologically identifiable as T cells. The evolving T-cell activities parallel the increasing structural complexity of thymus and of the T cells in these species.

Members of the order Urodela (salamanders and newts) have organized spleens and thymuses, although these lack discrete medullary and cortical regions. Salamanders have a lymphopoietic bone marrow, antigen-trapping cells in the liver, spleen, and kidneys, and cells which can mediate delayed-type hypersensitivity reactions. The toad has gut-associated lymphoid tissue and a well-differentiated spleen and thymus. The latter function as central lymphoid organs from which cells colonize the peripheral lymphoid organs.

Changes in amphibians represent critical links in the evolution of the lymphoid system; it is at this level of phylogeny that the macrophage appears. The macrophage "processes" particulate antigens prior to the ev-olutionary acquisition of the ability to respond to soluble antigens, and in the more advanced amphibians, it functions as an antigen-presenting cell. Thus, at the level of the more advanced amphibians, the macrophage takes its place as an active immune cell.

These various types of cells communicate with each other. Molecules with interleukin-1-like (IL-1-like) activity have been isolated from lizards and starfish. Starfish cells respond to their own IL-1-like "starfish factors" as well as to rabbit lymphokines, establishing the cross-species activity of the compounds. Carp produce IL-1-like activity and their lymphocytes respond to IL-1. Interleukin-2-like activity can also be demonstrated in the carp. IL-1 is phylogenetically much older than IL-2, as established by cross-species comparison of interleukin activities.

Natural killer cell (NK-cell) activity is measurable in certain fish, and cells morphologically resembling NK cells have been observed in the earthworm, coeval with the emergence of the protolymphocyte. Recent studies suggest that NK cells differentiate from the same precursor as T cells. NK cells may be more closely related to the protolymphocyte than are T cells; they may represent a transition between quasi-immunorecognition and regulation and the true immune response.

AGGLUTININS, PAST AND PRESENT

Antibodies homologous with human immunoglobulin are found only in vertebrate species, although recent evidence indicates that tunicates (prevertebrates) may have an immunoglobulinlike molecule. Coelenterates manufacture bacteriolysins, hemolysins, and opsonins in the coelomic cavity. Although demonstrating heterogeneity, none are specific for the immunizing substance, nor do they resemble immunoglobulin. Insect hemolymph contains molecules which are active as agglutinins, but do not increase phagocytosis. In the annelids, urn cells within the coelom secrete agglutinins. Upon rechallenge there is increased secretion of the agglutinins, but they do not mediate specific opsonization of the immunizing organism. In crustaceans, agglutinins also induce phagocytosis. The opsonin binds to specific oligosaccharides on the invading organism, a form of nonspecific, nonself-discrimination, i.e., quasi-immunorecognition. Alternatively, these molecules may be the first step on the road to humoral immunity and memory. Natural agglutinins are found in cyclostomes, sharks, and fish. The various molecules vary in structure and size, but one unifying feature is that all have a subunit structure; i.e., they are all multimers. They are not homologous with immunoglobulin, but many are homologous with C-reactive protein.

C-reactive protein (CRP) is a cyclic pentamer, the prototype of a recently described protein family known as the *pentaxins*. This family includes CRP, serum amyloid P component, the female protein of the hamster, and the hemolysins of limulus, the horseshoe crab. Pentaxins have been found in all vertebrate species studied. No human thus far studied has lacked CRP in the peripheral circulation (see Chap. 16 on the acute phase reaction).

CRP has significant homology with complement component C3a and with IgG heavy chain. CRP can interact with complement, apolipoproteins, and damaged tissue. CRP also binds to platelets, T cells, NK cells, and B cells, modulating the activity of these cells; serum amyloid P component shares many of these properties. Thus, the pentaxins have a variety of effects, and the conservation of structure for nearly 300 million years suggests that they have important functions. Thus, CRP may be an active aspect of quasi-immunorecognition still active in the human, providing a nonspecific defense system until antigen-specific cellular and humoral immune mechanisms can be invoked.

IMMUNOGLOBULIN

Approximately 600 million years ago, the oxygen concentration in the atmosphere reached 1 percent of current levels. It is at this oxygen concentration (the *Pasteur point*) that organisms can shift from fermentation to respiration, liberating 30- to 40-fold more chemosynthetic energy. About 420 million years ago, the oxygen concentration rose, providing more radiation protection so life could safely expand onto land. At about this time both vascular plants, the predecessors of modern plants and trees, and new animal phyla were developing in the increasingly friendly environment. This increasingly nurturing environment also favored further expansion of the number and species of bacterial flora. True immunoglobulin (Ig) appeared in evolution about 250 to 400 million years ago, in the cyclostomes or perhaps even in the tunicates. It may be more than coincidence that Ig appeared coincident with the great increase in bacterial growth. It is possible that nonspecific interactions mediated by agglutinins and cellular mechanisms were sufficient defense earlier, but that with the remarkable increase in variety and quantity of bacteria, a new means of specific immunorecognition was needed. Perhaps Ig was the evolutionary answer to the more complex polysaccharide and protein antigens which challenged the cyclostomes.

In the first vertebrates, the cyclostomes (hagfish and lamprey), two populations of lymphocytes, T cells and B cells, are discernible. These animals make true Ig, each molecule consisting of two heavy and two light chains. The basic building block of these peptide chains is the *domain*, defined as an approximately 100 to 110 amino acid sequence containing an internal disulfide bond. Each chain has one variable (V) region, involved in antigen recognition, and one or more constant (C) regions, each region being one domain subunit in size (Fig. B-3).

The cyclostomes have Ig molecules of two discrete sizes, 14 Sf (Svedberg flotation unit) and 7 Sf, also reported as 10.9 Sf and 6.6 Sf.

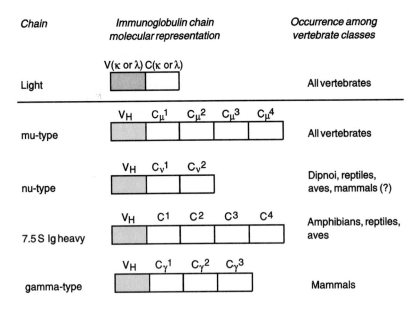

Chain	Immunoglobulin chain molecular representation	Occurrence among vertebrate classes
Light	$V(\kappa\ or\ \lambda)$ $C(\kappa\ or\ \lambda)$	All vertebrates
mu-type	V_H $C_\mu1$ $C_\mu2$ $C_\mu3$ $C_\mu4$	All vertebrates
nu-type	V_H $C_\nu1$ $C_\nu2$	Dipnoi, reptiles, aves, mammals (?)
7.5 S Ig heavy	V_H $C1$ $C2$ $C3$ $C4$	Amphibians, reptiles, aves
gamma-type	V_H $C_\gamma1$ $C_\gamma2$ $C_\gamma3$	Mammals

Figure B-3   Molecular representation of different immunoglobulin chains. The length of each chain is proportional to its carbohydrate-free molecular mass. Each chain is divided into domain regions, each of a molecular mass of approximately 11 kd; the variable region domain (V) is indicated by the dark or cross-hatched area and the constant region (C) by the clear areas.

The larger seems to be a dimer of the smaller molecule. This is characteristic of the Ig system: there is no species with only a single kind of Ig molecule, and except for the cyclostomes and elasmobranchs, the two types of Ig are dissimilar (Fig. B-4). The Ig V region, as early as the elasmobranchs, bears a close resemblance to the V region in mammalian Ig; and, as in mammals, the heterogeneity of V regions and Ig in the antigen-specific immune response has been noted.

The evidence to date suggests that IgM arose first in evolution. IgM is found in fish, both cartilaginous and bony, where both κ and λ light chains are found. No species has a light chain not identifiable as either κ or λ. This may be because at the level of the fish, most of the changes in heavy-chain structure have yet to occur, while most of the evolution of light chains has taken place; the two light-chain classes have already diverged and show little homology with each other. The J chain first appears in association with the IgM macroglobulin class of the shark, paddlefish, and gar. Although fish IgM is structurally like mammalian IgM, the IgM response does not mature at this phylogenetic level. Comparison of elasmobranch and rat antibody responses demonstrates that the

phylogenetically more advanced species can shift production to higher-affinity antibodies. The goldfish and the grouper make an early 19-Sf antibody response, followed by a later 7-Sf response; the 7-Sf heavy chain in the grouper may be different from that of the 19-Sf response. A second discrete class of Ig was recently found in the skate, a primitive cartilaginous vertebrate. It is a 9-Sf low molecular weight Ig with a dimer structure, antigenically different from the 19-Sf Ig and produced by different plasma cells. Thus, the first divergence of Ig heavy chains occurs very early in the evolution of the vertebrates.

A second, non-IgM, Ig molecule is found in a primitive fish, the lungfish (which also has IgM), and in certain reptiles, and is the predominant Ig in the duck. This Ig is known as IgN; its light chains are similar to those found in IgM, but its heavy chain is only three domains in size, two C and one V (Fig. B-3). A peculiarity of IgN molecules (and certain types of IgA) is that there are no disulfide bonds between the heavy and light chains.

Later in phylogeny Ig isotypes develop with larger molecular weights. The growth occurs at the C-terminal end, where increasingly complex functions and interaction potentials occur. All structural expansion occurs

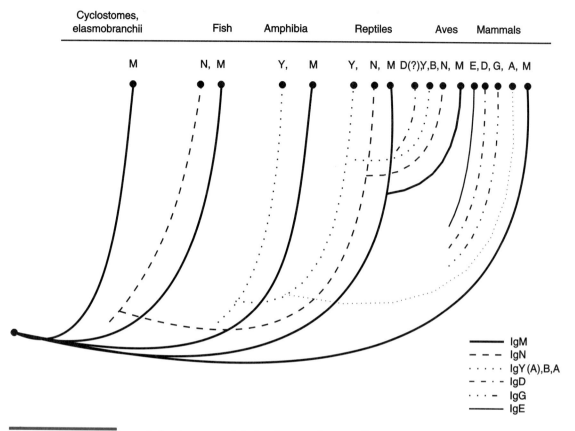

Figure B-4   Evolution of the immunoglobulin heavy chain. All species except the cyclostomes have two distinct isotypes. IgA and IgB are derived from IgY (also known as IgRAA), which in turn evolved from IgN.

in discrete units of domain size, suggesting that Ig growth was mediated by gene duplication.

In amphibians the first antibody response is 19 Sf, followed by a different, 7-Sf Ig which becomes the predominant Ig within 2 to 3 months. In the frog this second heavy chain is distinct; the new Ig is called IgY or IgRAA (R = reptile, A = amphibian, A = ave). The new heavy chain is essentially an elongated IgN consisting of five domains, four C and one V. It is from this new Ig class that IgA ultimately evolved. By lineage and by structure, IgA resembles IgM more than it does IgG (Fig. B-4). A true IgA-type Ig is first seen in the reptile, the first animals to need a unique extravascular surface-associated Ig.

Prior to the emergence of a primarily ter-

restrial lifestyle these surfaces would have been washed clean of adherent Ig, and perhaps of pathogens, in the primarily aquatic environment in which amphibians lived. Now, in primarily land-based animals, these body surfaces would need protection by Ig. The "IgA" class reported in chicken bile has come under closer scrutiny and is now known to be unrelated to the IgA of humans, mice, and pigs. This distinct class of Ig has been renamed IgB (B = bird or bile); like IgA, it seems to be an offshoot of the original IgY or IgRAA. Birds are closely related to the archosaurian reptiles and are more properly considered a subclass of reptiles rather than a separate class of chordates. The phylogeny of IgA and IgB is in agreement with this fact.

IgG appeared in the Therapsidae, the

reptile occurring phylogenetically immediately before mammals. IgG, probably derived from IgY, is present in the earliest of the mammals, with the various subclasses emerging after the divergence of the species in the last 70 million years. There are four IgG subclasses in humans, each with slightly different properties and functions within the immune system. For example, IgG1, IgG2, and IgG3 fix complement but IgG4 does not; IgG1, IgG2, and IgG4 are bound by rheumatoid factor and staphylococcal protein A, but IgG3 is not; mononuclear cells bind IgG1 and IgG3 better than IgG2 and IgG4. Mammalian Ig has a highly conserved structure; chimpanzee and gorilla Ig are more like human Ig than like rhesus and baboon Ig, in agreement with current evolutionary theory.

IgD-like molecules are found on the surface of primate, pig, mouse, and rat lymphocytes and possibly on chicken lymphocytes. Monomeric IgM seems to be the only phylogenetically conserved lymphocyte surface Ig. Homocytotropic antibodies, similar to human reaginic antibodies, with similar physicochemical properties have been found in the rat, rabbit, dog, mouse, monkey, guinea pig, and in cattle. Monkey reagins cross-react with anti-human IgE. IgE has only been demonstrated in mammals.

Two Ig-associated molecules are also members of this "Ig superfamily." Despite significant heterogeneity, the receptor for the constant region of Ig consists of extracellular and intracellular domains, homologous with other members of the Ig superfamily; ligand binding is encoded in one gene. Secretory component in the rabbit is much like that in the human and has been sequenced recently. It consists of 773 amino acid residues segregated into a signal peptide of 18 residues, a 629 amino acid extracellular Ig-binding site, a 23-residue membrane-spanning segment, and a 103 amino acid cytoplasmic tail. The Ig-binding site divides into five highly conserved domains of between 100 and 115 residues and a sixth, more distantly related, domain. There is homology with the Ig-variable region and with Thy-1 molecule; rabbit secretory component is more homologous

with rabbit κ chain. It may be that the secretory component–Ig interaction is analogous to the ability of IgA and IgM to self-associate into homopolymers, even in the absence of J chain. J chain, which first appears early in phylogeny, is not related to any Ig domain structure thus far described. It seems likely, therefore, that the Ig domain represents the fundamental structural unit which nature has developed for cell-cell and cell-antigen interactions. All of these molecules are described in more detail in Chap. 3.

As the environment and species changed, compensatory changes occurred in the immune systems of the species, including Ig development. IgN and IgY isotypes were deleted from the mammalian repertoire. IgM was retained, IgG continued to evolve into four distinct subclasses, and the new isotypes IgD and IgE appeared. In contrast to this diversification of the constant region, the variable-region structure, as determined by sequence and antigenicity, has been remarkably conserved through evolution. Ig molecules have become recognition molecules in B cells and antigen-specific effector molecules both in the body fluids and mucous membranes as well as on the surface of a variety of immune cells by means of various Fc receptors. Antigen specificity and the different functions are all mediated by domain structures which have been modified for each task.

MAJOR HISTOCOMPATIBILITY COMPLEX FUNCTION

As evolution proceeded, the internal structure of animals became more complex. Successful cell-cell cooperation required a more elaborate cell surface–bound communication system to assure that histogenesis would proceed smoothly—that ontogeny would be successful. Major histocompatibility complex (MHC) molecules may represent a system designed for the purpose of organogenesis. These molecules may act as anchorage sites for instruction molecules at critical points in organ development. Epithelial growth factor seems to do just this, using HLA antigens or closely associated molecules as binding sites. The expression of MHC correlates with stages of cell development and tissue origin; certain MHC molecules may actually be differentiation markers.

As the complexity of organisms increases, the need for control in internal variation increases. Presumably, genetic variation of somatic cells via mutation, crossover, or recombination would result in the breakdown of normal histogenesis in the individual; such changes may, however, be valuable in germ cells, introducing potentially salutary changes into the germ line. A method then would be required to eliminate variant somatic cells expressing new antigens, or modification of more familiar self-antigens. The maintenance of a stable internal milieu is a strong driving force for the complexity and conservation of the MHC, likely of more value than the identification of differences between individuals. It seems likely that the ability of the MHC to induce graft rejection and to kill virally infected cells was not the primary purpose of the MHC. In less advanced species, e.g., earthworms, only a chronic, low-intensity graft rejection occurs; only with the further evolution of the species and of the MHC does acute rejection develop.

A mutation causing deletion of part of the MHC might be disruptive to histogenesis. Cells which are semisyngeneic (i.e., have deleted some part of their MHC expression) do not grow as well as fully syngeneic cells when grafted into a syngeneic host. A truly immunologic mechanism cannot be implicated for this "syngeneic preference." Perhaps MHC deletions put cells at a disadvantage for binding growth or differentiation factors. "Allogeneic inhibition" of growth has been demonstrated where purified mouse H-2 antigens exert toxic effects if applied directly to growing cultures of nonidentical cells. This is not dependent upon the immunologic system of the host, but occurs via macromolecular interaction between H-2 antigen and the H-2-incompatible cells. These may be examples of quasi-immunorecognition mingling with the phylogenetically more sophisticated and specific MHC.

Classical teaching states that the MHC antigens are a means to detect the "altered self," e.g., to detect and destroy virally infected cells. However, viruses are several orders of magnitude faster in generation time than are their more complex host cells and so should always win a race for potentially advantageous adaptive change. In fact, viruses are capable of using the MHC surface glycoproteins as surface receptors for entry into cells. Evidence suggesting such an interaction includes the cocapping of H-2 and viral antigens on tumor cells and the coprecipitation of HLA class I heavy chains with adenovirus protein E19. Semliki Forest virus and lactate dehydrogenase virus, as well as certain bacteria, bind to HLA antigens or β_2-microglobulin. There is significant homology between the gene of the human immunodeficiency virus (HIV) envelope and HLA-B extracellular region gene segments. T-cell lines producing HIV display altered HLA antigens, suggesting an HIV-HLA interaction prior to transmembrane display.

Another example of the importance of the MHC is found in the relationship between diversity and the survival of the species. Fecundity increases with more MHC differences between the parents. Increased placenta and litter size and increased survival of newborn animals are seen in allogeneic pregnancies (hybrid vigor), perhaps because immunologic processes are crucial in implantation (see Chap. 27); with more viable offspring there is increased survival of genetic material and the potential for further improvement of the species.

Mice preferentially mate with H-2 dissimilar mice and are able to discern H-2 type by odor; it has been suggested that this sense is mediated by the vomeronasal gland, a second, independent, olfactory system in the rodent. Mice can detect differences at the H-2k and the Tla (thymus leukemia antigen, a thymocyte surface marker locus) regions. Urine of the heterozygotes at the H-2 region is not the equivalent of a combination of urines of individuals with the constituent types; detection of variations in the relative proportion and concentration of normal metabolites is felt to be crucial. Other examples of odor-chemosensory perception can be seen in the imprinting of young salmon for their home stream and in the yellow bullhead, a fish which recognizes other individuals and their standing in the bullhead community by scent.

In studies of human couples, evidence of preference for HLA loci is contradictory; the possibility that perfumes and hygiene might overwhelm such HLA-linked scent-mediated mate selection has been raised. Olfaction is a *direct* link between the external environment and the brain. It is a complex sense mediated by a population of cells which can replicate and, if transected, are capable of reestablishing specific connections with the brain. Boyse pointed out: "Olfaction and immunity both involve the recognition of a great range of chemical details. Whether this resemblance is more than superficial is a matter for speculation."

THE MHC: STRUCTURE AND EVIDENCE FOR MEMBERSHIP IN A SUPERFAMILY OF COMMUNICATION MACROMOLECULES

The human MHC system consists of class I and class II molecules. The class I molecule (HLA-A, HLA-B, and HLA-C) is a heterodimer of a polymorphic α chain with three domains and β_2-microglobulin; β_2-microglobulin is one domain in size and is monomorphic in humans and dimorphic in mice. The class II molecules (DP-SB, DQ, DR, and DZ) consist of an α and a β chain, each of which is polymorphic and contains two domains (see Chap. 4).

A molecule resembling β_2-microglobulin has been found on the surface of earthworm leukocytes and on goldfish visceral cells. At first, β_2-microglobulin was thought to be a product of a gene evolved from Ig, but it now seems that it represents a molecule closely related to the original domain gene. Thy-1, and its human analogue the surface glycoprotein p25, may be one step closer to the progenitor molecule than β_2-microglobulin. Thy-1 is a glycoprotein not associated with other membrane proteins. Its structure, two β sheets with antiparallel β strands, is close to that of the Ig domain (both variable and constant), more so than β_2-microglobulin; this suggests that Thy-1 is closer to the primordial domain than Ig or β_2-microglobulin. Thy-1 is conserved on neural cells (a Thy-1 homologue has been found in squid brain) and on fibroblasts, but varies in structure on lymphoid cells and is nearly absent on human thymocytes. Thy-1 may be concerned with general cell-cell communication rather than with immunologic mechanisms, consonant with the contention that the domain is the basic unit of such cell-to-cell interactions.

In examining MHC molecules, other homologies become apparent. HLA heavy chains show homology with Ig domains, as do H-2 heavy chains with murine Ig. Of the three domains of the HLA α chain, the one adjacent to the membrane, H-3, is homologous with Ig and β_2-microglobulin; H-1 and H-2 are related to each other, but not significantly to Ig. Mouse and human MHCs have several sites of conserved structure and heterogeneity.

Class II molecules are homologous with Ig as well. DR β chains show homology with Ig and HLA molecules, especially in the second, membrane-proximal, domain. The second domain of the DR α molecule is also related to Ig. Thus the membrane-proximal domains of all four of the MHC constituent chains show homology with Ig (Table B-2). Functionally, these domains might interact with each other in a manner similar to Ig in antigen binding. The class II restriction of the immunogenicity of certain peptides is probably due to the selective binding of those peptides by both the α and β chains of the class II molecule.

Functional similarity of β_2-microglobulin and the light chain of Ig may be seen in the

TABLE B-2 Major histocompatibility complexes of humans and mice. Extensive homology of class I and II molecules with immunoglobulin and β_2-microglobulin.

Class of Molecules	Human	Mouse	Chains	Domains	Homology
I	HLA-A,B,C	H$_2$,K,D,L	α	3	(1) and (2) distantly related to each other (3) β_2m and IgC
			β_2m	1	IgC
II	DP-SB,DQ, DR,DZ	I$_A$,I$_E$	α	2	(1) (2) Domain #2 of II β
			β	2	(1) (2) β_2m IgC Domain #3 of class I, α chain Distantly related to domains #1 and 2 of class I, α chain

ability of these two light chains to modify expression of the surface-bound heterodimers, HLA and Ig, respectively. The Daudi cell line derived from a human Burkitt lymphoma does not make β_2-microglobulin or express HLA. When these cells are fused with a β_2-microglobulin-producing cell (either murine or human), the fusion product can elaborate surface HLA markers. In analogous fashion, when mRNA or Ig heavy chain is injected into a *Xenopus laevis* oocyte, there is synthesis, but no secretion of the heavy chain. When light-chain mRNA is injected as well, tetrameric Ig is secreted. Light chains may solubilize the otherwise insoluble heavy chain, or they may induce conformational changes needed for transport, just as β_2-microglobulin–heavy-chain interaction is required to generate the quaternary structure needed for the expression of HLA antigenic determinants. The genes encoding Ig and class I MHC antigens may have been derived by recombinations within introns separating tandemly repeated primordial β_2-microglobulin. This divergence occurred 500 to 700 million years ago, based on sequence difference analysis. There is evidence that class II molecules are continuing to evolve, resulting in increasing complexity of the MHC; good examples of this are the subdivisions of HLA-DR4 and HLA-B27 defined in the

analysis of linkage with rheumatoid arthritis and ankylosing spondylitis, respectively.

T CELL–SPECIFIC (ANTIGEN) RECEPTORS

Mouse and human T cells have analogous function-specific surface markers: L3T4-Leu-3/OKT4 (now known as CD4) on the helper/inducer subset and Lyt-2, 3-Leu-2/OKT8 (now known as CD8) on the suppressor/cytotoxic subset; each of these pairs is homologous by size, charge, subunit structure, sensitivity to proteolysis, and density determination, but not so far by antigenic or sequence analysis. Expression of those surface antigens is related to the class of MHC molecule with which the cell interacts: CD4 with class II molecules and CD8 with class I molecules. These surface markers have homology with Ig and are part of the Ig superfamily. The sheep red blood cell receptor, a marker for T cells remarkably conserved since the protolymphocytes of the earliest vertebrates, provides a second nonspecific activation receptor in human T cells. This alternative means of activating T cells might be the cellular analogue of the alternative pathway for complement activation, providing global activation at a time when a specific immune response is still being developed. (Does this evoke a memory of "superantigens," described in Chap. 7—a means by which to activate a large number of T cells, a response with potential advantages for the organism and species?)

There has been an explosion of information concerning the previously elusive human T-cell-antigen receptor (TCR) described in more detail in Chap. 7. Such receptors have been isolated for study. The receptor is a 90-kd disulfide-linked heterodimer, with a 49- to 51-kd α chain and a 43-kd β chain associated with the monomorphic 20- to 25-kd T3 molecule. The mouse TCR is also a heterodimer, both α and β chains being 43 kd. The more basic β chain is more heterogenous, just as the human. Tryptic digestive patterns also suggest constant and variable regions.

Like Ig, these heterodimer constituents of the TCR can be divided into constant, joining, and variable regions. The constant and joining regions of the TCR are spaced on the genome much as are those of the Ig λ light chain. The TCR polypeptide is structurally similar to Ig. The predicted protein encoded thus bears a resemblance to a light chain and contains a leader segment followed by variable, joining, and constant sections; a hydrophobic, presumably transmembrane, stretch region; and a domain-sized extracellular region. The protein is no closer to the human light chain than to the murine light chain, suggesting that its development diverged before the species did. The human DNA clone hybridizes as well to murine as to human T cell mRNA, suggesting that the receptor gene is highly conserved between the species. There is gene rearrangement of T cell–specific cDNA in T cells but not in B cells, analogous to the Ig gene rearrangements seen in B cells but not in T cells. Two cDNA clones from a murine cytotoxic T-cell clone show just such rearrangement in T cells and both have similarities to Ig variable- and constant-region genes. The proposed structure of the TCR molecules consists of two disulfide-linked chains, each with one constant and one variable domain.

A second TCR has been identified, a heterodimer of two polypeptides known as δ and γ. The γ gene product is Ig-like, with variable, diverse, and joining segment rearrangement. The heterodimer is found associated with CD3 on cells with cytotoxic and NK-cell-like activities. γ-Chain genes are rearranged earlier in thymocyte development than are α and β chains. Cells which express the γ/δ heterodimer may represent a distinct lineage of cells. DNA sequence analysis of the δ gene reveals no such Ig homology, suggesting that it is not part of the Ig superfamily. Thus, TCR polypeptides, including α, β, and γ chains, are members of the Ig superfamily of cell-bound and circulating communication molecules (Fig. B-5), all derived from the ancestral domain molecule. The immunoglobulin superfamily is described in more detail in Chap. 3.

An alternative to the α/β heterodimer model is the antigen-binding surface molecule isolated from T-cell membranes which possesses serologic determinants related to Ig heavy-chain variable regions. This variable region heavy chain–related T-cell molecule (sometimes labeled V_TM) shares framework regions with Ig, is clonally restricted, and binds antigen. Further, in A/J mice immunized with arsonate, a small (<2 percent) subset of peripheral T cells expresses and synthesizes antigen-binding molecules which cross-react with antiarsonate idiotype and bear Fab-related determinants. Thus, V_TM may be an antigen-binding molecule which complexes with other, MHC-related, surface constituents.

CONCLUSIONS

The human immune system has evolved over the past billion years, developing the ability to react to changes in the environment, restructure its immune repertoire, reveal previous experience, and restrain itself. Specialization of cells and digestive enzymes has

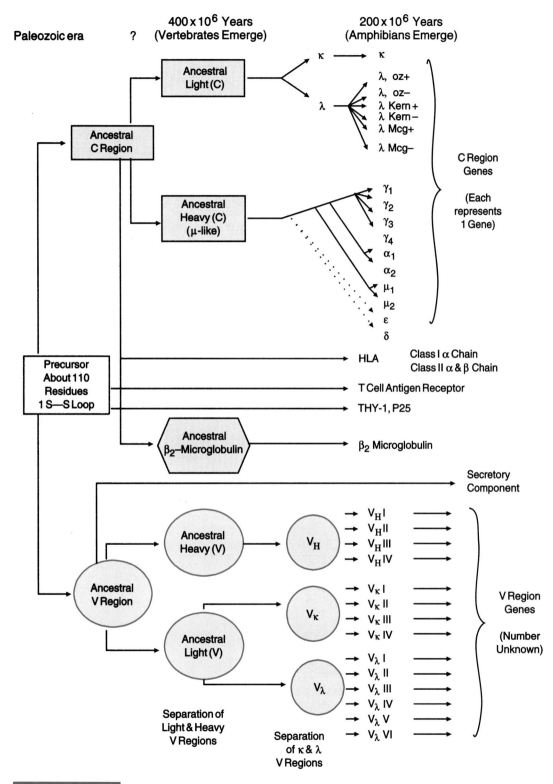

Figure B-5 Proposed phylogenetic tree of the superfamily of communicator molecules, including immunoglobulin, secretory component, β_2-microglobulin, HLA, Thy-1, p25, and TCRs.

745

occurred, with differentiation of nutritional and defensive capabilities. Immune cells have evolved to provide more and more specialized and efficient defense for the organism. The mechanisms involved have been added over the eons, but some of the more ancient, less sophisticated, and less precise defenses are still active in humans. The cells that were the sole defenders of the internal milieu have given rise to factors which either in themselves attack invaders or allow cells to do a better job in fighting invaders. Many of these molecules, although disparate in form, structure, location, and mechanism, are probably derived from a primordial domainlike molecule, perhaps best represented currently by the Thy-1 molecule. Modification of this original product has allowed diversification into a series of circulating and cell-bound molecules, which mediate immune cell–pathogen interactions and immune cell–immune cell communications. These many evolutionary steps have culminated in the immune response of mammals. Recalling the many layers of immune and quasi-immune mechanisms and the relatedness of many modern mechanisms may lead to new ways of analyzing and understanding the human immune response.

C
Immunologic Tests

ANTIGEN AND ANTIBODY DETECTION

Introduction to Gel Precipitation Reactions of Antibodies and Antigens

Antigen and antibody complexes form a precipitate at or near equivalence of each component. By allowing the precipitation reaction to occur in a semisolid medium such as agar, it is possible to distinguish separate antigen-antibody complexes produced by different antigens or antibodies. This is the basis for the following techniques (Fig. C-1).

Double Immunodiffusion

In double immunodiffusion type I, agar gels are poured onto slides and allowed to solidify. Two wells are cut out of the gel; the appropriate antigen solution is added to one well and an antibody solution to the other. The antigen and antibody are allowed to diffuse toward each other. If the antibody recognizes and binds an antigen, a precipitin line is formed. If two antigens are present which the antibody recognizes, two precipitin lines appear (Fig C-2).

In double immunodiffusion type II, the relationship between antigens and a particular antibody may be determined. Three wells are cut into an agar gel that form the apexes of an equilateral triangle. Into two of these wells antigen solutions to be tested are placed, and into the third well is placed the antibody. Three basic patterns can appear. With *identity*, the precipitin lines between the antibody and antigen wells fuse, indicating that the antibody precipitates identical epitopes on the antigens in each well. This does not mean that the antigens are identical, only that the antibody can not distinguish between them. In other words, there may be a family of antigens which the antibody will recognize because of similar common areas to which the antibody reacts. If there are different epitopes distinguished by the antibody, then a few precipitin lines may be

formed; this is *nonidentity*. Finally, in the case of *partial identity*, the antigens in wells one and two share a common epitope, but in addition a second epitope is present on one of the antigens that the antibody recognizes. This causes an extension of the line of identity, or a "spur," where the additional anti-epitope–epitope precipitin line has occurred (Fig. C-3).

Single Radial Immunodiffusion

Single radial immunodiffusion is a method for quantitative determination of the amount of antigen present. Agar containing a fixed

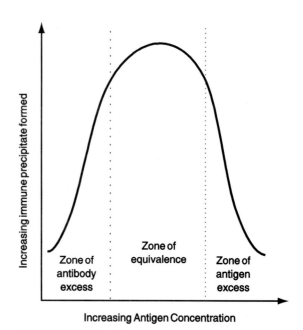

Figure C-1 This is a typical antigen-antibody precipitin curve where the antibody is kept constant and the amount of antigen is increased. The curve demonstrates the amount of immune complex produced with increasing antigen. Note that the most immune complex is formed at levels of antigen-antibody equivalence.

748

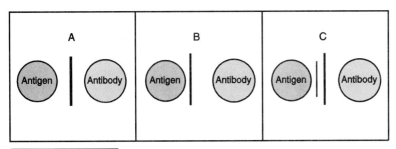

Figure C-2 Simple double immunodiffusion. In (a) both the antibody and antigen react intensely and at the midpoint where antigen and antibody equivalence occurred. In (b) the precipitin line is less intense and is closer to the antigen well. This may be due to the antigen being present in lesser amounts, or not diffusing as rapidly because of its charge or size. In (c) two lines have formed, indicating that there is a second antigen in the well that also reacts with the antibody.

and known amount of antibody is poured onto a plate. Wells are then cut into the agar and standard volumes of antigen of known concentration are placed into the wells and allowed to diffuse outward from the wells. The antigen and antibody combine to form soluble complexes (antigen excess) until a point of equivalence is reached between antigen and antibody (Fig. C-1). At the point of equivalence, the complexes are insoluble and form a precipitin ring. The area of the circle, measured as ring diameter squared, is proportionate to the amount of antigen present in the well. With the use of a standard curve derived by plotting area of the ring vs. the amount of antigen present in the wells, an unknown amount of antigen may be interpolated from the standard curve (Fig. C-4). This technique can be used to determine the amount of antigen or antibody present in a solution by means of semiquantitative double immunodiffusion (Fig. C-5).

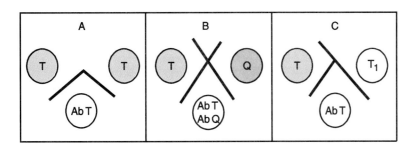

Figure C-3 Angular double immunodiffusion allows one to distinguish between identical, unrelated, and related antigens. T = antigen T, Q = antigen Q, T_1 = antigen T_1. Ab T and Ab Q are antibodies to antigens T and Q, respectively. In (a), where both antigens are the same, a sharp precipitin line that is identical for each well forms a sharp apex midway between the two wells. (b) shows crossing precipitin lines formed by two different antigen-antibody immune complex precipitin lines. Finally, in (c), one sees the intersection of the precipitin lines with a "spur," indicating that antibody T recognizes sites on both antigens T and T_1, but these antigens are not identical.

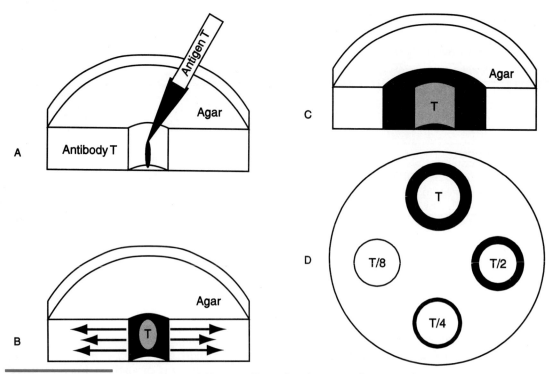

Figure C-4 Single radial immunodiffusion allows for the quantification of an unknown amount of antigen. In (a) a well is cut out of antibody-containing agar and an exact volume of unknown antigen is added. The antigen diffuses out of the well (b) for 24 to 48 h. The precipitin ring forms around the well. The size of the ring is proportional to the amount of antigen present in the test volume (c). (d) shows the amount of standard antigen T being diluted and treated in a manner similar to that shown in (a), (b), and (c). By measuring the sizes of the ring with each dilution of the known concentration of T, a standard curve can be constructed and the amount of antigen in the sample derived from the standard curve.

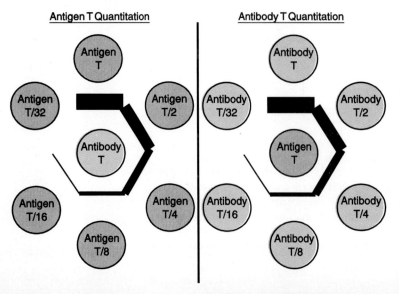

Figure C-5 In semiquantitative double immunodiffusion the antigen or antibody is held constant and the molecule of interest is serially diluted until no precipitin line is seen. With decreasing concentration of the molecule of interest, the precipitin line decreases in thickness. If only one precipitin line forms, most likely a single antigen-antibody complex is present.

An important use of single radial diffusion is the quantification of serum proteins, such as immunoglobulins. Inaccurate measurement can result if the antigen diffuses poorly because of aggregation (slowing its rate of diffusion) or if the antigen is smaller than expected and diffuses too quickly. In cases where the serum contains anti-immunoglobulin antibodies, reversed precipitation may occur: simultaneous diffusion and precipitation happen in two directions, leading to falsely high values.

Immunoelectrophoresis

Some antigen mixtures are too complicated to resolve by diffusion and precipitation alone. The pH of agar can be adjusted so that different antigens have different charges. When these antigens are placed in a gel with a specific pH and subjected to an electric field, the positively charged antigens move to the negative electrode and the negatively charged antigens move to the positive electrode. Once the antigens have finished moving in the gel after a fixed time (electrophoresed), a trough

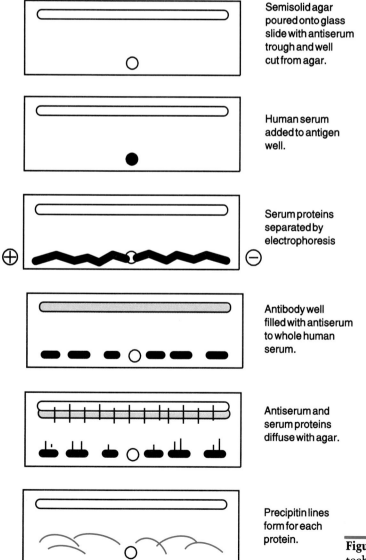

Semisolid agar poured onto glass slide with antiserum trough and well cut from agar.

Human serum added to antigen well.

Serum proteins separated by electrophoresis

Antibody well filled with antiserum to whole human serum.

Antiserum and serum proteins diffuse with agar.

Precipitin lines form for each protein.

Figure C-6 Immunoelectrophoresis technique. (See text for description.)

is cut next to the well parallel to the direction of the electric field. This well is filled with antibody and allowed to diffuse to form precipitin arcs. This technique operates effectively in the range of 20 μg/mL to 2 mg/mL of antibody or antigen, allowing qualitative comparisons of complex antigen mixtures, such as is found in serum (Fig. C-6).

Countercurrent Electrophoresis and Rocket Electrophoresis

Both countercurrent electrophoresis and rocket electrophoresis rely on the antigen and antibody having different charges at a selected pH. This difference in charge is true of most antigens, since most antibodies have a relatively high isoelectric point, pI (this means the antibodies are neutrally charged at a more alkaline pH than most antigens are). If an antigen and antibody cannot be made to carry a significantly different charge by adjusting the pH of the gel, then either one may be chemically modified in order to change its isoelectric point without changing the antibody-antigen binding.

In countercurrent electrophoresis (Fig. C-7), the pH of the agar is adjusted so that the antigen is negatively charged and the antibody is positively charged. The antibody is placed in a well at the positive side of the gel and the antigen in a well at the negative side of the gel, across from the antibody well.

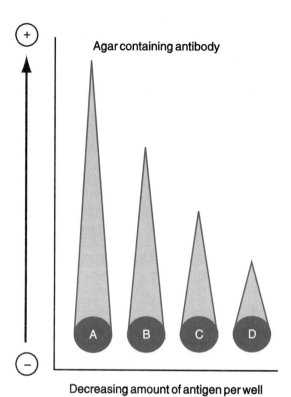

Figure C-8   Rocket electrophoresis. Several wells are cut into agar containing antibody and an increasingly diluted antigen sample is placed into each well. The antigen is electrophoresed into the agar, where it forms precipitin patterns with the antibody called "rockets." The height of the rocket is proportional to the amount of antigen in the well.

An electric voltage is applied, and the antigen and antibody move toward each other and precipitate in a precipitin arc between the two wells. This method, though similar in principal to double immunodiffusion, has a 10-fold to 20-fold greater sensitivity than double immunodiffusion.

Rocket electrophoresis (Fig. C-8) is similar to single radial immunodiffusion in that it quantifies amounts of antigen or antibody by finding a pH which immobilizes one (neutrally charged) and not the other. In general, for antigen quantification the pH of the agar is adjusted so that the antigen is charged and the antibody is neutral. The antigen is then

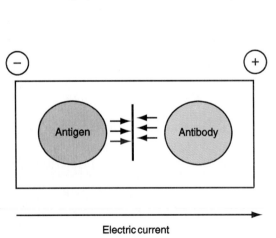

Figure C-7   Countercurrent electrophoresis. (See text for description.)

electrophoresed into the antibody-containing gel where it forms precipitin "rockets" whose height is proportional to the antigen concentration. A standard curve is made, and unknowns are interpolated from this curve.

Introduction to Agglutination Techniques

As discussed previously, precipitin reactions are quantitative techniques that are easy to perform. Agglutination techniques are only semiquantitative, and are more difficult to perform. Agglutination techniques (Fig. C-9) depend on insoluble antigens or antigen-coated particles (i.e., latex particles or red blood cells) clumping together after being cross-linked by antibody and precipitating from a suspension of the antigen or particles. This clumping may be visualized with or without the aid of a microscope. The chief advantages of agglutination techniques are their high degree of sensitivity and the tremendous diversity of substances detectable through the use of antigen- or antibody-coated particles.

In direct agglutination a cell or insoluble antigen particle is directly agglutinated (clumped) by the antibody. An example is the agglutination of red blood cells where the B blood group type is agglutinated by anti-B antibodies. In indirect (passive) agglutination antigen-coated cells or particles passively carry otherwise soluble antigens. An example is the agglutination of IgG-coated latex particles by rheumatoid factor. Reversed agglutination is accomplished by coating the cells or particles with antibody and having the antigen in solution.

Direct Agglutination Test

Many different particles including red blood cells, fungi, and other microbial agents can participate in direct agglutination (cross-linking) by serum antibodies. The amount of antigen is kept constant and the antigen titer is determined by serial two-fold dilutions of the antibody. After a few hours the reaction is completed and the particles are examined for clumping. The highest dilution of the antiserum (e.g., 1/128, 1/256, 1/512) at which agglutination occurs is reported as the titer. Because there is some variability in the test, a titer must differ by at least two-fold dilutions (a factor of 4) from any other given titer to be considered significantly different. Tests are carried out in small volumes to maximize sensitivity.

Indirect Agglutination

There are many soluble antigens that can be adsorbed to red blood cells or other particles,

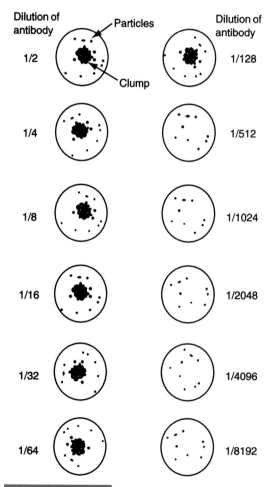

Figure C-9 In agglutination tests serial dilutions of the antibody of interest are added to plates containing a constant amount of antigen. The highest dilution where agglutination occurs is the reported result; in the example shown, it is 1:128.

such as synthetic beads, to allow antibody specificities to be detected by agglutination techniques. These antigens, such as penicillin and bacterial antigens (e.g., exotoxins) may adsorb spontaneously to the red blood cell (RBC). Other proteins and antigens may be chemically attached to red blood cells by using tannic acid, glutaraldehyde, chromic chloride, or other chemicals. These chemicals allow adsorption by changing the red blood cell membrane to allow adsorption of antigens after treatment, or by covalently binding the antigen to the red blood cell membrane. Once the red blood cells have been treated or "fixed" with glutaraldehyde, formalin, or pyruvic aldehyde, they may be stored for prolonged periods of time at 4°C. Other particles may be used for agglutination as long as antigens can be chemically coupled to the particles.

Agglutination tests are carried out in microtiter plates (multiple small wells in a plastic tray) or tubes. Using serial dilutions of the antibody to be tested decreases artifacts due to high antibody concentrations, thus reducing the number of false-negative results. Because IgM is about 750 times more efficient than IgG in agglutination (it is a pentameric antibody), the presence of significant amounts of IgM may influence the results of agglutination tests.

Latex Fixation
Latex particles may also have proteins adsorbed to them and participate in indirect agglutination reactions. Latex particles are most commonly adsorbed with 7-Sf IgG and then used for the detection of rheumatoid factor (IgM which binds to IgG).

Inhibition of Agglutination
Red blood cells are agglutinated by cross-linking with antibodies specific for an antigen found on the modified or unmodified red blood cell. A sensitive and specific method for the detection of small amounts of antigen found in serum or other fluids measures the inhibition of agglutination of red blood cells by first reacting the antibody with the serum or fluid sample.

Physicochemical and Immunochemical Methods

Zone Electrophoresis
Zone electrophoresis separates proteins on the basis of their surface charge in a specific buffer (Fig. C-10). Generally cellulose acetate strips are used as the supporting medium for the electrophoresis. This method allows rapid electrophoretic migration, adaptation to his-

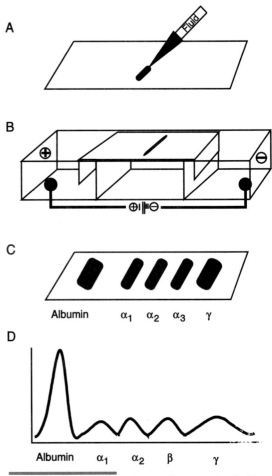

Figure C-10   In zone electrophoresis the fluid to be tested is placed on cellulose acetate and electrophoresed [(a) and (b)]. The cellulose acetate paper is then stained for protein, revealing characteristic bands (c). The bands are measured using a densitometer to give the characteristic peaks shown above.

tochemical staining, the use of microquantities of protein, and scanning with a densitometer (after staining the protein bound to the cellulose acetate).

In the clinical laboratory, the serum or other biologic fluid is placed as a vertical line perpendicular to the long axis of the cellulose acetate support. The proteins are separated by electrophoresis, the cellulose acetate is stained for protein, and scanned by a densitometer. The densitometer uses a beam of light that passes through the cellulose acetate with the stained proteins. The amount of light absorbed is proportionate to the amount of protein present. This variable absorption of light is reproduced on paper by an analogue recorder. The band pattern seen on the gel is converted into a series of peaks which can be measured. Normal human serum has five major electrophoretic bands, corresponding to albumin, α_1-globulin, α_2-globulin, β-globulin, and γ-globulin (Fig. C-10).

Zone electrophoresis is valuable in the detection of human paraprotein disorders such as multiple myeloma and Waldenström's macroglobulinemia. Here an electrophoretically restricted protein spike is seen most often in the γ-globulin region of the electrophoretogram, but may occasionally extend into the α and β regions. Other abnormalities of serum proteins may be detected, such as hypogammaglobulinemia, seen as a reduced peak; hypoalbuminemia seen in kidney, liver, and gastrointestinal diseases; and a reduced α_1-globulin peak seen in diseases such as α_1-antiproteinase deficiency. An elevation of the α-globulin peak may occur in inflammatory and neoplastic disorders while an increase in α_2-globulin often reflects the nephrotic syndrome or hemolysis with an increase in serum haptoglobin-hemoglobin complexes (Fig. C-11).

Column Chromatography

Chromatography allows for the separation of proteins and immunoglobulins by using the physical characteristics of protein molecules and of the chromatographic material to result in the differential retardation or

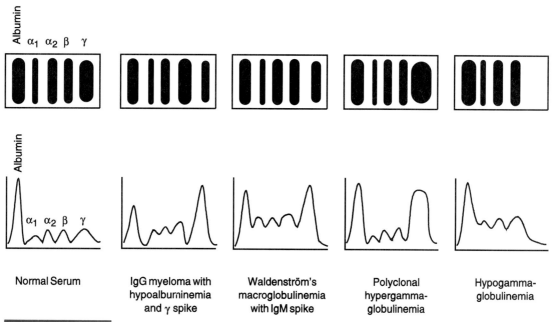

Figure C-11 Patterns of zone electrophoresis in some clinical diseases.

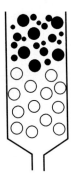 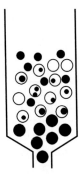 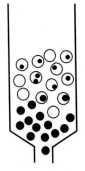

Solution placed on top of gel.

Largest molecules band and leave column first.

Smallest molecules are retained; larger molecules are retarded and leave column as another band.

Figure C-12 In gel filtration the molecules are separated on the basis of molecular size. Those molecules that are smaller than the bead pore size are retained within the pores; larger-sized molecules are excluded from the pores and retarded to different degrees, leaving the column in a band. Each band is a different size molecule.

retention of the various proteins by the chromatographic material. Chromatography is often performed by filling a glass cylinder with a synthetic gel and layering the sample over the top of the column, allowing the proteins to flow through the gel under the influence of gravity. The retained proteins of interest may then be eluted from the column material.

Gel Filtration Molecules can be separated according to their molecular size through the use of gel filtration (Fig. C-12). The gel is made of porous dextran beads or other polymers of predetermined pore size. Molecules larger than the pore size are excluded from the pores and are thus not retarded by the beads. They pass through the liquid phase of the column, leaving the column first. Smaller molecules will be retained to various degrees depending on their size and shape, with the same molecules traveling as a band through the column. This method can separate IgM from IgG, separate H and L chains of immunoglobulins, and separate Bence Jones proteins from the urine constituents in patients with multiple myeloma.

Ion-Exchange Chromatography The functional unit of an ion-exchange chromatography gel (Fig. C-13) is a charged moiety ad-

sorbed to an insoluble backbone such as acrylic copolymers, agarose, cellulose, or cross-linked dextran. This charged column separates proteins with different electrical charge. A cation-exchange column is used to fractionate negatively charged proteins while

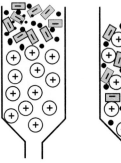 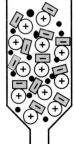 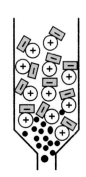

⊕ Positively-Charged Cellulose Bead
⊟ Negatively-Charged Molecule
● Uncharged Molecule

Figure C-13 The amount of charge that a protein molecule has determines the degree to which it is retarded by the column material in ion-exchange chromatography. Neutral particles pass through the column, while negatively charged particles are bound by the positively charged beads.

an anion-exchange column is used to fractionate positively charged molecules.

In order to release the retained molecules in ion-exchange chromatography, the pH and molarity of a buffer passing through the column are manipulated. In this way the proteins are eluted from the column in order of increasing protein charge. IgG may be removed in nearly pure form from serum using this method.

Affinity Chromatography   The specific and reversible biologic interaction between the substance to be isolated and the column material is the basis for separating molecules by affinity chromatography. This specificity is obtained by ligating an appropriate material covalently to an insoluble matrix such as agarose or dextran beads. The specific affinity for a particular molecule allows the column to adsorb and separate out that molecule from the rest of the substances in the solution that is flowing through the column. The unwanted materials are washed out of the column. The desired molecule is then eluted from the column by changing the buffer conditions (such as pH or ionic strength).

Many different materials are used to make an affinity column. If an antigen is bound to the column material, then its specific antibody may be purified from other proteins or antibodies. Alternatively, if an antibody is bound to the column, then its specific antigen may be purified in a similar manner.

This same method may be used to isolate specific subpopulations of cells using specific cell surface proteins, immunoglobulins, or receptors. Those cells having the specific surface material will be retained by the column, while other cells pass through. The cells of interest are eluted from the column by running a solution through the column containing the specific molecule bound by the column to compete with the same cell surface molecule retaining the cells.

Cryoglobulins

The common feature of a group of proteins known as *cryoglobulins* is the reversible precipitation that occurs when the protein is exposed to cold, i.e., the protein is a cryoprecipitate. Type I cryoglobulins consist of a single monoclonal immunoglobulin such as that found in Waldenström's macroglobulinemia, or multiple myeloma. Type II cryoglobulins are mixed cryoglobulins; that is, the cryoglobulin is made up of a monoclonal immunoglobulin which has as its antigenic specificity polyclonal immunoglobulin. An example is essential mixed cryoglobulinemia, where the antigenic specificity of the monoclonal antibody is most often the Fc portion of the IgG antibody, that is, the monoclonal antibody is a rheumatoid factor. Finally, type III cryoglobulins are a set of polyclonal antibodies directed against another set of polyclonal antibodies. Type III cryoglobulins, often found in rheumatic diseases like systemic lupus erythematosus, are not monoclonal antibodies.

Laboratory Analysis of Cryoglobulins   Blood and/or serum must be kept at 37° C during collection, clotting, and electrophoresis, since incorrect handling of the sample may result in precipitation prior to analysis and give a false-negative result. Once the blood has been collected and clotted at 37°C, it is stored at 4°C. When a cryoprecipitate forms, one may see a gel or white precipitate in the serum (usually within 24 to 72 h, though up to a week may be necessary).

The amount of cryoglobulin is quantified by several means. The protein concentration of the serum before and after cooling may be compared. The cryoprecipitate may be dissolved in an acidic buffer and the amount of protein measured using a spectrophotometer. Additionally, the cryocrit (the volume of the cryoprecipitate relative to the serum volume) may be measured.

Clinical Correlation   Type I and type II cryoglobulins contain monoclonal immunoglobulins and are often associated with paraproteinemias such as in patients with multiple myeloma. Type I and type II cryoglobulins are often present in high concentrations (often greater than 5 mg/mL), whereas type III cryoglobulins are often present in low concentrations (usually less than 1 mg/mL). Type III cryoglobulins are most often seen in the rheumatic diseases (e.g., rheumatoid arthritis) and in chronic infections (e.g., any of a number of chronic viral infections).

Signs related to any of the cryoglobulins may appear when the patient is exposed to cold. These signs include Raynaud's phenomenon, vascular purpura, cold-induced urticaria, bleeding tendencies, and even distal arterial thrombosis with gangrene.

Circulating soluble immune complexes are often associated with type I and type II cryoglobulins and may produce a variety of disease manifestations of serum sickness, such as glomerulonephritis, neurologic symptoms, vasculitis, and polyarthritis.

Cryoglobulins may interfere with a variety of laboratory tests, including platelet counts, immunoglobulin levels, and complement levels by precipitating at room temperature and removing substances from the blood or serum.

IMMUNE COMPLEX DETECTION

Immune complexes are found in a variety of diseases, and their accurate detection is an important aid in making a diagnosis. Because immune complexes are of various sizes and physical characteristics, no one method can detect all types of immune complexes.

Physical Methods

Ultracentrifugation and gel filtration are insensitive methods for immune complex detection and are usually used for separation of immune complexes from the rest of the serum.

Because of their large size, high molecular weight polymers such as polyethylene glycol are able to precipitate even low concentrations of immune complexes, leaving the smaller, soluble antigens and antibodies out of the precipitate. Once the immune complexes have been precipitated, they can be quantified by various methods including

spectrophotometry, radial diffusion, or their effect on complement consumption.

Interaction with Soluble Factors

Latex particles coated with aggregated IgG, can cross-link and agglutinate when Clq or rheumatoid factor is added to the suspension. Prior addition of immune complexes to the coated latex particles blocks the binding sites on the aggregated IgG, inhibiting the agglutination of the particles that result from the subsequent addition of Clq or rheumatoid factor. Thus, inhibition of coated-latex-particle agglutination serves as a test for immune complex detection.

When immune complexes bind Clq in vivo, the complement system is activated with subsequent depression of the hemolytic activity (CH_{50}). To measure the presence of immune complexes in a serum sample, the serum complement is first inactivated by heating it to 56°C. Several different dilutions of sample are then mixed with fresh normal serum which serves as a source of normal complement activity. The hemolytic activity of the normal serum and normal serum plus sample are compared. If the serum sample contains immune complexes, Clq and the rest of the complement cascade will be activated in proportion to the concentration of immune complexes in the sample. The anticomplementary activity of the sample is then reported as a percentage of reduction of the CH_{50}.

The conglutinin binding test uses conglutinin (a factor present in bovine serum that agglutinates red blood cells in the presence of complement) to bind the immune complex–C3 complex to a test tube, where the amount of immune complexes is measured by their uptake of an enzyme-conjugated or radiolabeled anti-immunoglobulin antibody.

Both solid-phase radioassay and liquid-phase radioassay may be employed to measure Clq binding. In the solid-phase radioassay, the Clq is adsorbed to a polystyrene tube. The amount of immune complexes in the sample bound to Clq is measured by the level of binding of a radiolabeled anti-immunoglobulin antibody or aggregated IgG to the remaining free Clq. In the liquid-phase assay, a radiolabeled Clq is employed, and either the free Clq or the Clq bound to the immune complexes may be measured.

Cell Receptor Assays

In the platelet aggregation test immune complexes interact with the platelet membrane, causing a measurable aggregation of platelets.

Immune complexes can be phagocytosed by macrophages. In the phagocytosis inhibition test radiolabeled aggregated IgG and the test sample are incubated with peritoneal macrophages. The sample's immune complexes interfere with the uptake of radiolabeled aggregated IgG by the macrophages. This interference in uptake is proportional to the amount of immune complexes in the sample.

B lymphocytes have C3 surface receptors which can bind complement-fixing immune complexes. The cells may be peripheral lymphocytes, certain lymphoblastoid B-cells, or Raji cells (which have C3 receptors but no surface immunoglobulins). The lymphoblastoid B cells and peripheral B cells, upon binding immune complexes, have fewer free complement receptors, which can be measured; fewer free receptors means more immune complexes in the sample being tested.

Nephelometry

When, in a dilute solution, antigen and antibody combine and precipitate, they cause an increase in the amount of light reflected from a light source shining through the solution. This scattering of light from a point light source can be measured using the technique called nephelometry.

The measurement of immune complexes by this method requires that the measurements be made in a state of antigen excess, since in cases of near equivalence and antibody excess, the relationship between light scattering and the amount of antigen present is not linear.

Nephelometry can also be used to measure antigen concentrations in a solution. Constant amounts of highly purified and optically clear specific antiserum are added to a variable amount of antigen. This reactant mixture is placed in a cuvette and the amount of light scatter from an incident light beam is measured and reported as the optical density of the reactant mixture. The higher the optical density, the higher the concentration of antigen in the solution.

Complement Fixation

The binding of antigen and antibody causes the activation of complement (fixation) which consumes the amount of available complement in a test system. If the amount of complement is kept constant, then either the amount of an antibody or an antigen can be determined if the other components of the system are kept constant. This measurement is done in a two-part system. First antigen and antibody are combined in a known amount of complement. A certain amount of complement is fixed by the resulting immune complexes. The remaining complement activity is then determined by adding antibody-coated RBCs in a hemolytic assay as described before. The result is expressed in terms of the highest serum dilution that shows antibody fixation or the concentration of antigen that limits fixation for determining antigen concentration.

MEMBRANE DETECTION METHODS FOR DNA, RNA, AND PROTEINS

Membrane support materials such as nitrocellulose and nylon are used to bind DNA, RNA, or proteins so that they may be detected using specific probes. These probes bind only those membrane-bound molecules of interest.

Single-stranded nucleic acids are able to bind to another nucleic acid that is complementary to its sequence. This is the basis of forming double-stranded DNA during replication and RNA from DNA to transcribe a message for manufacturing a protein. This also allows one to make probes that will bind only complementary DNA or RNA.

In the case of protein bound to a membrane, if the epitope of the protein is available and not changed by its binding to the membrane, it may be detected by using specific antibodies for that protein. Thus, an antibody probe can detect membrane-bound proteins.

In autoradiography, the localization of the complex formed by the labeled nucleic acid or antibody with its target is marked by the appearance of black dots in a photographic emulsion placed over a tissue section. The antibody may be chemically labeled with a number of radioisotopes, such as ^{125}I, ^{32}P, and ^{3}H. The radioisotope causes silver grains to appear in the developed photographic emulsion.

Southern Blot Analysis

Southern blot analysis, developed by E.M. Southern, allows for the detection of specific DNAs of interest by separating a sample of DNA by size in a gel electrophoretically, transferring the DNA to a membrane by capillary or electrophoretic means, and then probing the membrane with a specific piece of DNA or RNA (the probe) that has been radiolabeled. After nonspecifically bound probe has been washed away, the location of the probe on the filter is determined by exposing the membrane to the x-ray film. The developed film will have "bands" only where there is radiolabeled probe bound to membrane-bound DNA; this detection technique is called *autoradiography*. This method is used to detect the DNA of interest in genomic DNA (i.e., it is used in restriction-fragment-length polymorphisms for detection of abnormal genes) and in other applications in molecular biology.

Northern Blot Analysis

Northern blot analysis is similar to Southern blot analysis except that it is used to separate and identify RNA. Total or messenger RNA is run on a gel. The gel separates the RNA by size. The RNA is then transferred from the gel to a membrane. As in Southern blotting, a probe is used to detect specific RNA species. This method can be used to detect the presence of mRNA for a specific protein. Semiquantitative analysis of the amount of specific RNA can be performed in different cells or in cells treated in different ways.

Western Blot Analysis

Western blot analysis is similar to Southern and Northern blot analysis, the difference being that proteins are run on a gel and transferred to a membrane. The probe in this case is an antibody to a protein of interest. The antibody binds to its specific protein and is often detected by using a second labeled antibody that recognizes the first antibody. This protein band may be seen by autoradiographic means or as a colored band on the membrane when an enzyme-linked second antibody is used (as in ELISA; see below).

BINDER-LIGAND ASSAYS

Radioimmunoassay (RIA)

One of the most important analytical methods to be developed in the past 30 years is the ligand assay. The first binder-ligand assay to be used was the radioimmunoassay (RIA). This method has allowed accurate measurement of hormones, drugs, antibodies associated with allergy, and tumor markers. In the arena of infectious disease, bacterial and fungal infections can be detected quickly, as can the antibodies to such agents as hepatitis A, B and C viruses as well as the AIDS virus, HIV. The uses of ligand assays have been extended by modern methods using monoclonal and polyclonal antibodies.

In RIA (Fig. C-14) the molecule of interest is known as the *analyte*. The analyte is bound to a material called the *binder*. When the analyte reacts with the binder, it is referred to as a *ligand*. A radiolabeled analyte, the

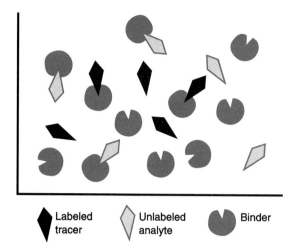

Labeled tracer   Unlabeled analyte   Binder

Figure C-14   Radioimmunoassay. The ability of antigen in the sample to block the binding of radiolabeled antigen (tracer) to the binder allows measurement of the unknown antigen.

tracer or *label*, is used to compete with the unknown concentration of unlabeled analyte. The more analyte present in a test solution, the more effectively it will compete with the tracer for the binder present in the assay system, leaving more tracer unbound. This relationship allows the concentration of an unknown analyte to be measured.

In all the ligand assay systems, one must establish a standard or calibration curve using known variable quantities of an analyte and fixed quantities of binder and tracer. As analyte in the ligand system increases, bound tracer decreases. The standard curve uses either the amount of free or bound tracer

present. One determines the amount of an unknown analyte concentration by comparing the measured tracer amount (bound or free) with the standard curve and estimating the amount of analyte by interpolation.

Measurement of IgE
There is only about 250 ng/mL of IgE in normal serum, with severely allergic individuals having IgE concentrations up to 700 ng/mL serum. Because of this low level, sensitive methods of detection are needed to measure serum IgE concentrations. In the radioimmunosorbent test (RIST) the total IgE concentration is measured by mixing the patient's serum with anti-IgE-coated particles and then with ^{125}I-labeled rabbit anti-IgE myeloma protein. After washing, the particles are counted in a gamma counter to determine the amount of bound radiolabeled IgE. In the radioallergosorbent test (RAST) the specific IgE concentration is measured by combining the patient's serum IgE with an antigen-bound immunosorbent, which is then washed and reacted with ^{125}I-labeled rabbit anti-IgE. The radioactivity of the immunosorbent is then measured and the amount of specific serum IgE antibodies to that allergen is determined.

Enzyme-Linked Immunosorbent Assay (ELISA)

In the enzyme-linked immunosorbent assay (ELISA) (Fig. C-15) an antigen is attached to a solid-phase material, usually a 96-well plastic plate (most proteins will bind to

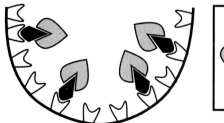
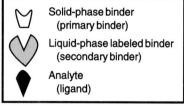

Solid-phase binder (primary binder)

Liquid-phase labeled binder (secondary binder)

Analyte (ligand)

Figure C-15   ELISA. A sandwich assay used for detecting the amount of antibody in a sample.

plastic noncovalently), and the solution containing the antibody to be detected is added to the well lined by the immobilized antigen. After the excess, unbound antibody is washed away, a second antibody, which is an anti-immunoglobulin antibody which is linked to an enzyme, is added to the reactants. Then the substrate for the enzyme is added to the above reaction mixture and the amount of altered substrate is measured. The enzyme and substrate are chosen so that enzymatic modification of the substrate produces a change in color of the substrate solution. The amount of changed substrate is proportional to the amount of antibody bound to the immobilized antigen.

Many modifications of the basic ELISA technique can be used. For example, one may use a biotinylated antibody followed by enzyme-conjugated avidin or streptavidin. The avidin-biotin method results in a multiplicative effect since many biotin molecules may be attached to a single second antibody molecule, with multiple avidin molecules binding subsequently to the second antibody. The avidin-biotin method is therefore particularly sensitive.

Another modification often used is the ELISA capture assay. In this assay, an antibody to antigen X is first immobilized on a plastic plate. A solution containing unknown amounts of antigen X is then added, followed by a second, enzyme-coupled antibody specific for a *different* determinant on antigen X. The amount of altered substance produced in the ensuing ELISA will now correlate to the amount of antigen X in the tested solution.

IMMUNOHISTOCHEMICAL METHODS

Immunohistochemical techniques are based on the detection of specific antigens by antibodies tagged by a fluorescent dye, an enzyme, or any other molecule that can be detected using chemical assays.

Fluorescent Staining Techniques

In *direct immunofluorescence* (Fig. C-16) the conjugated antibody is placed directly upon the tissue section or viable cell suspension. The fluorescence signal can be visualized directly on the treated specimen.

In *indirect immunofluorescence* (Fig. C-17) specific antiserum is placed upon the specimen and allowed to react and form immune complexes. The excess antiserum is washed off and a fluorescent-dye-conjugated antibody against the first antibody (e.g., goat antihuman IgG) is used to tag the immune complexes so that they fluoresce when exposed to the appropriate wavelength of light.

More than one antigen can be detected in a given section by using antibodies to each antigen conjugated with a different fluorescent dye. An example is the detection of immune complexes and complement deposited into tissues. An antibody to the immunoglobulin can be conjugated to the green-emitting dye fluorescein, while the antibody to complement can be conjugated to a red-emitting rhodamine dye derivative. Both colors can then be visualized in the microscopic section simultaneously.

The biotin-avidin immunofluorescent method makes use of the glycoprotein avidin, derived from egg albumin, which binds with great affinity to the vitamin biotin. Avidin can be labeled with a fluorochrome. Biotin may be conjugated to a protein such as an immunoglobulin. The material to be stained is treated with a specific biotinylated antibody to form an immune complex. Fluorescent avidin is then added to the biotin-antibody conjugate. Since many conjugated biotin molecules may be bound to an immunoglobulin, the resulting fluorescence can be particularly brilliant.

Immune Complex Detection in Tissues

Immunohistologic techniques using immunoperoxidase or immunofluorescence are used to detect immune complexes in tissue samples. By choosing the desired antisera,

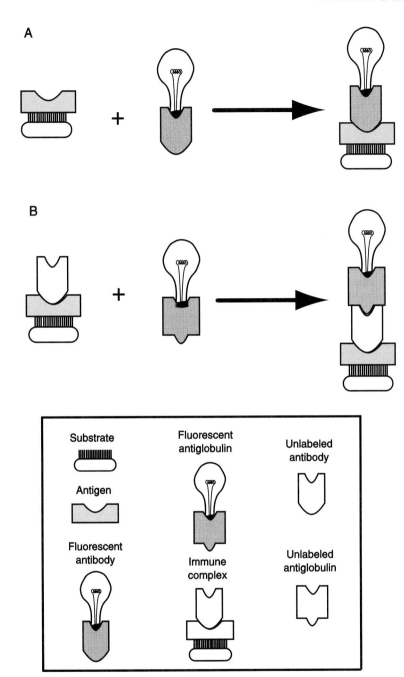

Figure C-16 Direct immunofluorescence. In direct immunofluorescence of an antigen in the substrate (a), an antibody that contains the fluorescent label and that is directed against the antigen is used. In order to visualize the immune complexes in the substrate (b), a fluorescent-dye-tagged anti-immunoglobulin is used.

A

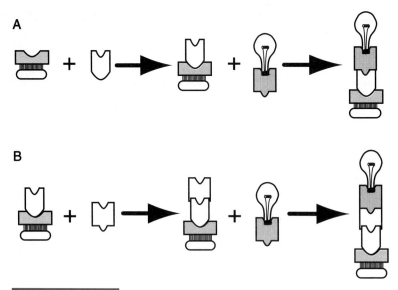

B

Figure C-17 Indirect immunofluorescence. Using the indirect immuno-fluorescence method, incubation of an unlabeled antibody with the antigen in the tissue sample forms an immune complex. This immune complex is then labeled with a fluorescent anti-immunoglobulin (*a*). When performing an indirect detection of the immune complex (*b*), an unlabeled anti-immunoglobulin is used to react with the immune complex, and this unlabeled anti-immunogloblin is then labeled with a second fluorescent anti-immunoglobulin that reacts to the added unlabeled anti-immunogloblin.

immunoglobulin classes, fibrin, fibrinogen, and complement components can be specifically visualized in the tissue.

Other Immunohistochemical Methods

In enzyme-linked antibody cytochemical techniques, instead of a fluorescent moiety coupled to an antibody, an active enzyme is bound to an antibody. The localization of antigen in a tissue section can be performed by direct or indirect methods. Once the antibody-enzyme complex is bound to the tissue section, the enzyme substrate is added. The altered substrate is then detected by microscopy. The most common enzyme coupled to antibody is horseradish peroxidase, which produces a black color when incubated with hydrogen peroxide and diaminobenzidine. Alternatively, autoradiography can be used to detect the antigen.

Metal-coupled antibody is electron-dense and is used with electron microscopy. The antibody can be attached to ferritin (an iron-containing protein), gold, or uranium and then used in either indirect or direct immunostaining of a tissue section. The localization of the immune complex is then seen as an electron-dense area in the electron micrograph.

COMPLEMENT ASSAYS

The complement factors C1–C9 as well as the various inhibitory complement proteins can be measured. Clinical laboratories can measure individual complement components, including some of the activated components such as C3a, C4a, C5a, and the total hemolytic complement CH_{50}. As mentioned previously, complement activation can occur with immune complex formation. This can be used in detecting antigens or antibodies in assay systems.

Hemolytic Assay

The CH_{50} is a general test employed to detect a depression of the serum complement components in patient samples. Substantial reductions in individual complement components are required to depress the value of the CH_{50}, making this an insensitive test in some situations. The hemolytic assay (determination of CH_{50}) combines red blood cells (RBCs), antibody to RBCs, and a source of complement. When combined, the RBCs will lyse, releasing hemoglobin which is measured spectrophotometrically and related to the number of RBCs lysed. In performing the assay, the number of RBCs, the amount of antibody, and other reaction conditions are kept constant. The CH_{50} value is set as the quantity of complement needed to lyse 50 percent of the RBCs. The results of the tests are reported as the reciprocal of the serum dilution that gave a 50 percent hemolysis of the RBCs.

Specific Complement Component Measurement

In order to cause hemolysis of antibody-coated RBCs the entire sequence of complement activation from C1 to C9 must be completed. To detect a depletion of any one component, two methods may be employed. First, one adds an excess of all the required purified components of the complement system, except the one to be measured, to antibody-coated RBCs. The test sample is then added and the subsequent hemolysis is related to the amount of the complement component to be measured. Another method is to use specifically deficient reagents from genetically defined complement deficiencies for estimating individual complement component activity in a sample.

Antibodies may be prepared against individual components of complement. These antibodies may then be used to quantify the amounts of individual complement components by rocket electrophoresis, quantitative immunofluorescence, and single radial diffusion. As in all complement measurement schemes, the sample must be stored at $-70°C$ or colder, since complement is labile at higher temperatures and may degrade with improper storage.

Coombs' Test

This test is used to detect antibodies and other proteins that are bound to RBCs. RBCs may have antibody attached to them, such as anti-Rh factor, which is insufficient to cause agglutination. With the addition of an antiglobulin antiserum (e.g., anti-IgG, anti-IgA) produced in another species, agglutination occurs. In addition, RBCs coated with complement components such as C3 and C4, as found in some autoimmune hemolytic anemias, may be agglutinated with antiserum directed against complement. The direct Coombs' test detects γ-globulin or other proteins coated onto RBCs directly from the sensitized person. The indirect Coombs' test requires that the patient's serum be incubated with test RBCs and that the possibly protein-coated RBCs then be agglutinated with a Coombs' antiserum.

METHODOLOGY FOR DETERMINATION OF CELLULAR IMMUNE FUNCTION

In the preceding section we reviewed the methods employed for the detection of soluble molecules and precipitates. In this section the techniques employed in the characterization and measurement of the immunocompetent cells will be considered. The cell types include neutrophils, lymphocytes (T and B), and monocytes and macrophages.

Delayed-Type Hypersensitivity (DTH) Skin Testing

DTH testing is a useful clinical test that is readily available to the clinician and is inexpensive to administer. The test examines the cutaneous hypersensitivity to an antigen or group of antigens. When using antigens from possible infectious agents, a positive test implies that the patient has been previously exposed to the agent and has developed an immune response, but not necessarily that he or she is currently infected by that agent. DTH testing may also be used in epidemiologic studies and as a guide to the integrity of the cellular immunity of a patient. There are a number of agents to which most people have been exposed in the course of their lives and to which they have developed a delayed hypersensitivity. An individual who reacts to none of these reagents is termed *anergic*, indicating a problem with the individual's cellular immunocompetence.

Skin testing is usually done by injection of a small amount of antigen intradermally using a 25- or 27-gauge needle. After 24 to 48 h, the largest dimension of erythema and induration is measured and recorded. A negative test can be interpreted as indicating a lack of exposure only if appropriate control antigens have been injected at separate sites to demonstrate that the patient has the ability to mount a DTH reaction, i.e., the patient is not *anergic*.

Patch Testing

Patch testing is used to determine whether a patient has delayed hypersensitivity to a variety of agents that may be responsible for contact dermatitis. The substance of interest is applied to the skin at a low concentration, and the area is covered with an occlusive dressing. After 24 to 48 h the area is examined for the presence of a superficial inflammatory reaction of the skin. A false-positive result may be obtained if too high a concentration of antigen is used, leading to irritation rather than an allergic reaction, or patients may react to the adhesive of the patch.

False negatives occur with too low a concentration of antigen or use of inadequate occlusion with poor skin penetration.

Separation of Mononuclear Cells from Whole Blood

Many of the specialized assays require that the mononuclear cells from peripheral blood be separated from the rest of the blood elements. The method of choice for separation of these mononuclear cells is Ficoll-Hypaque density gradient centrifugation, which allows a 70 to 90 percent yield of mononuclear cells, with a high degree of purity. Ficoll-Hypaque is a solution that produces a variable density within the solution when the Ficoll-Hypaque is subjected to centrifugal force. This variable density, or gradient, is able to separate white blood cells according to the cells' density.

The separation of mononuclear cells from blood is a relatively simple process. Whole blood is defibrinated with glass beads, and the blood elements are taken up into tissue culture medium and layered on top of a layer of Ficoll-Hypaque. After centrifugation, the more dense RBCs and granulocytes form a pellet on the bottom of the tube, while the less dense lymphocytes and monocytes are at the boundary of the Ficoll-Hypaque medium where they can be removed.

T-Lymphocyte Assays

Many monoclonal antibodies have been produced in murine hybridomas to T-cell surface antigens. Monoclonal antibodies coupled to fluorochrome may be used with live lymphocytes or in frozen tissue sections. A count of T-cell types and subtypes may be obtained by microscopy or flow cytometry.

Quantification of Lymphocyte Response to Stimulation

Most mitogens used to stimulate human T and B lymphocytes selectively stimulate either T or B cells. Concanavalin A (conA) and phytohemagglutinin (PHA) have stimulatory effects mostly on T cells, whereas lipopolysaccharide (LPS), purified protein derivative of tuberculin (PPD), and dextran sulfate specifically stimulate B cells in some systems.

In evaluating mitogenic effects on lymphocyte stimulation, the lymphocytes are often purified using Ficoll-Hypaque density gradient centrifugation. They are cultured in an appropriate medium with varying concentrations of mitogen. The amount of DNA synthesis is determined by the addition of a pulse of tritiated thymidine (^{3}H-Td), a nucleotide precursor that is incorporated into the cells' DNA. The amount of ^{3}H-Td incorporated is proportional to the amount of DNA being synthesized, and is counted in a scintillation counter. Results are usually given in counts per minute (cpm). This cpm value is used as the value for lymphocyte stimulation. The cpm value from the control cells is subtracted from the stimulated value, a result reported as *Δcpm*, or the stimulated value may be divided by the control cpm value to give a ratio called the *stimulation index*.

Antigenic stimulation of lymphocytes recruits far fewer lymphocytes to proliferate, since only those cells sensitive to the antigen are stimulated. These lymphocytes, which are usually T cells, proliferate to antigens usually used in skin hypersensitivity testing. This proliferation correlates well with the skin test, and may in some instances be more sensitive as an index of antigen-mediated cellular hypersensitivity.

Mixed Lymphocyte Reaction and Cell-Mediated Lymphocyte Lysis

In the mixed lymphocyte culture (MLC) (also known as the mixed lymphocyte reaction [MLR]) assay, one adds foreign lymphocytes to the lymphocytes under study. These foreign lymphocytes are defined by their foreign MHC antigens, the target antigens against which the lymphocytes to be studied respond. Lymphocyte proliferation is determined using the same tritiated thymidine uptake assay as is used in the antigen-stim-

ulation assays noted above. The MLC test can be performed as either a single proliferative response or as a two-way proliferative response. In the single proliferative response, the lymphocytes used as stimulators are treated with mitomycin C or irradiation, which prevents them from making DNA and proliferating. The detected DNA proliferative response is then solely due to the untreated responder cells. In the two-way MLR, both lymphocyte populations may react to each other, with one's contribution to the net proliferation unknown. The MLC assay is useful in determining the immunocompetence of T cells.

During the course of the single proliferative response assay MLC, cytotoxic effector cells are produced which recognize the MHC class I markers of the stimulator cells. These cytotoxic effector cells are drawn from a precursor population different from that which gives rise to the proliferating cells noted above. The stimulator cells can be labeled with ^{51}Cr and added to the cytotoxic study cells. The percentage of ^{51}Cr released from the sensitizing lymphocytes is compared with the percentage of ^{51}Cr released from control (nonsensitizing) target cells under the same conditions. This value is reported as the cytotoxicity measurement in an assay called *cell-mediated lympholysis (CML)*. The cytotoxic cells of the CML assay are responding to the class I HLA-A, HLA-B, and HLA-C antigens on target cells, whereas the class II antigens of the HLA-D locus are involved in lymphocyte proliferation in the CML assay.

B-Lymphocyte Assays

B lymphocytes can be easily detected and counted by detection of their surface transmembrane immunoglobulin (used as the antigen receptor on all B cells). Antibodies are very immunogenic proteins (recall the idiotype network control system), and one can make antisera against antibody molecules in many species and then label these xenogeneic antisera with a fluorescing tag. The total number of B cells in a sample can then be determined by using a polyspecific antisera against all the immunoglobulin classes or by using a mixture containing anti-κ and anti-λ immunoglobulins, i.e., sera binding to all heavy chains or all light chains. Alternatively, one can make an antiserum which identifies only a specific idiotype on the surface of B cells, by using that idiotype as the inoculant for the antiserum-producing animal.

Detection of B cells is then accomplished by mixing the lymphocyte suspension with the antiserum at 4°C for 20 to 30 min. The cells are then washed to remove unbound immunoglobulin, and the cells with surface fluorescence are counted using a fluorescent microscope.

In some cases one may see not only surface immunoglobulin, but also intracellular immunoglobulin which is identical to the surface antibody molecule. This is seen in some of the lymphoid malignancies, such as B-cell lymphomas with leukemia, and chronic lymphocytic leukemia. The method for optimum intracytoplasmic immunoglobulin detection requires the cells to be acetone- or ethanol-fixed prior to use of the above antisera with the purified lymphocyte preparation.

One may detect B lymphocytes by using a rosetting technique that utilizes the complement receptor of B cells. ox RBCs (which do not spontaneously bind to human lymphocytes) are coated with IgM in the presence of serum deficient in the complement factor C5 so that the RBCs are not lysed. These treated ox RBCs now have antibody and complement on their surfaces.

When these treated ox erythrocytes are incubated with separated lymphocytes, the treated ox RBCs attach to B lymphocytes via the B-cell complement receptor. A cell is considered positive when three or more treated ox erythrocytes are attached to the cell. Since both neutrophils and monocytes may form treated ox RBC rosettes, they must be distinguished from lymphocytes by other means. If one starts with a cell preparation first purified by Ficoll-Hypaque separation, there should be few if any neutrophils in the cells being studied. Ficoll-Hypaque purifi-

cation does not separate lymphocytes from monocytes, so other techniques must be used (see below). One finds a range of treated ox RBC rosetting cells of 10 to 19 percent from different laboratories.

One can identify antibody-producing cells by using hemolytic plaque-forming assays. Three modifications of this technique allow determination of cells producing IgG or IgM specific for an individual antigen, or identification of the total number of cells making antibody of any sort. Each of these assays starts with a mixture of the cell population being studied with antigen-sensitized RBCs plated in agar. Antigen-antibody complexes *on the surface of RBCs* can fix complement and cause RBC lysis, and this lysis appears as a clear area, or *plaque*, in the plate.

In the indirect hemolytic plaque assay, the production of antigen-specific IgG is detected by stimulating the B cells with the relevant antigen and coating the indicator RBCs with the same antigen. Only antibody to the specific antigen will bind to the indicator RBCs. Development of the plaque occurs when anti-IgG and complement are added to the plate. RBCs with antigen-specific IgG bound to their surface will be lysed (antibody plus anti-IgG plus complement yields lysis), and the clear plaques can be read.

In the direct hemolytic plaque assay, cells making antigen-specific IgM can be measured by RBC lysis without addition of the anti-IgG. The antigen-coated RBCs are bound by antigen-specific IgM, which then directly fixes the complement added in the development step.

In the reversed hemolytic plaque assay all B cells making immunoglobulin are measured, regardless of the antigenic specificity of the antibody being made. The lymphocytes to be tested are mixed with erythrocytes coated with goat or rabbit antihuman immunoglobulins in the same semisolid agar used above. Complement is then added to the plate, and the presence of hemolytic plaques indicates the location of immunoglobulin-producing B cells.

One may specifically (using antigen) or nonspecifically (using the mitogen staphylococcal protein A) stimulate B cells. Polyclonal antibody production after this stimulation can be detected by staining cultured cells for those containing intracellular immunoglobulins. The polyclonal antibody produced and released into the culture supernatant can be measured by RIA or ELISA techniques.

Flow Cytometry and Cell Sorting

One of the most revolutionary technologies in immunology is flow cytometry. In this technique, cells are labeled with a fluorescent tag (generally using a fluoresceinated monoclonal antibody to the cell surface marker of interest) and then passed through a very thin nozzle in front of high-intensity laser-emitted light which can activate the specific fluorescent tag used. The fluorescent light emitted by the stream of cells exiting the nozzle can be measured. The intensity of the fluorescent light increases with the amount of fluorescent antibody attached to each cell.

A second light source impinges on the stream of cells emerging from the nozzle. The amount of light scattered by the cells is measured by another detector to determine the number of cells passing through the beam. The information from the fluorescent and cell counter detectors can be analyzed to indicate the intensity of the light per cell as well as the number of positive cells present.

Two different fluorescent dyes can be used simultaneously, along with two different laser beams, in order to measure two different cell surface markers at the same time: cells which are positive for both, either one, or neither of the properties of interest can be measured.

Finally, flow cytometry can be used to purify different cell populations. Briefly, the stream of cells is broken up into tiny droplets, generally containing one or no cells. Each droplet is given a negative charge. Cells which are positive for the property of interest can then be deflected by positively charged panels in the apparatus and the cells of interest pooled for further studies.

Natural Killer Cells

With the use of monoclonal antibodies, natural killer (NK) cells can be identified using fluoresceinated antibodies to cell surface components, in the same manner as used for T and B cells. Differentiation antigens such as NKH-1, NKH-2, Leu-7, and HNK-1 are specific for NK cells and monoclonal antibodies are available to identify them. CD3/TCR is notably absent from natural killer cells.

The killer function of NK cells can be assess by the ^{51}Cr release assay as described earlier, using as a target cell line the K562 erythroleukemia cell.

Assays for Monocytes and Macrophages

In stained peripheral blood, monocytes and macrophages can be distinguished by their morphologic appearance and the presence of nonspecific esterase, which can be measured by a colorimetric assay. However, in tissues or in suspension other markers must be used. These additional markers include the antigens Leu-M3, OKTM1 (found at times on T cells), for which monoclonal antibodies are available. In addition, monocytes express MHC class II markers on their surface, along with receptors for complement components and the IgG Fc segment.

The functional capability of these cells can be tested by the monocyte's or macrophage's ability to phagocytose antibody-coated heat-killed microorganisms or other particles (like latex beads). This ability to engulf particles can be used to separate monocytes from the rest of a cell population. Monocytes will ingest iron filings; the use of a magnet can then remove these cells from the rest of the mononuclear cells isolated by Ficoll-Hypaque purification. Monocytes will nonspecifically adhere to plastic, and a cell population allowed to adhere to a plastic Petri dish can be enriched for monocytes by such an incubation. The cells gently washed from the dish will be monocyte-depleted; the remaining cells will be monocyte-enriched.

Polymorphonuclear (PMN) Cell Assays

Motility Testing

PMNs (neutrophils) are constantly in motion, which may be random or directed toward a specific stimulus; such purposeful movement is called *chemotaxis*, or movement down a chemotactic factor gradient. The chemotactic factors (chemotaxins) include a number of very different chemicals, such as endotoxins from microorganisms, lymphocyte chemotactic factor from lymphocytes, and activated complement components (i.e., C3a, C5a, C567). Both random and directed movement can be assessed by in vitro assays.

In testing for random motility a 5 × 10⁶/mL concentration of purified neutrophils in a 0.1% human albumin solution is placed in a siliconized microhematocrit tube. The tube is enclosed in a special chamber which is filled with immersion oil, and the chamber is then placed under a microscope where the leading edge of the neutrophil column is observed hourly. The motility is expressed as the number of millimeters of movement from the starting boundary of the neutrophil column.

Two methods for quantification of PMN chemotaxis are used in the clinical laboratory. The older method for detection of directed motion uses the Boyden chamber. Here the lower of two chambers is filled with a chemoattractant. A filter with a small pore size separates the lower chamber from an upper chamber, to which the neutrophils are added. After a suitable incubation time the filter is removed and stained. The number of neutrophils in the filter is then counted microscopically.

In the second method an agarose gel with wells is used in a fashion similar to the single-radial-diffusion method outlined earlier. Three wells are cut into the agar in a linear fashion. The neutrophils to be tested are placed in the center well. Into one of the outer wells a putative chemotactic substance is placed and into the other is placed a non-chemotaxin-containing control solution. Af-

ter several hours of migration, the distance from the center of the center well to the edge of the migrating neutrophils is measured. In this way, both the motility due to random motion as well as directed motility due to a chemoattractant can be quantified.

Recognition

Microorganisms or inert particles, like latex beads, may be coated with immunoglobulin and/or complement factors which enhance the phagocytosis of these materials by the neutrophil. This process of opsonization can then be measured by observing cells for phagocytosis.

Though complement and Fc receptors can be quantified on neutrophil surfaces, this remains a research tool and is not clinically available at this time.

Ingestion

A neutrophil must use energy to ingest a particle (e.g., a microorganism) after the neutrophil has recognized the particle. This recognition and ingestion occurs more rapidly when the particle has been opsonized with complement or immunoglobulin (Fig. C-18). The methods for quantifying the ingestion of particles by neutrophils include direct counting of ingested particle by microscopy, measurement of an easily stained lipid used for ingestion after extraction from cells, and the use of radiolabeled particles with estimates of cell-bound radioactivity after ingestion. Unfortunately, many noncontrolled variables interfere with these assays, and at present there is no commonly accepted standard assay for particle ingestion.

Degranulation

The neutrophil ingests particles through an invagination of its cell membrane which allows particles to be brought into the cell. This cell membrane pocket, once it is closed off to within the cytoplasm, is called a *phagosome*. In order to degrade and/or kill what is present in the phagosome, the contents of lysosomes are added to the phagosome. The contents of the lysosome and phagosome are combined by a process of membrane fusion.

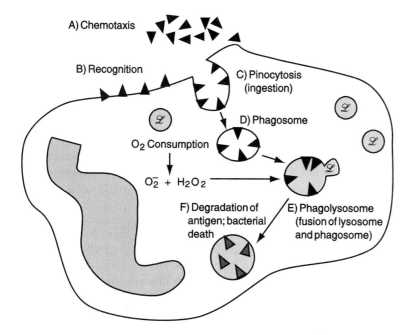

A) Chemotaxis

B) Recognition

C) Pinocytosis (ingestion)

D) Phagosome

O_2 Consumption

$O_2^- + H_2O_2$

F) Degradation of antigen; bacterial death

E) Phagolysosome (fusion of lysosome and phagosome)

Figure C-18 Stages in the phagocytosis and digestion of particulate matter. (a) The PMN is attracted to the area by a chemotactic stimulus. (b) Surface attachment is facilitated by opsonization by immunoglobulins and/or complement. (c) The cell membrane invaginates and the material is ingested. (d) The ingested material is retained in a phagosome. (e) The phagosome combines with a lysosome ($\mathscr{L}$) to form a phagolysosome. (f) There is bacterial killing and material degradation by the lysosomal enzymes and activated oxegen species.

The resulting *phagolysosome* is the organelle for killing and/or degradation of ingested particles. The process of lysosome fusion with the discharge of lysosomal contents into the phagosome is known as degranulation, which is an active process requiring energy expenditure by the cell. A process that interferes with the metabolic pathways of energy metabolism, such as oxygen consumption or the hexose monophosphate shunt (where glucose is metabolized) will impede degranulation.

The "frustrated phagocytosis" test (Fig. C-19) examines degranulation independent of ingestion. On a Petri dish heat-aggregated γ-globulins or immune complexes are attached to the Petri dish surface in such a manner that the γ-globulins or immune complexes can not be ingested by the phagocytic cell. A suspension containing neutrophils is added to Petri dishes with and without (control) attached γ-globulin or immune complexes. Cell receptors on the neutrophil's surface are activated, and the cells attach themselves to the bound γ-globulin or immune complexes. The cell is unable to engulf the dish-bound material and therefore is unable to form a phagosome, but the lysosomes within the cell move to these areas of the cell membrane and fuse, releasing their contents into the medium. The rate of degranulation is estimated by measuring the

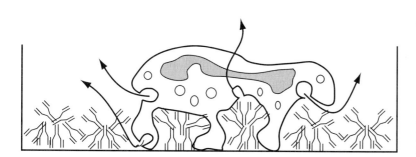

Figure C-19 The frustrated-phagocytosis test evaluates the ability of the neutrophil to degranulate independent of its ability to ingest. Lysosomal contents are discharged into the supernatant, which is then measured.

appearance of lysosomal enzymes such as acid phosphatase and α-glucuronidase in the medium.

The measurement of lactic dehydrogenase in the medium is a guide to the amount of nonspecific cytolysis, since this enzyme is found in the cytoplasm but not in lysosomes.

Intracellular Killing

Intracellular killing of microorganisms by the neutrophil involves the proper coordination of the previous steps as well as the constituents in the phagolysosome capable of killing microorganisms. Some of these consitituents are singlet oxygen, superoxide and hydroxyl radicals, hydrogen peroxide, acid pH, lactoferrin, cationic proteins, lysozyme, and the myeloperoxidase-halogenation system. Though there are many components for intracellular killing, a defect in any one of them may render killing inadequate for certain groups of microorganisms. Currently, only the nitroblue tetrazolium (NBT) dye reduction test and the intraleukocytic killing test are used in clinical practice to detect such defects.

The NBT dye reduction test measures the reduction of this clear yellow water-soluble compound to the deep blue dye formazan by mechanisms related to the metabolic events in the respiratory burst in the neutrophil. These events include hydrogen peroxide and superoxide radical formation, increased oxygen uptake, and an increase in the hexose monophosphate shunt. The neutrophil is induced to ingest latex or other particles with simultaneous uptake of NBT. Once the dye is reduced, it may be extracted from neutrophils with pyridine (organic solvent) and quantified photometrically at 515 nm. The NBT reduction test is a means of assessing the integrity of the metabolic burst pathways. Failure to reduce the dye is a finding in clinical diseases such as chronic granulomatous disease, where an inability of the neutrophil to produce hydrogen peroxide and superoxide radicals leads to an inability to kill some microorganisms ingested by the neutrophil.

Chemiluminescence occurs in certain chemical reactions when the excited electrons from chemically unstable groups relax to their ground state, releasing energy in the form of light. When the neutrophil undergoes its respiratory burst, it produces reactive oxygen species such as superoxide radicals, hydrogen peroxide, and singlet oxygen. When singlet oxygen in the lysosome combines with bacteria or other constituents, it forms unstable carboxyl groups, which emit light as their electrons return to the ground state. Neutrophil chemiluminescence requires that all steps prior to bacterial killing be intact. In fact, there is good correlation between microbiologic killing and the amount of chemiluminescence. This light emission may be intensified by an intermediate fluorescent compound, luminol, which is added to the balanced salt solution containing the ingestible particles and the neutrophils. The light emissions are then measured using a scintillation counter. Chemiluminescence is reduced in patients with granulomatous disease and patients who are myeloperoxidase-deficient.

In a number of diseases (such as chronic granulomatous disease, myeloperoxidase deficiency, Job's syndrome, acute leukemia, cryoglobulinemia, and acute infections) there may be defective intracellular microbial killing. To test for defective intracellular killing, neutrophils are mixed with a specific microbial organism, in the presence of opsonin, and incubated at 37°C. After an appropriate amount of time, an antimicrobial agent is added to the medium to kill extracellular organisms. The neutrophils are then sampled at different times and lysed with sterile water. An estimate of surviving viable previously intracellular bacteria is made by culturing diluted samples of the lysed neutrophils. One must independently assure ingestion of bacteria by neutrophils, since a false "normal" test may result if the bacteria are not ingested by the neutrophils but killed by the added antimicrobial agent.

D

Clusters of Differentiation (CD) Guide: Workshop Antigen Designation of Human Leucocyte Differentiation Antigens

CD Designation	Selection of Assigned Monoclonal Antibodies	Main Cellular Reactivity	Recognized Membrane Component
CD1a	NA1/34; T6; VIT6; Leu6	Thy, DC, B subset	gp49
CD1b	WM-25; 4A76; NUT2	Thy, DC, B subset	gp45
CD1c	L161; M241; 7C6; PHM3	Thy, DC, B subset	gp43
CD2	9.6; T11; 35.1	T	CD58(LFA-3) receptor, gp50
CD2R	T11.3*; VIT13; D66	Activated T	CD2 epitopes restr. to activ. T
CD3	T3; UCHT1; 38.1; Leu4	T	CD3-complex (5 chains), gp/p 26,20,16
CD4	T4; Leu3a; 91.D6	T subset	Class II HIV receptor, gp59
CD5	T1; UCHT2; T101; HH9; AMG4	T, B subset	gp67
CD6	T12; T411	T, B subset	gp100
CD7	3A1; 4A; CL1.3; G3-7	T	gp40
CD8	α chain: T8; Leu2a; M236; UCHT4; T811 β chain: T8/2T8; 5H7	T subset	Class I receptor, gp32, α/α or α/β dimer
CD9	CLB-thromb/8; PHN200; FMC56	Pre-B, M, Plt	p24
CD10	J5, VILA1, BA-3	Lymph. prog., cALL, Germ ctr. B, G	Neutral endopeptidase, gp100, CALLA
CD11a	MHM24; 2F12; CRIS-3	Leucocytes	LFA-1, gp180/95
CD11b	Mol; 5A4.C5; LPM19C	M, G, NK	C3bi receptor, gp155/95
CD11c	B-LY6; L29; BL-4H4	M, G, NK, B subset	gp150/95
CDw12	M67	M, G, Plt	(p90-120)
CD13	MY7, MCS-2, TÜK1, MOU28	M, G	Aminopeptidase N, gp150
CD14	Mo2, UCHM1, VIM13, MoP15	M, (G), LHC	gp55
CD15	My1, VIM-D5	G, (M)	3-FAL, X-Hapten
CD16	BW209/2; HUNK2; GLBFcGran1; 3G8	NK, G, Mac.	FcRIII, gp50-65
CDw17	GO35, Huly-m13	G, M, Plt	Lactosylceramide
CD18	MHM23; M232; 11H6; CLB54	Leucocytes broad	β chain to CD11a, b, c
CD19	B4; HD37	B, follicular DC	gp95, associated with membrane-bound Ig
CD20	B1; 1F5	B	p37/32, ion channel?, cell cycle regulation
CD21	B2; HB5	B subset, follicular DC	C3d/EBV-Rec. (CR2), p 140
CD22	HD39; S-HCL1; To15	Cytopl. B/surface B subset	gp135, homology to myelin assoc. gp (MAG)
CD23	Blast-2, MHM6	B subset, act.M, Eo, follicular DC	FcεRII, gp45-50
CD24	VIBE3; BA-1	B, G, epithelium	gp41/38?, signal transduction
CD25	TAC; 7G7/B6; 2A3	Activated T, B, M	IL-2R β chain, gp55
CD26	134-2C2; TS145	Activated T	Dipeptidylpeptidase IV, gp120
CD27	VIT14; S152; OKT18A; CLB-9F4	T subset	p55 (dimer)
CD28	9.3; KOLT2	T subset	gp44
CD29	K20; A-1A5	Broad	VLA β-, integrin β₁ chain, Plt GPIIa
CD30	Ki-1; Ber-H2; HSR4	Activated T, B; Reed-Sternberg	gp120, Ki-1
GD31	SG134; TM3; HEC-75; ES12F11	Plt, M, G, B, (T)	gp140, Plt, GPIIa
CDw32	CIKM5; 41H16; IV.3	M, G, B	FcRII, gp40
CD33	My9; H153; L4F3	M, Prog., AML	gp67
CD34	My10; BI-3C5; ICH-3	Prog.	gp105-120
CD35	TO5; CB04,J3D3	G, M, B	CR1
CD36	5F1; CIMeg1; ESIVC7	M, Plt, (B)	gp90, Plt GPIV
CD37	HD28; HH1; G28-1	B, (T, M), glial cells, epithel.	gp40-52
CD38	HB7; T16	Lymph. Prog., PC, Act. T, preB cells, plasma cells	p45
CD39	AC2; G28-2	B subset, (M), follicular DC	gp70-100, role in T cell signaling
CD40	G28-5	B, carcinomas	gp50, homology to NGF- and TNFα- receptor
CD41	PBM 6.4; CLB-thromb/7; PL273	Plt	Plt GPIIb-IIIa complex and GPIIb
CD42a	FMC25; BL-H6; GP-P	Plt	Plt GPIX, gp23

CD Designation	Selection of Assigned Monoclonal Antibodies	Main Cellular Reactivity	Recognized Membrane Component
CD42b	PHN89; AN51; GN287	Plt	Plt GPlb, gp135/25
CD43	OTH 71C5; G19-1; MEM-59	T, G, M, brain	Leukosialin, gp95
CD44	GRHL1; F10-44-2; 33-3B3; BRIC35	Leucocytes, brain, RBC	Pgp-1, gp80-95
CD45	T29/33; BMAC 1; AB187	Leucocytes	LCA, T200
CD45RA	G1-15; F8-11-13; 73.5	T subset, B, G, M	restricted T200, gp220
CD45RB	PT17/26/16*	T subset, B, G, M	restricted T200
CD45RO	UCHL1	T subset, B, G, M	restricted T200, gp180
CD46	HULYM5; 122-2; J48	Leucocytes	Membrane cofactor protein (MCP), gp66/56
CD47	BRIC 126; CIKM1; BRIC 125	Broad	gp47-52, *N*-linked glycan
CD48	WM68; LO-MN25; J4-57	Leucocytes	gp41, PI-linked
CDw49b	CLB-thromb/4; Gi14	Plt, cultured T	VLA-α2 chain, Plt GPla
CDw49d	B5G10; HP2/1; HP1/3	M, T, B, (LHC), Thy	VLA-α4 chain, gp150
CDw49f	GoH3	Plt, (T)	VLA-α6 chain, Plt GPlc
CDw50	101-1D2; 140-11	Leucocytes	gp148/108
CD51	13C2; 23C6; NKI-M7; NKI-M9	(Plt)	VNR-α chain
CDw52	097; YTH66.9; YTH34.5	Leucocytes	Campath-1, gp21-28
CD53	HI29; HI36; MEM-53; HD77	Leucocytes	gp32-40
CD54	7F7; WEHI-CAM1; RR1/1	Broad, activ.	ICAM-1, ligand for CD11a on T cells
CD55	143-30; BRIC 110; BRIC 128; F2B-7.2	Broad	DAF (decay accelerating factor)
CD56	Leu19; NKH1; FP2–11.14, L185	NK, activ. lymphocytes	gp220/135, NKH1, isoform of N-CAM
CD57	Leu7; L183; L186	NK, T, B sub, brain	gp 110, HNK1
CD58	G26; BRIC 5; TS2/9	Leucocytes, epithel.	LFA-3, gp40-65
CD59	YTH53.1; MEM-43	Broad	gp18-20
CDw60	M-T32; M-T21; M-T41; UM4D4	T subset	NeuAc-NeuAc-Gal-
CD61	Y2/51; CLB-thromb/1; VI-PL2; BL-E6	Plt	Integrin β3-, VNR-β chain, Plt GPIIIa
CD62	CLB-thromb/6; CLB-thromb/5; RUU-SP1.18.1	Plt activ.	GMP-140 (PADGEM), gp140
CD63	RUU-SP2.28; CLB-gran/12	Plt activ., M, (G, T, B)	gp53
CD64	MAb32.2; MAb22;	M	FcRI, gp75
CDw65	VIM2; HE10; CF4; VIM8	G, M	Ceramide-dodecasaccharide 4c
CD66	CLB-gran/10; YTH71.3	G	Phosphoprotein gp 180–200
CD67	B13.9; G10F5; JML-H16	G	p100, PI-linked
CD68	EBM11; Y2/131; Y-1/82A; Ki-M7; Ki-M6	Macrophages	gp110
CD69	MLR3; L78; BL-Ac/p26; FN50	Activated B, T	gp32/28, AIM
CDw70	Ki-24; HNE 51; HNC 142	Activated B,-T, Reed-Sternberg cells	Ki-24, Glycoprotein 32–40
CD71	138-18; 120-2A3; MEM-75; VIP-1; Nu-TfR2	Proliferating cells, Mac., plasma cells	Transferrin receptor
CD72	S-HCL2; J3-109; BU-40; BU-41	B, Mac	gp43/39, homology to CD 23
CD73	1E9.28.1; 7G2.2.11; AD2	B subset, T subset	ecto-5'-nucleotidase, p69, ligand of CD28 on T cells
CD74	LN2; BU-43; BU-45	B, M	Class II assoc. invariant chain, gp41/35/33
CDw75	LN1; HH2; EBU-141	Mature B, (T subset)	p53?
CD76	HD66; CRIS-4	Mature B, T subset	gp85/67
CD77	38.13(BLA); 424/4A11; 424/3D9	Resting B	Globotriaosylceramide (Gb3)
CDw78	Anti Ba; LO-pan8-a; 1588	B, (M)	?

Thy: thymocytes; DC: dendritic cells; B: B cells; T: T cells; M: monocytes; G: granulocytes; Plt: platelets; Prog.: progenitor cells; Germ. Ctr. B: germinal center B cells; ALL: acute lymphocytic leukemia; NK: natural killer cells; Mac.: macrophages; cytopl.: cytoplasmic; LHC: epidermal Langerhans cells; Eo: eosinophil; Reed–Sternberg: Reed–Sternberg cells; AML: acute myelogenous leukemia; lymph. prog.: lymphocyte progenitor cells; epithel.: epithelial cells. *Antibodies not submitted to workshop.

APPENDIX E: Answers to Self-Test Questions

Chap. 2:	1. C 2. A 3. E 4. D 5. D 6. B
Chap. 3:	1. c 2. e 3. d 4. b 5. a 6. b 7. c 8. a 9. d
	10. d 11. d 12. T 13. T 14. F
Chap. 5:	1. b 2. a+d 3. d 4. a+b 5. c 6. a+c
Chap. 8.	1. C 2. B 3. D 4. A 5. c 6. c
Chap. 10:	1. a 2. c 3. b/1; c/2; e/3; a/4; d/5 4. d 5. e 6. d
Chap. 11:	1 .a 2. c 3. e 4. a. T b. F c. F d. F e. T 5. a. T
	b. F c. F d. T 6. a. T b. T c. T d. T e. F
Chap. 12:	1. A and C 2. B and D 3. A, B, C, and D
Chap. 14:	1. d, e, f, g 2. d, e, h 3. b 4. a, c, e, f 5. c
Chap. 15:	1. B 2. B 3. B 4. B 5. D 6. C 7. B 8. D
Chap. 16:	1. (+) 2. (−) 3. (+) 4. (−) 5. (+) 6. (+) 7. (−)
	8. (c) 9. (d) 10. (a)
Chap. 17:	1. d 2. d 3. b 4. a 5. d 6. b 7. c 8. c
Chap. 18:	1. a 2. d 3. e 4. b
Chap. 20:	1. b 2. d 3. c 4. d 5. c 6. c 7. b 8. b 9. d
	10. d 11. c 12. b 13. e 14. a 15. c
Chap 21:	1. d 2. c 3. d 4. a 5. b 6. T 7. T 8. T 9. F
Chap. 22A:	1. c 2. a 3. b 4. c 5. d 6. a 7. b 8. c 9. d 10. b
Chap. 22B:	1. B 2. E 3. A 4. B 5. C 6. A 7. C 8. A
	9. C 10. A 11. D 12. B 13. E 14. B 15. C 16. A
Chap. 24A:	1. d 2. a 3. d 4. b
Chap. 26:	4. b 5. e
Chap. 27:	1. B 2. A 3. C 4. B
Chap. 29:	1. c 2. c 3. A 4. c 5. d 6. b 7. a
Chap. 30:	1. b 2. d 3. d 4. a 5. b
Chap. 32:	1. c 2. h 3. a 4. d 5. f
Chap. 33A:	1. e 2. d 3. 1/e; 2/c; 3/a; 4/d; 5/b; 6/e 4. f 5. c 6. f
Chap. 33B:	1. A 2. A
Chap. 34:	1. a 2. c 3. b

INDEX

Note: Page numbers in italics indicate figures; page numbers followed by t indicate tabular material.